COUNSELING THE NURSING MOTHER

A LACTATION CONSULTANT'S GUIDE

COUNSELING THE NURSING MOTHER

A LACTATION CONSULTANT'S GUIDE

FOURTH EDITION

Judith Lauwers, BA, IBCLC
Anna Swisher, MBA, IBCLC

JONES AND BARTLETT PUBLISHERS
Sudbury, Massachusetts
BOSTON   TORONTO   LONDON   SINGAPORE

World Headquarters
Jones and Bartlett Publishers
40 Tall Pine Drive
Sudbury, MA 01776
978-443-5000
info@jbpub.com
www.jbpub.com

Jones and Bartlett Publishers Canada
6339 Ormindale Way
Mississauga, ON L5V 1J2
Canada

Jones and Bartlett Publishers
International
Barb House, Barb Mews
London W6 7PA
UK

Jones and Bartlett's books and products are available through most bookstores and online booksellers. To contact Jones and Bartlett Publishers directly, call 800-832-0034, fax 978-443-8000, or visit our website www.jbpub.com.

Substantial discounts on bulk quantities of Jones and Bartlett's publications are available to corporations, professional associations, and other qualified organizations. For details and specific discount information, contact the special sales department at Jones and Bartlett via the above contact information or send an email to specialsales@jbpub.com.

The authors, editor, and publisher have made every effort to provide accurate information. However, they are not responsible for errors, omissions, or for any outcomes related to the use of the contents of this book and take no responsibility for the use of the products and procedures described. Treatments and side effects described in this book may not be applicable to all people; likewise, some people may require a dose or experience a side effect that is not described herein. Drugs and medical devices are discussed that may have limited availability controlled by the Food and Drug Administration (FDA) for use only in a research study or clinical trial. Research, clinical practice, and government regulations often change the accepted standard in this field. When consideration is being given to use of any drug in the clinical setting, the health care provider or reader is responsible for determining FDA status of the drug, reading the package insert, and reviewing prescribing information for the most up-to-date recommendations on dose, precautions, and contraindications, and determining the appropriate usage for the product. This is especially important in the case of drugs that are new or seldom used.

ISBN-13: 978-0-7637-2680-5
ISBN-10: 0-7637-2680-X

Production Credits
Acquisitions Editor: Kevin Sullivan
Production Director: Amy Rose
Associate Production Editor: Tracey Chapman
Associate Editor: Amy Sibley
Senior Marketing Manager: Ed McKenna
Marketing Manager: Emily Ekle
Manufacturing and Inventory Coordinator: Amy Bacus

Composition: GGS Book Services, Atlantic Highlands
Cover Design: Timothy Dziewit
Photo Research: Kimberly Potvin
Cover Image: © 2004 Chad Forsyth
Printing and Binding: Courier Westford
Cover Printing: Courier Westford

Library of Congress Cataloging-in-Publication Data
Lauwers, Judith, 1949–
    Counseling the nursing mother: a lactation consultant's guide /
Judith Lauwers, Anna Swisher. — 4th ed.
        p.;   cm.
    Includes bibliographical references and index.
    ISBN 0-7637-2680-X (casebound)
    1. Breast feeding.   2. Lactation.   3. Breast feeding promotion.
    4. Mothers—Counseling of.   I. Swisher, Anna.   II. Title.
    [DNLM: 1. Breast Feeding   2. Counseling—methods, 3. Infant
Nutrition.   4. Lactation—physiology.   WS 125 L391c 2005]
    RJ216.L354   2005
    649'.33—dc22
        2004026040

6048

Printed in the United States of America
10 09 08   10 9 8 7 6 5 4 3

TABLE OF CONTENTS

C H A P T E R

8

MATERNAL HEALTH AND NUTRITION   **133**

C H A P T E R

9

PROPERTIES OF HUMAN MILK   **157**

CHAPTER

10

IMPURITIES IN HUMAN MILK   **191**

C H A P T E R

13

INFANT ASSESSMENT AND DEVELOPMENT   243

C H A P T E R

14

GETTING BREASTFEEDING STARTED   273

C H A P T E R

15

INFANT ATTACHMENT AND SUCKING   289

C H A P T E R

16

BREASTFEEDING IN THE EARLY WEEKS   305

C H A P T E R

17

BREASTFEEDING BEYOND THE FIRST MONTH   335

C H A P T E R

18

PROBLEMS WITH MILK PRODUCTION AND TRANSFER   359

C H A P T E R

22

TEMPORARY BREASTFEEDING SITUATIONS   441

P A R T   5

ROLE OF THE IBCLC

C H A P T E R

26

PROFESSIONAL CONSIDERATIONS   527

CHAPTER

27

CRITICAL READING AND REVIEW
OF RESEARCH   **547**

C H A P T E R

28

BREASTFEEDING PROMOTION AND CHANGE   579

This fourth edition of *Counseling the Nursing Mother* is dedicated to all the members of the mother's healthcare team, in appreciation for all that you do to promote, protect, and support breastfeeding as we strive toward baby-friendly, and family-friendly, healthcare.

ACKNOWLEDGMENTS

As the lactation profession enters its 20th year, we wish to commemorate the profession's hallmark anniversary by acknowledging the contributions of all individuals who have guided the development of this and past editions of *Counseling the Nursing Mother*. There is always the danger of omitting the name of an important contributor. If any contribution has been omitted inadvertently we apologize.

James Akré, BA, MPIA
Pam Allyn, BSN, IBCLC
Tammy Arbeter, IBCLC, CD (DONA)
Helen Armstrong, MAT, IBCLC
Lois Arnold, MPH, IBCLC
Jan Barger, RN, MA, IBCLC
Genevieve Becker, DiplDiets, Msc, MEd, IBCLC
Cheston Berlin, MD
Debi Bocar, RN, PhD, IBCLC
Priscilla Bornmann, JD
Sarah Emery Bradley, MEd, IBCLC
Sandra Breck, RN, IBCLC
Cathy Carothers, BLA, IBCLC
K. Jean Cotterman, RNC, IBCLC
Sarah Coulter Danner, CNM, CPNP
Deanna Diodato, RN, IBCLC
Lee Anne Dobos, CPA
Patricia Donohue-Carey, BS, LCCE
Dianne Flury
Karen Foard, IBCLC
Scott Franklin, DDS
Teresa Gonzalez, MEd
Cynthia Good Mojab, MS, IBCLC
Anh Gordon, MD
Linda Gort-Walton, RN, MS
Thomas Hale, RPh, PhD
Peter Hartmann, PhD
Kay Hoover, MEd, IBCLC
Pat Houck, RN, IBCLC
Kathleen Huggins, RN, MS
Sharon Kelly
Connie Kishbaugh, RN, BSN, IBCLC
Kyle Knisely

Linda Kutner, RN, BSN, IBCLC
Miriam Labbok, MD, MPH
La Leche League of Blackburg, VA
Mary Grace Lanese, RN, BSN, IBCLC
Cathy Liles, MPH, IBCLC
Deanna Lockett, RN, LCCE, IBCLC
Margot Mann, BA, BEd, IBCLC
John Mann, MD
Becky Mannel, BS, BA, IBCLC
Lisa Marasco, MA, IBCLC
Chele Marmet, MA, IBCLC
Patricia Martens, BSc, IBCLC, PhD
Debbie Matisse
Carol Mavity
Valerie McClain, IBCLC
James McKenna, PhD
Valerie Mick, RN, IBCLC
Maureen Minchin, MA, IBCLC
Nancy Mohrbacher, IBCLC
Chris Mulford, RN, BSN, IBCLC
Jack Newman, MD
Jeanette Panchula, RN, IBCLC
Denise Parker, BA, IBCLC
Molly Pessl, BSN, IBCLC
Carole Peterson, MS, IBCLC
Ellen Petok, BS, IBCLC
Maureen Polivka, RN, BSN, JD
Donna Ramsay, DMU, PostGrad Dip PhD
Steve Rein, PhD
Jan Riordan, RN, EdD, IBCLC
Kathy Romberger, RNC, IBCLC
JoAnne Scott, MA, IBCLC
Debbie Shinskie, RN, IBCLC
Barbara Shocker, BSN, ICCE, IBCLC
Gina Solomon, MD, MPH
Ruth Solomon, RN, IBCLC
Amy Spangler, RN, MN, IBCLC
Marian Tompson, Founder, LLLI
Mary Toporcer, MD
Mary Rose Tully, MPH, IBCLC

Beverly Vaugh, BS, IBCLC
Marsha Walker, RN, IBCLC
Catherine Watson-Genna, BS, IBCLC
Nancy Williams, MA, MFT, CCE, IBCLC
Karen Wilson, RN
Barbara Wilson-Clay, BS, IBCLC
Michael Woolridge, BS, DPhil
Lisa Wyatt, PhD

Also, from the first and second editions published by Avery Publishing, we profoundly thank Candace Woessner, coauthor, mentor, and friend. We also acknowledge and thank M. Elaine Adams, Barbara Bernard, Celeste Marx, Gerry McKeegan, and Mary Jo Stine. Other individuals who were key in developing information that provided the basis of the first edition are Ditta and Frank Hoeber, Joanne Hill, Louise Stevens, and numerous volunteers in the Childbirth Education Association of Greater Philadelphia. We also thank the many mothers and babies from whom we have learned so much about the miraculous bonds of breastfeeding and parenting.

Finally, we wish to thank our families for their patience and support throughout the writing and editing process. We thank Judi's husband Dave, two sons Mike and Chris, and daughter-in-law Jenny, who is now beginning her own journey toward parenthood and breastfeeding. We thank Anna's husband David and their children, Travis, Faith, and Kristin. You ignited our passion for babies, mothers, and families.

PREFACE

I can't hear a word you're saying.
Who you are speaks too loudly.

                                        –Ralph Waldo Emerson

What an exciting time to be working in the lactation profession! This expanded fourth edition of *Counseling the Nursing Mother* goes to press amid a groundbreaking breastfeeding promotion campaign with far-reaching impact in the United States. The U.S. Ad Council's message, "Babies were born to be breastfed," resounds throughout the country in print and on television and radio. It is a gratifying time to be helping mothers and babies breastfeed.

Several underlying principles have guided our writing of this fourth edition. First and foremost, *Counseling the Nursing Mother* is unique among all other lactation texts in its focus on counseling. We hope you will gain an appreciation for the significance of counseling techniques and how your style and approach can enhance your interactions with mothers and thus your effectiveness. Topics are presented within a counseling framework, with practical suggestions for working with mothers. We hope you will gain insights into applying knowledge and research into day-to-day practice and that you will understand counseling challenges and how to meet them.

The text also serves as a significant tool for teaching interns and others in the healthcare profession. It is ideal as the first text in the journey to becoming an IBCLC, enabling the learner to understand lactation in easy-to-read terminology before advancing to more scientific texts. The extensive glossary and index and the key terms and *At a Glance* features in each chapter make the text a valuable study guide for the certification exam as well as a quick reference when counseling mothers.

The strong features from the third edition continue, with the popular chapter on critical reading of research that explains the process in easy-to-understand descriptions. Every chapter and every topic continues to interweave counseling technique with practical information. The text is written from a teaching perspective to help the reader grow professionally in the lactation field. The comprehensive glossary has been expanded to over 600 terms used in lactation practice, with each term presented in bold the first time it appears—a great study tool for the certification exam!

We are pleased to present several new features in the fourth edition:

◆ A new chapter on the sociological perspective of breastfeeding

◆ Autoimmune disorders and breastfeeding

◆ Dangers of baby training programs

◆ The latest in international promotion initiatives

◆ Groundbreaking research in breast anatomy

◆ Expanded sections on postpartum depression and HIV

◆ Special care recommendations for the near-term infant

◆ Key terms to let you know what to expect in the chapter

◆ "At a Glance" counseling applications at the end of every chapter

◆ Sample care plans and documentation forms that you may use in your practice

◆ ILCA's Spanish glossary of common terms you may use with mothers

Part 1 (Chapters 1–6) focuses on the IBCLC in action, beginning in Chapter 1 with a historical perspective of infant feeding and the growth of the lactation profession. Various work settings for IBCLCs are explored in Chapter 2. Chapter 3 presents new material on the sociological perspective of breastfeeding assistance and support. Chapters 4 and 5 focus on empowering mothers and using effective counseling strategies and techniques, which sets this text apart from others in the lactation field. Chapter 6 addresses practical elements in consultations with mothers and babies, including anticipatory guidance, problem solving, and documentation.

Part 2 (Chapters 7–10) covers the science of lactation. Chapter 7 describes the newest understanding of breast anatomy, growth and development, and variations in structure and function. Chapter 8 provides a basic understanding of nutrients, nutrition in pregnancy and lactation, and how to teach nutrition to mothers. Properties of human milk are studied in Chapter 9, with attention to its lifelong health benefits and a comparison to artificial feeding. Chapter 10 studies safety issues of medications, social toxicants, and environmental contaminants in the mother's milk.

Part 3 (Chapters 11–18) spans from the prenatal to postpartum phase, from the woman's decision to breastfeed through to weaning. Chapter 11 discusses issues involved with decision making, preparing for breastfeeding, and selecting a physician. Hospital practices are explored in Chapter 12, with an emphasis on early breastfeeding, a supportive climate, and comprehensive care plans. Chapter 13 examines newborn assessment, infant behavior and growth, and strategies for infant crying. Practical aspects of breastfeeding are presented in Chapter 14, including positioning, multiples, tandem nursing, and assisting with a feeding. Factors related to the baby's attachment and suckling are discussed in Chapter 15, with practical suggestions for assisting with problems. Chapter 16 presents common occurrences during the early weeks, including the establishment of lactation, leaking, nipple soreness, engorgement, plugged ducts, and mastitis. Chapter 17 relates factors inherent in breastfeeding beyond the first month, from patterns of growth, infant development, breastfeeding an older baby, and supplementary and complementary feedings, to weaning. Finally, Chapter 18 addresses the consequences of compromised milk production and transfer on the health outcome and growth of the infant.

Part 4 (Chapters 19–25) addresses special care situations and counseling challenges, beginning in Chapter 19 with changes that occur within the family in terms of parenting, sexual adjustments, fertility, and sibling reactions. Lifestyle variations such as low income, single parenting, adolescent mothers, and cultural differences are explored in Chapter 20, as well as dealing with opposition to breastfeeding. Chapter 21 discusses various breastfeeding techniques and devices and their appropriate use. Temporary breastfeeding situations such as jaundice, relactation, induced lactation, and delayed breastfeeding are presented in Chapter 22. Chapter 23 describes the special needs of high-risk infants, with a sensitive approach to counseling a mother whose baby has died. Interruptions in breastfeeding are explored in Chapter 24, with practical suggestions for managing feedings and combining working and breastfeeding. A wide variety of long-term special needs for mothers and babies are presented in Chapter 25, with advice on how to counsel mothers in these situations.

Part 5 (Chapters 26–28) examines the important role of the IBCLC as professional and advocate. Educational preparation and certification are emphasized in Chapter 26, along with standards of practice, promoting your services, educating other healthcare providers, and maturing in the role of IBCLC. Chapter 27 provides a clear and easy-to-understand review of how to read and review research critically, with illustrations provided through mock articles. The text ends with attention in Chapter 28 paid to the important role of the IBCLC in promoting breastfeeding and facilitating changes in policies and practices toward creating baby-friendly healthcare.

Lactation consultants, like other professionals, need to embrace change as the amount of new information accelerates. We must be lifelong learners! In *Counseling the Nursing Mother*, we have tried to accommodate that need by providing resources for your ongoing learning and research. We recognize the need to teach and mentor future lactation consultants and other healthcare providers. We urge our readers to accept that challenge and responsibility. This text provides a starting point for that journey.

Judith Lauwers
Anna Swisher

Anna Swisher, MBA, IBCLC, has a private practice, Abundant Blessings, in Austin, Texas. She also works part-time at an area hospital as a lactation consultant. Anna began helping mothers breastfeed in 1995 as a La Leche League Leader. She is active in her local ILCA affiliate, Heart of Texas Lactation Consultants. She has an MBA in business management.

Judith Lauwers, BA, IBCLC, is cofounder and retired Executive Director of Breastfeeding Support Consultants. She has worked in the lactation field since 1978 and is also coauthor of Breastfeeding Today. She served as conference planner and board member for the International Lactation Consultant Association (ILCA) and is currently ILCA's Education Coordinator.

PART

1

PROMOTION AND SUPPORT

CHAPTER 1

BREASTFEEDING PROMOTION IN THE MODERN WORLD

The promotion of breastfeeding among caregivers and parents is much more complex than it may seem on the surface. The superiority of **human milk** over substitutes is well documented and acknowledged by the scientific and medical communities and the general population. It is not easy to explain why parents choose artificial milk in spite of that knowledge. Many caregivers fail to recommend breastfeeding to their clients or provide questionable advice when complications arise. The reasons behind this are complex. To understand these contradictions requires examining the many issues involved with infant feeding practices that have evolved and will continue to evolve, along with other changes in society. Understanding the dynamics of this evolution, as well as the political and sociological factors involved, is essential to effecting tangible and enduring change that will enhance maternal and infant health.

KEY TERMS

Baby-Friendly Hospital Initiative
complementary feeding
exclusive breastfeeding
Global Strategy for Infant and Young Child Feeding
Innocenti Declaration
International Code of Marketing of Breast-milk Substitutes
lactation consultant
malnutrition
morbidity
mortality
osteoporosis

paradigm shift
protecting, promoting, and supporting breastfeeding
Ten Steps to Successful Breastfeeding
UNICEF
United States Department of Agriculture
U.S. Healthy People 2010
U.S. Surgeon General
wet nurse
WHO Global Data Bank on Breastfeeding
World Health Assembly
World Health Organization

INFANT FEEDING PRACTICES HISTORICALLY

Breastfeeding our young is so intrinsic to our existence that it defines humans as a class: *mammals*. Human milk historically has been the predominant means of nourishing infants—either the milk of the baby's mother or the milk of another woman (Figure 1.1). Throughout history, some women have made a conscious choice not to breastfeed. Women of wealth often chose to employ **wet nurses** or hand feeding in order to stay beautiful, get pregnant again, or as a status marker. As a result, **human milk substitutes** have been available for centuries. It has only been in recent history that more infants in the United States have received artificial baby milk than have been breastfed. Globally, breastfeeding still predominates as the method for feeding infants.

During the 18th and 19th centuries, the advent of modern medicine, science, and technology generated great changes in infant feeding. Feeding bottles and rubber nipples made it easier for infants to be raised on human milk substitutes. As cow's milk became available in increasing supply, parents turned to this as an acceptable substitute for human milk (Wolf, 2003). When the increase in **artificial feeding** caused greater numbers of infant deaths, efforts focused on improving **artificial baby milk** rather than increasing breastfeeding rates. Formula feeding continued to increase in popularity, with cow's milk products being promoted as the modern and civilized way to nourish infants. Breastfeeding conveyed low social status, and women who chose to breastfeed were given little support or encouragement. The prevailing cultural belief in many industrialized societies has evolved to one in which bottle-feeding is the norm and breastfeeding is the exception.

Increased Separation of Mothers and Babies

The advent of bottle-feeding provided women with new options. Although they still gave birth to babies, they did not have to invest themselves totally in feeding and raising their babies throughout infancy. Women were free to take a job or pursue other activities outside the home. Although their female ancestors had been bound by biology to nurture their young, modern women had a choice and the ability to determine their future. Feeding practices that liberated mothers from their babies were thus attractive to some women.

Dramatic changes took place in birth practices, which also affected infant feeding. By the early part of the 20th century, industrialized medicine had removed much of the danger from the birth process. Women traditionally had given birth at home with female family members and a midwife in attendance, enjoying a strong and continuous support system throughout labor and delivery. As medical technology advanced, childbirth moved from the home to the hospital, compromising both the mother's and baby's personal needs. Women now gave birth primarily in a sterile hospital setting surrounded by technology, without the support of female relatives that had been standard in the past. Birthing practices seperated mothers from their babies, regimented infant care, and interfered with the initiation of breastfeeding (Davis-Floyd, 1998; Leavitt, 1986).

Breastfeeding Revisited

Early in the 20th century, efforts increased within the medical community to question the wisdom of the prevalence of feeding babies artificial baby milk. In 1921, Julius P. Sedgwick advocated for students to spend more time in medical school observing and studying breastfeeding and less time studying artificial feeding and formula making (Sedgwick, 1921). The Brooklyn Pediatric Society addressed inclusion of breastfeeding instruction in postgraduate medical education in 1924. They concluded that breastfeeding was a matter of medical education and lay instruction (McKay, 1924). However, the scarcity of **lactation** education in medical and nursing schools continues to be a problem in the 21st century (Hillenbrand, 2002; Philipp, 2001; Moreland, 2000).

Researchers soon demonstrated a correlation between cognitive development and method of infant feeding. A 1929 report stated that breastfed babies walked more than two months earlier than artificially fed babies did. It also noted that all of the babies studied with IQs over 130 were breastfed (Hoefer, 1929). Recognition of the importance of breastfeeding to infant health led to books for parents, and professional articles on breastfeeding and infant feeding began to appear in the early 1950s.

Mother-to-mother breastfeeding support groups emerged around the same time. Grassroots efforts by La Leche League and other breastfeeding support groups actively promoted breastfeeding as the preferred method of infant feeding and it remains the preferred method today (Figure 1.2). By the 1960s, a movement had begun among women who advocated healthful living. These women regarded breastfeeding as the natural and culturally appropriate method of infant feeding.

Breastfeeding Rates

Despite a renewed interest in breastfeeding, there was still a general lack of encouragement and advice from the medical community. By the early 1980s, breastfeeding

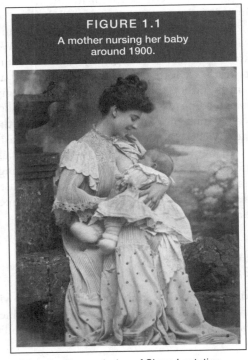

FIGURE 1.1
A mother nursing her baby around 1900.

Printed with permission of Sierra Lactation.

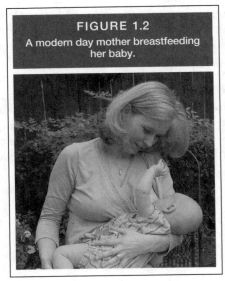

FIGURE 1.2
A modern day mother breastfeeding her baby.

Printed with permission of Anna Swisher.

rates reached a peak of 61.9 percent but then began to decline. In 1984, the U.S. Surgeon General convened a work group to study breastfeeding and human lactation. Yet breastfeeding rates continued to drop down to 51.5 percent in 1990, before rising again to initiation rates of between 65.1 percent (Li, 2003) and 69.5 percent in 2001 (Ryan, 2002). The latest marketing survey reported that 70.1 percent of U.S. mothers now initiate breastfeeding. Breastfeeding at 6 months increased from 18.9 to 33.2 percent in 1992 (Abbott, 2003).

The U.S. Healthy People 2010 initiative seeks to increase U.S. breastfeeding rates from the 1998 **baseline** rates. By 2010, the target rates of the initiative are 75 percent initiation, 50 percent at six months, and 25 percent at 12 months. The initiative reports that rates of breastfeeding are highest among college-educated women and women aged 35 years and older. The lowest rates of breastfeeding are found among those whose infants are at highest risk of poor health and development (those aged 21 years and under and those with low educational levels). However, many of these groups have shown the greatest increase in breastfeeding rates since 1989. Rates of breastfeeding among African American women during the **postpartum** period increased 65 percent. Rates of African American women breastfeeding at 6 months grew 81 percent between 1988 and 1997. Breastfeeding rates among women aged 20 years and under at both periods also increased substantially, as did those among women with a grade-school education (Healthy People, 2003).

Because definitions of **exclusive breastfeeding** varies from one country to another, compiling meaningful statistics presents a challenge. Exclusive breastfeeding as defined by the **World Health Organization** (WHO) means that breastfeeding babies receive no drink or food other than their mother's milk. WHO established a Global Data Bank on Breastfeeding in 1982. One of WHO's goals is to disseminate identical indicators and definitions worldwide to ensure consistent and comparable results in breastfeeding studies.

Breastfeeding rates vary significantly from one part of the world to another, and the quality of the data also varies. In the Sub-Saharan African region, approximately 29 percent of infants continue to breastfeed between 20 and 23 months. However, only 27 percent of infants younger than 6 months are breastfed exclusively in this region. The East Asia/Pacific region reports the highest rate, at 54 percent, for exclusively breastfed babies younger than 6 months (UNICEF, 2003a). Australia has an 87 percent initiation rate as of 2001. Initiation rates range as high as 99 percent in Norway for 2000, and as low as 31 percent in Ireland (LLLI, 2003).

The United Nations International Children's Emergency Fund (UNICEF) database for 2003 breastfeeding rates recalculated the rates to better reflect the recommendation of exclusive breastfeeding for the first 6 months of life. Because these data now include older infants, and exclusive breastfeeding tends to decline with age, the levels are lower than those previously reported for the younger, 0-to-4 months age range (UNICEF, 2003a).

UNICEF reported that 39 percent of infants in developing countries are exclusively breastfed for 6 months, and 52 percent continue to breastfeed with complementary foods at 20–23 months. Only 34 percent of infants in the least developed countries are breastfed exclusively for 6 months, but 63 percent continue to breastfeed with complementary foods at 20–23 months (UNICEF, 2003b). Current worldwide breastfeeding rates can be found at UNICEF's website: www.unicef.org; at WHO's Global Data Bank on Breastfeeding: www.who.int/ nut/db_bfd.htm; and at La Leche League International's Center for Breastfeeding Information: www. lalecheleague.org/cbi/cbi.html.

▶ BREASTFEEDING AS AN INFANT HEALTH ISSUE

Studies such as those discussed earlier illustrate the medical community's recognition of the impact of breastfeeding on infant **morbidity** and **mortality**. The medical community acknowledges that breastfeeding is healthiest for infants. Human milk is, in fact, a baby's first immunization as babies are born "autoimmune deficient" (Labbok, 2004). Its unique constitution fosters the infant's health and growth and makes it easily digested and efficiently used by the body. Human milk protects the baby from infectious diseases and reduces the chance of respiratory and digestive infections. The multitude of health benefits for the baby, discussed in Chapter 9, is a clear testimony to the significance of human milk in infant feeding.

Breastfeeding has been associated with a higher IQ of between five and eleven points (Anderson, 1999; Horwood, 1998). Researchers have debated whether the positive correlation between breastfeeding and intelligence results from human milk or from the inclination of breastfeeding mothers to be more nurturing toward their babies. Studies support the nutritional benefits of human milk and the contention that increased duration of breastfeeding correlates with higher IQ (Gomez-Sanchiz, 2004; Smith, 2003; Rao, 2002; Anderson, 1999; Horwood, 1998; Lucas, 1992).

Breastfeeding promotes optimal development of the oral cavity, which lowers the incidence of malocclusion (Labbok, 1987). It also develops a proper swallowing pattern that extends into adulthood. Both of these outcomes may reduce the risk of obstructive sleep **apnea** in adulthood (Palmer, 2004). With the greatest increment of craniofacial development occurring within the first four years of life (Shepard, 1991), the avoidance of bottles and artificial nipples during infancy can have far-reaching health consequences.

Breastfed children may have different early relationships with their mothers. Breastfeeding is a physical embodiment of the mother–baby relationship that continues long after birth. The **bonding** that accompanies breastfeeding fosters a special closeness and forms a deep and lasting attachment between the mother and child. A breastfeeding mother is able to respond quickly to her baby's hunger cries without the delay of preparing and heating a bottle. This immediate response to the baby's needs develops in him a sense of security and trust that may help him accept the demands of socialization later in life. The early sensory stimulation from skin-to-skin contact that takes place during breastfeeding helps develop the baby's perceptual and response mechanisms. It also aids respiration by stimulating blood flow. This may be one reason for the reduced incidence of respiratory ailments in breastfed babies (Bachrach, 2003).

▶ BREASTFEEDING AS A WOMEN'S HEALTH ISSUE

In many ways, breastfeeding is as much a women's health issue as an infant feeding issue. Women's health traditionally has received little attention in the U.S. health care agenda. Part of the challenge in promoting breastfeeding in today's climate stems from this persistent failure in the health care system. The health care arena needs to view breastfeeding as part of women's health and treat it as such. Whatever health care providers can do to help empower the women in their care will benefit women and their families for years to come.

Both giving birth and breastfeeding are empowerment issues for women (Davis-Floyd, 1998; Van Esterik, 1994). As women gain more control over their birth and breastfeeding experiences, they achieve a greater sense of power, self-esteem, and ego (Locklin, 1993). Medical technology often strips a woman of this power by placing external controls on pregnancy, birth, and breastfeeding, the three life functions that belong solely to women. Breastfeeding is a part of the entire childbearing cycle. The female body is designed to progress from pregnancy to birth and then on to breastfeeding. Interrupting this cycle by *not* breastfeeding interrupts the normal continuum. Breastfeeding is the normal transition from **intrauterine** maternal-based nutrition to **extrauterine** maternal-based nutrition. Anthropologist Ashley Montagu perceived an 18-month **gestation,** with a baby spending nine months in utero and nine months nurtured at the breast (Montagu, 1986).

In order for breastfeeding to be a real choice for all women, society needs to become more woman- and child-friendly (Heller, 1997). Breastfeeding and mothering are only two strands in the weaving of women's lives. To ignore the rest of the fabric is to fail to see how connected all the strands are. **Lactation consultants** and other caregivers help breastfeeding women by considering the total weaving. Van Esterik states that "breastfeeding is a holistic act and is intimately connected to all domains of life: sexuality, eating, emotion, appearance, sleeping, and parental relationships" (Van Esterik, 1994). It is an integral part of the whole fabric of women's lives.

Physical and Emotional Effects of Breastfeeding on Women

Breastfeeding has a significant impact on women's health. **Oxytocin** released during breastfeeding contracts the uterus and helps stop bleeding after delivery. It is, therefore, important that breastfeeding begin immediately after birth and that it continue frequently. Oxytocin, known as the "mothering" hormone, may pass to the infant (Lawrence, 1999). **Prolactin** and oxytocin play a role in maternal feelings of well-being, relaxation, and mothering. A positive breastfeeding experience can contribute to a woman feeling good about herself. This raises her self-esteem and empowers her as a woman.

Breastfeeding women are energy efficient (Illingworth, 1986) and can produce milk even with limited caloric intake. The increased caloric demand that accompanies breastfeeding allows the mother to supplement her usual eating pattern—provided that it is nutritionally sound—and still control her weight and return to her prepregnancy size more quickly. As discussed in Chapter 19, exclusive breastfeeding is 98 percent effective in delaying pregnancy naturally without the use of artificial contraceptives for the first four to six months postpartum.

The risk of premenopausal breast cancer is reduced, and the longer a woman breastfeeds, the greater the protection (Becher, 2003; Beral, 2002; Zheng, 2000; Newcomb, 1994). The risk of ovarian cancer is also decreased (Tung, 2003; Yen, 2003; Rosenblatt, 1993).

Continued research into the correlation between lactation and **osteoporosis** has provided reassurance to breastfeeding women that bone loss is regenerated after **weaning** and that lactation provides protection against osteoporosis (Paton, 2003; Carranza-Lira, 2002).

▶ CULTURAL INFLUENCES ON INFANT FEEDING

Most people acknowledge that breastfeeding is best for babies. Even the infant formula industry makes that declaration in its advertising. However, the messages that permeate the U.S. media do little to support breastfeeding. Despite a renewed interest in breastfeeding, bottle-feeding is still recognized as the cultural norm. Adolescent girls and boys, and indeed many adults, are generally uncomfortable with the topic or embarrassed at seeing a baby breastfed. However, it is common to see babies and toddlers of all ages in public with feeding bottles or pacifiers. Shelves in grocery stores, toy stores, and discount stores abound with bottle-feeding devices and infant formula. News media, children's books, parenting magazines, and medical journals carry scores of bottle-feeding messages. Several states even have found it necessary to pass legislation safeguarding the right to breastfeed in public or making it illegal to interfere with women breastfeeding in public.

A **paradigm shift** in the way society views infant feeding must accompany breastfeeding promotion efforts. For the past several decades, promotion efforts have focused defensively on the benefits of breastfeeding, enumerating all the reasons why mothers should breastfeed their babies. However, for healthful practices such as breastfeeding to be promoted more effectively, public awareness must shift to the hazards of *not* breastfeeding and the reasons mothers should *not* feed their babies artificial baby milk. The U.S. Ad Council adopted this approach in a 2004 breastfeeding awareness campaign (Merwood, 2004). Efforts to educate the American public date back to the late 19th century. Physicians "constantly decried the 'children with weak and diseased constitutions belonging to that generally wretched class called bottle-fed. . . .' Today's medical community recognizes what their predecessors knew a century ago—that the American propensity to shun human milk is a public health problem and should be exposed as such" (Wolf, 2003).

This shift in approach is illustrated with a study by Lucas (1992) who found that **preterm infants** receiving human milk have higher IQ levels than those receiving infant formula. However, the biologic norm is that infants receive human milk. Therefore, it is not the case that breastfed infants have higher IQs. They have *normal* IQs, and artificially fed infants have IQs *lower* than normal because they failed to receive human milk. Likewise, breastfed infants do not have lower rates of **otitis media**. Rather, formula-fed infants have *higher* rates. When the public makes this subtle shift in attitude, parents will make more informed and healthier choices.

▶ BREASTFEEDING AS AN ECONOMIC ISSUE

The economic costs of not breastfeeding for the United States alone are staggering. A March 2001 analysis from the **United States Department of Agriculture (USDA)** stated that a minimum of $3.6 billion would be saved if breastfeeding were increased from the 2001 levels of 64 percent in hospital and 29 percent at 6 months to 75 percent and 50 percent respectively, the levels recommended by the U.S. Surgeon General and Healthy People 2010. The analysis calculated cost savings from treating only three childhood illnesses: otitis media, **gastroentritis,** and **necrotizing enterocolitis** (Weimer, 2001). U.S. taxpayers would save $112 million in Medicaid costs and $478 million in government subsidy costs if **WIC** infants were breastfed for as little as 3 months. (WIC is the supplemental food program for low-income women, infants, and children.) A 50 percent reduction in pharmacy costs was also projected (Montgomery, 1997).

▶ INTERNATIONAL PROMOTION INITIATIVES

Beginning in 1981, several major global initiatives began to promote breastfeeding. Worldwide, the practice of substituting artificial baby milk, whether partially or fully, has resulted in greater incidents of **malnutrition,** infections, diarrheal diseases, impaired growth, and even infant deaths. By the mid-1970s, health experts realized a need for a global effort in order to stem the tide of these negative outcomes for children. This led to the adoption of the **International Code of Marketing of Breastmilk Substitutes** by the World Health Assembly in 1981.

The intent of the code is to regulate the advertising and promotional techniques used to sell infant formula and other human milk substitutes. It covers all foods marketed or otherwise represented to replace human milk, as well as feeding bottles and artificial nipples. A hospital that wishes to achieve the International Baby-Friendly Hospital designation must eliminate free and low-cost supplies of all artificial baby milks, feeding bottles, and teats. **Baby-friendly** hospitals use ordinary procurement channels to obtain artificial feeding supplies and do not accept free or low-cost supplies of formula.

Because of delays in national implementation of the code, as well as continued disregard of its provisions by manufacturers and distributors, the 1980s saw artificial feeding continue to increase and breastfeeding continue to decline. In an effort to improve breastfeeding rates throughout the world, UNICEF and WHO issued a 1989 joint statement entitled *Protecting, Promoting and Supporting Breastfeeding*. The statement led to the formation of the *Ten Steps to Successful Breastfeeding* (Figure 1.3) as a guide to promote sound breastfeeding practices and policies worldwide (WHO, 1989). In 1990, WHO and UNICEF reaffirmed their commitment to breastfeeding with the **Innocenti Declaration** *on the Protection, Promotion and Support of Breastfeeding*. The declaration called for national breastfeeding coordinators in all countries, use of the *Ten Steps to Successful Breastfeeding* by maternity services, implementation of the International Code,

---

FIGURE 1.3
Ten steps to successful breastfeeding.

Every facility providing maternity services and care for newborn infants should:

1. Have a written breastfeeding policy that is routinely communicated to all health care staff.
2. Train all health care staff in skills necessary to implement this policy.
3. Inform all pregnant women about the benefits and management of breastfeeding.
4. Help mothers initiate breastfeeding within a half hour of birth.
5. Show mothers how to breastfeed and how to maintain lactation even if they should be separated from their infants.
6. Give newborn infants no food or drink other than breastmilk unless medically indicated.
7. Practice rooming in—allow mothers and infants to remain together 24 hours a day.
8. Encourage breastfeeding in response to feeding cues.
9. Give no artificial teats or pacifiers (also called dummies or soothers) to breastfeeding infants.
10. Foster the establishment of breastfeeding support groups and refer mothers to them on discharge from the hospital or clinic.

---

and legal protections for employed breastfeeding women. The 1991 launch of the *Baby-Friendly Hospital Initiative* has resulted in over 15,000 baby-friendly hospitals in 134 countries. Chapter 28 contains elements of the initiative. In 2003, to strengthen world attention on infant feeding practices, WHO and UNICEF collaborated on the *Global Strategy for Infant and Young Child Feeding* (WHO, 2003).

Global Strategy for Infant and Young Child Feeding

The *Global Strategy for Infant and Young Child Feeding* builds on the 1981 *International Code of Marketing of Breastmilk Substitutes*; the 1990 *Innocenti Declaration on the Protection, Promotion and Support of Breastfeeding*; and the 1991 *Baby-Friendly Hospital Initiative*. The Global Strategy identifies essential interventions to ensure that children develop to their full potential, free from the adverse consequences of compromised nutritional status and preventable illness. The initiative charges governments, international organizations, and other concerned parties with ensuring that their collective action contributes to the attainment of these goals.

Breastfeeding promotion is a centerpiece of this strategy, which aims to reduce the global consequences of childhood undernutrition, specifically diarrheal disease, measles, malaria, and lower respiratory infection. The strategy reasserts exclusive breastfeeding for the first six months of life and breastfeeding with appropriate complementary foods for up to two years and beyond. Among its tenets, it calls for supporting working women, **culture**-specific nutrition counseling, skilled support to parents and caregivers, and appropriate response to global emergencies. Specific strategies within the health care system include skilled counseling, implementation of the *Baby-Friendly Hospital Initiative*, routine nutrition intervention, and guidance in appropriate **complementary feeding**.

▶ CURRENT BREASTFEEDING RECOMMENDATIONS

The ultimate goal of global promotion, protection, and support of breastfeeding is baby-friendly health care. Such a climate will empower and enable women to breastfeed exclusively for the first six months and will create circumstances that enable mothers to continue to breastfeed for two years or longer with complementary foods. Exclusive breastfeeding means that breastfeeding babies receive no drinks or foods other than their mothers' milk, with the exception of vitamin and mineral drops or medicines. For exclusive breastfeeding to go easily, infants receive no pacifiers or artificial teats (artificial nipples). The mother (or caregiver providing expressed milk) feeds the baby in response to **feeding cues**, and no limits are placed on frequency or length of feedings. When they are exclusively breastfed, most infants receive at least 8 to 12 breastfeedings in 24 hours, including night feedings.

The World Health Organization recommends that all babies around the world be breastfed with appropriate complementary food for up to two years and beyond (WHO, 2003). Optimal health of the mother and baby forms the basis of their recommendations, as well as minimal cost to the family, community, and environment. The American Academy of Pediatrics recommends that mothers breastfeed exclusively for six months and continue breastfeeding with appropriate complementary food through twelve months and beyond (AAP, 1997). The American Academy of Family Physicians supports breastfeeding past infancy, including **tandem nursing** (AAFP, 2001).

▶ SUMMARY

The infant feeding climate today is one in which many parents embrace the idea of breastfeeding. For the most part, healthcare providers share a conviction that breastfeeding is the optimal method for infant nutrition. Despite this intellectual agreement, breastfeeding women need support and advice in a society dominated by bottle-feeding messages, societal attitudes, and aggressive formula industry marketing. Caregivers, agencies, lactation consultants, and **breastfeeding counselors** can provide this support. They can educate parents about breastfeeding management and empower them to reach their breastfeeding goals. Breastfeeding is a basic right of all mothers and babies. The WHO and UNICEF initiatives will help ensure these rights. They provide a framework for real progress in breastfeeding promotion and the establishment of baby-friendly health care.

▶ CHAPTER 1—AT A GLANCE

Facts you learned—

The breastfeeding context:

- There is a cultural belief in many countries that bottle-feeding is the norm.
- There is a scarcity of lactation education in medical and nursing schools.
- Women with the lowest breastfeeding rates are 21 years old and under, with low education.
- Breastfeeding among African American women is increasing.
- Media in the United States do little to support breastfeeding.
- Breastfeeding could save billions of health care dollars.
- Babies should be breastfed exclusively for the first six months.
- Mothers should be empowered to breastfeed for two years or longer.

International promotion and support efforts:

- Baby-friendly Hospital Initiative
- Global Strategy for Infant and Young Child Feeding
- Innocenti Declaration
- International Code of Marketing of Breastmilk Substitutes
- Protecting, Promoting and Supporting Breastfeeding
- Ten Steps to Successful Breastfeeding
- UNICEF
- U.S. Healthy People 2010
- U.S. Surgeon General
- WHO Global Data Bank on Breastfeeding
- World Health Organization

Importance of breastfeeding for babies:

- Promotes cognitive development.
- Lowers the incidence of malocclusion.
- May reduce the risk of obstructive sleep apnea in adulthood.

- Forms deep and lasting attachment between mother and child.
- Helps develop the baby's perceptual and response mechanisms.
- Aids respiration by stimulating blood flow.
- Many other benefits, described in Chapter 9.

Importance of breastfeeding for mothers:

- Empowering.
- Contracts uterus and helps stop bleeding after delivery.
- Promotes maternal feelings of well-being, relaxation, and mothering.
- Returns her to prepregnancy size more quickly.
- Delays pregnancy.
- Reduces risk of breast and ovarian cancer.
- Reduces risk of osteoporosis.

▶ REFERENCES

Abbott Laboratories, Ross Products Division. New data show US breastfeeding rates at all-time recorded high. Press release, Columbus, OH; November 25, 2003.

American Academy of Family Physicians (AAFP). AAFP policy statement on breastfeeding. AAFP; 2001.

American Academy of Pediatrics (AAP). Work Group on Breastfeeding. Breastfeeding and the use of human milk. *Pediatrics* 100:1035–1039; 1997.

Anderson J et al. Breastfeeding and cognitive development: A meta-analysis. *Am J Clin Nutr* 70:525–535; 1999.

Bachrach VR, Schwarz E, Bachrach LR. Breastfeeding and the risk of hospitalization for respiratory disease in infancy: A meta-analysis. *Arch Pediatr Adolesc Med* 157(3):237–243; 2003.

Becher H et al. Reproductive factors and familial predisposition for breast cancer by age 50 years: A case-control-family study for assessing main effects and possible gene-environment interaction. *Int J Epidemiol* 32(1):38–48; 2003.

Beral V et al (Collaborative Group on Hormonal Factors in Breast Cancer). Breast cancer and breastfeeding: Collaborative reanalysis of individual data from 47 epidemiological studies in 30 countries, including 50,302 women with breast cancer and 96,973 women without the disease. *Lancet* 360(9328): 187–195; 2002.

Carranza-Lira S, Mera Paz J. Influence of number of pregnancies and total breastfeeding time on bone mineral density. *Int J Fertil* 47(4):169–171; 2002.

Davis-Floyd R, St. John G. *From Doctor to Healer: The Transformative Journey.* New Jersey: Rutgers University Press; 1998.

Gomez-Sanchiz M et al. Influence of breast-feeding and parental intelligence on cognitive development in the 24-month-old child. *Clin Pediatr* (Phila) 43(8):753–761; 2004.

Healthy People 2010: 2003 Available at: *www.healthypeople.gov/Document/HTML/Volume2/16MICH. htm#_Toc494699668.*

Heller S. *The Vital Touch.* New York: Henry Holt and Co.; 1997.

Hillenbrand K. Effect of educational intervention about breastfeeding on the knowledge, confidence, and behaviors of pediatric resident physicians. *Pediatrics* 110(5):e59; 2002.

Hoefer C, Hardy MC. Later development of breastfed and artificially fed infants. *JAMA* 92:615; 1929.

Horwood L, Fergusson D. Breastfeeding and later cognitive and academic outcomes. *Pediatrics* 101:1; 1998.

Illingworth PJ et al. Diminution in energy expenditure during lactation. *Br Med J* 292:437; 1986.

Labbok MH, Clark D, Goldman AS. Breastfeeding: Maintaining an irreplaceable immunological resource. *Nat Rev Immunol* 4(7):565–572; 2004.

Labbok M, Hendershot G. Does breastfeeding protect against malocclusion? *Am J Prev Med* 3:227–232; 1987.

La Leche League, International Center for Breastfeeding Information. *Breastfeeding Statistics.* September 15, 2003. *www.lalecheleague.org/cbi/bfstats03.html.* Accessed December 1, 2004.

Lawrence R. *Breastfeeding: A Guide for the Medical Profession.* St. Louis, MO: Mosby; 1999.

Leavitt J. *Brought to Bed: Childbearing in America, 1750–1950.* New York: Oxford University Press; 1986.

Li R et al. Prevalence of breastfeeding in the United States: The 2001 national immunization survey. *Pediatrics* 111(5 part 2): 1198–1201; 2003.

Locklin M, Naber S. Does breastfeeding empower women? Insights from a select group of educated, low-income minority women. *Birth* 20:30–35; 1993.

Lucas A et al. Breast milk and subsequent intelligence quotient in children born preterm. *Lancet* 339:261–264; 1992.

McKay F. Infant mortality in relation to breastfeeding. *New York State Journal of Medicine* 24:433–438; 1924.

Merewood A, Heinig J. Efforts to promote breastfeeding in the United States: Development of a national breastfeeding awareness campaign. *J Hum Lact* 20(2):140–145; 2004.

Montagu A. *Touching: The Human Significance of the Skin.* New York: Harper & Row; 1986.

Montgomery D, Splett P. The economic benefit of breastfed infants enrolled in WIC. *Am J Diet Assoc* 97:379–385; 1997.

Moreland J, Coombs J. Promoting and supporting breast-feeding. *Am Fam Physician* 61:2093–2100, 2103–2104; 2000.

Newcomb P et al. Lactation and a reduced risk of pre-menopausal breast cancer. *N Engl J Med* 330:81–87; 1994.

Palmer B. *Sleep Apnea from an Anatomical, Anthropologic and Developmental Perspective.* Presentation to the Academy of Dental Sleep Medicine, Philadelphia, PA; June 4, 2004.

Paton L et al. Pregnancy and lactation have no long-term deleterious effect on measures of bone mineral in healthy women: A twin study. *Am J Clin Nutr* 77(3):707–714; 2003.

Phillip B et al. Physicians and breastfeeding promotion in the United States: A call for action. *Pediatrics* 107(3):584–588; 2001.

Rao M et al. Effect of breastfeeding on cognitive development of infants born small for gestational age. *Acta Paediatrica* (91)3:267–274; 2002.

Rosenblatt KA, Thomas DB. Lactation and the risk of epithelial ovarian cancer. The WHO collaborative study of neoplasia and steroid contraceptives. *Int J Epidemiol* 22(2):192–197; 1993.

Ryan A et al. Breastfeeding continues to increase into the new millennium. *Pediatrics* 110(6):1103–1109; 2002.

Sedgwick JP, Fleishner. Breastfeeding in the reduction of infant mortality. *Am J Public Health* 11:153–157; 1921.

Shepard JWJ et al. Evaluation of the upper airway in patients with OSA/SDB. *Sleep* 14:361–371; 1991.

Smith MM et al. Influence of breastfeeding on cognitive outcomes at age 6–8 years: Follow-up of very low birth weight infants. *Am J Epidemiol* 158(11): 1075–1078; 2003

Tung K et al. Reproductive factors and epithelial overian cancer risk by histologic type: A multiethnic case-control study. *Am J Epidemiol* 148:629–638; 2003.

UNICEF. *The State of the World's Children, Statistical Tables. 2003. www.unicef.org/sowc03/tables/general-note.html.* Accessed December 1, 2004.

Van Esterik P. Guest Editorial. *J Hum Lact* 10(2):71; 1994.

Weimer J. Economic benefits: A review and analysis. Economic Research Service, USDA, *Food Assistance and Nutrition Research Report* 13: March 2001.

Wolf J. Low breastfeeding rates and public health in the US. *Am J Pub Health* 93(12):2001–2010; 2003.

World Health Organization (WHO). *Global Strategy for Infant and Young Child Feeding.* Geneva: WHO; 2003.

World Health Organization (WHO). *Protecting, Promoting, and Supporting Breastfeeding: A Joint WHO/UNICEF Statement.* Geneva: WHO; 1989.

Yen ML et al. Risk factors for ovarian cancer in Taiwan: A case-control study in a low-incidence population. *Gynecol Oncol* 89(2):318–324; 2003.

Zheng T et al. Lactation reduces breast cancer risk in Shandong Province, China. *Am J Epidemiol* 152:1129–1135; 2000.

▶ **BIBLIOGRAPHY**

Apple R. The medicalization of infant feeding in the United States and New Zealand: Two countries, one experience. *J Hum Lact* 10:31–37; 1994.

Carter C, Altemus M. Integrative functions of lactational hormones in social behavior and stress management. *Ann NY Acad Sci* 807:164–174; 1997.

Cummings N. Epidemiology of osteoporosis and osteoporotic fractures. *Epidemiol Rev* 7:178–208; 1985.

Cunningham A et al. Breastfeeding and health in the 1980s: A global epidemiologic review. *J Pediatr* 118(5): 659–666; 1991.

Cunningham A. *Breastfeeding, Bottlefeeding & Illness: An Annotated Bibliography.* Australia: Nursing Mothers Association of Australia and ALMA Publications, 2 volumes; 1986 and 1990.

Deering C. A review of infant feeding related messages in lay parenting magazines: July 1991–December 1991. Unpublished research; 1992.

Feldblum P et al. Lactation history and bone mineral density among perimenopausal women. *Epidemiol* 3:527–531; 1992.

Garret S. *Going It Alone.* Hampshire, England: Gower; 1991.

Hamosh M. Breastfeeding: Unraveling the mysteries of mother's milk. *Medscape Women's Health*; 1996.

Jackson EB et al. Statistical report on incidence and duration of breast-feeding in relation to personal-social and hospital maternity factors. *Pediatrics* 17:700–715; 1956.

Lawrence R. Breast-feeding trends: A cause for action. *Pediatrics* 88(4):867–868; 1991.

Liebman B. Breast cancer. *Nutrition Action Health Letter* 23: 4–7; 1996.

Ludington-Hoe S et al. Skin-to-skin contact beginning in the delivery room for Colombian mothers and their preterm infants. *J Hum Lact* 9:241–242; 1993.

McTiernan A, Thomas D. Evidence for a protective effect of lactation on risk of breast cancer in young women: Results from a case-control study. *Am J Epidemiol* 124:353–358; 1986.

Mepham TB. Science and the politics of breastfeeding: Birthright or birth rite? *Breastfeeding Review* 1(15):5–13; 1989.

Minchin M. *Breastfeeding Matters: What We Need to Know about Infant Feeding.* Victoria, Australia: Alma Publications; 1998.

Naylor A. Letter. *JAMA* 207:2300; 1993.

Newton N. *Maternal Emotions.* New York: Hoeber; 1955.

Pollock J. Long term associations with infant feeding in a clinically advantaged population of babies. *Dev Med Child Neurol* 36:429–440; 1994.

Rosenblatt K et al. Prolonged lactation and endometrial cancer. *Int J Epidemiol* 24:499–503; 1996.

Schanler R. Pediatricians' practices and attitudes regarding breastfeeding promotion. *Pediatrics* 103(3):e33; 1999.

Schneider AP III. Risk factor for ovarian cancer. *N Engl J Med* 317:508–509; 1987.

Silva PA, Fergusson DM. Socio-economic status, maternal characteristics, child experience and intelligence in pre-school children. *N Zeal J of Ed Stud* 2:180–188; 1976.

Van Esterik P. Breastfeeding and feminism. *Int J of Gynaecol Obstet* 47:S41–S54; 1994.

Whittemore A et al. Characteristics relating to ovarian cancer risk: Collaborative analysis of 12 US case-control studies. *Am J Epidemiol* 136(10):1184–1203; 1992.

Work Group on Cow's Milk Protein and Diabetes Mellitus. *Pediatrics* 94(5):752–754; 1994.

World Health Organization. *WHO Global Data Bank on Breast-Feeding.* Geneva: Nutrition Unit, WHO; 1996.

THE LACTATION CONSULTING PROFESSION

Contributing Authors: Linda Kutner, Jan Barger, and Carole Peterson

Until breastfeeding becomes the societal norm and several generations of women are comfortable with breastfeeding self-care and management techniques, breastfeeding care will be an integral part of maternal and infant health care. The mother and baby form a nursing **dyad**—one unit, each dependent on the other. The goal of breastfeeding is for the mother and baby to function smoothly as a team. Breastfeeding assistance is most effective when breastfeeding caregivers work collaboratively, both among one another and with parents. All members of the healthcare team must support the nursing dyad and provide consistent care in order for mothers to achieve their breastfeeding goals. The lactation consultant emerged in the mid-1980s and is the health care team member whose primary focus is breastfeeding. Volunteer lay counselors are important members of this team as well. They provide peer support and guidance as a complement to the assistance provided by health professionals.

KEY TERMS

certification
Clinical Competencies for
    IBCLC practice
community outreach
discharge planner
health consumer
ICD-9 code
International Board
    Certified Lactation
    Consultant
    (IBCLC)
International Board of
    Lactation Consultant
    Examiners
    (IBLCE)

International Lactation
    Consultant Association
    (ILCA)
lactation consultant
lay counselor
mother-to-mother support
    group
networking
outreach counseling
private practice
standards of practice
superbill
third-party reimbursement
warm line
WIC

THE LACTATION CONSULTANT AS PART OF THE HEALTHCARE TEAM

All caregivers—physicians, nurses, midwives, physician assistants, dieticians, physical therapists, occupational therapists, and childbirth educators—need to incorporate breastfeeding teaching and support into their existing practices. Although many mothers benefit from the services of a lactation consultant, women ideally would receive appropriate advice about basic breastfeeding management from all their health care providers.

As a lactation consultant, you are an advocate for the nursing dyad as well as, separately, for the infant, with the knowledge, skills, and willingness to work at the baby's pace. As the only member of the health care team whose primary focus is breastfeeding, you may need to suggest alternate plans of breastfeeding care if recommendations by other members of the health care team could affect breastfeeding negatively.

The Growth of a New Profession

During the past two decades, lactation consulting has become a profession in its own right. Many individuals working in maternal/child health have specialized in this new field (Figure 2.1). Their backgrounds are varied. Some possess advanced degrees in the healthcare field.

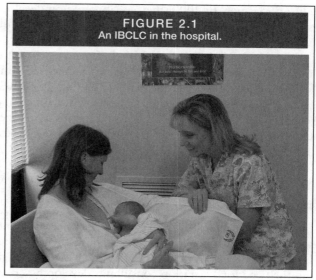

FIGURE 2.1
An IBCLC in the hospital.

Printed with permission of Anna Swisher.

Because of their professional education and experience, they are in a unique position to expand their services into lactation consulting. Some begin their careers as lay counselors and then acquire the advanced education and skills that enable them to work professionally as part of the health care team. Some enter lactation consulting from unrelated fields after breastfeeding their children and developing a desire to help other mothers achieve their breastfeeding goals.

Professional education for lactation management began in the early 1980s through various private programs. Texts on lactation management became available, some directed to the medical profession and others directed to practical aspects of counseling. In 1984, U.S. Surgeon General C. Everett Koop convened a *Workshop on Breastfeeding and Human Lactation*, which identified professional education as one of six core areas to be addressed.

A group of leaders in the profession established the **International Board of Lactation Consultant Examiners** (IBLCE) in 1985 to offer a **certification** examination. IBLCE later added "Registered Lactation Consultant" and "RLC" in the United Sates as additional trademark designations. Only an **International Board Certified Lactation Consultant** (IBCLC) may use the trademark.

The **International Lactation Consultant Association** (ILCA) formed in 1985 as an association for professional lactation consultants. ILCA developed **standards of practice** for the profession (Appendix D) that are available on the ILCA Web site. IBLCE developed a Code of Ethics (Appendix C) to guide IBCLCs in their practice. Directors of lactation courses throughout the world meet annually at the ILCA conference to address education issues. In 2002, they collaborated on development of a core curriculum (ILCA, 2002a) to establish educational standards for the lactation profession.

By 2002, clinical **internships** began to emerge for aspiring lactation consultants, providing supervised **clinical practice** with experienced IBCLCs. In 2003, IBLCE launched a pilot clinical pathway for qualifying to take the certification exam. The pathway utilizes *Clinical Competencies for IBCLC Practice*, a document developed by IBLCE in 2003 and endorsed by ILCA (see Appendix B).

Role in the Healthcare Team

Because the profession is so new, lactation consultants sometimes find it challenging to establish themselves as integral members of the health care team. Demonstrating the need for a lactation consultant, developing credibility, overcoming medical elitism, and addressing practical employment issues are some of the challenges you may face while trying to establish yourself in the profession. Your role as a lactation consultant may be new to many medical professionals. The services you offer and the manner in which you work with other health care providers will build your reputation and influence the cooperation you receive.

It is helpful to realize that those with whom you come in contact—parents, nurses, physicians, midwives, educators—all share your goal of ensuring the health of mothers and babies. Communicating with the nursing dyad's primary care practitioners will help establish you as part of the health care team. Inform caregivers of your services, and help them understand your role.

Sharing Information with Physicians

As a lactation consultant, you offer an adjunct service that builds on the physician–patient relationship. You can keep current by reading relevant research and literature from all disciplines that affect lactation and breastfeeding management. Exchanging information with medical professionals and working with them to provide parents with optimal healthcare can be personally rewarding, as well as a welcome contribution to your community. Sharing appropriate information among the various disciplines will help broaden your sphere of influence.

Many physician practices welcome research-based information and materials on lactation management. Most infant feeding literature that physicians receive pertains to the use of artificial formula. Similarly, most breastfeeding literature they receive is published by infant formula companies. Physicians need sound, unbiased breastfeeding information from a source that does not have a vested interested in women *not* breastfeeding.

When giving any information to patients, a physician relies on his or her background and training in a particular field. Unfortunately, little if any time in most medical schools is devoted to the practical management of breastfeeding. Biochemistry or breastfeeding problems of a medical nature are usually the focus, instead. Further, keeping up with the latest information in journal articles can be difficult in a busy practice. As a result, when it comes to breastfeeding management, many physicians rely on conferences, seminars, and the breastfeeding experiences of their own families and their patients. If these experiences were negative or problematic, it may bias the information and advice they give to patients.

Mother's Role in the Team

Encourage mothers to share the positive aspects of breastfeeding with their physicians. Because there is a tendency for mothers to concentrate on problems, physicians often react by prescribing unnecessary practices for what they perceive to be the mother's concern. If a mother mentions that her baby is fussy, her physician may respond by prescribing a formula supplement. The mother may not have considered a correlation between breastfeeding and her baby's fussiness. She may simply have general questions about caring for a fussy baby. Mothers need to be clear with the messages they send, and they need to be assertive regarding their wishes.

When mothers share the positive aspects of their breastfeeding experience, they can help modify or change physician attitudes, opinions, and practices. Remind mothers that physicians are usually very busy and may not recall all the details of a situation. A mother needs to be prepared to remind her physician of her desire to breastfeed as well as plans they previously discussed. She and her physician then can decide how to adapt the plans to her present situation.

Physician's Role in the Healthcare Team

Physicians generally are aware of the benefits of human milk as published in current literature. Their practices, however, may not reflect an understanding of the day-to-day management of breastfeeding. The best way to change physicians' practices is through the sharing of clinical data and positive comments from mothers.

Some physicians are reluctant to advocate breastfeeding in order to avoid causing mothers to feel pressured or guilty about their choice to bottle-feed. Adopting a middle-of-the-road stance regarding breastfeeding transmits a message to parents that artificial formula is equally healthy for their infant. There is no middle of the road when it comes to providing optimal nutrition and preserving an infant's health. Parents would not expect their infant's physician to be noncommittal about the importance of **immunizations**, car seat use, dental checkups, or avoidance of cigarette smoking and other **social toxicants**. Breastfeeding is no different.

You can help physicians recognize that mothers need support and validation in their decisions. Mothers need to be empowered as parents and welcomed as equal members of their baby's and their own health care team. Physicians need to understand the important role they play in protecting the continuation of breastfeeding for mothers and babies in their care. When they encounter a problem requiring specialized care, they can be encouraged to refer mothers to an IBCLC. They can also refer mothers to a support group that will provide mother-to-mother support.

Role with Mothers

If the mother's or infant's physician seems indifferent to breastfeeding or gives questionable advice, the mother will benefit from close contact with you or another breastfeeding support person. It therefore is important to recognize how your function in the health care system applies to the mothers in your care. Promoting **health consumerism** encourages parents to assume an active role in their family's health care. Parents may need guidance in assuming this new role. You can assist them by providing options and advice and by suggesting ways in which they can interact with their physicians. Your primary function is to coordinate the mother's breastfeeding care and empower her to breastfeed with minimal intervention or complications. Your role is to serve as a facilitator who educates and gently guides the mother. Acting as a true consultant, you use your scientific knowledge and practical experience to nurture and protect the relationship between the mother and her infant.

Several basic elements are important in developing a comprehensive program of breastfeeding education and support for parents. Ideally, you will provide prenatal and postpartum instruction. If you are a hospital-based IBCLC, you will be available to advise the mother during her hospital stay. Mothers benefit most from a program that provides the following range of services:

- ◆ Prenatal and postpartum classes
- ◆ Daily rounds to postpartum breastfeeding mothers in the hospital
- ◆ Assistance with breastfeeding problems before and after discharge
- ◆ Routine long-term **follow-up**
- ◆ Telephone **warm line** for counseling new mothers
- ◆ Periodic review and development of parent literature
- ◆ Referral to a mother-to-mother support group

Educating Mothers about Breastfeeding

Your primary role is to teach practical information about breastfeeding, point out options, and offer useful suggestions. Explaining why a certain technique works the way it does and giving the mother the reasons behind your suggestions will help her understand them, relate to them, and adapt them to her situation. Educating her in this manner will give her the tools to handle future similar circumstances.

In order for you to share information effectively, you must thoroughly understand the process of milk production, typical breastfeeding patterns, and factors that may affect them. If you are incorporating lactation consulting into a wider medical role, such as a hospital-based nurse or midwife, you may focus primarily on basic breastfeeding management. You will then need to be aware of potential complications and unusual circumstances, as well as resources for making appropriate referrals. If you are specializing in the lactation field as a board-certified lactation consultant, you will need expertise in more complicated and unusual breastfeeding circumstances.

Whatever your level of breastfeeding care, it is important to remain current with relevant literature and practices. Lactation research is dynamic and extensive, and continuing your lactation education will enable you to give appropriate advice to mothers. It is imperative in lactation, as in most fields today, that you become a lifelong learner and embrace change when warranted.

Sharing Medical Information

It is especially important that the information and advice you give to mothers is obtained from a reliable source. Anything beyond the scope of the lactation consultant must be presented in a manner of educating the mother, not prescribing treatment. (This is not the case for those who have prescriptive authority, such as a medical doctor, nurse practitioner, or physician's assistant.) Information on prescription drugs changes frequently based on current research, and you must be sure to have the most up-to-date information when you relate it to mothers. Although there may be no studies to show the ill effects of a particular drug, that does not rule out the possibility that such ill effects can exist for either the mother or infant. One authoritative source on medications and lactation is Hale's *Medications and Mothers' Milk* (Hale, 2004). When discussing drugs with a mother, always recommend that she consult her baby's physician concerning their advisability. The baby's physician ultimately should have the final decision.

Conflicting Advice and Informed Choice

There have been great strides in family-centered maternity care and breastfeeding in recent years. Breastfeeding advice in some situations may conflict with advice from other health care providers. This is not necessarily because one side is incorrect. Rather, it is because there is a variety of medical opinions concerning obstetrics and pediatrics. You can present information to the mother and urge her to make her own choices and to work toward suitable solutions with her physicians. When your advice contradicts the physician's, it can cause confusion and concern for the mother. Acknowledge this with her and help her to develop a plan.

When such a conflict exists, parents must resolve it with their other caregivers. Take care to avoid alienating people in your medical community. In some cases, you may communicate directly with the mother's or baby's physician. At other times, you may share information with the mother that she in turn will discuss with her physician. Polite assertiveness, a positive attitude, and a willingness to work with the physician to resolve the conflict to their mutual satisfaction will strengthen the parents' position. Informing and educating parents places

this responsibility on them. If parents fail to accept this active role, recognize that you have fulfilled your responsibility of informing them of their options, whether or not you agree with their decisions.

When you share information with mothers, be sure to communicate clearly and simply. Offer the least complicated explanation in lay terms. Relate the information in a friendly and low-key manner, neither overwhelming a mother nor making her appear uninformed. Relate only information that you are certain is up-to-date, correct, and evidence-based—not opinion or one person's experience. Whenever your information conflicts with information the mother has obtained from another source, check your sources for accuracy and try to help the mother resolve the conflict. Always check your sources if you are uncertain. If you cannot answer a question, tell the mother you will research it and follow up with her later.

▶ PRACTICE SETTINGS FOR LACTATION CONSULTANTS

Healthcare practitioners care for breastfeeding mothers and babies in a variety of settings. Lactation consultants work in hospitals, physicians' offices, public health clinics, home healthcare, and private practice. In some ways, the experience you bring to the job dictates the practice setting you choose. In many cases, hospitals, physicians' offices, and home health agencies prefer that the lactation consultant possess additional training in healthcare, such as nursing. Health clinics, especially those participating in the WIC program, may employ a lactation consultant who is also a registered dietician. A lactation consultant in private practice should have extensive experience with a great variety of babies and breastfeeding situations. The discussion in this chapter explores each of these practice settings.

Practicing in a Hospital

A large percentage of lactation consultants work in hospitals. Issues relevant to the role of the lactation consultant in a hospital setting are addressed throughout this text. One of the most important jobs of a hospital-based lactation consultant is ensuring that someone who is skilled in breastfeeding assessment observes every mother breastfeed her baby before discharge. That person is often a staff nurse who has learned about breastfeeding in order to provide optimal continuity of care.

The lactation consultant cannot be the only person responsible for helping mothers with breastfeeding. You have a responsibility to train other maternity staff in basic breastfeeding care and some of the more common challenges encountered in the immediate postpartum period. This permits the lactation consultant to respond to referrals for situations that are more complex. Chapter 12 discusses the lactation consultant's role in postpartum breastfeeding care.

Logistics of Hospital Practice

There are a number of factors to consider when choosing to practice in a hospital setting. As a member of the hospital staff, you will be part of a team and will have the support of peer relationships. Being a staff member carries the advantage of a steady income and work, as well as employment benefits. Work hours will depend on the amount of time allocated for lactation coverage. Ideally, the hospital should provide 24-hour assistance for breastfeeding mothers and babies. When there are limited numbers of lactation consultants on staff, coverage may occur only during the daily work week or for only one shift. Although you may not be able to see every breastfeeding mother, you will most likely see any who are having problems.

Working as a hospital-based lactation consultant may present some challenges. Many lactation consultants work longer hours than those in other staff positions in an effort to see every breastfeeding mother and baby. This is especially the case for those who are the sole lactation consultant on staff. When the staff learns how to provide basic breastfeeding care, you may see only mothers and babies with complicated problems. This can increase the potential for emotional **burnout**. There may be no other lactation consultant with whom to share problems or frustrations. Unsupportive staff or administrators may create obstacles or frustrations for you, especially when there is a conflict in philosophy or priorities.

Your role as a breastfeeding advocate may be restricted because of hospital policies and limitations. As a hospital employee, you are accountable to the administration, who may expect you to see all breastfeeding patients. The work schedule will be less flexible than if you were in private practice. When hospitals experience downsizing, administrators may regard the lactation consultant's position as less critical than other positions. Consequently, you may lose your job or assume duties unrelated to breastfeeding, especially if you have other clinical skills such as nursing, dietetics, or occupational therapy. That can be very frustrating to someone whose primary interest is breastfeeding support.

Despite these potential challenges, most lactation consultants work in a hospital setting. A wide group of colleagues can provide a source of reference as well as moral support. The rest of the staff will view you as an expert. Being on staff makes providing inpatient and staff education convenient. Your client base will be steady, and you will not need to seek referrals, as is the case in private practice.

Because necessary records and resources are readily available, you will not need to acquire them on your own. The hospital provides breastfeeding equipment and other necessary supplies. They bill for your services, which frees your time to see mothers. Hospitals may fund attendance at conferences as well as memberships to professional organizations. The hospital-based lactation consultant often has an opportunity to develop a strong lactation program and to be instrumental in designing and improving the care received by breastfeeding mothers and their babies.

Hospital Lactation Services

The hospital setting enables you to influence large numbers of people. How hospital-based lactation consultants function varies, based on the setting. You may provide services to both inpatients and outpatients and serve as a resource for hospital staff in the care of normal breastfeeding couples. This includes assisting with the care of couples who are having difficulty and providing inservice education and training for staff. You may make rounds on some or all breastfeeding mothers and babies, including those who are patients elsewhere in the hospital. On the other hand, you may see only those mothers and babies who other medical or nursing staff refer to you.

Administratively, you may develop breastfeeding policies and procedures, competency guidelines, performance evaluations, and patient documentation forms. You may also develop handouts and reading materials for breastfeeding parents. Patient follow-up is an essential element of breastfeeding care. It is important that contact with the mother continue after her discharge from the hospital, through follow-up telephone calls or outpatient visits. Some hospitals provide outpatient visits on a fee-for-service basis or as a billable service. Others provide it at no additional cost to the patient. Still others provide no outpatient lactation services and instead refer mothers to outside resources.

You will make referrals to mother support groups and, when necessary, to a community-based lactation consultant or other health professional. You can assist the mother in obtaining breastfeeding devices, when appropriate, and teach her how to use them. Another outpatient service provided by many lactation consultants is conducting prenatal education about infant feeding. This incorporates practical information about breastfeeding and the realities and risks of artificial infant feeding.

Financial Considerations

Lactation consultants in the hospital generally receive an hourly wage, although some may be salaried. The salary range for a hospital-based IBCLC often is comparable to that of a nurse clinician or a registered nurse certified in a specialty. You may work full-time or part-time; job sharing can be attractive to those who have small children at home. In order to keep the service viable, it is helpful to work with the billing department to determine the amount to charge patients for your services. The hospital may choose, for example, to charge only for outpatient services or for complex inpatient problems that you see.

Practicing in a Health Clinic

Public health clinics offer many avenues of employment for lactation consultants. You may provide information and education to agencies that deliver prenatal, labor and delivery, postpartum, pediatric, or day care services. Many health clinics offer one-on-one breastfeeding counseling, classes, and postpartum support groups. You may counsel mothers or supervise and train peer counselors. Many lactation consultants in public health participate in state breastfeeding workshops, consortiums, and committees.

You will encounter many diverse lifestyles when working in a public health clinic. It is important to be sensitive to families' cultural and socioeconomic values. Since lifestyles and priorities among clinic clients may be quite different from your personal experience, you need to remain flexible and adaptable. You can find common ground with mothers by focusing on their love and concern for their children. Many clients move frequently, making ongoing contact challenging.

In the United States, the Special Supplemental Food Program for Women, Infants and Children, commonly referred to as WIC, helps pregnant women choose nutritious foods and provides services to breastfeeding mothers, infants, and children up to five years of age. To qualify for WIC assistance, family income must be 185 percent of the poverty level. In other words, if the poverty level is $10,000/year, a WIC participant would need to make $18,500/year or less (USDA, 2004). Breastfeeding rates among WIC participants are increasing, whereas rates in the overall population remain unchanged. The WIC program has demonstrated that their programs save tax dollars by encouraging healthy eating, which, in turn, lowers health care costs.

The Canada Prenatal Nutrition Program (CPNP) provides many of the same services as the U.S. WIC program. A distinguishing feature of the Canadian program is that it provides no free formula except as a compassionate response to a woman who has run out of formula and cannot afford to buy more. CPNP believes that free supplies of formula affect women's choice of feeding method. They therefore place heavy emphasis on promotion and support of breastfeeding. One cross-generational study has found that free formula from WIC affected breastfeeding rates (Fooladi, 2001).

Breastfeeding Promotion in WIC

WIC's philosophy is to help participants become healthier and more self-sufficient through education and application of sound nutrition principles. At no cost to participants, the program provides nutritious foods to supplement the diet, information on healthy eating, and referrals for healthcare. WIC is engaged in extensive breastfeeding promotion efforts at the local, state, and national levels. The U.S. Department of Agriculture (USDA) encourages breastfeeding among WIC participants through regulatory provisions, publications, cooperative efforts with other federal agencies and private organizations, and funding of breastfeeding grants and studies.

A variety of approaches contributes to increasing the rates of breastfeeding among WIC participants. These include peer support counselors, special incentives, prenatal classes, toll-free telephone lines, and health professional training. WIC promotes the use of peer counselors in order to provide ongoing support to their clients. Peer counselors reach mothers on their own level, dispel cultural myths, and offer advice on other lifestyle issues based on personal experience. For that reason, WIC peer counselors must be representative of the community they serve (see Chapter 20 for a discussion of cultural issues).

WIC has access to a significant segment of America's low-income, at-risk mothers and infants. Therefore, the USDA has an opportunity to contribute toward achieving the Department of Health and Human Services Healthy People 2010 goals for breastfeeding as well as the program's own nutritional goals. The USDA's national breastfeeding promotion campaign augments breastfeeding efforts already underway in communities throughout the United States. The campaign promotes breastfeeding awareness and support among women of childbearing age, their families, and others who influence their infant feeding decisions.

Breastfeeding rates among WIC participants in 2002 were 58.8 percent initiation in the hospital and 22.1 percent at 5 to 6 months postpartum. This compares to the non-WIC population rates of 70.1 percent and 33.2 percent respectively (Ross, 2002). Many socioeconomic characteristics common among the WIC population are associated with lower rates of breastfeeding and may contribute to this discrepancy. These include race, age (younger than 20 years), and education (less than high school graduate).

A portion of WIC funding for breastfeeding goes toward salaries of healthcare professionals and peer counselors. This funding offers an ideal opportunity for the establishment of a lactation consultant position. Some states or agencies have breastfeeding promotion positions funded on a percentage basis. For example, a registered dietician's job position may be divided 80 percent for regular WIC job functions and 20 percent for breastfeeding promotion and support.

Most states designate a breastfeeding coordinator for each agency. Responsibilities are diverse, and backgrounds of potential coordinators vary as well. One position may require a lactation consultant certified through the IBLCE. Another may include non-breastfeeding functions that require a nursing or dietetic degree. Still another may require someone with experience in marketing, fundraising, or promotional activities to provide expertise in **community outreach**. A lactation consultant in WIC may train and supervise peer counselors or initiate a peer counselor program if none exists.

Practicing in a Physician Group

Working with an obstetrician, pediatrician, or family practice group offers an opportunity to care for mothers and babies through many stages of breastfeeding. In this type of practice, you will see healthy, normal babies as well as those who experience difficulties. Most of the practice is preventive rather than crisis management-based. Working with only a few physicians will make it easier for you to come to agreement on breastfeeding issues. Therefore, the potential for burnout is lower than in a hospital setting.

One challenge in this setting is that your client load will be dependent on the physician's patient load. Additionally, when you make rounds in the hospital, you may be there at a time when the baby is not ready for a feeding. Early discharge can make it difficult for you to see every breastfeeding mother in a timely manner. You may need to be creative with your schedule in order to visit all mothers and observe each one breastfeeding. Downsizing could eliminate your position, just as with a hospital-based lactation consultant. Be prepared, with documentation that illustrates your importance to the practice.

Lactation Services to a Physician Practice

Breastfeeding consultations can be time consuming. A lactation consultant frees up time that physicians and office personnel otherwise would spend with prenatal and postpartum calls about breastfeeding. Preventive education, hospital counseling, and telephone follow-up are far more effective than crisis management when problems surface. Being able to turn the care of a slow-gaining infant over to a lactation consultant relieves the physician's patient load. This approach identifies the cause of the problem and helps to preserve breastfeeding.

Offering the services of a lactation consultant attracts mothers to the practice. There is great marketing potential if yours is the first physician practice in the

community to have a certified lactation consultant on staff. If you wish to develop a lactation program for a physician or group practice, prepare a brief proposal outlining specific services you could provide for their patients. Chapter 26 contains further suggestions for developing a job proposal or job description. Services to the practice may include:

◆ TEACHING BREASTFEEDING CLASSES.
If you work with a group of obstetricians, nurse midwives, or family practice physicians, you will have many parents to whom you can offer breastfeeding classes. If you work with a pediatrician, you may be able to offer prenatal breastfeeding classes by sending a notice to the offices of the obstetricians who generally refer to that pediatric practice. Taking classes prenatally provides parents with a good start to learning about breastfeeding so that during postpartum time they can focus on reinforcing what they have already learned. See the sample class outlines in Chapter 11.

◆ MEETING WITH WOMEN DURING PREGNANCY.
Having contact with women prenatally offers tremendous benefits. You will have an opportunity to help them in their decision to breastfeed and to dispel any misconceptions that may cause them to consider bottle-feeding. During your visit, you can discuss a woman's breastfeeding goals, evaluate her previous history and the present condition of her breasts and nipples, and begin appropriate intervention, if necessary. This visit may take place in the office or in the context of prenatal breastfeeding or childbirth education classes.

◆ MAKING ROUNDS IN THE HOSPITAL.
If you work exclusively with a group of pediatricians, your first contact with mothers may be in the hospital when you make rounds. You will want to attempt to see every mother in the practice at least once before discharge and to observe her breastfeeding technique.

◆ PROVIDING FOLLOW-UP.
Ideally, follow-up calls occur at about two to three days after discharge, three to four days after that, and again at two weeks. Providing **anticipatory guidance** through follow-up telephone calls helps the mother avoid complications. Additional follow-up can take place more frequently as warranted. An office visit or **home visit** may be necessary to evaluate specific problems or concerns. You might consider installing a separate telephone line in your home to use for a warm line 24 hours a day. An answering machine or voice mail system will record calls that you can return. Depending on your service,

you may also wish to carry a pager or to be available by cell phone.

- ◆ SERVING AS A RESOURCE TO PHYSICIANS AND STAFF.

  You will be a valuable resource to the practice. You can update physicians and staff on new research and recommendations concerning the compatibility of medications with breastfeeding. Providing in-service programs for the nursing staff will help them in their discussions with breastfeeding patients. Encourage them to transfer telephone calls to you so that mothers receive accurate and consistent information.

- ◆ PROVIDING BREASTFEEDING PRODUCTS AND LITERATURE FOR PARENTS.

  You may find it helpful to write your own breastfeeding handouts to provide updated information from your health department, WIC, or La Leche League. See Appendix A for these and other resources. Breast pump rentals and other devices are also possible services to provide, either through the physician's office or directly from you.

- ◆ RECORDING BREASTFEEDING STATISTICS.

  Recording breastfeeding statistics within the practice will help you to document your effectiveness. You can record the number of mothers who initiate breastfeeding and those who continue to breastfeed for six weeks, three months, six months, and one year. You can also document the frequency and nature of problems and the assistance you provided. Such data can form the basis of a research article and benefit others in the lactation field as well.

- ◆ FACILITATING A SUPPORT GROUP FOR MOTHERS.

  Physicians in the practice may welcome having a postpartum support group for breastfeeding mothers. It will provide a needed service to their patients and set the practice apart from others in the community that do not offer breastfeeding support groups.

- ◆ MAKING TREATMENT RECOMMENDATIONS.

  Your expertise will be valuable to others in the practice who do not have time to research breastfeeding literature in order to be current with practice guidelines. You can make sure they have the latest information on breastfeeding management and treatment of problems.

Business Issues

You may choose to work specific hours, using the physician's office as your base, or you may decide to work on-call from home. In either case, you will contact the hospital in the morning to determine which mothers need a visit. You will then make follow-up calls and home or office visits as needed. You will need a private room with a comfortable chair, a variety of pillows, charting forms, a breast pump and other breastfeeding devices, literature, diapers, and other items discussed under private practice. You may wish to incorporate breast pump rentals and other breastfeeding devices into the physician's practice or provide them as a service separate from your arrangement with the physician.

Breastfeeding complications are not limited to specific hours. Just as with a private practice, you will need to be available around the clock. Mothers will need a way to contact you directly. A beeper or voice mail system allows you to contact clients at your convenience. It will also be important to provide coverage by another lactation consultant or other caregiver for times when you are unavailable.

Financial Issues

You can negotiate billing for your services with the physician at the time of your interview. A specific contract should be drawn up specifying your services and salary. You may want to renegotiate at the end of the first year to reflect any changes in your services. Wages in a physician's practice may range between those of an office staff nurse and a hospital-based lactation consultant. Compensation may be on a per-client basis to cover hospital rounds, follow-up telephone calls, establishment of a basic chart, and a warm line. The practice can bill breastfeeding classes and office or home visits separately or include it in the physician's fee. The practice may prefer to compensate for your services with an hourly salary. If the position is part-time, there may be no employment benefits such as health insurance or vacation time.

If clients pay you directly on a fee-for-service basis, they can submit the bill to their insurance company for reimbursement, or the physician can include your services on the bill submitted to the insurance company. Individual insurance companies will determine whether to reimburse for your services. This may be the least desirable arrangement, as many mothers will not use your services until they are in full-blown crisis to avoid the up front cost. Information on third-party reimbursement is available from ILCA.

Practicing in Home Healthcare

The home care lactation consultant provides follow-up to mothers and babies after discharge from the hospital. Home health services begin with discharge planning and continue through home visits and community referrals. It is essential that the home care nurse be well educated in breastfeeding management in order to give effective care and advice. Ideally, every home care agency that provides maternity services will have a lactation consultant on staff. Hospitals customarily contract with managed care companies to provide home care service. Home care staff see only mothers with insurance coverage.

In the context of short hospital stays, home care services are essential to mothers and babies. If the mother does not stay at least 48 hours after delivery, the hospital staff may not be able to observe a breastfeeding for every mother and baby. Many families elect to stay only 24 hours, especially when it is not their first birth. Knowing that a home care lactation consultant will visit the mother shortly after discharge provides greater assurance that these mothers receive the breastfeeding advice and care they need.

Breastfeeding advocates have varying degrees of success with health maintenance organization coverage of home care services. Some may be more likely to provide coverage for lactation services if the lactation consultant is also a registered nurse. In some places, home health staff see mothers only if they have a health problem. The American Alliance of Health Plans lists health plans with lactation coverage (www.aahp.org).

Home Health Lactation Program

This section provides a description of services provided through a home health agency in central Pennsylvania. Although other programs may vary, this agency can serve as a model for a continuum of breastfeeding support. The home healthcare staff received comprehensive instruction in breastfeeding management and support. The WHO/UNICEF "18-Hour Course for Breastfeeding Management and Promotion in a Baby-Friendly Hospital" was tailored to fit the needs of home care staff.

Discharge Planner

A maternity **discharge planner** reviews hospital charts every morning to identify which mothers will go home. This depends primarily on what the mother's particular insurance company will allow. In 1996, many American states reacted to the negative consequences of early discharge by passing legislation guaranteeing that new mothers and babies are kept in the hospital long enough to receive necessary care. Typically, this legislation ensures a 48-hour stay. The legislation, however, covered only about 50 percent of mothers. Federal legislation is now in place to protect all mothers in the United States.

The discharge planner sees every patient who will be leaving that day. She evaluates both the mother and baby and reviews their charts. She then gives the mother instructions to get her through until her first visit by the home care nurse. If the mother is breastfeeding, she asks how breastfeeding is going and discusses any concerns

the mother voices. Breastfeeding mothers receive a home visit by a lactation consultant who is also a nurse. The discharge planner documents sufficient information to provide to the home care lactation consultant in preparation for this visit.

The mother receives a packet of information with warning signs and symptoms to help her detect potential breastfeeding problems. A **breastfeeding diary** will help her track her baby's feedings, voiding, and stooling. Mothers eligible for home health services also receive information about the home care nursing and lactation consultant services. After hospital discharge of the mother, the lactation consultant contacts the home care department to arrange for follow-up.

Home Care Lactation Consultant

Agencies differ in their policies for determining which mothers are eligible for home visits, as well as the duration of the visits. The average length of a lactation visit in this home health agency is 90 minutes. Some agencies require that visits be no longer than 45 minutes. Some limit visits to mothers who are at risk, have given birth by cesarean, or have preterm babies.

The initial telephone call to schedule the patient's first visit is an opportunity to learn how the mother is doing. In preparation for the visit, the mother can be encouraged to think of herself still as a patient. She is not expected to dress or shower and is encouraged to not worry about a clean house or think of the nurse as a visitor. Helping the mother lower her expectations encourages her to continue getting the rest she needs.

The First Home Visit

Because a home environment will not be as controlled as a hospital environment, you will need to be flexible in your expectations and the manner in which you provide care. On the first visit, you may open the door to an excited **sibling** or to a frantic mother who needs reassurance. The visit may begin with social amenities and emotional support substantially different from that of a hospital setting.

Family dynamics may be different as well, with the baby's father, siblings, and grandparents often present. Although these people may be present during hospital visits, being on their home turf can create a more realistic and comfortable communication style. You are able to assess the mother's support system and capitalize on teaching opportunities with other family members. Often, speaking loudly enough for a family member in another room to hear what the mother is being told goes a long way in enlisting support from a skeptical relative.

A home visit should include observation and assessment of a breastfeeding, regardless of whether the provider is a lactation consultant or a nurse. The goal is to assess breastfeeding technique and build the mother's self-confidence. You can begin by asking the mother what she knows about breastfeeding. Check the mother's breastfeeding diary and discuss how everything is going. Asking about her labor and delivery will help you identify potential problems with breastfeeding, such as the possibility of a sleepy baby because of birth interventions. It also gives the mother an opportunity to talk through her birth experience. Encouraging the mother to get past her birth experience and to verbalize concerns or disappointments will help her to gain perspective and move on to other parenting issues such as breastfeeding.

The home care lactation consultant who is also a nurse will perform a complete assessment of both mother and infant, assess breastfeeding technique, and teach infant care. If a problem surfaces during the first visit, she will place an interim telephone call to monitor progress until the next visit. The infant assessment may take place on the couch, on the dining room table, or in the nursery—wherever the mother wishes. You may check the baby's **bilirubin** level according to the home care agency's guidelines. You will provide anticipatory guidance to avoid potential complications such as low milk production, nipple soreness, or **engorgement**. It is important to keep in mind that the mother may feel stressed and tired. She may not take in everything you say to her. If a nurse who is not a lactation consultant makes the first visit and encounters breastfeeding difficulties, the baby needs a referral to the agency's lactation consultant or a community-based lactation consultant.

The Second Home Visit

On the second home visit, the mother may seem more relaxed and reassured than she was on the first visit. She may feel more rested and her breasts may feel full, which brings a sense of confidence. She is now able to "take in and take hold," as described by Reba Rubin (1957). She may ask about long-term issues such as how to manage feedings after returning to work. The home care staff provides this vital link and helps the mother access community support.

The second visit includes another complete assessment of the mother and baby, including a breast exam. By this second visit, which occurs around day five or six, the mother should report at least six to eight wet diapers and three to five stools in 24 hours. Infant weight loss should be stabilized or less than seven percent of birth weight.

Working in Private Practice

Some lactation consultants elect to open a private practice in their community. Private practice is a reasonable option for a seasoned lactation consultant who has several years of experience working with a wide variety of breastfeeding mothers and infants. Some private practice

lactation consultants have another medical credential beyond their IBCLC (e.g., RN, MD, or RD). These credentials identify the lactation consultant as an expert, which can be important when working on a referral basis. Licensed credentials also make it more likely that insurance companies will provide reimbursement. The impetus for licensing board-certified lactation consultants is increasing so that more states will cover lactation services for Medicaid patients. Because *registered* is a more familiar term to many U.S. insurers than *certified*, IBLCE designated their lists of certificants in every country as a registry in 1999. This enables IBCLCs to state that they are registered with the IBLCE and to list "Registered Lactation Consultant" (RLC) after their IBCLC credential.

Challenges of Private Practice

Many private practice lactation consultants enjoy the autonomy of being their own boss. You are able to set your hours and arrange your schedule around family functions. Electing to go into private practice means that you will be dependent on referrals from other lactation consultants, hospitals, caregivers, and previous clients. Establishing a large referral base can take several years. However, because your referral base does not rely on a single source, you will be able to advocate for breastfeeding more assertively. It is easier to speak your mind when you are autonomous!

Working in private practice usually results in minimal contact with staff at the hospitals and thus limited opportunity for peer relationships. Working on community coalitions is an effective way for private practice lactation consultants to network with other professionals. They will learn more about you and your practice, and you will become acquainted with new colleagues. Some of the tips in Chapter 28 may help guide the manner in which you relate to other professionals.

You can subscribe to relevant journals in order to stay current on medical and practice issues. Membership in ILCA will entitle you to the *Journal of Human Lactation*. In addition, medical journal articles are available on the Internet, many at little or reasonable costs. You will also find it helpful to locate the nearest medical library in your area. Most medical disciplines have large numbers of Web sites that send out e-mail news updates. You can overcome the challenges of private practice, especially if you are a self-starter who enjoys autonomy. Ultimately, the key to your success will be sound business practices, time commitment to see clients, following through with necessary paperwork, and marketing your services.

Business Structure

Establishing a private practice is a serious business decision that will require work to succeed. It may be helpful to take a small-business course from your local community college if you do not have a business background. There are many books and seminars on starting small business and home offices. The U.S. Internal Revenue Service offers free business seminars to educate entrepreneurs about federal tax requirements. Although you will not have employee benefits, being self-employed may provide you with some tax benefits, which an accountant can help you identify.

Most private practice IBCLCs operate as sole proprietors. If you possess other professional credentials, establishing a professional association or S corporation may have tax advantages. For instance, an IBCLC may also be a marriage and family therapist or an occupational therapist. Establishing an S corporation may be more advantageous than a sole proprietorship. Limited liability corporations, or LLCs, are becoming more popular for entrepreneurs. They combine the personal liability protection of a corporation with the tax benefits and simplicity of a partnership. In addition, they are more flexible and require less paperwork than corporations require. Consulting with an accountant or tax attorney prior to beginning your practice can prevent potential tax and business pitfalls.

Financial Issues

Private practice will require you to process billing and collect fees. It is important that clients know what your charges will be before a consultation. When the nature of a telephone call requires a consultation, you can say to the mother, "I will be happy to see you. I have an opening at the following times . . . You will need to be here for about two hours and my fee is. . . ." If a mother says she cannot afford your services, it may help her to realize that she is paying the same fee for 1 hour of your time as she does for a ten-minute appointment with her primary caregiver. At that rate, your services are quite a bargain! You can help mothers be comfortable paying for your services by approaching the topic in a self-assured and practical manner.

You will need to bill for your services on a regular schedule. Few private practice lactation consultants have the luxury of relegating this task to another person. Plan a regular time monthly to update your records and mail bills for any outstanding accounts. If you do not have provider status with the mother's insurance carrier, you will want to collect the fee directly from the client rather than from the insurance company. The client can then send your receipt to her insurance company for reimbursement.

Financial Record Keeping

You will need to keep a monthly record of all business expenses and income. An inexpensive accounting software program such as QuickBooks or Quicken can simplify the process for you. These programs provide easy record retention and quick reference. Spreadsheets will enable you to note your profits and losses and assist you in business planning. Income records may include consultations and services, rental and sale of breast pumps and other devices, breastfeeding classes, and speaking engagements. It is important to include all expenses related to the business, such as office supplies and equipment, utilities, insurance, educational materials and programs, professional memberships, advertising, donations, and taxes. Software designed specifically for lactation practices is available.

Third-Party Reimbursement

Be sure to provide clients with appropriate forms with which they can seek reimbursement from their insurance companies. Third-party reimbursement is a legislative and policy issue related to healthcare insurance in the United States. A reimbursement tool kit is available from ILCA, with information about coding, coverage of lactation care and services, filing of claims, and a list of insurance commissioners in each U.S. state (ILCA, 2002b). A topic on third-party reimbursement is also on ILCA's Web site discussion board.

A three-part carbonless superbill, available from the UCLA Lactation Alumni Association, is designed specifically for reimbursement of lactation consulting services (see Appendix A for contact information). The copy the client submits to her insurance company must include your name and federal tax identification number. The second copy is for the client's records. She can use it to file as a tax deduction at the end of the year as a childcare expense if she works outside the home. The third copy is for your files in case you need it later. Some insurance companies require their own insurance form rather than the superbill. Encourage the client to contact her insurance carrier to learn its requirements.

Figure 2.2 illustrates a sample referral letter from the physician that may be helpful in seeking reimbursement for a breast pump rental. The mother can attach it as a cover letter to her insurer. It will help to attach a physician's prescription requesting your services, dated and made out in the client's name. You may create a form for the physician with information that needs to be reflected on the prescription, including specific **ICD-9** codes relevant to breastfeeding. The ICD-9 code is the International Classification of Diseases. Be aware that some codes may apply only if the physician is present for the consultation. Sample information to include on a prescription includes:

◆ For a consultation: Consult (your name) for evaluation, assessment and treatment of . . . (diagnosis and ICD-9 code).

◆ For breast pump rental: Feed baby mother's milk. Obtain the mother's milk by use of a hospital-grade

---

FIGURE 2.2
Physician letter for insurance coverage
for rental of a breast pump.

(Date)

To insurance carrier for: (client's name)

Name of policyholder:

Policy number: _____

The following explanation of medical need is provided in order to expedite insurance coverage for the rental of an electric breast pump.

(Name of mother) delivered the high-risk infant (name of baby) on (date). The child is too immature or ill to nurse directly at the breast. However, it is well established that human milk provides optimal infant nutrition for the first 6 months of life. Thus, the mother of a premature or high-risk newborn is encouraged to pump her breasts in order to supply milk for her hospitalized baby and to maintain lactation until the baby can nurse at the breast.

The intermittent electric breast pump is by far the most efficient, effective, and physiologic means of simulating the sucking action of a normal infant. Inexpensive manual, battery-operated, or small electric breast pumps are an adjunct to milk expression for occasional use when a large intermittent suction pump is unavailable. A piston-type electric breast pump is essential for the maintenance of an adequate milk supply whenever a child is unable to breastfeed normally. Such pumps cost approximately $1400 and thus are far more economical to rent.

The electric pump will be necessary until the baby is able to take all required nutrition by feeding at the breast. An electric breast pump is not a convenience for the mother; rather it is a medical necessity in the best interest of the child's health.

Sincerely,

(Pediatrician)

---

electric breast pump. Classified as durable medical equipment.

◆ For breast pump rental: Electric breast pump for treatment of . . . (diagnosis and ICD-9 code).

◆ For infant feeding supplies: To insure adequate caloric intake, use a . . . (name of device).

Location and Accommodations

You will need to arrange for adequate space for seeing clients and for office work, equipment, and supplies. The first decision is whether you will work from home or locate your office elsewhere in the community. If you base your practice in your home, check with your local zoning board to determine whether there are any restrictions on signs, parking, or storage of supplies. If you plan for clients to enter and leave your home, you may need additional coverage on your homeowner's insurance. Some insurance companies charge higher rates when pregnant women will be entering and leaving the home.

Home Office

You need a space where you and clients will have complete privacy for the entire consultation. The consultation should take place where the client cannot see or hear family members and where others cannot hear what you and the client discuss. Conversation between you and your client is confidential, and you do not want to risk others overhearing anything she says. You may discuss delicate issues such as abuse, rape, and sexually transmitted diseases. You will need an environment that is conducive to a mother who chooses to confide such sensitive issues. You will also need bathroom facilities, safe and easy access into and out of your home, and convenient parking. Some lactation consultants confine a home office to business aspects of their practice and see mothers only through home visits.

Off-site Location

A carefully selected office location can be your key to a successful practice. You need to be sure that clients will feel comfortable visiting you at this location. You will want good outdoor lighting for evening appointments, security, snow removal, and adequate parking. An office in a commercial building will require rent, insurance, utilities, a business sign, and maintenance. Many commercial offices offer secretarial services for small businesses, including copiers, fax machines, telephone, and voice mail systems. A commercial leasing service can help you determine if this is a viable option for your practice.

Office Equipment and Furniture

Equipment represents the highest capital expense for your business. You personally will need a desk, chair, filing cabinet, and any other furnishings that will provide for efficiency and comfort. A computer, fax machine, and printer will enable you to maintain accurate client records and produce professional reports and correspondence. A dedicated telephone line and a telephone with an answering machine or voice mail will ensure that you receive all calls and can answer them professionally. With the heightened presence of the Internet, mothers will appreciate e-mail access to your support and advice. Many lactation consultants have Web sites that provide personalized educational information for their clients. You will also need a reference library accessible to you during the consultation and when writing physician reports.

Lactation Provisions

Your business will require equipment and furniture specific to your profession. Select a comfortable chair or couch with arms for mothers to sit in to nurse, preferably one you can wipe clean. A footstool placed in front of the chair will help you teach mothers good body positioning. Pillows of various shapes and sizes will enable mothers to get comfortable for feedings and to position their babies at the breast. Using pillows with removable pillowcases will assure mothers of safe hygiene practices. A baby **sling** will allow you to hold the baby while the mother is pumping and to complete your paperwork for the visit at the same time.

You will need space where you can lay the baby for examining him and where you can secure the baby while you are assessing and working with the mother. A digital scale is standard equipment in a lactation consultant's office. If you cannot afford to purchase one, you can rent one from a distributor or the manufacturer. You will need either paper products or linens for use on your changing table and scale. Many lactation consultants provide toys for toddlers to keep them busy while they work with the mother and baby. If you do so, make sure you select toys you can clean adequately.

Breastfeeding Supplies and Inventory

You may wish to provide various breastfeeding devices for rental or purchase. Many private practice lactation consultants provide electric breast pumps for rental by clients. Appendix A contains the names of some breast pump companies. Rental programs for breast pumps usually allow clients to lease a pump at a daily, weekly, or monthly rate. There are often special rates for long-term use (i.e., five or six months). In the beginning, you may wish to serve as a rental station on consignment with a breast pump company. Later, after you have firmly established a rental station, changing to a flat rate may be a better option financially. In addition to large rental electric breast pumps, you can provide smaller electric pumps for purchase, motor adapters, power packs, feeding cups, and bottles. Providing replacement parts for breast pumps and breast pump kits is a convenience that mothers appreciate. You can also provide clients with instructions that address common questions regarding refunds for early returns, special rental rates, care of the pump, and arranging for its return.

Identify a place for supplies that is easily accessible. Make sure you have supplies you will use during consultations, such as nursing supplementers, a medicine dropper, small cups, and **nipple shields**. Some lactation consultants keep small amounts of formula in their office to feed babies who need calories when the mother's expressed milk is not available. If you use olive oil to improve the vacuum of the breast pump **flange**, make sure you have small medicine cups to provide individual amounts to mothers.

As you develop your practice, keep track of items you do not have that either would make a consultation go more smoothly or would make it more comfortable for the mother. Weigh the cost of such items with how quickly you will use or sell them. Ordering a small number of new items will allow you to test the market before making a large investment. If an item has a high turnover, you might consider purchasing it in quantity and prepaying to save money on shipping and handling.

Marketing Your Practice

Your marketing strategy can greatly affect the success of your practice. Decide *before* you open your practice how busy you want to be. Your life stage may determine the number of clients a day, week, or month you want to see. If you have small children or a nursling, you may want to limit your advertising to word-of-mouth to limit your practice to fewer clients. If your children are in school or no longer at home, you might market more assertively to attract more clients. Planning for the anticipated response of your target market will help you attract the number of clients you wish for your practice.

Talk with other lactation consultants who work in private practice to find out which marketing strategies work best for them. What mistakes did they make that you can avoid? Most lactation consultants will be happy to share their experience in setting up a private practice. Learn from the successes and mistakes of others. You do not have to reinvent the wheel!

Accessing Clients

Your clients will come primarily from medical referrals, referrals from past clients, and your listing in the telephone directory. Placing an ad in the yellow pages of your local directory is a good use of your marketing dollars. You may automatically get a listing in the white business pages and the yellow pages when you install a business telephone line. If so, check with your telephone company to ensure that your listing and category also appear online in the Internet yellow pages. Many IBCLCs have Web sites that offer basic breastfeeding information and links to other breastfeeding and parenting sites. IBCLCs who are ILCA members are listed in the association's Find A Lactation Consultant Web service at www.ilca.org.

Contact local practitioners, hospitals clinics, birthing centers, and childbirth educators to acquaint them with the services you provide. Letters to such groups and individuals will introduce your services to the community. A follow-up visit will allow them the opportunity to ask questions and get to know you. Be sure to keep a file of business cards, noting on the back of the card the date you received it and a brief note about the circumstances.

Ask for an e-mail address if one does not appear on the business card. Such contacts will prove helpful to you and your clients at various times in your practice. A press release in your local paper can garner you free publicity. Check with the program director of radio stations in your area as well. Often there are local call-in radio shows, especially healthcare shows, that will conduct on-air interviews about breastfeeding and lactation services.

Many aspects of your daily routine as a private practice lactation consultant provide marketing opportunities. You can meet with physicians and their staff at their offices to confer about clients and to discuss breastfeeding care. Offer to present a free in-service session on breastfeeding to the staff. After you have seen a client, send a report to the physicians involved (usually the pediatrician and the obstetrician). Some circumstances may warrant enclosing a copy of relevant research articles. These actions reinforce your credibility as a member of the mother's and infant's health care team and increase the likelihood that the physician will refer other mothers to you. Satisfied clients are the best sources of referrals. Your attention to meeting the needs of mothers in your care will reap marketing benefits as those satisfied clients recommend your services to friends and family and return with future babies.

Office Visits

In order to create a professional appearance, remove all family items from the area you use for your practice. A few attractively framed pictures of your family may be appropriate on your desk and confer credibility as an experienced mother. Invest in quality framing for your educational credentials, including your IBCLC certification. Framing local awards and certificates of appreciation reflects that you are a committed member of your community. Signs of academic and community achievement will help mothers feel secure in choosing you as a member of their healthcare team.

If you have a busy practice, paperwork and other items can clutter your office. Clear away any clutter before the client arrives so that you present an organized appearance. You can store items in a drawer or closet until after the consultation. You can save time by preparing several client charts ahead of time and giving the client a clipboard containing the consent form and intake form at the beginning of the consultation.

Home Visits

If your private practice includes visits to mothers' homes, you can equip your car with the necessary supplies and equipment. You will not be able to run back to your office easily for something you forgot. Mothers may not have items you need for teaching positioning, such as footstools or comfortable pillows. Take a cellular telephone in case

you become lost or if you expect to drive to an unsafe neighborhood. Always obtain clear directions to your client's home, including cross streets and landmarks. Use a new map or print a copy of the location from www.mapquest.com or another Internet map service.

Telephone Calls

As a private practice lactation consultant, you will need to be available to clients at established times. Telephone calls must be able to get through to your office at all times. You will therefore need either an answering machine or voice mail. Be aware that you are legally required to respond if a client leaves a message for you.

Maintain a professional demeanor during all telephone contacts with clients. This includes the manner in which you answer the telephone and the greeting you leave on your answering machine or voice mail. It is helpful in your recorded greeting to ask callers to say their telephone number twice, very clearly, or to ask for two separate telephone numbers. You may receive calls from distraught mothers whose telephone numbers are unintelligible, or not even given. You may want to add caller ID to your phone service. If you are unable to see a client because of a personal commitment, simply say that you are unavailable at that time and suggest the next available time. It is unnecessary and unprofessional to explain the reason you are not available. Make sure that family members know not to answer the business telephone.

You need to arrange coverage for times you are away from your practice. Carefully select the person who will cover for you in your absence. Agree ahead of time how she will respond to clients. You will want to know that she approaches breastfeeding with a philosophy that is compatible with yours. Also, learn if she has an answering machine and any times the practice may not be covered.

Documentation

It is important to document all aspects of a consultation in an organized and consistent manner. A signed consent form is important to obtain with every new client. You may wish to include in the consent form a statement granting permission for any photographs you may take for teaching purposes. As a courtesy, ask permission again before taking any pictures. You will also want to develop standard assessment forms that will elicit the information you need from each client. If you make it a practice to use these forms with all clients, you will avoid forgetting to ask an important question. See Chapter 6 for further discussion of documentation.

Physician Reports

At the end of the consultation, you will need to complete a report to the client's physicians, usually the pediatrician and obstetrician. Using the same format in this report as you do in the assessment forms will help you remember to include important elements. Schedule time to write the physician's report immediately after the client leaves. Do not consider your consultation completed until you have written and sent this important report.

Processing the physician report by computer produces a professional appearance and provides you with a permanent record. Always use the spell-check feature on your computer and proofread the document carefully. A medical dictionary will aid you in this process; you can access one online. Many caregivers take advantage of the timeliness, convenience, and cost savings of faxing or e-mailing reports rather than mailing them. Remember to include privacy notices on any report cover to protect your client's confidentiality.

Record Retention

Lactation consultants in private practice advise keeping records for at least seven years. This includes appointment books, client folders, telephone logs, financial records, and receipts. You can place everything for each calendar year in a separate box and label it clearly. If you maintain client files on your computer, be sure to back up these files on another storage medium frequently. At some time in the future, you may need a duplicate of a client's records, financial information for tax reporting, or other such paperwork. Your diligence in retaining files will facilitate locating material when you need it. See Chapter 26 for further discussion of documentation as it relates to legal liability.

▶ RELATIONSHIP WITH PEER COUNSELORS

A reciprocal and cooperative working relationship with breastfeeding counselors and other support people enhances your impact. As discussed earlier in this chapter, WIC employs peer counselors who receive training and who are usually of the same ethnic origin as the other women in the community. **Lay counselors** in La Leche League and Nursing Mothers groups provide mother-to-mother support and group meetings. Whether the counselor works for an agency or as part of a mother-to-mother support group, you can all work together toward accomplishing the breastfeeding goals for women in your community.

Mother-to-Mother Support Groups

Step 10 of the "Ten Steps to Successful Breastfeeding" from WHO and UNICEF calls for the establishment of breastfeeding support groups and the referral of mothers to them when they are discharged from the hospital or clinic (WHO, 1989). Support groups offer mothers emotional support and mother-to-mother contact through regular meetings and telephone counseling. Customarily, counselors acquire training in counseling and breastfeeding care. You will need to ascertain the degree of education and experience among the counselors with whom you plan to work and tailor your relationship accordingly.

The services provided to mothers by a support group are invaluable. Counselors contact mothers before difficulties arise to offer anticipatory guidance and emotional support. "The last of the Ten Steps is . . . breastfeeding support in its oldest, most enduring form—women learning without pressure, over time, from women they want to emulate. Step Ten is the medical model deferring to the role model" (Wiessinger, 2002).

Mothers benefit from a variety of resources. Participating in a support group's activities increases their satisfaction and self-confidence in their role as mothers. Mutual sharing and observing other mothers breastfeed their babies greatly enhances their breastfeeding and parenting experiences. Support groups often provide a lending library, as well as easy access to breast pumps and other devices. See Chapter 20 for further discussion of support groups for breastfeeding mothers. Mothers can also benefit from Internet support groups (see Appendix A).

Lay counselors are capable of dealing with many types of breastfeeding situations without a background of extensive lactation education. The **outreach counseling** and emotional support they provide contributes greatly to mothers' reaching their goals. Mothers are educated about their options and encouraged to participate actively in decisions about their baby's care. If a mother-to-mother support group does not exist in your community, you may wish to begin one among the women in your care. Through your association with a mother-to-mother support group, you can ensure that mothers receive continuing care and consistent information.

The Lactation Consultant's Services to the Support Group

Services you offer to mother-to-mother support groups generally will be voluntary. The value of good public relations often outweighs the benefit of monetary gain. Judge each service according to its impact and the scope of your commitment when deciding whether to charge a fee. Following are some suggestions for ways in which you can work with a mother-to-mother support group. These suggestions may increase your effectiveness as well as that of the group. Working together as a team, you can present a unified program of support to breastfeeding mothers.

◆ Maintain a reciprocal referral system. You refer mothers to the support group for continuing outreach support. The support group, in return, refers mothers to you and other IBCLCs when a special situation requires a higher level of expertise. This system ensures that a greater number of mothers receive necessary support and information.

◆ Maintain quality counseling and accurate information within the support group by training its counselors in counseling skills and breastfeeding information.

◆ Serve as an advisor to the group and be available to answer questions from counselors.

◆ Cosponsor and help organize outreach programs run by the group. Encourage community programs that address both parents and the medical community.

◆ Offer continuing education for counselors in the form of study nights, seminars, and workshops.

◆ Offer your services as a speaker at parent or counselor meetings.

◆ Serve as a liaison between the support group and the medical community. Maintain two-way communication when mothers have problems. Keep both physicians and the support group informed.

◆ Review written materials distributed by the support group for counselors and parents.

▶ SUMMARY

The professional lactation consultant has a variety of employment options to consider. Each particular work setting varies from others in many ways. A constant thread among all settings is the role of the lactation consultant as part of a strong health care team that provides consistent care to mothers as they establish breastfeeding. Mothers who receive support from a strong health care team will be empowered to participate as informed health consumers. Whether you work in a hospital, clinic, physician group, home health care, or private practice, a commitment to breastfeeding mothers and babies is the driving force. Volunteer counselors continue to play a valuable role in the mother's support. You can help coordinate this care by maintaining a reciprocal relationship with community support groups.

▶ CHAPTER 2—AT A GLANCE

Facts you learned—

Members of the healthcare team:

◆ Mothers share positive aspects of breastfeeding with physicians.

◆ Physicians empower parents as equal members of the healthcare team.

◆ IBCLCs provide lactation expertise:
  ◆ Read research and literature, and use evidence-based materials.
  ◆ Refer mothers to support groups.
  ◆ Teach prenatal and postpartum classes.
  ◆ Share medical information appropriately.
  ◆ Help mothers sort through conflicting advice.
  ◆ Teach and advise peer counselors.

IBCLCs in hospital practice:

◆ Make rounds with mothers.

◆ Provide inpatient and staff education.

◆ Provide equipment and supplies for mothers.

◆ Establish a hospital-based lactation program.

IBCLCs in WIC:

◆ Serve low-income mothers and infants.

◆ Counsel mothers with cultural, socioeconomic, and lifestyle differences.

◆ Teach classes and facilitate support groups.

◆ Teach and supervise peer counselors.

IBCLCs in a physician practice:

◆ See healthy mothers and babies and those with difficulties.

◆ Patient load depends on physician's patient load.

◆ Teach classes and facilitate support group.

◆ Meet pregnant women.

◆ Make rounds in hospital.

◆ Provide follow-up calls and warm line.

IBCLCs in home healthcare:

◆ Follow up with mothers after discharge.

◆ Assess the mother, baby, and breastfeeding.

◆ Provide anticipatory guidance on long-term issues.

IBCLCs in private practice:

◆ Seasoned IBCLC with extensive experience.

◆ Establish a small business and obtain office and lactation equipment.

◆ Market the practice and establish a referral base.

◆ Bill for services and facilitate third-party reimbursement.

◆ Provide office and home visits and telephone follow-up.

◆ Document consultations, send physician reports, and retain records.

▶ **REFERENCES**

Fooladi M. A comparison of perspectives on breastfeeding between two generations of Black American women. *J Am Acad Nurse Pract* 13(1):34–38; 2001.

Hale T. *Medications and Mother's Milk.* Amarillo, TX: Pharmasoft Publishing; 2004.

International Lactation Consultant Association (ILCA). *Core Curriculum for Lactation Consultant Practice.* Raleigh, NC: ILCA; 2002a.

International Lactation Consultant Association (ILCA). *Reimbursement Tool Kit for Lactation Consultants.* Raleigh, NC: ILCA; 2002b.

Ross Products Division, Abbott Laboratories. Ross Laboratories Mothers' Survey; 2002. Available at: http://www.ross.com/images/library/BF_Trends_2002.pdf. Accessed June 24, 2004.

Rubin R. Attainment of the maternal role. *Nursing Research* 16(3):237–245, 1957.

U.S. Department of Agriculture (USDA) Food and Nutrition Services, Women, Infants and Children, Frequently Asked Questions. Available at: www.fns.usda.gov/wic/FAQs/FAQ.HTM. Accessed December 1, 2004.

Wiessinger D. On behalf of breastfeeding: Last step first. *Cur Iss in Clin Lact* 69–73; 2002.

World Health Organization (WHO). Protecting, prompting, and supporting breastfeeding: A joint WHO/UNICEF statement. Geneva: WHO; 1989.

▶ **BIBLIOGRAPHY**

Bochinno C et al. *Advancing Women's Health: Health Plans' Innovative Programs in Breastfeeding Promotion.* Washington, DC: U.S. Dept of Health and Human Services; 2002.

Cadwell K. Using the quality improvement process to affect breastfeeding protocols in United States hospitals. *J Hum Lact* 13:5–9; 1997.

Elder S, Gregory C. The "lactation game:" An innovative teaching method for healthcare professionals. *J Hum Lact* 12: 137–138; 1996.

Hirschman J. Impact of the special supplemental food program on infants. *J Pediatr* S121–S122; 1990.

Howard C et al. Attitudes, practices and recommendations by obstetricians about infant feeding. *Birth* 24:240–257; 1997.

International Board of Lactation Consultant Examiners; August 1999. Available at: www.iblce.org/ibclc.htm.

MacGowan R et al. Breast-feeding among women attending Women, Infants, and Children clinics in Georgia, 1987. *Pediatrics* 87(3):361–366; 1991.

U.S. Department of Agriculture Breastfeeding Campaign. Available at: www.usda.gov/fcs/brfdcpgn.htm; 2004.

A SOCIOLOGICAL PERSPECTIVE ON BREASTFEEDING SUPPORT

The norms and perceptions of society determine much of what transpires in the context of breastfeeding promotion and support. This chapter explores breastfeeding support from a sociological perspective, with insights into the needs of breastfeeding women and the most effective strategies to help them meet those needs. Awareness of social thinking and social behavior will help you understand women's perceptions and processing of breastfeeding information and media messages. These insights will enhance your interactions with mothers and the assistance you provide.

Auguste Comte conceived the new academic discipline of "sociology" in 1838 as a formal study of society (Goodman, 1992). The term derives from Latin for *socius* and *ology* and reflects the scientific study of human society and social interactions (Tischler, 1999). Sociology examines the history, development, organization, and problems of people living together as social groups. It is a scientific study of social behavior, thought, and the manner in which we depend upon, interact with, influence, and are influenced by others.

KEY TERMS

attachment and bonding	intention
attitude	involvement theory
attribution	motivation
behavior	perception
cognitive learning	primary and secondary
compliance	groups
conformity	retention and recall
culture	role
decision making	self-image
demographics	sensory input
empowerment	social marketing
ethics	social thinking
evidence-based practice	split-brain theory
group behavior	status

ORGANIZATION OF A SOCIETY

Society is defined as a collection of people who share a common culture, territory, and identity. This commonality binds people together through relationships and interactions. The pattern of these relationships forms the social structure of a society. Culture, status, roles, groups, organizations, social institutions, and community are all elements of this social structure.

Culture

Culture involves all that we learn in the course of social life and transmit across generations. It is the "learned, socially transmitted heritage of artifacts, knowledge, beliefs, values, and normative expectations that provides the members of a particular society with the tools for coping with recurrent problems" (Goodman, 1992). Culture shapes and structures social life by defining the foods we eat, the clothes we wear, the language we speak, the values and beliefs we hold, and the practices we follow.

Societies differ in their values and in the norms that define appropriate behavior. Such cultural diversity demonstrates the flexibility and variability of human conditions. Subcultures are individual groups within a culture that vary by social class, ethnicity, race, religion, lifestyle, goals, and interests. The identity of a subculture may revolve around its ethnic heritage, economic circumstance, or geographic region. A subculture often has a distinctive language and form of communication. We tend to evaluate others' customs, practices, and behaviors in terms of our own culture and experience. However, we need to understand each cultural practice in terms of its place in the larger cultural context. Social values correspond to each individual subculture that exists within society. We cannot easily dismiss the worth of practices within each subculture merely based on what we consider to be "right" and "wrong." Rather, we need to approach and assess each culture individually and with an open mind.

When working with cultures different from your own, it can be easy to dismiss certain dietary or infant care practices as unimportant or senseless. For the mother in that culture, these practices may carry deep meaning or reflect familial tradition, and thus may contribute positively to her breastfeeding. A culture may promote beneficial practices of carrying a baby close, breastfeeding on demand, and long-term breastfeeding. Some cultures believe that pinning a band around the baby's abdomen will prevent an umbilical hernia. Such a practice is not harmful to the baby and does not need to change. The custom of restricting the mother's consumption of fresh fruit for several weeks postpartum may have some effect on her nutritional status. The belief that **colostrum** is harmful to the baby leads to delaying breastfeeding until the mother's milk transforms to mature milk. This practice can affect the health of the baby and the establishment of breastfeeding.

Chapter 20 explores cultural issues related to breastfeeding. The degree to which a mother merges into a new culture depends on how firmly she clings to traditional values. Mothers who wish to integrate into Western culture may perceive artificial formula to be the desired method of infant feeding. Despite the fact that breastfeeding is the norm in their native culture, they may choose to formula feed in order to fit in.

Status

We tend to think of status in terms of prestige, wealth, or power. In a sociological context, status refers to a person's position within a network of social relationships. Status may denote a place in the family, such as mother, father, daughter, or son. It can also refer to a position in the workplace, religious community, or other segment of society. The social statuses people occupy strongly influence the aspects of a culture they will experience. Although everyone occupies a variety of statuses within their social structure, people tend to identify themselves through one "master" status. Men traditionally define themselves in terms of their occupation. Women traditionally have defined themselves as mothers.

Definitions of self tend to evolve in response to societal changes. Over the past several decades, for example, women in Western culture increasingly have defined themselves through their personal professional role in society rather than their personal role within the family. It is important to consider this trend in your interactions with working mothers. When working with a professional woman who plans to return to work, it will help to recognize that she has invested heavily in her career. She may have conflicting feelings about leaving her baby versus losing her career "momentum." Acknowledging these conflicts and helping the mother explore her reservations will empower her both as a mother and in her career. Our motivations and goals change from childhood to old age as each season of our lives unfolds. The encouragement you can offer mothers to sequence their seasons of life may be a refreshing "new" thought for women who are merging motherhood with a career. By understanding this cultural dynamic, you will be able to tailor your approach and sensitively help women meet their needs and reach their breastfeeding goals.

Role

Social status determines our expectations and behavior or, in other words, the roles we play in society. Role differs from status in that a person occupies a status and performs a role within that status. Individuals who occupy the status of parent, for instance, hold certain values regarding the importance of children. Parents are subject to specific norms regarding the obligation to provide their children with emotional, physical, and financial support. These are their role expectations. The manner in which they perform their parental role—their role behavior—reflects on their status as a parent.

Parental norms vary widely between subcultures. Bottle-feeding is very much the norm among minority populations within the United States. Some immigrants consider the ability to provide formula as a status symbol, and the breastfeeding they would have done at home is denigrated. Well-educated, upper-middle-class, older parents tend to regard breastfeeding as the biologically superior way to feed infants. The expectation to breastfeed or at least "try" is a part of their parental status.

Groups and Organizations

The set of expectations shared by people with a common status and role forms the basis of their interactions with one another. Most activities take place in the context of groups such as families, teams, peer groups, and work groups. Social life, therefore, is group life. Members of a group have a sense of shared identity. This group membership may be figurative, or it may exist within an organized structure. By definition, an organization is a group created specifically to carry out a particular task. It has a formal structure through which it attempts to accomplish that task.

When a young couple begins a family, they become parents and thus part of the peer group of other parents, whether formally or informally. They may seek the company of other new parents. They may judge their parenting abilities against those of other parents. They may join a parenting group or a playgroup with their children. They may seek the formal structure of a parenting class, with specific goals for learning parenting skills. All of these group identities are important to the couple's perceptions of themselves as parents and to the manner in which they perform their parental role. Many first-time parents bond with other parents in their childbirth education classes. Mothers who join breastfeeding support groups often form long-term intimate friendships with other mothers who are also learning how to adapt to the parental role.

Social Institutions

Statuses, roles, and groups combine to form social institutions. Most societies are composed of five major institutions: economy, education, family, politics, and religion. A social institution has relatively stable clusters of values, norms, statuses, roles, social groups, and organizations that relate to a specific area of human activity. The institution of education, for example, satisfies society's need to provide its members with a basic set of knowledge and skills that will enable them to function in society.

Major institutions tend to base themselves on similar norms, values, and goals. When a change occurs in one institution, it usually triggers a change in others. Family structure, relationships, and mobility have changed tremendously over the past century. This transformation of the family represents a social change that has affected the nature of society as well as each person's childhood and adult experiences (Tischler, 1999).

Attitudes, beliefs, and values all play roles in future societal changes. Recognizing the interdependence among social institutions can provide insights into determining the needs of mothers and their families. For example, when working with a mother who is a member of a religious community, it will help you to understand that the high value placed on the family by the mother's community of faith will support her desire to stay home with her children, and probably to breastfeed.

Community

As a social group, the community shares an identity, a structured pattern of interaction, and a common geographical territory. This geographic proximity of members enhances the frequency of interactions as well as the consequences of those interactions. The **demographic** study of a population takes into account social, cultural, and environmental factors that influence behavior and change. The population within a particular community is a key defining element in its social structure and culture.

Understanding a community's demographics will assist you in framing your interactions with families. Most large population centers contain great diversity in family subcultures. An awareness of your city's characteristics will enhance your sensitivity to your clients'

cultural beliefs. For example, there is a burgeoning East Indian population in many U.S. cities. Educating yourself about Indian beliefs concerning childbirth and breastfeeding will help you establish credibility with the Indian mothers you serve. It is polite to remove your shoes when entering an Indian home. They prepare special foods for the postpartum mother and keep the baby warm. The **paladai**—a **cup feeding** device—has been used to feed babies in India for many years. It is gaining recognition in the Western world as a helpful lactation device (Sideman, 1999). If you are unsure about a cultural practice, do not hesitate to ask your client. Most families are receptive to explaining cultural practices to people who are sincerely interested.

▶ THE PROCESS OF SOCIALIZATION

Scholars argue the issue of "nature versus nurture," questioning whether our identity and behavior are determined biologically or by our social experiences. We all enter the world as potentially social beings dependent on others for survival. Heredity and environment contribute to the development of the person we become. Society teaches each new member how to think, feel, and live. This is the essence of socialization. Through social interaction, we develop an identity, a set of beliefs, and a range of skills that allow us to participate in society.

The process of socialization maintains social order. Socialization is a lifelong process in which our social development progresses through a series of stages. The quality of intellectual, social, and emotional behavior at one stage of development differs fundamentally from the next stage. Families, schools, and other socializing institutions instill members of society with socially acceptable values. Those who go against the majority opinion and challenge the dominant system of ideas are often deemed rebellious and perhaps even radical. Sometimes a challenge to a practice or set of beliefs evolves into a movement that creates real change. That is the case with promotional efforts to empower women to breastfeed in a climate that embraces bottle-feeding. It is also evident in many cultures when women breastfeed their children beyond the first year.

Social Thinking

Social behavior usually begins with social *cognition*, that is, social thinking. Most behavior results from deliberation, judgment, beliefs, and expectations. Through cognition, we form inferences from social information before we act. The study of cognition involves the manner in which we acquire, organize, and use knowledge and information, or data. It focuses primarily on perception, attention, memory, thought, and language. Within a social context, social thinking is a study of how we perceive, react to, and remember things about ourselves and other people. It involves how different social situations influence our thinking process, how we perceive ourselves, and how we form impressions of others.

People rarely collect social data with a truly open mind. Life experiences invariably lead to certain expectations that help us to sift through new information. These expectations can bias our interpretations, especially if they are based on few or single experiences. Additionally, negative expectations can cause us to reject the opportunity to collect new information. In order to arrive at a meaningful conclusion, we must recognize that prior expectations influence our beliefs and actions. We must select from among the data we collect, and judge which information is or is not relevant and useful.

The integration of our prior expectations and experiences helps us to interpret our social environment and evaluate new experiences and social encounters. Recognizing the impact of this cognitive process with those whom you counsel will help you to devise effective helping strategies. In a primarily bottle-feeding culture such as the United States, a young woman might react with distaste or discomfort when she sees a mother breastfeeding a toddler or older child in public. Her perceptions are based on a cultural belief of breasts as sexual objects, as evidenced by a preponderance of advertisements, commercials, television shows, and movies. Consequently, she may view breastfeeding as a sexual act, not a biological act of love and nurturing, and consider it inappropriate outside the home or with an older child.

Cognitive Learning

Learning is the process by which we acquire knowledge and experience that we apply to future related behavior. Newly acquired knowledge combines with experience to serve as feedback and provide the basis for future behavior in similar situations. The process of learning ranges from the most simple, almost reflexive responses to abstract concepts and complex **problem solving**.

When confronted with a problem, we sometimes see the solution instantly. More often, however, we are likely to search for information on which to base a decision and then carefully evaluate what we learn in order to make the best decision. This is the essence of **cognitive learning**. The process of problem solving enables us to gain some control over our environment and is pivotal to producing the desired response.

In order for learning to occur, four basic elements must be present: motivation, cues, response, and reinforcement. The process begins with a personal need or goal that is unmet. The motivation to satisfy this need or goal acts as a stimulus to learning. The degree to

which we are actively involved in learning will depend on our level of motivation. Cues are the stimuli that give direction to our motives and guide our actions toward the desired outcome. The way we respond to these cues—in other words, how we behave—constitutes our response. The response we choose depends greatly on previous learning and on responses reinforced in the past. Reinforcement increases the likelihood of a specific future response as the result of particular cues or stimuli. Such repetition increases the strength of the association and slows the process of forgetting.

For a new mother, learning how to hold her baby at the breast and practicing it with a skilled caregiver assists her in honing her technique. She will become increasingly more confident with each successive feeding as she is able to anticipate her baby's responses and feed him effectively. When a mother responds to her baby's hunger cues by putting him to the breast, she teaches her baby to anticipate that she will meet his needs for food and comfort. It also reinforces her future nurturing of her child. The repetition of breastfeeding throughout the child's nursing years reinforces the child's learning of parental concern and a mother's learning to put the child's welfare ahead of her own. This helps to set the pattern for lifelong maternal love and selflessness.

Processing Information

The human mind processes information it receives as input in much the same way as a computer processes data. The manner in which the brain processes information depends on our cognitive ability as well as the complexity of the information to be processed. Our ability to form mental images influences the degree to which we can recall information. Differences in the way we process images relates to our preference for and frequency of both visual and verbal processing. Figure 3.1 illustrates the process of receiving and retrieving **sensory input**, using an example of showing a mother how to position her baby at the breast.

Receiving and Storing Information

Processing information occurs in stages. A series of memory "storehouses" in the brain temporarily collect information. The image of a sensory input lasts for only one or two seconds in the mind's sensory store. It is lost immediately if it is not processed and transferred to the short-term store. The short-term store constitutes the working memory, where information is processed and held for a brief period. The amount of information that can be held in short-term storage is limited to about four or five items. At this stage, the information will be lost in about 30 seconds unless mentally repeated through the process of rehearsal. Information we rehearse transfers to the long-term store within two to ten seconds.

FIGURE 3.1
Pathway for sensory input.

Sensory input is received: Mother is shown how to position her baby at the breast. Input collects in the SENSORY STORE, where it is stored for 1–2 seconds.

When It Works	Why It Works	When Things Go Wrong	
Input is *processed* within 1–2 seconds. ⇩	Mother is alert. It is a teachable moment. Mother is motivated.	Input is not processed in time. ⟹	Information is lost immediately.
Input transfers to the *short-term store* and is retained for 30 seconds. ⇩	Process is described and demonstrated with a doll while mother brings baby to breast.	**Why It Went Wrong** Mother is tired or in pain. Mother lacks motivation. Mother is distracted.	
Input is *rehearsed* within 30 seconds.	Mother practices putting her baby to breast. Mother is given assistance and support in the early days.	Input is not rehearsed in time. ⟹	Information is not retained.
⇩		**Why It Went Wrong** Mother doesn't do a return demonstration. No one visits to reinforce. Mother forgets important features.	
Less than 5–6 items of input are received and rehearsed. ⇩	Mother is given printed and verbal instructions about what to expect in the first week: frequency, duration, feeding cues, number of stools and voids.	More than 5–6 items of input are received and rehearsed within 30 seconds. ⟹	Information overload. Information is not retained. Confusion takes place. Less effective choices. Poor decision making.

	RESULT FOR MOTHER ⬇	**Why It Went Wrong**	
Input is *encoded*. ⇩	Mother has a solid grasp of basic management.	Mother is given 2 pages of printed and verbal instructions that include: frequency, duration, feeding cues, number of stools and voids, what to eat, various positions for holding the baby at feedings, how to end a feeding, how to soothe a fussy baby, what to do about leaking, how to treat sore nipples and engorgement, when to start supplements, how and when to wean, how to express milk, how to manage breastfeeding and returning to work, how to increase milk production, and how to nurse in public.	
Input transfers within 10 seconds to *long-term store,* where 2–3 items are retained for days, weeks, or years. ⇩	Mother is ready to focus on additional factors for the next several months.		
Activation of input takes place to: ♦ Organize with new links. ♦ Expand network of relationships. ♦ Motivate search for more information. ⇩	Mother applies what she knows to new situations.		
Recoding of input takes place to: ♦ Accommodate more information. ♦ Interpret and elaborate. ♦ Match frame of reference. ♦ Match prior knowledge. ♦ Activate long-term memory. ⇩	Mother continues to learn more about breastfeeding at each stage of her baby's development and responds appropriately.	Does not match frame of reference or prior knowledge. ⟹	Retention and recall are hampered. Retrieval system fails. Forgetting takes place.

		RESULT FOR MOTHER ⬇	
Retrieval of information.	Mother feels confident about her breastfeeding knowledge and management techniques. Mother applies what she knows when she breastfeeds subsequent babies.	Mother doesn't know how to feed on cue; starts early supplements and solids. Mother doesn't get a good latch; gets sore nipples. Mother weans early. Mother doesn't breastfeed subsequent babies.	

At this stage, we can retain the information for days, weeks, or even years.

Retention and Recall of Information

The degree to which we repeat information or relate it to other data greatly affects retention. Rehearsal enables us to hold information in short-term storage long enough for encoding to take place. When we encode information, we select a word or visual image to represent an object we have perceived. Although both verbal and visual images are important in forming an overall mental image, verbal images take less time to learn than visual images (Goodman, 1992). Thus, one-on-one assistance with a breastfeeding mother produces better retention than asking the mother simply to watch a how-to video.

Information can be lost when the short-term store receives a great deal of input at the same time, which reduces its capacity to only two or three pieces of information. When receiving too much information—referred to as information overload—we find it difficult to encode and store it all. The result of this overload is confusion, less effective choices, and poor decision making. In the vulnerable immediate postpartum period, most parents receive an overwhelming amount of instruction on all aspects of maternal and infant care. This makes it unlikely the mother can even locate the breastfeeding information, much less process any of it!

Information in long-term storage is constantly organized and reorganized as new links are forged between chunks of information. As we gain more knowledge, we expand the network of relationships between data and sometimes are motivated to search for additional information. This process of activation relates new data to old data in order to make information more meaningful. It may involve re-encoding what we have already encoded to include larger amounts of information.

Chunks of information that do not match our frame of reference and prior knowledge hamper retention and recall. We are more likely to spend time interpreting and elaborating on information we find relevant to our needs, re-encoding this information and thus activating such relevant knowledge from long-term memory. Retrieval is the process by which we recover this information. When the retrieval system fails, forgetting takes place. New mothers often find it difficult to recall specific instructions regarding breastfeeding. Reinforcing verbal instruction with written materials and other visual aids will provide the necessary support at this time of change and confusion.

Involvement and Relevance

The way we process information depends on how relevant it is to us and our level of involvement. High involvement produces more extensive processing of information. Level of involvement is a critical factor in determining which method of persuasion is likely to be effective. As the message becomes more personally relevant and our involvement increases, we are more willing to spend the cognitive effort required to process the message. We seek information, weigh it carefully, and evaluate its merits. When we are highly involved or have a strong opinion about an issue, we may interpret something as being more positive than it actually is if it agrees with our opinion (Schiffman, 1997). Those who are uninvolved will be more receptive to arguments both for and against, or they will take no position at all. For these people, learning is enhanced by visual cues and repetition. Lactation consultants involved in complex cases often find that the health care provider (such as an endocrinologist or occupational therapist) least involved with the infant or mother's care may be the most willing to try new approaches.

Involvement theory evolved from a stream of research referred to as split-brain theory, which describes how the right and left hemispheres of the brain specialize in the kinds of information they process (Figure 3.2). The left brain involves cognition and is considered to be rational, active, and realistic. Cognitive information requires a high degree of active involvement. Conversely, the right brain is considered nonverbal, emotional, symbolic, impulsive, and intuitive, which all involve affect.

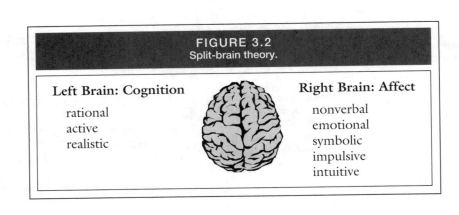

FIGURE 3.2
Split-brain theory.

Left Brain: Cognition

rational
active
realistic

Right Brain: Affect

nonverbal
emotional
symbolic
impulsive
intuitive

Affect refers to the manner in which a person projects his or her emotions. We process and store right-brain information passively—that is, without active involvement.

The right and left hemispheres of the brain work together to process information, and normally both hemispheres are engaged and integrated during the process. Integrated processors show greater overall recall of both verbal and visual input. Both sides of the brain are capable of high or low involvement. There is some initial engagement of the right brain in a high-involvement cognitive (left-brain) process; similarly, some engagement of the left brain is involved in a high-involvement affective (right-brain) process.

▶ SOCIAL BEHAVIOR

Human behavior is more than just the action of isolated individuals—it is social action. Perceptions and social norms govern our social behavior, even though much of the time we are unaware of these influences. The meaning individuals give to their action is what creates society. The foundations of most societies are intrinsically adaptable and durable and can accommodate people consciously making and altering the social order around them.

As a society increases in complexity, the individual parts of society grow increasingly dependent upon one another, becoming interconnected. Society sets boundaries for behavior. Our social surroundings either have helped to create or are affected by whatever we undergo as individuals. For example, a breastfeeding woman experiences resistance from her employer and fellow workers when she returns to work after having her first baby. She receives support from a breastfeeding counselor and ultimately becomes a counselor herself. She works with her employer to establish a lactation room and a positive work environment for mothers. When she returns to work after her second baby, her work environment is dramatically more supportive of her continuing to breastfeed. We each belong to a social group whose membership to a greater or lesser degree dictates our behavior. Other behavior determinants are personality, ethical values, and attitudes.

Personality

Our inner psychological characteristics both determine and reflect how we respond to our environment. Specific qualities, attributes, traits, and mannerisms distinguish one person from another. This unique combination of factors explains why no two individuals are exactly alike. Although personality is largely consistent and firmly grounded, specific needs, motives, attitudes, or reactions can influence a change in behavior. Thus, we may alter our personality as part of a gradual maturing process or because of major life events, such as childbirth. Becoming

a mother enables a woman to embrace unconditional love and learn unselfishness as she tends to her child's needs. The hormone oxytocin increases women's ability to do repetitive tasks, a vital ablity for daily child care (Taylor, 2000).

Self-Image

We all have an image of ourselves as having certain traits, habits, possessions, relationships, and ways of behaving. This self-image is likely to influence the manner in which we act with different people and in different situations. Our **self-image** is unique and is the outgrowth of our background and experience. It is influenced by how we see ourselves, how we would like to see ourselves, how we feel others see us, and how we would like others to see us. How we expect to see ourselves at some specified future time also influences our self-image and provides an opportunity for change. The manner in which these various self-images guide our attitudes and behavior depends on the specific situation. As a lactation consultant, you may see mothers who feel pressure by their spouse or peer group to breastfeed but who personally do not want to do it. The mother's self-image is in conflict. She sees her role as a mother as including breastfeeding, but internally (whether because of sexual abuse or social conditioning) she recoils from the physicality of feeding her baby at the breast.

Unconscious Needs

Unconscious needs or drives are at the heart of human motivation and personality. Freud believed that human drives are largely unconscious and that people are primarily unaware of the true reasons for their actions. In the case of the hypothetical mother above, she may feel discomfort with breastfeeding but not consciously know why. The unconscious reason could be repressed sexual abuse or a distorted understanding of breastfeeding due to sexual teasing. She may have an ill-defined self-image and believe that breasts are only sexual organs and that breastfeeding is therefore a sexual act.

Personality Types

There are many theories about personality types. We will discuss three of them here. Carl Jung, a contemporary of Freud, stressed the influence of personality on behavior. His personality types are used in the Myers-Briggs Type Indicators, a personality inventory that measures several psychological characteristics—sensing, intuiting, thinking, feeling, extroversion, introversion, judging, and perceiving. Each of these when paired with another reflect distinctly different personality characteristics. Identifying these proclivities offers a picture of how individuals will respond to their world.

The combinations of some of these indicators are especially useful in determining how people obtain and process information and how they make decisions. Learning how these particular personality types influence information processing and decision making enables us to better satisfy another person's needs. The four Myers-Briggs personality types describe personalities that combine Sensing and Thinking, Sensing and Feeling, Intuitive and Thinking, or Intuitive and Feeling (Figure 3.3).

A neo-Freudian approach to understanding personality contends that social relationships are fundamental to the formation and development of personality. Alfred Adler believed that human beings seek to attain various rational goals, which he termed "style of life." He placed emphasis on an individual's efforts to overcome feelings of inferiority. Harry Stack Sullivan believed that people continually attempt to establish significant and rewarding relationships with others. He was particularly concerned with an individual's efforts to reduce tension and anxiety.

Another premise, the trait theory, focuses on the measurement of personality in terms of specific psychological characteristics. A "trait" is defined as any distinguishing, relatively enduring way in which one individual differs from another. People who are inner-directed, for example, tend to rely on their own values or standards. They may respond favorably to an approach that stresses personal benefits. Those who are other-directed tend to look to other people for direction on what is "right" or "wrong." They will focus more on social acceptance, in keeping with their tendency to look to others for guidance. Specific personality traits can identify those who are more likely to be responsive to the influence of others. Individuals who are most susceptible to interpersonal influence tend to be less self-confident than those who are less susceptible. Lactation consultants may see both strong self-confidence and lack of confidence when working with teen mothers. The teen mother may be clearly inner-directed and strong beyond her years in advocating for her baby. On the other hand, she may be other-directed at the same time, looking to her mother, her caseworker, or another adult to make decisions for her.

Ethics

Morals and ethics greatly influence an individual's social behavior. "Ethics" derives from the Greek term *ethos*. Every culture develops its own form of ethics. In Western civilization, *ethics* is synonymous with *character* or *morals*. **Ethics** are principles or standards of human

	Thinking	Feeling
FIGURE 3.3		
Personality types and behavior.		
Sensing	Sensing-Thinking	Sensing-Feeling
	◆ Rational in decision making	◆ Practical and pragmatic
	◆ Driven by logic rather than values	◆ Driven by values rather than logic
	◆ Practical and pragmatic	◆ Makes decisions based on subjectivity
	◆ Expends considerable effort to search for information	◆ Likely to consider others when making a decision
	◆ Avoids risk	◆ Shares risks with others
	◆ Identifies with material objects	◆ Aware of how material objects influence others
	◆ Makes decisions for the short term	◆ Makes decisions for the short term
Intuitive	Intuiting-Thinking	Intuitive-Feeling
	◆ Takes a broad view of personal situation	◆ Takes a broad view of personal situation
	◆ Relies on imagination, yet uses logic to approach decisions	◆ Imagines a wide range of options in making a decision
	◆ Imagines a wider range of options in making a decision	◆ Highly people oriented and likely to consider views of others
	◆ Willing to take a risk	◆ Makes decisions based on subjectivity
	◆ Makes decisions for the long term	◆ Seeks risk
		◆ Makes decisions for an indefinite period of time

FIGURE 3.3
Personality types and behavior.

conduct. In an attempt to define the highest good, sociologists have identified three principle standards of conduct: happiness or pleasure; duty, virtue, or obligation; and perfection (MSN, 2005). Moral customs change with each new generation, but ethical values are enduring. They may or may not coincide with what is currently and locally moral.

Early Theories on Ethics

Philosophers first began to theorize about moral behavior in 6th century Greece, which led to the development of *philosophical ethics*. Pythagoras based moral philosophy on the beliefs that our intellectual nature is superior to our sensual nature and that the best life is one devoted to mental discipline. A century later, a group of Greek philosophers known as Sophists opposed moral absolutes and taught rhetoric, logic, and civil affairs. The Sophist Protagoras put forth the theory that human judgment is subjective and that an individual's perception of himself is valid only for him and cannot be generalized.

Socrates and his student Plato opposed the Sophist philosophy, teaching instead that virtue is knowledge and that people will be virtuous if they know what virtue is. They believed that education has the capacity to make people moral. Later Greek philosophers espoused these same beliefs, maintaining that the essence of virtue is self-control and that self-control can be learned.

Plato taught that good is an essential element of reality and maintained that human virtue lies in the fitness of a person to perform his proper function in the world. He described the human soul as having three elements: intellect, will, and emotion. Intellect leads to wisdom, will leads to courage or the capacity to act, and emotion leads to temperance or self-control. Of the three, Plato believed that intellect is the highest virtue and that emotion should be subject to intellect and will.

Plato's student Aristotle believed that happiness is the aim of life and that virtues are essentially good habits. One must develop two habits to attain happiness. The habit of mental activity consists of knowledge and contemplation. Practical action and emotion form the other habit, courage. Aristotle taught that moral virtues must be flexible to accommodate the differences among people and conditions. He saw intellectual and moral virtues as a means toward the attainment of happiness, which results when one realizes his full human potential.

The Stoics in 3rd-century Rome held that nature is orderly and rational and that only a life led in harmony with nature can be good. They believed that material circumstances influence life and that we should strive to be independent of such influences. They concluded that practical wisdom, courage, discretion, and justice could achieve independence. The Epicureans shared this philosophy and held that we should postpone immediate pleasure to attain more secure and lasting satisfaction in the future. They taught that self-discipline must regulate the good life.

The advent of Christianity revolutionized the concept of ethics. Western thought now had a *religious* notion of good, one in which man is totally dependent on God and can achieve goodness only with the help of God's grace, not by means of will or intelligence. Christianity gave rise to the "golden rule," teaching that we should treat others as we wish to be treated and that we should love others as we love ourselves.

Living an Ethical Life

The works of the early Greek, Roman, and Christian philosophers gave birth to the tenets that form the basis of modern ethics. John Locke believed in the natural goodness of humanity. He maintained that the pursuit of happiness and pleasure leads to cooperation when conducted rationally. He argued that private happiness and general welfare coincide, and that immediate pleasures must give way to a prudent regard for ultimate good.

This reveals the ultimate dilemma of trying to live an ethical life. Ethical living in its fullest sense is an aspiration we can only approach. In reality, none of us practices ethical habits all the time. Everyone has internal personal needs and external social needs—the challenge is to integrate these two selves. Individuals who seek power may not accept customary ethical rules, but may conform to rules that can help them become successful. They will seek to persuade others that they are moral. This is an attempt to mask their power seeking and to gain social approval of their actions, presenting them as morally motivated.

This is evident in recent actions by formula manufacturing executives, who pressured the American Academy of Pediatrics in an attempt to prevent a public service ad campaign promoting breastfeeding (Merewood, 2004). The formula industry acknowledges the superiority of breastfeeding in its advertising. Yet the industry strenuously lobbied against an advertising campaign that could dramatically increase breastfeeding rates. Their moral appeal for being recognized as supporting optimal health is eclipsed by their self-interests in selling their product.

We steer our lives by trial and error and by intuition and reason. Our assumptions about the world determine our direction, our identity, and ultimately the character of society. A community is composed of unique and interdependent beings who ideally relate to one another in such a way that elicits the best from every person. Our ethical values determine how we behave, how we treat one another, and how we create the social conditions and habits necessary for others to thrive, both individually and collectively.

Elements of an Ethical Culture

An *ethical culture* is one that creates a humane environment in which we treat others as unique individuals, value their worth, and treat them with respect. We elicit the best from each and every person. This enhances our personal growth, because when we see and encourage good in others, we discover it in ourselves. In an ethical culture, therefore, we live by habits that enable everyone to thrive. We reach beyond ourselves to decrease suffering and to increase creativity in the world. We allow others to make choices and to be accountable for their mistakes. Cultures that value mothering and children provide practices that support the worth of mothering and breastfeeding. Sweden, Norway, and several other European nations provide generous maternity leaves for mothers, enabling them to breastfeed without separation from their babies (European Commission, 2003).

Above all, we act with *integrity* in an ethical culture. A life of integrity is one in which we keep commitments. We are more open, honest, caring, and responsive to others. We make significant choices in our lives and build ethical relationships. We are committed to educating ourselves in order to grow, both in wisdom and socially. We remain true to our values and standards. We recognize that words have limited value without actions to support them, and that ultimately we are judged by what we do, not by what we say. Any lapse in ethics, or even the appearance of a lapse, can significantly harm one's reputation. IBLCE's Code of Ethics guides the behavior of lactation consultants. The IBLCE expects them to support the code and incorporate the code of ethics into their career (see Appendix C). Ethical issues relevant in the lactation profession are discussed further in Chapter 28.

Attribution

Sociology looks at how people attribute causes to their behavior and to the behavior of others. We want to know why we and others act or do not act in certain ways. We seek reasons for behavior, and we expect excuses and apologies when an error occurs or when we are disappointed. This process of explaining behavior is *attribution*. When we believe we understand the causes of behavior, we react with thoughts, feelings, and responses specific to those causes.

The manner in which we attribute causes and reasons for past events influences our expectations of the future. When we attribute cause, we search for and use information about the person and the social context in which the behavior took place. We seek to explain other people's behavior in an attempt to reduce uncertainty about what is likely to happen in the future, given similar conditions. This enables us to predict and to feel some measure of control over the world in which we live. A new mother may encounter this when she is told by her own mother, "I wanted to breastfeed you, but I didn't make enough milk." This may set the stage for the new mother to expect that she, too, will not "make enough milk."

It is important to recognize that how we perceive the cause of behavior may differ from its actual cause. Such discrepancies in perception are common and explain how individuals can draw such different conclusions about a particular event or behavior. What we expect to see often strongly influences what we do see. Our perception of the cause of a particular behavior depends on our personality, the features of the behavior, and the social context of the behavior. Our perception also influences the degree of responsibility we attribute to someone for his actions. For example, parents may ascribe conscious motivation to a baby's feeding behaviors with comments such as, "He's being lazy; he's just using me as a pacifier; he doesn't want to nurse."

Perception

Perception is the process by which an individual selects, organizes, and interprets stimuli into a meaningful and coherent picture of the world. An almost infinite number of stimuli bombard us during every minute and every hour of every day. A stimulus is any unit of input to any of the five senses of sight, hearing, sound, taste, and touch. We subconsciously add to and subtract from these raw sensory inputs to produce our private picture of the world. This picture is influenced by our own expectations, motives, and learning, which are all based on previous experience.

We consciously exercise a great deal of selectivity as to which stimuli—which aspects of the environment—we perceive. The stimuli we select depend on the nature of the stimulus, our previous experience, and our motives at the time. As mentioned before, we usually see what we expect to see. Familiarity, previous experience, and preconditioned expectations determine what we expect to see. We also tend to perceive things we need or want. The stronger the need or want, the stronger our awareness is of those stimuli and the greater our tendency to ignore unrelated stimuli. Our process of perception simply attunes itself more closely to elements in the environment that are important to us.

Preconditioned expectations mean that we tend to attribute the qualities we associate with certain people to others who may resemble them. We also tend to carry images in our minds of the meanings of various kinds of stimuli. Recognizing this can help us understand the implications of our perceptions and how they may influence our behavior and our expectations of others. It is important for you to "know thyself," and to recognize personality types that irritate or disturb you. When you encounter a mother with that personality, recognize your emotional reaction. You can consciously choose to interact with her in a respectful, healthy way and leave your "emotional baggage" at the door. Awareness strengthens your ability to help this mother and not react solely to her personality or allow her to "push your buttons."

It is important to note that people can be stimulated below their level of conscious awareness. In other words, we can perceive stimuli without being consciously aware that we are doing so. Stimuli that are too weak or too brief to be consciously seen or heard may nevertheless be strong enough to be perceived by one or more receptors. Such subliminal perception can result from a brief visual presentation, from accelerated speech in low-volume auditory messages, or from embedded or hidden imagery or words. Subliminal messages can motivate people to exhibit a certain behavior without being aware of why they are motivated to behave in that manner.

Infant formula manufacturers and other companies understand this. They spend millions of dollars on advertising to ensure that the image of a baby bottle or their particular logo connotes quintessential babyhood. Their advertising depicts a mother feeding a bottle to her baby, warmly portraying optimal eye contact and a wide smile. In the same ad they portray a breastfeeding mother with her eyes averted and minimal facial expression. They subliminally project the bottle-feeding mother as being more engaged with her baby and enjoying feeding time more completely.

Attitude

Attitudes are an expression of inner feelings that reflect whether we are favorably or unfavorably predisposed to something. We cannot observe others' attitudes directly. We infer them from what people say or do. Attitudes evaluate a message ("Do I want to do this?") and may either propel us toward or repel us away from a particular behavior. The process of trying and evaluating a behavior is the primary means by which we form attitudes.

Many health care professionals were trained in an era of formula feeding and schedules as the norm, and most of them bottle-fed their children. They often believe that formula is "just as good" as breastmilk. Formula manufacturers promote this attitude through aggressive marketing targeted specifically to the medical community.

In general, the more information we have about something, the more likely we are to form attitudes about it, either positive or negative. Individuals often use only a limited amount of the information available

to them and are not always ready or willing to process more. Therefore, it is important to focus on the few key points that are at the heart of your message. When you have the opportunity to interact with another health care professional, keep your message simple and succinct. He or she may be more open to one fact about breastfeeding than a barrage of emotional information. This is especially true for those in the medical field unfamiliar with the concepts of breastfeeding as the biological norm and artificial feeding as suboptimal and possessing health risks to the infant.

Determining Attitudes

Part of the information we use in developing attitudes are the mores and cultural norms of society. The rules of behavior within a peer group contribute to that group's uniformity. Cultural norms regarding personal conduct and ethical standards are responsible for a certain degree of uniformity. Attitude formation is linked to personal experience and the influence of family and friends. Our early childhood, family background, educational level, and subculture all contribute to differences among us and, consequently, to differences among our attitudes.

Direct marketing efforts and the mass media constantly expose us to new ideas, products, opinions, and advertisements and attempt to influence our attitudes through their messages. Parents are barraged with promotional messages about products they "must" have for their baby. We in the lactation profession must be careful not to send similar messages about the need for breastfeeding devices.

Predicting Behavior

Knowledge of people's attitudes provides insight into understanding and predicting behavior. Although attitudes are relatively enduring, they are easier to change than beliefs and values. Our central beliefs and values, those that influence and determine how we think and act, are resistant to change. Beliefs and values that are more peripheral have less influence on how we see the world and are more easily changed.

Attitudes are often influenced by circumstances. Individuals can have a variety of attitudes toward a particular behavior, each corresponding to a particular situation. Therefore, it is important to consider the situation in which a behavior takes place in order to interpret it correctly. A healthcare provider who espouses support for breastfeeding may be surprisingly quick to recommend supplementing with formula. You may understand this inconsistency better if you learn that the provider has adopted more aggressive protocols for treating **hyperbilirubinemia** in light of recent pediatric concerns (Ross, 2003).

FIGURE 3.4
Scale of intent.

- ◆ I definitely will
- ◆ I probably will
- ◆ I am uncertain whether I will
- ◆ I probably will not
- ◆ I definitely will not

Intention

The intention to act is the best predictor of behavior. A person's attitude toward something will occur at some point along a scale of intent (Figure 3.4) that ranges from positive to negative intentions (Schiffman, 1997). To understand intention, we must understand what influences our intent to act. We are primarily influenced by people who are significant and important in our life. These may be family, friends, or coworkers. We first consider how we believe they would respond to the decision and then whether their response will affect our motivation to act. The support of the child's father is one of the main determinants in whether a woman breastfeeds (Chang, 2003; Chen, 2003; Scott, 2001; Arora, 2000; Kessler, 1995). His attitude influences the mother's motivation, intention, and, thus, her behavior.

Attitude Changes

Attitudes can change because of personal experience and new sources of information. Personality plays a pivotal role in the speed with which attitudes are likely to change. Individuals who crave information and enjoy thinking (cognition) are likely to form positive attitudes in response to messages that are rich in information. Those who are relatively low in their need for cognition are more likely to respond to messages and impressions that appeal to their emotions.

An effective strategy for changing attitudes is to help the individual recognize how the new behavior serves a positive purpose and is superior to the alternative. If a woman can see that her attitude toward a behavior is in conflict with another attitude, she may change her evaluation of the behavior in question. Healthcare providers who receive education about the improved health outcomes of breastfed infants may change their early, less favorable attitudes. Another useful strategy is to change the individual's beliefs about the attributes of the alternative. The impetus behind advertising the risks of formula feeding instead of the benefits of breastfeeding exemplifies this (Merewood, 2004; Walker, 2001).

Motivation

As we have seen, motivation is a driving force. Our individual thinking and learning influences the specific goals we select, as well as the manner in which we act to achieve those goals. Experiencing an unfulfilled need, want, or desire creates internal tension. This tension provides the motivation to engage in behavior that will ultimately reduce the tension. In order to take action and exhibit this new behavior, we engage in a process of thinking, learning new information, and recalling previous learning. The new behavior, in turn, leads toward fulfilling the goal or need that initially provided the motivation. Reaching the goal reduces tension and enables us to manage the situation that precipitated these actions. Figure 3.5 illustrates this path (Weber, 1992).

Goals and Needs

All behavior is goal oriented, and all goals derive from some form of need. Needs and goals change in response to our physical condition, environment, experiences, and interactions with other people. We may actually be more aware of our goal than of the needs that lead us to seek that goal. We are usually more readily aware of physiological needs than psychological needs. The goals we select depend on our needs, personal experiences, cultural norms and values, self-images, physical capacity, and their accessibility within our physical and social environment.

The motivation for fulfilling needs can be either positive or negative. Positive drives take the form of needs, wants, and desires. Negative drives take the form of fears and aversions. Goals can be either positive or negative as well. We may wish to direct our actions toward a positive goal (**approach behavior**) or away from a negative outcome (**avoidance behavior**). Even babies exhibit

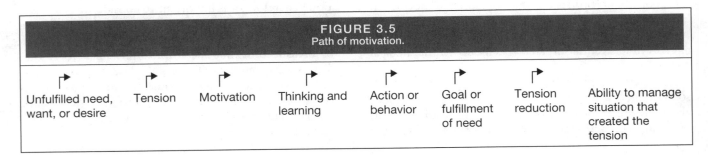

FIGURE 3.5
Path of motivation.

Unfulfilled need, want, or desire → Tension → Motivation → Thinking and learning → Action or behavior → Goal or fulfillment of need → Tension reduction → Ability to manage situation that created the tension

approach behaviors and avoidance behaviors that communicate their needs to parents and other caregivers. See Chapter 13 for more information about infant behavior.

A mother's desire to breastfeed based on her conviction that this offers her baby optimum health has a positive motivation. Her positive drive helps her persevere through initial soreness and engorgement to achieve her desired goal of a healthy, exclusively breastfed baby. A mother who has internalized horror stories of painful childbirth and breastfeeding may wish to prevent pain and be quick to ask for a nipple shield, nipple creams, and a bottle.

▶ RELATIONSHIPS

Relationships form the basis of our behavior with others. They occur through work-related contacts, social interactions, and our involvement with groups and organizations. The ways in which we interact will take on different forms depending on the setting. Sociology studies relationships among people—within the economy, the family, education, organizations, religions, corporations, government, and ethnic groups. How individuals and groups interact can help predict social change and how people will respond to social change.

Attachment and Bonding

Childhood forms a foundation for adolescent and adult functioning. The first two years of life are vital in determining personality, the ability to form relationships, and social behavior. Experiences during this critical time can set the stage for the manner in which we approach future social situations.

Many social psychologists regard a child's first relationship to be a prototype for future relationships and believe it determines the way a person approaches and interacts with other people (Ainsworth, 1978; Bowlby, 1982, 1975). Understandably, the study of this first relationship focuses on the quality of attachment between a mother and her infant. An infant's bonding with his mother describes the baby's tendency to seek proximity to his mother, to be receptive to receiving care from her, and to feel secure in her presence. Strength of attachment is positively associated with the ability and sensitivity of the mother to respond to her infant's verbal and nonverbal signals.

Attachment is strong when mothers respond consistently, regularly, and promptly. A parent's responsiveness to a baby's early hunger signs teaches the baby early trust. He realizes, "I'm hungry and Mom feeds me; I'm warm; I feel safe; Mom's milk is good; I'm full." Conversely, when a parent ignores hunger cues and crying, it teaches the baby, "I'm hungry; I'm upset; I'm lonely; where is Mom? Why doesn't she come?" These babies try self-soothing, but it does not relieve hunger. The world is not safe. The baby does not feel secure. Mom is unpredictable. Sometimes she answers and sometimes she does not. The stage is set for fear, anxiety, helplessness, and hopelessness.

Group Behavior

We all belong to a variety of groups, both formal and informal. These groups—familial, work-related, educational, religious, social, and recreational—influence how we communicate and interact with one another, how we perform tasks, and how we achieve goals. We are born into a social group, the family, where we gain our initial experiences. We grow and mature in social groups. We earn a living in a social group.

We have a defined role within each group structure, with our own specific degree of status and power. We exhibit our own form of group behavior, and we communicate with each other by sending and receiving messages. We conform to group norms to one degree or another. We are aware of each other, interact with each other, and exert influence on each other. Generally, people join a group to attain a goal or otherwise satisfy a need. Group participation addresses many social needs, such as approval, a sense of belonging, and friendship. Peer groups in similar life stages, such as young couples' bible classes in churches, play groups, or neighborhood associations can form long-term friendships as they move through adult life stages together.

In sociology, a "group" is usually defined as a collection consisting of a number of people who share certain aspects, interact with one another, accept rights and obligations as members of the group, and share a common identity. A group exhibits a degree of cohesiveness and may be loosely formed or have a formal structure. Like-minded people may form a formal association to accomplish a purpose based on shared interests and values. Most associations have some kind of document that regulates the way in which they meet and operate. Such an instrument is often called the organization's bylaws, regulations, or agreement of association. The group's policies guide the behavior and attitudes of its members. Associations such as ILCA and IBLCE have codes of behavior that are expected and encouraged.

Primary and Secondary Groups

Some groups to which we belong are basic to our social development and have a significant impact on us as individuals. Members of these primary groups often know a good deal about one another and care about one another's welfare. The family is an example of a primary group. We have close, personal, and enduring relationships in a family. Members typically spend considerable time together and share many activities and experiences. Relationships are deep because of the emotions invested in them.

Secondary groups tend to be temporary and may form for a specific purpose or task. Relationships are relatively impersonal with little emotional investment. Interaction between members tends to focus on activities that led the group to form rather than on the needs, desires, or concerns of the individual members. Members of a secondary group often have little personal knowledge of one another.

Some secondary groups may evolve to take on the characteristics of a primary group. The critical difference between the two types of groups is the degree of emotional investment in the group and the degree of relationships among the members. The degree to which members feel bound to one another will determine the group's stability and the likelihood that members will conform to its norms. Members of cohesive groups like each other more and support common goals more strongly than members of less cohesive groups do. Cohesive groups enjoy interactions more and tend to be better problem solvers.

Because mothers have to surmount cultural obstacles to breastfeeding, breastfeeding support groups tend to be cohesive. These mothers swim against the cultural norm. The empowerment they receive from breastfeeding makes them strong advocates for other areas of their children's welfare as their children grow. Many mothers remain involved in childbirth, breastfeeding, and other educational issues long after their children have weaned because of their strong beliefs.

The lactation profession is another example of a cohesive secondary group. La Leche League, ILCA, and IBLCE were all formed by women who were passionate about promoting healthy infant feeding practices. The strong beliefs and mutual commitment among the members of these groups has created a familial relationship of nurturing and loyalty.

Power and Empowerment

Power places controls within relationships. The center of power can shift in response to personal, interpersonal, and social changes. Power is dictated to a large degree by the social group within which the relationship exists. It occurs in various forms. *Expert* power derives from someone who has greater knowledge and skills than we do. *Coercive* power creates physical controls and coercion that is meant to limit our actions. *Reward* power takes the form of emotional or tangible rewards intended to alter our behavior. *Legitimate* power exists when another person or group has a genuine right to influence others. *Referent* power occurs when another person has attributes that we wish we had ourselves,

which alters our behavior. *Informational* power has the ability to transform a non-expert into an expert.

Medical professionals possess expert power made up of a specialized and exclusive body of knowledge, extensive vocational training, monopoly of practice, and self-regulation. The medical profession itself helps to maintain the social order, with benefits to both society and the individual. Within the medical profession is a wellspring of specialized professions. Each specialization possesses a unique body of knowledge, training, and area of practice. One consumer may be under the care of a primary physician, endocrinologist, cardiologist, gynecologist, orthopedist, rheumatologist, dermatologist, and physical therapist. It has become increasingly important for consumers to coordinate their care and to assume informational power that enables them to control their outcomes.

With wider access to medical information through the Internet and other resources, consumers are better informed and more demanding than ever before. As a result, the social distance between patient and medical practitioner is narrowing. Patient rights, health-related support groups, alternative therapies, and homeopathic practices permeate the health care arena. Ultimately, power is at the core of understanding a profession. With easy access to information, patients are transforming from nonexperts into experts. The center of power is shifting, and the face of the medical profession has been forever altered, evidence that professions, as social organizations, mutate as a result of social and scientific developments.

Nurses, physicians, other caregivers, and patients all have and use power in their relationships with one another. It should be the goal of all health care providers to empower individuals and encourage them to be active in their relationships with practitioners. True empowerment occurs only when health care providers transform the ways in which they relate to patients. When we relinquish coercive power and help mothers take more control over their health needs and the prevention of problems, we empower them to gain mastery over their lives. It helps them develop a critical awareness of the root causes of their problems and a readiness to act on this awareness.

▶ KNOWLEDGE AND CULTURE

The culture and times in which we live drive our knowledge. This knowledge may occur through folktales, religious and psychological beliefs, or science. Of these, scientific thought is currently the most predominant and successful premise for determining legitimate knowledge. Societal values, beliefs, and accepted wisdom often challenge the authenticity of scientific knowledge.

Science and Technology

Science and technology play central roles in the institutional structure of modern societies. Science is the systematic pursuit of reliable knowledge about the physical and social world. Through it, we obtain an understanding of the nature and operation of physical and social phenomena. The modern study of the natural and social world finds its roots among the ancient Greeks' logical and rational attempts to comprehend the origins of disease (Goodman, 1992). These same Greeks viewed their gods as all-powerful; yet they were the inventors of philosophy, mathematics, and science. A similar paradox exists for modern-day scientists who must reconcile Darwin's theory of evolution with their religious beliefs.

The sciences of sociology and anthropology can identify the origins of the family and anticipate future patterns from one generation to the next, but the public is not consciously aware of this cause-and-effect relationship between social phenomena. Nor do most people understand how modern technology works. We fly from one city to another, we watch television, and we communicate with one another by cellular telephones and computers. The emergence of computer technology and the Internet has created profound social change and links individuals collectively through cyberspace in a mass society. Yet, for the most part, we lack even a basic understanding of the scientific principles that make it all possible.

Subjective Nature of Science

Not all science is objective. Much of what is studied depends on the availability of funding. Funding, in turn, is often contingent on whether there is a perceived commercial or political benefit to the research. We would not expect a tobacco company to fund publicly available research that investigates the health risks of smoking. A brewery is unlikely to subsidize research on fetal alcohol syndrome or teenage death rates from alcohol abuse. Manufacturers of artificial baby milk are not likely to fund research examining the superiority of human milk except in their efforts to isolate and patent human milk components. Of course, there can be exceptions. A company may perceive that such financial support will lessen criticism of its business practices. Or they may wish to send a message that they promote practices or products that seem to be contradictory to their interests. Artificial infant milk manufacturers have honed this practice to the highest levels imaginable in their "promotion" of breastfeeding.

Another complicating factor is that scientists cannot agree on how to collect and test data (Goodman, 1992). One scientist may believe that establishing constant truths should form the basis of science. Another may approach science as an attempt to disprove apparent truths, believing that with good science it is possible to prove a **hypothesis** wrong. For example, a caregiver may recognize the importance of listening to patients and offering emotional support and finds that patients who are listened to seem to have greater self-esteem. The question becomes whether or not the **variables** of listening and self-esteem are dependent upon one another and whether heightened self-esteem always results from listening to a patient. The first scientist would theorize that the two variables always appear together and thus connect to one another. The second scientist would test alternative suppositions to disprove the connection, perhaps testing whether self-esteem increases on occasions when there is no communication between the patient and caregiver.

At times, researchers seem to accept the conclusions their predecessors have reached and address only certain puzzles that are inherent in those conclusions. Those conclusions form the paradigm within which most scientists operate. Inevitably, however, evidence accumulates that repudiates accepted practice and thinking. The evidence eventually becomes so great that the paradigm begins to fall apart.

What an individual thinks and does affects the way in which society is structured and, ultimately, what society accepts as reality. At the same time, society and the natural world create the circumstances through which we think and act. This illustrates the dynamic nature of the human condition. It continually changes in response to social influence and scientific fact, making it difficult to predict human behavior and social trends. Two hundred years ago, wealthy women were more likely to employ wet nurses and only the lower classes breastfed. Today, in developed countries such as the U.K., U.S., and Australia that practice has changed. Now the educated, upper middle class mother is more likely to breastfeed. Lower income and minority women disproportionately bottle-feed.

The pediatric profession arose in part from a desire to give artificial milk to infants whose mothers did not breastfeed. Mothers visited the new professional, a pediatrician, at periodic intervals in their babies' growth and acquired the appropriate recipe, or "formula" (Hess, 1923; Wolf, 2003). The age of infant formula feeding arrived, with its set of rules and scheduled feedings. Despite the introduction of commercial proprietary infant formulas in the 1920s, most parents continued to breastfeed or use home recipes because they were easy to prepare and affordable. It was not until the 1950s that commercial formulas began to slowly gain acceptance (Schuman, 2003).

The lactation profession arose several decades later to reverse the trend toward formula-feeding and return infant feeding to its biologic imperative. Researchers began to debunk many unsubstantiated practices that had carried over from formula-feeding to breastfeeding. Practitioners continue to correct misconceptions among the health profession and the public regarding breast-feeding care. As the paradigm continues to shift, previously accepted practices and thinking will change as well.

Evidence-Based Practice

A recent evolution in scientific thought has given rise to the pursuit of evidence-based practice. In an evidence-based society, scientific validation ultimately sways medicine. The media interpret research results, although these results are often couched in tentative terms, and the public relies on the media's interpretations rather than attempting to decipher the original research. As a lactation consultant, you hear "sound bites" of information in the popular press that cast breastfeeding in a negative light. Careful examination of the original studies may show, however, that the conclusions, in fact, do support breastfeeding. More tools for critical thinking and discernment are discussed in Chapter 27.

Although an evidence-based approach has merit, it cannot be at the exclusion of caring, intuition, and other "nonscientific" variables. Medicine receives its credibility through science, but it is also intuitive, humanistic, and behavioral. Much of what we do in breastfeeding care is experiential, based on anecdotal reports. The use of cabbage for engorgement was rediscovered from century-old practices that had been lost in a bottle-feeding culture (Rosier, 1988). Although modern research may not convincingly validate the effectiveness of this practice, the fact remains that many mothers have found it useful. Lactation consultants often observe trends among their clients that influence their care regimens. It is important that we balance such intuitive practices with those that are evidence-based.

▶ DECISION MAKING

We make decisions concerning every aspect of our daily lives. Generally, we make these decisions without stopping to think about how we make them and what is involved in the process. Motivation, perception, learning, personality, and attitudes influence our decision-making process. We begin the act of making a decision by recognizing a need or a new circumstance. We search for information, recall past experiences, and evaluate alternatives. We judge the information against each alternative, select from among the alternatives, and make a final decision. Figure 3.6 illustrates the decision-making process.

Mothers, whether they breastfeed or not, go intuitively through this process hundreds of times a day. A breastfeeding mother may notice her five-month-old is beginning to chew on her nipples, causing soreness. She may call a lactation consultant or an experienced breastfeeding mother or consult her breastfeeding book. She may learn that it is common for teething babies to change their nursing behavior. She evaluates the options, concluding that based on her baby's drooling and the buds in her baby's mouth that he is indeed teething. The mother may then try several comfort measures to minimize the baby chewing (e.g., breaking the latch herself or changing nursing positions). She will then select the one that best works for her and her baby (Mohrbacher, 2003). The same process occurs in deciding when to feed her baby, when she needs help with other breastfeeding issues, and a myriad of other parenting decisions.

Influencing Decisions

Influencing someone's decision making begins with an appeal to the needs and interests of that person. At times, objective, factual appeals are an effective method of persuasion. At other times, emotional appeals are more effective. In general, more-educated audiences respond better to factual appeals, and less-educated consumers respond better to emotional appeals. However, this is not always true. Healthcare professionals have been astounded and dismayed at the number of highly educated parents embracing scheduled feeding programs despite the abundance of medical information against these approaches (Aney, 1998).

Individuals are more likely to evaluate the pros and cons of a message when they are highly involved. Making the message memorable and persuasive begins by arousing interest in it and giving the other person a reason to listen. The U.S. Ad Council uses this method

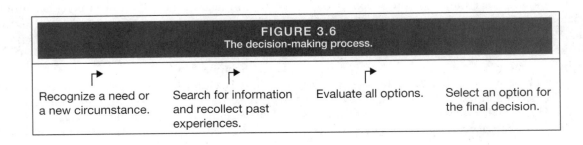

FIGURE 3.6
The decision-making process.

| Recognize a need or a new circumstance. | Search for information and recollect past experiences. | Evaluate all options. | Select an option for the final decision. |

effectively in its promotion campaigns. Asking questions generates involvement and helps to identify the points of interest and terminology that will be most effective. Interest ripens into desire only after we remove all lingering doubts from the other person's mind. Many lactation consultants increase participation in prenatal classes by asking parents to voice their questions about breastfeeding at the start of the class. If no one volunteers, several "ice breaker" questions can rhetorically draw out discussion.

It is important to be aware of any distractions that may impede the other person's receiving and retaining the key points of the message. If they are too engrossed in their thoughts or if they are emotionally unavailable, the message will not get through. The use of humor often increases the message's acceptance and persuasiveness. It attracts attention, increases comprehension, and enhances appreciation of the message. Consider demographic factors such as ethnicity and age when determining the appropriateness of using humor. Younger, better-educated, and professional people are generally more receptive to humorous messages. Lightening up your presentation, class, or other teaching with breastfeeding-related humor such as cartoons or anecdotes can both enliven the class and diffuse embarrassment.

The final step in influencing others' decision making is to involve them in forming a conclusion. You can ask them to voice their decision; if it conflicts with what you had hoped to convey, you can help them recognize the implications of their conclusion. When the consequences of a choice of action appear to be detrimental, people often begin to question the advisability of that decision. Verbalizing the implications of a positive decision can also serve to validate their choice and increase their self-confidence. Figure 3.7 shows the process of influencing a person's decision making.

If your message is to increase support for the use of human milk in the **NICU** and your audience is neonatologists, NICU nurses, and other neonatal healthcare professionals, you will use well-researched facts from respected sources. Hard data showing improved outcomes will arouse interest in your message (Sharpe, 2003). Distractors such as formula use need to be addressed and accounted for in your presentation. You can involve the audience by asking **open-ended questions** about what they would do or what they anticipate the results will be.

Compliance and Conformity

Social influence may be conscious or subconscious. It may be readily accepted, yielded to reluctantly, or resisted. Societal norms shape and influence our actions and result from social interaction. Social influence is greatest in face-to-face interactions. Group behavior determines what is popular, fashionable, and normal. These perceived group norms can influence behavior and effect social change.

Compliance

Acceptance is an internal process whereby we sincerely change because of social influence. **Compliance** occurs when we change our behavior or our expression of an attitude but do not accept the change completely. The degree to which we comply may depend in part on self-esteem and the fear of losing face. We may also be more likely to comply with a person who has previously done us a favor. Building influence is an effective way of increasing compliance. When we begin with a small request and follow with a larger request, people will be more likely to comply with the larger request. Another common approach is to begin with a large request that seems unreasonable and follow with a more reasonable request with which we actually wish the person to comply.

If you practice in a hospital or health care provider's office, you will have many opportunities to use the skill of increasing others' compliance. Lactation consultants can help their facilities take "baby steps" toward becoming baby friendly by using such approaches. Asking the purchasing department no longer to accept the "free" formula plied by marketing representatives may be too large a step initially. However, convincing the hospital to provide its own logo diaper bag as an advertising tool may enable you to remove the "free" formula gift bags as an interim step in becoming baby friendly (UNICEF, 2004). Mapping out a strategy for gradual change will help you build one change at a time.

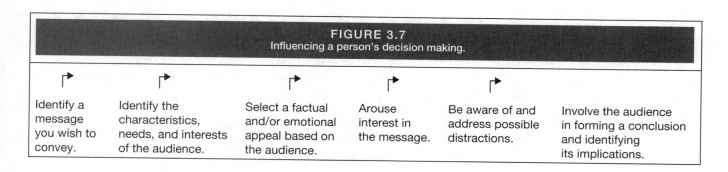

FIGURE 3.7
Influencing a person's decision making.

Identify a message you wish to convey. — Identify the characteristics, needs, and interests of the audience. — Select a factual and/or emotional appeal based on the audience. — Arouse interest in the message. — Be aware of and address possible distractions. — Involve the audience in forming a conclusion and identifying its implications.

Conformity

Whereas compliance primarily involves a request from an individual, *conformity* encompasses a wider range of influence. Conformity involves a change in attitude and behavior. It usually occurs in response to group pressure toward a social norm. People tend to conform to group norms when they find themselves in ambiguous or novel situations without prior experience to develop a frame of reference. Generally, the more ambiguous the situation and the less experience a person has, the more powerful the group influence will be.

The degree of appeal an individual feels toward the group and its perceived benefits affects conformity. People with high self-esteem tend to conform less from group pressure than do people who have low self-esteem. Groups we like and compare ourselves to are powerful sources of social influence. Conformity increases when the individual receives positive reinforcement, illustrating how the support of one person can have a considerable effect on another to comply with or to resist social pressure.

Many mothers benefit from joining breastfeeding support groups. Identifying with and networking with other breastfeeding mothers provides emotional and subcultural support that they may not receive from their extended family or friends. The moral support of mother-to-mother involvement encourages breastfeeding mothers to persevere through the predictable challenges of nursing a baby. It validates the importance of breastfeeding and the mother's choice to breastfeed.

Influences of Family and Society

Social influence refers to a change in attitude or behavior because of interactions with others. Others attempt to influence the way we think, feel, and behave throughout our lives. We, in turn, through our social interactions, attempt to influence others to think, feel, or act as we do. This encouragement of conformity is important in our society, which expects people to comply with requests and obey authority. At the same time, it is important for an individual to feel a unique sense of identity. Conflict can result from an attempt to maintain uniqueness and individuality while yielding to a certain degree of social influence.

Our family is often in the best position to influence our decisions. Because we generally have frequent contact with other family members, they are instrumental in establishing our values, attitudes, and behavior. The family serves as the primary agent for passing along basic cultural beliefs, values, and customs to society's newest members. Second to family, our friends are an important influence in our decisions. We are more likely to seek information from those friends who we believe have values or outlooks similar to our own. The greater the

similarity, the more likely we are to be influenced by their judgments. It is important to recognize these sources of influence when counseling mothers and considering what will be most helpful to them.

As mentioned earlier, society consists of a variety of subcultures, each of which interprets and responds to society's basic beliefs and values in a specific way. When a society undergoes constant change, as is the case in contemporary western culture, this rapid change makes it especially difficult to monitor changes in cultural values. The existence of contradictory values adds another dimension of confusion. There is considerable pressure to conform to the values of family members, friends, and other socially important groups, but it is often difficult to reconcile these seemingly inconsistent values.

The increase in public awareness of the importance of breastfeeding has led to many mothers choosing to breastfeed for the first time in two generations of their families. A mother may experience intellectual pressure to breastfeed, as well as negative feedback from family members. Lactation consultants deal frequently with the theme of regret versus guilt, and you can help the mother work through her feelings of being "disloyal" to her relatives if she breastfeeds.

Social Marketing

Behavior patterns determine our decisions and our responses to external influences. Marketing is a potentially powerful technology for bringing about socially desirable behaviors. This concept gave rise to the field of *social marketing*. The principles of social marketing can apply to a diverse set of social challenges, but the bottom line is influencing behavior. It applies commercial marketing strategies toward improving the personal welfare of a particular population. Social marketers analyze, plan, execute, and evaluate programs designed to influence human behavior. The premise of social marketing is to help individuals consider and choose a strategy that best fits their readiness for action and their resources.

Product, price, place, and promotion are the primary variables that determine people's likelihood of changing their behavior. Within the context of social marketing, the product is a commodity, service, or health practice. Price involves the barriers or costs associated with adopting a particular behavior. Place encompasses either the location where the product or services can be accessed or the channels of communication and distribution points for the messages. Promotion constitutes messages that are memorable and persuasive. Designing programs that reflect what consumers truly want and that influence positive behavior change requires careful analysis of each of these "4 P's" and how they interact.

An effective social marketing project for public or private health care typically begins with consumer-based research. A comprehensive social marketing plan is then designed, along with specific strategies and materials. An evaluation phase provides continuous monitoring and refinement of the plan. Ongoing monitoring allows social marketers and public health practitioners to modify products or services to meet consumers' expectations.

BestStart Social Marketing introduced the concept of social marketing for breastfeeding promotion in the early 1990s. Their mission is to help organizations that serve economically disadvantaged families to deliver sustainable, successful behavior change programs that are client centered and community based. The heart of their approach is utilizing consumer research to assist in developing programs, products, and practices that enable organizations to influence sustainable and positive behavior change. Their programs typically include mass media, print materials, personal counseling, and community-based activities (BestStart, 2003).

In 1997, the U.S. Department of Agriculture, Food and Consumer Service joined with BestStart in initiating the Loving Support Makes Breastfeeding Work© breastfeeding promotion campaign as part of the WIC National Breastfeeding Promotion Project. The goals of the campaign are to increase breastfeeding initiation and duration rates and to improve public support for breastfeeding. The campaign uses mass media, direct client education, staff training, and community outreach in a coordinated effort to provide breastfeeding support to the WIC community. BestStart has since expanded the Loving Support campaign materials to target Spanish-speaking and Native American communities and to provide strategy development support to states interested in expanding their use of Loving Support. See the description of the BestStart 3-Step Counseling Strategy in Chapter 5.

▶ SUMMARY

Society sets out boundaries for behavior. Each structure within society is interconnected. Humans can and do direct their own lives and alter the social order around them. Tension from an unsatisfied need motivates us toward action that will fulfill the need and reduce the tension. Positive drives take the form of needs, wants, and desires. Negative drives consist of fears and aversions.

Our specific qualities, attributes, traits, and mannerisms both determine and reflect how we respond to our environment. Unconscious needs or drives are at the heart of human motivation and personality. Personality types influence behavior; social relationships are fundamental to the formation and development of personality. Self-image influences our actions with different people and in different situations. Perception derives from sensory input and physical stimuli, as well as from our expectations, motives, and learning based on previous experience.

Learning occurs because of motivation, cues, response, and reinforcement. Through problem solving, we gain control over our environment. Processing information through a series of memory storehouses and repetition enables us to hold information in short-term storage long enough for encoding to occur. Information can be lost when the short-term store receives a great deal of input at once. Information in long-term storage is constantly reorganized as new links are forged between chunks of information. High involvement with an issue produces more extensive processing of information in both the right and left hemispheres of the brain.

The best predictor of behavior is the intention to act. Feelings about what family, friends, and coworkers would think of the action we contemplate influence our intent. The formation of attitudes is strongly linked with personal experience, the influence of family and friends, direct marketing, and mass media. An effective strategy for changing attitudes is to make the individual's new needs prominent.

Motivation, perception, learning, personality, and attitudes influence the decision-making process. A person's level of involvement is pivotal to the degree of attention paid to a message and the care taken in decoding it. The use of humor often increases the acceptance and persuasiveness of a message. Family, friends, and our position within our social class influence our decisions. Culture offers order, direction, and guidance by providing standards and rules of behavior.

Health care professionals and patients have and use power in their relationships with one another. The use of power places controls within these relationships. It should be the goal of health care providers to empower individuals and encourage them to be active in their relationships with practitioners. True empowerment will occur only when health care providers transform the ways in which they relate to patients.

▶ CHAPTER 3—AT A GLANCE

Applying what you learned—

◆ Empower women as both mothers and in their career choices.

◆ Learn your city's demographics and characteristics to assist you in framing your interactions with families and enhancing your sensitivity to clients' cultural beliefs.

◆ Help mothers with the challenge of going against the societal norm and breastfeeding.

◆ Reinforce verbal instruction with written materials, demonstrations, and other visual aids.

- Avoid making assumptions about teen mothers' motivations and goals.
- Empower mothers to make choices and to be accountable for their mistakes.
- Support the IBLCE Code of Ethics.
- Support the International Code of Marketing of Breastmilk Substitutes and subsequent resolutions.
- Incorporate ethics into your career and learn to integrate your internal personal needs with your external social needs.
- Respect cultural differences in foods, clothes, language, values, beliefs, and practices.
- Encourage parents to network formally and informally with other parents.
- Avoid overwhelming mothers with too much information.
- Elicit the best from mothers and colleagues.
- Make good first impressions.
- Use events or circumstances to help shape mothers' and colleagues' attitudes.
- Help mothers recognize infant signals to strengthen attachment and bonding.
- Respect the family as a mother's primary group.
- Help mothers link with a breastfeeding support group.
- Empower mothers to take control over their health needs.
- Combine evidence-based practice with caring, intuition, and other "nonscientific" practices.
- Influence decision making by appealing to the needs and interests of mothers and colleagues.
- Build one influence upon another to increase compliance.
- Help parents sort through messages they receive from the media.
- Use humor to increase a message's acceptance and persuasiveness.

▶ REFERENCES

Ainsworth MDS, Blehar MC, Waters E, Wall S. *Patterns of attachment: A psychological study of the strange situation.* Hillsdale, NJ: Erlbaum; 1978.

Aney M. Babywise advice linked to dehydration, failure to thrive. *AAP News* 14(4):21; April 1998.

Arora S et al. Major factors influencing breastfeeding rates: Mother's perception of father's attitude and milk supply. *Pediatrics* 106(5):E67; 2000.

BestStart. *BestStart Social Marketing*; 2003. Available at: http://www.beststartinc.org. Accessed March 12, 2004.

Bowlby J. Attachment. In *Attachment and Loss.* London: Hogarth Press; New York, Basic Books, 2nd edition of Vol 1; 1982.

Bowlby J. Separation: Anxiety and anger. In *Attachment and Loss.* London: Hogarth Press; 1973. New York: Basic Books; Harmondsworth: Penguin, Vol. 2; 1975.

Chang JH, Chan WT. Analysis of factors associated with initiation and duration of breast-feeding: A study in Taitung Taiwan. *Acta Paediatr Taiwan* 44(1):29–34; 2003.

Chen CH, Chi CS. Maternal intention and actual behavior in infant feeding at one month postpartum. *Acta Paediatr Taiwan* 44(3):140–144; 2003.

European Commission. *Dialogue with Citizens*; 2003. Available at: europa.eu.int/scadplus/citizens/en/d4.htm. Accessed May 15, 2004.

Goodman N. *Introduction to Sociology.* New York: Harper Collins Publishers; 1992.

Hess J. *Infant Feeding: A Handbook for the Practitioner*, pp. 64–126. Chicago: American Medical Association; 1923.

Kessler L et al. The effect of a woman's significant other on her breastfeeding decision. *J Hum Lact* 11(2):103–109; 1995.

Merewood A, Heinig, J. Efforts to promote breastfeeding in the United States: Development of a national breastfeeding awareness campaign. *J Hum Lact* 20(2):140–145; 2004.

Mohrbacher N, Stock J. *Breastfeeding Answer Book.* Schaumburg, IL: La Leche League International, pp. 478–480; 2003.

MSN Learning and Research. *Ethics*; 2005. Available at: encarta.msn.com/encnet/refpages/RefArticle.aspx?refid=761555614&pn=1&s=1#s1. Accessed January 10, 2004.

Rosier W. Cool cabbage compresses. *Breastfeed Rev* 1(12):28–31; 1988.

Ross G. Hyperbilirubinemia in the 2000s: What should we do next? *Am J Perinatol* 20(8):415–424; 2003.

Schiffman LG, Kanuk LL. *Consumer Behavior.* Englewood Cliffs, NJ Prentice Hall; 1997.

Schuman A. A concise history of infant formula (twists and turns included). *Contemporary Pediatrics* 2:91; 2003.

Scott JA et al. Factors associated with breastfeeding at discharge and duration of breastfeeding. *Paediatr Child Health* 37(3):254–261; 2001.

Sharpe G. *Milk Banking: An Investment in the Future Generations.* Presentation for the American Dietetic Association; San Antonio, TX; October 24, 2003.

Sideman A. American mothers to solve breast feeding problems with some help from India. *Rediff on the Net*; June 9, 1999. Available at: *www.rediff.com/news/1999/jun/09us2.htm.* Accessed October 6, 2004.

Taylor SE et al. Female responses to stress: Tend and befriend, not fight or flight. *Psychological Review* 107(3):411–429; 2000.

Tischler HL. *Introduction to Sociology*. Orlando, FL: Hartcourt Press; 1999.

UNICEF. *The Baby Friendly Hospital Initiative*; January 26, 2004. Available at: www.unicef.org/programme/breastfeeding/baby.htm. Accessed November 9, 2003.

Walker M. Selling out mothers and babies: Marketing breast milk substitutes in the USA. *NABA REAL*: 9–12; 2001.

Weber A. *Social Psychology*. New York: Harper Collins Publishers; 1992.

Wolf J. Low breastfeeding rates and public health in the US. *Am J Pub Health* 93(12):2001–10; 2003.

▶ BIBLIOGRAPHY

Abbott Laboratories, Ross Products Division. *New Data Show US Breastfeeding Rates at All-Time Recorded High*. Press release, Columbus, OH; November 25, 2003.

Barteck L, Mullin K. *Enduring Issues in Sociology*. San Diego: Greenhaven Press; 1995.

Ethical Culture Movement. *Eight Commitments of Ethical Culture*. Available at: www.aeu.org/8commit.html. Accessed July 29, 2004.

Ethical Society. *Ethical Culture as Philosophy*. Available at: www.ethicalsociety.org/philosophy.htm. Accessed July 29, 2004.

Gugliani E et al. Effect of breastfeeding support from different sources on mothers' decisions to breastfeed. *J Hum Lact* 10(3):157–161; 1994.

Infoplease. *John Locke*. Available at: www.infoplease.com/bio/8-29jlock.html. Accessed May 30, 2004.

International Business Ethics Institute. *Ethics in the New Millennium*. Available at: www.business-ethics.org/newsdetail.asp?newsid=17. Accessed May 30, 2004.

Losch M et al. Impact of attitudes on maternal decisions regarding infant feeding. *J Pediatr* 126:507–514; 1995.

Morrall P. *Sociology and Nursing*. London: Routledge; 2001.

Pennington DC. *Essential Social Psychology*. London: Edward Arnold; 1986.

CHAPTER
4

EMPOWERING WOMEN THROUGH YOUR ATTITUDE AND APPROACH

Those who demonstrate a sincere belief in breast-feeding as the natural and appropriate way to nourish an infant are the most effective in helping breastfeeding mothers. It is not enough to believe in theory that breastfeeding is best. Practitioners must put that theory into practice. Some health workers are reluctant to promote breast feeding for fear that they will create guilt in mothers who choose not to breastfeed. A caregiver who appears to be ambivalent about breastfeeding sends mixed messages and creates personal doubts in mothers. Those who promote and support breastfeeding enthusiastically serve as powerful motivators for mothers and staff alike.

The caregiver's approach with breastfeeding women determines the effectiveness of her support and advice. Establishing a partnership increases mothers' confidence and self-esteem. These characteristics, in turn, will foster parental independence and growth. Providing an effective learning climate will help you achieve the goal of actively involving mothers in problem solving and decision making. Using humor in your interactions with mothers will help them to gain perspective during challenging times and will increase your teaching effectiveness. Understanding the components of communication that affect the messages you send will enhance your interactions.

KEY TERMS

adult learning
body language
consumer responsibilities
consumer rights
empowerment
guilt
health consumerism
humor as a tool

imagery
informed consent
learning climate
learning style
mixed messages
relinquishing control
traits
voice tone

▶ EMPOWERMENT THROUGH BREASTFEEDING

Mothers who have a good self-image and feel confident in their parenting are more likely to form positive attachments with their children. Studies show that a

mother who lacks confidence has difficulty establishing a relationship with her baby (Zahr, 1991). Lactation consultants and other caregivers have the potential to enhance women's self-confidence and their growth as parents. Locklin reported in 1993 that achieving a positive and rewarding breastfeeding experience produces feelings of power and accomplishment in a woman. Women may view breastfeeding as the one thing they can control in their immediate postpartum environment. It is important that caregivers take a gentle approach that minimizes interventions and builds on the mother's confidence and self-direction (Auerbach, 1994).

The experience of giving birth is a major turning point in women's lives. Mothers often identify childbirth as their most significant learning experience. The act of creation brings to the woman a new awareness of her creative capacities. A mother will reassess her capabilities and her capacity to assume a new role as parent. One mother said as she found that she could hear, understand, and remember the things she learned about breastfeeding, she began to think of herself as a learner for the first time (Belenky, 1986). You and other caregivers can capitalize on this powerful time in a woman's life by helping her gain skills, knowledge, and confidence in breastfeeding.

Making the Breastfeeding Assumption

Because Western society has embraced artificial feeding as equal to and at times preferable to breastfeeding, some healthcare workers may be uncomfortable actively promoting breastfeeding as the normal and optimal way to nourish an infant. Research supports the health benefits of breastfeeding to mothers, babies, and society as a whole. Yet many healthcare practices today continue to convey a belief that artificial feeding is equally beneficial.

Caregivers need to adopt attitudes and language that send a positive message to parents about the superiority of breastfeeding. To ask a pregnant woman, "How are you going to feed your baby?" or "Are you going to breastfeed or bottle-feed?" implies that there is more than one alternative, one of which may be as good as the other. Unless you believe an alternative is equally healthy and an equally good choice, you would not want to phrase a question in a manner that leaves the door open for the less healthy choice. Asking instead, "What questions do you have about breastfeeding?" conveys the expectation that she will breastfeed in order to provide optimal nutrition for her baby. This approach underscores the health imperative implicit in breastfeeding and assumes that mothers will breastfeed unless they respond otherwise.

If a woman plans to bottle-feed, she may respond, "I'm not breastfeeding." If she is comfortable with that choice, there is no reason to worry about her having a negative reaction or guilt. On the other hand, if she is unsure about her choice she may start to question it. You can help her to discuss her concerns and options. She may be unaware of breastfeeding's importance to her baby's health and her own health. Helping her become an informed consumer will help lead her to make wise choices.

Addressing the Issue of Guilt

Although most health workers will tell you they consider breastfeeding superior to artificial feeding, the numbers of those who actively promote breastfeeding are much lower. The fear of provoking guilt presents an obstacle for many caregivers—fear of creating guilt in mothers who choose not to breastfeed, fear of causing guilt in mothers who choose to breastfeed but fail, and fear of pressuring mothers to choose to breastfeed. The common theme in all of these fears is the question of choice—the issue of informed consumerism and informed choice.

Informed choice implies rights and responsibilities. Parents have a *right* to the information necessary in making an informed choice about infant feeding. Caregivers have the *responsibility* to inform parents of their options. This is the basis of health consumerism. In teaching parents about the benefits of breastfeeding and the risks of artificial baby milk feeding, caregivers are not making a choice for parents. They, in fact, are fulfilling their responsibility of making parents aware of the issues involved in both feeding methods.

Believing in Breastfeeding's Superiority

If the medical community truly believes in the superiority of breastfeeding over artificial feeding and that it is the healthiest for babies and mothers, guilt should not be an issue. Guilt does not prevent caregivers from promoting other healthy practices. When a healthcare worker advises parents to use an infant car seat for their baby, there is no worry about offending a parent who elects to place their baby in danger by not using a car seat. A pediatrician does not consider guilt when informing parents of the need for immunizations. There is no guilt associated with advice against cigarette smoking or the use of drugs and alcohol for pregnant women. There is no fear of guilt in recommending diets that are low in cholesterol and fat, or advising good hygiene and dental care.

The issue of guilt can be quite complex and confusing relative to infant feeding choice. Many women feel a sense of personal failure at not breastfeeding that does not accompany the failure to stop smoking, the failure to use car seats, or the failure to meet immunization schedules. A woman assumes a risk in making her baby dependent on her ability to breastfeed. For some women, taking that risk can be more painful than the guilt of not breastfeeding. Consequently, although choosing to feed artificial baby milk may cause guilt, the mother may stay with that choice anyway.

Caregivers have a responsibility to help women feel confident in their ability to breastfeed. They cannot allow the fear of causing guilt to prevent them from promoting breastfeeding to their patients. Infant formula is, plain and simple, inferior to human milk. Caregivers have a responsibility to inform parents of this without reserve. You can help colleagues understand and appreciate this responsibility.

The driving force behind this issue is the caregiver's commitment and beliefs. Sending noncommittal messages compromises the mother's self-confidence and may cause her to question the wisdom of her decision. A noncommittal attitude by health workers also carries the danger of unwittingly promoting artificial baby milk. If parents do not learn the important differences between the two feeding methods, they are unable to make the necessary distinctions. An ambivalent approach does not advocate breastfeeding over the feeding of a **breastmilk substitute**. A positive and assertive approach to breastfeeding promotion will convey the appropriate message to parents.

Guilt About Past Actions

It is also important to dispel any guilt you may feel from your own past actions. Your past practices may have included formula supplementation, frequent use of pacifiers, strict rules about frequency and length of feedings, unsupervised use of a nipple shield, or sending a mother home with gifts of formula and bottles. Perhaps in the past you presented breastfeeding as being complicated and reliant on a variety of gadgets and special techniques. You may have bottle-fed your own children, either out of a lack of information or from receiving little help or encouragement to breastfeed. Perhaps your effort to breastfeed was brief because of hospital practices that led to lactation failure.

Be kind to yourself and recognize that you based what you did in the past on your level of knowledge and what you considered appropriate at the time. As you learn more about breastfeeding care and the negative consequences of past practices, you change the way you practice. The lactation field continues to evolve in its recommended practices. You cannot expect more from yourself than being willing to learn and to change based on what you have learned. Allow yourself to grow and change free from guilt or regret associated with past actions.

Guilt in Not Promoting Breastfeeding

Consider for a moment the consequences and guilt at *not* promoting breastfeeding to mothers. Family finances suffer because of the cost of infant formula feeding and accompanying devices. Formula-fed babies have a higher incidence of illness, sudden infant death syndrome, emotional neglect, and child abuse. They are at a greater risk for developing allergies and asthma. Learning deficiencies are higher and IQ levels are lower. The potential for contamination in artificial baby milk places an infant's health at risk. These are realities supported by scientific studies (Weimer, 2001; ILCA, 2002).

Perhaps the greatest potential for feelings of guilt lies in the disappointment of mothers who wanted to breastfeed but were unable due to lack of support and encouragement from a caregiver. Omitting information does not contribute to a trusting relationship with mothers. Consider the guilt a mother may feel later in her child's life after diagnosis of an illness for which breastfeeding affords protection. Perhaps, in order to spare a mother's guilt, her caregiver did not educate her about the risks of artificial feeding during her decision-making process. She does not choose to breastfeed, and later, her child develops recurrent otitis media, diabetes, or Crohn's disease, which are known to occur more frequently in infants fed artificial milk. Through the course of her research into her child's condition, the mother learns that breastfeeding decreases this risk. She may regard her caregiver unfavorably for not educating her about the risk associated with artificial baby milk.

Parents want to feel they have done the best they can for their baby. Learning that their baby is experiencing a condition that was potentially avoidable will very likely produce guilt and anger. The parents may question why no one told them about the relationship between their child's health and breastfeeding. This can erode their confidence in the caregiver and illustrates an important dimension of the healthcare worker's role in **informed consent**. The mandate of every health professional is to give information and responsible advice to parents, empowering them to make appropriate decisions.

Guilt in the Context of Parenting

Guilt or no guilt is not the issue. The issue for me is what is best for babies. If the truth makes mothers feel guilty and they develop some anxiety, perhaps the discomfort will tip the scales in favor of breastfeeding.

–Frank Oski, MD

Webster's Dictionary defines guilt as "the act or state of having done a wrong or committed an offense." A mother who feels guilty about her choice to not breastfeed most likely believes that she is not doing what is in the best interest of her baby. Oski (1995) suggests that guilt can actually serve a positive purpose for families. If parents feel guilty about their infant feeding choice, the caregiver can initiate a discussion of how they can use this sense of guilt to become better parents. Appropriate guilt can be a positive emotion within the realm of personal growth. It can serve as motivation to change a particular behavior or actions by parents on behalf of their children.

When you are open and honest with parents regarding the risks of artificial feeding, you will usually find that they appreciate learning what to watch for if they later introduce infant formula into their baby's diet. You can help parents make guilt work for them as a catalyst to become the best parents they can be. Make it work for you as well, helping you to provide the best advice and guidance possible.

▶ HEALTH CONSUMERISM

The healthcare system is a consumer-oriented operation concerned with attracting clients and keeping them satisfied and healthy. Those who serve the system must be alert to the needs and wishes of their clients and institute policies that will meet these needs. When a partnership forms between parents and their caregivers regarding decision making, parents accept responsibility for managing their lives.

As mothers learn about breastfeeding, they can clearly understand their options and develop necessary skills. This approach builds confidence and self-esteem. It promotes the mother's growth as both an individual and a parent. The process of each mother's education is a joint venture in which the mother helps determine what she needs to know. This philosophy of responsible and knowledgeable self-care forms the basis of the counseling approach promoted throughout this text.

Informed Consent

An informed parent is an advocate of health consumerism, either consciously or unconsciously. When weighing the risks involved in medications and medical procedures, caregivers may at times interject subjectivity into the decision. Based perhaps on tradition or accepted practice, this subjectivity is the cause, in part, for disagreement concerning the best course of treatment for a given situation. The fear of malpractice claims is a great motivator in such subjective approaches.

Informed consent benefits both the caregiver and the health consumer. By gaining as much information as possible about a recommended treatment and by exploring alternatives and possible outcomes, the consumer is able to offer knowledgeable and responsible input. Mothers then can be actively involved in making decisions and in guiding the course of treatment for themselves and their families. Healthcare providers benefit by having some of this responsibility shifted to the consumer. It reduces the risk of malpractice suits in the event of an unfavorable outcome. It also enables providers to broaden their perspectives based on consumer input. See Chapter 26 for further discussion of informed consent in relation to the lactation consultant's practice.

Informed consent means the consumer consents to treatment based on sufficient information and education. Consent given in an emergency is generally not considered informed consent, as the consumer has not had sufficient time to explore alternatives and to learn the implications involved in treatment. An informed consumer has adequate preparation and education before treatment. Informed consent is possible only when the consumer takes the initiative for self-education and the responsibility for informed decision making. The majority of medical situations allow adequate time for the consumer to achieve these goals. Even 20 or 30 minutes can permit time for consultation and research. Below are some suggestions to share with parents who wish to become informed healthcare consumers. You can incorporate these points into a handout for parents.

Suggestions for the Healthcare Consumer

◆ Acquire a medical vocabulary, subscribe to health magazines, acquire a small library of consumer-oriented medical references, research legitimate Internet medical sites, or use the public library.

◆ Attend courses for nonprofessionals, such as classes in first aid or home healthcare. Check local high schools, colleges, or civic organizations for such programs.

◆ Enlist the services of caregivers and hospitals who welcome and encourage actively informed patients.

◆ Select a **prepared childbirth** class that provides information on alternatives, enhances your understanding, and encourages active participation in medical decisions.

◆ Learn to recognize early symptoms of illness, and investigate appropriate methods of treatment before contacting the caregiver. This will enable you to have an informed and concrete discussion of the situation with the caregiver.

◆ If you are unfamiliar with a medical term or do not understand what was told to you, ask to have the point clarified and explained in simpler terms.

◆ Discuss alternatives with your caregiver, and ask why one course of treatment was chosen over another.

◆ If the situation warrants, seek a second (and even third) opinion. This is your right and your responsibility.

◆ Learn the cost for a recommended treatment, as well as alternative treatments.

◆ If you are uncomfortable or dissatisfied with your caregiver's advice, you are in most cases not legally committed to comply. However, you must be aware of the medical risks. You have the right to make your own choices. Even if it seems to the caregiver that you have made a wrong choice, the ultimate consequences and responsibilities are yours.

Informed consent is not a prerequisite for quality healthcare. However, it does increase the chances for positive outcomes for the consumer who has accepted the responsibility for becoming knowledgeable and actively involved in his or her own healthcare. The ultimate responsibility for informed decisions rests with the consumer, who should choose healthcare providers wisely and use them as resources.

A Parent's Role in the Healthcare System

Active health consumers are informed and responsible decision makers who are actively involved in the health care of all family members. Until recently, many parents have had few choices about their experiences, with hospital and physician policies dictating the course of their healthcare. Real change happens when an awareness and attitude shift occurs among caregivers and administrators. A healthcare delivery system that increases the incidence and duration of breastfeeding will create cost savings and better health outcomes over the life span of both the mother and child. If the system does not actively support breastfeeding, there will be a financial loss to the system and less optimal health outcomes.

If the healthcare system does not meet the needs of parents, a change of care providers may or may not be an option. In the years before managed care, consumers could express dissatisfaction simply by changing providers or hospitals. In managed care, the option to change providers is often limited to once-a-year enrollment through the client's employer. Consequently, consumer action has become more concentrated in written expression of both positive and negative experiences while continuing to receive care within the system. You can encourage positive change by urging parents to express their concerns and reinforce positive aspects of their care through written comments.

Consumer Rights and Responsibilities

Consumers and providers share a two-way relationship. Rights and responsibilities go hand in hand. Occasionally, parents may need information in order to grow as consumers. Parents who have not been accustomed to being actively involved in health care may need guidance from you in assuming a more active role. They will need to know their rights and accompanying responsibilities. In addition, they will need to know how to communicate their desires to physicians and hospital staff to ensure effective and positive interaction and a healthy working relationship between caregiver and patient.

A signed consent form is the consumer's best friend. Parents have used this as a means of obtaining their wishes, such as prohibiting a procedure for their hospitalized child without the parents being present. If a mother finds that the hospital is doing something she does not want, such as giving supplemental feedings to her baby, she can ask for the consent form and amend it. Urge mothers to check the patient's bill of rights in their hospital. Below are rights and responsibilities of every mother.

The Mother Has the Right:

- To understand what she is giving consent to.
- To receive information concerning a drug or treatment prior to its administration.
- To know alternative methods.
- To accept or refuse treatment or advice without pressure.
- To know if a procedure is medically indicated or elective.
- To have access to her complete medical records.
- To seek another medical opinion.
- To be kept informed of the most up-to-date information.
- To be treated as an equal partner in her health care.
- To have her questions answered completely and courteously.
- To be treated with respect.
- To be provided with the best care possible, with a focus on prevention.
- To make decisions regarding her treatment and that of her child.
- To care for herself and her child to the maximum extent she is able.

The Mother Has the Responsibility:

- To learn what is available and make an informed choice.
- To find caregivers who can help her reach her goals.
- To listen to her caregivers with an open mind.
- To let her preferences be known in a courteous manner.
- To carry through on an agreed plan of care.
- To learn the approximate cost of a procedure in advance.
- To state why she changes caregivers, if applicable.

The Lactation Consultant's Role in Health Consumerism

In defining your role as a consultant to consumers in the healthcare system, it is important to keep in mind that one of your primary goals is to encourage parents to take responsibility for their actions. This applies to areas of healthcare as well as parenting. In your role as an advocate for health consumerism, you may wonder how to educate parents about options you know they cannot have with their present provider. You may be limited to simply preparing them to deal with the healthcare available within the framework of their current medical relationships. In your caregiving role, you do not want to suggest to parents that they change providers. It is the parents' responsibility to select and work with their medical services.

Mothers will view a lactation consultant as a knowledgeable member of their healthcare team. You need to be tactful in counseling mothers regarding their relationships with caregivers. However, you can help parents with choices after they have established their medical relationships. Recognize, too, that parents may at times choose a course of action with which you disagree either personally or professionally. You will need to examine your position and decide to what extent it is appropriate for you to become involved.

Helping Parents Become Better Health Consumers

Parents are responsible for the health of their children as well as themselves, and so they have compound consumer roles and interests. Your primary means of helping parents become good consumers is by educating the mother about breastfeeding through reading, conversations, classes, and meetings. Guide parents to the many available consumer-oriented books and reputable Internet resources. Breastfeeding mothers can heighten awareness within the healthcare system. Encourage a mother to tell her caregiver how increasing feeding frequency helped increase her milk production, for example. Suggest that she convey how the importance of breastfeeding goes far beyond the milk she feeds her baby.

When you answer parents' questions, first determine whether they are informed consumers. They may be unaccustomed to questioning a statement made by their caregiver. Often, the first time a mother realizes that she disagrees with a caregiver is when she is told to supplement her milk with artificial baby milk or to introduce solid foods into her baby's diet after voicing a concern about whether her baby was receiving enough milk. You can help a mother gain confidence in herself and her maternal instincts regarding her baby's needs. Emphasize to her that she is the one who knows her baby best. Help her tune into her baby's behavior and understand his needs. She may perceive a newborn feeding every two hours as a problem unless she understands why. When she understands, she will be less likely to ask her baby's physician, "Do I have enough milk?" By helping mothers progress, you can help develop their awareness of their rights and responsibilities as health care consumers. They can then help educate their health care providers on appropriate breastfeeding care.

You can also help a mother understand the difference between parenting issues and medical advice. Parents often turn to medical professionals for answers to parenting concerns. If a mother asks a caregiver what to do about her baby waking at night and her caregiver suggests letting the baby cry or giving supplemental foods at 10 P.M., this is parenting advice, not medical advice. Most issues in the breastfeeding arena, in fact, are parenting concerns that do not require medical advice. What such concerns do require are informed parents who have faith in their abilities to determine what is best for their baby.

Presenting facts to parents will help them find the options that best suit their needs and goals. This pertains to all aspects of childbirth, breastfeeding, and parenting. You can teach parents the benefits of family-centered maternity care, prepared childbirth, **rooming-in**, exclusive breastfeeding for six months, and so forth. You are not establishing goals for parents. Rather, you are educating them about health practices that will help them establish and achieve their goals.

▶ RELINQUISHING CONTROL

Fostering informed consumerism and decision making among parents requires that the caregiver relinquish much of the control that has traditionally been associated with patient care. Most adults have experienced a hospitalization at some time in their life. The majority of hospitalized patients are ill or injured. This is not the case with a woman who enters the hospital to deliver her baby. Despite this, however, she loses varying degrees of control the moment she passes through the door. Her privacy is invaded, and she is placed in a dependent role. Often, hospital and physician policies impose unnecessary controls over a mother and her newborn. Other people make decisions about her care and that of her baby outside her control. Many parents choose birthing centers and home births because of these factors. In many countries outside the United States, traditional midwifery is still the norm. The medical community needs to regard a new mother differently than it does an ill or injured patient. New mothers need greater control and options regarding their care and that of their infants.

The caregiver's goal should be one of empowering the breastfeeding mother to be independent and self-reliant. If she feels controlled, she may not recognize ways to help herself. She needs the opportunity to use her own resources in order to become self-sufficient. If she becomes dependent on others, she may lose sight of her resources. She may expect others to solve her problems and find solutions; and she may blame those same people when they do not come through for her.

Medical intervention should never occur without a clear and specific purpose. Breastfeeding advice often imposes too many rules—always hold the breast during a feeding, wear a bra that gives good support, avoid certain foods, watch the clock, always use both breasts at a feeding, use only *one* breast at a feeding! These or other arbitrary rules about separating mothers and babies or giving supplements to breastfeeding babies are not well founded and interfere with establishing breastfeeding. A cavalier attitude about such practices is counterproductive to the goal of empowering the mother. London midwife Chloe Fisher (1996) tells us there is only one rule in breastfeeding. The rule is there are no rules!

Take care not to allow control issues to compromise the treatment mothers and babies receive. Control is important to a new mother. She may need to reestablish control following birth and may lack control for a new venture such as breastfeeding. Even if this is not her first child, it may be the first child she will breastfeed. She needs you and other caregivers to help her gain control or retain the control she has already established. Medical staff policies should model self-reliance and parental decision making from the very beginning. This requires a negotiation of control between the caregiver and patient. Caregivers need to become comfortable with relinquishing unnecessary control and placing control with babies and mothers where it belongs.

Trusting in Mothers and Babies

Relinquishing control requires caregivers to trust that mothers and babies are capable of assuming control. Newborns have amazing capabilities from the very moment of birth. When caregivers refrain from interfering with the process, and when mothers are taught how to read infant language, the baby can communicate effectively to have his needs met. Further, when mothers exercise legitimate control, they feel more independent, self-reliant, and confident. They learn to trust themselves and their babies. Consequently, they find it easier to adjust to their maternal role and they become responsible for their learning. They develop problem-solving skills, accept the consequences of their decisions and actions, and control their outcomes. You can help facilitate this growth by using words and actions that show you believe in the mother's abilities. Trust your instincts to put the mother and baby in control, not the caregiver.

▶ USING AN ADULT LEARNING APPROACH

A mother's control over her care increases when practitioners use an adult learning approach during consultations and discussions. The adult learning approach is one of active learning rather than passively being taught. In this approach, the practitioner serves as a facilitator rather than a teacher. Simply telling a mother what to do and prescribing a course of care is not as effective as including the mother in the learning process. *The sage on the stage is replaced by the guide on the side.* As a facilitator of the mother's learning, you explore options with her and guide her as she plans her course of care with you. This requires that she be an active participant in the learning. Your role is to provide choices and encourage the mother to select those that will work for her.

Your goal is to develop a partnership with the mother and baby, to form a problem-solving team. One of your most important functions is to observe at least one breastfeeding with every mother and baby in your care, watching how they learn to respond to one another (Figure 4.1). Observe how the first breastfeeding goes, realizing that the baby may want only to nuzzle at the breast in the early hours. There is no need to rush the first feeding. Remember that you are moving at the baby's pace—not your pace, and not the mother's pace. The mother's holding the baby near the breast, with ample skin contact between them, will help them bond and initiate breastfeeding when the baby is interested.

Hands Off

Make sure that any intervention is focused and that you have a good reason for becoming actively involved. Confine your interactions to guiding rather than directing unless a need for intervention becomes clear. Recognize times when you need to become more actively involved with a mother and times when you should keep your hands in your pockets. For instance, if the mother has not positioned the baby well enough to get a good latch, you can gently show her how to adjust her hold (Figures 4.2 and 4.3). This does not require that you take charge and put the baby to the mother's breast yourself. Rather, you can talk her through it, perhaps modeling it yourself with a teaching doll or cloth breast model.

Midwives in the United Kingdom learned this hands-off approach through a program that advocates teaching mothers about correct positioning and self-attachment without actually doing it for them. Mothers took greater ownership of their breastfeeding and had a higher rate of continuing to breastfeed when the midwife coached them but did not touch them (Fletcher, 2000). A hands-off approach puts the mother in control, actively involves her in the learning process, and contributes to her personal growth. Avoid a hands-off approach from becoming your mantra to the exclusion of times when appropriate intervention is required, however. Learn to recognize when you need to take a more active role in order to achieve a positive outcome for the mother.

Making Positive Impressions on Adult Learners

Adults respond to a learning experience in much the same way as adolescents. However, their expectations may be greater in some areas. The dynamics of interactions with adults are quite different from those with adolescents. Primary factors for this are the manner in which adults interact and the way they assess a facilitator's credibility.

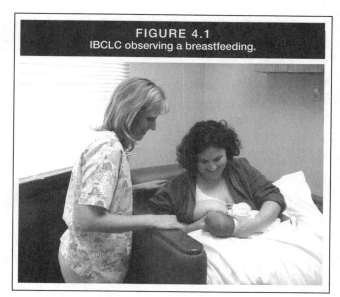

FIGURE 4.1
IBCLC observing a breastfeeding.

Printed with permission of Anna Swisher.

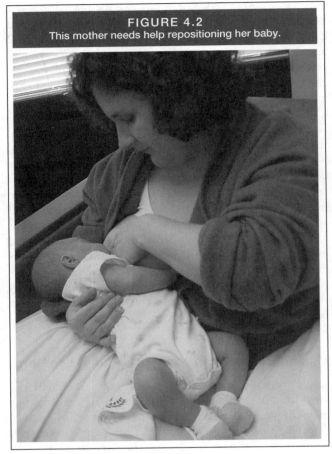

FIGURE 4.2
This mother needs help repositioning her baby.

Printed with permission of Anna Swisher.

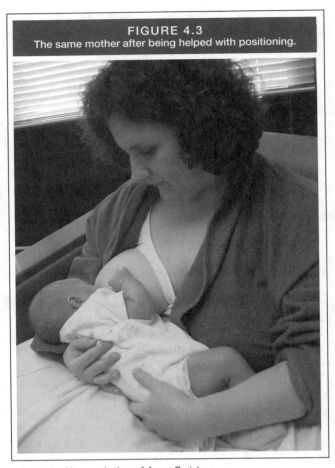

FIGURE 4.3
The same mother after being helped with positioning.

Printed with permission of Anna Swisher.

Guidelines for Making Positive Impressions

- A display of self-confidence
- A desire to share knowledge
- An ability to relate to people
- A willingness to be flexible and adapt
- A sense of humor
- A strong knowledge base
- A comfortable tone of informality
- Enthusiasm
- Respect for the learner
- Frequent eye contact
- Positive **body language**
- Neat, clean, and stylish attire
- A strong voice with carefully pronounced words

Creating an Effective Learning Climate

You will want to create an effective atmosphere for interactions with mothers. An effective learning environment is one that encourages the learner to be an active participant. Malcolm Knowles (1980) says, "People attach more meaning to learnings they gain from experience than those they acquire passively." Through your body language and the effective use of communication and counseling techniques, you can create a climate that is relaxed, trusting, mutually respectful, informal, warm, collaborative, and supportive.

Within this nurturing climate, you and the mother mutually accomplish planning, form a partnership, and explore issues together. This approach encourages self-direction and risk taking among mothers. The mother develops problem-solving skills and becomes more self-reliant. When the mother takes an active part in setting her goals, she has ownership for the plan and is responsible for the outcome.

As partners, you and the mother will mutually evaluate her needs and set objectives. You can present choices and ask, "What will work for you?" This approach actively involves the mother, as she practices techniques you have shown to her. Similarly, urge the mother to evaluate her learning, because she knows best what she has learned. You may ask, for instance, "How will you change your breastfeeding pattern when you get home?" With this approach, the mother develops increased competence and confidence, which fosters greater self-esteem and independence.

Individualize Your Approach

Recognize that every mother and baby is unique and that your approach will vary with each contact. Every mother you see will have an array of experiences and resources that make her needs different from others. Learning will be more effective and personalized when you respect the mother's background and tap into it. Mothers often offer rich resources for learning. You may find at times that the mother is the teacher and you are the learner! Remaining open to such opportunities will help you grow as a member of the healthcare team.

What Does She Need to Learn?

Be sure to assess each mother's learning needs before you enter into problem solving. Is this her first baby, or does she have previous parenting experience? What exposure has she had to breastfeeding? Does she have relatives or friends who breastfed? Has she breastfed before? What has she read or heard about breastfeeding? Inquire about her support system and resources. Does she have someone to help her with caring for her baby or with breastfeeding? Help the mother accommodate breastfeeding to her lifestyle. Will a return to work separate her from her baby for regular periods? Is she single? Is she a teen mother? Does she live with her extended family? Does she have an active social life? All of these areas will help you determine your approach with this particular mother and baby.

Is She Ready to Learn?

You need to assess the mother's readiness to learn. When is the **teachable moment** that will maximize her ability to learn and process information? How is her health and that of her baby? Is she in any physical discomfort? What is her confidence level and her emotional state? If she is anxious about her baby's health or discouraged because of difficulty with breastfeeding, you must address her emotional needs before addressing breastfeeding issues. She may be unable to focus on learning or problem solving until she works through these concerns.

Using this approach will help you individualize your objectives and your problem-solving techniques with each dyad. Avoid using an established agenda, and be ready to adjust your objectives based on input from the mother and baby. Remember, too, that you do not need to teach everything to every mother. Assessing her needs and her readiness to learn will help you recognize what each mother needs to learn.

What Will She Respond To?

Keep pace with the mother and slow down if you sense that she is not taking in what you are saying. Using her language style and imagery will help you relate to one another. Matching her intensity and her sense of humor will help you adopt an appropriate approach. Watch for responses and tailor your actions accordingly. Mothers typically respond well to such a personalized approach.

Each mother brings with her a rich background of experience and capabilities. Some appear confident and knowledgeable. Others have a greater need for increasing their self-esteem and confidence. Capitalize on each mother's strengths and build on her present capabilities. When she has learned a technique or overcome an obstacle, praise her for her accomplishment. Find something to praise about her baby as well, for example, "See how your baby looks at you!"

Relating to mothers on a personal level strengthens your helping relationship. Make it a point to use the mother's and baby's names. Focus on the mother as a whole person, rather than on her breasts or a particular condition. Regarding every mother and baby as a unique dyad and broadening your scope beyond the immediate situation will enhance your effectiveness as their caregiver.

Actively Involve the Mother

Involving the mother as an active participant in her learning will improve her outcome. Learning typically takes place at three levels. The lowest level of learning takes place when information is shared verbally. Learning increases when something visual is added to the verbal instruction. The level at which learning is most effective is one in which the learner participates actively in the learning process.

One way to characterize this learning curve is *I hear and I forget, I see and I remember, I do and I understand.* Stated in a similar fashion, the three levels are *Tell me and I may remember, show me and I may understand, involve me and I may master.* Some examples of breastfeeding teaching at these levels follow.

Tell Me and I May Remember

There will be times in your interactions with mothers when verbal instructions are sufficient and appropriate. You could approach a discussion of **contraception**, nutrition, or medications in this way. These types of information do not necessarily require visual or interactive reinforcement.

Show Me and I May Understand

Demonstrations of some sort will enhance much of the teaching you do with mothers. When you teach a mother how to position her baby at the breast, you can demonstrate this process with a doll. A chart showing the anatomy of the breast will also be helpful. In teaching **manual expression**, you can use a cloth breast to show expression technique. Use of a breast pump requires demonstration as well. Discussions such as engorgement, **mastitis**, nipple soreness, and **thrush** may also benefit by the use of a cloth breast and photographs (Figure 4.4). See Appendix A for sources of videos for teaching many aspects of breastfeeding, including positioning and hand expression.

Involve Me and I May Master

Although demonstrations are helpful, the mother enhances her learning even more when she practices the various procedures with you. While you are positioning the doll for feeding, at the same time the mother can position her baby at the breast. While you demonsrate manual expression or the use of a breast pump, the mother can practice with her breast. This learning method provides you with visual reinforcement that the mother has mastered the technique you taught. Such return demonstrations are essential to the mother's learning and growth (Figure 4.5).

Respond to the Mother's Learning Style

Match your approach to the mother's learning style, as discussed in Chapter 3. People tend to favor one side of the brain in their learning styles. Those with dominance in the left brain generally learn better from verbal instruction. They respond well to analytical and logical information. Right-brain learners respond more readily to images, symbols, intuition, and emotion. Although you may not be able to determine the learning style of every mother in your care, there are things you can do regardless of learning style to make your teaching more effective.

Tailor your approach to merge characteristics of both right-brain and left-brain learning into a more integrated style. Using a variety of teaching methods will help you achieve this integration. Written instructions, verbal instructions, visual aids, videotapes, and interactive learning in the form of demonstrations and verbal feedback are techniques you can use.

▶ USING HUMOR AS A COMMUNICATION TOOL

Humor serves as an indirect form of communication between caregivers and clients. It helps open both sides of the brain, making it more likely that integrative learning will take place. Therefore, infusing humor into your interactions with mothers will enhance their learning. It also makes your job more enjoyable!

When a woman enters the hospital or physician's office, many of the typical rules of society are suspended. She takes on a dependent role with her caregivers, who expect her to accept their concern and competency almost on faith. Humor can help the caregiver establish trust with the mother. With so little time to build a relationship in the healthcare setting, you will want to use any tools available to you to facilitate the process. The

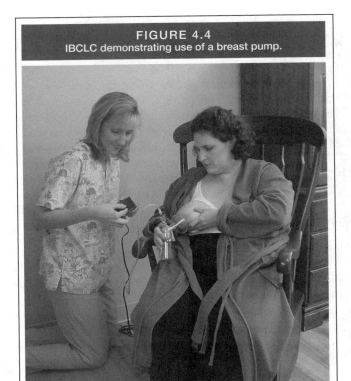

FIGURE 4.4
IBCLC demonstrating use of a breast pump.

Printed with permission of Anna Swisher.

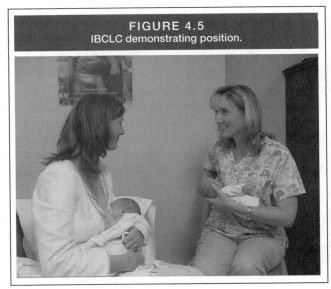

FIGURE 4.5
IBCLC demonstrating position.

Printed with permission of Anna Swisher.

relaxed atmosphere created through humor will help you develop relationships in which mothers heed your advice and follow through with their plan of care.

Your goal is to make learning fun for breastfeeding mothers. This sounds so simple. Yet mothers who lack self-confidence, who are anxious about their ability to breastfeed, or who have little support from family or friends may find it difficult to access their sense of humor and find enjoyment. You can help by approaching mothers in a friendly manner. When they first initiate breastfeeding or when they confront challenges, help them see humor in their situation so that they can learn not to take it too seriously. Incorporating laughter into learning helps ensure that the mother learns the lesson well. Humanizing your interactions will help you achieve your ultimate goal of a happy mother and baby.

Using humor as a tool may not be as easy as it sounds. We adults, and especially those who work in the medical profession, tend to take ourselves too seriously! As lactation consultants, we are often so intent on becoming better in our profession that we do not take the time to enjoy ourselves in the process. We need to become comfortable with having fun and incorporating humor in our work. Humor is something we choose, just as we choose to be in a foul mood or we choose to focus on the negative side of things. As members of the health profession, we need to be able to laugh at ourselves and learn to take ourselves more lightly. Learning to laugh at life and at the challenges we face will help us keep perspective and find solutions. Humor can help our clients as well. It can help them to deal with stress, tension, and frustration (Figure 4.6).

The Role of Humor in the Health System

In order to tap into our sense of humor, we first need to understand the nature of humor. Humor is more than an occasional witticism—it is a way of life, an attitude. Humor has a direct effect on both mental and physical health, and as such, it is important in all aspects of our life. A sense of humor helps you give the best of yourself to others. Humor in the health system is essentially *humanism*. Approaching clients in a humanistic manner shows each mother that you accept her as a person. It shows that you respect and care about her, and that you genuinely want to help her. You, in essence, are accepting the mother's humanness and offering your own in return.

Humor evolves naturally in a relaxed climate of support and acceptance. Such an atmosphere enhances a mother's self-concept and helps her be more tolerant and more understanding of herself and her baby. The warmth and caring you transmit to the mother will help her use humor to relieve the stresses of learning how to be a mother and how to breastfeed her new baby. She is better able to laugh at herself and shake off missteps as she and her baby learn to respond to one another.

Big stresses are not always the ones that get to us. Life is full of minor daily events and obstacles that pile up. We can choose to let those things make us miserable,

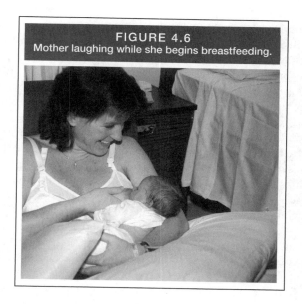

FIGURE 4.6
Mother laughing while she begins breastfeeding.

or we can choose to use our humor and a positive outlook to help us put it all into perspective. In health care, stresses may seem even more monumental, primarily because a loss of privacy and control often accompanies the stress. Traditionally, healthcare providers have intentionally avoided humor in their interactions with patients. However, humor has many faces. It may come through in the form of a warm and friendly approach, a smile, or a light touch. Such pleasantries are a valuable use of humor in your work as a lactation consultant.

The Health Benefits of Humor

Two useful resources are *Humor and the Health Professions: The Therapeutic Use of Humor in Health Care*, by Vera Robinson (1991) and *Anatomy of an Illness*, by Norman Cousins (1979). In *Anatomy of an Illness*, Cousins wrote about events in his life that were reported in 1976 in the *New England Journal of Medicine*. He used humor therapy to recover from a life-threatening disease that produced intense pain and paralysis. His health improved by eliminating all medications, taking heavy doses of vitamin C, and scheduling laughter sessions—watching videos of the television show *Candid Camera* and Marx Brothers movies and reading humorous books. Cousins found that ten minutes of genuine laughter had an anesthetic effect that gave him at least two hours of pain-free sleep. Gradually, he was able to regain movement and recover.

Humor actually causes a biochemical change in the body that is enormously healing and therapeutic. Eliciting laughter from a mother can produce positive effects in most of her body's major physiologic systems. Laughter speeds up heart rate, raises blood pressure, accelerates breathing, and increases oxygen consumption. It can stimulate muscles and relax muscle tension, thereby reducing pain and anxiety. Laughter stimulates the cardiovascular system, the sympathetic nervous system, and the production of catecholamines and endorphins, thus boosting the immune system. Laughter increases adrenaline in the brain, which stimulates alertness and memory and enhances learning and creativity. Following this arousal state, respiration, heart rate, and muscle tension actually return to below normal levels (Robinson, 1991). This may explain the growing popularity of Laughter Clubs in India and elsewhere. Members meet in a public place for a short period of sustained laughter before beginning the workday (Laughter Club Int'l, 2004).

Physiological benefits of laughter demonstrate that humor and a positive outlook can help in the healing process and disease prevention. Medical experts know that negative emotions can create organic changes within the body such as headaches and ulcers. It makes sense, therefore, that positive emotions can produce positive biochemical changes in the body.

Humor Enhances Learning

When mothers have a positive outlook, they will be more likely to meet new challenges with enthusiasm and optimism. Humor and laughter reduce tension and anxiety, increase productivity, and contribute to learning enjoyment, interest, motivation, and creativity. A humorous approach with mothers helps stimulate divergent thinking, increasing the mother's willingness to look at a situation in a new way. It frees the flow of ideas so that mothers can consider new alternatives and solutions. Humor stimulates both the right and left hemispheres of the brain at the same time, creating a level of consciousness and brain processing that enables the brain to work at its fullest capacity. When the right and left brain are integrated and functioning simultaneously, the capacity for learning is at its highest level. Humor helps achieve this goal.

As part of the mother's healthcare team, you can lighten the mood to facilitate a mother's learning and make the learning experience fun. Shared laughter will energize both of you and will increase a mother's ability to take risks. She will be more comfortable and will feel more welcome to ask questions and offer input. She will also be more receptive to your advice. Humor gets people to listen. Humor is graphic. It creates images in the learner's mind and helps the learner to remember better and longer.

The appropriate use of humor can help mothers gain perspective and see that a situation is not so serious. When humor blends with the right atmosphere, timing, and style, it will enhance your interactions with a receptive mother. You can learn to determine the need for humor and your purpose in using humor with breastfeeding clients. Humor is as much a form of preventive medicine as breastfeeding. It will help mothers to relax, which facilitates oxytocin release. It increases a mother's self-confidence and improves her frame of mind and perspective. Humor helps the mother enjoy her baby. Your use of humor will teach her to see and use humor herself.

Using Humor to Relieve Stress

Staff in the emergency room of St. Christopher's Hospital for Children in Philadelphia recognize the value of humor. In June 1992, *Pediatrics* reported on a retrospective review of their most interesting chief complaints over a 20-year period. "Some complaints that were charted and recorded in a notebook included 'Needs circumcision because his tonsils and adenoids are so big'; 'Can't find the baby's birthmark'; 'Drank the dog's milk—from the dog's nipple'; 'Lump down in his tentacle'; and 'Swollen asteroids.' Among the interesting telephone inquiries were 'Hello, I would like to schedule an emergency' and 'My little girl just kissed a dead chicken. Should I bring her in?' They keep a log of these statements to buoy the spirits of an emergency department staff stressed by long hours and a hectic work environment" (Nelson, 1992).

Lactation Humor

Lactation consultants might develop a similar notebook with humorous lactation situations. Using amusing terminology or a play on words may help you teach techniques to a mother. One lactation consultant makes it a point to use humor frequently with mothers. Linda Kutner (1996) refers to the **cross-cradle hold** as the chicken hold. "I show the mother how her elbow is pointed out like the wing of a chicken. I wave it up and down and go 'cluck, cluck.' This gets the mother laughing and relaxes her." The mother is also more likely to remember the technique she was being taught. People tend to remember stories more than any other form of teaching.

If a mother develops sore nipples, she may be very discouraged about the prospect of breastfeeding. To help lighten the mood, Kutner sympathizes that there are two things necessary for propagation of the species that should be pleasurable and not hurt—and the second one is breastfeeding. If a mother has had a long labor and her baby will not nurse, she will probably be very concerned that something is wrong, that her baby will starve, and that breastfeeding will not work for her. Kutner points out to this mother that her baby was standing on his head for 16 hours knocking at the door, and he probably has a headache! A humorous image can help the mother relax, chuckle, and realize that things will be okay.

You can share an amusing anecdote that may have happened to another mother in similar circumstances. Keeping a humor diary will help you capture such moments. The humor is out there, just waiting for you to capitalize on it in your interactions with mothers. For instance, when a mother was asked, "Why aren't you going to breastfeed?" she answered, "It doesn't run in my family." A mother at a dinner party had her baby pull off just as her milk let down. Her dinner partner, mystified by the sudden droplets on his sleeve, brushed them off and gazed at the ceiling to find the leak. A mother and father were in the recovery room following a cesarean delivery. The father turned to the nurse and asked, "Did they pierce her nipples yet to let the milk out?" When used appropriately, the use of humor in communication will enhance your effectiveness and enrich the lives of your clients and colleagues.

▶ COMPONENTS OF COMMUNICATION

The process of communication requires two basic elements: the delivery and the reception of a message. When delivering a message from one person to another, the way in which the message is received depends on a combination of three factors—body language, tone of voice, and the spoken message (Fast, 1970). Nonverbal language makes a far greater impression than the words that are spoken. Although you may be highly knowledgeable about every aspect of breastfeeding care and lactation, that knowledge will be lost if it is not transmitted effectively.

The Importance of the Spoken Word

The actual words you speak have a relatively low bearing on the message the mother receives. The message that is conveyed is determined only seven percent by the spoken word (Fast, 1970). You will study a variety of books, attend classes and conferences, and network with colleagues to learn all that is necessary about breastfeeding and lactation in order to help mothers. Yet, the verbal communication of that information alone has relatively little impact on the mother's receiving the intended message.

The words and phrases you use can influence the mother's emotional reaction to what you say. There are certain words and phrases that may convey negative messages unintentionally. It is important to avoid terminology that creates a negative impression or implies the mother is doing something incorrectly. Eliminating two specific words from your vocabulary can increase your effectiveness as a communicator with breastfeeding mothers.

Avoid the Use of "But"

Avoid use of the word "but" when you talk with mothers. When you join two thoughts together with *but*, you may not achieve your intended outcome. It actually negates the first half of the thought. Imagine how you would react if someone told you, "Your new hairstyle looks good on you, but it's a little outdated." You probably would not feel complimented. How might a child feel if his parent says, "Getting a *B* on your report is fine, but with a little more effort you can get an *A* next time."

Let's say you tell a mother, "You are holding your baby in a good position, but if you turn him slightly toward you he can get a better latch." Without intending to, you have told the mother that she was not holding her baby correctly. The mother might think, "I'm not holding my baby right. I feel so dumb!" As soon as the mother hears the word "but," it creates a negative impression and she forgets the first part of the statement. Your intention was to teach the mother how to hold her baby during breastfeeding. However, your phrasing has undermined her self-confidence as a new mother.

If you wish to connect two thoughts and at the same time correct the mother, you can simply replace the word "but" with "and." You could say, "You are holding your baby in a good position, and if you turn him slightly you will find that he can get an even better latch." Another way to phrase it is, "That's a good start. Now, you can turn him slightly toward you so that he can get a better latch." You have succeeded in helping the mother improve the manner in which she holds her baby and, at the same time, you have avoided any suggestion that the mother is doing something incorrectly. You have preserved her self-confidence and helped her to grow as a mother.

Avoid the Use of "Should"

Try to eliminate the word "should" from your vocabulary. Consider these statements by a caregiver who is attempting to teach the concept of **need feeding** and the avoidance of artificial nipples: "You should feed your baby whenever he wants." "You shouldn't give your baby a pacifier." Such phrasing may sound judgmental to the mother. The implication is that the mother should breastfeed in the way you consider correct and appropriate. To state that a mother *should* do something implies that she was doing something she should not have done or that she is doing something incorrectly.

You can offer advice in a more effective manner without diluting the message. Assume you want to teach the mother to feed her baby nothing but breastmilk and to give him no artificial nipples. You may tell her, "When you feed your baby in response to hunger cues, you will be meeting his needs. A baby **sucks** differently on an artificial nipple and the breast. If a breastfed baby receives a pacifier, it can confuse him when he tries to **suckle** at the breast." You are teaching correct practices and at the same time you are educating the mother about the reasons for the advice. You avoid sending a judgmental message or undermining the mother's confidence.

Negative Imagery

You also need to avoid words that create negative images. Such words abound in women's health—an *incompetent* cervix, *failure* to progress, *insufficient* **milk supply**, a baby who *fails* to thrive. Even words intended to be positive can suggest the possibility of something negative. If you refer to a mother as being *successful* with her breastfeeding, you raise the possibility that she may be *unsuccessful*. Talking to a mother about establishing an *adequate* milk supply may suggest that her milk supply might be *inadequate*. You can rephrase both of these messages by referring to the mother as reaching her breastfeeding goals and producing enough milk to meet her baby's needs.

Mixed Messages

Take care not to use phrases that create doubt in a mother's mind, send **mixed messages**, or compromise her self-confidence. Consider the message you may send to a mother with the following statements:

> Statement: *You need your rest. I'll take your baby to the nursery for you.* Message: You cannot get enough rest if you keep your baby with you. It does not really matter if you skip a feeding. We can give the baby a bottle of formula. Formula is just as good as your milk.

> Statement: *Are you going to try to breastfeed?* Message: You might not be able to breastfeed. A lot of mothers try and fail. You can go ahead and try, but do not be surprised if it does not work.

> Statement: *Do you have any milk yet?* Message: You might not have enough milk for your baby. We might need to give your baby a bottle. You should have more milk by now. Some women never establish a good enough supply of milk.

These clearly are not the messages you intend to send. Be certain that the words you use create the effect you want. You can tactfully help other caregivers recognize the effects of such phrases as well. Knowing that other elements of communication eclipse much of your spoken message, you can supplement your verbal messages with demonstrations, visual aids, written instructions, and careful attention to your voice tone and body language.

The Effect of Voice Tone

You can undoubtedly recall a time when you talked with someone on the telephone you hoped you would never confront again. You could tell by the tone of her voice and her speaking manner that she simply was not a pleasant person! You can probably recall a time as well when the sound of another person's voice was so pleasant that it enhanced your exchange. You sensed you would enjoy interacting with her again. Tone of voice has a dramatic effect on the manner in which others respond to you. In fact, your **voice tone** is responsible for 38 percent of the message a mother receives (Fast, 1970).

Make sure your voice tone matches the message you want to send, both in exchanges with mothers and with colleagues. Your manner of speech can create a warm, friendly, and even humorous atmosphere. In evaluating your speech, consider your volume. Many people speak either too loudly or too softly. Either extreme can irritate the other person and interfere with your message getting across. Your rate of speech is also a factor. If you talk too quickly, you may appear rushed and the other person may become anxious or nervous. Remembering to stop and breathe can keep you from running out of breath and seeming rushed. On the other hand, talking too slowly can irritate others, who will wonder if you will *ever* get your message across. Controlling the pitch of your voice may be a challenge. Often, our voice tends to get higher when we are angry or excited. Consciously trying to control it may help you to modulate the pitch and appear controlled. Moderating the rate and pitch of your voice and talking slowly enough to pause and breathe will help you achieve an effective voice tone. All of these aspects of your speech can have an effect on the message you convey.

The Effect of Body Language

Of the three components in communication, body language has the greatest effect on the manner in which a message is received—55 percent (Fast, 1970)! Body language describes the behavioral patterns of nonverbal communication. It is a study of the mixture of all body movements, including smiling, eye contact, posture, space, and touching. Body language ranges from deliberate gestures to unconscious ones. It may apply in only one culture or span across cultural barriers. In addition to sending and receiving messages, body language can serve to break through defenses. The manner in which you capitalize on your nonverbal messages will determine your effectiveness in the care you give to mothers.

Smile

A pleasant facial expression adds to a warm and inviting atmosphere. A calm, relaxed smile reflects that you enjoy your work and enjoy meeting people. That kind of smile will put mothers at ease. When you smile, you elicit a smile from the mother as well. It is almost impossible not to return a smile. She cannot help it—it is human nature to smile back! The warmth of a smile even comes through in your voice over the telephone.

Eye Contact

The eyes are the most important of all the body parts in transmitting information. When you interact with another person, try to maintain eye contact at least 85 percent of the time. You can avoid too much intensity or appearing to stare by blinking or by looking away and back again. Eye contact has a powerful impact on your message. Establishing eye contact with a mother conveys your desire to communicate with her. It establishes a warm, caring, and inviting climate.

Eye contact can be a powerful tool for influencing others. The next time you are competing for a parking place or trying to merge into traffic, establish eye contact with the driver in the other car. The driver will probably bend to your wishes. If you are standing in line for a movie and another person tries to cut into the line, look the other person straight in the eye. Chances are the other person will turn away and go to the back of the line.

Be aware of the power your eye contact has on the messages you send. Failing to establish eye contact also sends a message. We all use this tactic to avoid talking with others or being seen by them. Consider, therefore, the message you send if you talk to a mother with your back turned or your eyes focused on what you are writing (Figure 4.7). You have a powerful communication tool, in fact, two of them! Consciously engaging in eye contact with mothers in your care will enhance your interactions and your effectiveness.

Posture

Posture is another aspect of body language that sends a strong message. To create a warm and inviting climate, you want your body to be relaxed and comfortable. Try to avoid crossing your arms or legs, which can convey an attitude of disinterest and emotional distance. Instead, sit or stand squarely with both feet flat on the floor. Rest your arms at your side or, when sitting, on your knees. This open body posture shows your intent to communicate on a meaningful level. Leaning forward further conveys your interest in interacting with the mother.

Body Position

We all have a certain amount of personal space that creates our comfort zone. The amount of space people require to be comfortable varies. How we guard our personal zone and our reaction when others invade it affects how we relate to other people. Be careful not to invade a mother's comfort zone and cause her to feel uneasy or awkward. At the same time, if you position yourself too far away, you may convey a message that you are too busy or uninterested in engaging her in any meaningful way. Poking your head in the door and asking a mother how breastfeeding is going does not convey a willingness to help or an interest to interact (Figure 4.8). Neither does standing on the other side of the room. Establish a position that is comfortable for both of you—not too far away and not too close.

Another aspect of body position is altitude. When two people interact, the height each person assumes in relation to one another creates a perception of importance or control. When the mother's caregiver stands over her, it can be intimidating to the mother and does not empower her to be the one in charge (Figure 4.9). Placing the mother at an equal or greater height establishes that the mother is the person of greatest importance. It leads to greater self-reliance, which is one of the goals of your consultation with the mother. You can position a chair near the mother

---

FIGURE 4.7
Caregiver exhibiting poor eye contact.

Printed with permission of Anna Swisher.

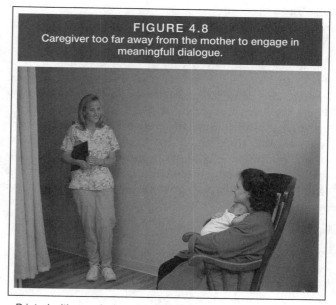

FIGURE 4.8
Caregiver too far away from the mother to engage in meaningfull dialogue.

Printed with permission of Anna Swisher.

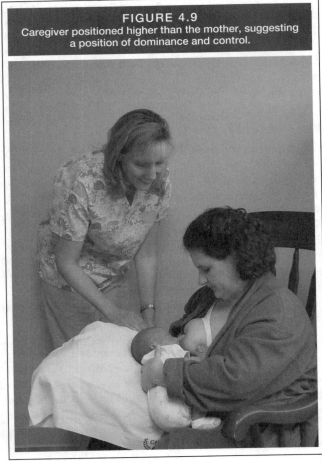

FIGURE 4.9
Caregiver positioned higher than the mother, suggesting a position of dominance and control.

Printed with permission of Anna Swisher.

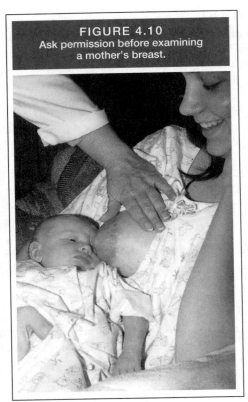

FIGURE 4.10
Ask permission before examining a mother's breast.

Printed with permission of Debbie Shinske.

or even kneel on the floor next her. Ask her permission and use her comfort as a guide.

Touch

Be judicious in your use of any posture that involves body contact. Some people are comfortable touching others, and some are not. Some will be receptive to being touched, and some will not. The touch of a hand, or an arm placed around someone's shoulder, can convey warmth, caring, and encouragement. However, such a touch must come at the appropriate moment and within the appropriate context. On your first contact with a mother, she may respond favorably to your arm around her shoulder as you observe her baby at the breast. However, if you were to touch her breast immediately, she may react in an embarrassed or negative manner. When you need to examine a woman's breasts, be sure to ask her permission first—"May I examine your breasts?"—and explain the purpose (Figure 4.10). These same rules apply to touching her baby. If you would like to examine the baby's mouth or help comfort

him, explain this to the mother and ask permission before invading her space and taking her baby from her.

Cultural Differences

Be aware that a particular body gesture may send different messages in different cultures. In Western culture, for instance, a person shakes his head up and down to indicate yes and from side to side to indicate no. However, in some societies the opposite is true. Side to side means yes and up and down means no! Smiling, eye contact, personal space, touching, and posture may vary greatly from one culture to another. Learn your clients' cultural backgrounds so that you send the messages you intend and interpret their body language correctly.

Reading the Body Language of Others

In addition to gaining an awareness of your own body language, you need to be alert for nonverbal messages the mother sends to you. Observe and respond to her body language. Determine whether she appears to be comfortable or in pain. Does she welcome eye contact, or does she avert her eyes? How is her tone of voice? Does she sound stressed or anxious (Figure 4.11)? Is her facial expression animated or listless? Is she comfortable being touched? Does her body sag, or does she sit or stand with

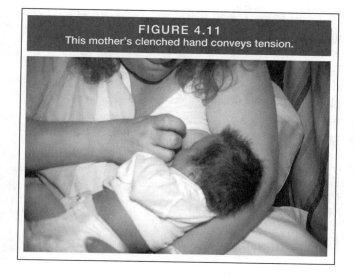

FIGURE 4.11
This mother's clenched hand conveys tension.

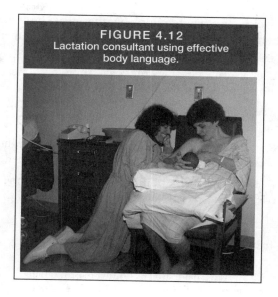

FIGURE 4.12
Lactation consultant using effective body language.

an erect posture? Does she have an air of self-assurance, or does she seem passive and unsure of herself? Does she shift her body and fidget? What is her posture while she is breastfeeding her baby? Are her shoulders hunched and tense? If so, perhaps she needs some pillows to help her get comfortable. Does she curl her toes when her baby is feeding? This may indicate that she is in pain and needs to reposition her baby. Paying careful attention to all of these nuances of the mother's body language will help you gather impressions about her situation.

▶ SUMMARY

The caregiver's commitment, beliefs, attitude, and approach are clearly a driving force behind a mother's ability to reach her breastfeeding goals. The caregiver who presents breastfeeding as the natural way to feed babies and who demonstrates a sincere belief in the superiority of breastfeeding over artificial feeding will increase the mother's self-image and confidence. When you serve as a facilitator, exploring options and developing a partnership with the mother in problem solving, the mother will grow as an active health consumer who is informed and responsible concerning her healthcare and that of her infant. She will continue to grow in a climate that relinquishes medical control, limits interventions, and trusts in the abilities of mothers and babies. A personalized approach with every mother—one that assesses her needs, capitalizes on her strengths, and praises her accomplishments—will lead to the mother's long-term satisfaction. Keeping a sense of humor and using effective communication skills will help you establish an optimal learning climate and develop a meaningful rapport with mothers (Figure 4.12).

▶ CHAPTER 4 — AT A GLANCE

Applying what you learned—

♦ Assume all mothers will breastfeed unless you are told otherwise.

♦ Recognize that your past actions were appropriate at the time and not a reason for guilt.

♦ Recognize guilt as a positive emotion that leads to personal growth.

♦ Form a partnership with parents and empower them to make decisions and accept responsibility for their actions.

♦ Help parents become informed health consumers.

♦ Place control and power with the mother and baby, not the caregiver.

♦ Lobby for reducing unnecessary medical interventions.

♦ Help parents recognize their newborn's capabilities.

♦ Confine interactions to guiding rather than directing unless intervention is needed.

♦ Create a learning climate that is relaxed, trusting, mutually respectful, informal, warm, collaborative, and supportive.

♦ Individualize your approach based on the mother's learning needs and readiness.

♦ Keep pace with the mother and baby.

♦ Actively involve the mother to heighten her learning and retention.

♦ Respond to the mother's learning style and use humor to enhance her learning.

◆ Avoid negative terminology that may undermine a mother's self-confidence or send a judgmental message.

◆ Use a smile and warm voice tone to appeal to mothers.

◆ Use body language that engages and empowers the mother.

◆ Recognize cultural differences in body language, personal space, and comfort with being touched.

◆ Read the mother's body language to determine her comfort and receptiveness.

▶ REFERENCES

Auerbach K. Maternal mastery and the assisting "hand" of the lactation consultant. *J Hum Lact* 10:223–224; 1994.

Belenky M et al. *Women's Ways of Knowing.* New York: Basic Books, Inc.; 1986.

Cousins N. *Anatomy of an Illness.* New York: Norton; 1979.

DeVito JA. *The Interpersonal Communication Book.* 5th ed. New York: Harper & Row; 1989.

Fast J. *Body Language.* New York: Pocket Books; 1970.

Fisher C. *Breastfeeding Basics.* Annual Conference, Breastfeeding: The Cross Cultural Connection, Kansas City, MO; July, 1996.

Fletcher D, Harris H. The implementation of the HOT program at the Royal Women's Hospital. *Breastfeed Rev* 8:19–23; 2000.

International Lactation Consultant Association (ILCA). *Core Curriculum for Lactation Consultant Practice.* Raleigh, NC: ILCA; 2002.

Knowles M. *The Modern Practice of Adult Education: From Pedagogy to Androgogy.* Chicago: Follett Publishing; 1980.

Kutner L. *Lactation Management Course.* Chalfont, PA: Breastfeeding Support Consultants Center for Lactation Education; 1996.

Laughter Club, International. Available at: www.laughteryoga. org. Accessed December 1, 2004.

Locklin M, Naber S. Does breastfeeding empower women? Insights from a select group of educated, low-income minority women. *Birth* 20:30–35; 1993.

Nelson DS. Humor in the pediatric emergency department: A 2-year retrospective. *Pediatrics* 89(6):1089–1090; 1992.

Oski F. In defense of guilt. *Contemporary Pediatrics* 12:9; 1995.

Robinson VM. *Humor and the Health Professions: The Therapeutic Use of Humor in Health Care.* Thorofare, NJ: Slack, Inc.; 1991.

Walker M. *Summary of the Hazards of Infant Formula.* Raleigh, NC: International Lactation Consultant Association; 1992.

Weimer J. Economic benefits: A review and analysis. Economic Research Service, USDA, *Food Assistance and Nutrition Research Report* 13; March 2001.

Zahr L. The relationship between maternal confidence and mother-infant behaviors in premature infants. *Res Nurs Health* 14:279–286; 1991.

▶ BIBLIOGRAPHY

Fine GA. Sociological approaches to the study of humor. In McGhee PE and Goldstein JH (eds). *Handbook of Humor Research*, Vol 1. New York: Springer-Verlag; pp. 159–181; 1983.

Foster S. Does your style block your message? *MCN* 13:207; 1988.

Fry WF Jr. Humor and the human cardiovascular system. In Mindess H and Turek J (eds). *The Study of Humor.* Los Angeles: Antioch University; 1979.

Fry WF Jr. *Mirthful Laughter and Blood Pressure.* Paper presented at the Third International Conference on Humor, Washington, DC; 1982.

Jackson M. The comedy of management. In Simms, Price, Ervin (eds). *The Professional Practice of Nursing Administration.* New York: Wiley; pp. 339–351; 1985.

Nahemow L, McCluskey-Fawcett K, McGhee P (eds). *Humor and Aging.* San Diego: Academic Press, pp. 81–98; 1986.

Meichenbaum D, Turk D. *Facilitating Treatment Adherence.* New York: Plenum Press; 1987.

Minchin M. Smoking and breastfeeding: An overview. *J Hum Lact* 7:183–188; 1991.

Mozingo J. Empowering women to breastfeed. *Advance:* 43–44, 46, 65; 1996.

Northouse PG. *Health Communication: A Handbook for Health Professionals.* Englewood Cliffs, NJ: Prentice-Hall; 1985.

Ziv A. Humor and creativity. *The Creative Child and Adult Quarterly* 5(3):159–170; 1980.

Ziv A. The influence of humorous atmosphere on divergent thinking. *Contemp Ed Psych* 9:413–421; 1983.

5

COUNSELING:
LEARNING TO HELP MOTHERS

▶ Helping mothers with breastfeeding goes far beyond book knowledge, research, scientific principles, and clinical practice. These are all important, indeed, essential to responsible healthcare. However, without effective communication and counseling skills, all of your knowledge and wisdom may fall on deaf ears. Whether you are a lactation consultant, other healthcare professional, or lay counselor, your primary role with breastfeeding mothers is that of a counselor. Counseling is the most basic element in the helping process. As a member of the mother's healthcare team, you have a responsibility to acquire the skills and techniques that will enhance your helping relationship.

KEY TERMS

active listening
attending
BestStart 3-Step
    Counseling Strategy
building hope
clarifying
emotional support
empathetic listening
evaluating
facilitating
focusing
follow-up method
guiding method

identifying strengths
influencing
informing
interpreting
leading method
open-ended questions
passive listening
physical comfort
problem solving
reassuring
reflective listening
summarizing

▶ UNDERSTANDING THE COUNSELING PROCESS

Basic counseling techniques provide the means for giving mothers the support they need to develop confidence in their mothering and breastfeeding abilities. Counseling skills involve encouraging the mother to express herself, educating her, and empowering her with problem-solving techniques. These skills are the essence of breastfeeding counseling. With effective counseling techniques, you can better use breastfeeding knowledge to work toward a positive outcome for the mother.

The ultimate goal of each individual counseling contact is increased satisfaction for the mother. When emotional stress and physical discomfort are relieved and you and the mother have talked through her situation, she will feel good about her participation in the outcome and her self-confidence will increase.

Increased self-awareness and understanding in turn will lead to the mother's personal growth. This enables her to take responsibility for her situation and to be self-sufficient. Table 5.1 lists the general skills that will assist you in helping the mother reach her goals. The mother's satisfaction comes about through your perception of her needs, your use of counseling skills, and your personality traits. These factors are explored in the following sections.

A variety of techniques are described that can be considered as part of your counseling "toolbox." You are not expected to go through a prescribed process with every contact. Rather, you are encouraged to assess each contact and use the skills appropriate to the situation. Practice the techniques presented in this chapter to learn which ones are compatible with your personality and approach. Use those that feel comfortable to you and that help you establish an effective and supportive relationship.

Counselor Traits

Your personality will have a direct effect on the rapport you establish with the mother. Mothers respond best to a person who has a warm and caring attitude and who shows deep and genuine concern and empathy. Positive regard and respect, which acknowledge the mother's individuality and worth without judgment, will give the mother freedom to be herself. It is important to accept mothers without judging their decisions based on your expectations. Show the mother that you approve of her and that you value what she has to say. Clear, accurate communication will reduce confusion and frustration. Flexibility will help you use a full range of skills so that you can respond appropriately to the mother at different stages in the counseling process.

TABLE 5.1			
Counseling Model to Meet the Mother's Needs			
Mother's Needs +	**Counseling Skills** +	**Counselor's Traits** =	**Satisfaction for Mother**
◆ Emotional support	◆ Listening	◆ Empathy and warmth	◆ Reduced stress
◆ Immediate physical comfort	◆ Influencing	◆ Concern	◆ Increased self-confidence
◆ Understanding	◆ Facilitating	◆ Openness	◆ Personal growth
◆ Positive action	◆ Informing	◆ Positive regard and respect	◆ Acceptance of responsibility
	◆ Problem solving	◆ Clear, accurate communication	
		◆ Flexibility	

You may have taken personality assessment tests in your educational or work experience. If not, there are many tests you can use to determine your primary style of communicating and relating to people. Common tests include Myers-Briggs (2004), DiSC (Inscape 2004), Birkman (2004), and Wilson Social Styles (Wilson Learning 2004). Many human resource departments use these tests in the hiring process. If you are presently working, check with your employer to see if these are available for you. Community colleges and adult continuing education programs frequently offer them, and they are also available through the Internet and self-help books. Insights into your personality will help you identify both your strengths and your weaknesses as you work with mothers and babies.

The Mother's Needs

The counseling process helps fulfill the mother's needs for emotional support, understanding, and action. Making sure you address all three of these with each contact will ensure that the mother is satisfied. A mother may need relief from physical discomfort as well. As shown in Table 5.1, you can use a variety of counseling skills as you interact with mothers (Brammer, 1973). The skills presented in each category provide tools for your interactions with mothers. Use those that you find comfortable and natural so you can blend them with your personal communication style.

Emotional Support

Providing emotional support to a mother validates her feelings, emotions, and concerns. It creates an atmosphere in which a mother feels validated, takes in information, and joins in problem solving. Visualize your grandmother preparing a stew in her pressure cooker. She knows that when the stew is cooked, she must slowly vent the steam to relieve the pressure before she

removes the top of the cooker. If she opens it too soon, the stew will end up on the ceiling instead of on the plate! This same principle can help you appreciate all the pressure and anxiety felt by mothers in your care. A flurry of emotions may be boiling and ready to explode. What will happen if you jump in to try to resolve a mother's engorgement or sore nipples before you have addressed these emotions?

You can use counseling skills to help the mother lower her pressure and stress. Help her verbalize her feelings, and validate her concerns. Show acceptance, and praise her actions or attempts. Listen to what she is saying as well as what she is *not* saying. Learn to read between the lines for her underlying message. When she is in a receptive state and able to process the information, you can then enter into educating and problem solving.

Factors that cause emotional distress can build up. Your emotional support will provide a sense of security and a climate that encourages the mother to express her feelings and anxieties. An important principle in a helping profession is: *People won't care how much you know until they know how much you care.* In providing emotional support, you send the message that you genuinely care about the mother's well-being and concerns. It shows that you are interested in helping the mother to achieve her goals. We all give support to those we love, unconsciously at times, simply as an outpouring of our care and concern for them. Likewise, support is an essential element in the care you give to a mother. It helps her feel secure and at ease, reduces her anxiety, and gives her someone with whom to share her concerns.

Use of listening and **influencing** skills—**attending, active listening, empathetic listening, reassuring, praising,** and **building hope**—provide emotional support. When you understand and become experienced in the use of these skills, you will find yourself giving support almost automatically. New mothers often feel inadequate at fulfilling all that is required of them as a mother, wife, professional, and homemaker. Frequently praise a new mother for how well she is doing with all her responsibilities. You may be the only person telling this mother she is doing a good job right now. Your interest in her and in her concerns, your frequent contacts with her, your enthusiasm for the things she is happy about, and your acceptance of her, her situation, and her decisions are all ways of showing support.

Immediate Physical Comfort

Often a mother needs to take some immediate action in order to reduce physical stress. Perhaps she is tired, her nipples are uncomfortable at the beginning of feedings, or her baby has slept through the night and her breasts are uncomfortably full or engorged. Before she can address ways to resolve her situation, she will first need immediate physical relief from her discomfort. In this case, you can first offer emotional support and then suggestions to help her feel better physically.

This approach temporarily deviates from the usual problem-solving process, in which you would carefully work toward defining the problem before suggesting any action. Intermediate actions to relieve the mother's discomfort will enable her to work with you to find the cause of the difficulty and eliminate it. After the mother is more comfortable, you can work with her to develop a better understanding of the problem. Figure 5.1 shows how immediate physical comfort fits into the counseling process as a temporary measure. Giving physical comfort is not always necessary. If a problem exists that is not urgent, or the mother seems calm and relaxed, then you can follow the usual counseling process.

Understanding

The mother's understanding is basic to the success of the counseling process. In order to develop satisfaction from a contact with you, the mother needs to understand herself and her feelings about a problem or concern. She needs to define and understand the problem clearly, as well as the events or actions that led to it and the actions that will help resolve it. She also needs to understand her options in order to make informed

choices and assume responsibility for her actions. Such understanding comes from your use of listening, influencing, **facilitating**, **informing**, and problem-solving skills.

Positive Action

After having received the appropriate support and gained an understanding of her situation, the mother may be able to take positive action in dealing with her concern. Even if a problem does not resolve immediately, she will gain satisfaction in actively working on it and can modify her action appropriately. You can initiate positive action with problem-solving and decision-making processes and skills. By developing a plan together, both you and the mother can mutually agree on what the mother will do.

Methods of Counseling

In order to meet the mother's needs for emotional support, physical comfort, understanding, and action, a systematic counseling process is used. In the context of breastfeeding support, counseling encompasses more than the typical definition of counseling as a "process of advising." The three distinct aspects that characterize this process are the methods of guiding, leading, and follow-up.

The Guiding Method

The **guiding method** will help you genuinely listen to the mother and empathize with her through understanding her feelings, goals, and other factors that influence her actions. Skills used in this method keep the conversation going and help you gather the information you need in order to determine the situation. Guiding skills encourage the mother to express her ideas and concerns openly. She is able to listen to herself so that she, as well as you, understands the situation better. Guiding skills help you hear what the mother is *not* saying, the hidden messages she does not verbalize. The other purpose of guiding skills is to help transmit a message of acceptance

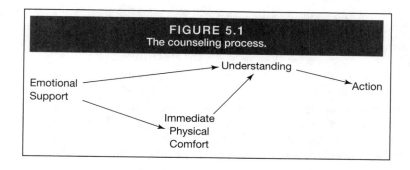

FIGURE 5.1
The counseling process.

of the mother's viewpoint and positive regard for her well-being. They help you say, "I care."

The Leading Method

The **leading method** requires you to take a more active role in directing the conversation. This method is useful when the mother has identified a problem or concern that she is unable to solve with her available resources. The skills used in this method help both you and the mother see her situation more accurately and define options open to her so that she can work with you to develop a plan of care. It is with these skills that you and the mother form a partnership in finding solutions.

The Follow-up Method

In order to be fully aware of the mother's progress, you need to analyze the effectiveness of every contact. You can then determine how and when to plan the next contact and what preparation is needed. Following up each counseling session with a subsequent contact will help you determine whether you have achieved your goal of increasing the mother's satisfaction and self-sufficiency. It will help you learn if your suggestions have been useful and if the mother needs further emotional support or assistance.

The follow-up method lets the mother know how actively concerned you are in helping her. It encourages you to review the situation and to research other sources of information. For IBCLCs who practice in fee-for-service situations, the mother's financial or insurance constraints may limit opportunities for follow-up. Appropriate referrals to community services or a breastfeeding support group can provide this component of follow-up and continuity of care.

▶ USING COUNSELING METHODS AND SKILLS

The individual skills within each method of the counseling process are tools you can develop to create a climate of acceptance that makes counseling possible. The numerous examples in this chapter will help you relate the skills to actual counseling concerns.

The most effective way to develop counseling skills and become proficient in their use is to practice them as frequently as possible. If you take the opportunity to practice counseling skills in conversations with your friends, colleagues, and family, you can soon develop an appreciation of their effectiveness and make them an important part of your communication style.

Table 5.2 presents an outline of the skills used in each of the three counseling methods. It gives an overview of the counseling process and can serve as a reference for you as you read the individual discussions of the methods and skills.

The Guiding Method

The guiding method is one in which the mother is helped through emotional support and limited direction from the counselor. Being aware of the mother's feelings, values, goals, and physical and emotional environment will enable you to understand her needs more clearly. The major responsibility for the direction of the discussion rests with the mother during this guiding process. She, therefore, does most of the talking. This allows you to concentrate on listening carefully to her message. There is a reason that you have two ears and only one mouth. During the guiding phase of your counseling contact, you should spend at least twice as much time listening as you do talking!

The aim of all counseling is self-help and self-sufficiency. By encouraging the mother to talk, reflecting her ideas and clarifying her concerns, you help her see a clear picture of her situation. This ideally results in the mother taking responsibility for what is happening and deciding her plan of care. Throughout the contact, continually evaluate the mother's capacity for independence and self-support. If she fails to take responsibility for herself, you may need to change your approach in order to encourage her to take the initiative while you continue to support her.

Listening skills that reinforce what she says will clarify the mother's statements, show acceptance of her situation, and encourage her to arrive at solutions. Effective listening lets the mother know that you care about her enough to give her your total attention.

While giving the mother the opportunity to hear herself and to sort out her feelings and concerns, listening also enables you to gather information. At times, you will need to be more actively involved in gathering information by directing the conversation so that the mother will focus on specific points. Facilitating the conversation in this way helps both you and the mother recognize and clearly define her situation. By facilitating, you act as a sounding board for the mother. As you gather information, you can use influencing skills to encourage her and give her emotional support if you feel the mother needs to increase her self-confidence or gain a new perspective. Influencing the mother's attitude in a positive way can help her view her circumstances more optimistically. This reduces stress so that she is able to think more clearly and work toward a solution.

Listening

Everyday listening usually takes place at one of four levels. The lowest level of listening is **ignoring**. No doubt, most adults have experienced this level of listening with a child or pet! The next level of listening is **pretending**, where the listener is trying to be polite but is not giving any attention to the speaker. It describes the non-committal response you might receive if you interrupt

TABLE 5.2
Counseling Methods and Skills

Method	Technique	Skills
Guiding	◆ Listening	◆ Attending
		◆ Active listening
		◆ Empathetic listening
	◆ Facilitating	◆ Clarifying
		◆ Interpreting
		◆ Asking open-ended questions
		◆ Focusing
		◆ Summarizing
	◆ Influencing	◆ Reassuring
		◆ Building hope
		◆ Identifying strengths
Leading	◆ Informing	◆ Presenting
		◆ Timing
		◆ Educating
	◆ Problem solving	◆ Listening to your first hunch
		◆ Looking for hidden factors
		◆ Testing your hunch
		◆ Exploring alternative hunches
		◆ Developing a plan
Follow-up	◆ Evaluating the session	◆ Analyzing
	◆ Arranging the next contact	◆ Use skills listed above as needed
	◆ Researching outside sources	
	◆ Renewing the counseling process	

someone who is deeply engrossed in reading or watching television. The third level is **selective listening**, in which the listener hears only certain parts of what is said. This can occur when you focus so much on how you plan to respond that you fail to listen carefully. The fourth level of customary listening is **attentive listening**, in which the listener actively focuses on the words and the message.

Learning to Listen

Developing skills beyond everyday listening is a consciously active process of responding to total messages and perceiving with your ears, eyes, and imagination. It means you must be silent much of the time and allow the mother to talk. We are all guilty of sometimes listening with half an ear to the speaker while busily figuring out what to say next or how to change the subject to something we would rather discuss. In order to help the mother, you need to listen carefully to what she is saying and avoid the temptation to interrupt. This requires that you put your thoughts and interests aside for the moment so that you can give yourself more fully to the job of listening.

Listening requires time and patience, and often means waiting until the mother develops an understanding of her feelings and concerns. Time is a valuable commodity for all of us. Few people take the opportunity to sit down with another individual and really listen to that person. Failure to help the mother is often a result of snap judgments and not taking enough time to hear the whole story. You need to give the mother enough time to collect her thoughts. If you ask a new mother how everything is going, she may quickly reply, "Fine." Ten minutes later, after you have talked about increases in the frequency of feedings at particular stages in her baby's growth, she may say, "No wonder my baby is nursing constantly!" She may then tell you she has been under great stress because of this and had begun to wonder if she has enough milk to satisfy her baby.

Many times a mother is not sure about how she feels and needs more time to talk and to feel at ease before you both communicate on the same level. When the mother has mixed feelings or several concerns, you will need time and ample conversation before you can be sure of how the mother really feels. Three listening skills that can give you this time are attending, active listening, and empathetic listening.

Attending

Attending is a **passive listening** skill that involves responses to assure the mother that you are listening, without asking questions or making comments. Examples include: "Yes," "I see," "I can appreciate that," "Oh," "Mmmmm," and "Really." The goal of attending behavior is to encourage the mother to continue talking freely. It has a strong reinforcing effect that helps the mother explore her way and be responsible for the course of the discussion. Attending minimizes your tendency to intervene unnecessarily. Silence is another effective attending technique. At times, pausing in the conversation and waiting for the mother to fill the silence may encourage her to take a more active role.

Other aspects of attending are visual observation and the use of eye contact, posture, gestures, and listening in a noninterfering manner. The absence of any type of attending behavior, whether verbal or nonverbal, may discourage the mother from pursuing a topic and cause her to feel that you are not interested in what she has to say. Your use of eye contact and other nonverbal behavior sends messages to mothers. If you avoid eye contact with a mother, cross your arms or legs, or seem otherwise unapproachable, you may send a message that you are disinterested. You cannot alter such a message with any verbal attempt to show interest. You can transmit a positive nonverbal message and show that you are genuinely interested through direct eye contact, leaning toward the mother with a natural relaxed posture, calm gestures, and a pleasant, engaged facial expression.

Active Listening

Active listening, also called **reflective listening**, is a very useful technique for gathering information from the mother. Active listening serves 3 distinct functions: It **clarifies**, shows acceptance of the mother's viewpoint, and encourages a response. With active listening, you paraphrase what the mother has said and reflect her message back to her. This type of exchange encourages the mother to respond and to feel free to explain her situation in detail. It provides an opportunity for the mother to recognize and solve her problem and creates an atmosphere in which she can grow and accept information.

Active listening clarifies a message and lets the mother know you received her message completely and correctly. It helps the mother hear what she is saying and think about it. Your response may involve some interpretation of her message. Her subsequent response lets you know that you understood correctly. This focuses the conversation and provides better mutual understanding.

Active listening is particularly useful when talking to a mother who has only some vague or as-yet unspoken thoughts on a situation. It is also useful with a mother who is emotionally upset and not sure what her concern is or how she feels about it. You cannot begin to offer suggestions until the mother is ready to accept them. She will be ready only after her situation and her feelings are clear. Listening and encouraging the mother to continue talking are crucial in defining her concerns.

Active listening shows acceptance of the mother's viewpoint and goes beyond a more passive type of attending response such as "I see" or "Really." In active listening, you send back what you believe the mother's message meant. This encourages her to continue discussing the issue further. You are letting the mother know that you understand how she feels, that you are interested in what she is saying, and that you validate what she is feeling.

Using the mother's and baby's names helps personalize the exchange and enhances the helping relationship between you and the mother. Make a conscious effort to use both of their names frequently. It is especially important that you use the baby's name with a mother who continually refers to her infant as "the baby" and does not refer to her infant by name. This could indicate that the mother is having difficulty bonding with her baby. Your use of the baby's name will help model bonding for the mother.

An example that illustrates clarification:

Mother: My nipples hurt.

Counselor: Your nipples are sore when you feed Michael. (Some interpretation that the soreness occurs during a feeding; and using the baby's name.)

Mother: Not just when I nurse, but after I wash them, too. (This is a correction, a clarifying message. Note that you have gathered some more information in her response that may help you in problem solving, i.e., the fact that she washes her nipples after a feeding.)

An example that shows acceptance:

Mother: I'm not sure I can breastfeed much longer. My nipples are so sore that breastfeeding is really unpleasant!

Counselor: It's no fun to feed Christopher when it hurts. We talked about how enjoyable breastfeeding is, and this isn't fun at all.

An example that encourages the mother to respond:

Mother: Jenny is four months old now and always looking around the room instead of nursing. I guess she's ready to wean.

Counselor: You're wondering if Jenny is ready to wean.

With an active listening response, you first accept what the mother feels. This usually encourages her to relax and respond openly. It is a warm, sincere, and considerate way of talking that most people cannot resist. Instead of informing the mother right away that a four-month-old does not usually self-wean and is probably just distracted, you first accept the mother's feelings, making no judgment. Later, after further discussion, you can offer the mother information about weaning and help her learn and grow. A mother may not feel comfortable sharing her personal feelings until you have talked for quite a while and trust develops. Active listening serves as an important means of developing trust and encouraging the mother to respond.

Empathetic Listening

Listening as part of the counseling process goes beyond merely reflecting someone's words. The highest and most effective level of listening is empathetic listening. Simple reflective or active listening conveys intent to reply or to manipulate the conversation. The empathetic listener goes even further, listening with the intent to understand emotionally and intellectually. You listen with your ears, eyes, and heart, tuning in to the feeling, meaning, and behavior conveyed. You integrate your right brain and left brain to sense and feel what is being said. When you reflect the message back to the mother, you rephrase both the content and the feeling of what she said. This will help you and the mother work through her feelings as well as her thoughts. When you reflect back what the mother seems to be saying, in your words, you reveal to her the emotions she has expressed.

Example of an empathetic listening response:

Mother: I don't know whether I should nurse my next baby. It might make my two-year-old child more jealous.

Counselor: You're afraid Joey will be more demanding if you nurse your new baby, Molly.

You may not be certain that this is the message the mother is sending. Hearing you say it back to her with your interpretation will help the mother know if she sent the intended message. She may say, "Yes, he already needs a lot of attention. I'm not sure how he'll react if I spend so much time nursing a new baby." If you misinterpreted her comment, she may say, "No, it's just that he is so sensitive and I don't want him to feel left out." Her response to your comment will help you determine the direction to take with your next comment.

Empathetic listening helps you gain information that will clarify the mother's situation. This makes it less likely that you will misinterpret her meaning. To illustrate the need to understand what the mother is saying before offering suggestions, Figure 5.2 contains a list of possible meanings for several statements. If you misinterpret the mother's initial statement, your explanation or suggestions will be inappropriate and unhelpful. The wide range of possible meanings reinforces the importance of coming to a common understanding with the mother. Be cautious when using empathetic listening and keep your feedback statements tentative. You cannot be sure you know exactly what a mother is feeling. Watch your tone of voice and avoid sounding like a mind reader.

When using empathetic listening, at times it may be difficult to think of words to express feelings. Figure 5.3 presents a list of "feeling words" to help you expand your vocabulary. You can add it to your counseling toolbox to assist you in reflecting the feelings of the mother you are counseling. Be specific in your responses. Avoid use of the general word "upset," which may communicate that you do not really understand the emotion the mother has expressed. When a mother sends you a "feeling" message, think to yourself, "What is she feeling?" Think of a word to describe the emotion she is expressing and then put that word into a sentence. If you concentrate on asking yourself this question, you will find that your empathetic listening responses come more easily and more spontaneously.

Facilitating

Facilitating skills actively encourage the mother to give more information and better define her situation. They also help to focus on specific concerns. Facilitating requires you to direct the conversation in order to help the mother pinpoint issues and feelings that need to be expressed. In addition to asking **open-ended questions**, facilitating helps you clarify and interpret meaning and focus and summarize the conversation.

Clarifying

Clarifying simply means to make a point clear. In counseling, you need to gather enough information from the mother in order to understand her message clearly. One way you can clarify a point is by admitting confusion about the mother's meaning and restating what you heard. You may also clarify what the mother has said by using other guiding method skills such as active listening, asking open-ended questions, and **interpreting**.

Examples of clarifying responses:

◆ "Are you saying that . . . ?"
◆ "Let me see if I understand what you said."
◆ "Can you tell me more about . . . ?"

FIGURE 5.2
Possible meanings from a mother's statements.

A mother says, "I think I'll have to give my baby a bottle in the evening so that my husband can do something for the baby."

Possible meanings:

◆ Mother wants to start a bottle.
◆ Husband wants to start a bottle.
◆ Husband feels left out.
◆ Mother wants father to take a more active role in child care.
◆ Mother wants baby to sleep through the night.
◆ Mother has other things to do in the evening and wants husband to care for baby.
◆ Husband doesn't think baby is getting enough nourishment.
◆ Mother is thinking of weaning her baby.
◆ Baby is fussy in the evening—mother thinks she doesn't have enough milk.
◆ Husband wants to help as much as possible.

A mother says, "I have to wean to go to a wedding."

Possible meanings:

◆ Mother wants to wean, and the wedding is a convenient excuse.
◆ Mother does not want to breastfeed baby at wedding.
◆ Father wants mother to wean.
◆ Mother doesn't realize she can miss a feed.
◆ Mother doesn't know how to collect and freeze milk.
◆ Mother is not comfortable breastfeeding in public.
◆ Mother wants more freedom.
◆ Mother cannot wear her favorite dress due to increased breast size.
◆ Mother's favorite dress will not accommodate breastfeeding in public.

A mother says, "My mother-in-law is here helping me these first 2 weeks, but she bottle-fed."

Possible meanings:

◆ Mother-in-law is not supportive of breastfeeding.
◆ Mother-in-law thinks baby isn't getting enough nourishment.
◆ Mother-in-law is helpful around the house but not with breastfeeding.
◆ Mother may be embarrassed breastfeeding in front of her mother-in-law.
◆ Mother-in-law envies her for being able to breastfeed.
◆ Mother-in-law is great. She wants to learn about breastfeeding and thinks it's wonderful.
◆ Mother-in-law is not familiar with differences between bottle-feeding and breastfeeding, and mother needs information to pass on to her.
◆ Mother needs support and mother-in-law may not know how to provide it.

A mother says, "I don't know how long I'll be able to breastfeed. My sister had to wean at 10 days because her milk dried up."

Possible meanings:

◆ Mother is worried that her milk may dry up.
◆ Sister may be unsupportive of breastfeeding.
◆ Mother may not know about growth spurts.
◆ Mother is worried about her baby getting enough milk.
◆ Mother is not getting enough encouragement to breastfeed.
◆ Mother fears that if she breastfeeds, it may make sister look like a failure.
◆ Mother has a ready excuse if anything goes wrong.
◆ Mother is not sure how long she wants to breastfeed.

Asking Open-Ended Questions

Asking open-ended questions is a useful skill for gathering information. It is the most direct way of finding out what you want to know. An open-ended question is one that cannot be answered by a simple "yes" or "no." Questions requiring only a *yes* or a *no* response are those that begin with words such as "are," "is," "do," or "does." These closed questions give you only minimal information and tend to shut down the conversation. Open-ended questions require answers that are more informative. They are the same questions a good reporter asks: "who," "what," "when," "where," "why," "how," "how much," and "how often."

If you ask, "Are you eating well?" the mother will probably answer, "Yes," and you gain no helpful information. You can change to an open-ended question by asking, "What did you eat today?" or "What do you usually eat for breakfast?" The mother's answers to these questions will tell you more about her diet and eating patterns.

In another example, you may suspect the baby is feeding infrequently and ask, "Does Rachel nurse often enough?" The mother can reply "Yes" or "No" and you will not have learned much. When you ask, "How many times does Rachel nurse in 24 hours?" you learn more about Rachel's breastfeeding pattern. Think about what you want to learn and then word the question in your mind before asking it, so that you get more information than a simple "yes" or "no." As with many counseling skills, asking open-ended questions becomes easier and more natural with practice.

When you use open-ended questions, take care not to pose too many questions in sequence. Avoid an interrogating manner that may cause the mother to feel threatened or irritated. Continually asking questions can establish a poor model for the relationship. The mother may learn to expect that when she describes symptoms and complaints you will provide a solution from your wealth of information. You can discourage this pattern from the very beginning of a conversation by setting up a

FIGURE 5.3
Words that reflect feelings.

Words that reflect "upset"	Words that reflect "happy"
angry	accepted
anxious	appreciated
defeated	better
difficult	capable
disappointed	comfortable
discouraged	competent
disrespected	confident
doubtful	empowered
embarrassed	encouraged
feel like giving up	enjoy
frightened	excited
guilty	glad
hate, hated	good
hopeless	grateful
hurt	great
inadequate	happy
left out	love, loved
miserable	pleased
put down	proud
rejected	reassured
sad	relieved
stupid	respected
unhappy	satisfied
unloved	validated
worried	wonderful
worthless	

FIGURE 5.4
Interpreting a mother's statements.

Mother: I'm 7 months pregnant, and I'd really like to breast-feed my baby. Everybody in my family thinks I'm crazy.

Counselor: It sounds like the idea of breastfeeding is new and unfamiliar to your family.

Mother: My mother can't understand why I'd even want to. It's kind of hard for me to explain it myself. It's just kind of a feeling I have.

Counselor: So you're saying you would like to breastfeed this baby.

Mother: Yes, I do really want to. But my husband kind of thinks of breasts, as something that belong in the centerfold of *Playboy*.

Counselor: Your husband doesn't want you to use your breasts to feed the baby.

Mother: No, it's not that exactly. I'm just not sure he understands what breastfeeding is all about.

---

friendly atmosphere that encourages the mother to talk on a conversational level rather than answer a series of questions. Your goal is to encourage the mother to talk freely and to develop her own solutions whenever possible. Balancing open-ended questions with other guiding skills promotes the mother's self-sufficiency, builds her self-confidence, and discourages her dependence on you.

Interpreting

Like active listening, the skill of interpreting clarifies, shows acceptance, and encourages a mother to respond. An interpreting response provides an analysis of what the mother says. It contains more of your thoughts and feelings than the simple rephrasing of what the mother said such as, "So you're saying that . . ." or "It sounds like you are saying . . ." or "That must mean. . . ." Drawing together several of the mother's statements and adding your tentative conclusions is a way to interpret what she said.

Leave the door open for the mother to process what you have said and correct you if she believes you have misinterpreted her message. The goal of interpreting is to reflect the meaning of the conversation so the mother can see her situation in new ways and learn to interpret events in her life. You can use this skill to listen and respond

empathetically. In the example in Figure 5.4, the counselor interprets each statement the mother makes. In an actual counseling session, you would not interpret one statement after another. This is simply an illustration of the technique. In the final response, the counselor misinterprets what the mother said and the mother corrects her.

Figure 5.5 presents further examples that distinguish between interpreting and active listening. These examples illustrate the similarity between the two skills. Essentially, interpreting is a form of empathetic listening, which we learned earlier is the highest level of active listening. Although you can use interpreting to analyze a conversation and to help a mother gain perspective, use it with discretion. Take care not to cause the mother to feel annoyed or offended by your interpretations. Use this technique when you have a clear impression of what she is saying and when the mother seems to need help in sorting out her feelings.

Focusing

Focusing is useful when a mother seems to be rambling or changing the direction to an unrelated topic. Typically, a mother will raise several topics during a conversation. When you believe the mother has touched on her main concerns, you can focus the conversation by pursuing one aspect you believe could be useful to her. The goal of focusing is to pursue a more meaningful dialogue that increases understanding for both of you.

To focus the conversation, you could select one particular point to repeat or could condense a number of points into a selective summary in order to concentrate on such things as how the mother feels and how the

---

FIGURE 5.5
Distinguishing between interpreting and active listening.

Mother of a 4-week-old infant: "I can't get anything done during the day because I'm nursing all the time." (Frustrated)

◆ You feel your housework is getting away from you. (*Interpreting*)

◆ You're surprised a newborn needs so much time. (*Active listening*)

◆ You wish you had more time to do other things. (*Interpreting*)

◆ You seem to be nursing all day. (*Active listening*)

Mother of a 2-month-old infant: "Johnny is still waking up 2 times during the night, and I feel like a zombie most days." (Yawning)

◆ You're wondering if you'll ever get a good night's sleep. (*Interpreting*)

◆ You feel tired because your sleep is interrupted. (*Active listening*)

◆ It seems as if this will go on forever. (*Interpreting*)

◆ You're wishing Johnny would sleep longer at night. (*Active listening*)

Mother of a 2-month-old infant: "My physician said Jimmy was doing very well, but then he said it was time to start cereal twice a day." (Confused)

◆ You're wondering if Jimmy needs solid foods at this time. (*Active listening*)

◆ You don't feel Jimmy needs solid foods yet. (*Interpreting*)

◆ You're wondering why your doctor suggested cereal at this time. (*Active listening*)

Mother of a 1-year-old child: "Tommy and I enjoyed breastfeeding so much, and now all of a sudden he would rather do other things than breastfeed." (Disappointed)

◆ You seem to miss the daytime feedings. (*Interpreting*)

◆ Nursing times were such happy and warm times for you and Tommy. (*Active listening*)

◆ Tommy seems to prefer his toys and other activities. (*Active listening*)

Pregnant woman: "I want to breastfeed but I'm not interested in classes. Natural childbirth is horrible." (Fearful)

◆ You don't want to go through that. (*Active listening*)

◆ You think natural childbirth is painful. (*Interpreting*)

◆ It sounds as though you've heard about some unpleasant experiences. (*Interpreting*)

◆ Natural childbirth is not what you want. (*Active listening*)

---

baby has been acting. Focusing is especially helpful with a very talkative mother. It is a way to bring her back to the important points that may really help her. You might say things like, "Tell me more about . . ." or "Can we talk about . . . again?" With focusing, you sort through the various issues to identify any topics you need to explore further. Consider the following conversation:

> Mother: Hi, Sue. I really liked the book you recommended on breastfeeding and the family. I just wish my husband would have been willing to read it. I gave it to my neighbor. She's going to have a baby next month. . . .
>
> Counselor: You say your husband needs to learn more about breastfeeding?
>
> Mother: He sure could. He's really kind of uptight about what our two kids are going to think when they see me breastfeeding. They're getting older now. My son Bobby is going out for Little League, and he's really a pretty good pitcher for a kid his age. And my daughter who's in nursery school only knows about bottles.
>
> Counselor: Let's get back to your husband. He's afraid of how your kids will react when they see you breastfeeding the new baby?

The mother had referred to her husband's attitude twice. It was also the first personal topic she mentioned. Often, the mother's first statement will give a clue about her concerns, as will the number of times she brings up a topic. You can use your feelings of confusion and sense of direction as a guide in deciding when and how to focus the conversation. With practice, this skill becomes almost second nature. After you have focused the conversation, you can be alert to feedback from the mother to make sure that she considers the topic worth pursuing.

Summarizing

Summarizing pulls together important points of a conversation. This is especially helpful when you and the mother have talked for a long time. It helps both of you to go over the highlights of the conversation and reinforce important aspects. The mother may need to hear the plan of care again, clearly and briefly, so that she is certain of what to try.

Summarizing reassures the mother that you hear her message and that you understand her. When possible, urge the mother to do the summarizing. This will indicate her understanding, as well as help her assume responsibility. You may say, for example, "Let's see. In order to change your baby's schedule from daytime to nighttime sleeping, which things will you try?"

Example of a summarizing response:

Counselor: "You have been having trouble expressing your milk at work. We talked about finding a more private place to pump, playing some soothing music, and trying to schedule a longer break so you don't feel so rushed. I will e-mail you my information sheet on working and nursing. How does that all sound?"

Influencing

Influencing the mother in a positive way can encourage her to continue to seek help and work toward a solution. A new mother often is unsure of herself. She may find that the reality of caring for her baby does not match her expectations. This may cause her to become discouraged or susceptible to poor advice. Heartening words from you can often counteract these negative factors to give reassurance, build hope, and identify her strengths.

Reassuring

Reassuring is an influencing skill that gives the mother perspective and lets her know that many babies act like her baby—they have fussy periods, do not sleep through the night, do not nap when you want them to, nurse frequently, and so on. Reassuring can help a mother see that her situation is normal.

Reassuring does have some limitations. Because it is easy to use, there may be a tendency to overuse it. Reassurance efforts sometimes come across as insincere sympathy or as a means of avoiding discussing the mother's concern. Be careful not to give the impression that you are minimizing the importance of her feelings or concerns. You can gently let her know that it is okay to feel the way she does and assure her that her situation will improve. Keep in mind that your goal is to build the mother's confidence. This will help you decide when reassuring is appropriate.

Example of reassuring responses:

Counselor: "Even though breastfeeding in front of relatives can be difficult, it gets easier the more you do it."

Counselor: "You are really going through a rough period. The first ten days of breastfeeding are the most challenging. It will get easier as you and your baby become more experienced."

Building Hope

Hope is the mother's main antidote to discouragement and is a source of relief from tension and unmet expectations. It gives the mother who is experiencing a bad time the feeling that the future may bring relief. Begin building hope by encouraging the mother to talk about her feelings. Help her see how her feelings relate to her present situation and how appropriate action can change that situation. Encouraging active participation helps the mother feel better and gets her functioning at an effective level. Mothers with such long-term conditions as persistent sore nipples, a fussy baby, an unsupportive family, or who has returned to work can usually benefit from your use of this technique.

Example of responses that build hope:

Counselor: "Your aunt really discourages you by giving your baby a bottle, doesn't she? Would it help to give her some information on the importance of exclusive breastfeeding?"

Counselor: "Since you returned to work, you seem to feel like you are not giving your baby enough attention. Maybe you could set aside the first hour when you get home for just nursing and being together."

Identifying Strengths

Identifying strengths is a form of praise that helps a mother focus on her positive qualities. It counteracts negative factors such as fatigue, a crying infant, or failure to meet preconceived expectations. Reminding the mother of how well she handled a situation or of a natural ability she has can encourage her to continue to work out an answer to her present concern. Reviewing past experiences from which the mother learned and grew can help her realize that she is capable of handling her present situation. It encourages her to develop and rely on her resources and is a step in the direction of self-sufficiency. Discussing how past problems were resolved is the essence of this technique. Other growth experiences such as childbirth offer fruitful discussions. Be careful to select experiences that you know had positive outcomes so that the discussion is uplifting.

Recalling peak moments can be another way to identify strengths for the mother. Happy, exciting times such as her baby's first smile, a sibling's helpfulness, or an enjoyable evening with other new parents are pleasant memories for the mother. They can help a new mother perceive her mothering experience as positive. She will see that she, her baby, and her family are special and that more memorable experiences will continue. Recalling peak experiences is a type of praise that gives the mother a positive outlook and lets her know that you have taken an interest in her by the fact that you can recall important events in her life.

Example of responses that identify strengths:

Counselor: "You handled that well."

Counselor: "You seem really tuned into your baby's needs."

Counselor: "You're the only one who can do that for your baby."

Practicing the Use of Guiding Skills

There are a number of listening, facilitating, and influencing skills that may be used in a given situation. The example in Table 5.3 illustrates the use of each of these skills. Table 5.4 presents less helpful responses to the same statement. The next section contains statements that you can use to practice your use of guiding skills. First read the types of responses that would be least helpful or encouraging to the mother. These may even be comments you have heard others make to mothers. They are followed by more positive and helpful responses based on the skills discussed in this chapter.

TABLE 5.3
Effective Use of Guiding Skills

A pregnant woman says, "I'm afraid that breastfeeding might make my child too dependent."

Listening responses	◆ Attending	*Hmmm, you do . . .*
	◆ Active listening	*You're worried that breastfeeding will make your child too dependent.*
	◆ Empathetic listening	*You want your baby to grow into an independent child and you're not sure that breastfeeding will make that possible.*
Facilitating responses	◆ Clarifying	*What do you mean by "too dependent?"*
	◆ Interpreting	*You believe the dependency associated with breastfeeding will keep your child from exploring his world.*
	◆ Asking open-ended questions	*In what ways do you think breastfeeding will make your child too dependent?*
	◆ Focusing	*Let's get back to your concerns about. . . . (This would be used later if it becomes necessary to focus on the mother's primary concern—dependence, or feelings of inadequacy as a prospective parent, or other concern.)*
	◆ Summarizing	*We talked about. . . . (This would be used later to go over the main points of this topic.)*
Influencing responses	◆ Reassuring	*Being a parent can be confusing. Many bottle-feeding mothers also wonder how the attention they give their baby relates to later independence.*
	◆ Building hope	*You know, research has actually shown otherwise. Babies given more attention and physical contact in the early years grow up to be more independent.*
	◆ Identifying strengths	*It's great that you are concerned about your baby's independence. How do you feel you can encourage him to become independent?*

TABLE 5.4
Unhelpful Responses to a Mother's Concern

A pregnant woman says, "I'm afraid that breastfeeding might make my child too dependent."

Unhelpful responses	◆ Disagreeing	*No, it makes him more independent.*
	◆ Criticizing	*That's because you don't know how babies learn to be independent.*
	◆ Ordering	*You need to read a book on parenting.*
	◆ Sharing experiences	*I used to think that way too. I remember when . . .*
	◆ Changing the topic	*I really wanted to talk to you about . . .*
	◆ Moralizing	*You really don't want your child to be so independent . . .*

My labor wasn't what I expected.

- Be glad you have a healthy baby.
- At least it's all behind you.
- That's why they call it labor!
- You're disappointed with the way it turned out.
- It didn't go the way you hoped it would.

I'm not sure what to do when the nurse brings my baby to me.

- Just hold him close to your breast and he'll figure it out.
- Haven't you read any books on breastfeeding?
- The lactation consultant will be here soon.
- You're unsure of yourself.
- You're feeling a bit overwhelmed.

I wish the doctor would spend more time with me.

- Doctors have a busy schedule.
- I can get you the doctor's telephone number.
- You have some unanswered questions.
- Are there any questions I can help you with?

I have to go back to work in six weeks.

- You're lucky to have a job.
- At least you can breastfeed until then.
- A lot of women combine breastfeeding and working.
- You're not sure you want to leave your baby.
- You're wondering how you can manage it.

My doctor says I have to give my baby formula.

- Your doctor knows best.
- A little formula won't hurt your baby.
- You don't want to give your baby formula.
- You don't understand why your baby needs formula.

My baby cries all the time.

- Try letting him cry himself to sleep.
- It will get better.
- You're worried you may not have enough milk.
- You're worried he doesn't want to breastfeed.

The Leading Method

The presence of a problem or concern the mother is unable to solve with her existing resources distinguishes the leading method in counseling from the guiding method. Through educating and problem solving, you provide her with additional resources to lead her toward a solution. The use of leading responses changes the nature of the relationship between you and the mother from what it was during the guiding phase. In guiding, you encourage the mother to do most of the talking. In leading, more responsibility for the direction of the discussion falls on you rather than the mother.

The goal of leading is for both you and the mother to understand her problem and to develop a plan of care.

During the guiding phase, you will have gathered sufficient information and impressions from the mother so that you are able to enter into effective problem solving. You can help the mother toward understanding by educating her and offering her two or three possible solutions. The mother then will decide which suggestions she will try, based on her perception of the situation.

During the leading phase, it is important that the decision of specific action rests with the mother in order to develop her self-sufficiency. The mother may need this kind of reinforcement, especially at a time when she is doubtful of her parenting abilities in other areas. "When do I pick up my baby?" "How warmly should I dress him?" "How do I care for him so that he will grow up to reach his potential?" Encourage mothers to make their own decisions on these issues.

The leading method works well when a mother clearly needs additional information or direction. When you have gathered enough information through listening and facilitating so that your leads are not premature or incorrect, your evaluation of the situation will be more accurate and you will be able to determine when leading is appropriate. You first need to take sufficient time to gain the mother's trust and clarify the situation so that you will know when leading will be helpful. Then you can intervene and educate the mother, working with her to overcome obstacles and find solutions.

Informing

Informing involves educating and explaining how something functions and why. It can range from stating a simple fact about nutrition to educating parents on the production of human milk. By providing parents with the proper information at the appropriate time, you help them grow as parents. Parents learn about breastfeeding at childbirth preparation and breastfeeding classes, at support group meetings, and from caregivers, friends, and relatives. Some of what they hear may be cultural myths or fallacies. You can educate them by suggesting appropriate reading material. Following up with discussions of parents' questions and ideas enhances the reading material and inspires parents to educate themselves further.

Explaining why things happen the way they do often makes basic facts more meaningful and more acceptable. For example, stating to a mother, "The more frequently you breastfeed, the more milk you will produce," may not convince her to feed her baby more frequently. Explaining briefly how nipple stimulation increases hormone production which in turn increases milk production will help her understand the process. When the mother develops understanding, she is more likely to institute changes that make her actions compatible with her new knowledge.

Before giving information to a mother, allow her enough time to explore her concerns and to determine what she needs to know. Ask yourself: "Does this mother need information?" If so: "How much information does she need?" Finally: "Is this the best time to educate her?" Determining the appropriate time—the teachable moment—for educating the mother can be critical to her accepting and processing the information. After you have determined what facts the mother needs, you can educate her, remembering to limit the amount of information so that it does not confuse or overwhelm her.

Example of responses that inform:

> Counselor: "Maybe it would help to understand what happens when a baby has a growth spurt. As your baby grows . . ."
>
> Counselor: "One way to tell if you are having letdown is by the leaking you're noticing from the other breast. When your baby suckles . . ."

Correcting a Misconception or Mismanagement

There will be times when you need to correct a mother's perception of something or correct the way she is managing her breastfeeding. If a mother is convinced that she will need to wean her baby when he gets teeth, you might first start with an active listening response such as, "It seems like it will hurt when your baby has teeth." Then continue with something like, "You will find that your baby's tongue covers his bottom teeth when he breastfeeds." You have cleared up the mother's misconception and at the same time, you are giving support by accepting her statement. Moreover, you corrected her perception without saying "but!"

Using a warm and friendly tone of voice, you can supply a mother with information without making her feel foolish or uninformed. Remember that you want to avoid telling a mother she "should" do something. Rather than saying, "You should . . ." or "I think . . . ," you can say "You may want to . . ." or "You may find that when you. . . ." These types of responses will educate her and preserve her self-confidence.

Example of a response to tactfully clear up a misconception:

> Mother: Isn't it great the way you don't get your period while you're breastfeeding?
>
> Counselor: Yes, that's true for some women. It doesn't always happen that way. There's a lot of variation among individuals. When you are lactating, . . . [You can then go on to explain about the effect of lactation on menstruation and ovulation. The mother had the general idea and just needed some clarification.]

Problem Solving

An important element in your role as a consultant to the mother is helping her when problems arise with her breastfeeding. As you gather information, you can sort through the facts and help her clarify her situation.

While guiding the mother, you may become aware that she has a problem. However, this is not always the case. Obtaining sufficient information and impressions will avoid your jumping in with irrelevant or unnecessary problem-solving advice.

To begin the problem-solving process, you will form your first hunch about what the mother's problem may be. Based on that hunch, you will look for additional factors to confirm that your hunch is correct. You can then test your hunch by suggesting to the mother what you consider her situation to be. If you both agree on the interpretation of the situation, you can go on to develop a plan of care together.

If the mother provides additional information that reveals your hunch to be incorrect, you will need to explore alternative hunches, reverting to guiding skills to gain more insight and information. After you and the mother have identified the problem, you are ready to develop a plan. Chapter 6 discusses each of the steps in the problem-solving process in more detail.

Combining the Guiding and Leading Methods

The most effective approach to counseling emphasizes the use of guiding skills. These skills best clarify the mother's message. You want to begin each contact with those listening techniques that help "feel mothers out" and provide them with emotional support. Guiding skills encourage the mother to determine the direction of the conversation. They will produce the information and impressions you need before going on to problem solving.

A conversation may reach a point where you realize the mother either has no problem or can handle her problem adequately. You can then end the conversation with a summary of what you talked about and any plan of care. When you determine that the mother needs further assistance, you can use your leading skills to educate or problem solve as needed.

By avoiding active participation early in the contact, you allow the mother the maximum opportunity to resolve her situation, which encourages her emotional growth and increased self-confidence. A conversation typically swings back and forth from guiding to leading as different topics arise. Achieving a balance between leading and guiding will help provide a clear picture of the situation and build the mother's confidence.

The counseling conversation in Table 5.5 concerns a mother and her three-month-old infant. It shows how the use of counseling skills defines a problem and progresses through the problem-solving process. Guiding and leading skills are intermingled, with the counselor taking the lead only when the mother's conversation wanders from the main concern or when she needs options pointed out to her. This nonassertive role of the

TABLE 5.5

Counseling Example of Guiding and Leading Skills

Mother	Counselor Response	Comments
(Sounding weary and discouraged) I'm so tired. My baby has been getting up three times a night for the last three nights.	You really sound discouraged, Linda.	Counselor uses *active listening* to provide emotional support. She personalize the exchange by using the mother's name.
Yeah. I thought we were really getting somewhere when Michael slept through the night last week. And now he acts starved at night. He eats and eats.	It seems to you like Michael is backsliding.	Counselor continues to give emotional support through *active listening*. She personalize the exchange by using the baby's name.
I'll say. And just when my sister and her three kids have come for a week's visit.	Mmmm. That's a lot of company.	Counselor uses an *attending* response and *forms a hunch* that the mother is too active and her milk production has decreased. The mother did not say anything about her activities with her sister, whether she's doing too much, and so on. So the counselor cannot assume immediately that the mother is too tired and the baby isn't getting enough milk. She needs to wait for the mother's response to know if this hunch is correct.
It *is* a lot of people, but my sister is very helpful. She's doing most of the cooking, and she keeps my house in better shape than I do!	That's great for you, Linda. So she's really more help than work for you.	Counselor learns that her first hunch was incorrect. She uses *active listening* to encourage the mother to give her more information. She uses the mother's name to personalize the exchange.
Definitely.	Let's get back to Michael. What's he like during the day?	Counselor *focuses* the mother back on the baby and uses the baby's name to personalize the exchange. She uses an *open-ended question* to seek additional information. She is *looking for hidden factors* that will help identify the problem.
Well, he eats around 8:00 when he wakes up, then again around 10:30 before his nap. He sleeps until 1:00, then eats again. He eats again around 3:00, then takes another nap until about 6:00. Then he fusses and eats a couple of times during the evening and goes to bed about 10:00. At least that's what he's done the last couple of days.	Let's see, Linda, that's about 6 feedings during the day, that's 9 in 24 hours. How does each feeding go?	Counselor uses the mother's name again to personalize the exchange. She *summarizes* what the mother has told her and asks an *open-ended question* to gain more information.

(continued)

TABLE 5.5 (CONTINUED)

Counseling Example of Guiding and Leading Skills

Mother	Counselor Response	Comments
Well, he fools around a lot, eating, looking around, and watching my sister's kids.	You know, Linda, this is the age when babies are easily distracted by people and motion and noise.	Counselor uses the mother's name and then responds with *interpreting* to test whether these distractions are the cause of the problem.
Michael is definitely distracted. Every time someone comes near he lets go and looks at them.	It's hard for Michael to pay attention to eating with so many people around.	Counselor uses the baby's name in an *active listening* response to voice an *alternative hunch*.
That's right.	So you're saying that Michael is distracted a lot during the day and seems really hungry at night.	Counselor uses the baby's name in an *interpreting* response to *test the hunch*.
Do you think he might be making up for not getting enough milk during the day? (This interpretation makes sense and she is pondering it.)	That seems to be a possibility.	Counselor uses an *attending* response to encourage the mother to add information that might shed more light on the situation.
That makes sense. When Michael and I were alone for a feeding yesterday, he ate for a long time and took an exceptionally long nap.	He seemed to sleep better when he ate with no distractions.	Counselor received confirmation that the *hunch* was correct and she uses an *interpreting* response.
Yeah. He did.	Linda, perhaps it might help if you breastfed Michael in a quieter place during the day.	Counselor uses the mother's and baby's names and *suggests an alternative action*.
I could go into the living room. The kids pretty much stay in the family room, and my sister and I could talk quietly.	Good idea. You might also try waking Michael sooner from his long afternoon nap and giving him an extra feeding in the afternoon.	Counselor uses the baby's name and *suggests an alternative action*. The mother has accepted the first suggestion and is trying to adapt it to her situation. The counselor will want to document this. It is the beginning of a *plan of action*.
Well, I could, but that would interfere with my making supper. I really like that quiet time to make supper, and I hate to work on supper in the morning.	It wouldn't work for you. Okay, so you're going to try to breastfeed Michael in a quieter place, to see if you can satisfy him during the day so he'll sleep better at night.	Counselor realizes the mother does not like the second suggestion and uses *active listening* as a graceful way to withdraw the rejected suggestion. By not pushing it, the counselor shows that she supports the mother and recognizes her right to make her own decisions on how to handle her situation. She uses the baby's name while *summarizing* what they have discussed and arriving at a *plan of action*. Although this example limits the plan to one option, there undoubtedly would be more suggestions in a real-life situation.
Yes.	Great, Linda! Please give me a call next week to let me know how this has worked. Feel free to call me before then if you need to.	Counselor uses the mother's name and *arranges follow-up*.

counselor encourages the mother to actively participate in the problem-solving process. It helps the mother understand and work out a solution that will suit her circumstance.

The Follow-up Method

Follow-up is an ongoing process that takes place during and after every counseling contact. By objectively analyzing the contact, you can determine what you and the mother accomplished and how to plan subsequent contact that will be most beneficial to her. You can also research outside sources such as literature and resource people to obtain information to meet the mother's special needs. You will then renew the counseling process with new information and a new perspective.

Generally, each individual contact requires some form of follow-up. The mother's level of need and the urgency of the situation will determine the nature of the follow-up and how soon and frequent it should be. The elements of follow-up—evaluation, planning and arranging for the next contact, researching outside sources, and renewing the counseling process—are discussed in the following sections.

Evaluating the Session

When **evaluating** a contact, ask whether the mother's needs were met for support, comfort, understanding, and action. Evaluate your use of counseling skills and the quality of information you gave to the mother. This approach enables you to determine the areas you need to explore further. The questions in Figure 5.6 will help you evaluate your contacts.

Evaluating can be very encouraging for you. It shows you how you have been helpful using counseling techniques such as supporting, clarifying, and educating. You will know that you have done a good job of counseling a mother if you can say some of these things to yourself:

◆ She freely talked about her concerns.

◆ She figured out what to do about her problem.

◆ She understood why the baby acted that way and what to do the next time.

◆ She seemed willing and eager to carry out the plan we developed.

It is especially important to evaluate yourself after you feel you have failed to help a particular mother. The best thing you can do is learn from such failures. You might find it helpful to discuss it with a colleague. You can plan how you will improve future contacts and recognize that as you gain more experience, you will increase your effectiveness and success. Be kind to yourself! It is through our failures and mistakes that we learn and grow. Bear in mind that you cannot always "fix" a breastfeeding problem. The problem belongs to the mother, and she owns the responsibility for resolving it. You offer your expertise; the ownership needs to be hers.

Arranging the Next Contact

As the final step in your evaluation, you will want to plan for your next contact with the mother. From your analysis of the mother's satisfaction and needs, you will be able to determine when the next contact needs to occur, if one is indicated. This may be through a follow-up telephone call or suggesting that she schedule a visit

---

FIGURE 5.6
Questions for evaluating a counseling contact.

1. What support did I give? In what other ways could I have supported the mother?

2. Did the mother require immediate physical comfort? If so, what suggestions did I offer?

3. Did I gather enough information so that the mother and I both understood the problem? If not, what further information do I need?

4. Did I give appropriate information? Did the mother understand it? If not, what information do I need to give to the mother during the next contact?

5. Did the mother seem relaxed and talkative? If not, what skills can I use in a new approach for the next contact in order to encourage her to talk freely?

6. What plan did the mother and I make? Is it workable? If not, what alternative actions could I suggest?

7. Did the mother seem satisfied with the contact? If not, what areas should I explore in future contacts?

8. What follow-up did the mother and I arrange? Is it adequate, or should I contact the mother sooner?

9. Did I take usable notes during or after the contact? How were notes from previous contacts with this mother helpful? How can I improve my method of documentation?

10. Did I form a partnership with this mother and empower her to be self-sufficient in her problem solving?

11. Am I satisfied in my helping role with this mother? If not, what can I do to bring about greater satisfaction?

with you. Also decide who will initiate the contact and what additional information or assistance you will need to provide.

You can judge how soon to get back to a mother by the urgency of her situation. If she is having difficulty at every feeding, daily or even more frequent support and information from you would probably be helpful. Whenever the mother needs emotional support, frequent contact is important. Less critical or short-term problems usually require less frequent contact. For example, a mother who is becoming discouraged trying to use an electric breast pump to get milk for her **premature infant** in the hospital might benefit from your contacting her every day for a while. A mother whose problem is a nonsupportive or interfering family member might prefer to talk with you periodically rather than daily.

Contact the mother any time you gain important new information, need to correct information you gave, or realize that you need to gather more information to resolve a problem. The mother will appreciate such concern about her welfare and that of her baby. Be sensitive to signals from the mother that she no longer feels the need for your continued follow-up.

Always make sure the mother understands that she may call you before the next prearranged contact. If you asked a mother to call you and she does not, you may want to contact her. Many lactation consultants use e-mail communication with mothers, which minimizes missed calls. If you work in a busy practice and are unable to initiate frequent contact with mothers, a referral relationship with a support group in your community can provide the needed follow-up. You may then refer mothers to the support group or give mothers the name of a contact person.

Researching Outside Sources

At times, you may need to gain further input and a fresh outlook on a problem. This is especially true if a situation is outside the realm of your usual counseling. It is important that you recognize your own need for assistance. There may be issues you have overlooked. You are not required to have every piece of information about breastfeeding immediately available. You should, however, know where to find the information and when to use your resources.

Contacting another experienced lactation consultant to discuss the issue may provide you with a new perspective. Your colleague may suggest additional information you need to obtain from the mother, such as how the baby is acting between feedings or what the baby's physician says about the weight gain. You can also gain valuable support from a colleague. Internet resources such as Lactnet, the e-mail list for lactation professionals, and lactation Web sites are invaluable. It is

important that you ask for help whenever you are involved in a situation that you are not able to resolve with your available resources.

Renewing the Counseling Process

The counseling process starts all over again with each successive contact. Begin with guiding skills and then progress to leading skills, just as in the original contact. You might start with an opening question such as, "Hi, Jen. This is Heather. How have things been going since we last talked?" Next, listen carefully to what the mother says. Perhaps everything you suggested worked and the problem is resolved. More likely, you can still help the mother work through a problem or concern.

▶ ## COUNSELING EXAMPLES

The counseling scenarios in the next section illustrate the use of counseling skills in a consultation. Pay particular attention to the lactation consultant's listening skills and use of emotional support for the mother. Note the plan of care and follow-up arrangements between the mother and lactation consultant. Guiding skills are interspersed throughout the contact. Abbreviations used to identify counseling skills are shown in Figure 5.7. The elements typically will progress roughly in the order in which they appear in the list.

Counseling Example with a Pregnant Woman

In Figure 5.8, Jan starts with open-ended questions to learn more about Kelly's situation. Then she uses active listening to clarify Kelly's feelings. She focuses on Kelly's main concern by asking why she felt that some women have difficulty breastfeeding. It becomes clear that a lack of information contributed to Kelly's hesitation to commit to breastfeeding. Jan begins to educate her and offer Kelly suggestions on how to learn more about breastfeeding.

FIGURE 5.7 Abbreviations for skills.	
ES	Emotional support
AL	Active listening
I	Interpreting
OEQ	Open-ended question
IS	Identifying strengths
F	Focusing
E	Educating
PS	Practical suggestion
S	Summarizing
FU	Follow-up

FIGURE 5.8
Counseling example with a pregnant woman.

Kelly, a pregnant woman, arrives for an appointment with Jan, the lactation consultant.

Jan: Hi Kelly! I'm glad you came to see me. When is your baby due? (OEQ)

Kelly: Oh, the baby's due in about 6 weeks. We are really getting excited!

Jan: It is exciting having a baby! (AL) Is this your first child?

Kelly: Yes, it is, and I wanted to talk to you about breastfeeding. I can't decide if breastfeeding is right for me.

Jan: You're not positive you want to breastfeed. (AL)

Kelly: Well, at first I kind of wanted to breastfeed, but my sister recently had a baby and she had so many problems that I just don't know. . . .

Jan: So, you would like to breastfeed, and you want to make sure you don't have the same problems. (I)

Kelly: Yes, it seems like I have talked with so many people who had problems that I don't think I want to even try.

Jan: That's understandable. Why do you think your sister had difficulty breastfeeding? (F) (LC acting on hunch that Kelly doesn't know much about breastfeeding.)

Kelly: I'm not sure. She didn't really know what to do.

Jan: It's true that many women have problems because they don't have the correct information about breastfeeding. (E) What kind of problems did your sister have? (OEQ)

Kelly: Oh, I can't exactly remember. It seems to me she had sore nipples, the baby was crying all the time, and she just didn't have enough milk. She just decided it wasn't worth it and then she quit. And then I have a friend who started breastfeeding and quit because her baby wanted to nurse all the time and she never could go anywhere. I really don't want to be tied down.

Jan: It's too bad your friend felt so hassled because it is possible for a mother to do a number of things to fit breastfeeding into your life. Would you consider postponing your decision about breastfeeding until you learn a little more about it?

Kelly: Well, I've got time to make a decision, and I would like to try breastfeeding if I could be sure that it wouldn't be an ordeal like my sister had.

Jan: There is no way to guarantee breastfeeding will be completely trouble free. Educating yourself will help you avoid most problems. You could start by reading some of our pamphlets on breastfeeding. Here's one on common questions mothers have and another one on how the breast makes milk. It would also help for you to attend a breastfeeding class. There is one coming up next week on Thursday night that you could attend with your husband. I can also give you the number of a support group near you. (PS) Where would you like to start? (OEQ)

Kelly: Well, these pamphlets look interesting. Do they cover how to keep from having problems?

Jan: Some problems are covered. See, sore nipples and low milk supply are in here. If you read this first, then we can talk about other concerns you have and I can suggest more reading if you like. What about the breastfeeding class? (OEQ/F)

Kelly: Yeah, that would probably be okay. I'll have to check with my husband and make sure he's free. Next Thursday night did you say?

Jan: Yes. The class meets right here in our office from 7:30 to 9:30, and because I'm teaching, we'll have an opportunity to talk again. There are several couples signed up for the class, so that will give your husband a chance to talk to some prospective breastfeeding dads, too. So, you are going to read the pamphlets, and then come to the class on Thursday night. (S) I will plan to see you then. If you have any questions before Thursday and you want to talk, don't hesitate to call me. (FU)

Kelly: Great. I'll see you next week. Thanks a lot!

Jan is careful not to overwhelm Kelly with information about the importance of human milk or reasons why she should breastfeed. Although that is important information, she can address it another time. Together, Jan and Kelly form a plan of reading and attending the breastfeeding class. Jan summarizes the plan and arranges for follow-up.

Comparison of Two Lactation Consultants

It is instructive to illustrate the differences between effective and ineffective counseling scenarios for the same mother. Figure 5.9 demonstrates the consequences of ineffective communication techniques. Figure 5.10 portrays the same scenario, with the lactation consultant using the counseling techniques presented in this chapter.

In Figure 5.9, Pam fails to provide emotional support and does not listen or respond to the mother's concerns about her emergency cesarean birth and failed birth plan. She does not pick up on Steph's feelings of inadequacy—that the nurses did such a good job and Steph feels as though she cannot do anything right. Steph needs to know that her feelings are normal and that a sleepy infant is normal. Pam may inadvertently contribute to underlying feelings of guilt by saying that Steph's pain medication caused the sleepiness.

FIGURE 5.9
Ineffective counseling technique.

Steph is in her hospital room with her 2-day-old infant Michael. Pam, the lactation consultant, comes to visit.

Pam: Hi, Steph! How are you doing today?

Steph: Oh, not very good.

Pam: Why? What's the matter?

Steph: I don't know. You know, I planned to have a natural childbirth with Bob in the delivery room, but I had to have an emergency c-section, and things just aren't going well.

Pam: Well, these things happen. You know the important thing is that you have a healthy baby, and my gosh, c-sections nowadays are almost as common as vaginal deliveries. It really isn't such a big deal any more.

Steph: I suppose. And I should just be grateful that he's healthy. But the other problem is that he isn't breastfeeding very well.

Pam: Really? Well, he sure looks content. Most c-section babies don't nurse very well the first couple of days anyway. He'll pick up.

Steph: All Michael wants to do is sleep all the time, and the nurses take real good care of him because I'm not moving around very well yet. His head is so floppy, and the nurses handle him so well. I'm afraid I might hurt him.

Pam: Isn't it great the nurses are so good with him! That saves you from having to do much, and you can get your rest. You'll have plenty of opportunity later on to take care of him.

Steph: Yeah, but I never get a chance to even hold him, and he's always too sleepy to nurse.

Pam: It's probably all the pain medication you are taking and the anesthesia you had during the c-section. Don't worry about it. He'll wake up and start breastfeeding better when you get home. You just take care of yourself and get plenty of rest while you have people around who can wait on you.

Steph: I guess you're right. I hope he'll do better. I'm really worried about him. I'm afraid he's starving.

Pam: Oh goodness, I'm sure they are giving him some formula in the nursery. Don't you worry. They won't let him starve. Well, listen. I've got to scoot. Nice seeing you. You look great! Give me a call if you need anything else.

Steph needs help learning to respond to her baby's feeding cues and wakeful times. She needs to see that she is capable of caring for and breastfeeding her baby. Pam could have accomplished this by offering specific suggestions on infant care and breastfeeding. Most of all, in this example, Pam is very impersonal and dismissive, failing to respond to Steph as an individual.

In Figure 5.10, as with many breastfeeding issues, the mother's state of mind and self-esteem are the factors that most influence her outcome. Pam listens to Steph and focuses on her concerns—disappointment over her birth experience and overall feelings of inadequacy. By building on Steph's ability to care for her infant and letting her know that awkwardness is common at first, Pam encourages Steph and helps her feel competent. By teaching Steph how to watch for Michael's cues and encouraging her to put Michael to breast on her own, she shows that she believes Steph can resolve her problem.

Best Start 3-Step Counseling Strategy©

Best Start Social Marketing teaches a comparable approach to counseling (Best Start, 2004). The Best Start 3-Step Counseling Strategy is divided into three components. The first step, asking open-ended questions, focuses on finding out as much as possible about the client's concerns. The second step is to affirm the client's feelings and to build a relationship with the client. Spending time on this step empowers the mother and helps to create an atmosphere of safety where she can feel confident sharing her concerns. It also serves as a bridge to the education the counselor will provide. The third step is to educate the client using the principles of adult education and offering information in small bites.

The Best Start approach is similar to the counseling method described earlier. It is designed to be simple, offering a three-step system that is easy for the clinician to remember. The technique places emphasis on listening and affirmation, both of which are prominent in the technique presented previously in this chapter. One difference is that the Best Start plan begins with questions and then moves to statements of affirmation. The guiding method described earlier begins with emotional support (affirmation) before gathering information through guiding statements and limited use of open-ended questions. It continues with affirming statements throughout the contact. Both systems follow these two steps with education and emphasize the avoidance of overwhelming the client with too much information. The leading method ends with a final step of follow-up, which the Best Start plan does not include. Both systems have the same goal of empowering the mother, validating her concerns, and equipping her with problem-solving skills.

FIGURE 5.10
Effective counseling technique.

Steph is in her hospital room with her 2-day-old infant Michael. Pam, the lactation consultant, comes to visit.

Pam: Hi, Steph! How are you doing today?

Steph: Oh, not very good.

Pam: Oh, Steph, that's too bad. (ES) What seems to be the problem? (OEQ)

Steph: I don't know. You know, I planned to have a natural childbirth with Bob in the delivery room, but I had to have an emergency c-section, and well, things just aren't going well.

Pam: What a disappointment! (ES) It is really hard when your birth experience doesn't go the way you planned. (AL).

Steph: I *am* disappointed. And I feel guilty for feeling disappointed, because Michael is beautiful and healthy, and that is all I should be concerned about. But I can't help wishing Bob could have been there to see him being born, and I feel as though both of us missed out somehow. To top it off, he isn't even breastfeeding well. He's too sleepy.

Pam: Steph, there is nothing wrong with feeling disappointed or even really angry. You need to have time to grieve your lost birth experience. Your feelings are part of the grieving process, and you need time to work it through. Being upset does not make you a bad person or ungrateful for your beautiful little boy. Expressing your feelings is healing. And this is important. (E/S) You feel as though you can't do anything right because first of all you had to have a c-section, and now he won't even breastfeed! (I/AL)

Steph: That's right. Talk about being inadequate. And I feel so awkward with the baby. The nurses all know just what to do. They make it look so simple to hold up his floppy head, and change his diaper. And they wrap him perfectly in that blanket, just like a cute little mummy! When I do it, the blanket just falls apart.

Pam: You feel that because you are Michael's mom, you should be able to care for him better than anyone else. (I)

Steph: Yeah.

Pam: Learning all the best ways of caring for Michael takes time. Most first-time mothers feel inadequate at first. You and Michael just need time to adjust to each other, time to learn to communicate with one another. You can trust your intuition about how to care for him and respond to his needs. (IS/E) For example, you seem upset about his sleepiness. Have you been wondering if you should wake Michael up to feed him?

Steph: Umhm. I wondered if I should, if it would be all right. I wanted to try feeding him again, but then I wasn't sure how or when to go about it.

Pam: One of the best things to do is what you are doing right now, and that is keeping Michael with you as much as possible. That way, you can watch for his feeding cues, things like bringing his hands to his mouth or around his head, making little sucking motions, rapid eye movement, or rooting toward the breast when you hold him. Sometimes unwrapping him completely will rouse him out of a light sleep and remind him that it might be time to nurse. (IS/E)

Steph: But won't he get cold if I do that?

Pam: Your breasts are the warmest part of your body, and when Michael is snuggled up to you with skin-to-skin contact, he will stay warm and cozy. You can put his blanket over the two of you after he starts breastfeeding. (E)

Steph: Well, he's beginning to stir and looks as though he wants to suck on his hands. Should I try feeding him?

Pam: Super. Using a position like this (demonstrates) that holds your baby to the side is especially good so you can avoid putting pressure on your incision. Hold your breast so your fingers don't touch the dark part of your nipple. Now, gently touch his upper lip with your nipple. Look, there, he's opening his mouth really wide. Pull him gently to your breast nice and tight. Gently pressing on his back brings him in close without touching his head. He's got it! By George, I think he's got it! See, you know just what to do! Notice those long, drawing sucks? He's having a lovely lunch. (E/PS/IS)

Steph: It really helped having you here to get us started. How long should I let him nurse?

Pam: As long as he continues to breastfeed with those long **nutritive** sucks. After he's feeling pretty content, his hands will probably relax, and he'll drift off to sleep or come off your breast spontaneously. In either case, you can then put him to breast on the other side. If he wakes up and breastfeeds some more, that's fine. If he continues to sleep, that's okay, too. (E)

Steph: He's really nursing well now. I think we'll be okay. Thanks so much for your help.

Pam: I think you'll both be fine. Just trust your judgment, and if you can't figure out what to do, don't hesitate to ask for help. I'll stop in again tomorrow to see how you're getting along. (FU)

▶ SUMMARY

With the use of basic counseling techniques, you can provide mothers with the support and teaching that will help them develop confidence in their mothering and breastfeeding. Approaching mothers with a warm, caring attitude will show deep, genuine concern and empathy that help the mother feel understood and will empower her to take positive action in dealing with her concern. Guiding skills help keep the conversation going while you gather information and provide emotional support. With leading skills, you will take a more active role in directing the conversation and help the mother work toward developing a plan of care. The final stage of a contact is arranging appropriate follow-up and analyzing the effectiveness of your assistance and support. Developing and continuing to improve your use of counseling skills will enhance your effectiveness in communicating with parents.

▶ CHAPTER 5—AT A GLANCE

Applying what you learned—

◆ Recognize how your personality affects your rapport with mothers.

◆ Validate a mother's feelings, emotions, and concerns through attending, active listening, empathetic listening, reassuring, praising, and building hope.

◆ Help mothers with immediate physical comfort before problem solving when needed.

◆ Practice using counseling skills with family and friends to become proficient.

◆ Avoid active participation early in the contact to allow maximum opportunity for the mother to provide information and insights.

◆ Develop listening skills that actively respond to both verbal and nonverbal messages.

◆ Perceive with your ears, eyes, and imagination.

◆ Use active listening to gather information, clarify messages, show acceptance, and encourage a response.

◆ Use empathetic listening to understand emotionally and help the mother work through her feelings.

◆ Use clarifying, open-ended questions, interpreting, focusing, and summarizing to get more information, define the situation, and focus on specific concerns.

◆ Ask open-ended questions rather than closed questions to receive more information.

◆ Influence the mother positively by reassuring, building hope, and identifying her strengths.

◆ Gather enough information so your problem solving is not premature or incorrect.

◆ Take time to gain the mother's trust and clarify the situation before problem solving.

◆ Give parents proper information at the appropriate time to help them grow as parents.

◆ Correct misconceptions or mismanagement with sensitivity.

◆ Form your first hunch based on information and impressions you gained.

◆ Use a nonassertive approach to encourage the mother to be active in problem solving.

◆ Arrange appropriate follow-up after every contact by evaluating the session, planning and arranging for the next contact, and researching as needed.

◆ Make sure the mother knows she may call you any time.

▶ REFERENCES

Best Start. Best Start Social Marketing. Available at: www.beststartinc.org. Accessed May 8, 2004.

Birkman International. Birkman Method®. Available at: www.birkman.com. Accessed April 3, 2004.

Brammer LM. *The Helping Relationship.* Englewood Cliffs, NJ: Prentice Hall; 1973.

Inscape Publishing. DisC. Available at: www.inscapepublishing.com. Accessed April 3, 2004.

Myers-Briggs. Myers-Briggs Type Indicator®. Available at: www.cpp.com. Accessed April 3, 2004.

Wilson Learning. Wilson Social Styles. Available at: www.wilsonlearning.com. Accessed April 3, 2004.

CLIENT CONSULTATIONS

Contributing Author: Linda Kutner

Women have more positive outcomes breastfeeding when they receive consistent encouragement, help, and guidance at appropriate times. Caregivers find a preventive approach to breastfeeding care to be a time-saving approach that is far more effective than crisis management. Some situations are suitable to telephone counseling, whereas others require a personal visit. Sometimes a problem has advanced by the time contact occurs, and requires more intense problem solving. By collaborating with mothers, you will help them recognize problems, possible causes, and practical actions. Using the counseling skills presented in Chapter 5 will help you determine the problem, gain insights into what caused the situation, and work toward a solution with the mother. This chapter describes a systematic process for consultations, as well as several methods of documentation.

KEY TERMS

alternative hunches	Infant Breastfeeding
anticipatory guidance	Assessment Tool
assessment	(IBFAT)
breastfeeding descriptors	LATCH method
consent	Mother-Baby Assessment
crisis intervention	(MBA)
documentation	outreach counseling
follow-up	physician report
hidden factors	plan of care
history	problem solving
hunch	telephone counseling

REACHING OUT THROUGH ANTICIPATORY GUIDANCE

Breastfeeding rates are higher when mothers receive consistent encouragement, help, and guidance prenatally, during their hospital stay, and throughout lactation (Guise, 2003). A mother's breastfeeding education needs to be viewed in the context of a preventive approach to healthcare, much in the same way that dental checkups

help prevent cavities. Practitioners are challenged by lack of time to provide anticipatory guidance and outreach in addition to their many other responsibilities in a busy hospital, clinic, or group practice.

By receiving continuing support and information prenatally and throughout lactation, the mother becomes prepared and knowledgeable. She is then better able to meet the challenges of mothering with confidence. Contacts at key times can diminish problems or avoid them entirely, and help establish a foundation of knowledge that leads to optimal breastfeeding practices. This investment of time and energy pays off in fewer problems and more positive outcomes for the mother and baby. An enjoyable experience for parents, coupled with less time spent in problem solving, makes this both a parent-friendly and timesaving approach.

The Timing of Anticipatory Guidance

Anticipatory guidance is as much a part of routine health supervision as the history and physical examination. It is an integral part of preventive healthcare for the breastfeeding mother. This guidance needs to occur at a teachable moment, when retention of information will be high and when decision making will occur. Women usually decide to breastfeed before the baby's birth, often prior to pregnancy (Guise, 2003; Earle, 2002). Therefore, earlier exposure is even more effective.

Several studies suggest that adolescents are interested in learning about breastfeeding during their high school years (Goulet, 2003; Ross, 2002; Alnasir, 1992; Neifert, 1988). This is an ideal time for correcting misconceptions early enough to help students form their perceptions of sexuality and parenthood (Volpe, 2000; Martens, 2001; Yeo, 1994). Anticipatory guidance and education at this critical stage in an adolescent's development promotes positive attitudes and establishes a sound knowledge base. When the adolescent approaches adulthood, reinforcement of these early concepts will guide her or him in sound decisions.

Contact with women during pregnancy helps build rapport and establish trust. The new mother then accepts advice more readily from the support person during breastfeeding. It is easier to address specific needs after you and the mother have established a comfortable relationship. A climate of acceptance, flexibility, and cooperation sets the stage for a positive breastfeeding outcome (Finch, 2002; Greenwood, 2002; Parker, 2000; Volpe, 2000; Sable, 1998; Valdes, 1993). After a program of comprehensive prenatal breastfeeding education, you can spend your valuable time with postpartum mothers and babies reinforcing and reviewing issues presented earlier.

Comparing Anticipatory Guidance and Crisis Intervention

An outreach approach of anticipatory guidance in the care of breastfeeding mothers is not a new concept. It forms the basis of breastfeeding counseling in support groups and breastfeeding programs throughout the world. All areas of the medical community engage in preventive medicine. Well-baby checkups, dental exams, routine breast exams, Pap smears, and routine eye exams are all examples of preventive care. Modern medicine clearly recognizes the benefits of early detection.

The breastfeeding mother is no exception when it comes to the need for preparedness. She often lacks role models, an experienced support person, practical and timely information, and the self-confidence to anticipate her needs. Her only source of breastfeeding information may be skimpy literature, formula company misinformation, or a brief discussion at a childbirth or postpartum class. At a time when her energies and concentration are centered on her infant's birth and her own changing role, retention of breastfeeding information may be minimal at best. She may combine half-remembered instructions with incorrect information from well-meaning friends and relatives, placing her breastfeeding at risk. A knowledgeable caregiver becomes a key to the mother meeting her breastfeeding goals.

Anticipatory guidance may save both the mother and infant from potential difficulties by guiding the mother one step at a time through her breastfeeding journey. When done on a timely basis, you can teach and inform a mother well in advance of critical periods. Her preparedness and self-confidence are often enough to prevent problems. Any problems, if they do occur, will be of shorter duration and the chances of recurrence decreased.

Crisis intervention occurs after a problem already exists. It may seem to some that crisis intervention is less time consuming than educating the mother before the delivery and supporting her throughout breastfeeding.

Yet, the time spent later in problem solving negates any time saved. Even more important, the results for the mother are less positive. Although the mother may alleviate her immediate problem, the crisis might not have occurred had she been educated and supported adequately beforehand. Additionally, the situation has compromised her sense of well-being and self-assurance. Breastfeeding is a normal part of childbearing and family life. A problem-oriented approach must be replaced with one of prevention and preservation of the healthy normal phenomenon—the breastfeeding dyad of mother and baby.

Counseling Examples of the Differences in Approach

The value of anticipatory guidance is illustrated by two women who attended the same prenatal breastfeeding class. In Figure 6.1, a mother-to-mother support counselor receives Lynn's referral and begins contacting her regularly one month before her due date. In Figure 6.2, Denise receives the telephone number of a lactation consultant and understands that she may call if she has questions or problems. The log of each mother's contacts illustrates how timing and frequency of contact can affect their results.

Over about a three-week period, compare the breastfeeding experiences for these two women. Lynn, who is equipped with information and support, is enjoying breastfeeding. She experiences a bit of nipple tenderness on the second day. Because her lactation consultant visited her the previous day, she feels comfortable calling her to ask for help. The soreness clears up after she is reminded about positioning her baby for a good latch and makes the necessary adjustments. Anticipatory guidance about **growth spurts** and her baby's first checkup helps Lynn anticipate these events. During her baby's growth spurt, the lactation consultant refers Lynn to the additional support of a breastfeeding counselor. Lynn is well on the road to long-term breastfeeding.

Denise's first contact with a lactation consultant is after her problems advance to a crisis. She lacks the knowledge and self-confidence to see her through the normal occurrence of a growth spurt and begins supplementing her baby with formula. She endures the discomfort of engorgement, sore nipples, and undiagnosed thrush. By the time she contacts a lactation consultant, she is discouraged and her baby prefers bottle-feeding over breastfeeding. Despite appropriate assistance, the lactation consultant is unable to help Denise return to her original plan of exclusive breastfeeding. Within three weeks after her baby is born, Denise is no longer breastfeeding.

With early contact, Denise would have felt comfortable calling her lactation consultant when she delivered.

FIGURE 6.1
Example of anticipatory guidance.

8/15   Saw Lynn at 9 A.M. in hospital. Baby was born at 1 P.M. yesterday. 3-hour labor. Apgars 9 and 9. Baby was put to breast within 1 hour. Feedings are on demand and going well. Baby has had 6 feedings. Lynn indicated a support counselor had called her several weeks ago. They discussed putting baby to breast as soon as possible after delivery. Suggested she read *Breastfeeding Today* and attend breastfeeding class, which she did. Counselor had given her my name as the LC who would see her in the hospital. Will return when baby is ready for the next feeding.

8/15   Visited Lynn at 10:30 A.M. Baby had good feeding needed some help with positioning. Reviewed basics of breastfeeding management while baby nursed.

8/16   Lynn called from home. Her nipples are tender. We discussed positioning and latch on again. Asked her to call tomorrow if no improvement.

8/18   Lynn called. Nipples are not as tender. She notices a difference with the way she positions baby. Realizes he wasn't getting a good latch before. Feels she finally has the hang of it. Breasts seem fuller. Reminded her to rest, and follow baby's feeding cues. Also discussed typical growth spurt at about 10 days.

8/25   Lynn called. Is having rough day. Baby nurses constantly. She's ready to give a bottle. Reminded her about growth spurts and gave encouragement. Lynn says she will hold off one more day. Suggested she contact her breastfeeding counselor to find out when the next support group meeting will be held.

8/27   Called Lynn. Baby is nursing less frequently now. Nipples no longer tender. She spoke with counselor and plans to attend a support group meeting in 2 weeks. Discussed what to expect at baby's first checkup. Asked her to call after checkup.

9/1   Lynn called. Weight gain is good and breastfeeding going great. Lynn in high spirits and enjoying breastfeeding.

12/6   Saw Lynn at the grocery store. Breastfeeding is going very well. She plans to become a counselor with her support group. Said, "I couldn't have done it without you!"

FIGURE 6.2
Example of crisis intervention.

8/12   Contacted by mother, Denise. Denise delivered her baby on 7/29 and began breastfeeding within 6 hours. She was given a lactation consultant's telephone number at the discharge. Baby was fussy at feedings for the first 2 days, and popped on and off the breast. Denise figured this was because she didn't have any milk yet. On day 3 Denise's nipples became very tender. She applied breast cream that was given to her by the hospital. Two days later, Denise's nipples were cracked and bleeding. Her breasts were full and uncomfortable. She remembered that she was given my phone number but could not find it. After another 5 days, baby wanted to nurse all the time. Denise began giving a bottle of formula two times a day. She believed that she did not have enough milk for her baby. Nursing was still painful at this time. After another 3 days, baby began to prefer the bottle and was still fussy when Denise tried to nurse. Denise contacted the hospital to get my phone number. Denise was in tears. Her baby is taking four bottles of formula a day. She wants to return to exclusive breastfeeding. Scheduled her for 3:00 appointment today.

8/12   Saw Denise and baby at office. Observed a feeding. Denise needed much help with positioning and attachment. Baby fussy, popped on and off frequently. Her nipples are red and tender. Evidence of thrush in baby's mouth. Advised her to contact her physician for appropriate treatment of nipples and baby's mouth. Gave her information sheet on treatment of thrush.

8/15   Called Denise. She cannot detect any increase in milk supply. Baby refuses the breast at most feedings. She is using medication for thrush on her nipples and in baby's mouth. Nipples are still tender but getting a little better. Denise is tired and frustrated at balancing bottle and breast. Discussed using nursing supplementer, to increase milk production, but Denise did not wish to use it. Reviewed positioning and treatment of her sore nipples.

8/18   Called Denise. She has decided not to continue trying to breastfeed. She is disappointed but resigned to bottle-feeding.

Learning about effective positioning and attachment would have increased her confidence and avoided prolonged nipple soreness. When she developed thrush, early treatment would have cleared the infection sooner. Not having made personal contact with the consultant before now, she put off placing a call until she was desperate. This type of scenario is all too common and can be easily avoided with appropriate anticipatory guidance by a lactation consultant or breastfeeding counselor.

Outreach Counseling

Prevention counseling requires more time during the early stages of breastfeeding. You can see from our example that Lynn received assistance and support twice as often as Denise did. This frequency of contact subsides,

however, after the first several weeks, by which time the mother and baby have developed together into a harmonious pair. You, the mother, and her infant will benefit from your guidance of the mother through her early stages, educating her in advance and building her self-confidence.

When outreach is not an option, a hotline, warm line, or e-mail may be the most practical method of ensuring contact with mothers. Referral to a community support group is essential when the caregiver is unable to initiate regular contact with mothers. Lay counselors will continue to remain important partners in the mother's breastfeeding support team. Lactation consultants can be instrumental in helping support groups establish effective outreach.

A 1970 study revealed that women who received information and support had significantly longer breastfeeding experiences with fewer problems. Although prenatal support was more effective than support given only after delivery, support both before and after delivery produced the best results. Lack of information correlated with all of the reasons why mothers stop breastfeeding prematurely (Ladas, 1970). Bottle-feeding mothers report they would have felt encouraged to breastfeed if they had received more information through prenatal class, the media, and books. Family support is also a factor (Arora, 2000).

Occasionally, a mother may not desire contact as frequently as anticipatory guidance suggests. Your sensitivity to the mother's cues will establish a graceful opportunity for the mother to make her wishes known. Some mothers prefer to handle the daily stresses of motherhood in a more private manner. The most effective approach in this case may be simply to let the mother know you are available and allow her to initiate any contacts.

Breastfeeding Support Counselor

Before the advent of the lactation consulting profession, mothers received breastfeeding support primarily from volunteer lay counselors who developed relationships with mothers through a series of contacts. This form of support continues to provide many mothers with day-to-day breastfeeding assistance. For the most part, contacts take place through telephone counseling. A counselor contacts the mother several weeks or months before delivery and continues to contact her through weaning. Some mothers attend monthly support group meetings as well. While the climate has changed with the emergence of lactation consultants, the method used by lay counselors serves as a noteworthy model for anticipatory guidance and support. If you do not incorporate such contact into your practice, referral to a support group can provide this guidance.

Prenatal Contact

Care providers and other support people need to make a concerted effort to contact women during pregnancy. Encourage the expectant woman to educate herself about breastfeeding through reading, attending meetings, observing other mothers breastfeeding, and having her questions and concerns addressed by a knowledgeable breastfeeding helper. Using listening skills, you can learn the mother's goals for breastfeeding, the extent of her breastfeeding knowledge, and her need for support. Be sure to give her an opportunity to ask questions.

In closing the initial contact, make certain that the mother does not have any unanswered questions or concerns. Be sure that she has your name, telephone number, and the best times to reach you. Remember that most mothers will be more comfortable receiving calls than initiating them. Initiating contact with a mother

shows your interest and concern. You and the mother can establish the most convenient times for subsequent contacts, taking into consideration family responsibilities and needs.

Continuing Regular Contact

A mother will benefit from frequent contact in the early weeks of breastfeeding. As she learns more about her baby and breastfeeding, the frequency of contacts can gradually diminish, unless she is experiencing problems. Initiating contact around times when the potential for problems typically occurs will give mothers the support and advice they need. Detailed records and thorough evaluations of each contact will help you determine appropriate follow-up.

During your conversations, check that every mother understands the basic information about breastfeeding management and the prevention of problems. Help her learn how to know if she has positioned her baby at the breast for optimal milk transfer and how to respond to feeding cues. Discuss ways to ensure ample milk production, responding to her baby's periods of increased hunger (growth spurts), and typical nursing patterns for babies of different ages. Help her learn to trust her baby and herself. Encourage her to look at him, to listen to him, and to watch his reactions. Table 6.1 shows some general guidelines for deciding how often to contact a mother and what to talk about at each stage.

▶ PROBLEM SOLVING WITH MOTHERS

Problem solving involves more than simply offering a suggestion to the mother. It requires gathering information and comparing it to the circumstances that fit known patterns of problem development. This kind of troubleshooting often involves using your intuition to develop hunches. You can use these hunches to focus your thinking and select suggestions that will be most helpful to the mother.

You may not always be in a position to help a mother prevent problems. Even when mothers practice sound breastfeeding techniques, problems may occur. You can help the mother recognize problems, as well as their possible causes and practical actions she can take in order to resolve them. There is no one universal solution to any breastfeeding problem. Suggestions may even contradict one another. It is up to you to decide which action to offer first to a particular mother, according to your perception of her situation and her ability to cope. If your first suggestion does not lead to the solution of her problem, you will need to suggest other actions until she finds the one that works for her.

	TABLE 6.1

Anticipatory Guidance from a Breastfeeding Counselor

Time Period	Anticipatory Guidance
◆ During pregnancy	Contact the pregnant woman once or twice during her pregnancy. You can recommend books and videos, and urge her to begin acquainting herself with breastfeeding. Invite her to attend a support group meeting. This is an opportune time to begin building rapport with the mother, perhaps discussing her expectations and preparation for childbirth.
◆ When the baby is born	Hopefully you will be in close enough contact to know when the mother delivers. You can ask her to call and let you know when she has the baby. Ask if she would like you to visit her if there is no lactation consultant support in the hospital. If you are unable to visit her in person, a telephone call will be a second best option. Encourage her to talk about her labor and delivery. You may be the only person who shows an interest in helping her verbalize any disappointments or concerns regarding the birth. Find out how she feels and how her baby is doing. Ask her baby's name and start referring to her baby by name. Be sure that she knows when you will contact her again. Because most mothers spend a short time in the hospital, it may be impractical to schedule a contact during her stay. This makes close prenatal contact with her even more critical, because she will be more likely to let you know when she delivers.
◆ Just home from the hospital	Contact the mother within 2 to 3 days after she returns home, and more frequently for specific problems. You can first ask, "How do you feel?" and then inquire about the number of feedings, voids, and stools in 24 hours. Discuss, as necessary, common concerns such as fatigue, positioning the baby during feedings, how to know the baby is getting enough milk, and how to avoid problems such as sore nipples and engorgement. Try not to overwhelm her with too much information at one time.
◆ Baby 1 week old	Call to remind the mother that babies typically seem more hungry and increase feeding frequency at approximately 10 days old. Also remind her that her breasts will reduce in size around this time as she responds to her baby's increased feedings. Make sure she understands how milk production depends on supply and demand, and encourage her to continue to respond to her baby's feeding cues. Discuss typical breastfeeding patterns for this age, and assure her that you welcome calls from her.
◆ Before baby's 2-week checkup	You can help the mother understand what her baby's physician will be looking for at this checkup. Discuss normal weight patterns and normal feeding patterns, and help her form questions to ask the physician. Call the mother again after the checkup, and ask about weight gain and any recommendations the physician has made. Help her integrate the physician's suggestions into her breastfeeding and clarify any possible misunderstandings.
◆ Baby 6 weeks old	At about 6 weeks, the mother will be returning for her postpartum checkup. Discuss the possible effects of oral contraceptives on her breastfeeding. She may be interested in resuming her prepregnant activity level. Caution her about overdoing. Remind her that her baby may go through another hunger spurt at this time. This may be prolonged if the mother has been very active and has been missing some feedings.
◆ After the first month	Continue to keep in touch with the mother as the need arises. If you feel confident that the mother will call you whenever she has a question or problem, you could discontinue initiating calls. Some mothers will benefit from routine calls all the way through weaning.

Using Counseling Skills to Determine the Problem

Often, breastfeeding problems are complex issues with more than a single cause and no specific "right" solution. The many factors that may affect breastfeeding—the infant's physical and medical status, his temperament and ability to suckle, the frequency and length of feedings, the condition of the mother's breasts, and hormonal and emotional influences, to name a few—make it inappropriate to offer information without first clearly defining her problem.

You can use the counseling skills presented in Chapter 5 to learn more about the circumstances surrounding the issue and to gather information about symptoms. By patiently listening and encouraging the mother to communicate openly, you show her that you value her perception of the problem and care enough about her to work with her conscientiously toward a solution. In doing this, you may gain additional insight into what caused her situation and thus more easily determine her needs. Providing her with emotional support can reduce her anxiety and allow her to be more patient and objective in working toward a solution.

Sometimes a mother needs to take immediate action in order to reduce physical discomfort before you can investigate the causes of her problem with her. You can first give her suggestions for physical relief and then continue with problem solving when she is more comfortable. If the mother does not receive comfort measures early in the contact, she may be unable to hear or accept the information you share with her.

In order to develop the most satisfaction from her contact with you and to decrease the likelihood of recurrences, the mother needs to understand her problem, the events and actions that led up to it, and the steps that will help her resolve it. Her understanding comes more readily when she is an equal partner in problem solving. By working with her to define her problem and explore possible actions, you help the mother understand her situation better and develop her confidence and skills.

Working Toward a Solution

When the nature of a problem begins to take shape through investigation with the mother, problem-solving skills will help you both move toward a solution. The problem-solving method should contain the elements that are essential to meeting the mother's needs. The consultation begins with gathering information and impressions before any intervention or active involvement by the helper. After gathering sufficient information and impressions, followed by taking a history and assessing the mother and baby, you can form a first hunch and begin to define the problem. While continuing to look for hidden factors, you eliminate related causes and test your hunch. In comparing your ideas with the mother's, you explore alternative hunches and look for other possible causes.

After you have defined the problem, you and the mother can examine the options, select one, and put it into action. Try to not give the mother more than 3 suggestions at a time so she is not overwhelmed with information. Ask the mother to indicate whether your suggestions suit her needs and how to adapt them to her

situation. Be prepared to offer further suggestions as needed. Involving the mother in the development of a plan will increase the likelihood that she will follow it.

Step 1. Form Your First Hunch

When a breastfeeding problem arises, you will first want to check with the mother to determine how she views the situation. What does she think is the cause, and what actions has she taken already? From this, you can form your hunch about the cause and possible solution to the problem. This is more an unconscious reflex than a carefully reasoned analysis. Concentrating on this preliminary hunch is an essential first step to working toward a solution. It helps focus observations and reduces aimless thinking. Your first hunch is only the beginning of the problem-solving process. You can think of it as a point of departure rather than a final destination. While forming your first hunch, you continue to use guiding skills to provide emotional support and to gather information and impressions to further clarify and define the problem.

Step 2. Look for Hidden Factors

Hidden factors often contribute to a problem. An infant who nurses all night may be sleeping for long periods during the day. A mother who thinks her milk is not rich enough may have expressed milk from her breasts and noticed the typical, thin, watery appearance of human milk. A mother who did not experience the sensation of her milk "coming in" and whose baby is not gaining weight may have significant **endocrine** problems. It is important to determine such hidden factors as early as possible in the process. Tuning in to the mother's needs, encouraging her to talk, and listening attentively will help you accomplish this. Guiding skills are essential to this process.

Step 3. Test Your Hunch

While gathering more information, you can continually evaluate your hunch to determine whether the situation is what you expected. New information may lead you to form a new hunch. Hidden factors and the mother's lack of breastfeeding information may obscure the problem unless you explore all possibilities. A mother who first complained that it hurt whenever she nursed may have led you to believe she had sore nipples. By exploring further, you might learn that she experiences pain when her milk lets down, which alters your hypothesis. To test your hunch, you can use interpreting, focusing, and summarizing: "So what you have told me is that . . . ," "Let me see if I understand . . . ," "You seem to be. . . ." When your hunch proves to be correct and the problem becomes clearly identified, you are ready to develop a plan of care with the mother.

Step 4. Explore Alternative Hunches

Based on additional input from the mother, your initial hunch may prove to be incorrect. You then need to pursue other hunches to resolve the problem. Perhaps when you tested your hunch, the mother corrected you and led you in another direction. Exploring alternative hunches may clarify the situation. Sometimes, a problem will remain ill defined throughout several contacts with the mother, perhaps over several weeks. At such times, you and the mother might develop a trial plan that addresses the most obvious symptoms or concerns. When the mother recognizes which actions are most effective, she may begin to identify the cause of the problem. You can also network with other lactation consultants and healthcare team members about a situation that puzzles you.

Step 5. Develop a Plan

Throughout the problem-solving process, you and the mother function as a team to come up with workable alternatives. *Workable* means that they fit the mother's situation and are specific to her problem. When you tell her why something is true, the mother is better able to work out her plan of how to do something. The way the mother responds to your facts and hints will give you important clues as to whether she feels they will help her. If she likes your suggestions and adapts them to her situation, you can be certain that she is likely to try them. You can then note them for your summary of the plan of care. If the mother seems noncommittal or replies with, "Yes, but . . . ," she may be telling you that she does not feel that your suggestions will address her problem adequately. Gathering further information will help define the problem more clearly.

After you and the mother have discussed the possible actions to take, you can develop a plan together. In order to eliminate confusion and to learn whether a particular action was helpful, it is best to develop a plan with only two or three actions for the mother. Asking the mother to summarize the plan will help you determine that she understands what you discussed. Be sure to follow up with her to learn if your plan worked. If it did not work, you can consider further suggestions.

Part of developing a plan is setting a time limit on the actions the mother will take and arranging for follow-up. Be sure to work this out with the mother: "So, you will try . . . for two days and will call me on Thursday afternoon to let me know how it worked. In the meantime, please call me if it gets worse or if something else develops." Always leave the door open for the mother to call you whenever she has a concern. Be sure to document any plan that you and the mother decide on. When you talk to the mother again, you can say, "Let's see, we talked about . . ." or, "You were going to try. . . ." This will show the mother that you are actively concerned about helping her and help you keep the situation clear in your mind.

Telephone Counseling

Many breastfeeding contacts occur over the telephone. It is important to recognize situations that require an in-person visit for assessment and advice and those that lend themselves to a telephone contact. Telephone counseling is sufficient for a good deal of follow-up that occurs after hospital discharge or subsequent to a clinic or office visit. Many breastfeeding contacts concern parenting issues that do not require a clinical assessment. A mother may be concerned that her baby is fussy or fails to sleep through the night. You can review her breastfeeding practices to determine if she is feeding frequently enough. If she describes engorgement, you can discuss adjustments in her breastfeeding routine. She may have questions about expressing her milk or returning to work. These issues generally do not require that you see the mother and baby in person in order to provide appropriate assistance.

Be aware of your telephone manner any time you rely on a telephone contact to assist a mother. Remember that body language is a great determinant of how the mother will receive your message. In the absence of any visual cues such as body language, you must rely on your tone of voice and your spoken words to relay a message that will be most effective and helpful for the mother. A smile and soothing voice tone will convey warmth and sincerity and enhance the exchange.

In-Person Visits

Circumstances sometimes require that you see the mother, her baby, or both of them. If the situation is after hospital discharge, you may need to see the mother in her home or in your office. Hospital staff has limited time to prepare mothers to care for their babies at home. Mothers will benefit from at least 1 home visit following discharge to ensure that breastfeeding is getting off to a good start. In addition, counseling is easier, more personal, and much more pleasant when you and the mother can see each other face-to-face. A variety of circumstances may indicate a need to see a mother in person:

◆ If a mother reports sore nipples, or difficulties that imply latch-on problems or incorrect positioning, you will need to assess her breasts and observe a breastfeeding in order to gain sufficient insight into the situation.

◆ Any time there is poor weight gain, you will need to examine the baby and observe a feeding. For legal protection, as well as the baby's safety, it is advisable that a lactation consultant insist on a consultation or refer the mother to her physician for any poor or slow weight gain.

◆ A mother who is using an electric breast pump will need to learn how to operate the pump and use it for the first time. If the need for the pump stems from a problem with the baby or with getting breastfeeding established, the mother may need help in dealing with the situation. It is for this reason that mothers should acquire breast pumps from a person experienced in caring for breastfeeding mothers whenever possible, rather than from a pharmacy or other business that does not provide assistance and support.

◆ If the mother seems to be shy or untalkative or if you sense she has difficulty relating her concerns to you in a telephone conversation, a face-to-face interaction may be necessary.

◆ Severe engorgement will require a visit in order to gain further insight into the cause and treatment.

These are only a few examples. Any time you feel uneasy about a situation or unable to obtain sufficient insight during a telephone contact, you need to see the mother. Make sure she understands that further consultation will be on a fee-for-service basis, or whatever payment policy you or your institution has established.

Last Resort Help

You may not always be in contact with a mother at an early stage of her problem. She may have received advice from various caregivers that was unhelpful, inappropriate, or contradictory. As a result, a mother may have lost hope when you see her for the first time (Auerbach, 1993). Although these conditions are less than ideal, the reality is that you will need to be prepared to enter into problem solving at various levels. You also will need to be sensitive to the frustrations and anxiety the mother brings with her to the consultation. There may be times when a problem advances to the point that your only recourse is to assist the mother in weaning and offer emotional support to her. When this happens, help the mother to recall with pleasure the positive aspects of her breastfeeding. She may need reassurance that breastfeeding can follow a more rewarding course for a subsequent baby.

▶ ELEMENTS IN A CONSULTATION

Regardless of the reason for the consultation, begin with guiding skills, obtain **consent**, and then gather information and assess the mother and baby. After the situation has been determined, your role becomes more active.

You will integrate problem solving into the logical flow of the consultation along with continued guiding skills. You and the mother will ultimately reach the point where you can discuss a plan of care that includes appropriate follow-up.

Example of the Consultation Process

A study at the Vancouver Breastfeeding Centre in British Columbia illustrates the consultation process (Ellis, 1993). The Vancouver model progresses through the process of assessment, analysis, diagnosis, care, and counsel. The assessment includes recording the mother's reason for the visit, a maternal and infant history, physical assessments of both the mother and infant, and any additional problems the mother reveals during the visit. The mother then initiates breastfeeding with no intervention by the staff in order to provide baseline data. Impressions gained through observing the feeding, the physical assessment, and information obtained from the mother enable the staff to analyze the situation and factors that contributed to the difficulty. The staff then makes a diagnosis that provides direction for the appropriate care and counsel for the mother. The mother participates in developing a plan of care and returns for a follow-up visit to evaluate its effectiveness. When necessary, the staff adjusts the plan of care to address continuing concerns.

Obtaining Consent

When you meet with a mother for the first time, it is good practice to obtain signed consent before initiating the consultation. This may not be required for a lactation consultant who works in a hospital, pediatric office, or clinic. You may need to determine whether consent is required in your work setting.

Elements of a consultation that require signed consent include:

◆ Working with the mother and infant at this and all subsequent visits.

◆ Examining her breasts or nipples.

◆ Performing an examination of the baby, including a digital oral examination.

◆ Observing a breastfeeding.

◆ Demonstrating or using equipment and techniques that may be necessary to ensure an adequate caloric intake for the infant and to improve breastfeeding.

◆ Releasing information to the insurance company.

◆ Sending reports to the mother's and infant's primary caregivers and consulting with them regarding their care.

◆ Using information obtained from the consultation for educational purposes.

◆ Taking photographs to be used for educational purposes.

◆ Receiving payment for the consultation and rental or sale of breastfeeding equipment.

Even after you and the mother have signed and dated the consent form, it is polite to ask before initiating physical contact. Ask, "May I examine your breasts now?" or "May I take your baby and examine him?" Continuing to ask the mother's permission helps give her some control over what occurs. If a mother refuses to sign a consent form or crosses out significant parts, such as allowing you to communicate with her or her baby's primary caregiver, you should not continue with the consultation. A signed consent form protects the lactation consultant, and a consultation should not occur without it. If you practice in a hospital or a medical group where a consent form for all care provided within that setting has been signed, you may be covered by that general consent and may not need the mother to sign a separate form. It is wise to discuss this with your employer in such a work setting. See Chapter 26 for further discussion regarding informed consent.

In 1996, the U.S. Department of Health and Human Services instituted the Health Insurance Portability and Accountability Act (HIPAA). Healthcare practitioners are required to have signed HIPAA consent forms for all their patients. HIPAA provides federal protections for the privacy of protected health information and prohibits use or disclosure of such information unless authorized by the patient. It recognizes there may be certain incidental uses and disclosures that occur as a by-product, such as a third party overhearing the exchange. You can avoid such incidental disclosure by speaking quietly and avoiding the use of patients' names in public areas. Locking file cabinets and using passwords on computer files provide additional safeguards. If patients have participated in research, you can ensure their privacy and confidentiality by protecting identifiers from improper use and by destroying them at the earliest opportunity. HIPAA does permit disclosure without authorization to public health authorities legally authorized to receive such reports for the purpose of preventing or controlling disease, injury, or disability, as in suspected child neglect or abuse.

Taking a History

When taking a history of the mother and baby, guiding skills will help you gather information and impressions when you use your history and assessment forms. Simply diving into a checklist of questions from your history form will do little to put the mother at ease. Active listening is a tool that helps you accept and validate her feelings. Remember that you are listening to both what she says and how she says it. Continue to provide feedback and give emotional support to the mother throughout the history taking.

As the discussion progresses, you will identify any problem the mother is experiencing. For the lactation consultant in private practice, the problem may be readily apparent; when the mother has initiated contact, she is often forthright about her situation. The lactation consultant working in an environment such as a hospital or clinic may see all the breastfeeding mothers present on a given day, and problems may not be so obvious.

History Forms

Many lactation consultants use a standard history form or develop their own. A sample history form appears in Appendix F. Using such forms will help you remember to ask all essential questions. Remember that the history needs to include all information regarding the health of the mother and infant, both past and present. Begin with how the mother perceives her problem and when it began. Document exactly what she says and obtain an appropriate history relevant to the situation.

Record any history of previous lactation and breastfeeding, as well as details about the present breastfeeding situation. Note any past or current medications taken by the mother and baby. Many mothers do not consider birth control pills, herbs, or food supplements to be medications. You may want to ask about these individually. Some mothers have been taking insulin or thyroid medication for most of their lives and again may not think of these as medications. It is also important to ask about the mother's diet, including the amount of fluids consumed daily.

Next, explore issues regarding the present situation, using open-ended questions and other guiding skills to gather more information. Be careful to word questions in such a way that will elicit the information you need. For example, ask, "How many times does your baby nurse in 24 hours?" rather than, "How frequently does your baby nurse?" Include the baby's feeding and growth patterns, as well as a review of his sleeping, crying, and ability to socialize. Record his pattern of stooling and voiding and obtain an estimate of the amounts in the past 24-hour period. Ask the mother if there has been any change in this pattern and, if so, when the change occurred. Learn what the mother has tried and the results of her efforts.

If you choose to omit an item on your history form, inserting "NA" (not applicable) in the space will indicate that you chose not to ask that question. To leave a question blank could imply that you forgot to address that particular issue. For the lactation consultant practicing within a hospital or medical group, history taking may not need as much detail. Charts for the mother and baby will include much of the information. Reading their charts before the consultation will familiarize you with the mother's and baby's histories. Any information relevant to lactation that is not already included on the charts can be noted on the mother's and baby's charts after the consultation.

Performing an Assessment

If you practice in a hospital, staff will have assessed the baby before your consultation. You can familiarize yourself with that information, particularly the baby's daily weight status, intake, and output. In a private practice setting, you may need to perform a more detailed assessment of the baby that includes his weight because you will not have access to nursery records. In either setting, you will want to look for signs of the baby's **hydration**, caloric status, and general health, as well as numbers of wet diapers and stools. You can then move onto assessing the mother's breasts and nipples. See Chapter 13 for further discussion of infant assessment.

You can then proceed to the feeding assessment. Flexibility is fundamental to assessing a feeding. You must be willing to move at the baby's pace. Depending on the situation, you may decide you need a full feeding assessment with pre-feeding and post-feeding weights. An electronic digital scale will enable you to measure milk transfer accurately. Weigh the baby naked. Then weigh the baby with a diaper on before nursing. This will be your pre-feed weight.

Help the mother into a comfortable position to nurse her baby, asking her to show you what her baby does while at the breast. This will focus the assessment on the baby and not on what the mother is doing. This approach is much less threatening and intimidating to the mother and avoids the impression that you are judging her. Allow the feeding to proceed without any suggestions or interventions on your part until you have a clear picture of what is going on. If you perceive a problem, it is then appropriate to suggest to the mother some alternative methods or interventions. Weigh the baby after feeding to determine the milk transfer amount.

While you observe the feeding, you have an opportunity to visit with the mother and gain further impressions. You can incorporate the insights you gain into your plan of care. Factors include:

◆ Interactions between the mother and baby

◆ The dynamics of the feeding process

◆ The baby's oral and facial structure

◆ The baby's and mother's temperaments, behavior, and emotional status

◆ The appearance and condition of the mother's breasts and nipples

◆ Evidence of milk transfer from the mother to the baby

◆ The mother's economic and employment status

◆ The mother's support network and cultural beliefs and practices

◆ The mother's breastfeeding goals

Once the physical and feeding assessments are complete, you will probably have developed a clear idea of whether a problem exists and, if so, of the nature of the problem. You can then begin to think about the overall goals for the mother and baby. If the mother has sore nipples, for example, the baby may not be receiving sufficient calories because the mother cannot nurse comfortably. Your overall goals will be to decrease the mother's pain while providing sufficient calories to the baby. From these general goals, you can develop a specific plan of care detailing all the steps necessary to achieving the final goal of having the mother nursing without pain and the baby nursing effectively and adequately from the breast.

Developing a Plan of Care

After you have determined the mother's situation, you will be prepared to take a more directive role in the consultation. Based on the identified problem, you next want to determine what the mother needs to know. You cannot enter into a consultation with a prescribed agenda. What this particular mother needs relative to the problem may be different from another mother with the same problem.

In developing a plan of care, begin with essentials such as feeding the baby, pain relief, and maintaining or increasing milk production. Help the mother understand what produced her situation and how she can avoid its recurrence. Brainstorm with her some of the available options. Be mindful of the mother's reactions to your suggestions. Although you may sense what would be most effective for this particular situation, the mother must be able and willing to follow your suggestions. For example, you are aware that cup feeding will provide sufficient calories to the baby while allowing the mother's nipples to heal. However, if this mother does not embrace the idea of cup feeding, you will need to offer an alternate solution that she will find more acceptable. Your role is to provide choices and encourage the mother to decide what will work for her.

After you and the mother have decided on a plan of care, you can ask her to repeat the suggestions that she accepted, reviewing them as necessary. After she has stated the plan of care, you can summarize it with her to avoid any confusion. If the baby's father is present for the consultation, be sure to include him in developing the plan of care. Remember that your goal is to empower the mother and to increase her self-confidence and self-reliance. At the end of every consultation, ask yourself if you have accomplished this.

Providing Follow-up

Before you end the consultation, learn what support may be available from the mother's family and friends. Refer her to a community support group, especially if you sense that she needs peer support. Provide the mother with a written plan of care and, when appropriate, other written materials, videos, or breastfeeding devices. Mothers tend not to remember much of the discussion from these consultations, so they will need something in writing for later reference.

Arranging the Next Contact

As discussed in Chapter 5, follow-up is important to the mother's outcome. Depending on the situation, the follow-up may be another visit in the next day or so, or perhaps in a week or more. If it is a self-limiting situation, following up by telephone or e-mail may be sufficient. The mother who comes in for a consultation regarding her return to work, for example, may not require a set time for follow-up and could be asked to call for any concerns or questions.

If you have arranged for the mother to call you and she does not call, you can try to contact her several times. Document each call and record whether you left a message on an answering machine or with a family member. If follow-up is critical, such as an infant who is failing to thrive, it would be wise to notify the pediatrician that the mother has not followed up as requested.

Writing Follow-up Reports

As a part of the mother's healthcare team, you will need to communicate regularly with other members of the team. This usually includes both the mother's caregiver (obstetrician, family practitioner, or midwife) and the baby's pediatrician or family practitioner. Regular communication is especially important if you work as an independent, community-based lactation consultant and do not have daily contact with other members of the mother's and baby's healthcare team. It is good practice to send reports to caregivers for both the mother and baby. Any time you have immediate concerns, you may want to contact the caregiver to discuss them.

Send a physician report to all appropriate primary care or referring physicians within 24 hours of seeing a client. You may also want to send a brief report if you rent a breast pump, sell **breast shells**, or help a mother over the telephone, after first obtaining the mother's permission to release the information. Take advantage of all opportunities to inform other members of the healthcare team of what you do. By your educating them through such reports, they in turn will be more likely to provide continuity of care and refer patients to you. Establish a routine of following up with documentation after every consultation. The follow-up report should be on professional letterhead listing contact information such as your name, credentials, address, telephone number, fax number, and e-mail address. See Figure 6.3 for

---

FIGURE 6.3
Elements of a physician report.

1. Date the patient was seen.
2. Names and addresses of mother's physician and baby's physician.
3. Regarding: Mother's and baby's names and baby's date of birth.
4. Dear Dr. . . . ,
5. Patient was seen at your request, was self-referred, was referred by (include name if possible).
6. If you called the physician's office to give a verbal report or faxed in a short report, you can mention this in your letter.
7. Because of . . . (reason for referral).
8. Brief description of the mother's history (general health, conception, pregnancy, and birth).
9. Assessment of the mother's breasts and nipples.
10. Brief description of the baby's history (birth, Apgar scores, in-hospital feeding, current feedings, output, weights, behavior, etc.).
11. Assessment and present status of the baby (muscle tone, activity, skin turgor, oral cavity, behavior, weight, and so on).
12. Assessment of the feeding (include feeding weights, if possible).
13. Your assessment of the situation.
14. Suggestions you made to the mother and the action plan that was developed.
15. Arrangements for follow-up with the mother.
16. If the patient was referred to you, thank the physician for allowing you to participate in the care of her/his patient. If the patient self-referred, you may comment about working with the physician with this couple ("It was a pleasure . . .").
17. Sincerely yours, . . . (use all your credentials behind your name).

TABLE 6.2

Main Parts of a Consultation

Situation: Nancy, the mother of a 2-week-old infant, says to you, "My son Justin just had his 2-week checkup. His doctor is concerned because his weight is still just under his birth weight. He thinks I may need to supplement with formula and I am so upset. I wanted to breastfeed exclusively and now I don't know what to do."

◆ Statement that shows emotional support	"You're upset because your pediatrician recommended that you supplement with formula."
◆ Consent	Ask Nancy to sign and date a consent form before proceeding with the consultation.
◆ Gather information through maternal-infant history and assessment	How often is Justin breastfeeding in 24 hours? Does he breastfeed during the day and night? What are his feeding cues to which Nancy responds? Does he swallow audibly during the feedings? Who ends the feedings? How does Justin react during and after feedings? How many voids and stools does he have in 24 hours? What does Nancy already know about breastfeeding? Did Justin's physician prescribe supplements now, or is that a future possibility if more immediate breastfeeding measures do not help Justin's weight gain? How is Justin's general appearance and hydration status? What is his present weight, birth weight, and hospital discharge weight? How are Nancy's breasts and nipples? What does she notice about her milk supply? How are latch, position, and milk transfer? Your hunch: Nancy is unfamiliar with normal feeding cues, and therefore, Justin is not breastfeeding frequently enough for adequate milk intake and weight gain.
◆ Develop a workable plan with the mother	Be sure Justin is nursing 10 or more times in 24 hours around the clock. Teach Nancy feeding cues and baby-led feeding. Instruct her to watch and listen for audible swallows at feedings. Teach her how to do breast compression to enhance milk transfer. Help Nancy identify sources of support and household help through this time.
◆ Follow-up	Call the next day to evaluate how the changes in Nancy's breastfeeding routine are going. See Nancy and Justin for a weight check in 2 days.
◆ Physician's report	If Nancy is unsure about the physician's exact request regarding supplements, a call to the physician's office may be warranted to clarify that issue. A report outlining the plan of care should be sent within 24 hours.

---

elements that need to be included in a physician report. Table 6.2 shows the steps in a counseling scenario.

Evaluating the Plan of Care

Any plan of care you and the mother establish needs to be reevaluated frequently. As the situation changes, the plan of care may also need to change. If you do not see resolution of a problem, it may be more complicated than you first thought, which calls for another complete assessment. Determine whether the mother is adhering to the plan of care. Perhaps you overwhelmed her or suggested things she is unable or unwilling to do. Family members may be interfering with her attempts. Evaluate whether your approach was too rigid and if other alternatives would work better. Remaining flexible, attending breastfeeding conferences, networking with colleagues, and reading current literature will help you offer the mother a variety of options. Following up with the mother will provide insights into the effectiveness of your consultation.

Reviewing Your Counseling Skills

Critically assessing your counseling skills is important to meeting the needs of mothers. Figure 6.4 contains a series of questions asked of dieticians. You can use it as a model to craft similar questions for your work setting (Isselman, 1993). Responses to the statements indicate the quality of the consultation. The questions in Figure 6.5 combine the use of counseling skills with elements of a consultation to help you assess your effectiveness with mothers. Both sets of responses can be rated on a scale ranging from *strongly agree* to *strongly disagree*.

▶ HOSPITAL DOCUMENTATION

Documentation does not need to be a time-consuming task. If you expect staff to provide complete and useful information about every mother and infant, you want to use a method that is user friendly and does not seem

---

FIGURE 6.4
Questions to measure the quality of a consultation.

1. My confidence in my counseling skills has increased over the past 6 months.
2. I have identified the counseling style in which I am most comfortable and effective.
3. I am able to adapt my counseling style to meet the needs of the patient.
4. I am now using more attending and listening skills in my counseling sessions.
5. I am now able to recognize when a patient is not attending or listening during the counseling process.
6. I am better able to acknowledge my feelings that arise during the counseling process.
7. I am better able to acknowledge the feelings of my patients during the counseling process.
8. I have altered the way I conduct the counseling session based on the recognition of my own or my patient's feelings.
9. I evaluate the counseling environment before beginning the counseling session.
10. I take steps to correct the environment before beginning the counseling session.
11. I have requested that management make changes in my work site counseling environment that will enhance the counseling process.
12. I need further instruction, encouragement, or evaluation to enhance my counseling skills.

FIGURE 6.5
Questions to evaluate counseling skills in a consultation.

1. Understanding of the problem: LC understood the mother and helped her.
2. Breastfeeding information: Information was correct and appropriate. Not too much or too little.
3. Clarity of instructions: The mother understood the information and advice.
4. Good counseling skills: LC put mom at ease, encouraged her to share feelings.
5. Partnership with mother: Mother was drawn into the problem-solving process.
6. Encouraged mother's self-reliance: LC fostered greater self-assurance in mother.
7. Balance: LC achieved balance between listening, educating, and problem solving with no lecturing.
8. Arrangements for follow-up: LC made it clear when any further contact will take place and who will initiate it.
9. Overall impressions of mother's satisfaction with consultation.

---

daunting to them. Teach the mother to chart much of her breastfeeding information. Giving her this responsibility is a step to her becoming self-sufficient and self-assured in her breastfeeding.

There are a variety of methods for charting hospital contacts with breastfeeding mothers and babies. The method you use needs to include essential information about the mother, the baby, and breastfeeding. Avoid using terms such as "good," "fair," or "poor" to evaluate the feeding. Used alone, these terms give very little information about progress for the mother and baby to another person who reviews the chart. Likewise, simply recording the duration of a feeding gives no indication of its quality. There are several methods for documenting breastfeeding. You can select one that works best for you in your practice setting.

Breastfeeding Observation Form

Figure 6.6 shows a form printed by UNICEF and WHO in their manual for training maternity staff throughout the world. It uses the acronym *B-R-E-A-S-T* to help health workers memorize how they can evaluate a breastfeeding (UNICEF, 1993). The main categories to evaluate are body position, responses, emotional bonding, anatomy, suckling, and time spent suckling. After having observed a complete breastfeeding, the clinician checks

off in the left column the signs that breastfeeding is going well. The right column identifies signs of possible difficulty. Hospitals may find this method convenient for helping staff recognize when a mother and baby need help. The intent of the checklist is for the elements to become ingrained in the clinician's memory so that noting the essential points when observing breastfeedings becomes second nature.

Charting with Breastfeeding Descriptors

Table 6.3 presents a useful method using descriptors that reflect the level of achievement by the mother and baby (BSC, 1998). When this method is used, it is important that all staff understand the definitions for each abbreviation. Each rating gives very specific information about the breastfeeding and is much more helpful than "good feed" with no definition of what a "good feed" is.

The LATCH Method

Figure 6.7 shows the LATCH charting system (Jensen, 1994). Each letter of the acronym *LATCH* represents the scored item: latch, audible swallowing, type of nipple, comfort (breast and nipple), and hold (positioning). LATCH assesses the infant's ability to latch onto the

---

FIGURE 6.6
UNICEF BREASTfeed observation form.

B-R-E-A-S-T FEED OBSERVATION

Mother's name _____ Date _____ Infant's age _____

[Bracketed items refer only to the newborn infant, not to the older infant who sits up.]

Signs that breastfeeding is going well:

BODY POSITION
___ Mother relaxed and comfortable
___ Infant's body close to mother
___ Infant's head and body straight
___ Infant's chin touching breast
___ [Infant's bottom supported]

RESPONSES
___ Infant reaches for breast if hungry
___ [Infant roots for breast]
___ Infant explores breast with tongue
___ Infant calm and alert at breast
___ Infant stays attached to breast
___ Signs of milk ejection: [leaking, after pains]

EMOTIONAL BONDING
___ Secure, confident hold
___ Face-to-face attention from mother
___ Much touching by mother

ANATOMY
___ Breasts soft and full
___ Nipples stick out, protractile
___ Skin appears healthy
___ Breast looks round during feed

SUCKLING
___ Mouth wide open
___ Lower lip turned outward
___ Tongue cupped around breast
___ Cheeks round
___ Slow deep sucks, bursts with pauses
___ Can see or hear swallowing

TIME SPENT SUCKLING
___ Infant releases breast
   Infant suckled for _____ minutes

Signs of possible difficulty:

___ Shoulders tense, leans over baby
___ Infant's body away from mother's
___ Infant must twist neck
___ Infant's chin does not touch breast
___ [Only shoulder or head supported]

___ No response to breast
___ [No rooting observed]
___ Infant not interested in breast
___ Infant restless or fussy
___ Infant slips off breast
___ No sign of milk ejection

___ Nervous, shaking, or limp hold
___ No mother/infant eye contact
___ Little touching between mother and infant

___ Breasts engorged and hard
___ Nipples flat or inverted
___ Fissures or redness of skin
___ Breast looks stretched or pulled

___ Mouth closed, points forward
___ Lower lip turned in
___ Cannot see infant's tongue
___ Cheeks tense or pulled in
___ Rapid sucks
___ Can hear smacking or clicking

___ Mother takes infant off breast

Notes:

From *Breastfeeding Management and Promotion in a Baby Friendly Hospital: An 18-Hour Course for Maternity Staff,* UNICEF/WHO, 1993.

---

breast and evaluates audible swallowing as a determinant of milk intake. Type of nipple indicates the shape, size, and texture of the nipple as an important factor in the baby's ability to latch on. Comfort of the breasts and nipples is an indicator of the possible need for adjustments in positioning or another aspect of breastfeeding care. Hold, the final component of the LATCH assessment, considers the breastfeeding position the mother uses and her ability to assume a comfortable position that enables her to achieve and maintain an effective latch.

TABLE 6.3
Breastfeeding Descriptors for Documenting a Feeding

You may chart two types of feedings in one session. For example, a mother and baby may need considerable assistance with attachment. After the latch is achieved, the baby demonstrates nutritive sucking with audible swallows. This would be charted as *FBF → GBF*. Another example: You observe a baby that has some difficulty latching and the mom is poorly positioned. After offering assistance, the mother and baby overcome the obstacles and have an excellent feeding with lots of swallows. This would be charted as *Initial → PBF after assistance EBF*. Any rating below Excellent Breastfeed or Good Breastfeed will require further documentation that describes the problem and any help that is given.

Descriptor	Meaning	Elements observed
EBF	◆ Excellent breastfeed Note: It would be unusual to see an excellent breastfeed in the first 24 to 48 hours of life.	◆ Baby can latch on without difficulty ◆ Sucks are nice and deep with a nice steady rhythm ◆ Pauses are brief, and baby quickly resumes sucking again ◆ Can hear baby swallowing frequently, sometimes with each suck ◆ Mother does not need assistance positioning the baby or latching him on ◆ No nipple discomfort
GBF	◆ Good breastfeed	◆ Baby can latch on without any difficulty ◆ Sucks are nice and deep with a nice steady rhythm ◆ Pauses are brief, and baby resumes sucking again without being moved or prodded ◆ Some swallowing is heard ◆ Mother requires a little help with positioning or latch-on ◆ No nipple discomfort
FBF	◆ Fair breastfeed	◆ Baby is able to latch on to the breast and once on is able to stay on ◆ Sucks are short and quick; only occasionally may there be a nice deep suck; no steady rhythm ◆ Mother has to stroke or prod infant to resume sucking ◆ An occasional swallow may be heard, but usually no swallowing is heard ◆ Mother requires a lot of assistance with positioning and latch-on ◆ Mother could be experiencing nipple discomfort
PBF	◆ Poor breastfeed	◆ Roots for the breast, licks the nipple ◆ Latches on, but has difficulty doing it ◆ Once latched-on he does not stay on the breast or if he does he does not suck ◆ No swallowing is heard ◆ Mother requires a lot of assistance with positioning and latch-on ◆ Mother could have nipple discomfort or pain
ABF	◆ Attempted breastfeed	◆ Roots and licks at the nipple ◆ Unable to latch on to the nipple ◆ Mother requires a great deal of assistance
0BF	◆ No breastfeed	◆ No effort at the breast (too sleepy, lethargic, no interest) ◆ Pushes away from the breast, fights or cries, or both ◆ Despite lots of assistance, unable to accomplish a feed

Printed by permission of Breastfeeding Support Consultants (Barger, Kutner, 1996).

	0	1	2
L Latch	Too sleepy or reluctant No sustained latch or suck achieved	Repeated attempts for sustained latch or suck Hold nipple in mouth Stimulate to suck	Grasps breast Tongue down Lips flanged Rhythmical sucking
A Audible swallowing	None	A few with stimulation	Spontaneous and intermittent <24 hours old Spontaneous and frequent >24 hours old
T Type of nipple	Inverted	Flat	Everted (after stimulation)
C Comfort (breast/nipple)	Engorged Cracked, bleeding, large blisters, or bruises Severe discomfort	Filling Reddened/small blisters or bruises Mild/moderate discomfort	Soft Nontender
H Hold (positioning)	Full assist (staff holds infant at breast)	Minimal assist (i.e., elevate head of bed; place pillows for support) Teach one side; mother does other Staff holds and then mother takes over	No assist from staff Mother able to position and hold infant

FIGURE 6.7
LATCH method.

Source: Jenson D, Wallace S, Kelsay P (1994). LATCH: A breastfeeding charting system and documentation tool. *JOGNN,* 23(1):29. Reprinted with permission of Lippincott-Raven Publishers and authors.

The Mother-Baby Assessment Method

Figure 6.8 presents a tool modeled after the Apgar system. The Mother-Baby Assessment (Mulford, 1992) evaluates the progress of a mother and baby as they learn to breastfeed. The five steps assessed are signaling, positioning, fixing, milk transfer, and ending. Signaling is the step in which the mother and baby reach agreement that a feeding will take place. Positioning refers to the placement of the mother's and baby's bodies in relation to one another. Fixing is the point at which the infant attaches to the breast and begins to suckle. Milk transfer occurs when the baby's suckling releases milk and the baby consumes the milk. The final step, ending, refers to the outcome of the feeding session. The caregiver evaluates the mother and infant on every step, with 10 possible points. The caregiver also documents any assistance the mother received.

The Infant Breastfeeding Assessment Tool

The **Infant Breastfeeding Assessment Tool** (IBFAT) in Figure 6.9 assesses the infant's behavior during a breastfeeding. A score of 0, 1, 2, or 3 is assigned to the level of stimulation required to coax the infant to the breast, the infant's **rooting** response, time lapsed from initiating the process until the infant latches, and the infant's sucking pattern. The mother also describes her baby's overall feeding behavior and how she feels about the feeding. The total score for a feeding ranges from 0 to 12. The IBFAT tool does not assess the mother's physical aspect of the

FIGURE 6.8
Mother-Baby Assessment (MBA) method.

	M	B	HELP
Signaling	x	x	
Positioning	x	x	
Fixing	x		
Milk Transfer			
Ending			

Total Score   5 (With Help)

This is an assessment method for rating the progress of a mother and baby who are learning to breastfeed.

For every step, each person—both mother and baby—should receive an *x* before either one can be scored on the following step. If the observer does not observe any of the designated indicators, score 0 for that person on that step. If help is needed at any step for either the mother or the baby, check *Help* for that step. This notation will not change the total score for mother and baby.

1. SIGNALING

◆ Mother watches and listens for baby's cues. She may hold, stroke, rock, talk to baby. She stimulates baby if he is sleepy, calms baby if he is fussy.
◆ Baby gives readiness cues: stirring, alertness, rooting, sucking, hand-to-mouth, vocal cues, cry.

2. POSITIONING

◆ Mother holds baby in good alignment within latch-on range of nipple. Baby's body is slightly flexed, entire ventral surface facing mother's body. Baby's head and shoulders are supported.
◆ Baby roots well at breast, opens mouth wide, tongue cupped and covering lower gum.

3. FIXING

◆ Mother holds her breast to assist baby as needed, brings baby in close when his mouth is wide open. She may express drops of milk.
◆ Baby latches-on, takes all of nipple and about 2 cm (1 inch) of areola into mouth, then sucks, demonstrating recurrent burst-pause pattern.

4. MILK TRANSFER

◆ Mother reports feeling any of the following: thirst, uterine cramps, increased lochia, breast ache or tingling, relaxation, sleepiness. Milk leaks from opposite breast.
◆ Baby swallows audibly; milk is observed in baby's mouth; baby may spit up milk when burping. Rapid "call up sucking" rate (two sucks/second) changes to "nutritive sucking" rate of about 1 suck/second.

5. ENDING

◆ Mother's breasts are comfortable; she lets baby suck until he is finished. After nursing, her breasts feel softer; she has no lumps, engorgement, or nipple soreness.
◆ Baby releases breast spontaneously, appears satiated. Baby does not root when stimulated. Baby's face, arms, and hands are relaxed; baby may fall asleep.

Mulford C (1992). The mother-baby assessment (MBA): An "Apgar score" for breastfeeding. *J Hum Lact*, 8:79–82. Reprinted with permission of Human Sciences Press, Inc., and the author.

FIGURE 6.9
Infant Breastfeeding Assessment Tool (IBFAT) method.

Check the answer which best describes the baby's feeding behaviors at this feed.

1. When you picked baby up to feed was he/she

(a) deeply asleep (eyes closed, no observable movement except breathing)	(b) drowsy	(c) quiet and alert	(d) crying
_____	_____	_____	_____

2. In order to get the baby to begin this feed, did you or the nurse have to

(a) just place the baby on the breast as no effort was needed	(b) use mild stimulation such as unbundling, patting, or burping	(c) unbundle baby; sit baby back and forward; rub baby's body or limbs vigorously at the beginning and during the feeding	(d) baby could not be aroused
3	2	1	0

3. Rooting (definition: at touch of nipple to cheek, baby's head turns toward the nipple, the mouth opens, and baby attempts to fix mouth on the nipple). When the baby was placed beside the breast, he/she

(a) rooted effectively at once	(b) needed some coaxing, prompting, or encouragement to root	(c) rooted poorly even with coaxing	(d) did not try to root
3	2	1	0

4. How long from placing baby at the breast does it take for the baby to latch-on and start to suck?

(a) starts to feed at once (0–3 min)	(b) 3 to 10 minutes	(c) over 10 minutes	(d) did not feed
3	2	1	0

5. Which of the following phrases best describes the baby's feeding pattern at this feed?

(a) baby did not suck	(b) sucked poorly; weak sucking; some sucking efforts for short periods	(c) sucked fairly well; sucked off and on, but needed encouragement	(d) sucked well throughout on one or both breasts
0	1	2	3

6. How do you feel about the way the baby fed at this feeding?

(a) very pleased	(b) pleased	(c) fairly pleased	(d) not pleased
_____	_____	_____	_____

(continued)

Source: Matthews MK (1988). Developing an instrument to assess infant breastfeeding behavior in the early neonatal period. *Midwifery,* 4(4), 154–165. Reprinted with permission of Churchill Livingstone and the author.

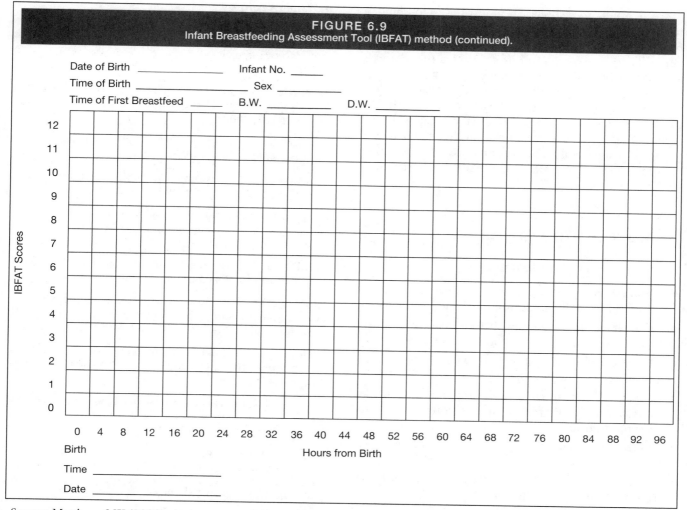

FIGURE 6.9
Infant Breastfeeding Assessment Tool (IBFAT) method (continued).

Date of Birth _____   Infant No. _____

Time of Birth _____   Sex _____

Time of First Breastfeed _____   B.W. _____   D.W. _____

IBFAT Scores

12 11 10 9 8 7 6 5 4 3 2 1 0

0   4   8   12 16 20 24 28 32 36 40 44 48 52 56 60 64 68 72 76 80 84 88 92 96

Birth

Hours from Birth

Time _____

Date _____

Source: Matthews MK (1993). Assessments and suggested interventions to assist newborn breastfeeding behavior. *I Hum Lact*, 9:243–48. Reprinted with permission of Human Sciences Press, Inc., and author.

feeding, nor does it specifically evaluate the baby's position and latch.

Developing a Plan of Care for Hospital Discharge

A final step in hospital documentation should include instructions that will help facilitate breastfeeding at home. For the mother and baby who are breastfeeding well on discharge, a diary to record the baby's feedings, voids, and stools with instructions regarding what is normal and where to get help will suffice. Appendix H presents an example of such a diary. When documenting a problem-oriented consultation, you will want to give the mother a written plan of care based on an assessment of her needs and her infant. There are a variety of care plans and other forms available. You do not need to

develop your own unless you wish to. See Appendix E for several examples of care plans. Using care plans such as these, you would check off the items that apply to a particular mother. Having a standard form will help you remember to include all essential information. See Appendix A for sources of additional care plans.

▶ SUMMARY

Using a preventive approach of anticipatory guidance will help parents achieve positive outcomes and actually will be less time consuming for the healthcare staff. The most effective method is early and continued contact so problems can be prevented or minimized. The nature of the situation will determine whether it lends itself to telephone contact or requires a consultation.

A consultation should begin with establishing a receptive climate. After you have established a supportive environment and obtained the mother's consent, you will gather information through taking the mother's and baby's histories and completing a physical assessment of both. You may then move on to sharing information and offering suggestions, working with the mother to develop a care plan. Part of that plan will include follow-up to evaluate the mother's and baby's progress. The consultation is completed after necessary documentation is recorded and a written report is sent to the caregiver.

▶ CHAPTER 6—AT A GLANCE

Applying what you learned—

◆ Provide anticipatory guidance at times when retention will be high and decision making can occur.

◆ Encourage initial learning before delivery so postpartum teaching can focus on reinforcement.

◆ Provide a hotline, warm line, or e-mail access to ensure contact with mothers.

◆ Arrange frequent contact during the early weeks postpartum, either personally or through referral to a support group.

◆ Recognize when a problem requires in-person rather than telephone help.

◆ Check for hidden factors that may contribute to the problem before forming a hunch.

◆ Be open to new information that may lead you to form a new hunch, and explore alternative hunches until you and the mother define the problem.

◆ Obtain signed consent before initiating a consultation.

◆ Take a complete history of the mother and baby.

◆ Assess the baby and the mother's breasts and nipples.

◆ Assess a breastfeeding, moving at the baby's pace and providing anticipatory guidance.

◆ Actively involve the mother in developing a plan of care.

◆ Give the mother a written plan of care and other necessary resources.

◆ Arrange appropriate follow-up and send reports to physicians for both the mother and baby.

◆ Teach the mother to chart her breastfeeding information.

◆ Use documentation that provides sufficient information for evaluating the quality of the feeding.

◆ Assess your counseling skills for areas of improvement.

▶ REFERENCES

Alnasir F. Knowledge and attitude of secondary school-girls towards breast-feeding in Bahrain. *J Bahrain Med Soc* 4(1):6–10; 1992.

Arora S et al. Major factors influencing breastfeeding rates: Mother's perception of father's attitude and milk supply. *Pediatrics* 106:e67; 2000.

Auerbach K. Last resort help-seeking and breastfeeding behavior. *J Hum Lact* 9:73–74; 1993.

Breastfeeding Support Consultants (BSC). Lactation Management Course. Chalfont, PA; 1998.

Earle S. Factors affecting the initiation of breastfeeding: Implications for breastfeeding promotion. *Health Promot Int* 17(3):205–214; 2002.

Ellis D et al. Assisting the breastfeeding mother: A problem-solving process. *J Hum Lact* 9:89–93; 1993.

Finch C, Daniel E. Breastfeeding education program with incentives increases exclusive breastfeeding among urban WIC participants. *J Am Diet Assoc* 102(7):981–984; 2002.

Goulet C et al. Attitudes and subjective norms of male and female adolescents toward breastfeeding. *J Hum Lact* 19(4):402–410; 2003.

Greenwood K, Littlejohn P. Breastfeeding intentions and outcomes of adolescent mothers in the Starting Out program. Review. *Breastfeed Rev* 10(3):19–23; 2002.

Guise J et al. The effectiveness of primary care-based interventions to promote breastfeeding: Systematic evidence review and meta-analysis for the US Preventive Services Task Force. *Ann Fam Med* 1(2):70–78; 2003.

Isselman M et al. A nutrition counseling workshop: Integrating counseling psychology into nutrition practice. *J Am Diet Assoc* 93:324–326; 1993.

Jensen D et al. LATCH: A breastfeeding charting system and documentation tool. *JOGNN* 23:27–32; 1994.

Ladas A. How to help mothers breastfeed: Deductions from a survey. *Clin Pediatr (Phila)* 9(12):702–705; 1970.

Martens P. The effect of breastfeeding education on adolescent beliefs and attitudes: A randomized school intervention in the Canadian Ojibwa community of Sagkeeng. *J Hum Lact* 17(3):245–255; 2001.

Mulford C. The mother-baby assessment (MBA): An Apgar score for breastfeeding. *J Hum Lact* 8:79–82; 1992.

Neifert M et al. Factors influencing breastfeeding among adolescents. *J Adolesc Health Care* 9:470–473; 1988.

Parker D, Williams N. *Lactation Consultant Series Two: Teens and Breastfeeding*. Schaumburg, Il: La Leche League International; 2000.

Piper S, Parks, PL. Predicting the duration of lactation: Evidence from a national survey. *Birth* 23(1):7–12; 1996.

Ross L, Goulet C. Attitudes and subjective norms of Quebecian adolescent mothers towards breastfeeding. *Can J Public Health* 93(3):198–202; 2002.

Sable M, Patton C. Prenatal lactation advice and intention to breastfeed: Selected maternal characteristics. *J Hum Lact* 14:35–40; 1998.

UNICEF/WHO. *Breastfeeding Management and Promotion in a Baby-Friendly Hospital: An 18-Hour Course for Maternity Staff*; 1993.

Valdes V et al. The impact of a hospital and clinic-based breastfeeding promotion programme in a middle class urban environment. *J Trop Pediatr* 39:142–151; 1993.

Volpe E, Bear M. Enhancing breastfeeding initiation in adolescent mothers through the Breastfeeding Educated and Supported Teen (BEST) Club. *J Hum Lact* 16(3):196–200; 2000.

Yeo S et al. Cultural views of breastfeeding among high school female students in Japan and the United States: A survey. *J Hum Lact* 10:25–30; 1994.

▶ BIBLIOGRAPHY

Axelson M et al. Primiparas' beliefs about breast feeding. *J Am Diet Assoc* 85:77–79; 1985.

Grossman L et al. The effect of postpartum lactation counseling on the duration of breastfeeding in low-income women. *Am J Dis Child* 144:471–474; 1990.

Matthews M. Assessments and suggested interventions to assist newborn breastfeeding behavior. *J Hum Lact* 9:243–248; 1993.

Matthews M. Developing an instrument to assess infant breastfeeding behavior in the early neonatal period. *Midwifery* 4:154–165; 1988.

Wiles L. The effect of prenatal breastfeeding education on breastfeeding success and maternal perception of the infant. *JOGNN* 13:253–257; 1984.

World Health Organization (WHO/CHD). *Evidence for the Ten Steps to Successful Breastfeeding*. Geneva: Division of Child Health and Development 98:9; 1998.

PART 2

THE SCIENCE OF LACTATION

CHAPTER
7

THE SCIENCE OF LACTATION

The breast, a marvelously complex mechanism, has ensured the survival of the human race. We humans, as mammals, continue to feed and nurture our babies. Mothers have always instinctively nurtured their young, confident in their natural abilities to produce milk. It is only in the past several decades that a study of the anatomy and physiology of the breast has become an issue in lactation. Today, health professionals study every detail of the breast, both externally and internally. The growth of functioning breast tissue, **milk synthesis** (production), the **letdown** reflex, and types of nipples all receive intense scrutiny. The information presented in this chapter will help you gain an understanding of these elements. Understanding of the breast and lactation function has changed dramatically within the past 10 years, thanks to ultrasound, computer imaging research, and increased public awareness of breast cancer and its prevention. It is imperative as you practice that you stay current on the ever-changing understanding of this amazing organ.

KEY TERMS

acinus
adhesion
afterpains
alveoli
areola
atresia
atrophy
augmentation
autocrine control
autonomic nerves
axilla
bactericidal
blood and lymph systems
capillaries
colostrum
connective tissue
Cooper's ligaments
dermis
duct system
ductule

edema
epidermis
epithelium
estrogen
evert
exocrine gland
fatty tissue
feedback inhibitor of
    lactation (FIL)
fibrocystic breast
fistula
foremilk
galactogogue
galactopoiesis
gestational ovarian theca
    luteal cyst
glandular tissue
hindmilk
Hoffman technique
hormonal imbalance

hormone pathways
hypopituitarism
hypoplasia
hypothalamus
inhibited letdown
innervation
insufficient mammary tissue
intercostal nerves
intraductal papilloma
inverted nipple
inverted syringe
involution
keratin
lactiferous
lactocyte
lactogenesis
lactose
leaking
letdown
lobule
lymph node
lymphatic system
lysozyme
malignant
mammary gland
mammary ridge
mammogenesis
mature milk
milk ejection reflex
milk synthesis
milk-producing tissue
milk-transporting tissue
Montgomery glands
myoepithelial cells

nerves
nipple pore
nipple preference
nipple shield
oxytocin
parenchyma
Paget's disease
pinch test
pitocin
pituitary
placenta
plugged duct
polycystic ovarian
    syndrome (PCOS)
progesterone
prolactin
prolactin inhibitory factor
    (PIF)
prolactinoma
protractility
reduction
resection
sebaceous gland
secretory
Sheehan's gland
sphincter
supernumerary nipple
supportive and sustaining
    tissue
Tail of Spence
transitional milk
transplantation
whey
witch's milk

▶ ANATOMY OF THE BREAST

The breast is part of the body's intricate system of reproduction. Although it is customarily referred to as a **mammary gland**, the breast is actually an organ. Each breast is an individual **exocrine** gland that functions and develops independently to extract materials from the blood and convert them into milk. Individuality in size and shape is especially evident during lactation, when a woman's breasts enlarge to accommodate milk synthesis. The rate of flow and the quantity of milk produced during lactation reveals the breast's uniqueness. The **nipple**, **areola**, and **Montgomery glands** are located within the surface layer of the breast. Knowledge of the components of the breast—skin, supportive tissue, and milk-producing and milk-transporting tissue—will enable you to help mothers understand the changes in their breasts during pregnancy and throughout lactation.

Skin

Most contact with our environment is through our skin, the body's largest organ. Skin helps hold us together and acts as a defensive covering for deeper tissue. It is flexible and elastic to allow for changes in tissue size. Skin acts as a screen against the damaging effects of light and performs respiratory and excretory functions—it breathes and perspires. Skin contains hair and **sebaceous** and sweat glands, and is composed of cells with many distinct layers. Dead cells lie on the surface, while living cells are underneath. The **dermis** and the **epidermis** make up two distinct layers.

Skin Layers

The dermis, composed of connective tissue, is the inner layer of the skin. It contains nerve endings, **capillaries** (small blood vessels), hair follicles, **lymph** channels, and other cells. Muscle cells are located under this layer, except in the area of the areola and nipple, where the two intermingle. The epidermis, made up of epithelial cells, is the outer layer of living cells. It covers and protects deeper skin layers from drying out and invasion by bacteria. Cells progress through the epidermis from initial growth in the germinating layer to loss of fluid in the transitional layer and on to the surface layer of dead skin, called **keratin** (Figure 7.1).

New cell growth in the germinating layer pushes dead cells outward toward the surface of the skin. As the cells move outward through the transitional layer, they undergo changes that cement them firmly together. This creates a tough, hard, waterproof barrier against bacterial invasion. The outer layer of the skin, the epidermis, protects the inner layer, the dermis, from abrasion and water evaporation.

Nipple

The nipple is the protruding part of the breast that extends and becomes firmer when stimulated, enabling the baby to latch onto the breast for nursing. The nipple is flexible and able to mold and elongate to conform to the baby's mouth during feeding. The tissue in the nipple is similar to the tissue in human lips, and is able to stretch and heal quickly. Sensory nerve endings in the nipple trigger milk release when the baby suckles.

The nipple is composed primarily of circular **smooth muscle** fibers that function as a closing mechanism for the milk ducts. The **ductule** openings, commonly called **nipple pores**, are located at the end of the nipple and enable the baby to receive the milk (see Color Plate 1). There are about 7 to 10 nipple duct openings (Ramsay, 2003).

During the last **trimester** of pregnancy, changes within the ducts may lead to a bloody discharge from the nipple (Lafrenier, 1990). It occurs when **epithelium** spurs that extend into the ducts are traumatized, resulting in bleeding (Dewitt, 1985; Kline, 1964). This phenomenon does not affect breastfeeding, and the bleeding often stops when the mother begins nursing. The cause may be excessive use of breast shells or breast expression late in pregnancy, or from edema during engorgement. Bleeding could indicate an intraductal papilloma, a growth in the duct. Occasionally, bleeding can be a sign of intraductal carcinoma (Matsunaga, 2004; Sauter, 2004).

Areola

The areola is the dark circular area surrounding the nipple. The size and color of the areola vary greatly from woman to woman. During puberty, menstruation, and pregnancy, it enlarges and becomes darker in color. Because the areola partially covers the underlying milk ducts, the baby's mouth needs to enclose a sizable portion. This enables his tongue to compress a large amount of breast tissue against his palate to facilitate milk release. Some older breastfeeding literature tells the mother to make sure the baby takes the entire areola into his mouth. However, some mothers' areolas can be very large. Suggest, instead, that the baby take in about one inch (diameter) of areolar tissue.

Montgomery Glands

The Montgomery glands, pimply in appearance, are sebaceous glands located around the areola. Also called Montgomery's tubercles, they secrete an oily substance that serves as a lubricant and a protective agent for the nipple. Because of this natural lubrication, the nipple and areola do not require creams and lotions to keep them soft and healthy. Montgomery gland secretions

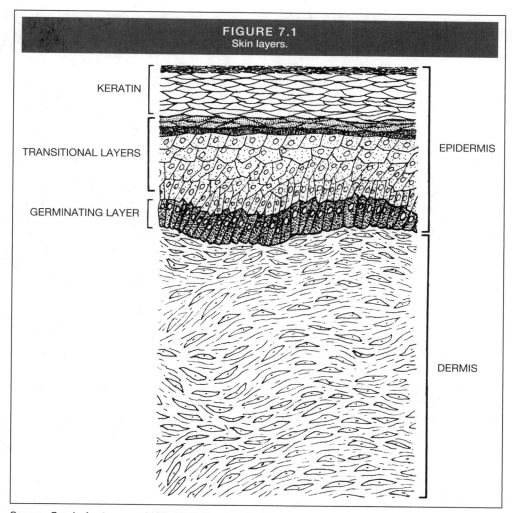

FIGURE 7.1
Skin layers.

KERATIN

TRANSITIONAL LAYERS

EPIDERMIS

GERMINATING LAYER

DERMIS

Source: Gray's Anatomy, p. 1137, 1977. Reprinted with permission from Lea & Febiger.

allow the skin to breathe and remain pliable. There is also some speculation that the secretions provide a taste and smell that enable the baby to find the nipple (Widstrom, 1993). Because they are rudimentary mammary glands, they may secrete a small amount of milk as well (Smith, 1982).

Washing the nipples with any substance other than plain water may remove this natural lubrication, dry out the breast skin, and reduce the scent. Lubricating the nipples with creams unnecessarily will coat the skin and reduce the amount of air reaching the tissue, making the skin less healthy. Creams may also introduce a scent or taste that the baby dislikes or does not recognize.

Supportive and Sustaining Tissue

Under the skin and between parts of the milk-producing and milk-transporting tissues lie other tissues that are vital to the function of the breast. Connective tissues support the breast, and **subcutaneous** fatty tissues give it shape. Nerves provide a triggering mechanism for milk synthesis and release. The blood and lymph systems bring nourishment to breast tissue, supply the nutrients for milk, and filter out bacteria and cast-off dead cell parts.

Nerves

The breast contains sensory nerves that trigger breast function for lactation. From the third, fourth, fifth, and sixth **intercostal** nerves, these sensory fibers innervate the smooth muscle in the nipples and blood vessels (Sarhadi, 1997; Silen, 1996). Intercostal nerves are located in the space between two ribs. **Innervation** is the distribution of nerve fibers or nerve impulses. Most sensation to the nipple and areola comes from the fourth intercostal nerve (Sun, 2004; Sarhadi, 1996).

There is extensive innervation of the nipple and areola complex, composed of both **autonomic nerves** and sensory nerves. Autonomic nerves have the ability to function independently, without outside influence. Innervation of the nipple differs from that of the areola. The areola has been believed to be the more sensitive of the two. However, a recent study suggests the opposite, maintaining that the nipple is more sensitive. It cites the higher density of the nipple as a possible explanation (Godwin, 2004). Another study reports that women with small breasts seem to experience more sensitivity than those with large breasts (Del Vecchyo, 2004).

A baby who grasps the breast well and suckles vigorously will stimulate the deeper nerves as well. This stimulation triggers oxytocin release and milk letdown. A baby who is weak or tired or who sucks on the nipple alone may not provide adequate stimulation to the deeper nerves. Ultimately, this factor may result in lower milk production and less effective letdowns. It explains why a mother whose baby cannot nurse and who must express milk from her breasts may notice a gradual decline in milk production.

Fatty Tissue

Fatty tissue within the breast cushions the organ and makes it comfortable and graceful. Fat cells are located throughout most of the breast, between lobuli (plural of **lobule**) and milk ducts, and under the skin. There is very little fat deposited immediately beneath the areola and nipple, an area dominated by muscular tissue and duct branching.

Fatty and glandular tissue determines breast size, not function. Fatty tissue does not contribute to milk synthesis or transport. Therefore, the amount of fat or size of the breast is little indication of the quality or quantity of milk the mother will produce. Women with large or small breasts are equally capable of breastfeeding. Some women may have large breasts consisting of mostly fatty tissue and sparse alveolar growth. Others may have smaller breasts in which there are ample alveolar lobes and little subcutaneous fat. Women with larger breasts may be more likely to have a larger storage capacity, explaining why some women deliver larger feedings at one time to their infants than other women (Kent, 2003; Cregan, 1999; Cox, 1996; Daly, 1995).

Connective Tissue

The breast contains fibrous connective tissue that supports and contains the fatty tissue and the milk-producing and milk-transporting tissues. Fibrous bands, called **Cooper's ligaments**, provide a framework to support the tissues of the breast. They attach the breast to the overlying skin and the underlying fibrous tissue enclosing the muscles. Fibrous tissue holds the segments of the breast together and supports the ducts as they fill with milk.

It is unclear whether fibrous tissue returns to its prepregnancy condition after pregnancy and lactation. Sagging breasts and protruding abdomens most likely result from the pregnancy, rather than lactation. Women who do not breastfeed their infants experience the same

effects. Some caregivers believe that breast sagging can be lessened by the wearing of a good support bra during pregnancy and lactation, especially at times when the breasts are enlarged and full. However, there is no research to support this belief. Mothers can wear a bra for comfort if they wish, but caution them against bras that are tight or have underwires or other stiff parts that can press on milk ducts.

Blood and Lymph Systems

Everything the breast cells need for nourishment—proteins, fats, carbohydrates, and other substances—is brought to them by the bloodstream. Fluids containing these nutrients pass through the capillaries to the tissue spaces, where they are absorbed. Capillaries are small blood vessels that link the arteries and veins. The body has amazing control over the amount of blood that flows into tissue, maintaining circulation at a level that meets the needs of each tissue. When the needs of the breast increase during menstruation and pregnancy, blood flow increases to support tissue building. Later, when frequent suckling signals a need to increase milk production, more blood becomes available to provide the nutrients needed to make milk.

The **lymphatic system** functions like the bloodstream in reverse. It is a complex network of capillaries, thin vessels, valves, ducts, nodes, and organs. Lymph is a thin, clear, slightly yellow fluid. It is about 95 percent water with a few red blood cells and variable numbers of white blood cells. The lymphatic system absorbs the excess blood fluids from the tissue spaces and eventually returns them to the heart.

Lymph nodes function as filters in the lymph vessels to trap bacteria and cast-off cell parts. Each node is a potential dam to arrest the spread of infection. At times, lymph nodes may swell and be painful. Most of the lymph produced within the breast flows into the nodes in the armpit. There, they trap bacteria that travel up the ducts from the nipple or bloodstream. The swelling of a lymph node in the armpit could suggest that an infection is present in the breast, arm, or hand.

During breast engorgement, increased pressure from milk in the ducts decreases the flow of blood and lymph. This condition can cause fluids to accumulate in the tissues, referred to as **edema** (Hill, 1994). With the lymphatic system at a standstill, the risk of local infection increases. The breast cannot remove bacteria and cell particles adequately, which leads to poor drainage of the ducts and alveoli.

Generally, bacteria multiply more easily in stagnant fluids than in moving ones. This predisposes a poorly drained breast to mastitis (breast inflammation characterized by pain, swelling, redness, and fever). A mother with mastitis must remove milk as effectively as possible to reduce pressure within the breast. She can do this by feeding her baby more frequently and thoroughly, or by expressing milk from the breast.

Glandular Tissue

The breast has highly efficient glands that take raw materials from blood and create new and essential nutrients for the baby. The breast **parenchyma** (functional parts of the organ) are composed of many smaller individual glands, or lobuli. These lobuli, in turn, consist of many milk-producing **alveoli**. The lobuli connect to a system of ducts that provide a passageway for the milk to flow out of the breast and to the infant. Glandular tissue is the functional part of the breast that produces and transports milk. Understanding the structure of the functioning tissue will help you assist mothers in preventing or treating breastfeeding problems.

Milk-Producing Tissue

The production of milk takes place in the breast in tiny individual glands called alveoli. The singular form is alveolus, also called **acinus**. The alveoli consist of epithelial cells (**lactocytes**) encased in a dense basketlike meshwork of smooth muscle, known as the **myoepithelial cells**. Numerous capillaries surround the alveoli and bring nutrient-rich blood from which the alveoli make milk.

Through this same system, the alveoli receive the hormones oxytocin and prolactin, which signal them to release and produce more milk. Like other smooth muscle cells in the body, such as those in the uterine wall and nipple, myoepithelial cells contract when exposed to oxytocin released during suckling. The contraction of these cells in the alveoli results in a squeezing effect on the lobule, forcing milk down the ducts. Myoepithelial cells multiply and greatly increase in size during pregnancy and lactation. They later decrease in size and number when breastfeeding ends. Color Plate 2 shows the interior of a milk-filled alveolus and its surrounding myoepithelial cells. Color Plate 3 illustrates the constriction of the myoepithelial cells that forces milk from the alveolus into the duct.

The alveoli are grouped together and form lobuli, often compared to a cluster of grapes. There is large variation in the distribution of lobuli in the breast. Computer image research indicates that there are fewer lobes than previously believed, probably seven to ten per breast (Ramsay, 2003). The **tail of Spence** describes the breast tissue that extends into the **axilla**.

Milk-Transporting Tissue

Milk flows through a system of **lactiferous** (mammary) ductules, secondary ducts, and nipple pores, as shown in Color Plate 1. In the young girl, the **duct system** begins with a few small basic ducts in childhood. They sprout and branch during puberty, forming tissue buds for the future development of alveoli and lobuli. With each ovulation, the ducts grow lengthwise as alveoli and lobuli develop. During the first four to five months of pregnancy, sprouting and growth of ducts and alveolar development intensify. In the second half of pregnancy, the duct and alveolar tissues become more specialized in preparation for their milk-related functions.

Previous texts called ducts beneath the areola the *lactiferous sinuses*. This evolved from cadaver work done by Sir Astley Cooper in 1840, in which he injected hot wax into the breast of a cadaver of a woman who had been lactating at the time of death. Scientists now hypothesize that the injection of the hot wax distended the cadaver's ducts, which led to the belief that lactiferous sinuses were larger than the rest of the ductule framework (Ramsay, 2003; Love, 2000). Real-time ultrasound, computer imaging now shows a temporary dilation of the ducts during letdown and the passage of milk through the ducts and out the ductule openings in the nipple. After this passage, the ducts collapse until the next surge of milk (Ramsay, 2003).

The mature lactating breast contains an intricate ductal system. These ducts bring the milk out of the breast through five to ten nipple pores. Each duct widens throughout the breast and in the area beneath the areola during the passage of milk through the ductule opening (Figure 7.2). The duct system is much more random and intricate than is usually presented in illustrations (Ramsay, 2004a). There is also great variance from mother to mother (Ramsay, 2004b).

Insufficient Mammary Tissue

Sometimes women will present with very small, poorly developed breasts, which is called **hypoplasia**. This is not the same as having small breasts. Widely spaced (over one and a half inches apart), tubular, thin breasts are markers for true insufficient glandular tissue. Color Plates 4–7 illustrate four common types of breasts (Huggins, 2000), including type 4, an example of hypoplasia. Whenever a mother has great difficulty producing enough milk and you have ruled out breastfeeding technique as a cause, consider the possibility of underlying hormonal problems or true insufficient glandular tissue. If a mother tries all means of increasing milk production and is unable to maintain an adequate supply, her baby may need supplements.

Signs of possible glandular insufficiency (Neifert, 1990):

♦ No noticeable change in breast size during pregnancy or lactation.
♦ One breast appreciably smaller than the other.
♦ Family history of lactation failure.
♦ Inadequate milk production despite appropriate feeding regimen.
♦ Ductal **atresia**, where the lack of a milk duct opening prevents milk from being ejected from that particular duct.

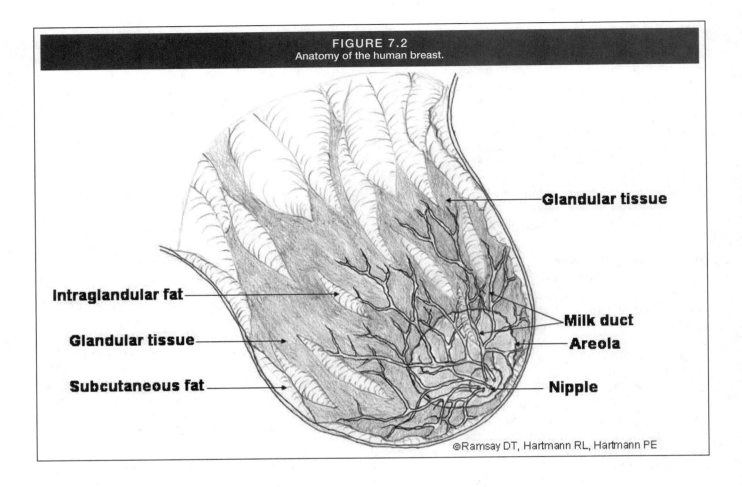

FIGURE 7.2
Anatomy of the human breast.

Glandular tissue

Intraglandular fat

Glandular tissue

Subcutaneous fat

Milk duct

Areola

Nipple

©Ramsay DT, Hartmann RL, Hartmann PE

Effects of Breast Surgery

A woman with a history of breast surgery of any kind, including biopsies, is advised to check with her surgeon to learn if any functional breast tissue was affected by the surgery. This applies to chest, back, and cardiac surgery as well. One technique measures blood flow and innervation to the nipple following surgery as a means of predicting a woman's ability to breastfeed (Hallock, 1992).

A quicker, less invasive measure is to breastfeed, evaluate intake, and monitor all signs of adequate production carefully, including the infant's feeding behavior, voiding, stooling, and weight gain indicators. If deficiencies are evident, early intervention to optimize milk production is crucial, such as with **galactogogues**, external oxytocin, increased stimulation, or supplementation.

Mothers who have had **augmentation** or **reduction** for cosmetic reasons may feel grief, guilt, regret, or disappointment over the surgery's impact on their ability to breastfeed. Listening to the mother and using reflective listening skills will help her process her feelings about the surgery's consequences. You can assure her that the breastfeeding she is able to do benefits her baby and contributes to responsive parenting that will meet her child's changing needs.

Types of Breast Surgery

Breast augmentation usually does not involve the destruction of functional breast tissue. It sometimes damages the nerves, particularly on the lateral side of the breast at the site of the incision. One study found that 28.6 percent of mothers who had breast augmentation and implant surgery experienced breastfeeding problems (Strom, 1997). Mothers who have had breast augmentation or reduction surgery need close follow-up to assure adequate milk production and infant weight gain.

Breast reduction is more intrusive and more often affects lactation. **Resection** of the breast with **transplantation** of the nipple severs all ducts. This free-nipple technique usually renders full lactation impossible. Another technique removes a portion of the breast with transposition of the nipple, areola, and ducts. This procedure may be more compatible with breastfeeding, as long as the nerve supply to the breast remains intact. Studies of breastfeeding after reduction report mixed results. One small cohort reported 7 out of 13 respondents breastfed without supplementation (Hefter, 2003). A German study reviewing five reduction studies found an average of about 31 percent breastfeeding (Zimpelmann, 2002). It is important to follow these mothers carefully and monitor infant intake and weight gain.

Women who have had surgery to remove cancerous cysts, or other growths need to contact a caregiver who is knowledgeable in lactation before their baby is born. Some health professionals believe that lactation hormones increase the probability that such conditions will recur. There is sufficient data, however, to encourage lactation after surgery for breast cancer. A review of ten years of breastfeeding and cancer studies concluded that "there is no evidence that breastfeeding increases the risk of breast cancer recurring. . . . Women previously treated for breast cancer, who do not show any evidence of residual tumour, should be encouraged to breastfeed their children" (Helewa, 2002). It is possible to breastfeed equally well from the untreated and treated breast after conservative surgery and radiation (Higgins, 1994). Women can breastfeed on the remaining breast after a mastectomy.

► MAMMARY GROWTH AND DEVELOPMENT

From the onset of puberty and throughout pregnancy, the mammary gland is in a stage of **mammogenesis**, when it develops to a functioning state. During the last trimester of pregnancy, it enters into **lactogenesis**, when milk synthesis and secretion are established. With the establishment of **mature milk** and throughout lactation, the breast is in a state of **galactopoiesis**. **Involution** occurs at the end of lactation, with the breast slowly returning to its prepregnant state. See Figures 7.3 and 7.4 for a comparison of the breast before and during pregnancy.

Mammary Growth during the Fetal Stage

The beginnings of breast development become noticeable in the fetus at five weeks of life. At this time, two **mammary**

ridges (also called "milk lines") are detectable, extending from the armpits to the inner thighs. The lower parts of the milk lines disappear after several weeks. By 20 to 32 weeks, the upper parts develop and form milk ducts. Sometimes, the lower ends of the milk lines fail to regress and the baby is born with one or more **supernumerary nipples** along this line. Toward the end of gestation, the ducts form openings in the nipples that are depressed below the surface of the skin. Just before birth, the nipples push outward and become level with the skin. In some cases, this step fails, resulting in a partially or completely inverted nipple.

Some babies (both male and female) are born with breasts that secrete a colostrum-like fluid, sometimes referred to as "witch's milk." This fluid consists primarily of shed epithelial cells and may result from an influx of hormones through the mother's **placenta** at birth. Babies who are born before term do not have this secretion. Left alone, witch's milk disappears in about 20 days.

Mammary Growth during Puberty

The majority of functional breast tissue development occurs during puberty and pregnancy, both periods of increased hormonal activity. Although the structural growth of the breast is very apparent during puberty, only a small amount of alveolar development takes place. During ovulatory cycles, the development of functional breast tissue is slight.

Because the breast covers the bony rib cage, it grows outward. The skin that covers and contains the breast expands and grows to accommodate it. The result is an evenly rounded organ with a protruding nipple. With the onset of menstruation, the body's hormonal balance alters because of an increased production of **estrogen**. This produces the growth of ducts and the connective tissue between them. A thick layer of fat is deposited

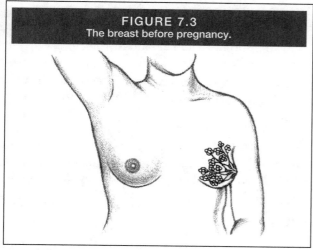

FIGURE 7.3
The breast before pregnancy.

Illustration by Marcia Smith.

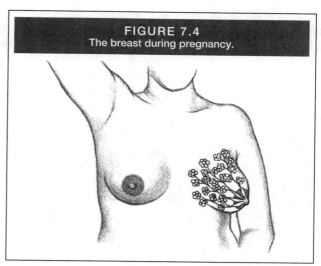

FIGURE 7.4
The breast during pregnancy.

Illustration by Marcia Smith.

under the skin and forms the firm and enlarged adolescent breast. The areola and the nipple grow and take on a deeper color during puberty and again in pregnancy.

The initial major changes in functional breast tissue are typically complete approximately 12 to 18 months after the first menstrual period. The formation of fibrous connective tissue and the laying down of fat continue to increase breast size during each adolescent menstrual period. Between the events of puberty and pregnancy, the mammary gland is relatively inactive. Around 12 to 16 days before the onset of each menses, the ovaries release an egg and estrogen releases. The reproduction of ductule tissue and the formation of alveolar cells begins to prepare the breast for pregnancy at this time. However, this proliferation is not significant in terms of breast size.

Breast fullness experienced by women just before menstruation is due to an increased blood supply and excessive fluid retained in the tissues. After each menstrual cycle is complete, tissue growth regresses and glandular cells degenerate. Loss of fluid from the tissues causes the breast to return to its previous size. Because regression of tissue growth is incomplete, the ovulatory cycle slightly enhances mammary growth for younger women (under approximately 30 to 35 years of age). However, in terms of overall breast development and preparation for lactation, breast tissue enhancement during pregnancy is far more significant than any total gain made during menstrual cycles.

Mammary Growth during Pregnancy

With the onset of pregnancy, the breast continues to progress through the stage of mammogenesis and further develops to a functioning state. It is at this time that hormonal changes cause a spectacular phase of growth and proliferation within the breast. During the first trimester of pregnancy (conception to three months), estrogen and **progesterone** levels cause the duct system to multiply. The skin begins to respond to internal enlargement, and circumference of the nipple and areola in particular increases. Increased pigmentation or darkening may make this growth seem more apparent.

Glands of Montgomery, often unnoticed before pregnancy, now enlarge or elongate. They give the area a rough pimply appearance, which is most noticeable if the breast is cool. The Montgomery glands begin to secrete an oily substance that protects the nipple and areolar skin. This protective lubricant continues to secrete throughout pregnancy and lactation. The Montgomery glands often become noticeable by the first missed menstrual period, giving the experienced mother an early sign of pregnancy.

In the second trimester (four to six months), the duct system continues to develop. Alveoli begin to appear because of placental prolactin (Figure 7.4). By the end of the trimester, the blood supply and body fluids (lymph) that support alveolar growth and the multiplying number of alveoli have increased the weight of the breast by as much as 1–1½ pounds. Production of colostrum is established, and at this point, a woman would lactate were she to deliver prematurely (Hartmann, 2003).

General breast development continues throughout the third trimester (seven to nine months). Stretch marks may appear as evidence of the stress on the skin. The nipple and areola continue to darken and enlarge. Their color may lighten somewhat when the mother gives birth and toward the end of lactation. This process repeats with each succeeding pregnancy. The change in color and size often appears more pronounced in younger women, perhaps because their breasts are not fully mature when pregnancy occurs. From the time the alveoli begin to proliferate during pregnancy, alveolar cells constantly wear out and replenish. This explains why adolescent mothers are able to lactate despite their recent pubescent changes. The replenishment cycle continues throughout lactation.

Lactogenesis

Lactogenesis occurs in 3 stages that establish milk synthesis and secretion. Understanding the physiology associated with lactogenesis will help you guide mothers in their daily breastfeeding routine. An awareness of the factors that influence milk synthesis will enable you to explain to mothers how frequent nursing increases milk production. In order to identify problems with milk letdown and to help mothers work out solutions, you need to recognize factors that initiate letdown, the function of hormones in the letdown process, and their effects on breast tissue.

Stages of Lactogenesis

◆ Stage I lactogenesis starts at the beginning of the third trimester of pregnancy. At this time, epithelial cells are converted to a secretory state and plasma concentrations of **lactose**, total proteins, and **immunoglobulin** increase. Sodium and chloride decrease. Substances needed for milk synthesis are drawn from the maternal bloodstream.

◆ Stage II lactogenesis occurs at around the second to fifth day postpartum. It is referred to as the time when the colostral phase ends and **transitional milk** is produced. Blood flow within the breast increases, and copious milk secretion begins.

◆ Stage III lactogenesis, also called galactopoiesis, marks the establishment and maintenance of mature milk. It occurs at about eight to ten days postpartum.

Involution

Lactogenesis is followed by a period of involution, which is a normal process marked by the decreasing

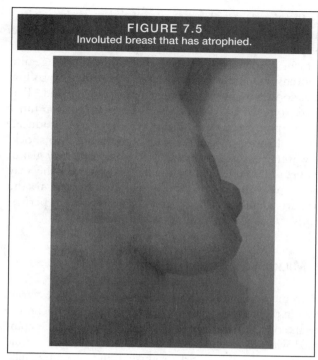

FIGURE 7.5
Involuted breast that has atrophied.

Printed with permission of Anna Swisher.

size—**atrophy**—of the breast. At this time, the breast slowly returns to its prepregnant state. The process takes about three months when accompanied by slow and gradual weaning. Abrupt weaning will cause marked involution in a matter of days or weeks.

After multiple pregnancies and extended breastfeeding, some women experience severe involution, in which fat deposits do not recur when the ducts regress (Figure 7.5). Normal breast shape usually returns within three years. Loss of fat and shape can also occur without breastfeeding. In the event of another pregnancy, the breast will regenerate and again lactate (Lawrence, 1999). Some mothers with severe involution, in which fat deposits do not regenerate, may choose to have breast augmentation.

▶ **HORMONAL IMPACT ON LACTATION**

A comprehensive understanding of lactation hormones and their function will help you identify problems with initiation and ongoing milk production. Lactation hormones affect letdown, milk production, breast tissue, and other aspects of a mother's physiology. Hormones are chemical products of the endocrine glands that regulate functions of specific organs or tissues. The growth, maturation, and function of the breast are the result of stimulation by four major hormones—estrogen, progesterone, prolactin, and oxytocin.

Estrogen

Estrogen is produced in the ovaries, adrenal glands, and placenta. It stimulates growth of the uterus, vagina, and other reproductive organs. Estrogen is responsible for the development of female secondary sex characteristics, such as the distinctive female skeleton, body contour, and mammary glands. In the breast, estrogen causes the growth of mammary ducts and the connective tissue between the ducts.

Progesterone

Progesterone is produced in the ovaries and placenta. The Latin word means *for gestation*. Progesterone works along with estrogen to maintain the reproductive tract and menstrual cycle. It is essential for the maintenance of pregnancy and aids in the development of the milk-secreting cells in the breast. Progesterone inhibits prolactin's effects during pregnancy. A retained placenta following delivery and its accompanying progesterone can impair stage II lactogenesis.

Prolactin

Prolactin is produced in the placenta and in the anterior **pituitary** gland in the brain. The Latin word means *for lactation*. Anterior pituitary prolactin stimulates alveolar growth in the breast during pregnancy. Prolactin levels in the mother's blood increase soon after initiation of the sucking stimulus. Prolactin signals the breast to speed up milk synthesis. It both serves as a natural tranquilizer and stimulates feelings in the mother of restlessness and yearning for her baby. This physiologically conditioned response stimulates the mother to interact positively with her baby. Thus, prolactin is often credited with inducing maternal behavior.

A mother can do several things to keep prolactin levels high. She can position her baby so he can attach effectively at the breast. She can avoid artificial nipples or pacifiers that may cause **nipple preference**. She can give her baby unlimited access to the breast, breastfeeding as frequently as he wants, usually every one to three hours, and as long as he wants at a feeding. Breastfeeding during the night, when prolactin release in response to suckling is greatest, will help to keep prolactin levels high as well.

Oxytocin

Oxytocin is produced in the **hypothalamus** and travels through nerve fibers to the posterior pituitary, where it is stored. The infant's suckling stimulates nerve endings in the nipple. Impulses travel through the hypothalamic region to the posterior pituitary and release oxytocin. The blood stream carries oxytocin to the breasts, where it causes smooth muscle cells to contract, thus producing the uterine contractions of childbirth, **afterpains**, and orgasm.

Oxytocin causes the muscle layer, or myoepithelial cell, around each milk-producing cell to contract during letdown. This is called the **milk ejection reflex**. In response, milk is pushed down the ducts and out through the nipple pores. The mother initially may need several minutes of stimulus to have a high enough level of oxytocin to be effective. She will notice when the milk ejects because the rhythm of her baby's suckling will change from rapid to regular deep, slow sucks (about one per second). **Pitocin** is a synthetic form of oxytocin, often used for induction or augmentation of labor.

Oxytocin is known as an affiliation hormone, or "mothering hormone." It plays a key role in the initiation of maternal behavior and the formation of adult pair bonds (Turner, 1999). Social stimuli may induce oxytocin release, and oxytocin may make positive social contact more rewarding. Some researchers believe oxytocin gives women a "tend and befriend" response to stress, encouraging bonding with other women and the tending of children (Taylor, 2000).

Hormonal Imbalances

Hormones in the mother's body regulate the lactation process. Therefore, a disturbance in her hormone levels has the potential to affect milk production and release. Pituitary, thyroid, and adrenal imbalances can alter a mother's hormone levels, as can certain medications. This imbalance may cause her to produce too little or too much milk, to release milk at inappropriate times, or to fail to release milk at all. Women who have difficulty conceiving or who have become pregnant by the aid of reproductive technologies are at a higher risk for hormone imbalance and milk insufficiency.

If a mother has breastfeeding problems accompanied by a vague feeling of physical discomfort or a history of previous thyroid problems or menstrual irregularities, she may have a hormone imbalance. Placental retention can inhibit the process of lactation by causing hormones to remain at pregnancy levels. The absence of breast fullness and changes in breast secretions can indicate the retention of placental fragments.

Hormone imbalances causing breastfeeding problems are becoming more common due to the increased number of women conceiving through infertility treatment. If a client fits the profile for hormone problems, refer her to her caregiver for a thorough hormonal screening—including measurement of progesterone, thyroid function, prolactin, and testosterone levels—to rule out hormone imbalance as a cause. See Chapter 25 for a discussion of pituitary and thyroid dysfunction and polycystic ovarian syndrome (PCOS).

Sheehan's syndrome, also known as **hypopituitarism** syndrome, postpartum hypopituitarism, and postpartum pituitary insufficiency, is a form of shock that can result from severe postpartum hemorrhage and hypotension. The mother's blood pressure drops so low that blood fails to circulate to the pituitary gland. This causes some or all of the cells in the gland to stop functioning permanently. The mother may have produced some colostrum in her breasts before going into shock. However, because of the malfunctioning pituitary gland, her breasts will remain soft after delivery and she may not be able to produce any milk. The damage to the pituitary gland is usually irreversible and may permanently rule out the prospect of breastfeeding.

▶ MILK SYNTHESIS

When the placenta is delivered, estrogen and progesterone levels in the body drop sharply, and prolactin production in the anterior pituitary rises. The high level of prolactin combined with decreased levels of estrogen and progesterone signals the alveoli to start producing and secreting milk. When the infant has free access to the breast, colostrum gives way to transitional milk. This is followed by increased milk production and breast fullness begin between the second and fifth day postpartum. With initial milk production, women typically experience a **normal fullness** in their breasts. Those who do not understand this normal physiologic response may mistake it for engorgement.

Colostrum Production

Colostrum is a unique substance that appears as a semi-transparent, thick, and sticky liquid ranging in color from pale to deep yellow. It contains water, minerals, fat droplets, **lymphocytes**, and similar cells. It also contains cast-off alveolar cells, which form a unique combination of nutrients designed to meet the nutritional and **immunologic** needs of the newborn. Colostrum acts as a natural lubricant and, because of its **lysozyme** content, it is **bactericidal** (destroys bacteria).

Alveoli begin producing colostrum in the fourth month of pregnancy. Only small amounts release into the center of the lobuli. As pregnancy advances, colostrum production continues to fill the alveoli. Some colostrum may leak out of the alveoli through the cell pores, and protruding portions of the alveoli may break away into the center of the lobule. Thus, some women find that their breasts leak colostrum during the later months of pregnancy.

Role of Prolactin

Prolactin is the hormone that promotes milk synthesis. It is present in small amounts in all humans, both male and female. Prolactin levels increase gradually during pregnancy and reach a peak of 20 times the normal value near term. Estrogen and progesterone levels during pregnancy act locally on the alveoli to inhibit milk production and secretion. After delivery, when estrogen and progesterone levels have dropped, the high prolactin levels stimulate initial milk production. Levels increase again tenfold in response to suckling. After three months postpartum, prolactin levels range three to five times above the level of a menstruating female. Further stimulation results in doubling of the level above the baseline through the second year of lactation (Lawrence, 1999).

Autocrine Control

Milk synthesis does not rely entirely on endocrine, or hormonal, control. Milk production becomes dependent on the frequency of drainage and the degree of drainage of each breast. Thus, milk production changes from endocrine control to **autocrine control**. Frequent breastfeeding is necessary in the beginning to ensure an increase in the number and sensitivity of prolactin receptors as prolactin levels drop after delivery. Both prolactin receptors and frequent infant feeding are necessary for long-term milk production.

Autocrine control is local control within the gland. In the case of the breast, the control agent is a **secretory** product from one type of cell that influences the activity of that type of cell. This suggests that milk that remains in the breast acts to inhibit the production of more milk. Thus, the mother produces only what her baby needs and protects her energy expenditure during lactation (Peaker, 1996; DeCoopman, 1993). This theory helps explain why women are able to nurse with one breast exclusively through the course of lactation and not develop chronic engorgement or mastitis in the other breast (Ing, 1977). Research on lactating goats has identified the apparent human **whey** protein, called **feedback inhibitor of lactation** (FIL), which enables autocrine inhibition of milk synthesis. Researchers believe a whey protein in humans provides a similar FIL function (Knight, 1998; Wilde, 1998).

Prolactin Inhibitory Factor

The **prolactin inhibitory factor** (PIF) prevents the release of prolactin at times when the baby is not nursing. Suckling inhibits PIF, thereby allowing the release of prolactin. The frequency of feeding and stimulation of the nipple significantly affect the level of prolactin that is released. It is important, therefore, to encourage frequent feedings, good positioning of the baby at the breast, and avoiding arbitrary use of nipple shields. In the absence of effective and frequent suckling to remove milk, prolactin production decreases and autocrine inhibition begins.

▶ MILK EJECTION REFLEX (LETDOWN)

Milk ejection, also referred to as letdown, is a reflex triggered by various stimuli. When the baby suckles, contact between his tongue and the mother's nipple stimulates nerve endings to send a message to the hypothalamus. The message then goes to the anterior pituitary, lowering the prolactin inhibitory factor and triggering prolactin release. As suckling continues, the posterior pituitary gland secretes oxytocin, causing the smooth muscles around the alveoli and the uterus to contract. The contraction forces milk down through the **lactiferous duct** system to the ductule openings behind the nipple (Figure 7.6). The milk is then available to the baby, who, through a combination of suction, rhythmic compression of the gums, and movement of the tongue, can nurse the milk out through the nipple pores.

Milk ejection is bilateral, occurring at the same time in both breasts. **Sphincters** at the end of the ducts prevent milk from flowing freely from the non-suckled breast. A sphincter is a circular band of muscle fibers that narrows a passage or closes a natural opening in the body. Letdown brings the milk into the ducts, thus making it accessible to the baby through the activity of suckling. Initially, letdown causes active expulsion of milk through pressure within the ducts. This lasts for a very short time, and then the flow subsides. Positive pressure continues within the breast, and milk flow will continue with further suckling. Letdown provides free flow of milk, which is essential to move fat globules down through the ducts. When milk does not flow freely, engorgement can develop, which could lead to a **plugged duct** or mastitis.

Signs of Letdown

A woman may become aware that her milk is letting down when her baby's swallowing pattern changes. He may begin gulping or be unable to control the flow of milk and pull away from her breast. Some women notice that milk drips from one breast while the baby is nursing on the other breast. Since letdown is bilateral, this **leaking** is a sign that milk has let down in both breasts. Letdown may cause a tingling or tightening sensation. This feeling is the result of thousands of alveoli contracting and of the pressure of milk forced through the duct system.

With letdown, the mother may experience increased thirst or sleepiness. In the first days postpartum, uterine contractions often accompany letdown due to oxytocin's action on the involuting uterus. Mothers experience several letdowns in a single feeding (Ramsay, 2004a, 2004b). The initial letdown is usually the only one the mother notices, because of the large quantity of milk moved at this time. She may not recognize the letdown reflex consistently in the first days and weeks of breastfeeding. This is especially the case for women who are breastfeeding for the first time.

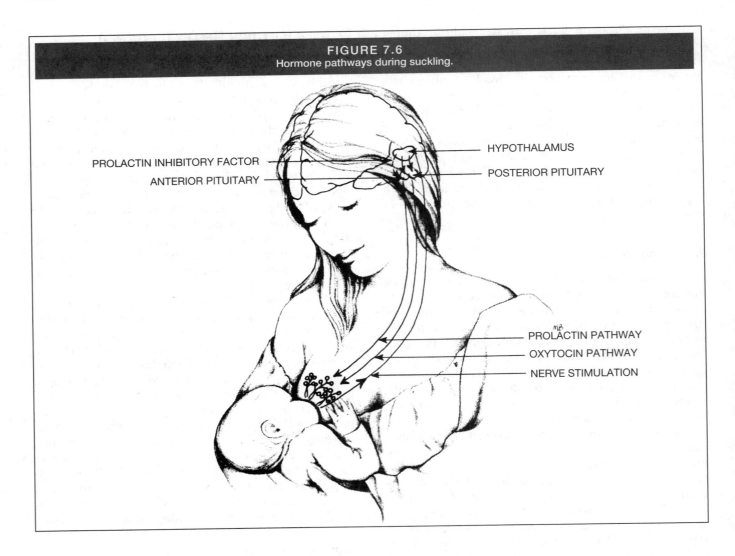

FIGURE 7.6
Hormone pathways during suckling.

PROLACTIN INHIBITORY FACTOR

ANTERIOR PITUITARY

HYPOTHALAMUS

POSTERIOR PITUITARY

PROLACTIN PATHWAY

OXYTOCIN PATHWAY

NERVE STIMULATION

Some mothers experience no physical sensations to signal that their milk is letting down. They can be encouraged to look for signs in the infant that their letdown reflex is functioning. The baby may begin gulping or even gagging from the sudden rush of milk and the mother will hear more pronounced swallowing. She can monitor the number of wet diapers and stools her baby has during a 24-hour period. From the end of the first week of life through the first six weeks, six or more wet diapers and three to five stools per day indicate that her milk is letting down and that her baby is well nourished. The mother's awareness of letdown may diminish as she and her baby become more experienced in breastfeeding and begin to focus on other aspects of their relationship.

Need for a Functioning Letdown

A functioning letdown reflex is crucial to nourishing an infant. In its absence, the infant receives an inadequate amount of milk. Letdown enables him to receive the majority of the fat content of the milk, which tends to stick to the duct lining. As letdown occurs, it forces this creamy **hindmilk** down into the ducts. The infant then receives more fatty milk after letdown as the feeding progresses.

It is important that the infant nurse long enough on each breast to receive sufficient calories. Limiting nursing time on one breast in order to switch to the other breast could cause the infant to receive a large volume of **foremilk**, which contains fewer calories. This practice may cause gastric upset, as well as low weight gain (Woolridge, 1988). In human milk, 50 percent of the calories come from the fat content. Therefore, an inhibited letdown can result in underfeeding an infant even if he consumes a fair amount of fluid.

Fat content correlates inversely with the amount of time between feedings (Daly, 1993). The percent of fat is higher when feedings are frequent, thus minimizing differences between hindmilk and foremilk. Restricting the number of feedings or limiting the baby's time at the breast can reduce fat intake. Because every dyad's pattern of nursing is unique, it is usually advisable to encourage a mother to let her baby finish nursing on one breast rather than switching arbitrarily to the other breast.

Inhibited Letdown

Fatigue, anxiety, fear, and pain can inhibit the letdown reflex. A new mother may be anxious about her breastfeeding and parenting. She may feel tense and pressured by work, family commitments, or unsupportive family and friends. She may be overtired due to lack of rest or overexertion. She may be in pain from childbirth or resulting surgery. Any of these circumstances could inhibit her letdown. Stress or fatigue may inhibit the secretion of oxytocin and may release adrenaline. This can negate the effects of oxytocin on the myoepithelial cell. Letdown also can fail to occur when nipple stimulation is weak, which may happen if the mother fails to attach the baby effectively.

Be cautious in discussing any concerns you may have about a mother's letdown reflex. You do not want to plant seeds of doubt that could further aggravate poor letdown. If you become reasonably certain that a woman's letdown reflex is not functioning well, you may need to see her in order to teach her relaxation techniques such as those presented in Chapter 14. You can also build her confidence in her ability to nourish her baby by explaining that her body is able to sustain her baby now, just as it did during pregnancy. A consultation will allow you to discuss emotional factors that may be involved and ways that she can cope.

Conditioning Letdown

Encourage mothers to relax both physically and mentally during the early weeks. The less tension a woman experiences, the more likely she is to let down her milk consistently during a feeding. Nursing in a quiet location and a comfortable position and setting up a routine to begin each feeding will help ensure that letdown becomes a firmly established part of each feeding session. This will condition the mother psychologically for letdown. These conditioning techniques are especially helpful to a woman who is separated from her baby during the day and is providing milk through **hand expression** or pumping. She may notice that her milk lets down when she picks up her baby, when she hears a baby cry, or whenever she thinks about her baby. See Chapter 14 for relaxation techniques.

▶ VARIATIONS IN BREAST STRUCTURE AND FUNCTION

Breastfeeding requires something essential from both mother and baby. The mother needs a desire to breastfeed and needs breasts that produce and release milk. The baby needs the ability to remove milk from the breast with effective suckling. How the mother attaches her baby at the breast helps determine the amount of milk the baby receives. The size and shape of her breasts are not usually indicators of how much milk they are able to produce, nor of how well her baby will thrive on her milk.

The ability to produce and release milk depends in part on the physical condition of the mother's breast. A wide variety of breast sizes and nipple shapes will accommodate breastfeeding. Only a few variations in structure will hinder or contraindicate breastfeeding. Mothers can overcome some differences in structure, such as nipple inversion. Other circumstances, such as previous breast surgery that has severed milk ducts, may make it necessary to supplement breastfeeding with other nutrition or to rely totally on an alternative feeding method.

Examining the Mother's Breasts

Caregivers do not need to examine every woman's breasts and nipples. However, if a difficulty arises that you suspect may be due to the mother's nipples or breasts, she should have a careful examination. Some women associate breast examination with illness or cancer prevention. Make sure that the mother knows that you are examining her breasts in preparation for breastfeeding. Ensure privacy to help the mother feel comfortable. Ask permission, and explain your purpose before you begin the exam. If you practice in a non-hospital setting, be sure the mother has read and signed a consent form granting you permission to examine her and her baby. Be aware of any customs of modesty that may make this procedure uncomfortable for the mother.

You can begin by asking the mother if both breasts became larger and the areolae became darker during pregnancy. If the answer is yes, there is probably sufficient functioning tissue in both breasts. Examining both breasts at the same time will enable you to observe the symmetry between them. Note the skin's elasticity as well as any engorgement, lumps, swelling, or redness. Look for evidence of past breast surgery, which may have severed some ducts (see Color Plate 8). Note the size and shape of the nipples and the size of the areolae. Learn how the mother's nipples respond to stimulation, in response to either cold or touching (see the discussion of nipple inversion that follows). Reassure the mother that small and large breasts alike will produce milk.

Discuss the shape of a woman's nipples sensitively and respectfully. If the message the woman hears seems negative, she may be unable to overcome that feeling in order to breastfeed. This type of phenomenon may explain why Alexander and associates (1992) found that recommending breast shells decreased breastfeeding duration. The researchers did not measure whether women actually used the shells and, if they did, for how many hours per day, nor for how many weeks before giving birth. They measured the recommendation to use shells and found that it was associated with a shortened duration of breastfeeding.

Differences in Nipples

Efficient milk transfer depends on a baby's ability to latch on to the breast, form it into a conical shape, and stretch it forward and then upward against the hard palate (roof of the mouth). Each woman's nipples are unique in shape, size, and the degree to which they protrude. A nipple that protrudes on stimulation aids the baby in finding and centering on the breast. It also provides tissue for him to grasp in order to draw sufficient breast tissue into his mouth.

There are many variations in types of nipples. For the convenience of discussion, Table 7.1 shows nipples classified into five types. Stimulation—such as touch, cold, or gentle compression—can reveal whether or not inversion is present. Color Plate 9 shows a nipple that appears normal and inverts, or retracts inward, when stimulated (Color Plate 10). The nipple in Color Plate 11 appears dimpled, and yet after pumping to release the adhesions, it **everts** (Color Plate 12). A **pinch test**, as described in Chapter 21, will help test the **protractility** of the mother's nipples.

Inverted Nipples

In order for the baby to receive milk, he needs enough breast tissue in his mouth to reach back almost to the hard palate. When the breast will not stretch to accommodate this pattern, the baby has difficulty maintaining suction. Only in the small percentage of women who have a truly inverted nipple will the problem be pronounced to the degree that the baby will have difficulty latching on. The degree of inversion decreases with each subsequent pregnancy.

Estimates of nipple inversion range from 3.26 percent (Park, 1999) to 9 percent (Kalbhen, 1998). Some mothers find the increased elasticity of skin during pregnancy decreases the inversion. Inverted nipples begin to respond to correction techniques during the last trimester of pregnancy. Some women may experience premature labor if their nipples are stimulated. Because of this, a woman should check with her caregiver before beginning any techniques that involve nipple stimulation.

With a good latch, the baby takes a large portion of the breast into his mouth and forms it into a cone-shaped teat. Milk transfer, therefore, often depends more on the pliability of the entire breast than on the configuration of the nipple itself. A recent study of suboptimal infant feeding behaviors included inverted nipples as a factor (Dewey, 2003).

Methods to Decrease Nipple Inversion

There are techniques to help evert nipples that are difficult for the baby to grasp. However, some are more effective than others. Some mothers have heard that wearing breast shells prenatally will improve nipple protrusion. Some also believe that wearing breast shells between feedings improves nipple protractility by gently placing pressure on the skin, stretching and pushing the nipple forward.

In the past, clinicians recommended the **Hoffman technique** for correcting nipple inversion. The forefingers would pull outward away from the nipple, in a pattern like rays of the sun, in order to break the **adhesions**. A study by the MAIN Trial Collaborative Group showed that neither the use of breast shells nor the Hoffman technique by randomly assigned women caused nipple elongation (MAIN, 1994).

A mother may be able to form the nipple by hand or with the aid of ice just before a feeding. **Inverted syringes** or devices marketed for this purpose such as the Nipplette or the Evert-It can help elongate the nipple as a preparation for breastfeeding (Arsenault, 1997; McGeorge, 1994; Kesaree, 1993). Another possibility to encourage protrusion of the nipple is the careful use of suction from a breast pump. Recommended times and frequency of use are similar to those for an inverted syringe. See Chapter 21 for detailed instructions on how to improve the graspability of the nipple with these methods. In using any of the techniques, mothers need to take care not to increase the suction to painful levels and to limit frequency of use to reasonable levels.

Some hospitals may use a nipple shield as a solution to inversion (see Color Plate 13). Nipple shields can be a useful transitional tool for breastfeeding when used wisely (Meier, 2000; Wilson-Clay, 1996). It is important that an IBCLC supervise use of a nipple shield to assure appropriate use. Considerations when using nipple shields include the following: selection of correct size and material (silicon, not rubber or latex), infant preference, possible breast tissue damage, adequate sucking stimulation, correct shield placement during feeding, and adequate milk transfer. See more on nipple shield use in Chapter 21.

Lumps in the Breast

The general population usually associates lumps in the breast with breast cancer. However, there are many breast lumps associated with lactation that are not a health risk. In fact, the normal state of the lactating breast is lumpy, due to the enlarged milk-filled alveoli distributed throughout the tissues. Other lumps may occur due to a plugged duct or breast infection (see Chapter 16). These two conditions are usually temporary, and after alleviating the cause, the associated lumps disappear.

TABLE 7.1		
Five Basic Types of Nipples		
Type of Nipple	**Before Stimulation**	**After Stimulation**
Common nipple		
The majority of mothers have what is referred to as a **common nipple**. It protrudes slightly when at rest and becomes erect and more graspable when stimulated. A baby has no trouble finding and grasping this nipple in order to pull in a large amount of breast tissue and stretch it to the roof of his mouth.		
Flat nipple		
A **flat nipple** has a very short shank that makes it less easy for the baby to find and grasp. In response to stimulation, this nipple remains essentially unchanged. Slight movement inward or outward may occur, but not enough to aid the baby in finding and initially grasping the breast on center. This nipple may benefit from the use of a nipple everter to increase **protractility**.		
Inverted-appearing nipple		
An **inverted-appearing nipple** may appear inverted but becomes erect after stimulation. This nipple needs no correction and presents no problems with graspability.		
Retracted nipple		
A **retracted nipple** is the most common type of inverted nipple. Initially, this nipple appears to be graspable. However, on stimulation, it retracts, making attachment difficult. This nipple responds well to techniques to increase nipple protrusion.		
Inverted nipple		
A truly **inverted nipple** is retracted both at rest and when stimulated. Such a nipple is more difficult for the baby to grasp. All techniques used to enhance protractility of breast tissue can be used to improve attachment. Even if the nipple remains retracted, the baby should be able to latch on if the mother helps form her breast into his mouth.		

If a lump does not move downward and begin to break up, consider a cause unrelated to breastfeeding. In this situation, the woman needs an examination by a caregiver to identify the cause of the lump. Lumps associated with **fibrocystic breasts** change with the menstrual cycle, shrinking and becoming less noticeable after menstruation. Other types of cysts may also be present within the breast.

Galactocele

A **galactocele**, caused by the closing or blockage of a milk duct, contains a thick, creamy milk-like substance that sometimes oozes from the nipple when the cyst is compressed. It can be aspirated, and some are removed surgically to prevent them from refilling. In a study of eight women with galactoceles, all eight galactoceles resolved spontaneously (Stevens, 1997). This suggests that surgical intervention may not always be required. The presence of a galactocele is compatible with breastfeeding. If surgery is required, breastfeeding does not need to be suspended.

Intraductal Papilloma

Intraductal papilloma is the second most frequent cause of bloody discharge. An intraductal papilloma is a benign, non-tender tumor within a milk duct. It is usually associated with a spontaneous bloody discharge from one breast. Breastfeeding may continue after serious disease has been ruled out and the discharge has stopped or surgeons have removed the involved duct.

Malignancy

When a lump is due to malignancy, breastfeeding may not be compatible with the treatments for breast cancer. A baby may refuse to nurse from a cancerous breast (Saber, 1996). You will want to explore breast rejection by the baby whenever you find a lump. Be careful not to confuse rejection with temporary refusal to nurse for a few feedings. A baby may reject breastfeeding for a number of reasons, such as a plug of milk expelled from the breast or a physical condition in the baby.

If the caregiver locates a lump and wishes to perform a biopsy to rule out cancer, breastfeeding can continue, as the procedure takes place under local **anesthesia**. In many cases, lumps are benign and breastfeeding is not interrupted. Mothers need to be aware that there is a small risk that a milk **fistula** may result from a biopsy. This can result in milk leaking from the biopsy incision site. Healing of the site may require temporary interruption of breastfeeding in that breast (Schackmuth, 1993).

Paget's disease is a rare form of malignancy of the breast that is usually unilateral (Color Plate 32). It produces a scaly, itchy skin condition on the nipple and areola that mimics **eczema**. There may be a bloody discharge from the nipple, and the nipple may appear flattened. In up to 30 percent of cases there are no visible skin changes. Almost half of all patients with Paget's disease have a lump in the breast felt at the time of diagnosis. It is important to see a healthcare provider about any of these symptoms (NCI, 2002).

Regular Breast Self-Examination

In the past, women were encouraged to check their breasts for lumps regularly and to notify the caregiver whenever they noticed unfamiliar lumps. There are now conflicting studies on the value of breast self-examinations in detecting breast cancer. Rather than recommending self-exams at only one time of the month, previously recommended on the seventh to tenth day after menses end, some specialists now recommend self-examination at different intervals. The emphasis is on a woman becoming familiar with her breasts overall in order to detect any changes over time (Love, 2000). Then, breastfeeding or not, women will develop a knowledge of their breasts and notice any changes more readily.

▶ **SUMMARY**

Although breasts vary from one woman to another in size and appearance, their basic anatomy makes it possible for the vast majority of women to nurture their babies in the manner nature intended. The breast is an intricate system of sensory nerves that trigger milk production, connective tissue that supports and contains fatty tissue, milk-producing glands, and milk-transporting tissues. Blood carries proteins, fats, sugar, and other substances needed for lactation to the breast. The breast takes raw material from blood to create nutrients for the infant. This nutrition travels through a system of lobuli and ducts to the nipple, where it discharges through several nipple pores. If a woman has undergone breast surgery that damaged the nerves or severed the ducts, her ability to breastfeed may be compromised.

Although puberty triggers the development of functional breast tissue, hormonal changes during pregnancy produce the majority of growth toward lactogenesis. The areola undergoes changes in size and color, and the Montgomery glands become more pronounced. Throughout the nine months of pregnancy, the breast experiences lactogenesis, transforming into a state of milk production and secretion. Estrogen, progesterone, prolactin, and oxytocin all play a role in altering the hormonal balance to stimulate milk production and release. Stress and fatigue can upset this balance of hormones, and mothers may need to learn measures to lower stress and stimulate milk letdown.

▶ **CHAPTER 7—AT A GLANCE**

Facts you learned—

Milk synthesis and breast development:

◆ The breast takes raw materials from blood and creates nutrients in the alveoli.

◆ Myoepithelial cells encompass the alveoli, contract when suckling releases oxytocin, and force milk down the ducts to the nipple.

◆ Most functional breast tissue development occurs during puberty and pregnancy.

◆ Increased estrogen during menstruation produces growth of ducts and connective tissue.

◆ In the absence of pregnancy, tissue growth regresses and glandular cells degenerate.

◆ In the first trimester of pregnancy the breast enters mammogenesis when the duct system multiplies, the skin stretches to accommodate internal enlargement, the nipple and areola increase in circumference, the areola darkens, and the Montgomery glands become noticeable.

◆ Colostrum is established by the end of the second trimester.

◆ At the beginning of the third trimester of pregnancy, the breast begins to gather the nutrients needed for milk synthesis (with increases in lactose, total proteins, and immunoglobulin and a decrease in sodium and chloride)—Stage I lactogenesis.

◆ Around the second to fifth day postpartum, transitional milk is produced, blood flow within the breast increases, and copious milk secretion begins—Stage II lactogenesis.

◆ About eight to ten days postpartum, establishment and maintenance of mature milk is achieved—Stage III lactogenesis (galactopoiesis).

◆ Lactogenesis is followed by a period of involution, when the breast slowly returns to its prepregnant state.

Hormones:

◆ Estrogen stimulates growth of the uterus, vagina, and other reproductive organs.

◆ Progesterone inhibits prolactin's effects during pregnancy.

◆ Prolactin stimulates alveolar growth and milk synthesis and induces maternal behavior.

◆ High prolactin levels can be maintained with unlimited, effective suckling and breastfeeding during the night.

◆ Oxytocin releases in response to suckling and causes myoepithelial cells to contract (milk ejection reflex).

◆ Pituitary, thyroid, and adrenal imbalances can affect milk production and release.

◆ Sheehan's syndrome (hypopituitarism) resulting from severe postpartum hemorrhage and hypotension can cause irreversible damage to milk-producing cells.

◆ Milk production depends on the frequency and degree of drainage of each breast.

◆ Autocrine control inhibits the production of more milk when milk is left in the breast.

◆ Suckling inhibits the prolactin inhibitory factor (PIF) to allow prolactin release.

◆ Letdown moves fat globules down through the ducts (hindmilk).

◆ Letdown can be inhibited by fatigue, anxiety, fear, or pain.

Breasts:

◆ Examining both breasts at the same time will enable you to observe symmetry.

◆ A small percentage of women have truly inverted nipples.

◆ An inverted nipple can be drawn out with an inverted syringe, commercial everter, breast pump, or nipple shield.

◆ The normal lactating breast is lumpy due to the enlarged milk-filled alveoli.

◆ A galactocele may resolve spontaneously or may be compressed, aspirated, or removed surgically.

◆ An intraductal papilloma produces a bloody discharge.

◆ Breast rejection can occur when malignancy is present.

◆ Paget's disease produces scaly, itchy nipples and areolas and sometimes bloody discharge.

◆ Widely spaced, tubular, and thin breasts are markers for insufficient glandular tissue.

◆ Women with a history of breast surgery should ask the surgeon if it involved functional tissue; their babies need to be monitored for appropriate intake and weight gain.

Applying what you learned—

Teach mothers:

◆ To preserve the keratin layer and lubrication of skin on the nipple.

◆ That the baby needs to take in about one inch or more in diameter of areolar tissue.

◆ To ensure the baby grasps the breast well and suckles vigorously to stimulate the nerves.

◆ That breast size is related to fatty and glandular tissue and does not predict how much milk she will produce.

◆ That breast sagging results from pregnancy, not lactation.

◆ That suckling signals milk production and that more blood becomes available to provide the nutrients needed to make milk.

◆ That engorgement decreases the flow of blood and lymph, causes edema, increases the risk of local infection, and leads to poor milk drainage.

◆ That frequent feedings, good positioning at the breast, avoiding arbitrary use of nipple shields, and using pumping in the absence of effective and frequent suckling will protect milk production.

▶ REFERENCES

Alexander J et al. Randomised controlled trial of breast shells and Hoffman's exercises for inverted and non-protractile nipples. *Br Med J* 304:1030–1032; 1992.

Arsenault G. Using a disposable syringe to treat inverted nipples. *Can Fam Physician* 43:1517–1518; 1997.

Cox D, Owens R, Hartmann P. Blood and milk prolactin and the rate of milk synthesis in women. *Experimental Physiology* 81:1007–1020; 1996.

Cox D, Owens R, Hartmann P. Studies on human lactation: The development of the computerized breast measurement system; 1998. Available at: http://biochem.uwa.edu.au/PEH/PEHRes.html. Accessed June 20, 2004.

Cregan M, Hartmann P. Computerized breast measurement from conception to weaning: Clinical implications. *J Hum Lact* 15(2):89–96; 1999.

Daly S et al. Degree of breast emptying explains changes in the fat content but not fatty acid composition of human milk. *Exp Physiol* 78:741–755; 1993.

Daly S, Hartmann P. Infant demand and milk supply. Part 2: The short-term control of milk synthesis in lactating women. *J Hum Lact* 11:27–37; 1995.

De Coopman J. Breastfeeding after pituitary resection: Support for a theory of autocrine control of milk supply? *J Hum Lact* 9:35–40; 1993.

DelVecchyo C et al. Evaluation of breast sensibility using dermatomal somatosensory evoked potentials. *Plast Reconstr Surg* 113(7):1975–1983; 2004.

Dewey K et al. Risk factors for suboptimal infant breastfeeding behavior, delayed onset of lactation, and excess neonatal weight loss. *Pediatrics* 12(3 Pt 1):607–619; 2003.

Dewitt JE. Management of nipple discharge by clinical findings. *Am J Surg* 149:789–792; 1985.

Godwin Y et al. Investigation into the possible cause of subjective decreased sensory perception in the nipple-areola complex of women with macromastia. *Plast Reconstr Surg* 113(6):1598–1606; 2004.

Hallock G. Prediction of nipple viability following reduction mammoplasty using laser Doppler flowmetry. *Ann Plast Surg* (5):457–460; 1992.

Hartmann P et al. Physiology of lactation in preterm mothers: Initiation and maintenance. *Pediatric Annals* 32(5):351–355; 2003.

Hefter W et al. Lactation and breast-feeding ability following lateral pedicle mammaplasty. *Br J Plast Surg* 56(8):746–751; 2003.

Helewa M. Breast cancer, pregnancy, and breastfeeding. *J Obstet Gynaecol Can* 24(2):164–184; 2002.

Higgins S, Haffty B. Pregnancy and lactation after breast-conserving therapy for early stage breast cancer. *Cancer* 73:2175–2180; 1994.

Hill P, Humenick S. The occurrence of breast engorgement. *J Hum Lact* 10:79–86; 1994.

Hoover K. Delayed lactogenesis II secondary to gestational ovarian theca lutein cysts in two normal singleton pregnancies. *J Hum Lact* 18(3):264–268; 2002.

Huggins K et al. Markers of lactation insufficiency: A study of 34 mothers. *Current Issues in Clinical Lactation*. Sudbury, MA: Jones and Bartlett, 25–35; 2000.

Ikegami H et al. Relationship between the methods of treatment for prolactinomas and the puerperal lactation. *Fertil Steril* 47:867–869; 1987.

Ing R et al. Unilateral breastfeeding and breast cancer. *Lancet* 2:124–127; 1977.

Kalbhen C et al. Mammography in the evaluation of nipple inversion. *AJR Am J Roentgenol* 170(1):117–121; 1998.

Kent J. *Breastfeeding Patterns: Variations on a Theme.* Presentation, Human Lactation Conference, Amarillo, TX; June 10, 2003.

Kesaree N et al. Treatment of inverted nipples using a disposable syringe. *J Hum Lact* 9:27–29; 1993.

Kline TS, Lash SR. The bleeding nipple of pregnancy and postpartum: A cytologic and histologic study. *Acta Cytolog (Phila.)* 8:336–340; 1964.

Knight C, Peaker M, Wilde C. Local control of mammary development and function. *Rev Reprod* 3(2):104–112; 1998.

Lafrenier R. Bloody nipple discharge during pregnancy: A rationale for conservative treatment. *J Surg Oncol* 43:228–230; 1990.

Lawrence R. *Breastfeeding: A Guide for the Medical Profession.* St. Louis, MO: Mosby; 1999.

Love S, Lindsey K. *Dr. Susan Love's Breast Book.* 3rd ed. Reading, MA: Addison-Wesley Publishing; 9–11; 2000.

MAIN Trial Collaborative Group. Preparing for breast feeding: Treatment of inverted and nonprotractile nipples in pregnancy. *Midwifery* 10:200–214; 1994.

Marasco L et al. Polycystic ovary syndrome: A connection to insufficient milk supply? *J Hum Lact* 16(2):143–148; 2000.

Matsunaga T et al. Intraductal biopsy for diagnosis and treatment of intraductal lesions of the breast. *Cancer* 101(10): 2164–2169; 2004.

McGeorge D. The "Nipplette": An instrument for the non-surgical correction of inverted nipples. *Br J Plast Surg* 47(1):46–49; 1994.

Meier P et al. Nipple shields for preterm infants: Effect on milk transfer and duration of breastfeeding. *J Hum Lact* 16(2):106–113; 2000.

National Cancer Institute (NCI). Cancer facts: Paget's disease of the breast: questions and answers. *cis.nci.nih.gov/fact/6_39.htm*; 2002. Accessed May 4, 2004.

Neifert M et al. The influence of breast surgery, breast appearance, and pregnancy-induced breast changes on lactation sufficiency as measured by infant weight gain. *Birth* 17:31–38; 1990.

Park H et al. The prevalence of congenital inverted nipple. *Aesthetic Plast Surg* 23(2):144–146; 1999.

Peaker M, Wilde C. Feedback control of milk secretion from milk. *J Mammary Gland Biol Neoplasia* 1(3):307–315; 1996.

Poppe K et al. Assisted reproduction and thyroid autoimmunity: An unfortunate combination? *J Clin Endocrinol Metab* 88:4149–4152; 2003.

Ramsay D et al. Breast anatomy redefined by ultrasound in the lactating breast. Conference proceedings of Australian Society for Ultrasound in Medicine. Perth, Australia; September, 2003.

Ramsay D et al. Ultrasound imaging of milk ejection in the breast of lactating women. *Pediatrics* 113(2):361–367; 2004a.

Ramsay D. *Ultrasound imaging of the sucking mechanics of the term infant.* Presentation, Human Lactation: Current Research & Clinical Implications, Amarillo, TX; October 22, 2004b.

Saber A et al. The milk rejection sign: A natural tumor marker. *Am Surg* 62:998–999; 1996.

Sarhadi NS, Shaw-Dunn J, Soutar DS. Nerve supply of the breast specific reference to the nipple and areola: Sir Astley Cooper revisited. *Clin Anat* 10(4):283–288; 1997.

Sarhadi N et al. An anatomical study of the nerve supply of the breast, including the nipple and areola. *Br J Plast Surg* 49(3):156–164; 1996.

Sauter E et al. The association of bloody nipple discharge with breast pathology. *Surgery* 136(4):780–785; 2004.

Schackmuth E et al. Milk fistula: A complication after core breast biopsy. *Am J Roentgenol* 161:961–962; 1993.

Silen W, Matory W, & Love S. *Atlas of Techniques in Breast Surgery.* Philadelphia/New York: Lippincott-Raven, 18–19; 1996.

Smith D. Montgomery's areolar tubercle: A light microscopic study. *Arch Pathol Lab Med* 106:60–63; 1982.

Stevens K et al. The ultrasound appearances of galactocoeles. *Br J Radiol* 70:239–241; 1997.

Strom S. Cosmetic saline breast implants: A survey of satisfaction, breast-feeding experience, cancer screening, and health. *Plast Reconstr Surg* 100(6):1553–1557; 1997.

Sun J et al. [The neuro-vascular anatomical study of breast and its signification in reduction mammaplasty] *Zhonghua Zheng Xing Wai Ke Za Zhi.* 20(4):277–9. Chinese; 2004.

Taylor SE et al. Female responses to stress: Tend and befriend, not fight or flight. *Psychological Review* 107(3):411–429; 2000.

Turner RA et al. Preliminary research on plasma oxytocin in normal cycling women: Investigating emotion and interpersonal distress. *Psychiatry* 62(2):97–113; 1999.

Ventz M et al. Pregnancy in hyperprolactinemic patients. *Zentralbl Gynakol* 118(11):610–615; 1996.

Widstrom A, Thingstrom-Paulsson J. The position of the tongue during rooting reflexes elicited in newborn infants before the first suckle. *Acta Paediatr* 82:281–283; 1993.

Wilde C et al. Autocrine regulation of milk secretion. *Biochem Soc Symp* 63:81–90; 1998.

Wilson-Clay, B. Clinical use of nipple shields. *J Hum Lact* 12:279–285; 1996.

Woolridge M, Fisher C. Colic, overfeeding, and symptoms of lactose malabsorption in the breast-fed baby: A possible artifact of feed management? *Lancet* ii:382–384; 1988.

Zimpelmann A, Kaufmann M. Breastfeeding nursing after breast surgery. *Zentralbl Gynakol* 124(11):525–528; 2002.

▶ BIBLIOGRAPHY

Brucker M, Scharbo-DeHaan M. Breast disease: The role of the nurse-midwife. *Breastfeeding Review* 18:342–350; 1993.

Daly S, Hartmann P. Infant demand and milk supply, Part 1: Infant demand and milk production in lactating women. *J Hum Lact* 11:21–26; 1995.

English J. Importance of breast awareness in identification of breast cancer. *Nurs Times* 13:99(40):18–19; 2003.

Harris L et al. Is breast feeding possible after reduction mammoplasty? *Plast Reconstr Surg* 89(5):836–839; 1992.

Mahon SM. Evidence-based practice: Recommendations for the early detection of breast cancer. *Clin J Oncol Nurs* 7(6):693–696; 2003.

Marshall D et al. Breast feeding after reduction mammoplasty. *Med J Aust* 159:428–429; 1993.

Matthews MK. Developing an instrument to assess infant breastfeeding behavior in the early neonatal period. *Midwifery* 4:154–165; 1988.

Matthews MK. Mothers' satisfaction with their neonates' breastfeeding behaviors. *JOGNN* 20(1):49–55; 1991.

Mulford C. The mother-baby assessment (MBA): An "Apgar score" for breastfeeding. *J Hum Lact* 8:79–82; 1992.

O'Connor ME, Burkle FM Jr, Olness K. Infant feeding practices in complex emergencies: A case study approach. *Prehospital Disaster Med* 16(4):231–238; 1991.

Semiglazof VF et al. Results of a prospective randomized investigation [Russia(St. Petersburg)/WHO] to evaluate the significance of self-examination for the early detection of breast cancer. *Vopr Onkol* 49(4):434–441; 2003.

Slavin J et al. Nodular breast lesions during pregnancy and lactation. *Histopathology* 22:481–485; 1993.

Soderstrom B. Helping the woman who had breast surgery: A literature review. *J Hum Lact* 9:169–171; 1993.

Stutte P et al. The effects of breast massage on volume and fat content of human milk. *Genesis* 10:22–24; 1988.

Tay C et al. Twenty-four hour patterns of prolactin secretion during lactation and the relationship to suckling and the resumption of fertility in breastfeeding women. *Hum Reprod* 11:950–955; 1996.

Uvnas-Moberg K, Eriksson M. Breastfeeding: Physiological, endocrine and behavioral adaptations caused by oxytocin and local neurogenic activity in the nipple and mammary gland. *Acta Paediatr* 85:515–530; 1996.

Vahabi M. Breast cancer screening methods: A review of the evidence. *Health Care Women Int* 24(9):773–793; 2003.

Widdice A, Thingstrom-Paulsson J. The effects of breast reduction and breast augmentation surgery on lactation: An annotated bibliography. *J Hum Lact* 9:161–167; 1993.

Wilde C et al. Breast-feeding: Matching supply with demand in human lactation. *Proc Nutr Soc* 54:401–406; 1995.

Wolfe JN. Breast cancer screening. *Breast Cancer Research and Treatment* 18:S89; 1991.

CHAPTER

8

MATERNAL HEALTH
AND NUTRITION

A basic understanding of nutrition and its effect on health leads to good eating practices. You can make nutrition information available to mothers and offer guidance in the selection and preparation of foods. Proper nutrition is vitally important to a woman during pregnancy and can have an effect on her breastfeeding. You can help women understand the nutritional factors that may cause them to feel hungry or fatigued. Prenatal and postpartum breastfeeding and parenting classes offer an excellent opportunity to discuss nutrition.

KEY TERMS

alcohol
allergen
amino acids
anemia
arachidonic acid
basal metabolic rate
body mass index
  (BMI)
caffeine
calcium
complex carbohydrates
fat stores
fats
fat-soluble vitamins
foodborne disease
food pyramid
hemoglobin

intrauterine growth
  retardation
iron
kcal
macrosomia
minerals
nutrients
proteins
salt
serum
simple carbohydrate
spina bifida
vegetarian diet
vitamin B$_{12}$
vitamins
water
water-soluble vitamins

NUTRITION EDUCATION

Her body reserves, plus the food she eats, provide a mother the energy and nutrients for her baby to grow and develop and for her body to cope with the changes taking place during pregnancy, delivery, and lactation. Maternal malnutrition, defined here as inadequate nutrition due to improper diet, can restrict healthy fetal growth by reducing the number or size of fetal cells, including brain cells. Severe maternal malnutrition due to critically low nourishment can contribute to fetal death.

Proper nutritional intake during pregnancy will help to produce healthy, full-term babies. It will also help mothers to keep their bodies in prime condition for labor, delivery, and lactation. Mothers often have questions about foods to eat or avoid when breastfeeding. An overly restrictive diet may put the mother or baby at nutritional risk. Occasionally, the IBCLC may be the first person to notice possible risk factors that require a referral for detailed assessment by a nutritionist or dietician. In order to counsel a mother about nutrition effectively, you need to use your counseling skills as well as a sound knowledge of nutrition.

Counseling Women Regarding Their Nutritional Needs

Nutritional education is frequently lacking in schools. There may be some information on the importance of the food pyramid, though often it is taught in the abstract. Food selection, meal planning, and the practical skills of food preparation are usually not included. Children may have few examples of healthy eating to serve as a good model to carry into adult life. In many cases, formal nutrition education ends in grade school, at a time when children do not have enough control over their diets to put the information into practice.

Much of what we learn about nutrition is through the media, and much of that information correlates to the marketing of a product rather than an independent analysis. An advertising campaign may tell us that a product has added vitamins, for instance, but does not explain that the additional vitamins replace the naturally occurring vitamins that were lost in processing. The combined effect of such marketing and limited education on nutrition is that many people reach adulthood with a mixture of information about nutrition and few skills to choose and prepare foods. Health practitioners and parents all need to distinguish between marketing promotion and unbiased information.

Pregnancy and lactation are times when women are especially receptive to nutrition education. During these peak periods of interest, women want to provide their babies with the best nourishment possible. Many wish to have children without a lasting change in their own body image. Others may begin to recognize the close relationship between what they eat and how they feel. Whatever the reason, this is a teachable moment—a time when the woman is most receptive to learning about nutrition. Tapping into the mother's motivating interests can influence a change in her eating habits.

Although your primary role is to assist women with breastfeeding, giving nutrition information is an important element in your counseling. Each mother has a history of food choices, eating patterns, and cultural beliefs about food. Some mothers may be well educated nutritionally, and you will need to determine a mother's nutritional awareness before offering suggestions. Tap into your listening skills, and ask relevant questions. Offer information and suggestions based on the woman's needs and situation. You can encourage parents to assume responsibility for their healthcare and that of their children without lecturing mothers about what they "should" eat. Health and well-being relate closely to nutrition. Education in this area helps parents to make responsible decisions.

One person's definition of a "healthy diet" may differ from that of another person. You need to give mothers nutrition information based on sound, accurate principles. It should not reflect your own individual preferences or dietary practices, fad diets, or unproven theories that can be detrimental to a woman's health, especially that of a pregnant or breastfeeding mother. By sharing basic nutrition information, you can minimize confusion or possible conflict and help her apply the information to her eating practices. The USDA's 2005 dietary guidelines emphasize reducing calorie consumption and increasing physical activity (USDA, 2005). This is sound advice for all of us!

▶ THE BASIC NUTRIENTS

All food contains nutrients. Nutrients are any nourishing substance in food released by digestion and then absorbed and used to promote body function. There are two types of nutrients—macronutrients (protein, fats, and carbohydrates) and micronutrients (vitamins and minerals). A basic understanding of nutrients and their functions in the body is necessary for realizing the importance of good nutrition. When counseling a mother about her diet, concentrate on foods rather than the individual nutrients that make up those foods. Eating all of the nutrients required by the body in proper quantities leads to good nutrition. Each nutrient has a specific function and relationship to the body. They must be present in proper quantities to maintain good health and a feeling of well-being.

Carbohydrates

Carbohydrates are the main source of energy for all body functions and activity. They also help to regulate protein and fat metabolism. The body needs carbohydrates in sufficient quantity to avoid relying on protein as an energy source. This allows protein to perform other important body functions. The body converts excess carbohydrates in the diet into fat and stores it.

Simple Carbohydrates

Simple carbohydrates include sugar, jams, honey, chocolate, and other sweets. They are found on the top of the food pyramid to indicate we need very little of these foods in our diet. Sugary foods can cause a sudden rise in blood sugar level. The level then drops again rapidly and can create a craving for more food. When consumed in the absence of nutritional foods, simple carbohydrate foods may cause fatigue, dizziness, nervousness, or headache.

Complex Carbohydrates

Complex carbohydrates include starches such as cereals, rice, breads, crackers, pasta, vegetables, and fruits. These are the foods on the bottom layers of the food pyramid. Complex carbohydrates take longer to digest than simple carbohydrates and do not stimulate a craving for more food. Whole-grain foods and unprocessed vegetables and fruit contain important vitamins and minerals often missing in processed foods. Fruits, vegetables, and whole-grain breads and cereals also provide needed fiber.

Proteins

Protein is the major source of building material for all internal organs, as well as for muscles, blood, skin, hair, and nails. Proteins are important to the formation of hormones that, among numerous other functions, control sexual development and the production of milk during lactation. They are a source of heat and energy for the body. It is better to provide adequate energy from carbohydrates and fat sources so protein can be used for functions other nutrients cannot perform.

Proteins consist of 22 building blocks called **amino acids**. The human body can synthesize 14 of these amino acids. The diet must supply the remaining 8 in proportions that allow the body to synthesize proteins properly. Foods containing all the essential amino acids are **complete protein** foods. Those lacking or extremely low in any of the essential amino acids are **incomplete protein** foods.

Most meats and dairy products are complete protein foods with high biological value, while most vegetable or plant proteins (such as beans and grains) are incomplete protein foods with low biological value. Meals need a balance of foods weak in an essential amino acid and those adequate in the same one. An incomplete protein food makes a complete protein complement when combined with others. Peanut butter and bread, pasta and cheese, breakfast cereal and milk, and beans and rice are examples of such combinations.

The body constantly builds and repairs tissues. At times of stress, such as surgery, hemorrhage, or prolonged illness, it is necessary to consume extra protein in order to meet the body's increased requirements for this function. The USDA recommended daily intake for an average adult woman is 50 grams of protein (now referred to as Dietary Reference Intake rather than Recommended Dietary Allowance). That same woman needs 60 grams during pregnancy and 65 grams during early lactation. In some countries, the recommendations are slightly lower. Most women may already be eating sufficient protein. In terms of food, the additional needs are quite low; a serving of baked beans with a slice of bread provides 10 extra grams of protein. Women should avoid high protein intakes, and intakes more than twice the recommended amount. Excessive protein intake can overload the kidneys and increase loss of calcium through excretion (Diet Information, 2004).

Fats

Fats are the most concentrated source of energy in the diet. They act as carriers for the fat-soluble vitamins A, D, E, and K. Fats prolong the process of digestion by slowing down the stomach's emptying. This creates a longer-lasting sensation of fullness after a meal. Fatty acids, which give fats their different flavors, textures, and melting points, are either saturated or unsaturated. Saturated fatty acids come primarily from animal sources, such as meat, milk products, and eggs. Unsaturated fatty acids come from vegetables, nuts, and seeds. A healthy diet should contain a greater amount of unsaturated fats than saturated fats.

Two particular fatty acids, linoleic and alpha-linolenic, which are known as essential fatty acids (EFAs), are converted into arachidonic acid (AA) and docosahexaenoic acid (DHA), respectively. Sufficient AA and DHA are important for neural and visual development in the fetus. Foods containing large amounts of EFAs include vegetable oils; margarines and salad dressings made from unsaturated oils such as canola; soybean oil for alpha-linolenic acid; and corn, sunflower, and peanut oils for linoleic acid. AA is directly available from beef, pork, poultry, and eggs. DHA is available in fatty fish such as mackerel, salmon, and sardines. Encourage women to use a variety of types of oil in addition to animal sources of AA and DHA. A very low-fat diet is usually not appropriate during pregnancy and lactation (WHO, 1993).

One U.S. artificial infant milk manufacturer has begun marketing a DHA supplement for pregnant and lactating women (Martek, 2004). This may play into women's fears that their own milk is inadequate. You can reassure questioning mothers that with essential fatty acids in their normal diet no additional DHA is necessary.

Vitamins

Vitamins are organic substances or groups of related substances that have special biochemical functions in the body. Vitamins convert fat and carbohydrates into energy and help to form bone and tissues. The diet must provide necessary vitamins. The body can synthesize some vitamins but needs adequate amounts of the precursor from the diet to do so. Table 8.1 lists the functions of each vitamin and its function during pregnancy and lactation.

Mothers who consider their foods inadequate in vitamin and mineral content may take prescribed or over-the-counter supplements. Encourage women to consult their caregiver before taking supplemental vitamins and minerals during pregnancy or lactation. These can be a valuable addition to the diet, if needed in special circumstances such as **anemia**, food intolerance, or allergies. However, supplements should not replace the proper intake of foods rich in vitamins and minerals. They should be supplements, not substitutes, for good nutrition. Excess amounts of some vitamins, such as vitamin A, can be harmful. High doses of vitamin B_6 (600 mg/day) may cause lactation suppression (Marcus, 1975; Foukas, 1973).

Water-Soluble Vitamins

The body cannot store **water-soluble vitamins** (the B vitamins and vitamin C). They need to be replenished daily. During lactation, water-soluble vitamins can move easily from maternal blood to milk, so maternal intake can affect the amount in milk for most of these vitamins. However, once mammary tissue reaches saturation, levels in the milk plateau for vitamin C, thiamin (B_1), and biotin.

Folic acid contributes to cell growth and reproduction. It functions with vitamins B_{12} and C in the breakdown of proteins and the production of **hemoglobin**. Folic acid, especially important to pregnant women in

TABLE 8.1

Nutrient and Vitamin Chart

Key Nutrient	DRI for Ages 23–50	Important Sources	Important Functions
Water and liquids	N 4 Cups P 6–8 Cups L 8+ Cups	Water, juice, milk	Carries nutrients to and waste products away from cells. Provides fluid for increased blood and amniotic fluid volume. Helps regulate body temperature and aids digestion. **Comments:** Often neglected. Is an important nutrient.
Protein amino acids	N 50 g P 60 g L 64 g	**Animal:** Meat, fish, eggs, milk, cheese, yogurt **Plant:** Dried beans and peas, peanut butter, nuts, whole grains and cereals, soy milk, meat substitutes	Constitutes part of the structure of every tissue cell, such as muscle, blood, and bone. Supports growth and maintains healthy body cells. Constitutes part of enzymes, some hormones, and body fluids. Helps form antibodies that increase resistance to infection. Builds and repairs tissues, helps build blood and amniotic fluid. Supplies energy. **Comments:** Fetal requirements increase by about ½ in late pregnancy as the baby grows.
MINERALS			
Calcium	N 800–1200 mg P 1200 mg L 1200 mg	**Animal:** Milk, cheese, yogurt, egg yolk, whole canned fish, ice cream **Plant:** Whole grains, almonds, filberts, green leafy vegetables	Combines with other minerals within a protein framework to give structure and strength to bones and teeth. Assists in blood clotting. Functions in normal muscle contraction and relaxation and normal nerve transmission. Helps regulate the use of other minerals in the body. **Comments:** Fetal requirements increase by about ⅔ in late pregnancy.
Phosphorus	N 1000 mg P 1200 mg L 1200 mg	**Animal:** Milk, cheese, lean meats	Helps build bones and teeth. **Comments:** Calcium and phosphorus exist in a constant ratio in the blood. An excess of either limits utilization of calcium.
Iron	N 18 mg P 30–60 mg L 18+ mg	**Animal:** Liver, red meats, egg yolk **Plant:** Whole grains, leafy vegetables, nuts, legumes, dried fruits, prune and apple juice	Aids in utilization of energy. Combines with protein to form hemoglobin, the red substance in blood that carries oxygen to and carbon dioxide from the cells. Prevents nutritional anemia and its accompanying fatigue. Increases resistance to infection. Functions as part of enzymes involved in tissue respiration. Provides iron for fetal storage. **Comments:** Fetal requirements increase tenfold in final 6 weeks of pregnancy. Supplement of 30–60 mg of iron daily recommended by National Research Council. Continued supplementation for 2–3 months postpartum is recommended to replenish iron.
Zinc	N 15 mg P 20 mg L 25 mg	**Animal:** Meat, liver, eggs, and seafood, especially oysters	A component of insulin. Important in growth of skeleton and nervous system. **Comments:** Deficiency can cause fetal malformation of skeleton and nervous system.
Iodine	N 150 μcg P 175 μcg L 200 μcg	**Animal:** Seafood **Mineral:** Iodized salt	Helps control the rate of body's energy use, important in thyroxine production. **Comments:** Deficiency may produce goiter in infant.

(continued)

TABLE 8.1 (CONTINUED)
Nutrient and Vitamin Chart

Key Nutrient	DRI for Ages 23–50	Important Sources	Important Functions
Magnesium	N 400 mg P 450 mg L 450 mg	**Plant:** Nuts, cocoa, green vegetables, whole grains, dried beans, peas	Co-enzyme in energy and protein metabolism, enzyme activator, tissue growth, cell metabolism, muscle action. **Comments:** Most is stored in bones. Deficiency may produce neuromuscular dysfunctions.
FAT-SOLUBLE VITAMINS			
Vitamin A	N 800 RE P 1000 RE L 1200 RE	**Animal:** Butter, whole milk, cheese, fortified milk, liver **Plant:** Fortified margarine, green and leafy vegetables, orange vegetables, fruits	Assists formation and maintenance of skin and mucous membranes that line body cavities and tracts, such as nasal passages and intestinal tract, thus increasing resistance to infection. Essential in development of enamel-forming cells in gum tissue. Helps bone and tissue growth and cell development. Functions in visual processes, thus promoting healthy eye tissues and eye adaptation in dim light. **Comments:** Is toxic to the fetus in very large amounts. Can be lost with exposure to light.
Vitamin D	N 5 μcg P 10 μcg L 10 μcg	**Animal:** Fortified milk, fish liver oils **Plant:** Fortified margarine, sun on skin	Promotes the absorption of calcium from the digestive tract and the deposition of calcium in the structure of bones and teeth. **Comments:** Toxic to fetus in excessive amounts. Is a stable vitamin.
Vitamin E	N 8 mg P 10 mg L 13 mg	**Plant:** Vegetable oils, leafy vegetables, cereals **Animal:** Meat, eggs, milk	Tissue growth, cell wall integrity, red blood cell integrity. **Comments:** Enhances absorption of Vitamin A.
WATER-SOLUBLE VITAMINS			
B vitamins and folic acid	N 400 μcg P 800 μcg L 600 μcg	**Plant:** Liver, green leafy vegetables, yeast	Hemoglobin synthesis, involved in DNA and RNA synthesis, co-enzyme in synthesis of amino acids. **Comments:** Water-soluble vitamins are interdependent. Deficiency leads to anemia. Can be destroyed in cooking and storage. Supplement of 200–400 μcg/day is recommended by the National Research Council. Oral contraceptive use may reduce serum level of folic acid.
Niacin	N 13 mg P 15 mg L 18 mg	**Animal:** Pork, organ meats **Plant:** Peanuts, beans, peas, enriched grains	Co-enzyme in energy and protein metabolism. **Comments:** Stable; only small amounts are lost in food preparation.
Riboflavin	N 1.2 mg P 1.5 mg L 1.7–1.9 mg	**Animal:** Milk products, liver, red meat **Plant:** Enriched grains	Aids in utilization of energy. Functions as part of a co-enzyme in the production of energy within body cells. Promotes healthy skin, eyes, and clear vision. Protein metabolism. **Comments:** Severe deficiencies lead to reduced growth and congenital malformations. Oral contraceptive use may reduce serum concentrations.

(continued)

TABLE 8.1 (CONTINUED)			
Nutrient and Vitamin Chart			
Key Nutrient	**DRI for Ages 23–50**	**Important Sources**	**Important Functions**
B₁-Thiamin	N 1.0 mg P 1.4 mg L 1.5 mg	**Animal:** Pork, beef, liver **Plant:** Whole grains, legumes	Co-enzyme in energy and protein metabolism. **Comments:** Its availability limits the rate at which energy from glucose is produced.
B₆-Pyrodoxine	N 1.6 mg P 2.2 mg L 2.1 mg	**Plant:** Unprocessed cereals, grains, wheat germ, bran, nuts, seeds, legumes, corn	Important in amino acid metabolism and protein synthesis. Fetus requires more for growth. **Comments:** Excessive amounts may reduce milk production in lactating women.
B₁₂	N 2.0 μcg P 2.2 μcg L 2.6 μcg	**Animal:** Milk, cheese, eggs, meat, liver, fish **Plant:** Fortified soy milk, cereals, meat substitutes	Assists in the maintenance of nerve tissue. Coenzyme in protein metabolism. Important in formation of red blood cells. **Comments:** Deficiency leads to anemia and central nervous system damage. Is manufactured by microorganisms in intestinal tract. Oral contraceptive use may reduce serum concentrations.
Vitamin C	N 60 mg P 80 mg L 100 mg	**Plant:** Citrus fruits, berries, melons, tomatoes, chili peppers, green vegetables, potatoes	Important tissue formation and integrity. "Cement" substance in connective and vascular substances. Increases iron absorption. **Comments:** Large doses in pregnancy may create a larger than normal need in infant.

N–nonpregnant; P–pregnant; L–lactating; DRI–Dietary Reference Intake.
From Worthington-Roberts B and Williams SR. *Nutrition in Pregnancy and Lactation*, 6th ed. New York: McGraw-Hill; 1996.
The Recommended Daily Allowance (RDA) or Dietary Reference Intake (DRI) refers to the intake of a nutrient that fulfills the needs of 97.5 percent of healthy people in the population. It does not necessarily reflect the lowest acceptable intake for the majority of the population. In fact, it exceeds the actual requirements of most individuals within a population. As individuals have a range of requirements, these amounts must be used with care when referring to an individual's diet.

preventing anemia, can be obtained from leafy green vegetables and whole grains. The U.S. Public Health Service advocates folic acid supplements during childbearing years for all reproductive-aged women in order to help prevent neural tube defects (**spina bifida**) (Charbonneau, 1993).

Excess water-soluble vitamins are excreted through the urine. In general, a varied diet that meets women's energy needs will provide sufficient water-soluble vitamins during lactation. Supplementation is unnecessary unless there is an established nutritional risk for the mother. Further information on vitamin B₁₂ and vegetarian diets appears later in this chapter.

Fat-Soluble Vitamins

Fat-soluble vitamins (A, D, E, and K) are stored in the body's fatty tissues. Vitamin A contributes to the growth of the skeleton and maintains the mucous membranes and vision. Vitamin K is essential for blood clotting. One form exists in green leafy vegetables, and another form derives from bacteria in the gut. Vitamin K deficiency in adults is rare. Newborn infants' stores at birth are low, which can lead to a risk of hemorrhagic disease of the newborn. Maternal supplementation during the final weeks of pregnancy may reduce the risk. Infants usually receive Vitamin K routinely at birth (Greer, 1997).

Vitamin D is unusual in that diet is not its only source. The body can manufacture vitamin D under the influence of sunlight. Low maternal levels of vitamin D during pregnancy can result in a deficiency in the infant. Women at risk are those who do not consume milk or fortified margarine, who regularly avoid sunlight or have little time outdoors, and who wear clothes that cover most of their skin. Women with dark skin coloring are at an even greater risk (Good Mojab, 2003). During pregnancy, the baby's body stores accumulate. If the mother has low levels of vitamin D, the baby will be born with low levels.

A regular short walk outdoors in sunlight, starting from pregnancy or before, can benefit both mother and baby. Supplementing pregnant women and mothers who are deficient improves the nutritional status of both the mother and baby. Supplementing the baby alone means the woman remains deficient, placing the next baby at risk for deficiency as well. Over-supplementation with vitamin D is a risk to the baby and can result in death. Recent American Academy of Pediatrics guidelines for infant supplementation with Vitamin D have caused concern in the lactation community (Gartner, 2003).

Many current recommendations for vitamin D occurred before scientists discovered that vitamin D is a pro-steroid, which the body converts into another form that circulates in the blood and is used in biological processes. Several researchers believe that the present DRI for vitamin D is inadequate, especially for the African American population, and they call for much higher doses during lactation than are presently recommended (Hollis, 2004a, 2004b). The human body is meant to produce vitamin D through sunlight exposure. Therefore, vitamin D deficiency is actually *sunlight* deficiency. See Chapter 9 for more information about vitamin D.

Minerals

Minerals contribute to a person's overall mental and physical well-being. They are involved in maintaining physiological processes, strengthening skeletal structures, and preserving the vigor of the heart, the brain, the muscles, and the nervous system. Minerals are important in the production of hormones and help maintain the delicate water balance essential to the proper functioning of mental and physical processes. The diet must supply essential minerals. A varied and mixed diet of animal and vegetable origin that meets energy and protein needs will typically furnish adequate minerals. Specific minerals and their functions appear in Table 8.1. Three minerals—calcium, iron, and salt—are especially important during pregnancy and lactation.

Calcium

Calcium is an important dietary mineral that gives bones their rigidity and teeth their hardness. It also has a role in blood clotting and in controlling the action of the heart, muscles, and nerves. Vitamin D promotes optimal absorption and use of calcium. Calcium maintains the mother's bones and provides for fetal bone development. Increased maternal intestinal absorption during pregnancy provides the additional calcium needed at that time.

Though pregnancy and lactation require high amounts of calcium, lactating women are no more prone to osteoporosis than those who have never been pregnant or have not lactated. Studies show that calcium mobilizes from the mother's bones during lactation, with a recovery of bone mass after weaning. Overall, breastfeeding appears to increase the mother's bone mineral density and, thus, helps prevent osteoporosis (Karlsson, 2001; Laskey, 1999; Henderson, 2000).

Pregnant women and mothers need to learn about adequate calcium intake, particularly women under the age of 25 who are still experiencing an increase in their bone content. Women who do not consume milk can obtain calcium through the sources listed in Table 8.2. Women who avoid all milk products must make up for the other nutrients available in milk—protein, vitamins, and calories—through other foods. Pregnant or lactating women who do not eat enough calcium-rich foods may

TABLE 8.2	
Good Sources of Calcium	
Food	**Calcium (mgs per serving)**
Yogurt, plain (8 oz)	415
Cheddar cheese (2 oz)	408
Sardines, drained (3 oz)	372
American cheese (2 oz)	348
Yogurt, fruit-flavored (8 oz)	345
Milk, whole, low-fat, or skim (8 oz)	300
Watercress (1 cup chopped)	189
Chocolate pudding, instant (½ cup)	187
Collards (½ cup cooked)	179
Buttermilk pancakes (3–4 inches)	174
Pink salmon, canned (3 oz)	167
Tofu (4 oz)	145
Turnip greens (½ cup cooked)	134
Kale (½ cup cooked)	103
Shrimp, canned (3 oz)	99
Ice cream (½ cup)	88
Okra (½ cup cooked)	74
Rutabaga, mashed (1/2 cup cooked)	71
Broccoli (½ cup cooked)	68
Soybeans (½ cup cooked)	66
Cottage cheese (½ cup)	63
Bread, white or whole wheat (2 slices)	48

need calcium supplements to provide 800–1200 mg per day. Calcium carbonate is the safest supplement. Several brands of bone meal and dolomite contain high levels of lead or other toxic metals; advise women to avoid these.

Iron

Additional iron is needed during pregnancy to support the growing fetus and placenta and to increase the mother's red cell mass. Low levels of iron can affect the oxygen-carrying capacity of the blood and cause a woman to feel tired constantly, even after adequate rest. An anemic woman has poor tolerance to blood loss and is at greater risk if she needs surgery. The effect of maternal iron deficiency on the fetus is unclear. Iron deficiency is most common in women with low socio-economic status, multiple gestations, and limited education. These women are also at risk of poor pregnancy outcome, independent of iron deficiency.

When iron stores are low, more iron is absorbed by the body. During pregnancy and the early months of breastfeeding when mothers are not menstruating, the reduced loss of blood partially offsets her additional needs. Recommended dietary intake of iron varies among different countries and so do practices regarding supplementation. Women who begin pregnancy with sufficient iron stores and eat a varied diet do not need iron supplements. Many doctors prescribe supplements routinely on the assumption that pre-pregnancy stores are low. If women were to have a blood test prior to conception, they could begin treatment for anemia before becoming pregnant.

Dietary iron exists in two forms. Heme iron comes from meat, poultry, and fish and is easily absorbed. Non-heme iron comes from vegetables, iron-enriched cereals, and whole grains. Adding small amounts of heme iron or foods containing vitamin C to the meal can improve iron absorption from non-heme sources. Iron absorption from non-heme food sources can be reduced with the consumption of tea, coffee, phyates in legumes and bran, and oxalates in spinach, beet greens, chard, rhubarb, and sweet potato. Excess calcium, both in food and supplements, can reduce iron absorption as well.

Some women avoid iron supplements due to gastrointestinal effects such as heartburn, nausea, constipation, and diarrhea. Effective dietary counseling can help these women improve their iron intake and absorption from foods. Supplements should be taken with water or juice, not with milk, tea, or coffee. They may be better tolerated when taken at bedtime. During lactation, iron levels in the mother's milk remain steady and are unrelated to maternal iron status. However, mothers should continue to pay attention to their iron intake to rebuild their stores.

Salt

As pregnancy progresses, the placenta needs increased blood flow to work efficiently. During a typical pregnancy, a woman's blood volume increases by more than 40 percent to meet this need. Salt usually causes the body to retain fluid in the bloodstream. Pregnancy is one condition in which the body actually requires more salt in order to function well. In the past, physicians placed restrictions on salt intake in an attempt to control weight and reduce water retention. Such routine salt restriction during pregnancy is not beneficial and may be harmful (Franx, 1999). Most pregnant women can continue to consume the same amount of salt as that recommended for the general population. It is not advisable that anyone have excessive salt intake, including pregnant women.

Water

Water is the most abundant and by far the most important nutrient in the body. It is responsible for and involved in nearly every body process. Most foods contain water, which is absorbed by the body during digestion. Fruits and vegetables are especially good sources of chemically pure water. The average adult female body contains 50–55 percent water (approximately 30 quarts) and loses about 2 quarts daily through perspiration and excretion.

A pregnant or lactating woman needs to consume adequate water in order to supply her fetus or infant with adequate fluids. The woman's consumption of additional water-containing foods as part of her normal increase in diet, as well as her natural sense of thirst, will usually provide the additional water she needs. Sometimes lactating women fail to respond to their increased thirst. Having a beverage next to them when they nurse their baby will remind them to drink to satisfy their thirst. During pregnancy and lactation, a woman needs about six to eight cups of fluid a day to ensure that her body has enough fluid to function and to avoid constipation. Table 8.1 advises that breastfeeding women consume eight or more cups of fluid daily. Thirst should dictate water consumption.

There is no data to support the suggestion that increasing a mother's fluid intake will increase milk volume. In fact, women who consume excessive amounts of fluid actually produce *less* milk and their babies gain less weight (Dusdieker, 1985). In addition, there is no research to show that restricting fluids decreases milk volume (Illingworth, 1986). When fluids are restricted, the mother will experience a decrease in urine output, not in milk (Lawrence, 1999). Mothers can monitor the adequacy of fluid intake by observing their urine. Except for the first morning void, the mother's urine should be clear to light yellow. If her urine appears more concentrated, she can increase her fluid intake throughout the day.

▶ NUTRITION IN PREGNANCY AND LACTATION

A woman's nutritional status prior to pregnancy and her nutritional intake during pregnancy contribute to a healthy pregnancy and baby. From infancy, the female body is developing toward childbearing. Undernutrition as a child can result in short stature and a small pelvis, thereby increasing the risk of pregnancy complications. The body's store of contaminants such as pesticides and heavy metals builds up throughout childhood. In an ongoing cycle, healthy babies need healthy mothers and healthy mothers result from a healthy childhood. Your influence can extend to increase the overall health of the community, not just that of pregnant women, mothers, and infants.

Pre-conception Nutrition

When you see women prior to conception or between pregnancies, encourage them to eat a healthy, varied diet and to aim for the recommended weight range. A very low weight or very high weight could decrease a woman's ability to conceive. Weight changes should be gradual—one to two pounds a week—rather than the result of a crash diet. Similarly, an adequate and varied diet, correction of grossly abnormal body weight, and at most a moderate alcohol intake by the male partner can assist in conception and a healthy baby. Maternal alcohol intake can have serious effects on the baby. Women planning a pregnancy can be encouraged to reduce or cease alcohol intake. By checking iron levels before pregnancy, treatment for anemia can begin if levels are low. A folic acid supplement is frequently recommended pre-conception and during the first three months of pregnancy to reduce the risk of neural tube defects.

Nutrition during Pregnancy

A woman needs an increased amount of most nutrients during pregnancy. Intake of folate, calcium, vitamin D, iron, and essential fatty acids needs special attention during pregnancy. There is potential for inadequate intake of these nutrients in some groups of women. A woman well nourished throughout her life may not need to make changes to her diet during pregnancy. For a woman poorly nourished prior to conception, pregnancy may provide an opportunity to improve her diet. Women can modify their nutrition to promote a healthy outcome for their pregnancy.

Fetal growth may affect later adult health. **Intra-uterine growth retardation** (IUGR) is associated with increased risk to the infant of coronary heart disease, stroke, diabetes, and high blood pressure in adult life. The underlying factor may be restricted growth followed by rapid postnatal catch-up growth (Robinson, 2002; Barker, 2002; Lumbers, 2001). Large size at birth, **macrosomia**, is also associated with increased risk of diabetes and cardiovascular disease in later life and an increased risk of some cancers. Optimal birth weight and length affects both immediate infant health and diet-related chronic disease (WHO, 2003).

Nutrition during Lactation

Sound nutrition practices will continue to enhance the well-being of the entire family long after pregnancy. The breastfeeding mother needs to recognize the effect her diet has on her health. An inadequate diet or irregular eating patterns can affect how a mother feels and acts and how she views herself and the world. This in turn may negatively influence milk production and letdown, as well as her ability to cope with her baby and other family members and friends.

High-quality milk production does not require special foods. The normal healthy diet recommended for an average adult should meet most needs. A very young mother, a pregnant woman who is carrying two or more babies, a mother nursing two or more babies, or a pregnant woman who is also nursing may need to increase her food intake significantly. Women can meet their needs with increased serving sizes, adding foods at meal times, or eating more foods between meals. Women in a wide variety of circumstances in the United States and elsewhere are able to produce milk of sufficient quantity and quality to support growth and promote the health of infants, even when the mother's supply of nutrients is limited (Institute of Medicine, 1991).

Weight Changes in Pregnancy and Lactation

Restricting weight gain in pregnancy can be harmful to the fetus and mother in some situations. There is a positive association between weight gain during pregnancy and fat concentration in the mother's milk. When **fat stores** laid down in pregnancy are minimal, milk fat content may decrease. The study that reported these results developed no parameters to assess the minimum level of acceptable weight gain (Michaelsen, 1994).

Prepregnancy weight should determine a woman's target weight gain in pregnancy. Underweight women with a **body mass index** (BMI) below 19.8 should gain 28–40 pounds. Women of normal weight with a BMI of 19.8 to 26.0 should gain 25–35 pounds. Overweight women with a BMI between 26.0 and 29.0 should gain 15–25 pounds. Obese women with a BMI over 29 should gain about 13 pounds (Institute of Medicine, 1991). Women over 35 years of age may have a lower **basal metabolic** rate and may not require as great an increase in energy intake.

Lactation uses energy from body stores and the mother's diet. The average weight loss during lactation is one to two pounds a month for a mother with a healthy diet and normal physical activity. If the mother's intake exceeds her needs, she will gain weight during lactation. Eating large amounts of sweet foods in place of more nutritious foods can contribute to weight gain. It can also prevent a woman from getting the vitamins, minerals, and other nutrients her body needs.

To reduce energy intake, the mother can substitute skim for whole milk, unsweetened yogurt for other dessert-type foods, and low-calorie fluids. The use of lean meat, fewer eggs, and less cheese will all help to reduce fat intake and thereby decrease calorie consumption. A mother can add more foods to her diet if she begins losing weight too rapidly or if she becomes easily fatigued.

Dieting While Breastfeeding

Several researchers express concern over the safety of maternal dieting while breastfeeding. Well-nourished women who modestly reduce caloric intake achieve gradual weight reduction and continued appropriate infant growth (Butte, 1984). Well-nourished, healthy women can safely lose up to one pound (0.45 kg) per week. They experience no adverse effect on milk production, fat content in the milk, or infant growth (Dusdieker, 1994). While this amount of weight loss is appropriate after lactation is established, caloric intake should not go below 1800 **kcal** per day. Liquid diets and diet medications should be avoided (Dewey, 1994b).

A healthy diet low in carbohydrates is compatible with breastfeeding. The mother should continue to eat fruits and vegetables and a limited amount of whole grains. She can eliminate high carbohydrate foods such as sugar, flour, breads, cakes, pasta, junk foods, desserts, potatoes, and rice. Limiting carbohydrates decreases appetite, and mothers need to ensure adequate caloric intake on this type of diet regimen.

A breastfeeding mother can be encouraged to increase her physical activity. She can use stairs instead of an elevator, park further from the door in the shopping center, go for a walk with the baby, or participate in more structured exercise programs. Moderate, regular physical activity is part of a healthy lifestyle that can be incorporated into the postpartum period. Exercising four to six times per week, beginning six to eight weeks postpartum, is safe for most women. The baby's acceptance of the

mother's post-exercise milk does not appear to be a problem in most cases (Dewey, 1994a). A mother who is considering a change in diet or exercise is encouraged to discuss her plans with her doctor or midwife prior to or at her postpartum check up. Women who restrict their food intake may need multivitamin and mineral supplements.

Breastfeeding appears to offer the mother assistance in her postpartum weight loss. One study noted larger reductions in hip circumference and greater weight loss at one month postpartum when mothers breastfed. At six months, changes were similar in all the groups studied, regardless of infant feeding method (Kramer, 1993). Another study found that in the first three months, breastfeeding mothers do not lose weight more rapidly than their formula-feeding counterparts. However, between three and six months, there was a significantly greater weight reduction when breastfeeding. Between months one and twelve, average weight loss was 2 kilograms more in breastfeeding mothers than in formula-feeding mothers. There was also a reduction in fat over the triceps area in breastfeeding mothers between months nine and twelve that was not seen in formula-feeding mothers (Dewey, 1993).

Postpartum weight loss should not occur too quickly. It occurs gradually and more easily in the normal course of breastfeeding. Weight loss can be a significant issue for women, particularly in the postpartum period. Women above the normal range for body mass index at one month postpartum have been found to stop breastfeeding sooner. There was no explanation for the early weaning (Rutishauser, 1992). However, overweight or obese women have a lower prolactin response to suckling and experience delays in stage II lactogenesis, especially first-time mothers (Rasmussen, 2004; Hilson, 2004). The higher progesterone levels contained in fat tissue may inhibit prolactin effects.

You may encounter women with eating disorders such as anorexia nervosa or bulimia nervosa. Recognize your limitations and refer these mothers to knowledgeable resources trained in treating such disorders. Anorexia is the deliberate restriction of calories, to the point of starvation. This condition may be indicated by very thin mothers who complain about being "fat" even though they are clearly underweight. Bulimics overfeed (binge) and then force themselves to vomit. They may use laxatives, diuretics, and extreme exercise to prevent gaining weight (NEDA, 2004).

▶ MAKING HEALTHY FOOD CHOICES

Women who receive practical, specific food suggestions are more likely to make healthy choices in their dietary practices. Basing their food selections and meal planning on the USDA food pyramid (Figure 8.1) will lead toward diet improvement. An awareness of food labels, additives, and processing will help them to avoid unhealthy choices. Understanding the nutritional causes of hunger and fatigue can motivate them to choose dietary practices that will enhance their health and well-being. Healthy eating is compatible with limited budgets and special diets such as vegetarianism. The information presented in this section will empower women to incorporate wise food choices into their lifestyles.

The Food Pyramid

The most widely used illustration of a healthy diet is the USDA's food pyramid, which groups foods with similar nutrient content (see Figure 8.1). The pyramid shows how much of each food group should be present in the diet relative to its size on the pyramid. In April 2005, the USDA released a new food pyramid, MyPyramid, which reflects a personalized approach to healthy eating and physical activity. Proportions of foods and oils are shown by the different widths of the vertical food group bands, which are considered general guides rather than exact proportions. The plan also calls for at least 30 minutes of physical activity a day, and discretionary calories to keep the body functioning and provide energy for physical activity. Visit www.mypyramid.gov for details about the new recommendations and to create a personalized plan.

Total daily food intake needs to contain a variety of foods from each group. While each meal may not contain all the pyramid groups, a balanced total daily intake will provide a nutritious, healthful diet. The pyramid food groups are especially helpful in planning daily food choices for meals. They can serve as a guide for evaluating diet and determining if a person is consuming enough of the right foods.

The food pyramid represents proportions of foods recommended for a healthy adult of normal weight. Pregnant or lactating women can increase amounts in the same proportions as needed to maintain an appropriate weight. Extremely overweight women will need to consume less food overall in the same proportions. Young adolescents who have not completed their growth cycle and women who are very active will require additional servings in each group to meet their energy needs. Refer to Table 8.3 for specific food selections.

Food Selection

During pregnancy, many women become more conscious of the foods they eat. They can be encouraged to continue their nutritional awareness during lactation. This may lead to gradual improvement in the eating habits of the entire family. Wise selection of foods is an

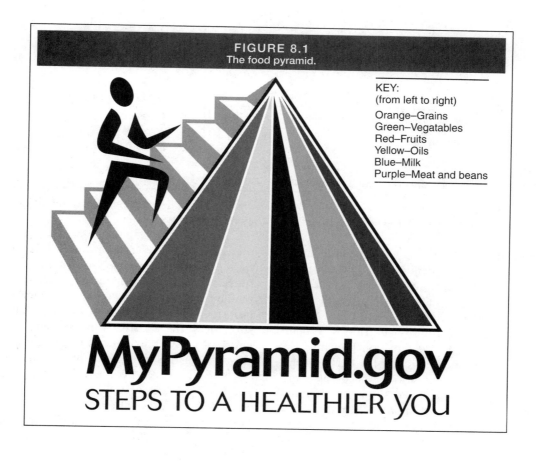

FIGURE 8.1
The food pyramid.

KEY:
(from left to right)
Orange–Grains
Green–Vegatables
Red–Fruits
Yellow–Oils
Blue–Milk
Purple–Meat and beans

MyPyramid.gov
STEPS TO A HEALTHIER YOU

TABLE 8.3

Menu Suggestions Using the Food Pyramid

Food Group	Sample Food Servings	Minimum Recommended Number of Servings Daily	
		Nonpregnant (1900 Calories)	Pregnant or Lactating (2200 Calories)
Milk or milk products	1 cup low-fat milk or yogurt 1½ ounces cheddar cheese 1 cup pudding 1¼ cups low-fat ice cream 2 cups cottage cheese 1 cup tofu (soybean curd)	2 servings	3 servings
Meats and meat substitutes	Cooked lean meat, fish, or poultry Cheddar cheese ½ cup cottage cheese 1 cup dried beans or peas 4 tablespoons peanut butter	5–7 ounces	7 ounces
Eggs		1 servings	1–2 servings
Fruits	(Include vitamin C–rich choice) ½ cup cooked or juice 1 cup raw 1 medium-sized fruit	2–4 servings	3–4 servings
Vegetables	(Choose from dark leafy and starchy vegetables. Variety is recommended.) ½ cup cooked 1 cup raw	3–5 servings	4–5 servings
Grains	(Whole grain, fortified, or enriched) 1 slice bread 1 cup ready-to-eat cereal ½ cup cooked cereal, pasta, or grits	6–11 servings	9–11 servings

Data from The Food Pyramid: How to make it work for you. *Consumer Reports on Health*, September 1996; Charbonneau, K. "Nutrition Continuum." *International Journal of Childbirth Education* 8:16–18; 1993.

important factor in good nutrition. Giving considerable thought to grocery shopping will help in the selection of foods with the highest nutritive values. Fresh, unprocessed foods are the most nutritious and most desirable choice. Food served directly after purchasing or picking is the most flavorful and nutritious. Proper food storage will help to preserve nutritional quality.

Home gardening is one way to get the freshest vegetables and fruits. Women can also be encouraged to look for fresh, crisp produce when shopping. Wilting indicates a lack of freshness and improper storage, both of which result in a loss of vitamins. Frozen produce is preferable to wilted fresh produce. Removing the skin of fresh fruits and vegetables robs them of much of their nutrients and fiber. Encourage mothers to select foods that are grown without, or with a minimum amount, of pesticides and heavy metals such as lead and mercury, substances that are stored in their fatty tissue and later enter into their milk. They can prevent this by limiting their intake of freshwater fish and animal fats and by washing all fruits and vegetables thoroughly.

Food preferences will affect a woman's food selection. She will most often choose foods that appeal to her, that are a part of her cultural heritage, and with which she is familiar. The person who does the shopping and cooking will greatly influence the nutritional value of foods consumed by the family. The available storage and frequency of shopping will also determine the variety and quality of the foods selected.

Reading Food Labels

Food labels are a source of nutritional information, with ingredients listed in order of weight. For example, in a can of chicken stew, the contents should have chicken rather than water as the main ingredient. Food labels include additives such as sugar, salt, preservatives, flavoring, and coloring. The label may also state if a product is kosher, organic, or free from particular ingredients such as nuts or wheat.

Package labels offer information on the percentage of the recommended daily allowances of nutrients the food provides. Nutritional claims on the label may need extra attention. For example, a food marketed as low in fat could be high in sugar and not a good food choice. Labels will also give information on preparation and storage. Learning to read labels will help women avoid additives such as corn syrup, sugar, and modified food starch, as well as large quantities of chemical preservatives and additives such as salt and fat.

Food Additives and Processing

Labels identify the foods and additives present in a product, with ingredients listed in descending order of quantity. When comparing ingredients in several foods, the most nutritious product will list fewer highly refined or artificial ingredients at the beginning of the list. Chemical additives that color the food, enhance flavor, or preserve freshness may alter the nutritional quality. While some changes may improve the quality, it is important to weigh the benefits of each ingredient against its possible harmful effects.

Handling and preserving techniques may alter food quality. Foods such as fresh fruits and vegetables may contain additives that are not obvious to the consumer. Mushrooms may be bleached, and other vegetables may be treated with fungicides to retard mold growth. Some foods, such as peppers, cucumbers, and tomatoes, are waxed to preserve freshness during long transport and storage times. Other foods, such as some oranges, are colored to enhance their visual appeal.

The methods used to treat foods often are beneficial because they make it possible to store or ship the foods and make them available to the consumer throughout the year. It is nearly impossible for the consumer to avoid purchasing treated foods. By washing or peeling such foods, the consumer can reasonably avoid the consumption of undesirable ingredients. Washing with water and mild dish detergent can reduce pesticide residues in fruits and many vegetables. A report on cumulative body burden found an average of 91 industrial compounds, pollutants, and other chemicals in the 9 volunteers (Williams-Derry, 2004). Information on **environmental contaminants** and ways to avoid them is at the Environmental Working Group Web site: www.ewg.org. See also ILCA's position statement on contaminants and breastfeeding at www.ilca.org. Additional information about toxins is found in Chapter 10.

Effect of Processing on Nutritional Value

Processing foods can change their nutritional value either favorably or unfavorably. Their natural state may change through bleaching, removal of fiber, soaking, drying, heating, canning, or freezing. Frozen food is a better choice than canned, since the freezing process preserves more nutrients than canning. There are nutritional differences among canned foods as well. Fruits canned in heavy syrup contain many more empty calories than those canned in natural fruit juices. Fortifying some foods, such as enriched breads or cereals, replaces nutrients removed during processing. Fortifying other foods, such as iodized salt, provides nutrients needed by the general population that are difficult to obtain. Whole-grain products are richer sources of vitamin E, vitamin B_6, folic acid, phosphorus, magnesium, and zinc than are enriched refined products.

Some forms of processing can be especially beneficial. For example, popcorn that is "popped" is in a more digestible state than in its natural form. Home canning or freezing of fruits and vegetables make it possible to store them safely for longer periods. Consumers need to be aware of the benefits and the disadvantages of various methods of processing and try to select foods processed by methods that will provide the most nutrients at an affordable price.

Cooking food for as short a time and in as little liquid as possible, as with stir-frying and pressure cooking, helps preserve nutrients. Steaming is preferable to boiling, since the nutrients are not lost in the water needed for boiling. Raw food is even more desirable, as cooking destroys some vitamins. Raw spinach, for example, contains more B vitamins than cooked spinach. However, some foods, such as meat, may contain harmful bacteria that cooking can destroy.

Vegetarian Diets

Some families follow a vegetarian diet due to cultural, philosophical, ecological, health-related, and economic factors. It is therefore very likely that you will encounter pregnant and lactating women who are on various forms of a vegetarian diet. There are several types of vegetarian

TABLE 8.4

Classification of Vegetarian Diets

Type of Vegetarian Diet	Types of Foods Consumed
Vegan	Foods from plant sources only (no animal products are consumed.)
Lacto-vegetarian	Milk and milk products, such as cheese and ice cream, in addition to plant foods.
Ovo-vegetarian	Plant foods and eggs.
Lacto-ovo-vegetarian	Plant foods, dairy products, and eggs.
Fruitarian	Fruits, nuts, olive oil, and honey.

Reprinted with permission of *The New England Journal of Medicine*, Vol. 299, 317–323, 1978.

diets; Table 8.4 classifies them by the types of foods consumed.

A vegetarian diet that includes animal products such as milk and eggs can easily supply the pregnant or lactating woman with the necessary nutrients to support her body functions and provide for the healthy growth of her baby. Indeed, the majority of the world's population consumes this type of diet. A rice and bean combination has been a staple in China, India, Africa, and South America for centuries. In some ways, a balanced vegetarian diet may be more healthful than a meat-based diet. Vegetarians consume more volume and fiber with fewer calories and fats, thereby aiding digestion and decreasing the likelihood of accumulating excess weight.

Balancing Foods in a Vegetarian Diet

Your guidance may be helpful to a woman who is new to a vegetarian diet, who has little nutritional knowledge, or whose access to food choices is limited. A teenage mother living with her parents may eat the vegetables served at the family meal and avoid the meats. The key to successful management of a vegetarian diet is to plan combinations of foods that will provide the essential amino acids. Without the proper balance of amino acids, the body is unable to synthesize the proteins essential for building tissues. A poorly managed vegetarian diet, or one that severely restricts the types of foods eaten, can be deficient in protein and minerals. This may result in inadequate growth of the fetus and breastfed infant and inadequate nourishment of the mother. A basic understanding of nutrition, careful meal planning,

and selective food shopping are prerequisites for a woman on a vegetarian diet.

Many vegetarians become well-versed in nutrition through years of practice. They may be knowledgeable about balanced diets or may feel they are knowledgeable but yet do not actually understand the basics of a healthful vegetarian diet. If you encounter a woman who you believe needs help with her diet, you may be able to motivate her to make changes by explaining the effect diet has on her well-being and on her baby's growth. You can build on the woman's present knowledge of nutrition to help her understand what additional foods she needs. Open-ended questions will help you learn what she knows about nutrition and how she plans meals.

Table 8.1 will help you offer the mother suggestions for selecting foods to fulfill her nutrient needs. Specific food suggestions are the most helpful to women. Combinations of bread or crackers with nut spreads or tofu (soybean curd) spreads are healthy snack foods. If dairy products are not part of her diet, calcium needs can be met by large quantities of green leafy vegetables, broccoli, almonds, molasses, tofu, and fortified soymilk. Iron requirements can be the most difficult to meet. Food containing vitamin C—citrus fruit or juice and fresh vegetables eaten at the same meal with legumes and whole grains—helps the body absorb the iron from these foods. Drinking coffee or tea, including herbal tea, with the meal will decrease the amount of iron absorbed (Hurrell, 1999).

Be watchful for extremely strict vegetarian regimes such as a macrobiotic diet, raw foods diet, fruitarianism, or any other arbitrarily adopted pattern that may be harmful to a woman's pregnancy or lactation. These diets tend to be unbalanced, emphasizing one specific food group while neglecting others at the expense of needed proteins, vitamins, minerals, and calories.

Vitamin B$_{12}$ Intake

Because vitamin B$_{12}$ is available primarily from animal sources, women on vegetarian diets that avoid animal products such as milk, cheese, and eggs may be deficient in this vitamin. A small amount of B$_{12}$ is present in fermented products and some seaweed, but these foods may not be incorporated into the diet frequently enough to provide adequate amounts. Even mothers with low consumption of animal foods may be at risk for deficiency (Allen, 1994). Levels of vitamin B$_{12}$ are similar in both **serum** and human milk.

Low vitamin B$_{12}$ intake by the mother leads to low levels in her milk. Be alert for signs in the 4- to 8-month-old infant that suggest a deficiency. These signs include anemia, growth failure, neurological delay, tremors, and excess skin pigmentation. Vitamin B_{12} supplementation during pregnancy and lactation is essential when the mother's diet limits or excludes sources of the vitamin (Kuhne, 1991). A caregiver who is knowledgeable about the woman's diet can prescribe these supplements.

Avoiding Feelings of Hunger and Fatigue

Food consumption should respond to hunger. Understanding the causes of hunger may help a mother plan and control her selection of foods. An empty feeling in the stomach, discussing or seeing an appealing food, or a drop in the body's blood sugar level can activate hunger. The body absorbs foods at varying rates, and food affects blood sugar in different ways. It is, therefore, possible to feel hungry even after consuming a large amount of calories.

Refined sugar is absorbed directly and quickly, causing the blood sugar to rise and fall rapidly and resulting in hunger soon afterward. The body converts complex carbohydrates like potatoes and grains into sugar. They enter the bloodstream more slowly than when sugar is consumed alone, leading to a slower rise and more gradual fall in blood sugar.

Proteins and fats, by contrast, digest more slowly than carbohydrates. Blood sugar rises slowly and steadily, remains sustained for a longer period, and falls slowly. Therefore, although many foods will result in a full stomach, fluctuating blood sugar levels will continue to cause feelings of hunger and lack of energy unless adequate protein and fat are consumed. A breakfast consisting primarily of such refined carbohydrate foods as presweetened cereal, doughnuts, or sweet rolls will cause blood sugar to rise rapidly and then swoop downward. Fatigue will follow two or three hours later, hence the mid-morning break, with more sugar to continue the blood sugar swings.

Nonfood stimulants or suppressants may affect appetite as well. Caffeine and tobacco tend to suppress the appetite, while marijuana promotes indiscriminate snacking. Alcohol can stimulate the appetite. However, when consumed in large amounts, the empty calories from alcohol take the place of more nutritious foods, often resulting in nutritional deficiencies. Various over-the-counter and prescription medications can affect appetite, either suppressing or stimulating it, depending on the drug.

Consuming a sufficient amount of protein and complex carbohydrates at breakfast will avoid mid-morning and mid-afternoon fatigue. Peanut butter on whole-grain toast, bread and cheese, yogurt and fruit, or whole-grain cereal and milk are breakfast meals that do not require much preparation. Breakfast should provide about one-third of the day's needs in order to provide a feeling of well-being throughout the day as well as the highest degree of efficiency in terms of attentiveness, performance, and endurance.

Pregnant or lactating women need at least three well-balanced meals and two snacks daily, chosen from the food pyramid and distributed throughout the day. You can offer suggestions for high-quality foods that supply needed nutrients without excessive calories. You can also encourage women to read food labels carefully. The information on labels can help them make better decisions on healthy foods for their family.

Healthy Eating on a Budget

Women who are concerned about proper nutrition and who have a limited food budget can employ cost-saving methods in purchasing, storing, and preparing foods for their families. Supermarket sales and coupons can help control grocery costs. Advance meal planning and a well-written shopping list help to avoid impulse buys. Unit pricing labels can help reveal better buys, and store-brand items are generally the same quality as popular brand names at substantially lower prices. The U.S. Center for Nutrition Policy and Promotion offers USDA food plans based on low-cost, moderate-cost, and liberal budgets (USDA, 2003).

Larger-sized packages are usually cheaper per serving and are practical when adequate storage is available and when the extra food in the house does not result in eating more. An alternative may be to shop with a friend and divide large packages. Convenience foods can be more expensive than the individual ingredients. In these cases, women can purchase individual items and make their own dishes. Shopping wisely helps to limit spending and enables families to purchase high-quality foods at a lower cost.

Proper storage and careful menu planning will help minimize food waste and fuel costs, factors often overlooked in food costs. Stir-frying for a short time will use less fuel than boiling. Baking several items in the oven at the same time, such as a casserole, baked potatoes, and a dessert saves on fuel costs as well. Careful storage of fruits and vegetables will reduce bruising and waste.

A meal can be based on starchy foods such as pasta, rice, potatoes, or bread rather than building the meal around a higher-priced meat portion. Adding beans or vegetables to the main course will help it serve more people with less meat. Families who enjoy steak can purchase a beef chuck roast and slice it to half the thickness, making two steaks. When marinated and cooked with care, this can be an appealing substitute for higher-priced cuts of beef. Canned fish is usually cheaper than fresh fish.

In addition to these suggestions, you can direct women to a local health or welfare office for nutrition assistance. The Supplemental Program for Women, Infants, and Children in the United States (WIC) provides supplemental foods and nutrition counseling to pregnant and postpartum women, breastfeeding mothers, and children from birth to age five if they meet basic requirements of low income or nutritional risk. If you are counseling a low-income woman, you can suggest this option for acquiring the nutritional assistance she will need during pregnancy and lactation. Other U.S. programs available are the food stamp program and Aid to Families with Dependent Children (AFDC). The Canada Prenatal Nutrition Program provides many of the same services as the U.S. WIC program. IBCLCs in other countries can check with their local health authority for similar programs.

Foods to Limit or Avoid

Many cultures have a wide variety of foods that are thought to cause problems while breastfeeding. The list can include high-fiber foods, acidic fruits, gas-forming vegetables and beans, milk, spices, and chocolate. However, foods that one culture avoids may be highly valued for breastfeeding women in another culture. Women sometimes believe they must avoid certain foods that cause gas, or **flatulence**. However, foods that affect the mother do not have the same effect on the baby (Lust, 1996).

Essential oils in foods such as garlic and some spices may have odors and smells that pass into the milk and are noticeable to the infant. Sensitivity to flavors in the mother's milk may increase acceptance of foods when the baby starts solid foods, as the baby is already accustomed to a variety of tastes (Mennella, 1995). In general, most mothers find they can eat a wide variety of foods. If a mother suspects a particular food is causing a problem, she can omit that food for a week and then reintroduce it. A dietician can help determine exclusion of a major food such as wheat or milk and ensure replacement of the nutrients provided by the excluded foods.

Alcohol

A safe level of alcohol consumption for breastfeeding women has not been determined. Alcohol enters the bloodstream and quickly migrates to the milk. Human milk metabolizes alcohol at about the same rate as the body metabolizes it—1½ to 2 hours per ounce of absolute alcohol. Occasional alcohol use timed around breastfeeding does not seem to have any harmful effects on the breastfed infant (Hale, 2004). Moderate amounts of alcohol consumed over time by the nursing mother may slow brain growth in her child. Large amounts delay brain growth even more dramatically and limit parental effectiveness. Excessive amounts of alcohol can cause life-threatening conditions in both the fetus and the breastfed infant. Chapter 10 further discusses alcohol consumption during lactation.

Caffeine

Caffeine passes to the infant through his mother's milk. Very young infants cannot eliminate it easily from the body. Particularly susceptible infants may experience fussiness or excessive wakefulness. Consult Chapter 10 for a more detailed discussion of substances found in human milk and their effect on the infant.

Allergens

There is some evidence that a fetus and breastfed infant can be sensitized to **allergens** in utero and through breastfeeding. A baby born to parents with a history of allergies has a greater possibility of developing the same allergies. Maternal avoidance of potentially allergenic foods as cow's milk, eggs, and fish during late pregnancy and lactation suggests a lower incidence of allergy (Lovegrove, 1994; Sigurs, 1992). However, most foods are acceptable in the mother's diet unless they cause allergic reactions in the parents or the mother consumes them in excessive amounts. Consult Chapter 10 for a more detailed discussion of substances found in human milk.

Foodborne Disease

Food poisoning can be serious during pregnancy. To reduce risks, any reheated foods should be piping hot all the way through. Raw eggs should not be consumed, and eggs should be cooked until both the white and the yolk are solid. Raw foods should be stored separately from cooked foods, and hands and utensils should be washed between preparing these foods. Food should be stored in a clean, dry, cool area away from flies, vermin, and household pets. Pregnant women should drink only milk that is pasteurized and discard food not used prior to its expiration date. Wearing gloves when gardening or changing cat litter adds further protection. All family members should wash their hands after using the toilet or changing diapers and before eating.

Pregnant women and women considering pregnancy should not eat shark, swordfish, king mackerel, or tilefish. These fish could contain enough mercury to harm a fetus's nervous system, according to a 2004 advisory by the U.S. Department of Health and Human Services and the U.S. Environmental Protection Agency. The advisory warns that young children and nursing women also should avoid those species of fish, which tend to live longer and have higher mercury concentrations in their tissues than other fish. The guidelines suggest it is permissible to eat up to twelve ounces a week of shrimp, canned light tuna, salmon, pollock, and catfish. The FDA warns against eating more than six ounces of white albacore tuna, which contains more mercury than light tuna (USDHHS, 2004).

▶ OFFERING NUTRITION SUGGESTIONS TO MOTHERS

When you have a solid understanding of nutrition and its impact on pregnant and lactating women, you can incorporate nutrition suggestions in your counseling and educate women about the basic elements of proper nutrition. After a woman accepts what she has learned about nutrition, it is yet another step for her to realize that what she actually eats may conflict with her new beliefs. For example, many of us know it is important to eat breakfast, yet we continue to skip this essential meal. Women need to recognize that where they shop, what they buy, how they plan meals, and what they keep on hand for snacks all affect their eating habits.

Nutrition education can be a positive experience that promotes a continued interest in further education. Suggestions that result in an immediate improvement may catch a mother's interest. For example, women who are sensitive to the effects of caffeine will find that eliminating caffeinated beverages before bedtime will help them sleep better. Take care not to burden women with irrelevant information or unrealistic goals. For example, cooking tips for women who eat out frequently, suggesting expensive foods to a low-income family, or suggesting that a working mother avoid convenience foods altogether probably would not be practical.

Some women fear they cannot breastfeed because they do not eat "well enough." Good nutrition need not become a barrier to breastfeeding. You can help mothers see the strengths in their diets and see that small changes can lead to big improvements. They will learn how both they and their babies will be healthier, and that the human body is very flexible and can make good milk out of many combinations of foods.

Learn the Mother's Dietary Habits

Before suggesting diet improvements to a woman, you need to learn why she chooses certain eating patterns and what factors influence her food choices. You can tactfully investigate a woman's diet practices by finding out her usual eating habits. Remember that a closed question such as, "Do you eat a good breakfast?" will not give you much information about what and how the mother eats. Few people would answer "No" to such a question! Open-ended questions or statements such as, "What have you eaten today?" or "It sounds like you

haven't had a chance to eat breakfast yet," will provide you with information that is more specific. Taking time to gather information will give you insights into factors that influence the woman's dietary habits. After exploring these influences, you will be ready to offer meaningful and appropriate suggestions.

A woman's understanding of nutrition and attitudes about eating will affect her food practices significantly. She may eat impulsively, using food to try to satisfy other needs. If she is sensitive about her appearance, she may ignore her hunger in order to lose or control her weight. Alternately, she may pay close attention to her eating practices in order to look and feel her best. Some overweight and underweight women may not see themselves as others do and therefore will not be motivated to change their eating habits. Providing accurate nutritional information will often help women avoid fad diets and improve poor eating patterns such as skipping meals.

A woman's living situation and lifestyle will affect the types of food that are available to her and the regularity of her meals. Women on limited incomes, particularly those on assistance programs, may have a narrow selection of foods from which to choose. When new parents live with their relatives or in a cooperative arrangement with others, other people may determine the food they eat and its preparation. A woman may eat in a desire to please someone who has prepared food for her, or she may eat with someone without really being hungry or needing to eat at that time. Work and school schedules often dictate whether family members share regular meals together and where they dine—at home, in restaurants, at fast food chains, from vending machines, or as bagged lunches at work. Even for the highly motivated woman, outside influences can make it difficult to obtain the well-balanced diet she needs for lactation.

A few women in your care may have health conditions that require special diet considerations. These may include food allergies or intolerances, diabetes, **hypertension**, anemia, ulcers, or weight problems. When these conditions exist, you can help the woman work within the guidelines suggested by her caregiver in order to plan a diet that is suitable for lactation. She may also benefit from a referral to a dietician.

Practical Suggestions for Diet

As you discover a mother's food practices, you can begin helping her to recognize the positive results of diet improvement. Women's interest in learning about nutrition may increase when they understand how they will feel better or how their lives will become easier with sound dietary practices. After you gain a general idea of the woman's eating patterns and the kinds of food she typically eats, you can begin suggesting diet changes. If she usually eliminates breakfast and consumes empty calories the rest of the day, as a first step you can suggest a quick protein food such as peanut butter on toast and a glass of milk for breakfast. An additional suggestion of whole-grain bread may be premature at this point. Help her to change one step at a time, making sure she understands the purpose for each change.

A realistic goal is one of diet improvement in the direction of three well-balanced meals a day with snacks as needed. If such changes are gradual, the family may be more receptive and the woman will not feel she has had to change her whole lifestyle to accommodate pregnancy and breastfeeding. After one change has become second nature, women will be more receptive to further change. You may move someone only a short way on the spectrum of food attitudes during the time she is in your care. Even the slightest improvement is worth your efforts.

Pregnancy and Postpartum Nutrition

Pregnant women can be encouraged to begin working on good eating habits by learning the relationship of nutrition to the way they feel. Issues may include doing the best thing for the baby, having a healthy pregnancy, maintaining a safe weight during pregnancy, and losing weight more easily after delivery. If a woman experiences morning sickness and nausea, she can eat a cracker or a protein such as a piece of turkey or a cube of cheese before getting out of bed. Following this with a high-protein breakfast and continued access to simple and healthy foods throughout the day will avoid an empty stomach and the return of the nausea. It may also help to open a window or turn on a fan to remove food odors.

Encourage pregnant women to eat small frequent meals, avoid fatty foods, and drink plenty of liquids. They may need to avoid highly spiced and very rich foods. She can relieve constipation with regular exercise, drinking plenty of fluids, and consuming a sufficient amount of fiber in the form of fresh fruits and vegetables, whole grains, nuts, seeds, and bran. Avoiding refined foods may also help.

After the baby arrives, you can help the mother understand how a good diet will help her overcome problems with a fussy baby, recurring breast problems, infections or nipple soreness, depression, and lack of energy. You can use the woman's problem or concern as a way of encouraging her to change her eating habits. It is important for the health of both the mother and baby that a woman embrace good nutrition during pregnancy, and that she continue healthful habits throughout lactation. One of the most effective ways of encouraging such healthful eating is to provide specific food suggestions to accompany the teaching of the basic principles of nutrition.

Specific Food Suggestions

Suggestions that mention specific foods are easier for people to accept and adapt to their eating practices. Instead of, "You need 60 grams of protein a day," translate the advice into a food practice, with specific food selections that provide protein. For example, "You can keep a couple of containers of yogurt on hand for mornings when you don't feel like making breakfast."

Suggest to women that they limit their consumption of animal fats and use vegetable or olive oils instead. All the vitamins and minerals necessary to a balanced diet are available by selecting a variety of foods from the food pyramid in forms as near as possible to their natural state. For example, a woman can use whole-wheat bread rather than white bread, bake with whole-wheat flour mixed half and half with unbleached flour, use whole-grain cereals and crackers, and use brown rice rather than polished, instant, or converted rice. See Table 8.1 for other suggestions.

Because many vitamins are water soluble, suggest that she cook vegetables in a minimal amount of water, tightly covered, and until just tender. Cooking them in their skins will further help to preserve nutrients. Water saved from cooking vegetables can form the basis of soups and gravies. She can serve something raw at every meal, such as carrots, celery, peppers, cauliflower, broccoli, spinach salad, cabbage, cucumbers, grapefruit sections, apple slices, or fresh pineapple.

Purchasing fruits canned in juice rather than heavy syrup will help reduce sugar intake. One hundred percent fruit juices are superior to fruit drinks or other beverages that are high in sugar. Homemade popsicles with fruit juice provide a nutritious substitute for commercial popsicles that contain high levels of sugar. Other nutritious snack ideas include a bran muffin with cream cheese, cheese with crackers, yogurt dip with raw vegetables, fresh fruit, custard, popcorn, cottage cheese and fruit, and hard-boiled eggs.

Meal Planning

Giving forethought to meals during pregnancy can help the woman's meal planning for the first days or weeks after the baby arrives. Stocking up on staples in the last few weeks of pregnancy can help limit repeated trips to the store when she is home with her newborn. In addition, she can prepare meals and freeze them to reheat on days when time is at a premium.

Translating the number of servings required from the food pyramid into meals with the proper number of calories may seem like a difficult task, especially to a new mother. You can help the mother eliminate that step by offering her the sample meal plans in Table 8.5. They contain the proper number of calories and all the necessary nutrients to support the baby's growth and the

TABLE 8.5
Sample Meal Plans

	Sample Menu One			Sample Menu Two	
Breakfast	Cereal, Honey Nut Chex + skim milk, 4 oz	157 calories	Breakfast	1 English muffin	134 calories
				Peanut butter, 2 tablespoons	190 calories
	Fruit juice (100%), apple, 6 oz	88 calories		Jelly, 2 teaspoons	35 calories
				Skim milk, 8 oz	86 calories
Snack	1 medium banana	133 calories	Snack	4 rye crackers	146 calories
				Low-fat swiss cheese, 1 oz	50 calories
				Orange juice (100%), 6 oz	84 calories
Lunch	Sliced turkey	73 calories	Lunch	Bowl chicken vegetable soup	166 calories
	Whole wheat bread, 2 slices	140 calories		4 saltine crackers	59 calories
	Low-fat mayonnaise, 2 tablespoons	50 calories		Apple	52 calories
	Lettuce	13 calories		Skim milk, 8 oz	86 calories
	Tomato slice	6 calories			
	Vegetable juice, 6 oz	31 calories			
Snack	Low-fat or nonfat yogurt, 1 cup	114 calories	Snack	¼ cup raisins	125 calories
Dinner	Hamburger (lean ground beef), 2 oz	150 calories	Dinner	Broiled chicken, 3 oz	165 calories
				Broccoli, ½ cup	32 calories
	Whole grain bun	120 calories		Rice, brown, ½ cup	107 calories
	Tomato slice, lettuce, onion	16 calories		Dinner roll	100 calories
	Spinach and tomato salad	41 calories		Spinach and tomato salad	41 calories
	w/low-fat dressing	20 calories		w/low-fat dressing	20 calories
	Skim milk, 8 oz	86 calories		Skim milk, 8 oz	86 calories
Snack	2 full sheets low-fat graham crackers	120 calories	Snack	½ cup nonfat ice cream	110 calories
	Skim milk, 8 oz	86 calories			
TOTAL		1,449 calories	TOTAL		1,874 calories

Source: Medela, Inc., *Rental Roundup*, Vol. 10, Number 1, Winter 1993. www.nutribase.com.

FIGURE 8.2
Nutrition topics for group meetings.

There are many interesting and entertaining ways to present nutrition information during group discussions. It is hoped that those listed below will interest mothers in nutrition and help them understand how it relates to their daily food selection and preparation.

◆ At a discussion on the "First Days of Breastfeeding," you can emphasize good nutrition as a necessity for pregnant women and new mothers. Avoid overwhelming mothers with healthy food ideas. Stress two or three basic points, and explain why they are important.

◆ Diet recall: Ask mothers to record everything they have eaten that day. Have them analyze their diets according to food groups, or ask them to hand in their recall lists anonymously for the group to analyze. Look for foods that supply specific nutrients such as protein, vitamin C, iron, calcium, and so on.

◆ At a discussion on "Starting the Baby on Solid Foods," present a buffet of homemade infant foods, including finger foods for mothers to sample. For comparison, also provide a taste of the same food prepared commercially.

◆ To highlight a nutrition discussion, serve several complete protein dishes made with meat substitutes and show a variety of milk servings in nutritionally equal amounts (milk, cheese, yogurt, sesame seeds, soy products, and so on).

◆ Approach an old topic with a new point of view. For example, the health benefits of breastfeeding, delaying solid foods, and how to introduce solid foods can be approached from the perspective of avoiding food intolerances and entitled "Food Intolerances and Healthier Babies."

◆ Have a recipe swap, and ask everyone to bring a nutritious snack and recipe for all to sample and enjoy.

---

mother's well-being. Substituting most sweets with more nutritious selections results in very generous amounts of food.

The specific foods listed in the sample meal plans are suggestions for diet planning. A mother can substitute foods that suit her preferences, group foods into smaller, more frequent meals, or eat the lunchtime apple as a midmorning snack. In addition to the fluids suggested, she will want to drink water according to her thirst.

Group Instruction in Nutrition

Example is the best teacher, so any refreshments served at support group meetings and classes should be nutritious. You can encourage healthful snacking and eating habits either by bringing nutritious refreshments yourself or by requesting that volunteers bring specific foods to serve. Nutritious snacks might include natural fruit juices, fresh fruit, raw vegetables and dip, wholesome cookies and breads, cheese and crackers, and other snacks discussed in this chapter. Figure 8.2 suggests topics on nutrition for group meetings.

▶ SUMMARY

A responsible part of counseling is making sure that breastfeeding women have the opportunity and the necessary information to improve their health through nutrition. Poor dietary habits are widespread and continually promoted by the advertising of nutritionally empty high calorie foods. Most mothers can benefit from sound practical suggestions. Becoming familiar with basic nutrition principles and, more specifically, the food practices of the women in your care will help you to understand influences on their diet. This, in turn, will provide insight into helping them to institute changes.

You can be a positive force in helping women improve nutrition for themselves and their families. Educating them about their nutritional needs and the effects of their nutrition on their health and the way they feel will help to influence dietary changes. Offering practical food suggestions rather than theoretical dietary requirements will make it easier for women to embrace these changes. Pregnancy and lactation are milestones in a woman's life when she is most receptive to nutrition counseling. Helping families integrate sound nutrition gradually into their lifestyles increases the likelihood that these practices will continue to benefit family members for years to come.

▶ CHAPTER 8—AT A GLANCE

Facts you learned—

Nutrition in pregnancy and lactation:

◆ Pregnancy and lactation are times when women are receptive to nutrition education.

◆ A mother's body stores and the food she eats provide energy and nutrients for her baby.

◆ Sugary foods cause erratic blood sugar, fatigue, dizziness, nervousness, and headache.

◆ Complex carbohydrates take longer to digest and prevent cravings for more food.

◆ Protein is needed for formation of hormones and milk production during lactation.

◆ Fats create a longer feeling of fullness.

◆ Folic acid helps prevent anemia in pregnancy and neural tube defects.

- A newborn's vitamin K levels are low and are typically supplemented.

- Low levels of vitamin D in pregnancy result in low levels in the baby.

- Pregnancy and lactation require increased calcium, iron, and water intake.

- Consuming excessive fluid can reduce milk production.

- A normal, healthy diet will meet the mother's needs during lactation.

- Lactation uses energy from body stores and from diet.

- Well-nourished, healthy women can safely lose up to one pound per week.

- Food additives and processing alter nutritional quality favorably and unfavorably.

- Vegetarian diets that include milk and eggs supply necessary nutrients.

- Occasional alcohol timed around breastfeeding has not proven harmful to breastfed infants.

- Infants sensitive to caffeine may experience fussiness or excessive wakefulness.

- Most foods are acceptable unless they cause allergic reactions in the mother or father or are consumed in excessive amounts.

Applying what you learned—

- Strive for diet improvement of three well-balanced meals a day with snacks as needed.

- Encourage pregnant women to eat small frequent meals, avoid fatty foods, drink plenty of liquids, and avoid highly spiced and very rich foods.

- Teach mothers about practical food choices rather than nutrients.

- Teach mothers to base their meal planning on the food pyramid.

- Teach mothers how to balance complete protein and incomplete protein foods.

- Teach mothers how to consume more unsaturated fats than saturated fats.

- Teach mothers to respond to thirst for necessary additional fluids.

- Teach mothers that protein and complex carbohydrates at breakfast will avoid later fatigue.

- Teach mothers to read food labels for nutritional information.

- Teach mothers that a healthy diet helps overcome a fussy baby, recurring breast problems, infections or nipple soreness, depression, and lack of energy.

REFERENCES

Adair LS, Pollitt E. Outcome of maternal nutritional supplementation: A comprehensive review of the Bacon Chow study. *Amer Clin Nut* 41(5):948–978; 1985.

Allen L. Vitamin B_{12} metabolism and status during pregnancy, lactation and infancy. *Adv Exp Med Biol* 352:173–186; 1994.

Barker D. Fetal programming of coronary heart disease. Review. *Trends Endocrinol Metab* 13(9):364–368; 2002.

Beal VA. Nutritional studies during pregnancy: Dietary intake, maternal weight gain and size of infant. *J Am Diet Assoc* 58:321; 1971.

Butte N et al. Effect of maternal diet and body composition on lactation performance. *Am J Clin Nutr* 39:296–306; 1984.

Charbonneau K. Folic acid and neural tube defects. *Int J Childbirth Education* 8:42–44; 1993.

Chesley L. *Testimony to U.S. Food and Drug Administration.* Rockville, MD: Bureau of Drugs, OB Gyn Advisory Committee; July 17, 1975.

Dewey K et al. A randomized study of the effects of aerobic exercise by lactating women on breastmilk volume and composition. *N Engl J Med* 330:449–453; 1994a.

Dewey K, McCrory M. Effects of dieting and physical activity on pregnancy and lactation. *Am J Clin Nutr* 59(supp):446s–453s; 1994b.

Dewey KG et al. Maternal weight-loss patterns during prolonged lactation. *Am J Clin Nutr* 58:162–166; 1993.

Diet Information. How much protein do you need to eat in your daily diet? Available at: www.diet-i.com/protein-intake-in-daily-diet.htm. Accessed December 16, 2004.

Dusdieker L et al. Is milk production impaired by dieting during lactation? *Am J Clin Nutr* 59:833–840; 1994.

Dusdieker LB et al. Effect of supplemental fluids on human milk production. *J Pediatr* 106:207; 1985.

Foukas MD. An antilactogenic effect of pyridoxine. *J Obstet Gynaecol Br Commonw* 80:718–720; 1973.

Franx A, Steegers EA, de Boo T, Thien T, Merkus JM. Sodium-blood pressure interrelationship in pregnancy. *J Hum Hypertens* 13(3):159–166; 1999.

Fukushima Y et al. Consumption of cow milk and egg by lactating women and the presence of B-lactoglobulin and ovalbumin in breastmilk. *Am J Clin Nutr* 65:30–35; 1997.

Gartner LM. Prevention of rickets and vitamin D deficiency: New guidelines for vitamin D intake. *Pediatrics* 111(4):908–910; 2003.

Good Mojab, C. Sunlight deficiency: A review of the literature. *Mothering.* 117:52–55; 57–63; 2003; Available at: www.mothering.com/articles/new_baby/breastfeeding/sunlight-deficiency.html. Accessed January 30, 2005.

Greer F et al. Improving the vitamin K status of breastfeeding infants with maternal vitamin K supplements. *Pediatrics* 99(1):88–92; 1997.

Hale T. *Medications in Mothers' Milk*, 11th ed. Amarillo, TX: Pharmasoft Pub; 2004.

Henderson P et al. Bone mineral density in grand multiparous women with extended lactation. *Am J Obstet Gynecol* 182(6): 1371–1377; 2000.

Hilson J et al. High prepregnant body mass index is associated with poor lactation outcomes among white, rural women independent of psychosocial and demographic correlates. *J Hum Lact* 20(1):18–29; 2004.

Hollis B, Wagner C. Assessment of dietary vitamin D requirements during pregnancy and lactation. Review. *Am J Clin Nutr* 79(5):717–726. 2004a.

Hollis B, Wagner C. Vitamin D requirements during lactation: High-dose maternal supplementation as therapy to prevent hypovitaminosis D for both the mother and the nursing infant. *Am J Clin Nutr* 80(6 Suppl):1752S–1758S; 2004b.

Hurrell RF, Reddy M, Cook JD. Inhibition of non-haem iron absorption in man by polyphenolic-containing beverages. *Br J Nutr* 81(4):289–295; 1999.

Illingworth PJ et al. Diminution in energy expenditure during lactation. *Br Med J* 292:437; 1986.

Institute of Medicine (National Academy of Sciences). *Nutrition During Lactation*. Washington, DC: National Academy Press; 1991.

Jelliffe DB, Jelliffe EFP. *Human Milk in the Modern World*. Oxford: Oxford University Press, 62; 1978.

Karlsson C et al. Pregnancy and lactation confer reversible bone loss in humans. *Osteoporos Int* 12(10):828–834; 2001.

Kramer FM et al. Breastfeeding reduces maternal lower-body fat. *J Am Diet Assoc* 93:429–433; 1993.

Kritz-Silverstein D. Pregnancy and lactation as determinants of bone mineral density in postmenopausal women. *Am J Epidemiol* 136:1052–1059; 1992.

Kuhne T et al. Maternal vegan diet causing a serious infantile neurological disorder due to vitamin B_{12} deficiency. *Euro J Pediatr* 150:205–208; 1991.

Lappe FM. *Diet for a Small Planet*. New York: Ballantine Books; 1992.

Laskey M, Prentice A. Bone mineral changes during and after lactation. *Obstet Gynecol* 94(4):608–615; 1999.

Lawrence R. *Breastfeeding: A Guide for the Medical Profession*. St. Louis, MO: Mosby; 1999.

Liebman B. Folic acid for all. *Nutrition Action Healthletter* 19(10):4; December 1992.

Lipsman S et al. Breastfeeding among teenage mothers: Milk composition, infant growth and maternal dietary intake. *J Pediatr Gasteroenterol Nutr* 4:426; 1985.

Lovegrove JA et al. The immunological and long-term atopic outcome of infants born to women following a milk-free diet during late pregnancy and lactation: A pilot study. *Br J Nutr* 71:223–238; 1994.

Lumbers E et al. The selfish brain and the barker hypothesis. *Clin Exp Pharmacol Physiol* 28(11):942–947; 2001.

Lust K et al. Maternal intake of cruciferous vegetables and other foods and colic symptoms in exclusively breast-fed infants. *J Am Diet Assoc* 96(1):46–48; 1996.

Marcus, RG. Suppression of lactation with high doses of pyridoxine. *S Afr Med J* 49:2155–2156; 1975.

Martek Biosciences Corporation. Mead Johnson launches prenatal and nursing supplement containing Martek DHA(TM); *Press Release*. Columbia, MD; October 6, 2004.

Mennella J. Mother's milk: A medium for early flavor experiences. Review. *J Hum Lact* 11(1):39–45; 1995.

Michaelsen K et al. The Copenhagen Cohort study on infant nutrition and growth: Breast-milk intake, human milk macronutrient content, and influencing factors. *Am J Clin Nutr* 59:600–611; 1994.

Munoz LM et al. Coffee consumption as a factor in iron deficiency anemia among pregnant women and their infants in Costa Rica. *Am J Clin Nutr* 48:645–651; 1988.

Naeye RL. Cigarette smoking and pregnancy weight gain. *The Lancet* 1(8171):765–766; 1980.

National Eating Disorders Association (NEDA). *Eating Disorders Information Index*. www.nationaleatingdisorders.org. Accessed December 15, 2004.

Prentice A. Calcium requirements of breast-feeding mothers. *Nutr Rev* 56:124–130; 1998.

Rasmussen K, Kjolhede C. Prepregnant overweight and obesity diminish the prolactin response to suckling in the first week postpartum. *Pediatrics* 113(5):e465–e471; 2004.

Robinson S, Barker D. Coronary heart disease: A disorder of growth. Review. *Proc Nutr Soc* 61(4):537–542; 2002.

Rutishauser L, Carlin J. Body mass index and duration of breastfeeding: A survival analysis during the first six months of life. *J Epidemiol Community Health* 46:559–565; 1992.

Sigurs N et al. Maternal avoidance of eggs, cow's milk and fish during lactation: Effect on allergic manifestations, skin-prick tests and specific IgE antibodies in children at age 4 years. *Pediatrics* 89:735–739; 1992.

Specker BL. Changes in calcium homeostasis over the first year postpartum: Effect of lactation and weaning. *Obstet Gynecol* 78:56–62; 1991.

US Department of Agriculture (USDA). New dietary guidelines will help Americans make better food choices, live healthier lives. News release; January 12, 2005. Available at www.usda.gov. Accessed January 25, 2005.

US Department of Agriculture (USDA). The low-cost, moderate-cost and liberal food plans. USDA CNPP; 2003. Available at:www.usda.gov/cnpp/FoodPlans/FP2003/FoodPlans2003. pdf. Accessed March 5, 2004.

US Department of Health and Human Services (DHHS) and US Environmental Protection Agency (EPA). What you need to know about mercury in fish and shellfish: 2004 EPA and

FDA advice for women who might become pregnant, women who are pregnant, nursing mothers, young children. March 2004. Available at: www.cfsan.fda.gov/~dms/admehg3.html. Accessed December 15, 2004.

Williams-Derry C. Flame retardants in Puget Sound residents. *Northwest Environmental Watch*; 2004. Available at: www.northwestwatch.org. Accessed October 5, 2004.

World Health Organization (WHO). *The International Pharmacopoeia*, 3rd ed., Vol 5. Geneva: WHO; 2003. Available at: www.who.int/medicines/library/pharmacopoeia/itoxviii.pdf. Accessed April 8, 2004.

WHO/UNICEF. *Breastfeeding Management and Promotion in a Baby-Friendly Hospital*. New York: UNICEF; 1993.

Worthington-Roberts B, Rodwell-Williams S. *Nutrition in Pregnancy and Lactation*, 6th ed. New York: McGraw-Hill; 1996. Available at: www.usda.gov/cnpp/FoodPlans/FP2003/FoodPlans2003.pdf. Accessed April 8, 2004.

 BIBLIOGRAPHY

Brewer S, Brewer T. *What Every Pregnant Woman Should Know: The Truth about Diets and Drugs in Pregnancy*. New York: Penguin Books; 1979.

Food and Nutrition Information Center. National Agricultural Library/USDA. Nutrition during pregnancy and breastfeeding resource list for consumers; April 2000. Available at: www.nal.usda.gov/fnic/pubs/bibs/topics/pregnancy/pregcon.html. Accessed May 20, 2004.

Grains and Cereals Module. Oregon State University: Corvallis, OR. Available at: www.oregonstate.edu/instruct/nfm236/cereals/#a. Accessed May 20, 2004.

Institute of Medicine. Subcommittee for a Clinical Applications Guide. *Nutrition During Pregnancy and Lactation: An Implementation Guide*. National Academies Press; 1992.

Liebman B. Do you know your vitamin ABCs? *Nutrition Action Health Letter*. Center for Science in the Public Interest; September 1999.

Mennella JA, Beauchamp GK. Maternal diet alters the sensory qualities of human milk and the nursling's behavior. *Pediatrics* 88(4):737–744; 1991.

Motil K et al. Lean body mass of well-nourished women is preserved during lactation. *Am J Clin Nutr* 67:292–300; 1998.

Mughal M et al. Florid rickets associated with prolonged breast feeding without vitamin D supplementation. *Br Med J* 318:39–40; 1999.

Spurr G et al. Increased muscular efficiency during lactation in Colombian women. *Eur J Clin Nutr* 52:17–21; 1998.

Tinkle M. Folic acid and food fortification: Implications for the primary care practitioner. *Nurse Pract* 22:105–114; 1997.

CHAPTER
9

PROPERTIES OF HUMAN MILK

Human milk is a marvelous substance that is more than just nutrition for the child. The breast initially secretes protein-rich colostrum that provides the infant with antibodies and other protection against disease. Colostrum is exactly what the newborn needs, both in amount and composition, during his transition from intra- to extra-uterine life. During the first few days after birth, colostrum mixes with increasing quantities of newly formed milk and eventually transforms to mature milk (Hartmann, 2003; Humenick, 1994; Viverge, 1990). The composition of human milk is ideally suited to the human infant. Its components are studied continually, and despite efforts by the manufacturers of artificial baby milk substitutes, no parallel can be found to this perfect infant nutrition.

KEY TERMS

acrodermatitis
  enteropathica
active immunity
alpha-lactalbumin
amylase
antibacterial
antibody response
antigen
antimicrobial
antiparasite
antiviral
assimilate
atopic dermatitis
bifidus factor
bioavailability
calories
carbohydrates
casein
Centers for Disease Con-
  trol (CDC)
cholecystokinin (CCK)
colicky behavior
colostrum
congenital

cow's milk
creamatocrit
cytokines
dehydration
diarrhea
donor milk
dopamine
eclampsia
ELBW
enteral feeding
enzyme
exogenous
fat
flora
fluoride
growth factors
hemorrhagic disease
human milk bank
human milk fortifier
humoral factors
hypocalcemia
IgA
immunologic properties
iron

lactobacillus bifidus
lactoengineering
lactoferrin
lactose intolerance
LBW
lipase
long-chain polyunsaturated
  fatty acid
lysozyme
macrophages
mature milk
meconium
mineral
mucin
myelin
necrotizing enterocolitis
neurological development
neurotransmitter
nosocomial
nucleotide
oligosaccharide

otitis media
passive immunity
pathogen
peptide
phagocytic cells
phthalates
product recall
prostaglandin
protein
rickets
rotavirus
sepsis
SGA
tube feeding
vaccine
virus
vitamin D
vitamin K
VLBW
vomiting
whey

COLOSTRUM: THE EARLY MILK

Colostrum can be secreted prenatally and for several days postpartum. It is a thick, sticky, rich-looking substance, yellowish in color. Colostrum is concentrated with protein suited to early rapid growth of the newborn. It is actually the residual mixture of materials present in the mammary glands and ducts, which started production at about 120 days' gestation. This substance mixes with the newly formed milk and is the thick, clear to golden-yellow fluid that the infant first receives.

Colostrum contains approximately 67 kcal/dl (18.76 kcal/oz). Compared with mature milk, colostrum is richer in sodium, potassium, chloride, protein, fat-soluble vitamins, and minerals. It also contains less fat (2 percent) and lactose than mature milk (Wagner, 1996; Jelliffe,

1978). Colostrum contains the appropriate level and balance of the essential fatty acids required by the newborn (Ronneberg, 1992).

Colostrum is a baby's first immunization against many bacteria and **viruses**. It contributes to the infant's health as artificial baby milk cannot, which makes it the baby's ideal first food. Colostrum plays an important role in protecting the infant against infection. It contains many living cells that engulf and digest disease organisms. Colostrum aids in rapid gut closure, or resistance of the baby's intestinal wall to penetration by disease organisms and **antigens**. Thus, the infant who receives colostrum is less likely to develop diseases and infantile allergies.

The mother produces antibodies to all the diseases to which she has already acquired relative **immunity**. Colostrum contains many antibodies produced by the body in response to a threat by a particular microbial invader, or antigen. The mother passes many antibodies to her fetus through the placenta and to her newborn through colostrum and her milk.

Three specific antibodies that are highly concentrated in colostrum and human milk are immune globulin A (IgA), immune globulin G (IgG), and immune globulin M (IgM). An immune globulin, or immunoglobulin, is a group of proteins that provides immunity. Of these immunoglobulins, IgA occurs in the highest concentrations in colostrum and human milk and is the most biologically active. **Secretory IgA** is available only through the mother's milk. The baby cannot produce it until approximately six months of age. Secretory IgA is not present in artificial baby milks.

The infant receives most of his circulating antibodies from the placenta. The very high levels of IgA and other antibodies in colostrum provide further protection to his gastrointestinal tract against organisms that might otherwise invade it. Colostrum facilitates the establishment of bifidus **flora** (normal bacteria and other microbes) in the digestive tract. Bifidus flora promotes the growth of beneficial bacteria, primarily **lactobacillus bifidus**, and facilitates the passage of **meconium**.

Colostrum provides protection against some **pathogens** (disease agents), including polio, Coxsackie B virus, several staphylococci, and *Escherichia coli*, the intestinal bacteria that can cause serious intestinal, urinary, and other infections in infants. Health professionals have found colostrum so effective in preventing disease that they give it to premature infants, older children, and teenagers with compromised immune systems or metabolic disorders (Arnold, 1995). Mature milk also is ideal for these needs (Tully, 2004).

In addition to providing disease protection and superior nutrition during the infant's first days of life, colostrum produces a laxative effect that results in the elimination of meconium from the infant's bowels. Meconium is a thick, black, sticky substance present in the newborn infant's first stools. Stimulating bowel function is necessary for the infant's body to begin excreting waste products effectively. This elimination can be a critical factor in reducing the severity of jaundice.

In the first 24 hours, total infant intake of colostrum can range from 3 to 32 ml/kg of weight, or 10.2 to 108.8 ml based on a 7½ pound baby (Casey, 1986). This amount corresponds with the newborn's small stomach. It is reassuring to a mother to know that her newborn is receiving nourishment in addition to other important health benefits until her milk production increases and transforms to mature milk. The removal of colostrum by the infant stimulates further production of colostrum and milk in the breast. Any water or artificial milks the baby receives will dilute colostrum's effects. Additionally, a baby's kidneys are not capable of handling large volumes of fluid and are stressed by additional water. Breastfed newborns do not need water.

▶ TRANSITION TO MATURE MILK

Colostrum changes to transitional milk by about the sixth day. During that time, volume increases until production typically ranges from 556 to 705 ml (14 to 19 oz) in a 24-hour period (Hartmann, 2003).

The color and consistency of human milk varies according to the type of milk and specific additives in the mother's diet. Transitional milk appears at about 6 to 13 days postpartum and gradually changes to mature milk. As the baby's suckling stimulates the nipple, oxytocin releases and activates letdown. The milk then travels from the alveoli through the ducts, washing the fat from the walls of the ducts and ductules. This process results in hindmilk, which is much higher in fat and thus richer looking than the initial milk, or foremilk.

Fat content varies from mother to mother and from feeding to feeding (Lai, 2004). It is inversely proportional to the length of time between feedings and correlates with the degree of breast fullness. Although there is not a clear demarcation between foremilk and hindmilk, allowing a baby to finish at the first breast and not restricting feeding time ensures the baby has access to the fat available in that feeding (Daly, 1993a).

Appearance of Mature Milk

Human milk has a naturally watery appearance that looks even more dilute when the supply is more plentiful. If the mother expresses milk at the end of a feeding when fat content is higher, she will note a thicker and denser consistency.

Human milk often appears bluish and may take on other colors. The typical bluish cast results from the presence of **casein**, a component of the proteins in milk. A greenish color may be caused by additives in vitamin or iron supplements taken by the mother. Excessive amounts of vitamin A, either in foods or as a supplement, may color the milk yellow. Black milk can result from use of the drug minocycline (Hunt, 1996). It is helpful to inform a mother to expect these variations so that she is not concerned unnecessarily.

Milk Volume

The volume of milk is dependent on regular removal of milk from the breast, whether it be through nursing, manual expression, or pumping. It also depends on the degree of drainage at each feeding or pumping session. Volume does not decrease because of supplemental milk removal. It is more likely to increase, because removing milk signals the breast to make more milk. Removal of milk at one feeding signals the amount of milk available at the next feeding (Daly, 1993b).

Minor variations may occur in the volume produced by each breast, on different days, or in response to the infant's suckling pattern. Milk often seems most plentiful in the morning hours, especially immediately after the mother awakens. She can express milk at that time and throughout the day without decreasing the amount of milk available to her baby.

Milk volume is most dependent on the baby's removal of milk from the breast. Babies have the ability to self-regulate their feedings to meet their individual needs for optimal growth (Cox, 1998; Woolridge, 1990). They determine their supply on a feeding-to-feeding basis through the amount of milk they remove.

Although milk volume is most dependent on regular milk removal from the breast, it is to a much lesser extent influenced by the mother's nutrition and water intake. There is little scientific evidence to support substantial effects of maternal nutritional status on lactation. Lactation consultants should therefore not overemphasize the importance of diet during lactation, especially among first-time mothers who may be unsure of their bodies' ability to nourish newborn children properly (Greiner, 1994). When a woman's diet includes the Dietary Reference Intake (DRI) of all nutrients, there is no significant decrease in milk volume. This helps explain why women are able to nourish their babies under varied nutritional conditions. Their babies have growth patterns similar to the baby of a well-nourished mother.

COMPOSITION OF HUMAN MILK

The composition of human milk changes throughout lactation as the child grows and even during any given day or feeding. Scientists continually study the many components in human milk, including fat, protein, lactose, vitamins, and minerals. Each component has a specific function in ensuring optimum nourishment of the infant.

Human milk continues to change to meet the needs of the growing child from the first few days of colostrum to beyond the second year. The milk is high in immunoglobulins and protein during the first several weeks postpartum, yielding to a relatively dilute state by the first month. In the later months of lactation, the fat content decreases. From six to twelve months of age, the infant receives three-quarters or more of his nutrient needs from human milk. During the second year of lactation, the output of human milk is equivalent to at least one 8-ounce glass daily. Thus, human milk is still valuable to the toddler's diet in both quantity and composition.

Protein and fat content are usually higher at the end of a feeding, with 4 to 5 times as much fat and 1½ times as much protein than at the beginning. The baby may consume nearly ⅙ of his calories between minutes 11 and 16. Therefore, it is important that mothers place no limits on the amount of time the baby is at each breast (Hall, 1997). In order for the baby to obtain important fats, proteins, and calories, the mother should continue to nurse until he decides he is ready to end the feeding.

Clearly, human milk provides appropriate changes in composition to meet the child's needs. It varies in sensory qualities as well. Human milk provides the exclusively breastfed infant with richly changing experiences in taste and odor that are not provided to the artificially fed infant, whose formula has a consistent taste and smell. Mennella (1991a) noted in her research that babies demonstrated a preference for garlic-flavored milk.

Calories

The caloric content of human milk is ideally suited to the human infant, so much so that formula companies design their products around the average calories found in human milk. Colostrum contains about 17 kcal/oz. By 2 weeks, the average caloric content of mature human milk is 20 kcal/oz. At around 4 months, the caloric content is about 26 kcal/oz. Differences in caloric content of mature milk result from variations in fat. If a feeding is not long enough for the baby to receive the fatty hindmilk, he may not receive sufficient calories. In severely malnourished mothers, both volume and fat may be lower. In the vast majority of women, however, this is not an issue.

Fat

Human milk fat provides up to 50 percent of the infant's energy needs. It is the main source of fat-soluble vitamins and essential fatty acids needed for growth and development of the infant's central nervous system. Fat is an extremely variable constituent in human milk (Mitoulas, 2002). The amount of available fat seems dependent on maternal body fat stores (Koletzko, 2001; Martin, 1993; Nommsen, 1991). Maternal fat stores laid down during pregnancy are easier to mobilize for lactation than other fat stores in the mother's body (Michaelsen, 1994). If the mother is severely malnourished, not usually an issue in developed countries, the level of fat in her milk may be lower.

Fat content changes during feeding as well. If a mother's milk fat content decreases, the baby will stay at the breast longer in order to gain a higher fat yield. This yield is comparable to a mother with higher milk fat (Tyson, 1992), which illustrates the importance of baby-led feeding (Perez-Escamilla, 1995).

Short-chain, medium-chain, and long-chain fatty acids are very important. Like milk fat, fatty acids in human milk are also dependent upon maternal stores (Del Prado, 2001; Sauerwald, 2000). Linoleic and linolenic acids, essential fatty acids, have significance in the quality of **myelin** laid down. One study showed that multiple sclerosis (MS) is rare in countries where breast-feeding is common. The development of myelin in infancy may be critical to preventing degradation later (Dick, 1976). Another study described a rise in MS in Mexico as breastfeeding rates decreased (Tarrats, 2002). Arachidonic acid (AA) from linoleic acid and docosahexaenoic acid (DHA) from linolenic acid are essential for development of visual acuity (Williams, 2001; Innis, 2001; Carlson, 1996).

The amount of fat a breastfed infant receives depends on the length of suckling time at the breast. A baby who is not gaining sufficient weight may not be nursing long enough at each feeding or frequently enough throughout the day and night. If the mother removes the baby from one breast too early, before he receives the fatty hindmilk, he will fill up on foremilk from both breasts. This could lead to behavior resembling **colic** and poor nourishment. Fat content decreases after five or six months and may be lower when the let-down reflex is inhibited.

Carbohydrates

Lactose is present in human milk in high levels (7 percent) and represents almost all of the carbohydrate in the milk (Jelliffe, 1978). Lactose provides 40 to 45 percent of the energy in human milk. Lactose concentration increases by approximately 10 percent over the first 6 months of lactation (Coppa, 1993). It is specific for newborn growth and performs 3 unique functions that benefit the infant. Lactose enhances calcium absorption, thereby helping prevent **rickets**. It helps supply energy to the infant's brain and it helps check the growth of harmful organisms in the intestine. It also is essential to development of the central nervous system.

Lactose is the major sugar in mammalian milk and appears nowhere else in nature. It is the most constant of all the constituents in human milk and remains constant throughout the day and despite dietary fluctuations (Jelliffe, 1978). Lactose digests slowly, producing a steady release of glucose into the bloodstream. Sucrose, the sugar often used in milk substitute formulas such as soy, is sweeter and splits rapidly, resulting in a high peak of glucose in the infant's bloodstream. Sucrose probably plays a significant role in tooth decay, whereas lactose does not (Erickson, 1999, 1998). Additionally, the consequences of feeding an infant a food without lactose such as soy formula and milk-based lactose-free formula are not clear.

Oligosaccharides, a type of carbohydrate, are the third largest solid in human milk. There have been more than 80 identified. Oligosaccharides protect the baby from pathogens by preventing them from binding to receptor sites in the gut (Newburg, 1996). They survive passage through the baby's digestive system and provide protection throughout his digestive system (Chaturvedi, 2001b). They protect against urinary tract infections in both the child and the mother (Hanson, 2004a; Pisacane, 1992; Coppa, 1990) and against diarrhea (Newburg, 2004). Oligosaccharides vary among mothers and over the course of lactation (Chaturvedi, 2001a).

Protein

All animal species have growth and development needs that determine their milk composition. Within the animal kingdom, human milk contains the least amount of protein, which results in the slowest rate of growth. Protein in human milk digests easily and is well absorbed. The distribution of specific proteins in human milk is ideally suited to the growth of the human infant. It enables him to use the proteins with extremely high efficiency. Colostrum contains about three times more protein than does mature milk. The protein content of human milk seems to remain relatively constant regardless of the mother's nutritional status or dietary practices.

Manufacturers of artificial baby milk substitutes have attempted to adjust their products to equal the protein content of human milk as closely as possible. Infant formula, however, lacks certain proteins found in human milk, such as **lactoferrin**. The infant does not use lactoferrin completely and passes some amino acids in his stool. Cow's milk curd is tough and rubbery, whereas the curd of human milk is soft, small, and less compact, making it easier for the infant to digest.

Whey and Casein

The ratio of whey to casein changes throughout lactation. Whey is the clear fluid in the milk, and casein is the curd portion. The ratio changes from 90:10 in early milk to 60:40 in mature milk and to 50:50 in late lactation. Ratios in formula vary depending on the manufacturer. Ratios in Carnation Good Start are 100:0—there is no casein (Nestle, 2004). Ratios are 60:40 for Enfamil and Enfamil Lipil with iron (Mead Johnson, 2004). In Similac, ratios are 82:18, 48:52 for Similac with iron, and 48:52 for Similac Advance with iron (Ross, 2004).

Lactoferrin

Lactoferrin, the iron-binding protein in whey, inhibits the growth of iron-dependent bacteria (*E. coli*) in the gastrointestinal tract. This protects the baby against gastrointestinal infections. Lactoferrin renders intestinal iron unavailable to pathogens in the baby's gut, thus protecting him from such infections as salmonella, *E. coli*, and **Candida albicans**. One study terms the elevated bifidobacterial count from lactoferrin "one of the greatest advantages that breastfed infants have over infants fed with milk formulas" (Chierici, 2003). Giving iron supplements to newborns may saturate lactoferrin, thus allowing proliferation of *E. coli*. Protection from lactoferrin is not present if the baby receives any other type of feeding.

Researchers have been exploring various methods to commercialize human lactoferrin. Lactoferrin, largely purified from human milk, costs over $3,600 per gram at 90 percent purity. One company markets recombinant lactoferrin, genetically engineered from fermented aspergilus, a fungus (Agennix, 2002). Aggressive patenting of human milk components is one more demonstration of the value of human milk.

Lysozyme

Another whey protein found in human milk is lysozyme. Lysozyme, one of the more than 20 active **enzymes** present in human milk, provides an **antimicrobial** factor against enterobacteriaceae and gram-positive bacteria. Human milk also contains 8 essential amino acids, including taurine. Taurine is important for vision and general development and improves fat absorption in preterm infants.

Long-chain Polyunsaturated Fatty Acids

Human milk contains at least 160 different long-chain polyunsaturated fatty acids (LCPUFA). Although their purpose is not fully understood, LCPUFAs are linked to optimal neural and visual development. Two of these acids known to benefit vision and brain development are docosahexaenoic acid (DHA) and arachidonic acid (AA). Studies have demonstrated this very conclusively, and two major formula companies are marketing the additives of synthetic DHA and AA to their products, claiming that this makes them "similar to breast milk" (Williams, 2001). See the discussion of infant formula later in this chapter for more information.

Vitamins

Generally, all vitamins are available in human milk in sufficient quantities (note the following discussion of vitamins D and K). Excessive doses of vitamin B_6 (300 to 600 mg/day) can reduce milk production (Hale, 2004). Strict lacto-ovo-vegetarians may be deficient in vitamin B_{12}, which can result in megoblastic anemia and neurological malfunction in the newborn (see the discussion of vegetarian diets in Chapter 8). Colostrum is particularly rich in vitamin E, and mature milk levels are high as well. Since a deficiency in vitamin E in infancy can result in anemia, breastfeeding is a preventive measure against anemia in infancy. See the discussion below for more details about vitamin D and vitamin K.

Vitamin D

Vitamin D is a steroid hormone produced in the body from a pro-steroid that results from direct exposure of the skin to ultraviolet B (UVB) radiation in sunlight (Good Mojab, 2003). Vitamin D is present in both water- and fat-soluble portions of human milk (Lakdawala, 1997). Vitamin D deficiency in childhood can cause rickets, which is marked by abnormal bone growth, muscle pain, and weakness. In infancy, it can lead to "developmental delays, failure to thrive, respiratory distress, tetany, and heart failure" (Good Mojab, 2002).

Supplementing the Infant

There are no national data on the incidence of rickets in the United States (Scanlon, 2001). Reports of increased rickets in breastfed infants resulted in the AAP recommending that breastfed infants receive 200 IU/day of vitamin D. Studies that led to the AAP's recommendation involved primarily non-Caucasian babies who rarely had sun exposure (Kreiter, 2000; Pugliese, 1998; Sills, 1994). There is an increased risk of vitamin D deficiency for those who have darkly pigmented skin, live in the northern hemisphere, receive little outside exposure, or reside in an inner-city home, among other risk factors (Good Mojab, 2004, 2003a, 2003b; LLLI, 2003; Bhowmick, 1991). Babies in day care often see very little sunlight, remaining indoors during the day and arriving and leaving when it is already dark. Rather than there being a vitamin D deficiency in human milk, the deficiency lies in a lifestyle that does not allow for sufficient vitamin D through sun exposure.

Exposure to Sunlight

Previous studies recommend exposing babies to adequate sunlight (Greer, 2001b; Specker, 1994). Specker suggested 30 minutes per week wearing only a diaper, or 2 hours per week if fully clothed without a hat (Specker, 1985). A World Health Organization (WHO) recommendation states, "It is now understood that the optimal route for vitamin D ingestion in humans is not the gastrointestinal tract, which may permit toxic amounts to be absorbed. Rather, the skin is the human organ designed, in the presence of sunlight, both to manufacture vitamin D in potentially vast quantities and to prevent the absorption of more than the body can safely use and store" (Akre, 1989).

Data on appropriate amounts of sunlight for adults with varying degrees of skin pigmentation are conflicting (Good Mojab, 2003a, 2004). Some studies show that adults with darker skin pigmentation require more UVB exposure to produce the same amount of vitamin D as adults with lighter skin pigmentation (Harkness, 2004; Scragg, 1995; Holick, 1995; Clemens, 1982). Other studies suggest that skin pigmentation makes little difference (Malvy, 2000; Matsuoka, 1991; Brazerol, 1988; Lo, 1986). There is no data on the effect of skin pigmentation on vitamin D production in infants.

No research exists examining the relationship between the risk of skin cancer and a lifetime of minimal levels of sun exposure sufficient for endogenous production of adequate levels of vitamin D. Recommendations of small amounts of sun exposure are at odds with the **Centers for Disease Control (CDC)** and the AAP advice to avoid sun exposure for older babies and children by keeping them out of direct sunlight and by using sunscreen. The WHO currently recommends no sun exposure for babies under one year of age. Sunscreen impedes the synthesis of vitamin D.

Supplementing the Mother

Mothers can increase the level of vitamin D in their milk by supplementing their diet. One study showed that supplementing the mother with 50 µg (2000 IU) of vitamin D per day was as effective for maintaining the baby's vitamin D levels as supplementing the baby with 10 µg (400 IU) per day (Ala-Houhala, 1986). Some researchers believe mothers need higher levels of supplementation to maintain adequate infant vitamin D levels.

U.S. government health agencies believe levels of 1000 IU per day and greater exceed human requirements. Hollis and Wagner (2004a, 2004b) believe that limited scientific methods and small sample sizes form the basis for many vitamin D recommendations. They state that present guidelines for vitamin D requirements are very inadequate for adults deprived of sun exposure, especially for people with darkly pigmented skin and women during pregnancy and lactation. In the absence of adequate exposure to UVB rays, vitamin D supplementation can increase vitamin D concentrations to be equal to those of people living in sun-rich environments. A study supplemented 18 lactating mothers with either 2000 IU or 4000 IU daily for 3 months. It concluded that the higher supplementation of 4000 IU safely increased vitamin D levels in both mothers and babies (Hollis, 2004b).

Bone mineral content and markers for bone turnover are similar in breastfed and formula-fed infants, even if breastfed infants have low vitamin D status. This suggests that mineral absorption may occur from a passive transport mechanism that is somewhat independent of vitamin D (Park, 1998).

Vitamin K

Vitamin K is present in small amounts in human milk. Additionally, fetal stores of vitamin K protect the infant, as well as the prophylactic dose usually given at birth, until he receives sufficient milk from his mother and his intestine matures enough to manufacture its own. There has been much debate regarding the use of prophylactic vitamin K in newborns. It raises the question of whether human milk is sufficient to provide adequate vitamin K for the newborn. Some experts question why supplemental doses of vitamin K are necessary, and if so, how they are most effectively given.

Protection from Hemorrhagic Disease

Newborns routinely receive vitamin K to promote blood clotting and avoid hemorrhagic disease of the newborn (HDN). Presently, babies are not screened routinely for hemorrhagic disease. IBCLCs should be aware that symptoms of hemorrhagic disease include convulsions, feeding intolerance and poor sucking, irritability, and pallor. It may cause bulging or full **fontanels**, diminished or absent neonatal reflexes, and ecchymosis (Bor, 2000).

Increasing the mother's dietary intake of vitamin K to over 1 mg a day during the final weeks of pregnancy may reduce the risk of hemorrhagic disease (Greer, 1997). Breastfed infants may benefit from increased maternal vitamin K intake during lactation as well. A supplement of 5 mg of vitamin K to lactating mothers will increase the concentration in human milk and significantly increase infant plasma vitamin K (Nishiguchi, 2002; Greer, 2001a).

Dosage Method

Vitamin K is administered by either **intramuscular** (IM) injection or oral dose. There is some debate about the use of IM injection versus an oral dose of vitamin K to the newborn. Oral dosing is much less distressing to the newborn than an injection, which carries the added risk of nerve damage. Recent studies suggest that oral administration (initial dosing at birth, plus two to four follow-up doses) is as effective as an IM injection in providing protection (Arteaga-Vizcaino, 2001; Wariyar, 2000; Greer, 1997). The Danish practice of parents providing weekly doses for the first three months for primarily breastfed infants revealed high parental participation and no reports of hemorrhagic disease in an 8-year period (Hansen, 2003).

Minerals

The mineral balance in human milk is more favorable to the baby's needs than that in cow's milk. Human milk has a lower percentage of minerals and minimizes the load on the baby's immature kidneys. The calcium in human milk is absorbed much more efficiently (Rudloff, 1990). The higher ratio of phosphorus to calcium present in cow's milk can interfere with calcium absorption. Therefore, artificially fed infants are more likely to develop late neonatal **hypocalcemia** than their breastfed counterparts (Specker, 1991). In addition, under stress situations such as hot weather or diarrhea, the higher mineral content of an infant formula based on cow's milk is a significant contributor to **dehydration**.

The higher solute load of infant formulas may require additional water intake by the infant to expel the solutes. Mothers often misinterpret the thirst induced by this type of food as hunger. Consequently, they feed more formula to their baby instead of the water he needs. Babies who are breastfed exclusively require no water supplements—not even in hot climates—because there is little waste to flush through the kidneys (Ashraf, 1993). Increased feedings will satisfy the need for more fluids when it is hot. Part of the higher weight gains in artificially fed infants may result from greater sodium and water retention.

Iron

During the final six to eight weeks of pregnancy, a healthy nonanemic mother lays down iron stores to provide her baby with enough iron through her milk for the first few months postpartum. Blood from the umbilical cord also contributes iron that the infant stores in his liver. Although iron is present in human milk in small quantities, the level is sufficient to meet the iron requirements of the exclusively breastfed full-term infant until he is about six months old. A premature infant may need iron supplementation due to receiving insufficient iron in utero.

The iron in human milk is absorbed more efficiently than that of cow's milk, partially because of the high vitamin C level present in human milk. The baby absorbs 60 percent of iron in human milk, compared with only 4 percent of iron in artificial baby milk. He does not begin to deplete his iron stores until 4 to 6 months after birth or even later.

Lactoferrin loses its ability to inhibit the growth of bacteria when saturated with **exogenous** iron (Chan, 2003). Routine supplementation of iron is questionable and may be detrimental to the breastfed infant. A longitudinal study found that infants who were iron deficient at 12 months had been breastfed a shorter time than those who had sufficient iron levels (Thorsdottir, 2003).

The healthy infant's hemoglobin is high at birth (18 to 20 g/dl) and decreases rapidly as his body adjusts to extrauterine life. Hemoglobin is the portion of the red blood cell that carries oxygen to all parts of the body. At 4 months of age, the typical range is between 10.2 and 15 g/dl. Over this same period, there is also a change in the type of hemoglobin, from fetal to adult, which is more efficient in delivering oxygen to the tissues. Therefore, although the actual grams of hemoglobin decrease, the efficiency of each gram increases as this change takes place.

Fluoride

Breastfed infants have fewer dental caries and better dental health. Conclusive studies have shown that during the development of primary and secondary teeth, fluoride supplements ingested by the infant reduce cavities by 50 to 60 percent. In communities with fluoridated drinking water, breastfed babies receive fluoride through their mother's milk. If the family's water supply contains less than 0.3 **ppm** of fluoride, infant fluoride supplementation is recommended after the age of 6 months (CDC, 2001; Institute of Medicine, 1997).

Babies who receive supplementary fluoride may occasionally exhibit allergic reactions, described by mothers in the form of fussiness, irritability, refusal to take the fluoride, and spitting it up (Jelliffe, 1978). Excessive fluoride may cause fluorosis, a condition in which teeth become mottled or discolored. Breastfeeding beyond six months may protect children from developing fluorosis in their permanent teeth (Brothwell, 2003). One study concluded that infant formulas prepared with fluoridated water increase the risk of fluorosis in primary teeth (Marshall, 2004).

Other Constituents

Human milk contains over 200 known components, including the trace elements copper, zinc, manganese, silicon, aluminum, and titanium. Scientists continue to study the significance of these components. Zinc deficiency in infancy can cause **failure to thrive** and skin lesions. In the inherited zinc deficiency disorder **acrodermatitis enteropathica**, human milk can be life saving, due to the increased **bioavailability** of the zinc. Cow's milk formula has no effect (Lawrence, 1999).

Researchers have identified more than 20 human milk enzymes, as well as prolactin and steroid hormones (Lawrence, 1999). One enzyme, **lipase**, is essential for the digestion of fat so the fat will be available to the infant as energy. Another enzyme, **amylase**, is important for carbohydrate digestion (Dewit, 1993). Artificial baby milk lacks these digestive enzymes.

Nitrogen compounds in human milk are being investigated. **Nucleotides** are a nonprotein nitrogen that is relatively absent in cow's milk. Nucleotides are an integral part of the immune system. They act as the host defense against bacteria, viruses, and parasites, as well as various malignancies. Other components under study include **prostaglandins**, bile salts, and epidermal growth factor. Epidermal growth factor (EGF), which is present in colostrum, preterm and term milk, promotes the growth and healing of gut mucosa. In preterm babies, epidermal growth factor may be significant in helping their guts mature more efficiently. (Dvorak, 2003; Xiao, 2002). Artificial baby milks do not contain this growth factor.

Cytokines are proteins secreted by cells, especially the immune system, including granulocyte colony-stimulating factor (G-CSF). Concentrations are higher for two days postpartum and are lower in the milk of mothers with preterm infants. G-CSF receptor cells are present in the intestinal cells of breastfed infants (Calhoun, 2000).

Cholecystokinin (CCK) is a digestive hormone found in the digestive tract and brain. Triggered by the baby's suckling, CCK may be responsible for the sleepiness mothers and babies experience while nursing. It also may create the feeling of satiety in babies (Marchini, 1992).

Not only does human milk contain a vast number of components, studies of specific components also show that each mother's milk differs slightly due to individual genetic codes. In other words, each breastfed infant receives a unique product! Table 9.1 compares the major elements in human milk with those present in cow's milk.

TABLE 9.1

Comparison of Components in Human Milk and Cow's Milk

Component	Human Milk	Cow's Milk
Water (ml/100 ml)	87.1	87.2
Energy (Cal/100 ml)	60–75	66
Total solids (g/100 ml)	12.9	12.8
Protein (%)	0.8–0.9	3.5
Fat (%)	3–5	3.7
Lactose (%)	6.9–7.2	4.9
Ash (minerals) (%)	0.2	0.7
Protein (% of total protein)		
Casein	40	82
Whey	60	18
Ash, major components per liter		
Calcium (mg)	340	1170
Phosphorus (mg)	140	920
Sodium (mEq)	7	22
Vitamins per liter		
Vitamin A (IU)	1898	1025
Thiamin (μg)	160	440
Riboflavin (μg)	360	1750
Niacin (μg)	1470	940
Vitamin C (mg)	43	1.1

▶ HEALTH BENEFITS OF HUMAN MILK

Human milk is a species-specific first food that offers biologically natural nutrition for the child as well as health protection to support his developing immune system. The mother gives her child the specific protection he needs for the environment in which they live, both in terms of allergens and infection protection. Human milk further protects the infant through its packaging. It does not spoil, the temperature is always correct, it is not subject to mixing errors, there are no omissions of components, and there are no product recalls! Research continues to confirm new health benefits of human milk for the newborn, older child, and mother.

Intelligence and Neurological Development

Several studies demonstrate that human milk confers greater intelligence to human babies. In other words, artificially fed babies are not as smart as their biologically normal peers. Noteworthy among these studies is Lucas' work with premature infants fed human milk via **tube feedings**, away from the breast (Lucas, 1992, 1990a, 1990b). These studies revealed a dose-related response, with an average of 8.3 IQ points higher at ages 7½ to 8 years. At 18 months, there was increased neuromotor development of 15 motor development index points, and 23 points for infants born small for gestation (**SGA**).

A Spanish study measuring infants at 18 months found that breastfeeding longer than 4 months resulted in an average 4.6-point advantage on mental development scores (Gomez-Sanchiz, 2003). An IQ increase of as little as 3 points from 100 to 103 moves a person from the 50th to the 58th percentile of the population (ILCA, 2002). The ease of learning, abstract thinking, and complex problem-solving abilities are skills each child deserves. Breastfeeding gives children the optimal start for learning.

A study that examined breastfeeding and adult IQ found that breastfeeding is dose-dependent. Adults who had been breastfed 9 months or more as infants measured an average of 4.6 IQ points higher on the Weschler Adult Intelligence Scale (WAIS) and 2.1 points higher on the Borge Priens Prove (BPP), two standard intelligence tests (Mortensen, 2002). A **meta-analysis** of 11 studies found a difference in cognitive function of 3.16 points at ages between 6 and 23 months and years later. It was concluded that the cognitive developmental benefits of breastfeeding increases with duration (Anderson, 1999). A study measuring verbal cognitive IQ found an adjusted score of 3.56 points higher for babies breastfed beyond 6 months compared to non-breastfed babies (Oddy, 2003a). A 2002 **prospective study** predicts an 11-point IQ advantage for children born small for **gestational age** and exclusively breastfed for 24 weeks (Rao, 2002).

In a study of children aged 6 through 8 years who had been very low birth weight (**VLBW**) infants, breastfed children scored 5.1 IQ points higher for visual-motor integration, 3.6 IQ points higher for overall intellectual function, and 2.3 IQ points higher for verbal ability (Smith, 2003). Another study found that at only 8.5 days old, breastfed infants outperformed artificially fed infants on orientation, motor, range of state, and state regulation dimensions on the Brazelton newborn assessment scale. Breastfed infants had fewer abnormal reflexes, signs of depression, and withdrawal. It was concluded that breastfeeding benefits newborns' neuro-behavioral organization (Hart, 2003).

There are also dissenting voices. Jain (2002) surveyed 40 studies on the link between breastfeeding and IQ. Although 68 percent of these studies concluded that breastfeeding increased intelligence, the "higher quality" studies were less persuasive. Jain's 40 studies did not include the newer studies listed above. The information presented in Chapter 27 will help you learn to read research with a critical eye and determine the **validity**, strengths, and weaknesses of a study.

Disease Protection

Perhaps the most spectacular advantage of human milk over commercially prepared infant formula is its lifelong protection against disease. Human milk contains a wide variety of soluble, cellular, and **humoral** factors that protect the infant against a host of diseases. As the baby grows, he develops his own **active immunity** as his body begins to produce antibodies. He is protected against bacterial infections, viral infections, protozoa, and allergies (Newburg, 2004; Silfverdal, 2002; Tellez, 2003; Van Odijk, 2003). Table 9.2, Table 9.3, and Table 9.4 identify these factors.

Studies show higher death rates for babies not fed human milk. Research from developed countries sometimes concludes that breastfeeding is not important for protection from infection for babies in wealthy nations (Rubin, 1990; Bauchner, 1986). However, these studies are flawed both methodologically and by improper grouping of partially breastfed and exclusively breastfed babies. Breastfeeding could prevent an estimated 720 infant deaths per year in the United States (Chen, 2004). Preventable infant deaths in Brazil range from 33 to 72 percent for deaths from respiratory infections and 35 to 86 percent for diarrheal infections (Escuder, 2003). The longer an infant breastfeeds, the greater protection he receives (Chen, 2004; Habicht, 1986). Chapter 27 discusses research and statistics to help you read and analyze all studies with discernment. These tools will be especially

TABLE 9.2
Antibacterial Factors Found in Human Milk

Factor	Shown in Vitro to Be Active Against
Secretory IgA	*E. coli* (also *pili*, capsular antigens, CFA1), *C. tetani*, *C. diphtheriae*, *K. pneumoniae*, *S. mutans*, *S. sanguins*, *S. mitis*, *S. agalactiae*, *S. salvarius*, *S. pneumoniae*, *C. burnetti*, *H. influenza*, *H. pylori*, *S. flexneri*, *S. boydii*, *S. sonnei*, *C. jejuni*, *N. meningitidis*, *B. pertussis*, *S. dysenteriae*, *C. trachomatis*, Salmonella (6 groups), *Campylobacter flagelin*, *S. flexneri* virulence plasmid antigen, *C. diphtheriae* toxin, *E. coli* enterotoxin, *V. cholerae* enterotoxin, *C. difficile* toxins, *H. influenza* capsule, *S. aureus* enterotoxin F, *Candida albicans*
IgG	*E. coli*, *B. pertussis*, *H. influenza* type b, *S. pneumoniae*, *S. agalactiae*, *N. meningitidis*, 14 pneumococcal capsular polysaccharides, *V. cholerae* lipopolysaccharide, *S. flexneri* invasion plasmid–coded antigens, major opsonin for *S. aureus*
IgM	*V. cholerae* lipopolysaccharide
IgD	*E. coli*
Free secretory component*	*E. coli* colonization factor antigen I (CFA1)
Bifidobacterium bifidum	Enteric bacteria
Growth factors (oligosaccharides, glycopeptides)	
Other bifidobacteria growth factors (alpha-lactoglobulin, lactoferrin, sialyllactose)	
Factor-finding proteins (zinc, vitamin B$_{12}$, folate)	Dependent *E. coli*
Complement C1-C9 (mainly C3 and C4)	Killing of *S. aureus* in macrophages
Lactoferrin*	*E. coli*, *E. coli*/CFA1, *Candida albicans*
Lactoperoxidase	Streptococcus, Pseudomonas, *E. coli*, *S. typhimurium*
Lysozyme	*E. coli*, Salmonella, *M. lysodeikticus*, growing *Candida albicans* and *Aspergillus fumigatus*
Unidentified factors	*S. aureus*, *B. pertussis*, *C. jejuni*, *E. coli*, *S. typhimurium*, *S. flexneri*, *S. sonnei*, *V. cholerae*, *L. pomona*, *L. hyos*, *L. icterohaemorrhagiae*, *C. difficile* toxin B, *H. pylori*
Nonimmunoglobulin (milk fat, proteins)	*C. trachomatis*, *Y. enterocolitica*
Carbohydrate	*E. coli* enterotoxin, *E. coli*, *C. difficile* toxin A
Lipid	*S. aureus*, *E. coli*, *S. epidermis*, *H. influenzae*, *S. agalactiae*
Ganglioside GM$_1$	*E. coli* enterotoxin, *V. cholerae* toxin, *C. jejuni* enterotoxin, *E. coli*
Ganglioside GM$_3$	*E. coli*
Phosphatidylethanolamine	*H. pylori*
Sialyllactose	*V. cholerae* toxin, *H. pylori*
Mucin (milk fat globulin membrane)	*E. coli* (S-fimbrinated) sialyloligosaccharides on sIgA(Fc), *E. coli* (S-fimbrinated) adhesion
Glycoproteins (receptor-like) + oligosaccharides	*V. cholerae*

(continued)

TABLE 9.2 (CONTINUED)
Antibacterial Factors Found in Human Milk

Factor	Shown in Vitro to Be Active Against
Glycoproteins (mannosylated)	E. coli
kappa-Casein*	H. pylori, S. pneumoniae
Casein	H. influenza
Glycolipid Gb₃	S. dysenterae toxin, shigatoxin of shigella and E. coli
Fucosylated oligosaccharides	E. coli heat-stable enterotoxin, C. jejuni, E. coli
Analogues of epithelial cell receptors (oligosaccharides)	S. pneumoniae, H. influenza
Milk cells (macrophages, neutrophils, B and T lymphocytes)	By phagocytosis and killing: E. coli, S. aureus, S. enteritidis
	By sensitized lymphocytes: E. coli
	By phagocytosis: Candida albicans[†,‡], E. coli
	Lymphocyte stimulation: E. coli, K antigen, tuberculin
	Spontaneous monokines: simulated by lipopolysaccaride
	Induced cytokines: PHA, PMA + ionomycin
	Fibronectin helps in uptake by phagocytic cells

*Factors found at low levels in human milk can be antibacterial at higher levels, e.g, secretory leukocyte protease inhibitor (antileukocyte protease) has antibacterial (E. coli, S. aureus) and antifungal (growing C. albicans and A. fumigatus) activity.
†Fungi.
‡Contain fucosylated oligosaccharides.

From Proceedings of Breast Milk and Special Care Nurseries: Problems and Opportunities Conference. August 1995. Melbourne. Copyright J. T. May and Australian Lactation Consultants Association Victorian Branch, 1995. Updated August, 1998. Reprinted by permission of Department of Microbiology, La Trobe University, Bundoora Victoria 3083, Australia.

helpful when you read a popular media report of a study that has an apparent negative focus on breastfeeding.

In light of what has already been learned about human milk, the AAP (2005) recommends that all mothers breastfeed their infants for at least one year. They cite both the psychological value afforded the breastfeeding mother and infant and the protection against disease received by the maturing infant. WHO (2001) recommends exclusive breastfeeding for six months and breastfeeding for two years and beyond. The AAFP (2001) supports breastfeeding beyond infancy and tandem nursing.

Anti-infective Agents

Although human milk is not sterile, it contains a number of anti-infective agents that maintain a very low bacterial level for many hours. It can destroy bacteria in the infant's GI tract before they affect the infant. Milk components also coat the GI tract, thus preventing other offending organisms and molecules from entering the infant's system. Many researchers have reported a lower incidence of infection in breastfed babies (Wold, 2000).

At birth, the infant is suddenly exposed to a variety of microorganisms to which the mother is already immune. She passes this **passive immunity** to her baby, both across the placenta before birth and in her colostrum and milk after birth. When a new microorganism enters the environment, the mother most likely produces corresponding antibodies and passes them to the baby through her milk (Hanson, 2004b).

In addition to this internal mechanism, it seems that the breast itself also produces antibodies to the organisms passed into it by the suckling infant. The mammary gland produces immunoglobulins locally and passes them to the infant in the mother's milk, protecting him from the harmful effects of disease organisms.

IgA

The presence of IgA in colostrum and human milk protects the gastrointestinal tract of the infant against penetration by organisms and antigens. It is probably the most important of the antiviral defense factors and is at its highest level immediately after birth. IgA continues to remain

TABLE 9.3

Antiviral Factors Found in Human Milk

Factor	Shown in Vitro to Be Active Against
Secretory IgA	Polio types 1, 2, 3; Coxsackie types A9, B3, B5; echo types 6, 9; Semliki Forest virus; Ross River virus; rotavirus; cytomegalovirus; reovirus type 3; rubella varicella-zoster virus; herpes simplex virus; mumps virus; influenza; respiratory syncytial virus; human immunodeficiency virus; hepatitis C virus; hepatitis B virus; measles
IgG	Rubella, cytomegalovirus, respiratory syncytial virus, rotavirus, human immunodeficiency virus, Epstein-Barr virus
IgM	Rubella, cytomegalovirus, respiratory syncytial virus, human immunodeficiency virus
Lipid (unsaturated fatty acids and monoglycerides)	Herpes simplex virus, Semliki Forest virus, influenza, dengue, Ross River virus, Japanese B encephalitis virus, sindbis, West Nile, human immunodeficiency virus, respiratory syncytial virus, vesicular stomatitis virus
Non-immunoglobulin macromolecules	Herpes simplex virus, vesicular stomatitis virus, Coxsackie B4, Semliki Forest virus, reovirus 3, poliotype 2, cytomegalovirus, respiratory syncytial virus, rotavirus
alpha2-macroglobulin (-like)	Influenza haemagglutinin, parainfluenza haemagglutinin
Ribonuclease	Murine leukemia
Hemagglutinin inhibitors	Influenza, mumps
Mucin (glycoprotein/lactadherin)	Rotavirus
Chondroitin sulphate (-like)	Human immunodeficiency virus
Secretory leukocyte protease inhibitor (colostrum levels)	Human immunodeficiency virus, *Bifidobacterium bifidum*, rotavirus
sIgA + trypsin inhibitor	Rotavirus
Lactoferrin	Cytomegalovirus, human immunodeficiency virus, respiratory syncytial virus, herpes simplex virus type 1, hepatitis C
Milk cells	Induced interferon: virus, PHA, or PMA and ionomycin
	Induced cytokine: herpes simplex virus, respiratory syncytial virus
	Lymphocyte stimulation: rubella, cytomegalovirus, herpes, measles, mumps, respiratory syncytial virus

Factors found at low levels in human milk, known to be antiviral at higher levels:

prostaglandins E2, F2 alpha (parainfluenza 3, measles)

gangliosides GM1-3 (rotavirus, respiratory syncytial virus)

heparin (cytomegalovirus, respiratory syncytial virus)

glycolipid Gb4 (human B19 parvovirus)

From Proceedings of Breast Milk and Special Care Nurseries: Problems and Opportunities Conference. August 1995. Melbourne. Copyright J. T. May and Australian Lactation Consultants Association Victorian Branch, 1995. Updated August, 1998. Reprinted by permission of Department of Microbiology, La Trobe University, Bundoora Victoria 3083, Australia.

at a significant level for at least six or seven months. IgA and sialic acid survive passage through the GI tract and are much higher in breastfed infants' stools than in artificially fed infants' (Kohler, 2002; Fernandes, 2001). Colostrum and human milk also contain living white cells—lymphocytes and **macrophages**—that engulf and digest bacteria and synthesize IgA and other protective substances.

Growth Factors and Enzymes

Growth factors enhance the infant's development and the maturation of the immune system, the central nervous system, and organs such as skin. Digestive enzymes **lactase** and lipase, as well as many other important enzymes, protect babies born with immature or defective enzyme systems. Lactase is necessary for

TABLE 9.4
Antiparasite Factors Found in Human Milk

Factor	Shown in Vitro to Be Active Against
Secretory IgA	*Giardia lamblia*
	Entamoeba histolytica
	Schistosoma mansoni (blood fluke)
	Cryptosporidium
	Toxoplasma gondii
	Plasmodium falciparum (malaria)
IgG	*Plasmodium falciparum*
Lipid (free fatty acids and monoglycerides)	*Giardia lamblia*
	Entamoeba histolytica
	Trichomonas vaginalis
	Giardia intestinalis
	Eimeria tenella (animal coccidiosis)
Unidentified	*Trypanosoma brucei rhodesiense*

From Proceedings of Breast Milk and Special Care Nurseries: Problems and Opportunities Conference. August 1995. Melbourne. Copyright J.T. May and Australian Lactation Consultants Association Victorian Branch, 1995. Updated July, 1996. Reprinted by permission of Department of Microbiology, La Trobe University, Bundoora Victoria 3083, Australia.

converting lactose into simple sugars that the infant can **assimilate** easily. A deficiency in lactase can result in **lactose intolerance**. This generally occurs because of diminishing activity of intestinal lactase after weaning. A person who is lactose intolerant is unable to digest milk sugar (lactose). The condition is more prevalent in adults and is rare in children under three years of age. As discussed earlier, lactose helps prevent rickets and aids calcium absorption and brain development.

The enzyme lysozyme protects the breastfed infant by breaking down bacteria in the bowel. The bowel receives protection from lactoferrin, an iron-binding protein that acts together with specific antibodies to inhibit the growth of *E. coli*, the major cause of bowel infection in infants (Kelly, 2000; Orrhage, 1999). Human lactoferrin is 100 times more resistant to breakdown than bovine lactoferrin (Van Veen, 2004). If a baby receives too much iron, through supplements or enriched foods, the effectiveness of this protein will be significantly diminished (Chan, 2003).

Bifidus Factor
A carbohydrate called the **bifidus factor** discourages the growth of undesirable organisms such as *E. coli*. The factor, lactobacillus bifidus, is present in high concentrations in both colostrum and mature milk. Human

milk contains seven times as much of this factor as does cow's milk. The bifidus factor works with the low pH of the stool to help special bacteria grow in the infant's intestine and prevent harmful bacteria from growing.

Thymus
The thymus in breastfed babies is larger than that of artificially fed babies (Jeppesson, 2004; Hasselbalch, 1999). The thymus is a gland active in infancy and childhood. Its main function is to develop immature lymphocytes into immunocompetent T-cells. The larger size in breastfed babies suggests that breastfeeding helps the developing immune system.

Specific Protection

Human milk protects the infant and the breast by providing anti-infective agents and minimizing inflammation. It protects against infections outside the GI tract as well. Protection includes upper and lower respiratory infections, including **respiratory syncytial virus** (RSV) (Oddy, 2003b; Levine, 1999; Bulkow, 2002), otitis media (see separate discussion that follows), urinary tract infections (Marild, 2004), **sepsis** (Meinzen-Derr, 2004), **rotavirus** (Gianino, 2002; Mastretta, 2002), and meningitis (Hylander, 1998).

Breastfeeding has been shown to protect against childhood cancers (Smulevich, 1999), leukemia and lymphoma (Perrilat, 2002; Bener, 2001; Shu, 1999), Hodgkin's disease (Davis, 1998), and neuroblastoma (Daniels, 2002). Having been breastfed lowers women's risk of breast cancer in adulthood (Potischman, 1999; Freudenhim, 1994).

Breastfeeding reduces the risks for chronic and autoimmune diseases, including inflammatory bowel disease such as Crohn's and ulcerative colitis (Thompson, 2000; Corrao, 1998), juvenile diabetes (Young, 2002; Monetinti, 2001; Kimpimaki, 2001), juvenile arthritis (Mason, 1995), multiple sclerosis (Tarrats, 2002; Pisacane, 1994), celiac disease (Ivarsson, 2002), hypertension (Singhal, 2001), and high cholesterol and heart disease (Singhal, 2004; Owen, 2002; Ravelli, 2000). Childhood and adult obesity is a major health problem worldwide. Breastfeeding protects against obesity (Martin, 2004; Grummer-Strawn, 2004; Toschke, 2002).

Otitis Media

One of the most common infant infections—otitis media, or middle ear infection—occurs more frequently in the absence of breastfeeding. Aniansson (1994) observed this link and noted that the first episode of otitis media occurs earlier in children weaned before 6 months of age. In this study, both mixed feedings and the absence of human milk in the diet increased the risk of infection.

The best protection against otitis media appears to be exclusive breastfeeding for at least 4 months (Duncan, 1993). The longer a baby breastfeeds, the greater protection he receives. In one study, infants who were breastfed for at least 12 months had otitis media rates 19 percent lower than formula-fed infants (Dewey, 1995).

Even after weaning, the protection against otitis media afforded by human milk is at work. Human milk stimulates the breastfed infant's immune system, reducing the risk of otitis media for several years after breastfeeding ends (Hanson, 2002). A study by the Centers for Disease Control and Prevention (CDC) states that "when compared with exclusively breastfed infants, infants who received only formula had an 80 percent increase in their risk of developing diarrhea and a 70 percent increase in their risk of developing an ear infection" (Scariati, 1997).

Necrotizing Enterocolitis and Sepsis

Human milk decreases the occurrence of necrotizing enterocolitis (NEC). NEC is characterized by inflammation of the intestinal wall, often causing the tissue to die. It is frequently associated with prematurity, respiratory disease, and early **enteral** feedings of formula in premature babies (Lucas, 1990b). NEC occurs in 2 to 7 percent of premature babies (Buescher, 2004, 1994; Udall, 1990). Lucas found that NEC is 6 to 10 times more likely to occur in artificially fed babies than those fed human milk exclusively. Among babies born after 30 weeks' gestation, the risk of NEC was 20 times higher for the artificially fed babies. He further noted that NEC was 3 times more likely to occur in babies receiving mixed feedings than in those receiving feedings of human milk alone (Dugdale, 1991; Lucas, 1990b).

Research indicates that this same protection against NEC is found with pasteurized **donor milk**. A meta-analysis of 4 studies found infants who received donor human milk were 3 times less likely to develop NEC and 4 times less likely to have confirmed NEC (McGuire, 2003). Researchers theorize that human milk's secretory IgA and **phagocytes** help protect against NEC (Buescher, 2004, 1994). Preventive therapy using human milk feedings has reduced NEC in trials (Caplan, 1993).

Another protection offered by human milk to hospitalized babies is a decreased incidence of **nosocomial** (hospital-acquired) sepsis. Researchers at George Washington University Hospital found that even though babies who received expressed human milk had bacterial colonies like those in formula-fed babies, they had a significantly lower incidence of infection (El-Mohandes, 1997). Although preterm infants grow more slowly with human milk, they leave the hospital an average of 15 days earlier because of reduced sepsis and NEC (Schanler, 1999).

Diarrhea

In developing countries, 5 million children a year die from diarrheal disease. Study data suggest that the risk of dying from diarrhea could decline 14 to 24 times by breastfeeding. Even babies in the industrialized world would benefit (Brandtzaeg, 2003). A Brazilian study found non-breastfed infants were 82 percent more likely to experience diarrhea than infants who were exclusively breastfed for the first 6 months of life (Vieira, 2003). Exclusive breastfeeding also protects infants against diarrhea caused by *Giardia* (Tellez, 2003; Mahmud, 2001) and *E. coli* (Clemens, 1997).

Protection from Maternal Antigens

Protection from human milk extends beyond common childhood illnesses and illnesses of the mother to the infant in his immediate environment. Antibodies in human milk are highly targeted against infectious agents in the mother's environment, those to which the infant is likely to be exposed shortly after birth (Brandtzaeg, 2003). Whenever a mother contracts an infection, whether it be a cold, fever, or more serious illness, her body responds by producing antibodies in her milk that help protect her breastfed baby.

Although some viruses pass into the mother's milk, the presence of antibodies to counteract them offsets potential harm to the baby. In fact, there is evidence that milk responds to and "remembers" for years specific infections it has encountered. Asian mothers in the United Kingdom showed antibodies to pathogens they had encountered in their home countries several years earlier (Nathavitharana, 1994). Researchers believe this transmission may confer passive immunity to the infant, as in the case with cytomegalovirus (Hamprecht, 2001).

A more likely mechanism of disease transmission from mother to baby is through close contact such as touching and through close mouth and nose contact, rather than through the mother's milk. When a breast-feeding mother does contract an illness, it is likely that her baby was exposed through contact with her during her most contagious period. Therefore, the most effective treatment for the infant is to continue breastfeeding while receiving any necessary medication. The mother can decrease the infant's exposure to the disease with careful handwashing before contact and, in extreme cases, by wearing a mask over her nose and mouth. A mother who develops a cold or fever need not worry about infecting her baby through her milk. Encourage her to practice good hygiene and limit facial contact with her baby during the infectious period. Advise her to rest and follow the treatment plan prescribed by her caregiver in order to return to good health quickly and not compromise her milk production.

Immunization Response

Human milk contains antibodies capable of enhancing infant **antibody** response (Van de Perre, 2003). Studies show higher immune responses to **vaccines** in breastfed infants. Some researchers believe that breastfed and artificially fed infants have similar levels of protection after immunization (Scheifele, 1992). However, continued studies have concluded that breastfeeding offers both current and long-term immune-modulating effects on the child's developing cellular immune system (Jeppesen, 2004; Pickering, 1998; Pabst, 1997).

Other Immunologic Factors

Countless unidentified factors in human milk aid in the protection of the infant from disease. Ongoing research continues to uncover these protective factors. **Mucins** found in human milk play a role in protection against bacterial infections, including such severe illnesses as neonatal sepsis and meningitis (Schroten, 1993, 1992). They also are linked to protection against rotavirus, an acute GI infection (Mastretta, 2002; Gianino, 2002).

Human milk contains three essential thyroid hormones that are totally lacking in cow's milk and conventional infant formulas. These hormones may be responsible for preventing **hypothyroidism**, masking

diagnosis, and protecting the baby until he weans. **Alpha-lactalbumin** acts as a bactericide against *Streptococcus pneumonaiae*. A **peptide** in human milk similar to human k-casein inhibits bacteria and yeast growths (Hakansson, 2000). Xantine oxidase is an antibacterial enzyme that, when combined with nitrites, creates nitric oxide, which inhibits *Enterobacteriaceae, E. coli*, and *Salmonella enteritidis* (Hancock, 2002).

Nucleotides are compounds derived from nucleic acid and secreted by mammary epithelial cells. They play key roles in many biological processes, including optimal function and growth of the gastrointestinal and immune systems. Human milk contains much higher amounts of nucleotides than cow's milk formulas (Carver, 1999). Formula manufacturers now add nucleotides to most artificial baby milks.

Allergy Protection

There are almost no antibodies in the immature intestine of a newborn infant, which leaves the wall of the intestine susceptible to invasion by foreign proteins. Human milk contains high levels of antibodies, especially IgA, which provides an antiabsorptive protection on the lining of the infant's intestine. This shields the surface from the absorption of foreign protein as well as from bacterial invasion. The infant's GI tract develops more quickly when he receives human milk. This prevents foreign proteins from entering his system. Nutrients such as zinc and the long-chain polyunsaturated fatty acids aid in the development of the infant's immune response.

Cow's Milk Allergy

Giving babies even a single feeding of artificial baby milk in the first days of life can increase the rates of allergic disease. All formulas, including soy formulas, carry a risk of allergy. Studies consistently reveal increased allergies among formula-fed infants (Van Odijk, 2003; Tariq, 1998). Symptoms of allergy are more prevalent in infants fed cow's milk-based formula than in breastfed infants. A Finnish long-term study revealed evidence of reduced allergy in the breastfed group at age 17 (Saarinen, 1995). There is also the possibility that other food antigens cause allergy responses in these infants, because solid foods frequently are introduced at an earlier age in formula-fed infants. Exclusive breastfeeding for 4 months can postpone the onset of cow's milk allergy (Yinyaem, 2003).

Giving formula in the first week of life is the first of several factors in allergy development (Marini, 1996). Cow's milk is the most common food allergen in infants, with an estimated allergy rate between 3 and 5 percent in industrialized countries (Infante, 2003). One researcher suggests that 25 percent of colic is in response to cow's milk allergy (Lindberg, 1999). Most infants with cow's milk allergy develop symptoms before one month of age, often within one week after introduction of cow's milk protein-based formula (Host, 2002). Cow's milk formulas do not contain the antibodies necessary to protect the infant's intestines. The foreign protein of cow's milk passes through the intestinal wall and causes allergic reactions in sensitive infants. These reactions may manifest themselves as colicky behavior, diarrhea, **vomiting**, malabsorption, eczema, ear infections, or asthma.

Atopic dermatitis, including eczema, is much more common in artificially fed infants. One large meta-analysis of 18 studies found that exclusive breastfeeding during the first 3 months of life is associated with significantly lower rates of atopic dermatitis in children with a family history (Gdalevich, 2001a). A 5-year study showed a lowered rate of atopic disease in infants who were breastfed or fed whey hydrosolate formula compared to cow's milk and soy formula groups (Chandra, 1997). Exclusive breastfeeding for 4 to 6 months and delaying supplemental foods reduces the incidence of atopic symptoms, especially eczema, as well as gastrointestinal symptoms attributable to cow's milk (ESPGN, 1993).

Other Allergies

An infant is rarely, if ever, allergic to his mother's milk. However, he may show allergic symptoms in response to foods ingested by the mother and passed through her milk (Hill, 2004; Saavedra, 2003). Allergens pass through the mother's milk and may cause reactions such as spitting, vomiting, gas, diarrhea, colicky behavior, or skin rash. See Chapter 13 for a discussion on causes and treatment of colic.

Human milk is best able to protect any infant, with or without allergic tendencies, until his intestinal tract and immune system mature. While breastfeeding does not eliminate food allergies, it greatly reduces their incidence and delays their onset. In addition, it reduces the incidence of asthma, a respiratory disease. Allergies cause half of all asthma cases. One study showed that exclusive breastfeeding for less than 4 months was a "significant risk factor for recurrent asthma, with an **odds ratio** of 1:35" (Oddy, 2002). "A large cohort study found a dose-response effect, with a longer breastfeeding duration being protective against the development of asthma and wheeze in young children" (Dell, 2001). A meta-analysis of 12 studies found that exclusive breastfeeding during the first months is associated with lower asthma rates during childhood and especially benefits the child with a family history of allergy (Gdalevich, 2001b).

Human Milk for the Preterm Infant

The medical community has become increasingly aware that human milk is vital to the premature infant. The milk of women who deliver prematurely has special properties that are particularly beneficial to the infant (Butte, 1984). Such milk contains higher concentrations of sodium, chloride, and nitrogen, as well as immunoprotective factors. This may be of great significance for the immature GI tract of the preterm infant. Human milk also helps prevent NEC (Bisquera, 2002).

Preterm infants fed human milk, including mature donor milk, have better neurodevelopment than their artificially fed counterparts (Lucas, 1994). Human milk is also associated with higher IQ scores during childhood (Smith, 2003). Thus, many caregivers recommend that the preterm infant receive his mother's milk regardless of whether the mother had planned to breastfeed. The next best choice is donor milk from a **human milk bank** (Wight, 2001).

Human Milk Fortifiers

Some debate remains over whether the mother's milk requires supplementation for her preterm infant. The concern is with keeping up with the missed intrauterine growth through increased protein and energy in the preterm diet (Klein, 2002). The question of optimal brain growth receives little attention (Ebrahim, 1993).

Human milk has the ideal protein balance for babies who weigh 1500 g or more (about 3 lbs, 5 oz). For infants who weigh less than 1500 g, and especially those under 1000 g (2 lbs, 3 oz), the mother's milk is not considered adequate as the sole source of nutrition. However, recent clinical practice guidelines in Canada state, "Breast milk is used preferentially" (Premji, 2002). **Human milk fortifiers (HMF)** contain protein, calcium, potassium phosphate, carbohydrates, vitamins, and trace minerals. They may be necessary in these cases and can be added to the mother's milk for feedings.

Preterm infants who receive no supplementation may experience fractures of the long bones during rapid growth phases. Supplements are not without concern, however. Quan (1994) found that some additives, particularly cow's milk–based infant formulas, have an adverse effect on the anti-infective properties of human milk. This effect was not seen in his study with soy-based infant formulas nor with HMF. Soy-based formulas, discussed later, contain other problematic components. Preterm human milk protects against *E. coli*, *Staphylococcus*, *Enterobacter sakazaki*, and Group B *Streptococcus*, but this effect was not present if iron was added (Chan, 2003).

Another study revealed lower lymphocyte counts in formula-fed infants versus those fed with human milk alone or human milk with HMF (Tarcan, 2004). A Cochrane review found preterm infants fed human milk with HMF had improved short-term weight gain and linear and head growth (Kuschel, 2004). There was insufficient data to evaluate long-term neurodevelopmental and growth outcomes.

Lactoengineering

Researchers have long proposed using mothers' hind-milk to increase calories, carbohydrates, and proteins for preterm infants. This is termed **lactoengineering**. One researcher added isolated human milk protein to mothers' milk for four babies with good results (Lindblad, 1982). NICUs are now able to perform **crematocrits**, a test to measure fat and calories in human milk (Meier, 2002). A recent study examined this method for infants in Nigeria and found that **LBW** infants grew well without human milk fortifier. (It did not include VLBW infants.) The study concluded that hindmilk feedings were "effective and feasible for . . . infants in developing countries" (Slusher, 2003). Researchers are working to separate the crucial components of human milk for very preterm babies, including the fat, protein, and calcium, so that these infants can be supplemented with human, not bovine, milk fortifier (Lai, 2004; Kent, 2004).

▶ DIFFERENCES BETWEEN HUMAN MILK AND INFANT FORMULA

Breastfed babies are significantly healthier than those raised on artificial baby milk. A baby has a 20 percent lower risk of dying in the first year of life if breastfed at all. Longer breastfeeding is associated with lower risk (Chen, 2004). Human milk contains a host of immunologic agents that protect the infant against infections and allergens until his defenses are more fully developed. Research increasingly demonstrates that infant feeding has a lifelong effect on the immune system (Kelly, 2000; Hanson, 1998; Hamosh, 1996). The individualized characteristics of each mother's milk provide her baby with nourishment that is ideally suited to his specific needs for health and growth. Donor milk is always the best alternative for babies whose mother cannot breastfeed or provide her milk.

During and after World War II, cow's milk formula came to be the routine source of infant nutrition in the United States and many other developed countries. With a growing reliance on scientific achievements and new technology, breastfeeding knowledge and skills decreased, especially in Western hospitals. Intense and unscrupulous marketing of artificial milks by formula manufacturers ensued. Today, America is one of the largest markets for infant formula. Over half of all formula sold in the United States is obtained through WIC (Oliveira, 2004; Weimer, 2001).

Uncontrolled Marketing

Artificial baby milk feeding is described as one of "the largest uncontrolled in vivo experiments in human history" (Minchin, 1998). Studies show that artificial baby milk carries with it serious risks for infants, young children, and their mothers (Chen, 2004; Raisler, 1999). In 1981, an awareness of these dangers prompted the World Health Organization to adopt the International Code of Marketing of Breastmilk Substitutes.

The Code, as it is referred to by breastfeeding advocates, attempts to restrict the unethical marketing and promotion of food and drink, such as infant formula, used to feed babies inappropriately, as well as all associated paraphernalia, such as bottles and teats. When the World Health Assembly considered the Code, the United States cast the lone dissenting vote, which stirred a wave of controversy throughout the world. In 1994, the United States finally approved the Code. See Chapter 28 for more information.

The United States is not immune to the dangers associated with infant formula. The potential dangers of misuse are dramatic in any impoverished community with substandard conditions and low education levels. Incorrect and inadequate use of infant formula accounts for about 1½ million deaths each year worldwide (Walker, 2001). Some of these deaths occur even in affluent communities with access to clean water and education, and in highly specialized intensive care nurseries. It is intrinsically hazardous to deprive any infant of his mother's milk (Lucas, 1990a, 1990b).

Dangers in Artificial Feeding

There are substantial differences between human milk and artificial baby milk. The composition of human milk makes it far superior to any artificial baby milk on the market. A mother's milk continually changes to meet her baby's needs. Nature has produced a product composed of hundreds of components, each with a specific function in ensuring optimal nourishment of the human infant.

Artificial formulas are deficient in many of the constituents that are essential for optimum infant growth and health. They do not benefit from nature's consistency of quality and adaptability to the baby's age and unique needs. They provide no protection against allergies and confer no immunity to the baby. All formulas are slightly different and yet are intended to meet the universal needs of infants. Logic dictates that nature's sole "formula"—human milk—eclipses any "ideal" substitute.

Individual companies compete to advertise that their brand contains more of one element than that of another manufacturer. Theirs, they argue, is "closest to mother's milk" in that particular element. These pronouncements can be confusing to parents, who may worry that they must select one advantage over another. Try as they might, these companies can never replicate all the bioactive, immunologic, nutritional, and other health benefits of human milk (Goldman, 1998; Hamosh, 1996; Hanson, 1998).

Clearly, artificial feeding is not without its risks to infants, young children, mothers, and their families. Yet parents fail to learn of these hazards, and the media promotes human milk substitutes as safe, acceptable, and the social norm (Walker, 2001; Hawkins, 1994; Sawatzki, 1994). In order for parents to be responsible health consumers, they need all the facts. You can assist parents in acquiring necessary information so that they can make an informed choice about infant feeding.

Too Little or Too Much

Artificial baby milk can contain micronutrients or macronutrients in either excessive or deficient amounts. It may also be completely lacking in essential elements. One of the more alarming deficiencies in infant formula are essential fatty acids that are important to proper brain development and visual acuity. No current formula has replicated human milk's complex fatty acid pattern, even after adding fats derived from a variety of sources, including fish heads, egg yolks, and genetically engineered marine algae.

Benefits to the infant's brain development and visual acuity from these formulas remains controversial. One formula manufacturer removed those claims from its advertisements in Canada (Sterken, 2004). However, U.S. companies continue to stress their formulas' "enhancement" of brain and vision development. The addition of fatty acids now has led to other concerns, such as the effect on infant growth. In a study of human milk versus formula with added long-chain polyunsaturated fatty acids (LCPUFA), breastfed infants had significantly higher developmental scores at 9 and 18 months than the formula groups. They also weighed more and were taller at 18 months than the group fed LCPUFA formula (Fewtrell, 2002).

These additives presently are made from algae and fungus (Agennix, 2002). In one study, lower levels of nervonic acid (NA), docosapentaenoic (DPA) acid, and DHA were found in all infants fed formula compared with levels in the human milk–fed infants, regardless of the source of the formula supplement (Sala-Vila, 2004). In another study, formulas containing DHA resulted in higher DHA blood levels but did not result in significantly increased visual acuity (Horby, 1998). Current concentrations of DHA in infant formulas are considered inadequate (Sarkadi-Nagy, 2004). There is concern about the potential for too much or an unbalanced intake of n-6 and n-3 fatty acids with the increased addition of LCPUFA to other infant foods (Koo, 2003a). The levels of palm olein needed to provide a fatty acid profile similar to human milk can lead to lower bone mineralization (Koo, 2003b).

Vitamin D, which is toxic in high doses, appears in excessive amounts in many formulas. Some formulas are deficient in chloride. Any formula that contains high levels of iodine could affect neonatal thyroid function. Some formulas are marketed as "hypoallergenic." One study found that these extensively hydrolyzed formulas are usually effective, but intolerance to hydrolysates recently has been observed (Smith, 2003).

Concerns About Soy Formula

Infants who consume soy formula receive the equivalent of 6 to 11 times the normal dose of isoflavones. This amount, if given to women, would change their menstrual patterns (Kumar, 2002). **Congenitally** hypothyroid infants receiving soy formula have demonstrated elevated thyroid stimulating hormone (TSH) levels even when taking thyroid medication (Conrad, 2004). Soy milk contains about 80 times more manganese than human milk. Research on rats showed behavioral changes and lowered levels of the **neurotransmitter dopamine**, suggesting a possible correlation between heavy soy intake and neurological deficits (Tran, 2002).

Aluminum levels in soy formula are 36 times higher than in human milk. Aluminum competes with calcium receptors and is associated with renal problems. An AAP study concluded that "continued efforts should be made to reduce the aluminum content of all formulas used for infants, but especially soy formulas and formulas tailored specifically for premature infants" (AAP, 1996). The British Dietetic Association issued a position statement discouraging the use of soy formulas for infants (BDA, 2003). There may be additional hormonal effects from other estrogen-mimicking compounds known as **phthalates**, which are present in various plastics that infants can be exposed to, often by artificial feeding (Densley, 1996).

Infant and Maternal Health Risks

ILCA's *Core Curriculum for Lactation Consultant Practice* (ILCA, 2002) provides a comprehensive review of the risks associated with artificial feeding. IQ levels may be 8 points lower in formula-fed babies than in breastfed babies. One bottle of formula can change the baby's gut flora for 3 weeks. Formula sensitizes the baby to cow's milk protein and can provoke an allergy later in the first year if the baby is exposed again to cow's milk. Compounding the risk is the fact that formula-fed infants are more likely to receive cow's milk at an earlier age than are breastfed infants. Bovine protein sensitivity can lead to serious malabsorption problems, even in affluent communities. Table 9.5 shows some of the ratios reported in studies of infants who are fed artificial baby milk compared with those who are breastfed.

Women who do not breastfeed experience an earlier return of fertility. This can result in shorter birth intervals, maternal depletion, and a higher number of pregnancies over their life span. These factors often result in earlier maternal death. Women who do not breastfeed are at

TABLE 9.5

Health Risks Associated with Artificial Feeding

	Ratios Reported in Studies			
Health Risk as Identified in Studies	**Study**	**Not Breastfed**		**Breastfed**
Infant hospitalized more often	Study 1	15	to	1
	Study 2	10	to	1
Infant sick more often and to a greater degree	Study 1	21	to	8
Infant more likely to develop childhood cancers	Study 1	6	to	1
	Study 2	8	to	1
Infant more likely to develop gastroenteritis	Study 1	6	to	1
Infant more likely to develop ulcerative colitis and Crohns disease	Study 1	3	to	1
Infant more likely to develop bronchitis and pneumonia	Study 1	5	to	1
	Study 2	2	to	1
Infant more likely to die from SIDS	Study 1	3	to	1
	Study 2	5	to	1
Premature infant more likely to develop necrotizing enterocolitis (NEC)	Study 1	20	to	1
Infant more likely to develop juvenile diabetes	Study 1	2	to	1
	Study 2	7	to	1
Women at greater risk for breast cancer	Study 1	2	to	1
Women at greater risk for ovarian cancer	Study 1	1.6	to	1

increased risk for developing premenopausal breast cancer, ovarian cancer, and thyroid cancer. They also have a higher rate of developing osteoporosis in later life.

Dangers in Manufacturing

Artificial milks carry hazards for the formula-fed infant. Most parents are unaware of what is actually in the formula they give their babies. Cultural conditioning and trust in the health care field foster the belief that "My doctor wouldn't recommend it if it weren't safe." Therefore, most bottle-feeding parents do not question what they feed their babies.

Aluminum has contaminated some formulas. Parents need to wash the formula can and can opener to avoid residue of pesticides and animal droppings in the warehouse from entering the formula. In 2003, tragedies involving formula resulted in the deaths of 15 infants within months of each other. The absence of vitamin B_1 (thiamine), mistakenly omitted from formula in Israel, resulted in brain damage in 17 infants and at least 2 deaths (Siegel-Itzkovich, 2003). The sale of fake formula caused malnutrition in at least 171 infants and the death of at least 13 infants in China (Chinaview, 2004). One manufacturer was charged with relabeling animal feed containing dirt and flies as baby formula and selling it to Mexican food manufacturers (Gilot, 2004). These cases demonstrate the lack of oversight, lack of product assurance, and opportunity for fraud in the infant formula industry.

Product Recalls

There have been over 47 formula or infant food recalls in the past 22 years in the United States alone. Recall reports are available at the U.S. Food and Drug Administration Web site, www.fda.gov. Manufacturing problems range from incorrect preparation to incorrect packaging. Contamination with bacteria, including *Enterobacter sakazakii*, has occurred frequently (FDA, 2002; Walker, 2001). *E. sakazakii* can cause severe illness and death, especially in preterm babies or babies with compromised immune systems (NABA, 2004).

Ironically, the most expensive formula, Nutramigen, was one of Mead Johnson's many recalls. The manufacturer's press release states, "If not properly prepared, Nutramigen® 16-oz. powder infant formula and Nutramigen® 32-oz. ready-to-use infant formula have the potential to cause serious adverse health effects such as seizures, irregular heart beat, renal failure or in extreme cases, death. Symptoms to look for include vomiting, diarrhea, decreased urine output, irritability, decreased activity or sunken eyes" (Mead Johnson, 2001).

Multiple Burdens With Formula Use

The use of artificial baby milks can have an adverse impact on all members of a family. It affects the family's time because they must always carry infant formula in sufficient quantity, along with its paraphernalia to prepare and feed it. The preparation of the infant formula by the mother or other family member includes time for shopping, storing, preparing, and cleaning up—all time taken away from interacting with the baby or each other.

The impact on attachment between the mother and her baby is also a factor. A 14-year study found that, compared with babies breastfed for 4 or more months, non-breastfed babies were $4\frac{1}{2}$ times more likely to experience mistreatment from their mothers. Babies separated from their mothers for more than 20 hours per week had about a threefold increase in risk (Strathern, 2003). Fergusson and Woodward found that breastfed children reported higher levels of parental attachment at ages 15 to 18 (Fergusson, 1999).

Drain on Family Finances

The family of a baby who is not breastfed will experience the economic burden of purchasing infant formula and the equipment needed for artificial feeding. The financial burden imposed on families for the purchase of infant formula is significant. The San Diego Breastfeeding Coalition's 2001 study found an annual range in formula costs between $648 for a store brand and $2,800 for Nutramigen, a hydrolized formula.

Impoverished families could spend as much as 100 percent of their cash income for these products if they were to use them appropriately, especially in developing countries. In an attempt to stretch their supply of formula, parents may dilute it or supplement their baby's diet with inappropriate foods such as coffee, tea, sugared fruit drinks, and soy milk. The women and family members may go hungry, with food money going toward artificial formula and medications to deal with illnesses associated with formula feeding. Such malnutrition can have serious long-term effects. Families also have the increased cost of medical expenses when the baby lacks the health protection of human milk. One study found the average additional healthcare cost for formula-fed infants ranged between $331 and $475 (Ball, 1999).

Drain on Community Resources

The community's burden from the use of artificial baby milks is far reaching. The production and packaging consume valuable land and resources. Production errors, such as contamination and mishandling, create a burden on society as a whole, as well as on the individual child. Once packaged, the distribution process takes additional resources for fuel and contributes to environmental pollution. Even the disposal of waste products such as infant formula tins taxes the environment. The ever-increasing need to improve the infant formulas is a burden to research. It drains time and resources that could go toward unavoidable health concerns, helping women breastfeed and making safe human milk available for infants whose mothers cannot provide it.

Drain on Healthcare

Educating parents in the proper use of infant formula consumes valuable healthcare resources and time healthcare workers could spend with other health issues. It is the healthcare industry's responsibility to make sure parents understand the nuances of purchasing, storing, mixing, and feeding formula. Additionally, the many errors, omissions, and purposeful rationing that occur with regularity impose harmful health consequences on the child, some subtle and some not so subtle. Parents' time goes toward caring for children who are acutely and chronically ill due to the lack of human milk. This leads to an increase in the spending of healthcare dollars, which is a burden passed along to the consumer.

Legitimate Need for Formula

Step Six of the Ten Steps to Successful Breastfeeding states that newborn infants should be given "no food or drink other than breastmilk, unless *medically* indicated." This recommendation recognizes there will be times when a mother cannot breastfeed or feed her milk to her baby. If she is not a candidate for or does not wish to use donor human milk, she will need education regarding the use of human milk substitutes. There may be circumstances in which a mother specifically refuses to breastfeed. She, too, will need instructions in the use of an alternative feeding method. Until the baby is one year of age, it is important that he receive infant formula rather than cow's milk.

Ideally, parents select an infant formula carefully, in conjunction with the baby's healthcare provider, with consideration given to the family's life circumstances and health history. Infant formula should be the choice of last resort after exhausting all other options to provide human milk. Unfortunately, this is usually not the case.

Maternal Circumstances That Preclude Breastfeeding

Some medical conditions prevent a mother from breastfeeding her baby. As discussed in Chapter 25, a mother with a physical condition such as Sheehan's syndrome, long-term drug therapy, severe congestive heart failure, or true insufficient milk supply may need to feed her baby artificial milk. In addition, because tuberculosis spreads through close contact, it may be dangerous to a breast-feeding infant. After the mother receives appropriate treatment for at least 1 week and is no longer infectious, she can return to breastfeeding (Lawrence, 1999).

If a mother is infected with **HIV** prior to the birth of her baby and if she has access to a sanitary water supply, current health guidelines state she should not breastfeed her baby unless she can pump and pasteurize her milk to kill the HIV virus (WHO, 2003; Jeffery, 2001, 2003; Black, 1996). If the mother's infection with HIV occurs after delivery, she should not breastfeed; her baby had not been exposed to HIV in utero, so breastfeeding would present an unnecessary risk. The presence of HIV does not mean, however, that the baby cannot receive human milk. The mother's milk can be heat-treated, or she can feed him banked human milk.

A mother who has an active herpes lesion on her breast where the baby will come in contact with it should not breastfeed on the affected breast until the lesion heals. The baby may continue to nurse on the other breast, and the mother can express her milk and discard it from the affected side. If a mother is severely ill with a condition such as psychosis, **eclampsia**, or shock, she may be unable to breastfeed until her healing is sufficient to begin or resume breastfeeding. Mothers who must take certain medications, such as cytotoxic or radioactive drugs, may need to stop breastfeeding while the drug is present and active (Hale, 2004). See Chapter 25 for more discussion of maternal circumstances.

Infant Circumstances That Require Formula

Human milk supplementation is required in situations such as hypoglycemia or dehydration, when the condition has not improved through increased breastfeeding or increased intake of human milk. Babies with very low or extremely low birth weight or who are born preterm, less than 1000 grams or 32 weeks' gestation, may require supplementation with HMF (Morton, 2003; Landers, 2003; Klein, 2002). If it is determined that the baby needs supplementation, an alternative feeding method must be chosen that will interfere the least with the return to breastfeeding and fit most comfortably into the family's lifestyle.

Galactosemia is an extremely rare condition that requires the use of a special formula. A baby with galactosemia is unable to metabolize lactose, the main carbohydrate in human milk. Therefore, use of human milk by any means is not possible. Be aware that babies with Duarte's variant, a variation of galactosemia, can breastfeed with precautions (see Chapter 25 for a further discussion). Although other inborn errors of metabolism, such as **phenylketonuria** (PKU) or maple syrup urine disease, require the use of milk substitutes, they also allow for carefully monitored intake of the mother's milk.

Selecting a Brand and Type of Formula

When selecting a particular artificial baby milk, the family's health history must be considered with respect to allergies and problems with past use of such substitutes. The allergy history of the entire family—siblings, parents, and other close blood relatives—needs to be considered. Symptoms of those allergies need investigation. In theory, parents should make the choice of a human milk substitute together with the baby's caregiver, mindful of the health implications for that particular family. The reality is that parents' brand choice often depends on which company left a case on their doorstep, which discharge pack they received at hospital discharge, and which cents-off coupon is available. The caregiver's choice may be a formula whose company sales representative is the best salesperson or gives the "best gifts." Some caregivers rotate brands on a 4-month cycle. Consideration is not always given to which brand will agree best with a particular baby.

Careful attention to expiration dates and label instructions are important. Some clinicians advise mothers to record the lot number of each can in the event of a recall or class action lawsuit. Another consideration that dictates the choice of a formula is the family's financial circumstance. Formula may be ready-to-feed, concentrated, or powdered.

Powdered Formula

Powdered formula is the least expensive of the 3 types. In 2004 dollars, cost in the U.S. southwest averaged about $130 per month (based on Ross Lab's estimate of 14,500 oz required in the first 12 months of life). It is the most portable and has the longest shelf life.

Concentrate

At about $144 per month in the U.S. southwest, concentrate is more costly than powdered formula but is easier to mix. Like powdered or ready-to-feed, parents must discard any unused portion within one hour after they have opened and mixed it.

Ready-to-Feed

Ready-to-feed formula is the most convenient of the 3 forms. One of the advantages of ready-to-feed formula is that the mother does not need to make decisions about whether to use tap water or bottled water. Nor would there be changes to the baby's system when traveling, as there might be when various water supplies are used. However, ready-to-feed formula is the most expensive of the 3 types, at an average of $176 per month in the U.S. southwest, and parents must discard any that remains after the specified period.

Dangers in Preparation

Aggressive marketing of infant formula, together with modeling of its use in wealthy countries where infant mortality is generally low, contributed to a massive shift away from breastfeeding (Wolf, 2003). This change occurred both in developed countries and among women in developing countries who cannot use artificial baby milk safely and whose babies become ill and malnourished (Michels, 1995). In communities where the mother cannot afford to purchase sufficient quantities of infant formula, families may attempt to stretch the supply by diluting it. There may be no access to refrigeration, clean water, or adequate waste facilities. Additionally, parents may not understand directions well enough to mix the infant formula properly.

Unsafe Water Supply

The American Academy of Pediatrics cautions mothers to check their water supply to make sure that it is safe for the baby to drink. Families with well water should have it tested. If there is any concern about unsafe water supply, they should purchase bottled water. When traveling, parents will want to consider the safety of the water en route.

If the mother is unsure about bacterial level in the water supply, she can use bottled water or boil the tap water for five minutes (boiling longer may cause the lead to concentrate). To prevent lead poisoning, parents should obtain the water used for formula from the cold-water tap only. In older homes and in some newer ones, the water pipe joints contain lead solder, which leaches out more easily in hot water. The AAP recommends that parents run the cold water for at least one minute before collecting it, and longer if no one has run the water for several hours.

Another concern with the water used to mix formula is the extra fluoridation that occurs with the addition of fluoride to the community water supply. Excessive fluoride may cause fluorosis, a condition in which teeth are mottled or discolored. One study concluded that infant formulas prepared with fluoridated water increase the risk of fluorosis in primary teeth (Marshall, 2004). The possibility of nitrites, sodium, bacteria, and parasites in the water is another consideration. Babies are susceptible to methemoglobinemia from water containing nitrates.

Unsafe Mixing and Use

A systematic review in the United Kingdom found that feedings were not prepared accurately. Reviewers stressed the urgent need to minimize the risk of incorrect preparation (Renfrew, 2003). Mixing errors do not occur only within the less educated population. One college-educated father failed to read mixing directions carefully and fed his newborn concentrated infant formula.

Even when parents mix formula according to the directions on the can, there may be wide variations in the final composition of the product. This is partly because the composition of formula in the can varies from season to season, depending on the cow's diet. In addition, powder can pack down in the can over time, so that a scoop of powder may contain a greater or lesser quantity by weight.

Powdered formula is the most prone to mixing errors. Parents may not follow package directions or use the specific scoop provided with the can. Each company has a particular set of instructions, and the size of the scoop is not uniform between manufacturers. Parents need to read the instructions carefully and use the scoop that came with that particular brand of formula. Caregivers should ask the mother to prepare the formula in the hospital as a return demonstration to ensure that she understands the correct procedure.

It is easy for parents to confuse concentrate with ready-to-feed. Even the most educated parents run the risk of misreading the label and feeding their infants with straight concentrate. The higher cost of ready-to-feed formula may tempt parents to save unused portions rather than discard them after the specified period. Oral water intoxication resulting in seizures is becoming more common in the United States when parents dilute expensive formula with more water than is called for (Keating, 1991).

Precautions for Parents

Parents need to consider the length of time the substitute remains at room temperature and how long it may be stored in the refrigerator after the can is open. Parents often mix several bottles at one time. They need to understand that artificial baby milk is an **inert** substance. Unlike human milk, it is not **bacteriostatic** and does not contain anti-infective properties to fight bacteria. Bacteria can multiply rapidly in formula that remains at room temperature. Formula must be refrigerated or chilled if it is stored in the diaper bag.

Parents should use a clean bottle and sterile utensils for every feeding. They should wash the can opener and top and bottom of the can with hot soapy water before opening the can. Advise mothers to open the can from the bottom, because the bottom is less likely to have the same level of pesticide sprays as the top (Kutner, 1996). They should check the expiration date on each can of formula carefully before use to ensure that it has not expired.

Parents must discard formula mixed from concentrate after 48 hours and discard formula mixed from powder after 24 hours. They must discard formula removed from the refrigerator after one hour (Barger, 1997). When a feeding is finished, they cannot save any unused portion for a later feeding. This prevents the baby from receiving any contaminated milk substitute and preserves his health.

▶ SUMMARY

Human milk is the perfect nutrition for the human infant. Health benefits to the infant resulting from the immunologic properties of the mother's milk are irrefutable. Human milk is specific to the infant's age and changes throughout lactation to meet his changing needs. Researchers continue to uncover newfound benefits of the many components in this rich and complex substance. There are also lifelong benefits to mothers who breastfeed. Caregivers have a responsibility to promote the use of human milk for all babies. The American Academy of Pediatrics, World Health Organization, American Academy of Family Physicians, and American Dietetic Association, among others, have translated this responsibility into strong statements in support of breastfeeding through the first year of a child's life and beyond. Artificial baby milks are an inferior substitute for mother's milk.

▶ CHAPTER 9—AT A GLANCE

Facts you learned—

Colostrum:

◆ Consists of residual materials in the breast that mix with newly formed milk.

◆ Is richer than mature milk in sodium, potassium, chloride, protein, fat-soluble vitamins, and minerals.

◆ Contains less fat and lactose than mature milk.

◆ Engulfs and digests disease organisms and aids in rapid gut closure.

◆ Has high concentrations of IgA, IgG, and IgM (as does mature milk).

Fat content:

◆ Varies from mother to mother and from feeding to feeding.

◆ Is inversely proportional to the length of time between feedings.

◆ Is related to the degree of breast fullness.

◆ Decreases in later months of lactation.

◆ At the end of a feeding may be up to four to five times higher than at the beginning.

Lactose:

◆ Enhances calcium absorption (preventing rickets).

◆ Supplies energy to the infant's brain.

◆ Protects the infant's intestines from the growth of harmful organisms.

◆ Is essential to development of the central nervous system.

◆ Is the most constant among mothers of all the constituents in human milk.

Composition and volume:

◆ Composition changes throughout lactation and during a given day or feeding.

◆ Milk is high in immunoglobulins and protein during the first several weeks.

◆ Milk often seems most plentiful in the morning hours.

◆ Volume of milk is dependent on regular removal of milk from the breast.

◆ Three-quarters of nutrient needs through twelve months can be met by human milk.

◆ Daily output during the second year is at least eight ounces.

Other properties of human milk:

◆ Oligosaccharides prevent pathogens from binding to receptor sites in the gut.

◆ Protein level is relatively constant, regardless of the mother's diet.

◆ Curd is soft, small, less compact, and easy to digest.

◆ Lactoferrin inhibits growth of *E. coli*; its effects decrease when saturated with exogenous iron.

◆ Lysozyme protects against enterobacteriaceae and gram-positive bacteria.

◆ Long-chain polyunsaturated fatty acids promote optimal neural and visual development.

◆ All vitamins are present in sufficient levels, when combined with sun exposure for additional vitamin D.

◆ Healthy nonanemic mothers lay down sufficient iron stores for the first few months.

◆ Suckling triggers cholecystokinin (CCK) and causes sleepiness in mothers and babies.

◆ IgA protects the GI tract and is the most important of the antiviral defense factors.

◆ Lactase and lipase protect babies born with immature or defective enzyme systems.

◆ Lactase converts lactose into simple sugars that can be assimilated easily by the infant.

◆ A deficiency in lactase can result in lactose intolerance.

◆ Lysozyme breaks down bacteria in the bowel.

◆ Lactoferrin inhibits the growth of *E. coli*.

◆ Bifidus factor works with the pH of the stool to discourage the growth of *E. coli*.

◆ Antibodies in human milk enhance infant antibody response.

◆ Mucins in human milk protect against bacterial infections.

◆ Thyroid hormones prevent hypothyroidism, mask diagnosis, and protect the baby until he is weaned.

◆ Alpha-lactalbumin inhibits bacteria and yeast growth.

◆ Xantine oxidase combined with nitrites inhibits *E. coli* and *Salmonella enteritidis*.

◆ Nucleotides promote optimal function and growth of the GI and immune systems.

◆ High levels of antibodies provide antiabsorptive protection on the lining of the infant's intestine.

Specific health benefits:

◆ Fewer dental caries and better dental health.

◆ Dose-dependent in increasing IQ.

◆ Provides lifelong protection against disease.

◆ Destroys bacteria in the GI tract before they affect the infant.

◆ Protects the infant against upper and lower respiratory infections, otitis media, diarrheal disease, urinary tract infections, sepsis, rotavirus, meningitis, leukemia, lymphoma, Hodgkin's disease, and neuroblastoma.

◆ Lowers risk of breast cancer, chronic and autoimmune diseases, hypertension, high cholesterol, and heart disease.

◆ Decreases the risk of NEC and the incidence of asthma.

◆ Antibodies are produced against organisms passed into the breast by the suckling infant.

◆ Maternal antigens to a cold, fever, or more serious illness protect her breastfed baby.

Milk of women who deliver prematurely:

◆ Higher in sodium, chloride, nitrogen, and immunoprotective factors.

◆ Human milk fortifiers (HMF)—protein, calcium, potassium phosphate, carbohydrates, vitamins, and trace minerals—are used to supplement very low birth weight (VLBW) infants.

◆ Lactoengineering offers an alternative to HMF by isolating hindmilk to increase calories, carbohydrates, and proteins for preterm infants.

Artificial formula:

◆ Composition of human milk makes it far superior to any artificial baby milk.

◆ Formulas are slightly different from one another, yet are intended to meet universal needs of infants.

◆ Formula is deficient in many constituents essential for optimum infant growth and health.

◆ Formula has been found to:

　◆ Have excessive or deficient amounts of micronutrients or macronutrients.

　◆ Be completely lacking certain essential elements.

　◆ Have lower levels of nervonic acid (NA), docosapentaenoic (DPA) acid, and DHA.

　◆ Have excessive vitamin D, which is toxic in high doses.

　◆ Be deficient in chloride.

　◆ Be contaminated with aluminum or bacteria.

◆ Soy formula can cause neurological deficits and renal problems.

◆ Formula use drains family finances, community resources, and healthcare dollars.

◆ Babies are at risk for contaminated water, mixing errors, and bacteria from formula left at room temperature for too long.

◆ Infants fed cow's milk are more likely to develop late neonatal hypocalcemia and dehydration.

◆ A single feeding of cow's milk in the first days of life can increase rates of allergy.

◆ Cow's milk is the most common food allergen in infants.

◆ Most infants with cow's milk allergy develop symptoms before one month of age, often within one week after introduction of cow's milk protein-based formula.

◆ Atopic dermatitis and eczema are more common in artificially fed infants.

◆ Babies should receive formula only if there is a legitimate need:

　◆ In the mother: Sheehan's syndrome, long-term drug therapy, severe congestive heart failure, insufficient milk supply, tuberculosis (until after treatment), HIV (in the U.S.), active herpes lesion, eclampsia, cytotoxic or radioactive drugs.

　◆ In the infant: Hypoglycemia or dehydration if unimproved by increased breastfeeding and no donor milk is available, prematurity, galactosemia, PKU, or maple syrup urine disease.

REFERENCES

Agennix, Inc. Recombinant Human Lactoferrin 2002. Available at: www.rhlf.com. Accessed February 14, 2005.

Akre J. Infant feeding: The physiological basis. *WHO Bulletin Supplement* 67:29; 1989.

Ala-Houhala M et al. Maternal compared with infant vitamin D supplementation. *Arch Dis Child* 61(12):1159–1163; 1986.

American Academy of Family Physicians (AAFP). AAFP Policy Statement on Breastfeeding; 2001. Available at: http://www.aafp.org/x6633.xml. Accessed February 8, 2004.

American Academy of Pediatrics (AAP) Committee on Nutrition. Aluminum toxicity in infants and children. *Pediatrics* 97(3):413–416; 1996.

American Academy of Pediatrics (AAP). Breastfeeding and the use of human milk. *Pediatrics* 100:1035–1039; 1997.

American Dietetic Association (ADA). Breaking the barriers to breastfeeding. *J Am Diet Assoc* 101:1213; 2001.

Anderson J et al. Breastfeeding and cognitive development: A meta-analysis. *Am J Clin Nutr* 70:525–535; 1999.

Aniansson G et al. A prospective cohort study on breastfeeding and otitis media in Swedish infants. *Pediatr Infect Dis J* 13:183–188; 1994.

Arnold L. Use of donor milk in the treatment of metabolic disorders. *J Hum Lact* 11:51–53; 1995.

Arnold R et al. A bacteriocidal effect for human lactoferrin. *Science* 197:263–264; 1977.

Arteaga-Vizcaino M et al. Effect of oral and intramuscular vitamin K on the factors II, VII, IX, X, and PIVKA II in the infant newborn under 60 days of age. *Rev Med Chil* 129(10):1121–1129; 2001.

Ashraf R et al. Additional water is not needed for healthy breast-fed babies in a hot climate. *Acta Paediatr* 82:1007–1011; 1993.

Ball T, Wright A. Health care costs of formula-feeding in the first year of life. *Pediatrics* 103(4 Pt 2):870–876; 1999.

Barger J, Kutner L. Teaching parents safe formula feeding. *Clinical Issues in Lactation* 2(2):1–2; 1997.

Bauchner H et al. Studies of breastfeeding and infections: How good is the evidence? *JAMA* 256:887–892; 1986.

Bener A et al. Longer breast-feeding and protection against childhood leukaemia and lymphomas. *Eur J Cancer* 37(2):234–238; 2001.

Bhowmick S et al. Rickets caused by vitamin D deficiency in breastfed infants in the southern United States. *Am J Child Dis* 145:127–130; 1991.

Bisquera J et al. Impact of necrotizing enterocolitis on length of stay and hospital charges in very low birth weight infants. *Pediatrics* 109(3):423–428; 2002.

Black R. Transmission of HIV-1 in the breast-feeding process. Review. *J Am Diet Assoc* 96(3):267–274; 1996.

Bor O et al. Late hemorrhagic disease of the newborn. *Pediatr Int* 42(1):64–66; 2000.

Brandtzaeg P. Mucosal immunity: Integration between mother and the breast-fed baby. *Vaccine* 24(21):3382–3388; 2003.

Brazerol W, McPhee A, Mimoumi F et al. Serial ultraviolet B exposure and serum 25 hydroxyvitamin D response in young adult American blacks and whites: No racial differences. *J Am Coll Nutr* 7(2):111–118; 1988.

British Dietetic Association (BDA). Paediatric group position statement on the use of soya protein for infants. *J Fam Health Care* 13(4):93; 2003.

Brothwell D, Limeback H. Breastfeeding is protective against dental fluorosis in a nonfluoridated rural area of Ontario, Canada. *J Hum Lact* 19(4):386–390; 2003.

Buescher S. Host defense mechanisms of human milk and their relations to enteric infections and necrotizing enterocolitis. *Clin Perinatol* 21:247–262; 1994.

Buescher S. Anti-infective Properties of Human Milk with Special Reference to the Pre-term Baby. Presentation, Human Lactation: Current Research and Clinical Implications. Amarillo, TX; October 21, 2004.

Bulkow L et al. Risk factors for severe respiratory syncytial virus infection among Alaska native children. *Pediatrics* 109(2):210–216; 2002.

Butte N et al. Longitudinal changes in milk composition of mothers delivering preterm and term infants. *Early Hum Dev* 9(2):153–162; 1984.

Calhoun D et al. Granulocyte colony-stimulating factor is present in human milk and its receptor is present in human fetal intestine. *Pediatrics* 105:e7; 2000.

Caplan et al. Necrotizing enterocolitis: A review of pathogenetic mechanisms and implications for prevention (review). *Pediatr Pathol* 13(3):357–369; 1993.

Carlson S et al. Visual acuity and fatty acid status of term infants fed human milk and formulas with and without docosahexaenoate and arachidonate from egg yolk lecithin. *Pediatr Res* 39:882–888; 1996.

Carver J. Dietary nucleotides: Effects on the immune and gastrointestinal systems. Review. *Acta Paediatr Suppl* 88(430):83–88; 1999.

Casey C et al. Nutrient intake by breast-fed infants during the first five days after birth. *Am J Dis Child* 140(9):933–936; 1986.

Centers for Disease Control and Prevention (CDC). Recommendations for using fluoride to prevent and control dental caries in the US. *MMWR* 50(No RR-14); 2001.

Chan G. Effects of powdered human milk fortifiers on the antibacterial actions of human milk. *J Perinatol* 23(8):620–623; 2003.

Chandra R. Five-year follow-up of high-risk infants with family history of allergy who were exclusively breast-fed or fed partial whey hydrolysate, soy, and conventional cow's milk formulas. *J Pediatr Gastroenterol Nutr* 24(4):380–388; 1997.

Chaturvedi P et al. Fucosylated human milk oligosaccharides vary between individuals and over the course of lactation. *Glycobiology* 11(5):365–372; 2001a.

Chaturvedi P et al. Survival of human milk oligosaccharides in the intestine of infants. *Adv Exp Med Biol* 501:315–323; 2001b.

Chen A, Rogan W. Breastfeeding and the risk of postneonatal death in the United States. *Pediatrics* 113(5):e435–e439; 2004.

Chierici R et al. Advances in the modulation of the microbial ecology of the gut in early infancy. *Acta Paediatr Suppl* 91(441):56–63; 2003.

Chinaview. 22 detained for fake milk products. Chinaview; April 26, 2004. Available at: www.chinaview.cn. Accessed July 10, 2004.

Clemens J et al. Breastfeeding and the risk of life-threatening enterotoxigenic Escherichia coli diarrhea in Bangladeshi infants and children. *Pediatrics* 100(6):E2; 1997.

Clemens TL, Adams JS, Henderson SL, Holick MF. Increased skin pigment reduces the capacity of skin to synthesise vitamin D_3. *Lancet* 1(8263):74–76; 1982.

Conrad SC et al. Soy formula complicates management of congenital hypothyroidism. *Arch Dis Child* 89(1):37–40; 2004.

Coppa G et al. Changes in carbohydrate composition in human milk over 4 months of lactation. *Pediatrics* 91:637–641; 1993.

Coppa G et al. Preliminary study of breastfeeding and bacterial adhesion to uroepithelial cells. *Lancet* 335:569–571; 1990.

Corrao G et al. Risk of inflammatory bowel disease attributable to smoking, oral contraception and breastfeeding in Italy: A nationwide case-control study. *Int J Epidemiol* 27(3):307–404; 1998.

Cox D et al. Studies on human lactation: The development of the computerized breast measurement system; 1998. Available at: http://biochem.uwa.edu.au/PEH/PEHRes.html. Accessed March 12, 2004.

Daly S et al. Degree of breast emptying explains changes in the fat content but not fatty acid composition of human milk. *Exp Physiol* 78:741–755; 1993a.

Daly S et al. The short-term synthesis and infant-regulated removal of milk in lactating women. *Exp Physiol* 78:209–220; 1993b.

Daniels J et al. Breast-feeding and neuroblastoma, USA and Canada. *Cancer Causes and Control* 13(5):401–405; 2002.

Davis M. Review of the evidence for an association between infant feeding and childhood cancer. *Int J Cancer* (Suppl 11): 29–33; 1998.

Del Prado et al. Contribution of dietary and newly formed arachidonic acid to human milk lipids in women eating a low-fat diet. *Am J Clin Nutr* 74(2):242–247; 2001.

Dell S, To T. Breastfeeding and asthma in young children—findings from a population-based study. *Arch Ped Adolescent Med* 155(11):1261–1265; 2001.

Densley B. Phthalates in formula: A report. *ALCA Galaxy* 7(3):34–37; 1996.

Dewey K et al. Differences in morbidity between breast-fed and formula-fed infants. *J Pediatr* 126(5 Pt 1):696–702; 1995.

Dewit O et al. Breastmilk amylase activities during 18 months of lactation in mothers from rural Zaire. *Acta Paediatr* 82:300–301; 1993.

Dick G. The etiology of multiple sclerosis. *Proc R Soc Med* 69:611; 1976.

Dugdale A. Breast milk and necrotising enterocolitis. *Lancet* 337:435; 1991.

Duncan B. et al. Exclusive breastfeeding for at least 4 months protects against otitis media. *Pediatrics* 91:867–872; 1993.

Dvorak B et al. Increased epidermal growth factor levels in human milk of mothers with extremely premature infants. *Pediatr Res* 54(1):15–19; 2003.

Ebrahim G. Feeding the preterm brain. *J Trop Pediatr* 39:130–131; 1993.

El-Mohandes A et al. Use of human milk in the intensive care nursery decreases the incidence of nosocomial sepsis. *J Perinatol* 17:130–134; 1997.

Erickson P et al. Estimation of the caries-related risk associated with infant formulas. *Pediatr Dent* 20:395–403; 1998.

Erickson PR, Mazhare E. Investigation of the role of human breast milk in caries development. *Pediatr Dent* 21:86–90; 1999.

Escuder M et al. Impact estimates of breastfeeding over infant mortality. *Rev Saude Publica* 37(3):319–325; 2003.

European Society of Paediatric Gastroenterology and Nutrition (ESPGN) Committee on Nutrition. Comment on antigen-reduced infant formulae. *Acta Paediatr* 82:317; 1993.

Fergusson D, Woodward L. Breast feeding and later psychosocial adjustment. *Paediatr Perinat Epidemiol* 139(2):144–157; 1999.

Fernandes R et al. Inhibition of enteroaggregative *Escherichia coli* adhesion to HEp-2 cells by secretory immunoglobulin A from human colostrum. *Pediatr Infect Dis J* 20(7):672–678; 2001.

Fewtrell M et al. Double-blind, randomized trial of long-chain polyunsaturated fatty acid supplementation in formula fed to preterm infants. *Pediatrics* 110(1 Pt 1):73–82; 2002.

Food and Drug Administration (FDA) Center for Food Safety and Applied Nutrition Office of Nutritional Products. Labeling and Dietary Supplements. Health professionals letter on *Enterobacter sakazakii* infections associated with use of powdered (dry) infant formulas in neonatal intensive care units; April 11, 2002; Revised October 10, 2002. Available at: www.cfsan.fda.gov/~dms/inf-ltr3.html. Accessed January 10, 2004.

Freudenheim J. Exposure to breast milk in infancy and the risk of breast cancer. *Epidemiology* 5:324–331; 1994.

Gartner L et al. Prevention of rickets and vitamin D deficiency: New guidelines for vitamin D intake. *Pediatrics* 111(4): 908–910; 2003.

Gdalevich M et al. Breast-feeding and the onset of atopic dermatitis in childhood: A systematic review and meta-analysis of prospective studies. *J Am Acad Dermatol* 45(4):520–527; 2001a.

Gdalevich M et al. Breast-feeding and the risk of bronchial asthma in childhood: A systematic review with meta-analysis of prospective studies. *J Pediatr* 139(2):261–266; 2001b.

Gianino P. Incidence of nosocomial rotavirus infections, symptomatic and asymptomatic, in breast-fed and non-breast-fed infants. *J Hosp Infect* 50(1):13–17; 2002.

Gilot L. Plant's Baby Formula Called 'filthy'. *El Paso Times*, El Paso, TX; November 2, 2004.

Goldman AS. The immunological system in human milk: The past—a pathway to the future. In Woodward WH, Draper HH (eds). *Advances in Nutritional Research*. New York: Plenum Press, 106; 1998.

Gomez-Sanchiz M et al. Influence of breast-feeding on mental and psychomotor development. *Clin Pediatr (Phila)* 42(1): 35–42; 2003.

Good Mojab C. Sunlight deficiency and breastfeeding. *Breastfeeding Abstracts* 22(1):3–4; 2002.

Good Mojab C. Sunlight deficiency: A review of the literature. *Mothering* 117:52–55, 57–63; 2003a.

Good Mojab C. Sunlight deficiency: Helping breastfeeding mothers find the facts. *Leaven* 39(4):75–79; 2003b.

Good Mojab, C. *Sunlight Deficiency, Vitamin D, and the Breastfed Baby: Helping Mothers Make Informed Decisions.* Texas WIC 2004 Nutrition and Breastfeeding Conference. Austin, TX; April 21, 2004.

Greer F et al. Improving the vitamin K status of breastfeeding infants with maternal vitamin K supplements. *Pediatrics* 99(1):88–92; 1997.

Greer F et al. A new mixed micellar preparation for oral vitamin K prophylaxis: Randomised controlled comparison with an intramuscular formulation in breast fed infants. *Arch Dis Child* 79(4):300–305; 1998.

Greer F. Are breast-fed infants vitamin K deficient? *Adv Exp Med Biol* 501:391–395; 2001a.

Greer F. Do breastfed infants need supplemental vitamins? *Pediatr Clin North Am* 48(2):415–423; 2001b.

Greiner T. Maternal protein-energy malnutrition and breastfeeding. *SCN News* (11):28–30; 1994.

Grummer-Strawn L et al. Does breastfeeding protect against pediatric overweight? Analysis of longitudinal data from the Centers for Disease Control and Prevention Pediatric Nutrition Surveillance System. *Pediatrics* 113(2):e81–e86; 2004.

Habicht J et al. Does breastfeeding really save lives, or are apparent benefits due to biases? *Am J Epidemiol* 123(2):279–290; 1986.

Hahn-Zoric M et al. Antibody responses to parenteral and oral vaccines are impaired by conventional and low protein formulas as compared to breast-feeding. *Acta Paediatr Scand* 79:1137–1142; 1990.

Hakansson A et al. A folding variant of alpha-lactalbumin with bactericidal activity against Streptococcus pneumoniae. *Mol Microbiol* 35:589–600; 2000.

Hale T. *Medications and Mother's Milk*. Amarillo, TX: Pharmasoft Publishing; 2004.

Hall B. Changing composition of human milk and early development of appetite control. *Keeping Abreast—Journal of Human Nurturing* 12:3; 1997.

Hamosh M. Breastfeeding: Unraveling the mysteries of mother's milk. *Medscape Womens' Health*; 1996.

Hamprecht K et al. Epidemiology of transmission of cytomegalovirus from mother to preterm infant by breastfeeding. *Lancet* 357(9255):513–518; 2001.

Hancock JT et al. Antimicrobial properties of milk: Dependence on presence of xanthine oxidase and nitrite. *Antimicrob Agents Chemother* 46:3308–3310; 2002.

Hansen K et al. Weekly oral vitamin K prophylaxis in Denmark. *Acta Paediatr* 92(7):802–805; 2003.

Hanson L et al. Breast-feeding, a complex support system for the offspring. *Pediatr Int* 44(4):347–352; 2002.

Hanson L. Breastfeeding provides passive and likely long-lasting active immunity. *Ann Allergy Asthma Immunol* 5:178–180; 1998.

Hanson L. Protective effects of breastfeeding against urinary tract infection. *Acta Paediatr* 93(2):154–156; 2004a.

Hanson L. *Immunobiology of Human Milk: How Breastfeeding Protects Babies*. Amarillo, TX: Pharmasoft Publishing; 2004b.

Harkness L, Cromer B. Low levels of 25-hydroxy vitamin D are associated with elevated parathyroid hormone in healthy adolescent females. *Osteoporos Int*; 16(1): 109–113; 2005.

Hart S et al. Brief report: Breast-fed one-week-olds demonstrate superior neurobehavioral organization. *J Pediatr Psychol* 28(8):529–534; 2003.

Hartmann P et al. Physiology of lactation in preterm mothers: Initiation and maintenance. *Pediatr Ann* 32(5):351–355; 2003.

Hasselbalch H et al. Breast-feeding influences thymic size in late infancy. *Eur J Pediatr* 158(12):964–967; 1999.

Hawkins N. Potential aluminum toxicity in infants fed special infant formula. *J Pediatr Gastroenterol Nutr* 19:377–381; 1994.

Hill D et al. Sensitivity to dietary proteins released in breast milk causing colic in infants. 2004 AAAAI Annual Meeting San Francisco; March 25, 2004.

Holick MF. Environmental factors that influence the cutaneous production of vitamin D. *Am J Clin Nutr* 1(3 Suppl): 638S–645S; 1995.

Hollis B, Wagner C. Assessment of dietary vitamin D requirements during pregnancy and lactation. *Am J Clin Nutr* 79(5):717–726; 2004a.

Hollis B, Wagner C. Vitamin D requirements during lactation: High-dose maternal supplementation as therapy to prevent hypovitaminosis D for both the mother and the nursing infant. *Am J Clin Nutr* 80(6 Suppl):1752S–1758S; 2004b.

Horby J. Effect of formula supplemented with docosahexaenoic acid and gamma-linolenic acid on fatty acid status and visual acuity in term infants. *Pediatr Gastroenterol Nutr* 26(4):412–421; 1998.

Horne RS et al. Comparison of evoked arousability in breast and formula fed infants. *Arch Dis Child* 89(1):22–25; 2004.

Host A. Frequency of cow's milk allergy in childhood. *Ann Allergy Asthma Immunol* 89(6 Suppl 1):33–37; 2002.

Humenick S et al. The maturation index of colostrum and milk (MICAM): A measurement of breast milk maturation. *J Nurs Meas* 2(2):169–186; 1994.

Hunt M et al. Black breast milk due to minocycline therapy. *Br J Dermatol* 134:943–944; 1996.

Hylander M et al. Human milk feedings and infection among very low birth weight infants. *Pediatrics* 102(3):E38; 1998.

Infante P et al. Use of goat's milk in patients with cow's milk allergy. *An Pediatr (Barc)* 59(2):138–142; 2003.

Innis S, Gilley J, Werker J. Are human long chain polyunsaturated fatty acids related to visual and neural development in breast-fed term infants? *J Pediatr* 139(4):532–538; 2001.

Institute of Medicine. *Dietary Reference Intakes for Calcium, Phosphorus, Magnesium, Vitamin D and Fluoride.* Washington, DC: National Academy Press, 288–313; 1997.

International Lactation Consultant Association (ILCA) (Walker M ed.). *Core Curriculum for Lactation Consultant Practice.* Sudbury, MA: Jones and Bartlett; 2002.

Ivarsson A et al. Breast-feeding protects against celiac disease. *Am J Clin Nutr* 75(5):914–921; 2002.

Jain A et al. How good is the evidence linking breastfeeding and intelligence? *Pediatrics* 109(6):1044–1053 Review; 2002.

Jeffery B et al. Determination of the effectiveness of inactivation of human immunodeficiency virus by Pretoria pasteurization. *J Trop Pediatr* 47(6):345–349; 2001.

Jeffery B et al. The effect of Pretoria pasteurization on bacterial contamination of hand-expressed human breastmilk. *J Trop Pediatr* 49(4):240–244; 2003.

Jelliffe DB, Jelliffe EP. *Human Milk in the Modern World.* New York: Oxford University Press; 1978.

Jeppesson D et al. T-lymphocyte subsets, thymic size and breastfeeding in infancy. *Pediatr Allergy Immunol* 15(2):127–132; 2004.

Keating J et al. Oral water intoxication in infants: An American epidemic. *Am J Dis Child* 145(9):985–990; 1991.

Kelly D, Coutts A. Early nutrition and the development of immune function in the neonate. *Proceedings of the Nutrition Society* 59(2):177–185; 2000.

Kent J. Breastmilk Calcium for the Pre-term Baby. Presentation, Human Lactation: Current Research and Clinical Implications, Amarillo, TX; October 22, 2004.

Kimpimaki T et al. Short-term exclusive breastfeeding predisposes young children with increased genetic risk of Type 1 diabetes to progressive beta-cell autoimmunity. *Diabetologia* 44(1):63–69; 2001.

Klein C. Nutrient requirements for preterm infant formulas. *J Nutr* 132(6 Suppl 1):1395S–1577S; 2002.

Kohler H et al. Antibacterial characteristics in the feces of breast-fed and formula-fed infants during the first year of life. *J Pediatr Gastroenterol Nutr* 34(2):188–193; 2002.

Koletzko B et al. Physiological aspects of human milk lipids. *Early Hum Dev* 65:S3–S18; 2001.

Koo W. Efficacy and safety of docosahexaenoic acid and arachidonic acid addition to infant formulas: Can one buy better vision and intelligence? Review. *J Am Coll Nutr* 22(2):101–107; 2003a.

Koo W et al. Reduced bone mineralization in infants fed palm olein-containing formula: A randomized, double-blinded, prospective trial. *Pediatrics* 111(5 Pt 1):1017–1023; 2003b.

Kreiter SR et al. Nutritional rickets in African American breast-fed infants. *J Pediatr* 137:153–157; 2000.

Kumar N et al. The specific role of isoflavones on estrogen metabolism in premenopausal women. *Cancer* 94(4):1166–1174; 2002.

Kuschel C, Harding J. Multicomponent fortified human milk for promoting growth in preterm infants. *Cochrane Database Syst Rev* 1:CD000343; 2004.

Kutner L. *Lactation Management Course.* Chalfont, PA: Breastfeeding Support Consultants Center for Lactation Education; 1996.

Lai C. *Variation in the composition of breastmilk and its fortification for pre-term babies.* Presentation, Human Lactation: Current Research and Clinical Implications. Amarillo, TX; October 22, 2004.

Lakdawala DR, Widdowson EM. Vitamin D in human milk. *Lancet* (8044):167–168; 1997.

La Leche League, International (LLLI). *Sunlight Deficiency, "Vitamin D," and Breastfeeding.* Schaumburg, IL; April 2003.

Landers S. Maximizing the benefits of human milk feeding for the preterm infant. *Pediatr Ann* 32(5):298–306; 2003.

Lawrence RA. *Breastfeeding: A Guide for the Medical Profession.* St. Louis, MO: Mosby; 1999.

Levine O et al. Risk factors for invasive pneumococcal disease in children: A population-based case-control study in North America. *Pediatrics* 103(3):E28; 1999.

Liepke C et al. Purification of novel peptide antibiotics from human milk. *Jnl Chromatogr Biomed Sci Appl* 752:369–377; 2001.

Lindberg T. Infantile colic and small intestinal function: A nutritional problem? *Acta Paediatr Suppl* 88(430):58–60; 1999.

Lindblad BS et al. Blood levels of critical amino acids in very low birthweight infants on a high human milk protein intake. *Acta Paediatr Scand* Suppl 296:24–27; 1982.

Lo C, Paris P, Holick M. Indian and Pakistani immigrants have the same capacity as Caucasians to produce vitamin D in response to ultraviolet irradiation. *Am J Clin Nutr* 44(5):683–685; 1986.

Lonnerdale B. Effects of maternal nutrition on human lactation. In Hamosh M and Goldman AS, (eds). *Human Lactation 2: Maternal and Environmental Factors.* New York: Plenum Press, 301–323; 1986.

Lucas A et al. A randomized multicentre study of human milk versus formula and later development in preterm infants. *Arch Dis Child* 70:F141–F146; 1994.

Lucas A et al. Breastmilk and subsequent intelligence quotient in children born preterm. *Lancet* 339:261–264; 1992.

Lucas A et al. Early diet in preterm babies and developmental status at 18 months. *Lancet* 335(8704):1477–1481; 1990a.

Lucas A. Breastmilk and neonatal NEC. *Lancet* 336:1519–1523; 1990b.

Mahmud M et al. Impact of breast feeding on *Giardia lamblia* infections in Bilbeis, Egypt. *Am J Trop Med Hyg* 65(3): 257–260; 2001.

Malvy DJ, Guinot C, Preziosi P et al. Relationship between vitamin D status and skin phototype in general adult population. *Photochem Photobiol* 71(4):466–469; 2000.

Marchini G, Linden A. Cholecystokinin, a satiety signal in newborn infants? *J Dev Physiol* 17(5):215–219; 1992.

Marild S et al. Protective effect of breastfeeding against urinary tract infection. *Acta Paediatr* 93(2):164–168; 2004.

Marini A et al. Effects of a dietary and environmental programme on the incidence of allergic symptoms in high atopic risk infants: Three years' follow-up. *Acta Paediatr Suppl* 414:1–21; 1996.

Marshall TA et al. Associations between intakes of fluoride from beverages during infancy and dental fluorosis of primary teeth. *J Am Coll Nutr* 23(2):108–116; 2004.

Martin J et al. Dependence of human milk essential fatty acids on adipose stores during lactation. *Am J Clin Nutr* 58:653–659; 1993.

Martin L et al. *Presence of Adiponectin and Leptin in Human Milk.* 2004 Pediatric Academic Societies' Annual Meeting, San Francisco; May 2, 2004.

Mason T et al. Breast feeding and the development of juvenile rheumatoid arthritis. *J Rheumatol* 22(6):1166–1170; 1995.

Mastretta E et al. Effect of lactobacillus GG and breast-feeding in the prevention of rotavirus nosocomial infection. *J Pediatr Gastroenterol Nutr* 35(4):527–531; 2002.

Matsuoka L, Wortsman J, Haddad JG, Kolm P, Hollis BW. Racial pigmentation and the cutaneous synthesis of vitamin D. *Arch Dermatol* 127(4):536–538; 1991.

McGuire W, Anthony M. Donor human milk versus formula for preventing necrotising enterocolitis in preterm infants: Systematic review. *Arch Dis Child* 88(1) SI:11–14: 2003.

Mead Johnson Inc. Nutramigen 16-oz. powder infant formula and Nutramigen 32-oz. ready-to-use infant formula recalled due to Spanish-language labeling error that could result in adverse health effects; 2001. Available at: http://www.mead johnson.com/about/pressreleas/nutramigenengpr.html.Access ed August 10, 2004.

Mead Johnson Inc. Enfamil with iron. Milk-based infant formula for the first 12 months; 2004. Available at: http://www. meadjohnson.com/products/hcp-infant/penfaml1.html. Accessed September 6, 2004.

Meier P et al. Mothers' milk feedings in the neonatal intensive care unit: Accuracy of the creamatocrit technique. *J Perinatol* 22(8):646–649; 2002.

Meinzen-Derr J et al. *The Role of Human Milk Feedings in Risk of Late-Onset Sepsis.* 2004 Pediatric Academic Societies' Annual Meeting, San Francisco, CA; May 1, 2004.

Mennella J, Beauchamp G. Maternal diet alters the sensory qualities of human milk and the nursling's behavior. *Pediatrics* 88:737–744; 1991a.

Mennella J, Beauchamp G. The transfer of alcohol to human milk. *N Engl J Med* 325:981–985; 1991b.

Michaelsen KF et al. The Copenhagen cohort study on infant nutrition and growth: Breastmilk intake, human milk macronutrient content and influencing factors. *Am J Clin Nutr* 59:600–611; 1994.

Michels D, Baumslag N. *Milk, Money and Madness: The Culture and Politics of Breastfeeding.* Westport, CT: Greenwood; 1995.

Minchin M. *Breastfeeding Matters: What We Need to Know about Breastfeeding.* Victoria, Australia: Alma Publications, 360; 1998.

Mitoulas L et al. Variation in fat, lactose and protein in human milk over 24 h and throughout the first year of lactation. *Br J Nutr* 88(1):29–37; 2002.

Monetini L. Bovine beta-casein antibodies in breast- and bottle-fed infants: Their relevance in Type 1 diabetes. *Diabetes Metab Res Rev* 17(1):51–54; 2001.

Mortensen E et al. The association between duration of breast-feeding and adult intelligence. *JAMA* 287(18):2365–2371; 2002.

Morton J. The role of the pediatrician in extended breastfeeding of the preterm infant. *Pediatr Ann* 32(5):308–316; 2003.

Nathavitharana K et al. IgA antibodies in human milk: Epidemiological markers of previous infections. *Arch Dis Child* 71:F192–F197; 1994.

National Alliance for Breastfeeding Advocacy (NABA). FDA alerts public regarding recall of powdered infant formula. Available at: www.naba-breastfeeding.org. Accessed May 18, 2004.

Nestlé. Nestlé Infant Formulas. Available at: www.verybestbaby. com/content/article.asp?section=bf&id=200192815178157571 7469. Accessed December 15, 2004.

Newburg D et al. Innate protection conferred by fucosylated oligosaccharides of human milk against diarrhea in breastfed infants. *Glycobiology* 14(3):253–263; 2004.

Newburg D. Oligosaccharides and glycoconjugates in human milk: Their role in host defense. *J Mammary Gland Biol Neoplasia* 1(3):271–283; 1996.

Nishiguchi T et al. Improvement of vitamin K status of breastfeeding infants with maternal supplement of vitamin K2 (MK40). *Semin Thromb Hemost* 28(6):533–538; 2002.

Nommsen L et al. Determinants of energy, proteins, lipid and lactose concentrations in human milk during the first 12 months of lactation: The DARLING study. *Am J Clin Nutr* 53: 457–465; 1991.

Oddy W et al. The effects of respiratory infections, atopy, and breastfeeding on childhood asthma. *Eur Respir J* 19(5):899–905; 2002.

Oddy W et al. Breast feeding and cognitive development in childhood: A prospective birth cohort study. *Paediatr Perinat Epidemiol* 17(1):81–90; 2003a.

Oddy W et al. Breast feeding and respiratory morbidity in infancy: A birth cohort study. *Arch Dis Child* 88(3):224–228; 2003b.

Oliveira V, Prell M. Sharing the economic burden: Who pays for WIC's infant formula? *USDA/ERS Amber Waves*, September 2004. Available at: www.ers.usda.gov/Amberwaves/September04/Features/infantformula.htm. Accessed December 8, 2004.

Orrhage K, Nord C. Factors controlling the bacterial colonization of the intestine in breastfed infants. *Acta Paediatr Suppl* 88(430):47–57; 1999.

Owen C et al. Infant feeding and blood cholesterol: A study in adolescents and a systematic review. *Pediatrics* 110(3): 597–608; 2002.

Pabst H et al. Differential modulation of the immune response by breast- or formula-feeding of infants. *Acta Paediatr* 86(12): 1291–1297; 1997.

Pabst H, Spady D. Effect of breast-feeding on antibody response to conjugate vaccine. *Lancet* 336(8710):269–270; 1990.

Park MJ et al. Bone mineral content is not reduced despite low vitamin D status in breast milk-fed infants versus cow's milk based formula-fed infants. *J Pediatr* 132(4):641–645; 1998.

Perez-Escamilla R et al. Maternal anthropometric status and lactation performance in a low-income Honduran population: Evidence for the role of infants. *Am J Clin Nutr* 61:528–534; 1995.

Perrilat F. Day-care, early common infections and childhood acute leukaemia: A multicentre French case-control study. *Brit Jnl Canc* 86(7):1064–1069; 2002.

Pickering L. Modulation of the immune system by human milk and infant formula containing nucleotides. *Pediatrics* 101(2):242–249; 1998.

Pisacane A et al. Breast-feeding and urinary tract infection. *J Pediatr* 120(1):87–89; 1992.

Pisacane A et al. Breastfeeding and multiple sclerosis. *Br J Med* 308:1411–1412; 1994.

Pizarro F et al. Iron status with different infant feeding regimens: Relevance to screening and prevention of iron deficiency. *J Pediatr* 118:687–692; 1991.

Potischman N, Troisi R. In-utero and early life exposures in relation to risk of breast cancer. *Cancer Causes and Control* 10(6):561–573; 1999.

Premji S et al. Evidence-based feeding guidelines for very low-birth-weight infants. *Adv Neonatal Care* 2(1):5–18; 2002.

Pugliese MF et al. Nutritional rickets in suburbia. *J Am Coll Nutr* 17:637–641; 1998.

Quan R et al. The effect of nutritional additives on anti-infective factors in human milk. *Clin Pediatr (Phila)* 33(6):325–328; 1994.

Raisler J et al. Breast-feeding and infant illness: A dose-response relationship? *Am J Public Health* 89(1):25–30; 1999.

Rao M et al. Effect of breastfeeding on cognitive development of infants born small for gestational age. *Acta Paediatr* 91(3):267–274; 2002.

Ravelli A et al. Infant feeding and adult glucose tolerance, lipid profile, blood pressure, and obesity. *Arch Dis Child* 82(3):248–252; 2000.

Renfrew M et al. Formula feed preparation: Helping reduce the risks; a systematic review. *Arch Dis Child* 88:855–858; 2003.

Ronneberg R, Skara B. Essential fatty acids in human colostrum. *Acta Paediatr* 81:779–783; 1992.

Ross Products Division (Abbott Laboratories). Customer service response to inquiry. 800-227-5767; March 2004.

Rubin D et al. Relationship between infant feeding and infectious illness: A prospective study of infants during the first year of life. *Pediatrics* 85:464–471; 1990.

Rudloff S, Lonnerdal B. Calcium retention from milk-based infant formulas, whey-hydrolysate formula, and human milk in weanling rhesus monkeys. *Am J Child Dis* 144:360–363; 1990.

Saarinen U, Kajosaari M. Breastfeeding as prophylaxis against atopic disease: Prospective follow-up study until 17 years old. *Lancet* 346:1065–1069; 1995.

Saavedra M et al. Infantile colic incidence and associated risk factors: A cohort study. *J Pediatr (Rio J)* 79(2):115–122; 2003.

Sala-Vila A et al. The source of long-chain PUFA in formula supplements does not affect the fatty acid composition of plasma lipids in full-term infants. *J Nutr* 134(4):868–873; 2004.

San Diego Breastfeeding Coalition (SDBC). Breastfeeding facts: Costs of infant feeding; December 2001. Available at: www.breastfeeding.org/bfacts/costs.html. Accessed November 10, 2003.

Sarkadi-Nagy E et al. Formula feeding potentiates docosahexaenoic and arachidonic acid biosynthesis in term and preterm baboon neonates. *J Lipid Res* 45(1):71–80; 2004.

Sauerwald T et al. Polyunsaturated fatty acid supply with human milk. Physiological aspects and in vivo studies of metabolism. *Adv Exp Med Biol* 478:261–270; 2000.

Sawatzki G. et al. Pitfalls in the design and manufacture of infant formulae. *Acta Paediatr* 402(Suppl):40–45; 1994.

Scanlon K, ed. *Final Report*. Vitamin D Expert Panel Meeting, Atlanta, GA, Oct. 11–12, 2001. Available at: www.cdc.gov/nccdphp/dnpa/nutrition/pdf/Vitamin_D_Expert_Panel_Meeting.pdf. Accessed June 2, 2004.

Scariati P et al. A longitudinal analysis of infant morbidity and the extent of breastfeeding in the US. *Pediatrics* 99(6): E5–E7; 1997.

Schanler R et al. Feeding strategies for premature infants: Beneficial outcomes of feeding fortified human milk versus preterm formula. *Pediatrics* 104(6 Pt 1):1150–1157; 1999.

Scheifele D et al. Breastfeeding and antibody responses to routine vaccination in infants. *Lancet* 340:1406; 1992.

Schroten H et al. Inhibition of adhesion of S-fimbriated *Escherichia coli* to buccal epithelial cells by human milk fat globule membrane components: A novel aspect of the protective function of mucins in the nonimmunoglobulin fraction. *Infect Immun* 60:2893–2899; 1992.

Schroten H et al. Inhibition of adhesion of S-fimbriated *E. coli* to buccal epithelial cells by human skim milk is predominantly mediated by mucins and depends on the period of lactation. *Acta Paediatr* 82:6–11; 1993.

Scragg R, Holdaway I, Singh V, Metcalf P, Baker J, Dryson E. Serum 25-hydroxyvitamin D3 is related to physical activity and ethnicity but not obesity in a multicultural workforce. *Aust N Z J Med* 25(3):218–223; 1995.

Shu X et al. Breast-feeding and risk of childhood acute leukemia. *J Natl Cancer Inst* 91(20):1765–1772; 1999.

Siegel-Itzkovich J. Police in Israel launch investigation into deaths of babies given formula milk. *BMJ* 327:1128; 2003.

Silfverdal S et al. Long term enhancement of the IgG2 antibody response to Haemophilus influenzae type B by breastfeeding. *Pediatr Infect Dis J* 21(9):816–821; 2002.

Sills I et al. Vitamin D deficiency rickets: Reports of its demise are exaggerated. *Clin Pediatr* (Phila) 33:491–493; 1994.

Singhal A et al. Early nutrition in preterm infants and later blood pressure: Two cohorts after randomised trials. *Lancet* 357(9254):413–419; 2001.

Singhal A et al. Breastmilk feeding and lipoprotein profile in adolescents born preterm: Follow-up of a prospective randomised study. *Lancet* 363(9421):1571–1578; 2004.

Slusher T et al. Promoting the exclusive feeding of own mother's milk through the use of hindmilk and increased maternal milk volume for hospitalized, low birth weight infants (< 1800 grams) in Nigeria: A feasibility study. *J Hum Lact* 19(2):191–198; 2003.

Smith M et al. Influence of breastfeeding on cognitive outcomes at age 6–8 years: Follow-up of very low birth weight infants. *Am J Eped* 158(11):1075–1082; 2003.

Smulevich V et al. Parental occupation and other factors and cancer risk in children: 1. Study methodology and non-occupational factors. *Int J Cancer* 83(6):712–717; 1999.

Specker B et al. Sunshine exposure and serum 25-hydroxyvitamin D concentrations in exclusively breastfed infants. *J Pediatr* 107:372–376; 1985.

Specker B et al. Low serum calcium and high parathyroid hormone levels in neonates fed "humanized" cow's milk-based formula. *Am J Dis Child* 145:941–945; 1991.

Specker B. Do North American women need supplemental vitamin D during pregnancy or lactation? *Am J Clin Nutr* 59(2 Suppl):484S–490S; discussion 490S–491S; 1994.

Sterken E. Director, INFACT, Canada. Personal e-mail correspondence; April 27, 2004.

Sterling L, Richardson J. Does breastfeeding protect against viral GI infections in children < 2 years old? *J Fam Pract* 52(10):805–806; 2003.

Strathern L. *Breastfeeding Status and Mother-Infant Separation Are Independent Predictors of Maternal Maltreatment.* American Academy of Pediatrics National Conference and Exhibition; November 3, 2003.

Tarcan A et al. Influence of feeding formula and breast milk fortifier on lymphocyte subsets in very low birth weight premature newborns. *Biol Neonate* 86(1):22–28; 2004.

Tariq S et al. The prevalence of and risk factors for atopy in early childhood: A whole population birth cohort study. *J Allergy Clin Immunol* 101(5):587–593; 1998.

Tarrats R et al. Varicella, ephemeral breastfeeding and eczema as risk factors for multiple sclerosis in Mexicans. *Acta Neurol Scand* 105(2)88–89; 2002.

Tellez A et al. Antibodies in mother's milk protect children against giardiasis. *Scand J Infect Dis* 35(5):322–325; 2003.

Thompson N et al. Early determinants of inflammatory bowel disease: Use of two national longitudinal birth cohorts. *Europ Jnl Gastroenter Hepatology* 12(1):25–30; 2000.

Thorsdottir I et al. Iron status at 12 months of age: Effects of body size, growth and diet in a population with high birth weight. *Eur J Clin Nutr* 57(4):505–513; 2003.

Toschke A et al. Overweight and obesity in 6- to 14-year-old Czech children in 1991: Protective effect of breast-feeding. *J Pediatr* 141(6):764–769; 2002.

Tran T et al. Effects of neonatal dietary manganese exposure on brain dopamine levels and neurocognitive functions. *Neurotoxicology* 23(4–5):645–651; 2002.

Tully M et al. Stories of success: The use of donor milk is increasing in North America. *J Hum Lact* 20(1):75–77; 2004.

Tyson J et al. Adaptation of feeding to a low fat yield in breastmilk. *Pediatrics* 89:215–220; 1992.

Udall J. Gastrointestinal host defense and necrotizing enterocolitis. *J Pediatr* 117:S33–S34; 1990.

Van de Perre P. Transfer of antibody via mother's milk. *Vaccine* 21(24):3374–3376; 2003.

Van Odijk J et al. Breastfeeding and allergic disease: A multidisciplinary review of the literature (1966–2001) on the mode of early feeding in infancy and its impact on later atopic manifestations. *Allergy* 58(9):833–843; 2003.

Van Veen H et al. The role of N-linked glycosylation in the protection of human and bovine lactoferrin against tryptic proteolysis. *Eur J Biochem* 271(4):678–684; 2004.

Vieira G et al. Child feeding and diarrhea morbidity. *J Pediatr* (Rio J) 79(5):449–454; 2003.

Viverge D et al. Variations in oligosaccharides and lactose in human milk during the first week of lactation. *J Pediatr Gastroenterol Nutr* 11:361–364; 1990.

Wagner C et al. Efficacy of maternal vitamin D (VitD) supplementation during lactation. *ABM News & Views* 9(3):19; 2003.

Wagner C et al. Special properties of human milk. *Clin Pediatr* 35:283–293; 1996.

Walker M. *Selling Out Mothers and Babies: Marketing of Breast Milk Substitutes in the USA*. Weston, MA: NABA REAL; 2001.

Walker-Smith J. Hypoallergenic formulas: Are they really hypoallergenic? Review. *Ann Allergy Asthma Immunol* 90(6 Suppl 3):112–114; 2003.

Wariyar U et al. Six years' experience of prophylactic oral vitamin K. *Arch Dis Child Fetal Neonatal Ed* 82(1):F64–68; 2000.

Weimer J. Economic benefits: A review and analysis. Economic Research Service, USDA. *Food Assistance and Nutrition Research Report* 13; March 2001.

Wight NE. Donor human milk for preterm infants. *J Perinatol* 21(4):249–254; 2001.

Williams C et al. Stereoacuity at age 3.5 y in children born full-term is associated with prenatal and postnatal dietary factors: A report from a population-based cohort study. *Am J Clin Nutr* 73(2):316–322; 2001.

Wold AE, Adlerberth I. Breast feeding and the intestinal microflora of the infant: Implications for protection against infectious diseases. *Adv Exp Med Biol* 478:77–93; 2000.

Wolf J. Low breastfeeding rates and public health in the US. *Am J Pub Health* 93(12):2001–2010; 2003.

Woolridge MW et al. Do changes in pattern of breast usage alter the baby's nutrient intake? *Lancet* 336:395–397; 1990.

World Health Organization (WHO). *Infant and young child nutrition*. WHA54.2, agenda item 13.1; 2001. Available at: www.who.int/gb/EB_WHA/PDF/WHA54/ea54r2.pdf. Accessed September 13, 2004.

World Health Organization (WHO). *HIV and Infant Feeding: Framework for Priority Action*. WHO; 2003.

World Health Organization (WHO)/UNICEF. *Breastfeeding Management and Promotion in a Baby-Friendly Hospital*. New York: UNICEF; 1993.

Xiao X et al. Epidermal growth factor concentrations in human milk, cow's milk and cow's milk-based infant formulas. *Chin Med J (Engl)* 115(3):451–454; 2002.

Yinyaem P et al. Gastrointestinal manifestations of cow's milk protein allergy during the first year of life. *J Med Assoc Thai* 86(2):116–123; 2003.

Young T et al. Type 2 diabetes mellitus in children—prenatal and early infancy risk factors among native Canadians. *Arch Ped Adol Med* 146(7):651–655; 2002.

▶ BIBLIOGRAPHY

Ainsworth MDS. Blehar MC, Waters E, Wall S. *Patterns of Attachment: A Psychological Study of the Strange Situation*. Hillsdale, NJ: Erlbaum; 1978.

Angier N. Mother's milk found to be potent cocktail of hormones. *New York Times* B5; May 24, 1994.

Arnold L. Human milk for premature infants: An important health issue. *J Hum Lact* 9:121–123; 1993.

Bowlby J. Separation: anxiety and anger. In *Attachment and Loss*. London: Hogarth Press; 1973. New York: Basic Books; Harmondsworth: Penguin, Vol. 2; 1975.

Bowlby J. Attachment. In *Attachment and Loss*. London: Hogarth Press; New York: Basic Books, 2nd edition of Vol 1; 1982.

Calvo E et al. Iron status in exclusively breast-fed infants. *Pediatrics* 90:375–379; 1992.

Chang Y et al. Hypocalcemia in nonwhite breast-fed infants. *Clin Pediatr* 31:695–698; 1992.

Ellis M et al. Anaphylaxis after ingestion of a recently introduced hydrolyzed whey protein formula. *J Pediatrics* 118:74–77; 1991.

Estrada B. Human milk and the prevention of infection. *Infect Med* 20(6):270; 2003.

Genze, Boroviczeny O et al. Fatty acid composition of human milk during the first month after term and preterm delivery. *Eur J Pediatr* 156:142–147; 1997.

Gessner B et al. Nutritional rickets among breast-fed Black and Alaska native children. *Alaska Med* 39:72–74, 1997.

Grover M et al. Effect of human milk prostaglandins and lactoferrin on respiratory syncytial virus and rotavirus. *Acta Paediatr* 86:315–316; 1997.

Grulee CG et al. Breast and artificial feeding. *JAMA* 103(10):735; 1934.

Haschke F et al. Iron nutrition and growth of breast- and formula-fed infants during the first nine months of life. *J Pediatr Gastroenterol Nutr* 16:151–156; 1993.

Heiskanen K et al. Risk of low vitamin B_6 status in infants breast-fed exclusively beyond six months. *Pediatr Gastroenterol Nutr* 23:38–44; 1996.

Hey B. Tap-water supply safety questioned. *AAP News* 11(11):1; 1995.

Hopkinson J et al. Milk production by mothers of premature infants: Influence of cigarette smoking. *Pediatrics* 90:934–938; 1992.

Horwood L, Fergusson D. Breastfeeding and later cognitive and academic outcomes. *Pediatrics* 101:1; 1998.

Institute of Medicine (National Academy of Sciences). *Nutrition During Lactation*. Washington, DC: National Academy Press; 1991.

Irvine C et al. The potential adverse effects of soybean phytoestrogens in infant feeding. *N Z Med J* 108:208–209; 1995.

Jensen RG. *The Lipids of Human Milk*. Boca Raton, FL: CRC Press; 1989.

Kuhne T et al. Maternal vegan diet causing a serious infantile neurological disorder due to vitamin B_{12} deficiency. *Eur J Pediatr* 150:205–208; 1991.

Kunz C et al. Nutritional and biochemical properties of human milk, part 1: General aspects, proteins, and carbohydrates. *Clin Perinatol* 26(2):307–333; 1999.

Lebenthal E ed. *Textbook of Gastroenterology and Nutrition in Early Infancy.* 2nd ed. Raven Press, chapter by Goldman & Goldblum; 1989.

Lin T et al. Longitudinal changes in Ca, Mg, Fe, Cu and Zn in breast milk of women in Taiwan over a lactation period of one year. *Biol Trace Element Res* 62:31–41; 1998.

Lucas A et al. Randomized outcome trial of human milk fortification and developmental outcome in preterm infants. *Am J Clin Nutr* 64:142–151; 1996.

Lucas A, Cole T. Breastmilk and neonatal necrotising enterocolitis. *Lancet* 336:1519–1523; 1990.

Malpas T et al. Neonatal abstinence syndrome following abrupt cessation of breastfeeding. *N Z Med J* 112:12–13, 1999.

Nettleton JA. Are N-3 fatty acids essential nutrients for fetal and infant development? *J Am Diet Assoc* 93:58–64; 1993.

Oldaeus G et al. Extensively and partially hydrolyzed infant formulas for allergy prophylaxis. *Arch Dis Child* 77:4–10; 1997.

Ortega R et al. Ascorbic acid levels in maternal milk: Differences with respect to ascorbic acid status during the third trimester of pregnancy. *Br J Nutr* 79:431–437; 1998.

Quinsex P et al. The importance of measured intake in assessing exposure of breast-fed infants to organochlorines. *Eur J Clin Nutr* 50(7):438–444; 1996.

Rodriguez-Palmero M et al. Nutritional and biochemical properties of human milk: II. Lipids, micronutrients, and bioactive factors. *Clin Perinatol* 26(2):335–359; 1999.

Sankaran K et al. A randomized, controlled evaluation of two commercially available human breast milk fortifiers in healthy preterm neonates. *J Am Diet Assoc* 96:1145–1149; 1996.

Setchell K et al. Exposure of infants to phytoestrogens from soy-based infant formula. *Lancet* 350:23–27; 1997.

Silfverdal S et al. Protective effect of breastfeeding on invasive Haemophilus influenzae infection: A case-control study in Swedish preschool children. *Int J Epidemiol* 26:443–450; 1997.

Voepel-Lewis T et al. Evaluation of simethicone for the treatment of abdominal discomfort in infants. *J Clin Anesth* 10:91–94; 1998.

Williams C. *Milk and Murder.* Speech to Singapore Rotary Club, 1939. Papers of Cicely Williams in Wellcome Library for the History and Understanding of Medicine, 183 Euston Road, London NW1 2BE, PP/CDW/B.2/2.

Wright A et al. Breastfeeding and lower respiratory tract illness in the first year of life. *Br J Med* 299:946–949; 1989.

Yolken R et al. Human milk mucin inhibits rotavirus replication and prevents experimental gastroenteritis. *J Clin Invest* 90:1984–1991; 1992.

CHAPTER
10

IMPURITIES IN HUMAN MILK

Much concern and confusion exist when a lactating woman consumes medications or social toxicants or when she is exposed to environmental contaminants. When impurities are present in the mother's milk, the most important consideration is the effect a particular substance has on the breastfeeding infant. The molecular weight or binding capacity of some impurities does not allow them to enter the mother's milk. In many cases, substances are excreted into the milk in low concentrations and pose no danger to the infant. When a substance passes into the milk, the infant's GI tract often offers protection by either not absorbing it or by altering it. The infant may experience some adverse effects, however, from contaminants that pass into the milk and are not altered or eliminated by his GI system.

Drugs ingested by the mother can travel through her milk to the baby, as can social toxicants such as tobacco, caffeine, alcohol, marijuana, cocaine, and other mood-changing drugs. Any environmental contaminants present in the mother's milk can pass on to her baby. The International Lactation Consultant Association has issued a position statement on breastfeeding and environmental contaminants in human milk. It is available on the ILCA Web site at www.ilca.org.

KEY TERMS

alcohol	half-life
amphetamines	heroin
breast implants	marijuana
caffeine	nicotine and tobacco
cocaine	over-the-counter
DDE	phencyclidine hydro-
DDT	chloride
detoxify	polybrominated diphenyl
drugs of abuse	ethers
environmental contaminant	social toxicant

MEDICATIONS

Almost any substance that is present in the mother's blood will also be present in some amount in her milk. Not long ago, experts believed that if a woman was breastfeeding she should take no medications. If she needed medications, she should not breastfeed. As experts have learned more about breastfeeding and human milk, they have adopted a more moderate approach toward medications and breastfeeding.

When reviewing the advisability of a particular substance, the degree to which it is excreted into the mother's milk and its possible effects on the infant should be considered. Potential risk to the infant will depend on whether pediatric medicine uses the same drug. Additionally, a medication considered safe during pregnancy is not necessarily safe during lactation. During pregnancy, the maternal liver and kidney **detoxify** and excrete substances for the fetus through the placenta. During lactation, the infant must handle the drug on his own.

Among the drugs on which information is available, few are **contraindicated** in breastfeeding according to the AAP (2001). Generally, a relative infant dose of under ten percent is considered safe (Hale, 2004). A breastfeeding mother does need to use caution in taking medications, however. She should consult the baby's caregiver before taking any prescription drug, over-the-counter medication, or supplemental vitamins. A drug that is safe for the fetus and the breastfeeding infant may still affect the mother's letdown reflex, milk production, or milk secretion. The mother can remind the prescribing caregiver that she is breastfeeding and confirm the drug's advisability.

Infant Exposure

The effect of any substance on the breastfed infant is of primary importance when the mother needs medication. One consideration is whether the medication will pass into the mother's milk and be absorbed in the baby's GI tract. Another is whether the infant can be exposed safely to the substance as it appears in the milk. Understanding the substance's characteristics can help resolve the dilemma of both healthcare worker and mother when the need for a medication arises.

FIGURE 10.1
Potential for infant exposure to substances in human milk.

Factors to consider

◆ Size of the molecules in the substance (molecules over 800–1000 daltons have difficulty passing through alveolar cells).
◆ Solubility of the substance in water or fat (fat diffuses more easily into milk).
◆ Binding capacity of the substance with protein.
◆ pH of the substance.
◆ The milk/plasma ratio.
◆ Route of administration (oral, intramuscular, intravenous).
◆ Short- or long-acting version of the drug.
◆ Activity or inactivity of components of the substance.
◆ Rate of detoxification in the mother's system.
◆ Whether the substance accumulates in the mother's system.
◆ Duration of use.
◆ Time substance is ingested relative to a feeding.
◆ Number of days postpartum when substance is consumed.
◆ Age and size of the infant (preterm, full-term, older baby).
◆ Amount of milk the infant consumes (exclusively breastfed or supplemented).
◆ Absorption of the substance in the infant's gut.
◆ Safety in giving the substance to the infant directly.

Figure 10.1 shows the factors that influence the complex process by which a substance passes from the mother's bloodstream into her milk and eventually reaches the infant. Many factors influence the level of a substance found in the infant's bloodstream. Some relate to the infant and others to characteristics of the drug itself.

How Soon After Birth

One consideration is how soon after birth the mother takes a medication. The junctures between the alveolar cells in the mammary glands are open for several days postpartum. Thus, more of a medication can penetrate the mother's milk at that time than in later weeks (Hale, 2002b). The amount of milk a baby consumes relates directly to the amount of a substance he will receive through the milk. The newborn consumes small quantities of colostrum in the first few days, so the amount of other substances ingested would be small. A baby who additionally receives artificial baby milk or solid foods will receive a lesser amount of a substance than will an infant who is breastfed exclusively. The volume of human milk consumed by a supplemented infant is less and possibly is diluted by the supplemental food in the infant's system.

Gestational Age

The baby's age and size are also factors. A premature infant assimilates substances received through the mother's milk differently than does a full-term infant or older baby. An older and larger baby may be able to metabolize a substance more effectively, and therefore the substance will have less effect on his system. The baby's age will also determine his ability to detoxify a substance with his liver and excrete it in the urine or stool. Because an infant's liver is immature in the early days postpartum, it may be difficult for him to excrete even small amounts of a substance. A drug that depends on the liver for detoxification could pose a risk if not metabolized effectively.

Resistance to Detoxification

If a substance is particularly resistant to being destroyed in the infant's GI tract, it would pose a danger to the infant as it accumulates to toxic levels. On the other hand, some drugs must be administered by injection because they are destroyed in the infant's GI tract when taken orally. These drugs may reduce the infant's **systemic** absorption of the drug but could cause GI symptoms such as diarrhea. Some substances compete for protein-binding sites, displacing other toxic substances that then can migrate to other parts of the body. Sulfadiazine, an antibacterial agent, may displace bilirubin and cause it to flow freely in the infant's blood during the first weeks postpartum. This increases the risk of jaundice for the baby.

Over-the-Counter Medications

Questions often arise about over-the-counter medications such as pain relievers, cough medicines, cold remedies, suppositories, antacids, diarrhea remedies, and herbal preparations. Because these medications are more accessible than prescription drugs, there is a greater possibility mothers will use them. You may receive calls questioning their potential risk to the baby and to breastfeeding. Many cold remedies contain antihistamines to dry up nasal secretions. Products containing pseudoephedrine can lower mothers' milk production by up to 24 percent (Aljazaf, 2003). Antihistamines also may enter human milk and produce sedation in the baby.

Any person taking over-the-counter medications needs to exercise caution in taking drugs and other substances when there is the possibility of interaction among prescription drugs, over-the-counter medications, herbs, and vitamins. Mothers are encouraged to discuss this potential with their baby's caregiver to determine the safety in taking an over-the-counter drug. Physicians need to know the mother's present consumption of drugs, vitamins, herbs, or other substances before prescribing any additional medication.

Minimizing Effects of Medications

Drugs present in the mother's milk may affect milk production or secretion. Some may lower production, and others may stimulate it. They can also cause reactions in the infant. The mother can watch for unusual changes in her baby's behavior, feeding, and sleeping patterns such as fussiness, lethargy, rash, vomiting, or diarrhea. A mother can minimize the effects of drugs in her milk in a number of ways.

Schedule Around Breastfeeding

Adjusting her schedule for taking the drug will result in the least amount of drug possible entering the milk. Because of the usual absorption rates and peak levels of most drugs, the mother will want to take the medication toward the end of the dose cycle. A general rule may be to take the drug immediately after nursing or three to four hours before the next feeding. Depending on the drug, she may need to stop breastfeeding while the drug is at its peak level in her milk. She can take a fat-soluble drug at bedtime, when the baby usually does not feed as often.

Avoid Long Half-Life

Advise mothers to avoid medications with long plasma **half-life**. This form is more difficult for the baby to eliminate and could build up over time to higher concentrations in the baby's plasma. It usually requires enzyme action in the liver in order to metabolize it, thus increasing the possibility of its accumulation in the baby.

Select Least Offensive Drug

When possible, the caregiver can choose a drug that produces the least amount in the milk and has the least potential for causing problems. If a mother must take a medication that has not been tested for safety during lactation, she can discuss her options with her baby's caregiver. You can also provide her with information from a source such as Hale's *Medications and Mother's Milk* or *Clinical Therapy in Breastfeeding Patients*. See Table 10.1 for the safety of various drugs.

TABLE 10.1
Safety of Medications with Breastfeeding

◆ Breastfeeding contraindicated.	◆ Anticancer drugs (antimetabolites). ◆ Radioactive substances (stop breastfeeding temporarily).
◆ Continue breastfeeding: Side effects possible; monitor the baby for drowsiness.	◆ Psychiatric drugs and anticonvulsants.
◆ Continue breastfeeding: Use alternative drug if possible. ◆ Continue breastfeeding: Monitor baby for jaundice.	◆ Chloramphenicol, tetracyclines, metronidazole. ◆ Quinolone antibiotics (e.g., ciprofloxacin). ◆ Sulphonamides, dapsone. ◆ Sulfamethoxazole + trimethoprim (co-trimoxazole).
◆ Continue breastfeeding: Use alternative drug (may inhibit lactation).	◆ Estrogens (including estrogen-containing contraceptives). ◆ Thiazide diuretics. ◆ Ergometrine.
◆ Continue breastfeeding: Safe in usual dosage; monitor baby.	◆ Most commonly used drugs. ◆ Analgesics and antipyretics—Short courses of paracetamol, acetylsalicylic acid, ibuprofen; occasional doses of morphine and pethidine. ◆ Antibiotics—Ampicillin, amoxicillin, cloxacillin, and other penicillins. Erythromycin. ◆ Antituberculars, antileporotics (see dapsone earlier). ◆ Antimalarials (except mefloquine), anthelminthics, antifungals. ◆ Bronchodilators (e.g., salbutamol), corticosteroids, antihistamines, antacids, drugs for diabetes, most antihypertensives, digoxin. ◆ Nutritional supplements of iron, iodine, and vitamins.

Source: Breastfeeding and Maternal Medication, Recommendations for Drugs in the Eight WHO Model List of Essential Drugs, Division of Diarrhoeal and Acute Respiratory Disease Control, UNICEF/WHO, 1995. Printed with permission.

Counseling Mothers about Medications

Your role with mothers is to share information and point out options. Mothers will often contact you with questions and concerns about the safety of a particular medication while they are breastfeeding. Unless you have prescribing privileges, confine your role to encouraging the mother to be an active health consumer. She needs to take responsibility for making decisions and taking specific action. You can help the mother pose questions and stimulate her thinking so that she will explore the facts and base her decisions on accurate and sound information. It is important that you present all drug information objectively and not in a manner that appears to be recommending or advising the mother about the safety of a particular medication. Encourage the mother to consult her physician regarding these questions and to share any concerns or questions she may have.

In the absence of appropriate medical licensure, it is extremely important that you use caution in how you share drug information with a mother. You run the risk of placing yourself in a vulnerable legal position if you deviate from facts or attempt to interpret them. When a mother expresses doubts or fears about a medication, you can discuss objectively the options available to her. After clarifying her situation, issues to consider may include:

◆ Is there an alternative course that would avoid any medication?

◆ Can she use other, safer medications or medical procedures?

◆ Do the benefits of the medication to the mother outweigh possible risk to the baby?

◆ Does exposure to the medication pose less risk to the baby than the use of artificial baby milk?

◆ Would another medical opinion be helpful?

FIGURE 10.2
Factors to consider in drug literature.

Factor	Comments
Newness of the data	There is much case reporting of drugs used during breastfeeding that provides newer data, whereas most original data regarding drugs in human milk were published between 1920 and 1960.
Human versus animal data	Animal data may or may not apply to human lactation. The peer review process will assist in determining this relevance.
Completeness of screening	The reader should always look for whether the researcher mentions studying metabolites of the particular drug in question. If metabolites were not studied, justification is needed. Usually, researchers will justify that within their study. Consulting a pharmacologist will help you understand the significance and quality of a study about drugs.
Isolated cases	Much of the original data about a particular substance may be based on only 1 or 2 case reports, with insufficient controls. This results because ethics prevent experiments on humans. Clinicians are left to make decisions without complete data to guide them. If a mother needs a medication and wants to continue breastfeeding, physicians sometimes allow it, monitor it, and then write up the experience to share with colleagues. Such case reports have no control, but the medical community has at least a small amount of information instead of none. One cannot conclude universal safety from one case report. However, physicians who support breastfeeding even in difficult circumstances may be less reluctant to try a drug instead of stopping breastfeeding. You can encourage mothers taking newer or little-used medications to register at the International Registry for Lactation Research to benefit other mothers and babies by providing milk samples for research. Mothers can register at www.neonatal.ttushc.edu/lact/.
Sampling technique	Older studies may show random sampling of milk rather than samples based on drug peak and trough levels. Trough is the lowest blood or milk level achieved by the drug during its dosing period. Women who are given gentamicin, for instance, are tested every 3 days or so to see what the highest and lowest levels of the drug are in the blood. This is done by testing an hour after a dose and an hour before the next dose is due. The timing of testing is different in different drugs. Some drugs have a narrow safety range, so it is important to keep the dose within that range. Although newer research is less problematic in this area, it is still important that you consider this when reading such research.
Personal correspondence	Although much personal correspondence is useful, the reader should be aware that the data may not be available for public inspection and could be biased. Often, personal correspondence is research in progress that lends support to the article at hand.
Speculation	Speculation by the author of the original article may be interpreted as fact after several review articles have been written. This can be a problem, and readers should always beware of speculation.

Locating Drug Information

Information about the advisability of taking a drug during breastfeeding needs to come from a reliable source. Become acquainted with each drug group and its potential risks and benefits. You will usually need to determine the drug's generic name in order to locate it in a drug listing. Recommended sources are *Medications and Mothers' Milk*, Hale (2004) mentioned above; *Clinical Therapy in Breastfeeding Patients*, Hale and Berens (2002); *Drug Therapy and Breastfeeding*, Hale and Ilett (2002); and *Drugs in Pregnancy and Lactation*, Briggs, Freeman, and Yaffe (2003).

When presenting information to mothers, read the facts to her exactly as they appear on the page, citing the reference for the information. As an IBCLC, you are not medically qualified to interpret the data unless you are also a prescribing clinician. Confine yourself to the facts only. If you have a personal experience or opinion that conflicts with the research, do not share this with a mother. When you share studies and research in an appropriate, objective manner, mothers can use the information to make informed decisions.

Critical Reading of Drug Studies

A legitimate evaluation of medical information must go beyond personal observation and stand the test of scientific criticism. The effectiveness of a drug or treatment should be compared with other treatments, and its safety should be determined after large numbers of observations over long periods. The burden of proof rests with the researcher—the one who is recommending a particular drug or treatment—especially if it involves a substance that is not well established in medical practice.

Many review articles written in both lay and professional publications are helpful in providing background information on lactation and impurities in human milk. When reading such articles, carefully consider each study's methods and conclusions. Figure 10.2 identifies factors to consider when reading literature about drugs. See Chapter 27 for an in-depth discussion of research methods.

▶ SOCIAL TOXICANTS

Social mood-changing toxicants—tobacco, coffee, tea, alcohol, marijuana, and other drugs—are used in varying degrees in most cultures. It is important to recognize that the use of recreational drugs is not an issue of class, race, or economics. Caution mothers about substances that can negatively affect the quality or quantity of their milk.

Nicotine and Tobacco

A breastfeeding mother who smokes cigarettes, even if only occasionally, may possibly affect her baby more by the smoke the baby inhales than by the small amount of nicotine present in her milk. If a mother chooses to continue smoking, she should not smoke in the baby's presence. She can time her breastfeeding to minimize the baby's exposure in her milk, for example, smoking after a feeding rather than just before it. Smoking is not just an issue if a mother is breastfeeding. Babies who receive artificial baby milks are also exposed to undesirable chemicals in their parents' cigarette smoke without the protective benefits of their mother's milk (Minchin, 1991; Newman, 1990).

Effects on the Baby

Children whose parents smoke in the home have a greater susceptibility to respiratory ailments, including asthma, than do children of nonsmokers (Jang, 2004; Rizzi, 2004; Shiva, 2003). Exposure to secondhand cigarette smoke is linked to increased incidence of otitis media (Owen, 1993). Babies whose mothers smoke are at increased risk of sudden infant death syndrome (SIDS) (Kahn, 2003; Daltveit, 2003; L'Hoir, 1998). The mother and other members of the baby's household need to be discouraged from smoking.

Nicotine in the mother's milk can cause fussiness, diarrhea, shock, vomiting, rapid heart rate, and restlessness in an infant. The mother may experience a decrease in milk production due to lowered prolactin levels, leading to poor infant weight gain. Twenty cigarettes daily can lead to relatively high levels of fat-soluble nicotine in the mother's milk, which can be harmful to the baby and cause vomiting and nausea. It can also diminish the mother's milk secretion, lower the fat concentration in her milk, or inhibit her letdown reflex if the mother smokes immediately before feeding her baby (Hopkinson, 1992; Vio, 1991).

Any of these factors could be a cause of slow infant weight gain. Ask mothers of slow-gaining babies if they smoke, if they have not already volunteered the information. Those who smoke should be encouraged to quit or to reduce the amount of cigarettes they smoke. Mothers who smoke should be told that they will need twice the usual intake of vitamin C because smoking interferes with the body's ability to use that vitamin (Kim, 2004; Valachovicova, 2003).

Smoking cessation programs, such as the use of a nicotine patch and chewing gum for nicotine withdrawal, can be used by nursing mothers (Hale, 2002a; Ilett, 2003). The nicotine level is about one-third that of cigarettes. In order to continue nursing safely, mothers who are on such a program cannot smoke while using a

TABLE 10.2

Common Sources of Caffeine

Product	Caffeine in Milligrams	Product	Caffeine in Milligrams
Hot Drinks		**Soft Drinks (cont.)**	
Coffee (16 oz) Starbucks	550	Diet Dr. Pepper	37
Coffee (12 oz) Starbucks	375	Pepsi Cola	37
Coffee (8 oz) Starbucks	250	Royal Crown Cola	36
Coffee, non-gourmet (8 oz)	136	Diet Rite Cola	34
Maxwell House (8 oz)	110	Diet Pepsi	34
Coffee, instant (8 oz)	95	Coca-Cola	34
Caffe Latte or Cappuccino Starbucks	70	Sunkist Orange	0
Espresso, double (2 oz) Starbucks	70	7-Up	0
Coffee, decaf (16 oz) Starbucks	15	Diet 7-Up	0
Coffee, decaf (8–12 oz) Starbucks	10	RC-100	0
Coffee, decaf, nongourmet (8 oz)	5	Diet Sunkist Orange	0
Espresso, decaf (1 oz) Starbucks	5	Patio Orange	0
Tea, leaf or bag (8 oz)	50	Fanta Orange	0
Tea, green or instant (8 oz)	30	Fresca	0
Tea, bottled (12 oz)	15	Hires Root Beer	0
Tea, decaf (8 oz)	5	**Pain Relievers (standard dose)**	
Chocolate, dark, bittersweet, or semi-sweet (1 oz)	20	Excedrin	130
Chocolate milk mix (1 oz)	5	Anacin	65
Cocoa or hot chocolate (8 oz)	5	Midol	65
Water, caffeinated (Edge20) (8 oz)	70	Plain aspirin (any brand)	0
Nonprescription Stimulants (standard dose)		**Diuretics (standard dose)**	
Caffedrine capsules	200	Aqua-Ban	200
NoDoz tablets, maximum strength	200	Pennathene H20ff	200
Vivarin tablets, maximum strength	200	Pre-Mens Forte	100
NoDoz, regular strength	100	**Cold Remedies (standard dose)**	
Soft Drinks		Coryban-D	30
Mountain Dew	55	Triaminicin	30
Mello Yello	51	Dristan	32
Tab	44	**Weight-Control Aids (daily)**	
Shasta Cola	42	Dexatrim	200
Dr. Pepper	38	Dietac	200
		Prolamine	280

As tested by Consumers Union for the October 1981 issue of *Consumer Reports.* Formulations can change.
Sources: Consumers Union of United States, Inc., Mount Vernon, NY 10550—reprinted by permission of *Consumer Reports,* October 1981; Caffeine: The Inside Scoop, Nutrition Action Newsletter, December 1996.

nicotine patch or chewing gum because this would further increase the baby's level of exposure to nicotine.

Caffeine

Caffeine is present in coffee, tea, cola, and chocolate—substances often consumed in large quantities in Western culture. Breastfeeding mothers can safely ingest moderate amounts of these foods. The amount of caffeine present in human milk varies dramatically from mother to mother and according to the timing of ingestion. Some women appear to have low absorption and efficient metabolism and excretion, so that levels of caffeine in their milk remain low. Therefore, each mother-infant pair is unique with respect to caffeine response. Acceptable levels of ingestion for the mother depend on her baby's reaction.

Effects on the Baby

Mothers can watch for signs of sensitivity in their babies, such as wakefulness, hyperactivity, and colicky behavior. These symptoms may indicate an excessive amount of caffeine in the mother's milk. Newborn and preterm babies are particularly susceptible to caffeine's effects, because their immature digestive systems take longer to eliminate caffeine from the body.

Some breastfeeding infants have reacted to their mothers' consuming 6 to 8 servings of caffeinated beverage daily. Symptoms disappeared within 1 week after caffeine was discontinued (Rivera-Calimlim, 1987). Ryu found in a study that as many as 5 cups of coffee with 100 mg of caffeine each did not result in detectable infant caffeine levels (Ryu, 1985b). However, in another study with mothers consuming 750 mg of caffeine, there were traces of caffeine as late as 9 days afterwards (Ryu, 1985a).

Sources of Caffeine

Table 10.2 identifies the most common sources of caffeine. Caution women about high intake of herbal tea as a substitute for caffeinated drinks. Herbal teas may contain active ingredients that can pass into human milk and cause toxic effects. Cathartics such as buckhorn bark and senna may result in cramps and diarrhea in the infant. Chamomile tea may sensitize the infant to ragweed pollen and cause an allergic reaction. Sage, parsley, and peppermint inhibit lactation; women often use them for weaning (Humphrey, 2003).

Alcohol

Alcohol rapidly enters a woman's bloodstream, and subsequently her milk. Experts have not defined a safe level of alcohol consumption for the breastfeeding mother. We do know that alcohol achieves the same level in the mother's milk that it does in blood (Silva, 1993). Excessive amounts completely block the release of oxytocin and prevent letdown from occurring.

Generally, the consumption of one or two drinks socially is not a contraindication for breastfeeding. A mother may ask when it is safe to nurse again after having consumed alcohol. She can be told that she can breastfeed when she feels normal again, that is, when the effects of the alcohol have worn off. By this time, levels will be quite low (Hale, 2004). Elimination guidelines for Motherisk, a Canadian maternal health program, recommend that mothers wait at least two hours per drink to avoid unnecessary infant exposure (Ho, 2001).

Of greater concern than an occasional drink is the mother's pattern of drinking. Excessive alcohol consumption can limit parental effectiveness and result in life-threatening conditions for the infant. If the mother reports drinking frequently or drinking more than one or two drinks in succesion, or if you suspect alcohol is a problem for her, she may need to be referred for help. Local alcohol and substance abuse treatment centers, drug abuse counselors, and Alcoholics Anonymous meetings are valuable resources. Impairment of her judgment and her ability to care for her baby may have risks to the baby just as serious, if not more so, as the actual physical exposure to alcohol in her milk.

Effects on the Baby

Alcohol consumption can cause sleepiness in the baby and affect his development and linear growth. One study found that babies of mothers who consumed the equivalent of four drinks daily had psychomotor scores one standard deviation below the **mean** (Little, 1989). A later study was not able to replicate these results and recommended studying older children to better determine outcomes (Little, 2002). Babies consume less milk after mothers ingest an alcoholic beverage (Mennella, 1991). They also have significantly less active sleep after exposure to alcohol in their mother's milk (Mennella, 2001).

Drugs of Abuse

Substance abuse is a concern to neonatologists, who see an increasing number of infants suffering from the damaging effects of drug exposure. Prenatal use of recreational drugs is associated with fetal distress, lower Apgar scores, impaired fetal growth, impaired neurodevelopmental outcome, and acute infant withdrawal (Wagner, 1998).

Breastfeeding mothers should avoid all drugs of abuse. The AAP Committee on Drugs (2001) categorizes drugs of abuse as contraindicated during breastfeeding. These drugs include marijuana, amphetamines such as ecstasy, cocaine, heroin, and phencyclidine hydrochloride (angel dust). Drugs of abuse are hazardous both to the breastfeeding infant and to the health of the mother.

Marijuana

Marijuana can have a direct effect on the mother's ability to produce sufficient quantities of milk by lowering or inhibiting prolactin levels. There are no documented long-term effects for breastfed babies whose mothers use marijuana. Infants exposed to marijuana through their mothers' milk may test positive for up to three weeks (Hale, 2004). The AAP categorizes marijuana as contraindicated in breastfeeding mothers.

Amphetamines

Amphetamines are stimulants that quickly transfer into human milk. Amphetamines include popular street drugs such as ecstasy, harmony, and love. Most studies on the effects of these drugs have occurred with laboratory animals, primarily rats. One study on the levels of amphetamines in human milk found higher levels of amphetamine (taken prenatally) in the breastmilk than in the mother's plasma up to the forty-second day after delivery. Small amounts were present in the baby's urine (Steiner, 1984).

Hallucinations, extreme agitation, and seizures in the baby could occur from his exposure to these drugs. The mother should wait 24 to 48 hours after taking them before breastfeeding (Hale, 2004). As with all illicit drugs, the key concern is that a mother using these drugs may not be exercising prudent judgment and may not be aware enough to care for her baby appropriately. The AAP classifies amphetamines as contraindicated in breastfeeding mothers.

Cocaine

Cocaine is a powerful central nervous stimulant. Effects of cocaine intoxication in the infant include irritability, jitteriness, tremors, increased heart and respiratory rate, and convulsions or seizures. Cocaine's "high" is brief, but excreting the inactive metabolite from the body takes a long time. Traces may be present in exposed infants' urine for over a week.

There are no studies with precise measurement of the amount of cocaine transmitted through the mother's milk. However, significant secretion is probable, along with a high **milk/plasma ratio**, since cocaine is so easily absorbed (Hale, 2004). The mother should pump and discard her milk for a minimum of 24 hours to be safe. The AAP classifies cocaine as contraindicated for use by breastfeeding mothers.

Heroin

Heroin is a highly addictive drug that converts to morphine in the body. Although it is illegal in the United States, it is used medically in the United Kingdom and elsewhere. Heroin passes to the infant through the mother's milk. It can cause increased sleepiness and poor appetite in the infant, resulting in an undernourished baby. An uncoordinated and ineffective suckling reflex may also result from heroin ingestion, as well as tremors, restlessness, and vomiting. The AAP categorizes heroin as contraindicated for use by breastfeeding mothers.

Methadone is an opiate given to heroin addicts in recovery. Research has shown that amounts of methadone in the mother's milk appear to be small, and breastfeeding therefore seems to be safe (Jansson, 2004; Begg, 2001). Infant levels are dependent on maternal dosage, however. The AAP placed methadone in the approved category for breastfeeding women (Hale, 2002a). Buprenorphine is a newer treatment for heroin addiction. One case study found that the amount in the mother's milk was small and probably had little effect on the baby. The baby had no withdrawal signs when later abruptly weaned (Marquet, 1997). However, a study evaluating the use of buprenorphine for postpartum cesarean pain found a correlation with low infant weight gain and the amount of breastfeeding done, suggesting a suppressant effect (Hirose, 1997). The AAP has not reviewed buprenorphine.

Phencyclidine Hydrochloride

Phencyclidine hydrochloride (PCP) is a powerful hallucinogen known as angel dust. Studies found very high concentrations of this drug (ten times maternal plasma levels) in infant mice (Nicholas, 1982). PCP is stored in fat tissue and excreted very slowly from the body. The AAP categorizes it as contraindicated in breastfeeding mothers.

Counseling Implications

Regardless of the pharmacologic effects or safety to the infant of illicit drugs, there is also concern about the mother's ability to care for her baby when she is abusing drugs. One study showed that mothers intending to breastfeed are more likely to decrease or stop their substance abuse (Frank, 1992). Another study revealed that the fear of passing "dangerous things" to their babies through breastmilk prevented 25 percent of at-risk women in the study from breastfeeding (England, 2003).

Given the number of risks, both known and unknown, mothers should be educated whenever possible about the dangers of using such drugs, both prenatally and while breastfeeding. They also need to recognize the dangers involved due to the inhibition of effective parenting skills while under the influence of these drugs, whether breastfeeding or not.

Although you can educate a mother and warn her about harmful practices, you cannot take responsibility for her actions. If she chooses to ignore your advice, you can remind her of the potential danger to her baby and urge her to tell her baby's caregiver about the substance she is using. If you see signs of child endangerment, abuse, or neglect, most governments require that you report your observations to the child protective services agency in your area. Familiarize yourself with the reporting requirements where you live, and add relevant contact information to your list of resources.

 ## BREAST IMPLANTS

Silicone breast implants and perceived risks to the breast-feeding infant made media headlines in the 1990s. One study described a connection between an infant's esophageal swallowing **dysfunction** and having been breastfed (Levine, 1994). This controversial study involved a small, selective group of infants and did not apply the same standards to the control group and the study group. The study also did not take into account the large amount of data available that demonstrate significant health benefits afforded the child through breastfeeding (Williams, 1994). The author of these controversial studies was an expert witness for the plaintiffs in a lawsuit against Dow Corning. Some of the mothers in these studies were the plaintiffs in the class action litigation. Levine later revised his study (Levine, 1996).

Berlin (1994), in his commentary to this study, noted that the compound used in breast implants, poly-dimethylsiloxane (PDMS), was not present in the few samples of milk from mothers with implants. He also noted that Mylicon drops, frequently recommended for infant colic, contain PDMS. There are no reports of side effects after decades of use. Berlin suggests that there should be no contraindication to breastfeeding with silicone implants based on this one study. Greater amounts of silicone are present in other substances, such as cow's milk formulas!

A large cohort study of children of mothers with silicone implants and children of mothers with reduction surgery found no significant increases in connective tissue diseases or congenital malformations (Kjoller, 1998). Another study compared levels of silicon in cow's milk, cow's milk formula, milk from mothers with implants, and milk from mothers without implants. It found similar silicon levels between the breastfeeding mothers. Silicon levels were ten times higher in cow's milk and even higher in infant formulas (Semple, 1998).

ENVIRONMENTAL CONTAMINANTS

While mothers can take measures to avoid the ingestion of social toxicants, they probably do not have such control over exposure to contaminants in their environment. Many chemicals are strongly resistant to breakdown, which has led to environmental pollution. Toxins primarily deposit in fat and a mother's milk is naturally rich in fat. Therefore, human milk contains traces of many contaminants that pass on to the breastfeeding infant. Hundreds of studies document the presence of contaminants in human milk. Maternal diet, especially the consumption of fish, is a major factor in levels of certain pollutants in her milk (Solomon, 2002).

Mothers generally are not discouraged from breastfeeding because of exposure to environmental contaminants. Most studies conclude their reports by reaffirming the superiority of breastmilk. As the author of one study states, "The findings of this study should not discourage women from breastfeeding. Women deserve the ability to choose to nourish and protect their children by breastfeeding, without having to fear that environmental pollution has compromised the value or safety of their milk. The real solution is to pass policies that will reduce the levels of these toxic chemicals in the environment to safeguard babies in the womb and protect breastmilk" (Williams-Derry, 2004).

PBDEs

Of recent concern are flame-retardant chemicals, or poly-brominated diphenyl ethers. PBDEs are flame-retarding chemicals used in many computer plastics, foam cushions, textiles, and other products. Some PBDEs accumulate in animals and people. PBDE levels in people and the environment have risen, especially in Americans, who have levels from 10 to 100 times that of Europeans. PBDEs cause learning, memory, and behavior problems in laboratory animals. They also affect thyroid hormones and other bodily functions in laboratory studies (Schecter, 2003).

PBDEs are very similar to a class of chemicals known as polychlorinated biphenyls (PCBs). PCBs, banned in the late 1970s, can impede a child's mental development. Scientists have found that PBDEs and PCBs work in similar ways and may even act together to impair development (Williams-Derry, 2004). It is unclear whether a relationship exists between postnatal PCB exposure through breastfeeding and neurological development (Ribas-Fito, 2001). An Inuit study calculated 36 percent of the PCB traces in breastfed infants to be due to breastfeeding and the remainder to prenatal exposure (Ayotte, 2003).

DDT and DDE

DDT has been a concern for years. Restrictions on its use have resulted in a decline in the levels of DDE, the main breakdown product of DDT, in human milk since 1950. Despite this, a 1995 Australian study found DDT in nearly all samples of study milk. The study showed a number of infants had daily intakes above acceptable levels for chlordane, DDT, dieldrin, heptachlor epoxide, and PCB (Quinsey, 1995). Several studies have found that women with higher levels of DDE in their milk have more difficulty with milk production and are more likely to stop breastfeeding earlier, which implies that this chemical may interfere with lactation (Rogan, 1987). A Michigan study found that high levels of DDE in the mother's milk reduce protection against atopic disorders such as asthma, eczema, and hay fever (Karmaus, 2003).

Geographic Concentrations

Contaminants vary somewhat depending on local pollution sources, diet, and occupation. Kazakhstan, for example, has the highest documented concentrations of tetrachlorodibenzo-p-dioxin (TCDD) in the world for women in their childbearing years. Yet their levels of many other toxins are lower than in Europe (Lutter, 1998). Mothers in the Netherlands have four times the amount of PCBs and dioxins in their milk than mothers in Hong Kong (Soechitram, 2003). Breastmilk contamination by lead and organochlorines such as PCB and DDT actually declined by 50 to 70 percent or more in Germany during the last decade (Schaefer, 2003). Where countries ban or regulate these chemicals, trends show a decline in pollutants such as organochlorine pesticides, PCBs, and dioxins in breastmilk (Solomon, 2002).

Exposure at Home or Work

Today, large numbers of women continue to breastfeed after returning to work. Some of these women have jobs that expose them to such chemical pollutants as lead, mercury, cadmium, pesticides, plastics, or solvents. Mothers need to be aware of these contaminants in the same way they are aware of drugs and alcohol. Offer anticipatory guidance to pregnant and new mothers by asking about any chemical exposure they may have at work or home. Healthcare practitioners who suspect that a contaminant in the mother's milk may be the cause of illness in a child should ask about occupational exposure. Mothers sometimes inquire about having their milk tested. This is usually not necessary unless the caregiver suspects illness in the mother or baby that may be due to chemical exposure.

Reducing Exposure to Environmental Toxicants

Mothers can take precautions to reduce their exposure to contaminants and the potential for chemical pollutants in their milk. They can avoid occupations that involve possible exposure to chemicals. If that is not possible, they may wish to consult with an expert in occupational medicine to evaluate whether the exposure is safe. Avoiding hobbies that involve exposure to oil-based paints, paint or varnish removers, glues, and other solvent-based chemicals will reduce exposure to these chemicals. Recommend avoidance of mothproofed garments, which may contain chemicals that can be absorbed through the skin or inhaled. Limiting the use of domestic sprays such as pesticides and household cleaners will also reduce chemical exposure.

Dietary precautions can lower the risk of contaminants. Limiting consumption of freshwater fish will reduce exposure to chemical wastes that wash into lakes and streams and become concentrated there. The U.S. Food and Drug Administration advises pregnant women, nursing mothers, and young children to avoid eating shark, swordfish, king mackerel and tilefish in order to keep mercury intakes low. They also advise eating no more than six ounces per week of canned albacore tuna, or twelve ounces per week of a variety of other fish. Because toxins concentrate in fatty tissue, mothers should avoid fatty meats and remove excess fat. They can also avoid eating organ meats, where toxins are stored. Thoroughly washing or peeling fresh fruits and vegetables will remove many chemicals that are present. Mothers can also use certified organic produce when practical and economically feasible.

▶ COUNSELING A MOTHER ABOUT IMPURITIES

The guidelines in Figure 10.3 and Figure 10.4 will help you when you are counseling a mother concerning the potential for impurities in her milk. They can remind you of the proper procedures concerning these questions and guide you when you are talking to a mother.

FIGURE 10.3
Issues to address about impurities.

- Give well-documented facts in an objective manner.
- Make a mother aware of her options concerning potential impurities.
- Remind a mother that infant formula may sometimes be contaminated with impurities, as may water.
- Urge a mother to seek her caregiver's advice and to share her concerns openly.
- Urge a mother to remind her caregiver that she is breastfeeding.
- Cite references for facts that you give a mother.
- Discuss drug substitutes in a neutral manner, citing reliable sources.
- Suggest ways a mother can minimize the effects of drugs.
- Advise a mother to avoid unnecessary consumption of or exposure to contaminants.

FIGURE 10.4
Precautions in discussing impurities.

- Refrain from giving personal opinions.
- Do not interpret drug information for a mother unless you have prescriptive privileges.
- Do not advise a mother about a drug's safety; read straight from the literature.
- Do not indicate to a mother that you disagree with advice from her caregiver or other medical resource unless you are medically qualified.
- Do not suggest that a mother refuse a drug when it is needed.
- Do not encourage a mother to act against her caregiver's advice.

The guidelines apply to any of the substances that may compromise the safety or quality of a mother's milk. They are especially important when discussing medications with a mother.

▶ SUMMARY

Almost any substance in the mother's blood will be present to same degree in her milk. The question is whether it will be absorbed in the baby's GI tract and whether the infant's exposure to the substance as it appears in the milk is safe. Factors that influence the level of a substance found in the infant's bloodstream include how soon after birth the mother takes a medication, how it is metabolized, and the baby's age and size.

Drugs in the mother's milk may increase or decrease milk production and secretion. They may also cause changes in her baby's behavior, feeding, and sleeping patterns such as fussiness, lethargy, rash, vomiting, or diarrhea. A mother can minimize the effects of drugs in her milk by selecting the least offensive drug, adjusting her schedule for taking the drug, and avoiding medications with long plasma half-life. Drug information must be presented objectively from well-documented sources, and the IBCLC must not appear to be recommending or advising the mother about the safety of a particular medication.

Environmental toxins deposit primarily in fat and are excreted through the mother's milk. Maternal diet, especially fish consumption, is a factor in breastmilk levels of certain pollutants. Mothers can take precautions to reduce their exposure to contaminants and the potential for chemical pollutants in their milk. Silicone implants do not appear at this time to present a problem. All recreational drugs are contraindicated for use by breastfeeding women.

▶ CHAPTER 10—AT A GLANCE

Facts you learned—

Medications:

- Few medications are contraindicated in breastfeeding.
- In general, a relative infant dose of fewer than ten percent is considered safe.
- Use drug information from well-documented sources.
- Become acquainted with drug groups and their risks and benefits.
- Questions to ask about a particular medication:
  - Will it pass into the mother's milk and be absorbed in the baby's GI tract?
  - Can the baby safely be exposed to the substance as it appears in the milk?
  - How soon after birth will it be taken?
  - What is the baby's gestational age?

Social toxicants:

- Newborn and preterm babies are susceptible to caffeine because it takes them longer to eliminate it.
- Generally, one or two drinks socially is not a problem.
- A mother may breastfeed when the effects of alcohol have worn off.
- All recreational drugs are contraindicated.

Environmental contaminants:

- Silicone breast implants have not been proven dangerous when breastfeeding.
- Toxins are primarily deposited in fat and are found in breastmilk.
- Flame-retarding chemicals affect learning, memory, behavior, thyroid hormones, and other bodily functions.
- PCBs affect mental development.
- DDE affects protection against atopic disorders such as asthma, eczema, and hay fever.

Applying what you learned—

- Recommend that mothers minimize effects of a medication by:
  - Taking it immediately after nursing or three to four hours before the next feeding.
  - Avoiding breastfeeding when the medication is at its peak level in the milk.
  - Avoiding drugs with a long half-life.
  - Selecting the least offensive drug.

◆ Recommend that mothers:

- ◆ Consider alternatives that do not involve medication or substitute a safer medication.
- ◆ Weigh benefits of a medication against possible risk to the baby.
- ◆ Weigh risk of a medication to the baby against the risk of artificial baby milk.
- ◆ Avoid nicotine and tobacco or time breastfeeding to minimize exposure in the milk.
- ◆ Avoid excessive alcohol consumption.
- ◆ Avoid all drugs of abuse.
- ◆ Avoid occupations, hobbies, and fabrics that involve possible exposure to chemicals.
- ◆ Avoid eating shark, swordfish, king mackerel, and tilefish.
- ◆ Limit consumption of canned albacore tuna and other fish.
- ◆ Avoid eating organ meats.
- ◆ Wash or peel fresh fruits and vegetables.
- ◆ (See additional counseling tips in the chapter tables.)

▶ REFERENCES

Aljazaf K et al. Pseudoephedrine: Effects on milk production in women and estimation of infant exposure via breastmilk. *Br J Clin Pharmacol* 56(1):18–24; 2003.

American Academy of Pediatrics (AAP) Committee on Drugs. The transfer of drugs and other chemicals into human milk. *Pediatrics* 108(3):776–789; 2001.

Ayotte P et al. Assessment of pre- and postnatal exposure to polychlorinated biphenyls: Lessons from the Inuit cohort study. *Environ Health Perspect* 111(9):1253–1258; 2003.

Begg E et al. Distribution of R- and S-methadone into human milk during multiple, medium to high oral dosing. *Br J Clin Pharmacol* 52(6):681–685; 2001.

Berlin C. Silicone breast implants and breast-feeding. *Pediatrics* 4(Pt 1):547–549; 1994.

Briggs G, Freeman R, Yaffe S, *Drugs in Pregnancy and Lactation: A Reference Guide to Fetal & Neonatal Risk*, 6th ed. Baltimore, MD: Lippincott Williams & Wilkins; 2003.

Daltveit A et al. Circadian variations in sudden infant death syndrome: Associations with maternal smoking, sleeping position and infections. The Nordic epidemiological SIDS study. *Acta Paediatr* 92(9):991–993; 2003.

England L et al. Breastfeeding practices in a cohort of inner-city women: The role of contraindications. *BMC Public Health* 3(1):28; 2003.

Frank D et al. Cocaine and marijuana use during pregnancy by women intending and not intending to breast-feed. *J Am Diet Assoc* 92:215–216; 1992.

Hale T, Berens P. *Clinical Therapy in Breastfeeding Patients*. Amarillo, TX: Pharmasoft Publishing; 2002a.

Hale T, Ilett K. *Drug Therapy and Breastfeeding: From Theory to Clinical Practice*. New York: The Parthenon Publishing Group, 4–6; 2002b.

Hale T. *Medications and Mother's Milk*. Amarillo, TX: Pharmasoft Publishing; 2004.

Hirose M et al. Extradural buprenorphine suppresses breast feeding after caesarean section. *Br J Anaesth* 79(1):120–121; 1997.

Ho E et al. Alcohol and breast feeding: Calculation of time to zero level in milk. *Biol Neonate* 80(3):219–222; 2001.

Hopkinson J et al. Milk production by mothers of premature infants: Influence of cigarette smoking. *Pediatrics* 90(6):934–938; 1992.

Humphrey, S. *The Nursing Mother's Herbal*. Minneapolis, MN: Fairview Press, 42:229–230; 2003.

Ilett KF et al. Use of nicotine patches in breast-feeding mothers: Transfer of nicotine and cotinine into human milk. *Clin Pharmacol Ther* 74(6):516–524; 2003.

International Lactation Consultant Association (ILCA). Position on breastfeeding, breastmilk, and environmental contaminants; 2001. Available at: www.ilca.org. Accessed May 10, 2004.

Jang A et al. The effect of passive smoking on asthma symptoms, atopy, and airway hyperresponsiveness in schoolchildren. *J Korean Med Sci* 19(2):214–217; 2004.

Jansson L et al. Methadone maintenance and lactation: A review of the literature and current management guidelines. Review. *J Hum Lact* 20(1):62–71; 2004.

Kahn A et al. Sudden infant deaths: Stress, arousal and SIDS. *Early Hum Dev* 75 S147–S166; 2003.

Karmaus W et al. Atopic manifestations, breast-feeding protection and the adverse effect of DDE. *Paediatr Perinat Epidemiol* 17(2):212–220; 2003.

Kim S et al. An 18-month follow-up study on the influence of smoking on blood antioxidant status of teenage girls in comparison with adult male smokers in Korea. *Nutrition* 20(5):437–444; 2004.

Kjoller K et al. Health outcomes in offspring of mothers with breast implants. *Pediatrics* 102(5):1112–1115; 1998.

L'Hoir M et al. Sudden unexpected death in infancy: Epidemiologically determined risk factors related to pathological classification. *Acta Paediatr* 87(12):1279–1287; 1998.

Lawrence R. A review of the medical contraindications to breastfeeding. *Technical Information Bulletin*. Washington, DC: National Center for Education in Maternal Child Health, USDHHS; October, 1997.

Levine J et al. Esophageal dysmotility in children breast-fed by mothers with silicone breast implants: Long-term follow-up and response to treatment. *Dig Dis Sci* 41:1600–1603; 1996.

Levine J, Ilowite N. Scleroderma-like esophageal disease in children breastfed by mothers with silicone breast implants. *JAMA* 271:213–216; 1994.

Little R et al. Maternal alcohol use during breast-feeding and infant mental and motor development at one year. *N Engl J Med* 321:425–430; 1989.

Little R et al. Alcohol, breastfeeding, and development at 18 months. *Pediatrics* 109(5):e72; 2002.

Lutter C et al. Breast milk contamination in Kazakhstan: Implications for infant feeding. *Chemosphere* 37(9–12):1761–1772; 1998.

Marquet P et al. Buprenorphine withdrawal syndrome in a newborn. *Clin Pharmacol Ther* 62(5):569–571; 1997.

Mennella J, Beauchamp G. Maternal diet alters the sensory qualities of human milk and the nursling's behavior. *Pediatrics* 88:737–744; 1991.

Mennella J, Garcia-Gomez P. Sleep disturbances after acute exposure to alcohol in mothers' milk. *Alcohol* 25(3):153–158; 2001.

Minchin M. Smoking and breastfeeding: An overview. *J Hum Lact* 7:183–188; 1991.

Newman J. Drugs and breastmilk (Letter to the Editor). *Pediatrics* 86:148; 1990.

Nicholas J et al. Phencyclidine: Its transfer across the placenta as well as into breast milk. *Am J Obstet Gynecol* 143(2): 143–146; 1982.

Noble L et al. Factors influencing initiation of breast-feeding among urban women. *Am J Perinatol* 20(8):477–483; 2003.

Owen M et al. Relation of infant feeding practices, cigarette smoke exposure, and group child care to the onset and duration of otitis media with effusion in the first two years of life. *J Pediatr* 123(5):702–711; 1993.

Quinsey P et al. Persistence of organochlorines in breast milk of women in Victoria, Australia. *Food Chem Toxicol* 33(1): 49–56; 1995.

Ribas-Fito N et al. Polychlorinated biphenyls (PCBs) and neurological development in children: A systematic review. Review. *J Epidemiol Community Health* 55(8):537–546; 2001.

Rivera-Calimlim L. The significance of drugs in breast milk. *Clin Perinatol* 14:51; 1987.

Rizzi M et al. Environmental tobacco smoke may induce early lung damage in healthy male adolescents. *Chest* 125(4): 1387–1393; 2004.

Rogan WJ, Gladen BC, McKinney JD et al. Polychlorinated biphenyls (PCBs) and dichlorodiphenyl dichloroethane (DDE) in human milk: Effects on growth, morbidity, and duration of lactation. *Am J Public Health* 77(10):1294–1297; 1987.

Ryu J. Caffeine in human milk and in serum of breast-fed infants. *Dev Pharmacol Ther* 8(6):329–337; 1985a.

Ryu J. Effect of maternal caffeine consumption on heart rate and sleep time of breastfed infants. *Dev Pharmacol Ther* 8:355–363; 1985b.

Schaefer C. Recreational drugs and environmental contaminants in mother's milk. Review. *Zentralbl Gynakol* 125(2):38–43; 2003.

Schecter A et al. Polybrominated diphenyl ethers (PBDEs) in US mothers' milk. *Environ Health Perspect* 111:1723–1729; 2003.

Semple J et al. Breast milk contamination and silicone implants: Preliminary results using silicon as a proxy measurement for silicone. *Plast Reconstr Surg* 102(2):528–533; 1998.

Shaker I et al. Infant feeding attitudes of expectant parents: Breastfeeding and formula feeding. *J Adv Nurs* 45(3):260–268; 2004.

Shiva F et al. Effects of passive smoking on common respiratory symptoms in young children. *Acta Paediatr* 92(12):1394–1397; 2003.

Silva DA et al. Ethanol pharmacokinetics in lactating women. *Braz J Med Biol Res* 26:1097–1103; 1993.

Soechitram S et al. Comparison of dioxin and PCB concentrations in human breast milk samples from Hong Kong and the Netherlands. *Food Addit Contam* 20(1):65–69; 2003.

Solomon G et al. Chemical contaminants in breast milk: Time trends and regional variability. *Environ Health Perspect* 110(6):A339–A347; 2002.

Steiner E et al. Amphetamine secretion in breast milk. *Eur J Clin Pharmacol* 27(1):123–124; 1984.

Valachovicova M et al. Antioxidant vitamins levels: Nutrition and smoking. *Bratisl Lek Listy* 104(12): 411–414; 2003.

Vio F et al. Smoking during pregnancy and lactation and its effects on breastmilk volume. *Am J Clin Nutr* 54:1011–1016; 1991.

Wagner CL, Katikaneni LD, Cox TH, Ryan RM. The impact of prenatal drug exposure on the neonate. *Obstet Gynecol Clin North Am* 25(1):169–194; 1998.

Williams A. Silicone breast implants, breastfeeding and scleroderma. *Lancet* 343:1043–1044; 1994.

Williams-Derry C. Flame retardants in the bodies of Pacific Northwest residents. Northwest Environmental Watch; September 29, 2004. Available at: www.northwestwatch.org. Accessed December 16, 2004.

▶ **BIBLIOGRAPHY**

Batagol R. *Drugs and Breastfeeding*. London: British National Formulary; 1994.

Blackwell A, Salisbury L. Administrative petition to relieve the health hazards of promotion of infant formulas in the US. *Birth and the Family Journal* 8(4):290; 1981.

Chasnoff I et al. Cocaine intoxication in a breast-fed infant. *Pediatrics* 80:836–838; 1987.

Hansen B, Moore L. Recreational drug use by the breastfeeding woman. Part I: Illicit drugs. *J Hum Lact* 5:178–180; 1989.

Harvard Medical School, Department of Continuing Education. Evaluating medical information. *Harvard Medical School Health Letter* 7(1):6; 1981.

Howard C, Lawrence R. Breast-feeding and drug exposure. *Obstet Gynecol Clin North Am* 25:195–217; 1998.

Ito S et al. Maternal noncompliance with antibiotics during breastfeeding. *Ann Pharmacother* 27:40–42; 1993.

Ito S et al. Prospective follow-up of adverse reactions in breast-fed infants exposed to maternal medication. *Am J Obstet Gynecol* 168:1393–1399; 1993.

Kacew S. Adverse effects of drugs and chemicals in breastmilk on the nursing infant. *J Clin Pharmacol* 33:213–221; 1993.

Lanting C et al. Neurological condition in 42-month-old children in relation to pre- and postnatal exposure to polychlorinated biphenyls and dioxin. *Early Human Dev* 50:283–292; 1998.

Mennella J. Infants' suckling responses to the flavor of alcohol in mothers' milk. *Alcoholism: Clin Exp Res* 21:581–585; 1997.

Nahas GG et al. Inhibition of cellular mediated immunity in marijuana smokers. *Science* 193:419; 1974.

Nutrition Action Newsletter. Caffeine: The inside scoop. December 1996.

Ortega R et al. Influence of smoking on vitamin E status during the third trimester of pregnancy and on breastmilk-to-tocopherol concentrations in Spanish women. *Am J Clin Nutr* 68:662–667; 1998.

Rubow S et al. The excretion of radiopharmaceuticals in human breast milk: Additional data and dosimetry. *Eur J Nucl Med* 21:144–153; 1994.

Schulte P. Minimizing alcohol exposure of the breastfeeding infant. *J Hum Lact* 11(4) 317–319; 1995.

World Health Organization. *The International Pharmacopoeia.* 3rd ed., Vol 5. Geneva: WHO; 2003. Available at: www.who.int/medicines/library/pharmacopoeia/itoxviii.pdf. Accessed December 16, 2004.

PART
3

PRENATAL THROUGH POSTPARTUM

PRENATAL CONSIDERATIONS

Parents face many choices regarding the care of their new babies. Some choices, such as dress or daily routines, have little or no impact on the health of the child. However, healthcare choices directly affect the health and well-being of children in both the short term and the long term. Such choices include the use of a car seat, immunizations, and breastfeeding. Just as there are serious risks to the child of parents who choose not to use a car seat or immunize, so are there consequences in choosing not to breastfeed. Because breastfeeding often involves lifestyle adjustments, parents may benefit from your guidance in blending breastfeeding into their lives.

The healthcare profession has an obligation to provide true informed consent to women and their families prenatally. In order to make an informed decision, they need to understand the consequences of not breastfeeding. IBCLCs can look for ways to educate parents prenatally so they can make informed feeding decisions. Contacting local groups that offer prenatal classes, childbirth educators, obstetricians' offices, and family practice groups is an excellent start. If sound breastfeeding education is unavailable, you can provide breastfeeding classes to your clients. You might also provide breastfeeding updates to physicians, nurses, and other caregivers who see prenatal women.

KEY TERMS

caregiver	hospital affiliation
cesarean birth	nipple correction
continuing education	standing orders
decision to breastfeed	

▶ MAKING THE DECISION TO BREASTFEED

A belief in breastfeeding is the underlying motivator in a woman's infant feeding decision. Although brochures can provide information, they have little influence on the incidence of breastfeeding. A positive attitude toward breastfeeding prior to pregnancy has the greatest influence. One study found that 63 percent of women made the choice to breastfeed prior to pregnancy,

26 percent during pregnancy, and 11 percent after delivery. A significantly greater number of experienced mothers decided to breastfeed prior to pregnancy compared with first-time mothers (Noble, 2003). A study of 10,548 women in the United Kingdom showed that prenatal intention to breastfeed influences duration as well as initiation rates. Women who intended to breastfeed for 1 month had a mean duration of 2.5 months, whereas women who intended to breastfeed for at least 5 months had a mean duration of 4.4 months (Donath, 2003).

Research shows that women most likely to breastfeed are in their mid-thirties, college educated, white, married, and in the middle-income level. Statistically, black and teen mothers are least likely to breastfeed (Ryan, 2002), although these groups have seen the largest increase in breastfeeding initiation. A study of African American mothers found that mothers who chose to breastfeed were more educated, employed prior to birth, married, and using postpartum contraception. Breastfeeding was associated with a higher awareness of preventative healthcare (Sharps, 2003). A woman also is more likely to breastfeed if she has received positive prenatal information about breastfeeding (Guise, 2003; Noble, 2003).

Influence from Other People

Significant people in a woman's life can exert a substantial influence over her decision to breastfeed. A woman is more likely to breastfeed if other family members have either breastfed or are supportive of breastfeeding (Ekstrom, 2003). Friends and acquaintances who breastfeed provide additional role models. Support from the baby's father plays a pivotal role in her decision. Likewise, the attitude and knowledge level of her healthcare practitioners influence a mother's choice.

Influence from the Baby's Father

One of the strongest influences on the breastfeeding decision among American women is that of the child's father. Pregnant women frequently say, "But if I breastfeed, my husband won't be able to feed the baby." Fathers want to be involved in caring for their infant, and they often see feeding as an important interaction. In a **qualitative study**, 14 fathers identified the process of postponing their feeding the baby as a significant issue (Gamble, 1993). These men's experiences can form the basis for your prenatal education of parents.

A 1994 study by Littman noted that the father's approval of breastfeeding was the single most **statistically significant** indicator of whether or not women in the study breastfed. Other studies reveal that fathers' approval and support are key influences in both breastfeeding initiation and breastfeeding beyond four months (Chang, 2003; Kong, 2004). A study conducted by Freed (1992) among expectant mothers revealed that women do not always correctly predict the attitudes of the father regarding breastfeeding.

IBCLCs can encourage more discussion by couples and more sharing of information with fathers. The quality of a couple's relationship does not seem to be a factor in early breastfeeding termination. However, a good relationship is associated with more breastfeeding support and more involvement in the baby's care from the father (Falceto, 2004). In another study, mothers received greater partner support for breastfeeding, as well as greater family knowledge and positive attitudes about breastfeeding (Rose, 2004). This is further evidence for the importance of including fathers in education. See Chapter 19 for ways fathers can be involved with their babies.

Influence from the Caregiver

Caregivers exert a tremendous influence on a parent's choice of infant feeding. Frequently, knowledgeable professionals are unaware of or may even openly dispute the value of breastfeeding in spite of evidence to the contrary (Walker, 2001). The approach taken with women can move them in the direction of breastfeeding. A positive approach assumes that all pregnant women intend to breastfeed unless they indicate otherwise. Asking a woman if she plans to breastfeed or asking how she plans to feed her baby implies equality between a mother's milk and substitutes. Asking how you can help with breastfeeding conveys belief in the superiority of breastfeeding. If the woman indicates that she does not plan to breastfeed or if she seems uncertain, it provides an opportunity to discuss concerns or misconceptions.

Lu (2001) found that encouragement from a healthcare professional increased mothers' breastfeeding initiation fourfold. He found provider encouragement to breastfeed had a major impact on the segment of women least likely to breastfeed. There was a threefold increase among low-income, young, and less-educated

women, a fivefold increase among black women, and nearly an elevenfold increase among single women (Lu, 2001).

A review of 20 trials involving over 23,700 mother-infant pairs suggests that extra professional support increases exclusive breastfeeding and duration (Sikorski, 2002). Caregivers can help instill in women a belief in their ability to breastfeed and an understanding of its superiority over artificial baby milk. It's all about confidence, and the mother's confidence is determined in large part by her caregivers.

One study tested the perceptions of clinicians who felt they spoke about breastfeeding and mothers who felt their caregivers rarely discussed breastfeeding with them. It identified significant communication gaps in terms of discussing breastfeeding duration and ways to breastfeed after returning to work (Taveras, 2004a). African American women were less likely to have received breastfeeding advice from WIC counselors than white women were, and they were more likely to receive bottle-feeding advice. However, African American and white women were equally likely overall to report having received breastfeeding advice from medical care providers (Beal, 2003). Prenatal parenting support and postpartum visits increase the likelihood that families will continue breastfeeding, read to their three-month-old, and provide other appropriate parenting (Johnston, 2004).

Social Influence on the Decision to Breastfeed

Many social barriers are in place in developed countries, which, at best, fail to recognize breastfeeding as the natural way to nourish babies. At worst, barriers openly discourage breastfeeding. In prenatal contact with mothers, it is important that the caregiver is aware of these barriers and addresses them with clients. You can help women verbalize and address the conflicting feelings that sometimes are involved in the decision to breastfeed (Kitzinger, 1992).

Separation of generations, frequent relocation, little experience caring for children, and lack of breastfeeding as the cultural norm can leave new mothers with little confidence in their ability to breastfeed or little understanding of how the process works. Few women have breastfeeding role models. You can help women recognize the important contribution they make to society in their role as a mother and nurturer of the next generation.

Bottle-feeding as the model in Western culture influences professionals and lay persons alike. When media and advertising portray the breast as a sexual object, they ignore nature's intended use of breasts for infant nutrition. Much of the healthcare system bases routines, policies, education, and even the facility's architectural layout on artificial feeding. Although the maxim "Breast is best" is freely spoken, many infant feeding messages imply equality between human milk and artificial baby milk (Taveras, 2004b). When parents receive such mixed signals, they become even more confused.

Because over half of women make their infant feeding choices before pregnancy and 26 percent during pregnancy, public education is imperative. A Scottish study revealed that breast and bottle-feeders had the same goals regarding infant feeding. However, they differed in their perception of barriers to breastfeeding, including embarrassment at nursing in front of others and inconvenience (Shaker, 2004). During prenatal teaching, it helps to ask women to share their goals and concerns and then specifically discuss these barriers.

A variety of issues may affect a woman's decision to breastfeed. Most women know breastfeeding is best for the baby. Health and nutrition benefits for her and her baby may motivate a woman to breastfeed. She may be concerned about the increased risk to her baby of substituting artificial milks.

Breastfeeders perceive breastfeeding as more convenient. Interestingly, women who choose to bottle-feed tend to perceive breastfeeding as less convenient, perhaps associating it with a loss of freedom. They believe that if they bottle-feed, someone else can feed the baby and they will be able to resume outside activities earlier than if they breastfeed. Among low-income women, other factors identified as barriers to the decision to breastfeed include modesty, privacy, work or school conflicts, lack of confidence, and lifestyle issues such as diet, stress, substance abuse, and inadequate sleep (England, 2003; Bryant, 1993).

Another cultural trend in the infant feeding decision mirrors trends in the management of labor and birth. Women often fear being totally responsible for their baby's weight gain and health, much as they fear embracing the responsibility of laboring and birthing. Women describe a need to have **epidural anesthesia** or a need to have their caregiver "deliver" the baby. After birth they may reject the next step of motherhood—breastfeeding—for fear of failure. The need for control in one's life may influence this. Women who view control as a priority are more likely to rely on bottle-feeding. Fear of failure may be due to the woman's lack of confidence that her body can produce a superior product that will provide sufficient food for her baby.

Customs in the home environment may influence a woman to feed her baby artificially if that is what most women in her culture do. Her knowledge of infant care or lack of knowledge about breastfeeding may cause her to believe that it will not fit into her lifestyle. Commercial messages about human milk substitutes and bottle-feeding may be so strong that she is convinced

that there is little difference between breastfeeding and artificial feeding.

Mixed images of the breasts as sexual as opposed to a means of nurturing babies may be confusing (Harris, 2003). An aversion to having her breasts touched may make it emotionally painful for a woman to breastfeed. Such an aversion is common in women who are survivors of sexual or physical abuse (Prentice, 2002; Kendall-Tackett; 2001). Often, a woman may not even be aware of past abuse until birth and breastfeeding trigger memories. See Chapter 19 for a discussion of abuse survivors.

When discussing infant feeding with pregnant women, the risks of not breastfeeding provide a sound basis for informed decision making. A breastfeeding mother need not purchase special equipment or incur daily expenses of infant formula. While breastfeeding, the mother has a free hand to attend to other needs or activities such as reading, snacking, and helping other children. Because breastfeeding is possible virtually anywhere, travel and other activities are more convenient when the baby accompanies the mother. Give mothers examples of how they can breastfeed modestly in front of others. Mothers are often pleased to find that their breastfed baby's stools and spit-up have a less offensive odor than those of formula-fed babies; spit-up and stools also do not stain clothing. Presenting the idea of traveling "with" the baby, instead of "away from" the baby can be very empowering and liberating for mothers whose cultural messages suggest they "need" to leave their baby.

Realistic Expectations

Fear of instilling guilt is not an acceptable excuse for failing to inform women of the potentially negative outcomes of formula use. Bottle-feeding artificial milk falls far short of the biological norm of breastfeeding. Bottle-feeders often choose artificial feeding because of a perceived disagreeable aspect of breastfeeding. You can help a mother develop realistic expectations about breastfeeding by acquainting her with some of the realities. In the early days of breastfeeding, she may experience a degree of breast fullness and nipple tenderness. Because of the more frequent feedings required by a breastfed baby, she will need to be available to her young baby for nourishment.

It is important that you neither minimize nor dismiss a mother's concerns regarding these issues. You can encourage her to consider that this is the normal, expected postpartum course. Remind her, too, of the many health, emotional, and financial benefits of breastfeeding. Help her see that there are ways to decrease discomforts and minimize inconveniences. Address specific concerns by offering ways of coping and including her baby in her activities. This type of support may be all she needs to build her confidence and help her overcome perceived obstacles. Learning how to fit breastfeeding into their lifestyle will be the first of many accommodations parents will make as they blend their new child into their family.

Misconceptions That Influence the Decision to Breastfeed

A number of misconceptions about breastfeeding may cause a woman to choose not to breastfeed. You can help dispel these misunderstandings and increase a woman's confidence in her decision to breastfeed. Below is a list of some common misconceptions.

The baby will be too dependent if he breastfeeds.
Breastfed babies actually seem to display more independence because their needs are met. See Chapter 13.

Breastfeeding is too time-consuming.
There is actually less work involved for a mother in breastfeeding than in bottle-feeding, if the mother is doing the bottle-feeding. Breastfeeding frees the mother to spend valuable time with her baby and other family members. See Chapter 19.

My mother didn't have enough milk, so maybe I won't, either.
A well-nourished woman produces the amount of milk her baby needs. The breastfeeding experience of the woman's mother has no bearing on her ability to breastfeed. Between 1930 and 1970, healthcare practitioners gave women little effective advice or support to breastfeed. See Chapter 1.

Maybe my milk won't agree with my baby.
Each mother's milk is ideally suited to her baby. Breastfed babies rarely experience negative reactions to their mother's milk. On the other hand, many babies are not able to tolerate cow's milk. See Chapter 9.

My breasts are too small to breastfeed.
The size of a woman's breasts depends primarily on the amount of fatty tissue, not functional breast tissue. Size usually has little bearing on her ability to produce sufficient milk. See Chapter 7.

I am too high-strung to breastfeed.
Breastfeeding can actually be calming to a high-strung woman because of the hormones activated by nursing.

The added skin contact with the baby can have a calming effect on a mother as well. See Chapter 7.

If I breastfeed, my diet will be too restricted.
Breastfeeding babies generally can tolerate the same foods the mother tolerates. The only foods a mother may need to restrict are those that seem to produce signs of intolerance in her baby. See Chapter 8.

If I have a cesarean birth, I won't be able to breastfeed.
The type of birth a mother experiences has no effect on her ability to breastfeed, although it may delay the onset of stage II lactogenesis. Mothers who deliver by cesarean birth are able to breastfeed. See Chapter 12.

Breastfeeding will drain my energies too much.
All mothers find caring for a newborn infant tiring, regardless of feeding method. Breastfeeding encourages a mother to relax during feeding times. This permits her to get even more rest than a mother who bottle-feeds her baby, if the mother is a sole caregiver. A mother can recoup her energies by making it a practice to rest while her baby is sleeping. Breastfeeding seems to be nature's way of ensuring that the mother gets the rest she needs in the postpartum period. The formula-feeding mother spends more time purchasing and preparing formula and caring for the child, who will be sicker more often than a breastfed child. See Chapter 9.

Breastfeeding mothers lose their figures and get sagging breasts.
The sagging in a woman's breasts results from pregnancy and loss of muscle tone as a woman ages, not from having breastfed. See Chapter 7. The caloric demands of breastfeeding can actually help mothers control their weight. See Chapter 8.

Artificial baby milk is just as healthy as human milk.
There are substantial differences between infant formula and a mother's milk. Human milk is a live substance that provides immunities and antibacterial properties. See Chapter 9 for a detailed discussion about the properties and health benefits of human milk.

Breastfeeding is essentially an alternative to infant formula.
Breastfeeding is much more than the milk the baby receives. It is a dynamic process, a bonding relationship between a mother and her baby. Breastfeeding involves people, not simply food for the baby. See Chapter 4.

Mothers will have to wean before they return to work.

Mothers who are separated from their babies, whether for a return to work, school, or other activity, have many options. They can express milk for the caregiver to feed to the baby or provide formula for the baby during the separation. Unrestricted breastfeeding at times when the mother and baby are together will help maintain milk production. Many employers and insurance companies support employees who breastfeed, as it lowers absenteeism and health insurance claims (see Chapter 24).

Conditions That Contraindicate Breastfeeding

It is extremely rare for a mother to be unable to breastfeed her baby. Sheehan's syndrome, as discussed in Chapter 7, prevents the mother from producing milk. Long-term drug therapy such as lithium rules out breastfeeding, as the substance or treatment would be dangerous to the infant. Severe illness in the mother, such as unresolved congestive heart failure or chemotherapy treatment of cancer, may contraindicate breastfeeding. Mothers can breastfeed after at least two weeks of treatment for active tuberculosis (Lawrence, 1997). Women who test positive for the human immunodeficiency virus (HIV) and live in a developed country with a sanitary water supply are presently advised by WHO not to breastfeed. See Chapter 25 for a discussion of these conditions.

▶ PREPARATION FOR BREASTFEEDING

Women throughout history have breastfed their babies without the aid of recent scientific knowledge and special devices. Many modern women, however, benefit from education about breastfeeding techniques and preparation for breastfeeding. Although women historically have nurtured their babies primarily with their milk, the past several decades have experienced an increase in the popularity of bottle-feeding and a decline in breastfeeding. Consequently, fewer family members are knowledgeable enough about breastfeeding to offer mothers the practical information and support they need in order to breastfeed. The educational process and the mother's active participation in planning for her breastfed baby are effective means of preparing psychologically for breastfeeding. Her self-confidence will increase, enabling her to overcome minor discomforts and obstacles she may experience that are associated with nursing her baby.

Learning about Breastfeeding

A woman who plans to breastfeed will benefit from learning about it early in her pregnancy. The earlier she receives information, the greater the likelihood that she will breastfeed for a substantial period. The woman's attentiveness and retention of the information may be greater in the later months of pregnancy, as she gets closer to her delivery date. Keeping this in mind, you may want to focus early discussions on the decision-making process. You can then discuss the practical aspects of breastfeeding management closer to the time she will deliver.

One way for pregnant women to obtain such information is through attending a prenatal breastfeeding class. They can also begin attending meetings of a community support group for breastfeeding mothers. These meetings can enhance women's confidence and increase their knowledge of breastfeeding. They also provide an opportunity for mothers to share common interests with others in the community.

In your contacts with a woman during her pregnancy, you can discuss her individual goals for breastfeeding. What is her vision of breastfeeding in her everyday life? How important are feeding issues to her and her partner? What do they expect breastfeeding to be like? Answers to these questions provide a foundation for her breastfeeding education.

Give the mother information to help her blend breastfeeding into her life. Helping her identify aspects that will be useful to her personally leads to the development of useful strategies that she can apply postpartum. Education is the most important tool for increasing breastfeeding rates (Guise, 2003) and helps form an effective relationship between you and the mother (Pridham, 1993). See Figure 11.1 for questions that are helpful in gathering the information necessary to assess a woman's need for breastfeeding education and support. Open-ended questions encourage mothers to respond with information that is more descriptive.

In order to prepare for breastfeeding, the women in your care can educate themselves in several ways. By obtaining information from literature, classes, and meetings, they will be able to develop a firm base for sound breastfeeding practices. This will help them avoid or minimize problems. A woman can familiarize herself with baby care and breastfeeding by associating with mothers of young babies and occasionally caring for babies during her pregnancy. In this way, she will develop proficiency in handling babies and build confidence in her mothering abilities, which will enable her to overcome worries she may encounter when her baby arrives.

FIGURE 11.1
Questions to ask about breastfeeding prenatally.

Assessing a woman's need for breastfeeding education

◆ How does she feel about the prospect of breastfeeding?

◆ What practical knowledge does she have about breast-feeding?

◆ What prior experience or exposure does she have to breast-feeding?

◆ How many friends or relatives have breastfed?

◆ What reading has she done on breastfeeding? What videos has she seen?

◆ Has she attended a breastfeeding information class?

◆ Is she attending prepared childbirth classes?

◆ What has her physician discussed with her about breast-feeding?

◆ What has she done to prepare for breastfeeding?

◆ Has she checked for inverted nipples?

◆ What has she learned about breast care?

◆ What clothing does she have that will allow her baby easy access to her breast?

◆ What arrangements has she made for help at home?

◆ Has she arranged for rooming-in if she is delivering in a hospital?

◆ Is she interested in attending group discussions with other breastfeeding mothers?

◆ What are her specific questions or concerns?

Attending childbirth classes and practicing relaxation techniques can enhance a woman's awareness of her body and help her learn ways to overcome tension and discomfort. The information and skills she obtains during pregnancy will be especially useful to her when she and her baby go through the trial-and-error period of establishing a comfortable breastfeeding routine.

Breastfeeding Classes

A large part of breastfeeding teaching occurs through group instruction. Breastfeeding classes are an important part of your practice. Through classes, you are able to reach large numbers of women at various stages. The purpose of the class will determine its content. Ideally, the couple's childbirth classes include breastfeeding discussions. Early in the series, couples benefit from a discussion that helps them make the decision regarding infant feeding. After they make the decision, a discussion of expectations and getting off to a good start with breastfeeding is helpful. A postpartum class after the baby begins breastfeeding will provide continued support and information to parents.

Guidelines for Teaching a Breastfeeding Class

The most important rule in teaching a parent class is to keep it simple. If you are fortunate to have more than a couple of hours for parent classes, dividing your teaching into three separate classes, as described below, will give short information pieces to parents. Most of what you accomplish during the prenatal period is in the area of attitude and expectations. Expectant parents may remember little of the particulars for establishing breastfeeding. They will recall, however, the impressions they gained in class regarding the health benefits and long-term ease of breastfeeding, as well as the risks of not breastfeeding. These perceptions will reinforce their decision after the baby is born.

Teach parents that the only rule in breastfeeding is that there are no rules! All that is required is that the baby gains weight appropriately and the mother is comfortable in the process. Encourage parents to trust their instincts and to respond to their baby's cues. Identify the teachable moment for class participants, and tailor your teaching methods to adult learners. During a prenatal class, parents may focus on their anticipated delivery and find it difficult to think beyond that point. Use activities that will involve them actively in order to enhance their learning. Recognize that much of what they learn prenatally may be lost, and reinforce learning with handouts on specific issues. Visual learning from other breastfeeding parents and short videos may also be effective. Help parents to focus on the positive aspects of breastfeeding and to regard it as a learning and growth process for both the mother and the baby. Help couples recognize that any problems that arise are usually resolvable.

Infant Feeding Class

Advertising a class as an "infant feeding" class rather than a breastfeeding class will make it clear that it is open to everyone. Because fathers are instrumental in the mother's decision to breastfeed, be sure to encourage them to participate in classes. Often, couples express a concern that fathers will feel left out if the mother breastfeeds. Help fathers recognize the importance of their participation in making the decision to breastfeed, and discuss ways they can be involved with the baby (see Chapter 19).

In this early class, you may help some undecided couples choose breastfeeding. You can dispel any misconceptions the couples may have and address information they will need for making their decision. Discuss the health benefits of breastfeeding for both the mother and the baby, as well as the convenience, economics, and ease of travel. Addressing the short-term and long-term risks of *not* breastfeeding will also be useful.

Prenatal Breastfeeding Class

In a prenatal class, you can address issues that will help parents prepare for establishing breastfeeding. Identify babies' cues and behaviors as they relate to feeding. Point out to parents that babies communicate through distinct cues before, during, and after feedings. Help them identify how these cues can enable them to understand and best meet their babies' needs (Delight, 1991). See Chapter 13 for a discussion of infant feeding cues.

Use visual examples to demonstrate the usual positions mothers use for holding their babies for feeding. Give parents dolls to practice positioning. Show them through videos and slides how to recognize when their baby has a good latch and positioning at the breast. Explain how an effective latch is the key to milk transfer and avoiding nipple soreness.

Help parents learn how to determine if their baby is receiving enough milk. Discuss milk production in the context of **supply and demand**. Help them learn to watch for other signs of good intake, such as audible swallows and the number of wet diapers and stools. Provide them with a feeding diary to use during the first two weeks of breastfeeding to identify the appropriate number of feedings, voids, and stools. Characterize the first two weeks as a learning time for both the mother and baby.

Explain the importance of eating when hungry and drinking when thirsty without strict dietary regimens. Encourage mothers to rest with their babies to facilitate recovery after childbirth. All of these issues will help parents achieve a smooth transition to initiating breastfeeding. See Figure 11.2 for a sample outline for a prenatal breastfeeding class.

Postpartum Breastfeeding Class

You may want to have a separate postpartum class to give mothers support and information after the baby is born. Pregnant women can be encouraged to attend this class as well. It might even be developed into a mother-to-mother support group in which pregnant women have an opportunity to talk with breastfeeding mothers and to see babies breastfeed. At this time, you can discuss what the new parents expect in the next several months. Help them anticipate typical infant behavior, growth spurts, crying, and teething. Discuss planning of activities, breastfeeding in public, and returning to work or school. You can also address complementary foods and weaning at this time.

Allow some time for group problem solving and prevention of problems such as engorgement, plugged ducts, and mastitis. Review the importance of exclusive breastfeeding and the question of supplementing with infant formula. Make sure that mothers know where they can go for help with questions or concerns. See Figure 11.3 for a sample outline for a postpartum breastfeeding class.

Prenatal Breast Care

Mothers often ask what breast preparation is needed prenatally. During pregnancy, hormones act on the breast to prepare it for lactation. The skin stretches and

---

FIGURE 11.2
Sample outline for a prenatal breastfeeding class.

I. Welcome and introductions (5 minutes)
II. Infant feeding and cultural expectations (30 minutes)
   A. Use and overuse of infant formula
   B. What our culture says about formula
   C. What our culture says about breasts
   D. Risks to mother and baby of not breastfeeding
III. How were we fed? (15 minutes)
   A. Our parents and grandparents did their best at that time (lecture and discussion)
   B. Guilt for us and those around us (lecture)
   C. How guilt helps us (lecture)
BREAK (10 minutes)
IV. Our babies (10 minutes)
   A. Speaking their language (lecture)
     1. Sleep states
     2. Feeding cues
   B. What the baby human needs (discussion and lecture)
     1. Relating baby's nutritional needs and growth to adult eating paterns
     2. Relating baby's nighttime needs to the adult
V. Breastfeeding basics (30 minutes)
   A. Milk supply (lecture)
     1. Milk removed is replaced
     2. Getting started, rooming-in, and the first week
     3. How to know baby is getting enough milk
     4. Feeding diary
   B. Positions for mom and baby (lecture and video)
     1. Basics: How to achieve good position and why it is important
     2. Options
     3. Comfort
   C. Attachment and suckling (lecture and video)
     1. Why it is important
     2. Works with good position
     3. Steps to a good latch
     4. Normal suckling
VI. Breastfeeding myths you may hear (lecture and discussion—10 minutes)
VII. How to find breastfeeding help and why you may need it (lecture—10 minutes)

Used with permission of Debbie Shinskie.

---

becomes more pliable in order to accommodate internal breast development. Increasing pigmentation protects the nipple and areola, which have enlarged. Pigmentation is due to increased melanin in the skin, which "toughens" the skin. The Montgomery glands lubricate the nipple and areola, protecting the keratin from drying out and flaking off.

Near the beginning of the third trimester, the mother can determine whether her nipples will need any assistance for a good latch. She can do this by performing the pinch test described in Chapter 21. A nipple that protrudes when stimulated makes it easiest for the baby to get a good mouthful of breast tissue. A nipple that remains flat or inverts may require assistance to improve latch. The last trimester is the best time for the woman

---

FIGURE 11.3
Sample outline for a postpartum breastfeeding class.

  I. Welcome and introductions (5 minutes)
 II. Breastfeeding's continued importance (lecture and discussion—15 minutes)
　　A. Review of risks of not breastfeeding
　　B. AAP breastfeeding recommendations
III. Growing baby milestones and issues (lecture and discussion—20 minutes)
　　A. Growth spurts
　　B. Crying
　　C. Sleep
　　D. Baby's new abilities
　　E. Teething
IV. New parents' issues (lecture, discussion, and video—20 minutes)
　　A. Resuming activities, prioritizing, and not overdoing
　　B. Ideas for including baby
　　C. Staying healthy—rest, diet, and exercise
BREAK (10 minutes)
 V. Returning to work or school (lecture, hands-on, and discussion—30 minutes)
　　A. Options
　　B. Planning ahead—talk with employer, prioritize needs
　　C. How you will feed baby in your absence
　　D. Pumps and other devices
　　E. Troubleshooting and realistic expectations
VI. The family table and weaning (lecture and discussion—10 minutes)
VII. Where to find breastfeeding help (lecture—10 minutes)

Used with permission of Debbie Shinskie.

---

to manipulate flat or inverted nipples because at that time the skin has gained elasticity and stretches more easily than earlier in her pregnancy.

Nipple Correction

When a woman has flat or inverted nipples, she first needs to establish whether intervention is appropriate or necessary. A woman with a history of prematurity or a tendency toward miscarriage or false labor should discuss with her caregiver the advisability of nipple preparation, breast foreplay, or intercourse. Such stimulation may trigger oxytocin release, which can cause the uterus to contract and induce labor.

Mothers need to know that some babies breastfeed on an inverted nipple without any difficulty. However, some babies will have difficulty with an inverted nipple that does not stimulate the baby's palate in a way that elicits his response. If a mother needs to increase the nipple's eversion, she may want to wear breast shells during the first few weeks of breastfeeding. Breast shells exert gentle pressure around the nipple, making the skin more pliable and the breast easier to grasp. When the infant suckles on the breast, this process further increases skin elasticity. Some women use an inverted

syringe to pull out the nipple before a feeding. Recommendations for the use of breast shells are mixed. See Chapter 21 for a discussion of breast shells, including the drawbacks, and the use of nipple everters.

Colostrum During Pregnancy

Colostrum production begins during pregnancy. Some mothers leak copious amounts of colostrum; others cannot express any. Prenatal leakage of colostrum is not a predictor of how much milk a mother will produce. Infrequently, some women's breasts become uncomfortably full with colostrum. These women can gently express it, only to the point of comfort. If they experience leaking, they can blend the colostrum into the areola. If colostrum causes the bra to stick to the nipple, moistening the bra with warm water before attempting to remove it will prevent skin irritation.

Many mothers breastfeed during pregnancy and go on to tandem nurse the newborn and older baby. During the last trimester, the mother's milk changes to colostrum. Many children will wean when the taste of the milk changes and the quantity decreases. See Chapter 14 for more discussion on tandem nursing.

Practices to Avoid

Make sure mothers know that they should not rub their nipples with a towel to toughen them. Rubbing of any kind damages breast tissue and should not be practiced. Mothers also will want to avoid wearing tight bras and other clothing that binds the breasts. Such localized pressure on breast tissue can cause discomfort and result in plugged ducts. Advise women to avoid these practices:

◆ Use of any drying agent on the nipples and areola.
◆ Use of plastic liners in breast pads.
◆ Use of artificial lubricants unless they are needed.
◆ Use of lubricants that do not allow the skin to breathe or that must be washed off (read labels on lotions or creams carefully).
◆ Rubbing the nipples with a towel or washcloth.
◆ Wearing tight, restrictive clothing.

Practical Planning Suggestions

An expectant woman can prepare her family, home, and wardrobe for breastfeeding. Suggest that she plan a quiet place in her home for feedings. She will want to consider initial sleeping arrangements for the baby, as well as clothing in her wardrobe that will accommodate breastfeeding. You can also encourage her to arrange household help for her early weeks home with her newborn. These plans and preparations, as well as learning about breastfeeding, can be instrumental in building the woman's confidence.

Planning a Nursing Area

Planning a particular space that will be convenient for feedings will help the mother get a comfortable start with breastfeeding. She will want a quiet spot where she can relax undisturbed for 20 to 30 minutes at a time. Whether she decides to nurse in a chair or on a sofa or bed, she will want several pillows available for support so that she is able to relax and find a comfortable position. A comfortable chair with armrests will assist the mother in supporting her baby during feedings. A footstool will enable her knees to be high enough to provide additional support. Placing a small table within arm's reach will provide a place for a beverage, snack, reading materials, telephone, and any other items she may need. Just as planning for the baby's wardrobe helps a woman prepare mentally for the arrival of her baby, planning a cozy nursing corner can help her feel confident and prepared for feeding her newborn at home.

Clothing Suggestions

Many representations of breastfeeding women show their upper chest area uncovered. In truth, mothers can breastfeed discreetly with little of their body visible. Suggest that the mother choose clothing that will cover her upper torso and allow her baby easy access to the breast. Her baby will obstruct her lower chest and abdomen from view.

The wardrobes of most women already include many items suitable for breastfeeding. Very few clothing purchases are necessary. One type of clothing is a loose-fitting item the mother can open midway. Two-piece outfits, blouses, pullovers, sweaters, and dresses with front or side openings are ideal. Blouses that button in the front can be unbuttoned from the bottom for good coverage. During feedings, the mother can drape any exposed area of the breast with an open sweater, jacket, blanket, or diaper. Dark-patterned materials hide spots caused by milk leakage, and natural fiber materials are the most comfortable. Synthetic materials are less desirable because they tend to hold in moisture and do not allow the skin to breathe. Half-slips make breastfeeding less cumbersome for some mothers, and other mothers adapt full slips by altering the straps. For nighttime feedings, the mother can select front-opening gowns, pajamas, or special nursing nightgowns with layered bodices.

There are many nursing apparel manufacturers, including several that are Internet-based. Nursing fashions have openings such as flaps or zippers to make breastfeeding easy and discreet in public. However, these clothes tend to be very expensive. Suggestions for altering clothing the mother already has are more cost-effective. Expectant mothers can find good values in maternity and nursing clothes at resale stores and garage sales, especially those benefiting nursing mothers' groups.

Selecting a Nursing Bra

The mother may select a nursing bra during her last trimester of pregnancy, or she may choose to wait until after her mature milk has come in. An expectant mother who experiences significant breast growth during pregnancy will need new bras during that time. She will want a bra that provides support and does not bind. Suggest that the mother try on bras for proper fit before making a purchase and that she buy only one bra initially. After she wears the new bra for a while, she can decide whether it meets her needs before purchasing another one. It will also save her money should the new bra not fit postpartum.

Mothers should avoid underwires and elastic around the cups, which can prevent sufficient drainage by pressing on milk ducts. For the same reason, the seams of the bra need to be well past the front of the breast, toward the underarm. Bra cups need to be cotton or a cotton-polyester blend. The mother can place breast pads, handkerchiefs, or diapers inside the bra to absorb leaking. A bra with simple cup fasteners will allow easy access to the breast. The mother can try on the bra and practice unfastening and fastening the cup several times to decide whether she will be able to manage it easily with one hand. Velcro fasteners, although convenient, are sometimes noisy. This may attract attention when breastfeeding in public and may make the mother uncomfortable. Some mothers find that sports bras provide enough support while accommodating changes in breast size during the early days of lactation. Mothers can try a variety of bras and decide which type best fits their needs.

Planning for Help at Home

Expectant parents often receive offers of help for the first several weeks after delivery. They will want to clarify the roles of potential helpers before accepting any offers of assistance. Family and friends who offer to help can do household chores so the mother can relax, rest, and care for her baby. Perhaps the father can arrange vacation time for several days while the mother and baby settle in at home. It is important that helpers understand that the parents will be caring for and bonding with their baby. The helpers can perform household tasks, run errands, shop for groceries, and ensure that the mother gets adequate rest and nutrition.

Dana Raphael devotes an entire book, *Breastfeeding: The Tender Gift*, to the topic of a helper for the mother. She offers practical suggestions for parents in determining what they would like the role of their helper to be. Marshall Klaus describes the role of the **doula** in labor and delivery in his book, *Mothering the Mother*. The Greek word *doula* refers to an experienced woman who helps other women either during the birth process or in the early postpartum period. Many times, a birth doula extends her services to the postpartum period as well, assisting the mother at home. A postpartum doula typically provides services to the mother at home rather than attending the birth.

Sleeping Arrangements

Parents will need to consider sleeping arrangements for their breastfed baby, especially during the early weeks. Keeping the baby in the parents' bed or in a separate bed in the same room makes nighttime feedings easier. The mother needs to make only minor adjustments for the baby to latch on. Limiting disruptions will make it more likely that both mother and baby quickly return to sleep.

The practice of **cosleeping** is increasing in the United States. If parents do not wish for the baby to remain in their bed, they might place an extra bed or mattress on the floor. When the baby falls asleep after nursing, the mother can return to her bed and leave him undisturbed on the mattress (depending on his age and degree of mobility). Some mothers prefer a rocking chair in the baby's room for nighttime feedings. See Chapter 13 for further discussion of cosleeping and other sleep issues.

▶ SELECTING A PHYSICIAN

Women will need to select a caregiver for both themselves and their baby. In the United States, the insurance company that provides coverage for the mother and child largely dictates the choice of caregiver. Women most likely will have established a relationship with a gynecologist before pregnancy. They can consider whether that same caregiver can meet their needs regarding prenatal care and birth. Perhaps an even more important decision is that of selecting a caregiver for their baby, especially for a woman who plans to breastfeed. She will want to know that her baby's caregiver will support her plans and provide appropriate advice.

Factors to Explore with a Potential Caregiver

Parents can investigate a number of things when they select caregivers for the mother and her baby. They need to be comfortable and secure in their decision and have confidence in their caregiver's ability. The parents and caregiver must be able to develop an adult working relationship. Parents want a caregiver who is willing to listen, will respond to questions, and demonstrates flexibility in decisions. Their goal is to form a partnership with their caregiver to develop a health plan that will result in the most favorable outcome.

Background

Parents can check the caregiver's credentials and background by contacting the local hospital, requesting information from the caregiver's receptionist, or calling the county medical society. They may also question friends who use this caregiver's services. The *Directory of Medical Specialists*, available in any public library, will indicate whether a physician graduated from a fully accredited medical school. Parents may also want to ask whether the caregiver is board certified and what his or her hospital standings are. These items can reflect a physician's qualifications and professional standing.

Continuing Education

Parents can check literature around the caregiver's office to see if current information about breastfeeding is available. They can ask about any continuing education by the caregiver in breastfeeding and other activities, such as teaching at a nearby hospital or medical school. In a recent survey, four out of ten obstetricians felt their training in breastfeeding management was inadequate (Power, 2003). Other studies have found consistent deficits in practitioners' knowledge of breastfeeding (Freed, 1995a, 1995b, 1995c; Saenz, 2000). Saenz provides a helpful model for a lactation management rotation for medical residents in her article.

Hospital Affiliation

Parents will want to know whether the caregiver has privileges at the facility they have chosen to give birth. Is it family centered? Have they heard positive reports from people who have used the facility, including women who have breastfed?

Accessibility

The caregiver should be easily accessible for scheduled visits and emergencies. Many times, a nurse, medical assistant, or receptionist can answer parents' questions. However, when there is a pressing medical concern, parents have the right, after describing a problem to the nurse, to talk directly with the physician. They also will want to choose someone who, when not on duty, provides coverage by someone who is acceptable to the parents. They can ask how much time the caregiver allots for office visits, whether there is a specific telephone hour, and how prompt the caregiver is in returning calls.

Standing Orders

Most physicians have standing orders that apply to all patients under their care. These are orders the nursing staff follow unless directed otherwise. Parents will want to learn their particular physician's standing orders relative to breastfeeding and postpartum care in the hospital. Such orders may concern the administration of certain medications, routine water or formula for infants, or other practices that parents may want to discuss with the physician before delivery.

The nursing staff has special instructions, referred to as nursing protocol, in all areas, including breastfeeding. Parents will want to be alert to the possibility of scheduled feeding times, routine use of nipple shields or pacifiers, or routine supplementation with water or formula for all babies. If the mother and physician develop a plan that is different from the standing orders or nursing protocol, advise that they put it in writing. Both the parents and physician should sign it and keep a copy. Hospital personnel also need a copy to help ensure compliance with the parents' wishes.

Relationship with the Patient

Parents will want a caregiver who genuinely listens to patients, gives understandable explanations, welcomes questions, and returns calls. Will the caregiver openly discuss alternatives and welcome a second opinion? What is the caregiver's position regarding prepared childbirth and breastfeeding? Parents may want to talk to friends who use this caregiver's services and discuss his or her strengths and weaknesses.

Mother's Choice of the Baby's Caregiver

The choice of a baby's caregiver is an important decision for parents. Encourage them to give the selection careful consideration and investigation. Most parents in developed countries choose either a pediatrician or a family practice physician for their baby's care. A pediatrician is a medical doctor who specializes in pediatric care for children from newborn through adolescence. A family practice physician, similar to a general practice or family doctor of the past, is now considered a specialty. A family physician is able to treat the entire family. More information about each specialty is available at www. aap.org for pediatricians and www.aafp.org for family physicians.

Many pediatric offices have pediatric nurse practitioners (PNPs) on staff. These nurses have extra education and certification in pediatrics, have prescriptive privileges, and can handle routine well-child check-ups. One study found that although PNPs were more knowledgeable about lactation than pediatricians were, 38.2 percent reported they never counseled women about breastfeeding in their practices. Another 17.1 percent never assisted mothers with breastfeeding technique. Just under a third of respondents

frequently counseled prenatal patients and assisted mothers with breastfeeding technique and lactation problems (Hellings, 2004). Many PNPs provide medical care for indigent or welfare patients in clinics and are often the primary caregiver for these populations. Suggest that the parents arrange a prenatal visit with the caregiver to discuss the issues listed below:

- How soon after birth the first office visit will be scheduled
- The number of times the caregiver expects to see the baby for health maintenance
- The caregiver's staff privileges at the hospital where the baby will be delivered and, if none, would the caregiver give a referral to another pediatrician or family practitioner
- Degree to which parents are encouraged to make non-medical decisions such as feeding schedule, sleep patterns, supplemental foods, and weaning
- Treatment of jaundice in the newborn
- Viewpoint on circumcision
- Hospital policy regarding delay of antibiotic ointment in the baby's eyes, to enhance initial bonding between parents and baby
- Policy on vitamin, iron, and fluoride supplements
- Percentage of breastfeeding babies in the practice and the average duration of breastfeeding
- Hospital policy regarding how soon the mother and baby can breastfeed after delivery
- Hospital's encouragement of rooming-in
- Breastfeeding protocol in the hospital
- Policy on water and formula supplementation
- Willingness to support the mother's breastfeeding practices
- Management of breastfeeding problems
- The person who answers breastfeeding questions
- Whether there are IBCLCs on staff
- Whether mothers are referred to an IBCLC if there is not one on staff
- Criteria for starting solid foods
- Guidelines for weaning, including support for child-led weaning
- Relationship with breastfeeding support groups in the community

Communicating with the Caregiver

Make sure mothers know that it is never too late to discuss a concern with her caregiver. If she has second thoughts after a visit, suggest that she call their office. While in the hospital, a mother may have questions that cannot wait until the scheduled rounds. She can ask the nursing staff to contact the caregiver. If the staff is busy, they may not get to this as quickly as the mother would like. She can place the call herself rather than wait. When the mother and the caregiver have a plan, she can ask that the baby's chart reflect the change. Many times, caregivers will be flexible when a mother explains her position with confidence and self-assurance.

If the mother decides to contact her caregiver with a concern, you can help her formulate her questions and clarify the caregiver's response. Ask the mother what the exact words were. Did her caregiver say, "You *must* start solid foods now" or "You *can* start solid foods now"? Encourage her to share any confusion tactfully. Most caregivers enjoy educating receptive parents. Encourage the mother to communicate her commitment to breast-feeding and to appeal for support through difficulties.

Conflicting Advice

When mothers are knowledgeable about breastfeeding, they are more aware of advice from their caregiver that seems questionable. You can offer suggestions to prepare a mother for times when advice seems detrimental to breastfeeding. Provide her with a solid basis of information and give her literature to take to her caregiver. Encourage the mother to work with and inform her caregiver about her day-to-day breastfeeding. If she is under the care of a medical team, suggest that she try to work with the most supportive and knowledgeable member.

It is important that mothers understand that their caregiver's advice is simply that—advice. When a caregiver advises a patient to have her cholesterol checked, the patient can decide whether to act on the advice. The caregiver cannot make a patient comply with the advice. Physicians advise; they do not command. Parents must comply only when there is clear and definite danger to the child. Responsible parents can make responsible decisions regarding the care of their baby. This includes breastfeeding decisions that are, for the most part, not medical in nature.

Working through Conflicts

If a mother encounters conflicts with her caregiver, you can support her while being careful not to drive a wedge between them. Prepare her before a visit by reminding her of typical breastfeeding patterns at her baby's present stage of development. Encourage her to prepare specific questions prior to office visits.

When seemingly detrimental advice is given, urge the mother to ask for the reason behind the advice and whether alternative treatment is possible. Help her work out solutions. Never encourage a mother to go against her caregiver's medical advice, either openly or by implication. Help a mother adapt the advice to breastfeeding

if you can. If the caregiver insists that her baby receive supplements or solid foods, you can suggest that the mother give the supplements after a breastfeeding and that she limit the quantity of the supplements. You could suggest that she use a device for supplementing at the breast to stimulate milk production.

You might suggest that the mother ask for a trial period during which she can nurse more frequently in an effort to increase her milk production. Perhaps she can schedule a weight check for a short time later and postpone supplements until then. When a mother has successfully overcome breastfeeding challenges, such as low milk supply or thrush, encourage her to share her success with her caregiver. This way, both the caregiver and the mother can learn and benefit from her experience. The caregiver will then be better able to help mothers with similar problems in the future.

Recommending Caregivers to Mothers

If a mother finds she is always at odds with her caregiver, she may decide she wants to change to a new provider. On the other hand, she may be satisfied with her caregiver in other areas and only wants a consultation on a specific breastfeeding issue. If a woman asks you to recommend a caregiver, you can suggest the names of three local providers. In this way, it does not appear that you are recommending a particular one. This provides the woman with a choice of caregivers to suit her personality and her needs. It also helps ensure that the breastfeeding women in your community will work with a variety of caregivers. This increases the caregivers' practical experience with breastfeeding care. In addition, it helps you remain professional and objective in making recommendations and contacts with the medical profession.

In addition to the caregivers' names, you can be prepared to give women as much factual information as is practical about each caregiver. At the same time, avoid any personal opinions. You may want to keep an accurate updated file on caregivers, including office hours, call hours, practices related to breastfeeding, and standing orders for hospital and office procedures. Many medical practices provide information brochures and maintain Web sites. Practices that accept new patients will usually be happy to provide you with brochures.

You can provide mothers with pertinent questions to ask a prospective caregiver. You may also use your information about caregivers to help prepare mothers for their hospital experiences and pediatric checkups. ("Dr. _____ usually tells mothers to _____ at the first checkup. You may want to think about this before you go so that you can have any questions or concerns ready.") An informed and prepared mother is more likely to be satisfied with the outcome of her visit. She is more likely to understand and follow recommendations and less apt to need to call the caregiver for clarification.

▶ **SUMMARY**

You can be instrumental in helping parents in their decision to breastfeed. Parents are entitled to facts that will enable them to make informed choices. Teaching and counseling parents prenatally will help them acquire this information at a time when they are considering a method of infant feeding. Help couples distinguish between breastfeeding facts and possible misconceptions that can cause confusion and concern. Provide practical suggestions prenatally regarding breast care and preparations at home. Be available to expectant parents who may need assistance in selecting a caregiver who is knowledgeable and supportive of breastfeeding.

Consider offering a series of classes on breastfeeding to provide relevant information at key times. A prenatal class on infant feeding will help in the decision-making process. A later prenatal class on practical breastfeeding management will help parents prepare for their baby's arrival. A postpartum breastfeeding class will reinforce effective practices and address any questions the parents may have as they continue breastfeeding. All of these early interventions will form a strong foundation for parents as they approach the birth of their baby and the beginning of breastfeeding.

▶ **CHAPTER 11 — AT A GLANCE**

Facts you learned—

Deciding to breastfeed:

- Women most likely to breastfeed are in their mid-30s, middle income, college educated, white, and married.
- Statistically, African American and teen mothers are least likely to breastfeed.
- Over half of women make their infant feeding choices before pregnancy.
- Support of the baby's father is pivotal to the decision.
- Attitude and knowledge level of caregivers greatly influences parents' decision and confidence.
- Prenatal support and postpartum visits increase the likelihood of continuing breastfeeding.
- Modesty, privacy, work or school conflicts, lack of confidence, diet, stress, substance abuse, and inadequate sleep create barriers to breastfeeding.
- Commercial messages about formula imply little difference with breastmilk.
- Sexual images of breasts may be confusing.

- Aversion to breasts being touched is common in survivors of sexual or physical abuse.

Prenatal preparation for breastfeeding:

- The last trimester is the best time for manipulating flat or inverted nipples.
- Discourage nipple stimulation when there is a history of prematurity, miscarriage, or false labor.
- Cosleeping with the baby can make early feedings easier.
- Confidence in and a working relationship with their physician are important to parents.
- Parents can ask about physicians' background, breastfeeding knowledge, hospital affiliation, accessibility, and standing orders regarding breastfeeding.

Applying what you learned—

- Encourage discussion by couples and sharing of information with fathers.
- Explain the risks of not breastfeeding.
- Point out the health, emotional, and financial benefits of breastfeeding.
- Explain the convenience of caring for other children and traveling when breastfeeding.
- Acquaint mothers with the realities of breast fullness, nipple tenderness, and the need to be available to the baby for nourishment.
- Offer ways to cope with concerns and to include the baby in her activities.
- Dispel misconceptions and increase confidence in her decision to breastfeed.
- Be aware of circumstances in which a mother may not breastfeed her baby.
- Discuss practical aspects of breastfeeding closer to baby's due date.
- Encourage prenatal breastfeeding classes.
- Discuss individual goals for breastfeeding, and give mothers information that will help them blend breastfeeding into their lives.
- Teach infant feeding classes, and keep it simple.
- Teach parents to trust their instincts and how to respond to their baby's cues.
- Actively involve parents in learning, and reinforce it with visual aids.
- Encourage fathers to participate in classes.
- Demonstrate positioning for feeding, and have parents practice with dolls.
- Teach how to know when the baby is receiving enough milk.

◆ Discuss the basis of supply and demand in milk production.

◆ Offer a support group with time for problem solving and prevention of common problems.

◆ Talk with mothers about planning a nursing area, clothing that allows easy access for feedings, how and when to select a nursing bra, and arranging for help at home.

◆ Encourage mothers to be open with their physician about their breastfeeding.

◆ Be careful not to drive a wedge between a mother and her physician.

◆ When recommending physicians, give at least three names and information about their breastfeeding practices and standing orders.

▶ **REFERENCES**

Beal A et al. Breastfeeding advice given to African American and white women by physicians and WIC counselors. *Public Health Rep* 118(4):368–376; 2003.

Bryant C. Empowering women to breastfeed. *Int J Childbirth Education* 8:13–15; 1993.

Chang J, Chan W. Analysis of factors associated with initiation and duration of breast-feeding: A study in Taitung Taiwan. *Acta Paediatr Taiwan* 44(1):29–34; 2003.

Daneault et al. Psychosocial determinants of the intention of nurses and dietitians to recommend breastfeeding. *Can J Public Health* 95(2):151–154; 2004.

Delight E et al. What do parents expect antenatally and do babies teach them? *Arch Dis Child* 66:1309–1314; 1991.

Donath SM, Amir LH, ALSPAC Study Team. Relationship between prenatal infant feeding intention and initiation and duration of breast feeding: A cohort study. *Acta Paediatr* 92:352–356; 2003.

Ekstrom A et al. Breastfeeding support from partners and grandmothers: Perceptions of Swedish women. *Birth* 30(4): 261–266; 2003.

England L et al. Breastfeeding practices in a cohort of inner-city women: The role of contraindications. *BMC Public Health* 3(1): 28; 2003.

Falceto O et al. Couples' relationships and breastfeeding: Is there an association? *J Hum Lact* 20(1):46–55; 2004.

Freed G et al. Accuracy of expectant mothers' predictions of fathers' attitudes regarding breast-feeding. *J Fam Pract* 37: 148–152; 1992.

Freed G et al. Breast-feeding education and practice in family medicine. *J Fam Pract* 40(3):263–269; 1995a.

Freed G et al. National assessment of physicians' breast-feeding knowledge, attitudes, training, and experience. *JAMA* 273(6): 472–476; 1995b.

Freed G et al. Pediatrician involvement in breast-feeding promotion: A national study of residents and practitioners. *Pediatrics* 96(3 Pt 1):490–494; 1995c.

Gamble D, Morse J. Fathers of breastfed infants: Postponing and types of involvement. *JOGNN* 22:358–365; 1993.

Guise J et al. The effectiveness of primary care-based interventions to promote breastfeeding: Systematic evidence review and meta-analysis for the US Preventive Services Task Force. Review. *Ann Fam Med* 1(2):70–78; 2003.

Harris et al. Breasts and breastfeeding: Perspectives of women in the early months after birthing. *Breastfeed Rev* 11(3):21–29; 2003.

Hellings P, Howe C. Breastfeeding knowledge and practice of pediatric nurse practitioners. *J Pediatric Health Care* 18(1): 8–14; 2004.

Johnston B et al. Expanding developmental and behavioral services for newborns in primary care: Effects on parental well-being, practice, and satisfaction. *Am J Prev Med* 26(4): 356–366; 2004.

Kendall-Tackett K. *The Hidden Feelings of Motherhood.* Oakland, CA: New Harbinger; 2001.

Kitzinger JV. Counteracting, not reenacting, the violation of women's bodies: The challenge for perinatal caregivers. *Birth* 19:219–220; 1992.

Klaus et al. Maternal assistance in support in labor: Father, nurse, midwife or doula? *Clinical Consultations in Obstetrics and Gynecology* 4; 1992.

Kong S, Lee D. Factors influencing decision to breastfeed. *J Adv Nurs* 46(4):369–379; 2004.

Lawrence R. A review of the medical contraindications to breastfeeding. *Technical Information Bulletin.* Washington, DC: National Center for Education in Maternal Child Health, USDHHS; October 1997.

Li L et al. Factors associated with the initiation and duration of breastfeeding by Chinese mothers in Perth, Western Australia. *J Hum Lact* 20(2):188–195; 2004.

Littman H et al. The decision to breastfeed. *Clinical Pedatrics* 33(4):214–219; 1994.

Lu M et al. Provider encouragement of breast-feeding: Evidence from a national survey. *Obstet Gynecol* 97(2):290–295; 2001.

Marchand L, Morrow M. Infant feeding practices: Understanding the decision-making process. *Fam Med* 26:319–324; 1994.

Noble L et al. Factors influencing initiation of breast-feeding among urban women. *Am J Perinatol* 20(8):477–483; 2003.

Power M et al. The effort to increase breast-feeding: Do obstetricians, in the forefront, need help? *J Reprod Med* 48(2): 72–78; 2003.

Prentice J et al. The association between reported childhood sexual abuse and breastfeeding initiation. *J Hum Lact* 3: 219–226; 2002.

Pridham K. Anticipatory guidance of parents of new infants: Potential contribution of the Internal Working Model construct. *Image* 25:49–56; 1993.

Rose V et al. Factors influencing infant feeding method in an urban community. *J Natl Med Assoc* 96(3):325–331; 2004.

Ryan A et al. Breastfeeding continues to increase into the new millennium. *Pediatrics* 110(6):1103–1109; 2002.

Saenz R. A lactation management rotation for family medicine residents. *J Hum Lact* 16(4):342–345; 2000.

Shaker I et al. Infant feeding attitudes of expectant parents: Breastfeeding and formula feeding. *J Adv Nurs* 45(3):260–268; 2004.

Sharps P et al. Health beliefs and parenting attitudes influence breastfeeding patterns among low-income African-American women. *J Perinatol* 23(5):414–419; 2003.

Sikorski J, Renfrew MJ, Pindoria S, Wade A. Support for breastfeeding mothers (Cochrane Review). *Cochrane Database Syst Rev* 1: CD001141; 2002.

Taveras E et al. Mothers' and clinicians' perspectives on breastfeeding counseling during routine preventive visits. *Pediatrics* 113(5):e405–e411; 2004a.

Taveras E et al. Opinions and practices of clinicians associated with continuation of exclusive breastfeeding. *Pediatrics* 113(4): e283–e290; 2004b.

Walker M. *Selling Out Mothers and Babies: Marketing of Breast Milk Substitutes in the USA*. Weston, MA: NABA REAL; 2001.

BIBLIOGRAPHY

Heinowitz J, Horn W. *Fathering Right from the Start*. Navato, CA: New World Library; 2001.

Izatt S. Breastfeeding counseling by health care providers. *J Hum Lact* 13:109–113; 1997.

Jordan P, Wall V. Breastfeeding and fathers: Illuminating the darker side. *Birth* 17:210–213; 1990.

Jordan P, Wall V. Supporting the father when an infant is breastfed. *J Hum Lact* 9:31–34; 1993.

Lawrence R. *Breastfeeding: A Guide for the Medical Profession*, 5th ed. St. Louis, MO: Mosby; 1999.

Leff E et al. Maternal perceptions of successful breastfeeding. *J Hum Lact* 10(2):99–104; 1994.

Raphael D. *Breastfeeding: The Tender Gift*. New York: Schocken Books; 1976.

Ryan A et al. Recent declines in breastfeeding in the United States, 1984–1989. *Pediatr* 88(4):719; 1991.

Sears W et al. *Becoming a Father*, 2nd ed. Schaumburg, IL: La Leche League International; 2003.

Smith L. How to teach great breastfeeding classes. Bright Futures Lactation Resource Centre; 1996. Available at: www.bflrc.com/ljs/teaching/bf_class.htm. Accessed January 8, 2004.

Weissinger D. A breastfeeding teaching tool using a sandwich analogy for latch-on. *J Hum Lact* 14:51–56; 1998.

HOSPITAL PRACTICES THAT SUPPORT BREASTFEEDING

Contributing Author: Jan Barger

Most countries use the midwifery model of family-centered care, with families giving birth in birth centers or at home. This chapter addresses hospital practices, which are the focus of the Baby-Friendly Hospital Initiative. Hospital practices directly influence a mother's breastfeeding experience. An environment that is supportive and accepting and that builds the mother's self-confidence enhances the establishment of breastfeeding. Institutional routines need to reflect a belief in breastfeeding as the norm and to facilitate sound breastfeeding care. Policies must be evidence based, rather than based on personal experience or tradition. Developing hospital policies based on the *Ten Steps to Successful Breastfeeding* (WHO/UNICEF, 1989) is the first step in providing a supportive environment. The *Ten Steps to Successful Breastfeeding* presented in Figure 12.1 forms the basis of this discussion. Using the Ten Step protocol has an extended positive impact on breastfeeding rates in a hospital setting (Philipp, 2003).

SETTING THE STAGE PRIOR TO BIRTH

Women typically view their caregivers as authority figures and value their opinions because of their extensive training and experience. Their caregiver's attitudes about breastfeeding will greatly influence the mother's attitude and, indirectly, the quality of her breastfeeding (Taveras, 2003). A hospital that is baby friendly fosters a climate of acceptance and support for breastfeeding mothers through supportive policies and supportive healthcare professionals.

KEY TERMS

analgesia
artificial teats
baby friendly
bonding
cesarean
cluster feeding
clutch hold
discharge planning
Duarte's variant
edema
epidural anesthesia
episiotomy
feeding cues
finger-feeding
football hold
forceps
galactose
hydration

interventions
kangaroo care
mother-to-mother support
　group
natural childbirth
nipple shield
nonnutritive sucking
phenylalanine
phenylketonuria
phototherapy
red flags
rooming-in
self-appraisal tool
supplementary feeding
Ten Steps to Successful
　Breastfeeding
vacuum extraction
vernix

FIGURE 12.1
Ten steps to successful breastfeeding.

Every facility providing maternity services and care for newborn infants should:

1. Have a written breastfeeding policy that is routinely communicated to all health care staff.
2. Train all health care staff in skills necessary to implement this policy.
3. Inform all pregnant women about the benefits and management of breastfeeding.
4. Help mothers initiate breastfeeding within a half hour of birth.
5. Show mothers how to breastfeed and how to maintain lactation even if they should be separated from their infants.
6. Give newborn infants no food or drink other than breastmilk unless medically indicated.
7. Practice rooming in—allow mothers and infants to remain together—24 hours a day.
8. Encourage breastfeeding in response to feeding cues.
9. Give no artificial teats or pacifiers (also called dummies or soothers) to breastfeeding infants.
10. Foster the establishment of breastfeeding support groups and refer mothers to them on discharge from the hospital or clinic.

Establish Supportive Breastfeeding Policies

STEP ONE OF THE TEN STEPS
Have a written breastfeeding policy that is routinely communicated to all health care staff.

Developing a set of breastfeeding policies based on current scientific knowledge will help eliminate unnecessary and intrusive interventions that negatively affect the initiation of breastfeeding. Policies do not need to be extensive. In fact, staff will follow policies more closely if they are brief and cover only the salient points. Staff often read policies at orientation and look at them again only when there is a specific question. Posting policies where staff can review them frequently will improve compliance. One of the first responsibilities of the IBCLC at a hospital may be to develop or review current breastfeeding policies in order to improve the quality of care given to breastfeeding mothers and to decrease obstacles that hamper the smooth initiation of breastfeeding.

Polices need to be communicated to all healthcare staff who encounter breastfeeding mothers and infants. This extends beyond the nursing staff on the mother-baby unit to include physicians, ancillary staff, patient care technicians, and administrative staff of all units that care for mothers and babies. Staff in the NICU, labor and delivery, pediatrics, and to a certain extent, the emergency room and medical-surgical units all have contact with breastfeeding mothers.

Teach Breastfeeding Care to Staff

STEP TWO OF THE TEN STEPS
Train all healthcare staff in skills necessary to implement this policy.

An important job of the IBCLC will be to educate the healthcare staff in how to implement breastfeeding policies. Understanding the rationale and scientific basis behind them will increase acceptance by the medical and nursing staff. Training in basic breastfeeding care will free the IBCLC to concentrate on cases that are more difficult. Basic instruction should include positioning and latch, evaluating the quality of a feeding and when and how to supplement infants. It will also ensure that mothers will receive appropriate and consistent help when the IBCLC is not available.

Educate Pregnant Women

STEP THREE OF THE TEN STEPS
Inform all pregnant women about the benefits and management of breastfeeding.

All women need to know about the benefits and management of breastfeeding in order to make an informed decision about how they will feed their baby and to dispel any misconceptions. Many hospitals offer prenatal breastfeeding classes. If one does not exist in your hospital, you can initiate one. You can work in cooperation with childbirth education classes to ensure that information about breastfeeding is included in every class. This will reach women who may not otherwise receive it. Work with obstetric and family practice physicians and health clinics to make sure they include correct and consistent information about breastfeeding during prenatal visits.

▶ LABOR AND DELIVERY PRACTICES THAT SUPPORT EARLY BREASTFEEDING

A woman's labor and delivery experience can affect early breastfeeding and whether or not she breastfeeds her baby for a long period. It is very difficult to initiate normal postpartum breastfeeding after intrusive labor and delivery practices. Policies that routinely separate mothers and babies and interfere with the process of breastfeeding are not in the best interest of mothers and babies and need to be changed. A mother needs a warm, reassuring, and caring atmosphere that supports her goals and helps her develop the self-confidence that will enable her to be comfortable with making decisions concerning her baby.

Provide Labor Support

A 1991 study showed that women who receive support during labor are more likely to be breastfeeding at six weeks than are those who receive no support. Despite the fact that the support was specific to breastfeeding, women felt they had coped well with the birth and thus were more confident. This self-confidence carried over to their feelings about mothering and breastfeeding (Hofmeyer, 1991).

Ideally, hospitals will encourage women to have an experienced labor support person, often referred to as a doula, with them throughout the entire labor and delivery. This results in fewer medications, less anesthesia, and fewer complications. Babies are more alert and responsive after an unmedicated birth, and an unmedicated birth is much more likely when the mother has doula support. Babies are then better able to breastfeed within 1 to 2 hours after birth.

The presence of a doula during labor and birth provides the laboring woman with continuous physical, emotional, and informational support. The doula does not replace the baby's father or other support person chosen by the mother from her family or friends. Rather, the doula enhances the mother's support system. She is experienced in the use of comfort measures that will decrease the pain of labor without using medications or anesthesia. She provides ongoing support in a manner different from the baby's father.

Studies show that the presence of a doula will result in fewer interventions for the mother and baby. It can reduce the overall cesarean rate by 50 percent, the length of labor by 25 percent, pitocin use by 40 percent, pain medication by 30 percent, the need for forceps by 40 percent, and requests for epidural anesthesia by 60 percent (Klaus, 1992).

Limit Interventions

The use of medications, anesthesia, and other interventions during labor and birth can affect early breastfeeding and influences whether a baby is breastfed for a long period. It can be difficult to achieve normal and optimal postpartum breastfeeding management after a labor and delivery that involves intervention. Any policy that routinely separates a mother from her baby interferes with breastfeeding and contradicts good medical care.

Non-Essential Routine Interventions

Between 1975 and 1982, the United States experienced the peak of the "natural childbirth" movement. During that same period, the breastfeeding initiation rate increased from approximately 25 percent to 62 percent. This was followed by more than a decade during which birth interventions increased by more than 50 percent— interventions such as medications, epidural anesthesia, IVs, electronic fetal monitors, and cardiac monitors. In the same period, breastfeeding initiation declined from 62 percent to 51 percent. Between 1991 and 2003, the breastfeeding initiation rate rose from 51 percent to 70.1 percent.

Labor and birth are normal biological processes. However, most U.S. hospitals do not treat them as such. The events that surround birth clearly have an impact on breastfeeding (Kroeger, 2004; Hofmeyer, 1991). American hospitals have evolved to rely on an increased use of technology. In order for breastfeeding to get off to a good start, parents can try to limit the routine use of technology surrounding birth. Mothers need opportunity and assistance to put the baby to breast within

1 hour of birth unless there is a clearly identifiable and justifiable reason for intervention.

Medications Used in Labor

Medications the mother receives during labor may cause babies to become drowsy and to have difficulty suckling (Hale, 2004). They may also make mothers less responsive to their babies. Mothers can avoid these drugs when possible. They can educate themselves about techniques and drugs that are least likely to interfere with breastfeeding, such as the use of support persons, walking, showers, bathing, birthing balls, and other comfort measures (Bond, 1992).

Analgesia

Mothers frequently receive **analgesia** such as nalbuphine, alphaprodine, butorphanol, and meperidine to "take the edge off" labor pain. One study found that the babies of mothers who received Nisentil 1 to 3 hours prior to delivery took an average of 21.2 hours to establish effective breastfeeding (Matthews, 1989). Only 66 percent were effectively breastfeeding by 24 hours. On the other hand, babies whose mothers received no central nervous system depressants in labor took only 11.8 hours to establish feedings, and 93 percent were effectively breastfeeding by 24 hours. Pain relief medications diminish early suckling (Riordan, 2000). Consequently, mothers who receive medication during labor are more likely to leave the hospital without having established breastfeeding. Mizuno (2004a) demonstrated that sucking behavior during the early newborn period affects breastfeeding rate and duration. Any practice that delays early suckling therefore can have long-lasting consequences.

Epidural Anesthesia

Epidural anesthesia compromises a baby's ability to breastfeed by diminishing early suckling (Riordan, 2000). Additionally, women who receive epidural anesthesia in labor receive significantly more pitocin, are more likely to have forceps deliveries, and spend less time with their babies while in the hospital (Sepkoski, 1992). The babies of these mothers have poorer behavioral outcome and recovery, have less alertness and ability to orient over the first month of life, and are less mature in their motor function. Traces of bupivucaine, an anesthesia used in epidurals, is present in the babies' **cord blood** and in the neonate's blood up to three days after delivery. Sepkoski suggests that the depressed performance of infants may be a direct result of the anesthetic on the neonatal central nervous system.

A later study showed that mothers who receive epidurals during labor have an increased incidence of intrapartum fever. The baby may then also be worked up for sepsis, receive antibiotics, and be transferred to the

NICU (Liberman, 1997). The earlier a mother receives epidural anesthesia, the greater her risk of cesarean section (Morton, 1994). Mothers who have epidural anesthesia and do not breastfeed within the first hour are at high risk for having their babies receive supplementation. In one study, 81 percent of unmedicated mothers achieved 2 effective breastfeedings within 24 hours of delivery, compared to 69.6 percent of the mothers who had received epidural anesthesia (Baumgarder, 2003).

Other Interventions During Labor and Delivery

Frequent and routine medical intervention during labor and birth increases the risk of interference with breastfeeding. Many of these interventions result from the overuse of central nervous system depressants and epidural anesthesia. Women need to be empowered to birth their babies without the use of medications and anesthesia and should receive the support to do so.

Episiotomy

Women who have had an **episiotomy** often find it difficult to get comfortable, particularly when they sit upright. An episiotomy increases the risk of a fourth-degree laceration, which is a tear through the rectal mucosa. If the mother is not comfortable when she is sitting, it is difficult for her to relax enough to focus on getting the baby positioned well at the breast. Because pain can inhibit the mother's milk ejection reflex, she may need more analgesia, which can pass through her milk in small doses to her baby.

Suctioning

Hospital staff may be inclined to put a baby to breast in an attempt to soothe him immediately after deep suctioning and visualization of the **larynx**. However, this can have disastrous consequences for breastfeeding. Some babies appear to associate breastfeeding with the pain that preceded their first experience at the breast and to react negatively whenever put to breast.

Mechanical Devices

Forceps and **vacuum extraction** both carry increased risk of bruising and sensitivity to the infant's head. This will limit the ways in which he will be comfortable when positioned for early breastfeedings. Bruising also increases the risk of jaundice, thereby causing sleepiness and a lack of interest in feeding.

Pitocin

Pitocin, used to induce or stimulate labor, has an antidiuretic effect. Edema may result, particularly in extremities such as the breast and nipple tissue. The result may be "meaty" and "flat" nipples that are difficult for

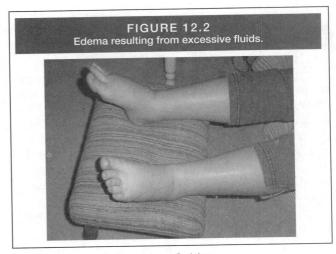

FIGURE 12.2
Edema resulting from excessive fluids.

Printed with permission of Anna Swisher.

the infant to latch onto until the edema is relieved, generally in about 3 days. Refer to Chapter 21 for the use of reverse pressure softening (RPS) to help soften these mothers' areolas in order for their babies to latch on effectively (Cotterman, 2004). IBCLCs have noted edema in women who receive many liters of IV fluids in conjunction with epidurals and pitocin. These women often experience a delay in milk production, perhaps due to an overload of edema in the breast. Figure 12.2 shows edema in a mother's ankles and feet.

Removing the Baby to a Radiant Warmer

Hospital staff often place babies in radiant warmers because of babies' inability to self-regulate their temperatures. However, warmers are unnecessary if the mother and baby remain together. Babies who are snuggled skin to skin with their mothers kangaroo style (**kangaroo care**) warm faster, stay warm longer, and have less risk of dehydration than babies placed under radiant warmers (Christensson, 1992). Skin-to-skin contact allows for adequate temperature maintenance without increased fluid loss. The infant's nose is near the mother's skin and thus he breathes warm, humidified air, rather than dry hospital air. The heat from the mother's body is humid, unlike the dry air from artificial warmers.

Several studies support the benefits of kangaroo care. A study in Nepal showed that the mother's body successfully prevents hypothermia in the newborn (Johanson, 1992). In another study, infants with kangaroo care slept longer, were mostly in a quiet sleep state, exhibited more flexor movements and postures, and showed less extensor movements (Ferber, 2004). A review of 17 other studies correlated skin-to-skin care with increased breastfeeding duration, maintenance of infant temperature, reduced infant crying, stable blood glucose levels, and expressions of maternal love and touch (Anderson, 2003). Another study suggests that skin-to-skin contact for more than 50 minutes immediately after birth results in enhanced infant recognition of their own mother's milk odor and longer breastfeeding duration (Mizuno, 2004b). See Chapter 23 for further discussion of kangaroo care.

Delayed First Breastfeeding

The longer a mother waits to initiate breastfeeding, the more likely she will be to feed her baby infant formula in the first few days of life and the more likely the hospital staff will be to use formula. Kurinij (1991) reports, "This implies that hospital staff and routines, centered on a formula-feeding mode, can by suggestion influence maternal infant feeding behavior. These nonverbal hospital routines may be responsible for the observed differences in exclusive breastfeeding rates between hospitals." The routines cited include delayed first feeding, rising cesarean rate, decreased mother-baby contact, and feeding on a schedule. The labor and delivery staff can preserve and protect breastfeeding by reducing these obstacles. Avoiding episiotomies and other technological assistance increases comfort for the mother and her baby.

Promote Bonding Immediately After Birth

Ideally, parents will spend the initial moments with their baby, hugging, smiling, loving, and nursing. They will flourish in their transition to parenthood in a supportive environment that enables them to begin their new family in privacy—an environment that is both baby friendly and mother friendly. When an infant leaves the comfortable secure confines of his mother's womb, he finds himself in an unfamiliar and perhaps unsettling environment. When placed in the comfort of his mother's arms, he feels the warmth of her body heat and can nuzzle at her breast.

Bonding between the mother and her baby is strongest in the first one or two hours. Skin-to-skin contact enhances bonding even further. A newborn's rooting and sucking reflexes are particularly strong in the first hours after an unmedicated delivery. The mother's normal body bacteria will colonize her baby's body—but only if she is the first person to hold him, rather than a nurse, physician, or other caregivers. Keeping the mother and baby together will accomplish this.

Soon after birth, staff will observe and assess the baby and determine his Apgar score, which ranges from 0 to 10. The Apgar score evaluates the baby's heart rate, respiratory effort, body tone, grimace, and color. The score indicates his overall state of health and assists caregivers in determining if any intervention is necessary. It is performed at 1 minute of life and again at 5 and 10 minutes. The process need not interfere with bonding, as staff can perform it while the mother holds her baby.

U.S. state laws require treatment of all newborn infants' eyes with an antibiotic to safeguard against the effects of sexually transmitted disease. Staff can delay this procedure to allow the parents and baby at least one hour of uninterrupted time together. Postponing antibiotic treatment of the baby's eyes will allow eye contact and enhance bonding between the parents and baby.

The Bonding Process

John Kennell and Marshall Klaus popularized the term "bonding" in their book, *Maternal-Infant Bonding* (Klaus, 1982). They later incorporated the concepts into a new book, *Bonding: Building the Foundations of Secure Attachment and Independence* (Klaus, 2000). They stress the importance of close physical contact between the mother and baby soon after birth, as well as the detrimental effects of routine hospital practices that separate them. Delayed contact following birth and strict feeding schedules with the baby spending the majority of time in the nursery discourage the development of attachment. The most favorable time to initiate bonding is in the first minutes after birth when the baby is alert and the parents are most eager to see and touch him.

The process of bonding begins with the first parent-infant contact in the hours following birth and continues as parent and infant interact to form a unique lasting relationship. This close emotional tie develops through exchanging messages and feelings with all five senses— sight, touch, smell, taste, and sound. Parents often express attachment through touching, fondling, talking to, and kissing their babies while holding them face to face. Babies reciprocate through recognizing and responding to the parents' overtures. They smile, follow their parents' image with their eyes, and show signs of contentment and acceptance. The skin and eye contact and the pattern of the parent speaking and the baby responding, as well as other interchanges, are essential to building a loving relationship. Time spent together soon after birth encourages affectionate contact between parent and child throughout the child's formative years.

The Positive Results of Bonding

Studies cited by Kennel and Klaus show that extended infant contact with the mother beyond regular feeding times during the first three days of life results in behavioral and developmental advantages during the child's early years. Mothers with extended contact show a higher incidence of breastfeeding and are more responsive to their children, with more fondling and face-to-face contact.

At three months, these mothers perceived their adaptation to their infants to be easier and expressed fewer problems with nighttime feedings, despite these feedings lasting almost twice as long as those in the control group. When observed during a ten-minute play period at three months of age, early contact babies and mothers smiled and faced one another more. At five years, the children had significantly higher IQs and better-developed skills (Klaus, 1982).

Bonding encompasses the affectionate attachment of both mother and father to their newborn infant. Fathers who touch, fondle, and talk to their newborn babies form close emotional ties. Fathers can experience a hormonal response to their babies' cries, as evidenced by a rise in prolactin and testosterone levels. They are more responsive to infant cues than are non-fathers (Fleming, 2002). The father's fascination with his baby may mix with some jealousy about the more intimate relationship between the mother and her breastfeeding baby. Bonding and the building of love for the baby helps the father adjust to new family relationships.

Help Mothers Initiate Breastfeeding

STEP FOUR OF THE TEN STEPS
Help mothers initiate breastfeeding within a half-hour of birth.

Baby-friendly healthcare facilitates early breastfeeding for mothers and babies. The duration of breastfeeding is higher for mothers who breastfeed immediately after birth. A 2001 study showed that mothers who initiate breastfeeding later than 1 hour after birth are more at risk for early termination of breastfeeding (DiGirolamo, 2001). A 1994 study revealed that mothers who took no medication in labor established effective breastfeeding within 6.4 hours, compared to 50.3 hours for those who breastfed immediately and received analgesia. Mothers who received no analgesia and whose first breastfeeding was 1 hour or more after delivery took 49.7 hours to establish effective breastfeeding. Male infants took longer to establish effective feeding than female infants. Infants who experienced a delay in the first feeding and who received analgesia took 62.5 hours (Crowell, 1994). This finding has implications for mothers who leave the hospital at 24 or 48 hours, as they may not yet have established effective feedings by the time of discharge.

There are many health advantages to initiating breastfeeding as early as possible. Breastfeeding duration is higher for mothers who breastfeed in the delivery room (Anderson, 2003). Increased oxytocin secretion from suckling contracts the uterus more quickly and controls bleeding. Routine use of synthetic oxytocin is not necessary when mothers breastfeed after delivery. Colostrum clears meconium from the baby's gut and provides immunologic protection. Delaying the first bath until after the first breastfeeding allows the **vernix** to soak into the baby's skin, lubricating and protecting it. It also prevents temperature loss that could interfere with the first breastfeeding.

Helping mothers maintain hydration during labor can support their early breastfeeding. Dehydration can deplete a woman's energy, which in turn may have a subtle impact on her birth and early feeding experiences. Policies should allow women to labor in any position they choose rather than requiring that women labor lying down. A woman who labors while lying down may experience more difficulty during second stage labor because gravity is not assisting her. Following a difficult second stage and delivery, she may then experience further difficulty with the initiation of breastfeeding.

Let the Baby Lead the Way

It is unnecessary, and sometimes harmful, to rush or compel babies to breastfeed. A better approach is to leave a mother and her unwrapped baby alone until they both are ready to breastfeed. A warmed blanket placed over both of them will prevent heat loss. When the mother and baby remain together quietly, skin to skin, the baby typically will work through pre-feeding behaviors such as bringing his hands to his mouth and making sucking motions. This is an excellent time to teach feeding cues and encourage mothers to respond to them. See Chapter 13 for a discussion of infant feeding cues.

A 1987 study, repeated in 1990, showed that babies who remained on their mother's abdomen undisturbed accomplished breastfeeding on their own. They would crawl up the mother's abdomen, search out the nipple, latch on, and suckle—all within about 1 hour of birth. Babies who were left with their mother for 20 minutes and then taken to another part of the delivery room to be bathed, suctioned, and have other procedures had a great deal of difficulty remembering what to do (Righard, 1990; Widstrom, 1987).

Widstrom advises that suckling and feeding develop in a predictable and organized way after birth. Drugs given to the mother in labor that depress the central nervous system adversely affect nutritive sucking. Mothers who received medication in labor (pethidine, in this case) had babies who could not suck correctly. Babies taken from their mothers after 20 minutes and whose mothers were given pethidine during labor were unable to latch onto the breast in the delivery room. According to Widstrom, it takes an average of 55 minutes for most babies to move to the breast, attach, and begin to suckle. To facilitate this process, hospital practices need to allow mothers and babies to stay together for at least 2 hours with no interference (Righard, 1990).

Help with the First Breastfeeding

Birth attendants can help this natural process by placing the baby in skin-to-skin contact with the mother's abdomen or chest immediately after birth and covering both the mother and baby with a warm blanket. The mother can make the breast available close to the baby's mouth and allow him to lick and explore the breast. A caregiver can be available to help with attachment if the baby wishes to breastfeed and has not started spontaneously within one hour. The mother can initiate the rooting reflex by gently stroking her baby's mouth area with her nipple. In response, her baby will turn toward the nipple and open his mouth. Mothers who move to a different room for the rest of their postpartum care can remain with their babies during transport to allow this continued contact.

Breastfeeding After a Cesarean Delivery

Cesarean delivery does not preclude early breastfeeding. A mother who delivers surgically may breastfeed as soon as the repair is completed and she is in recovery. Occasionally a mother may receive general anesthesia for the cesarean. Use of general anesthesia does not preclude breastfeeding. In this case, she may breastfeed as soon as she is awake and able to respond.

You can help the cesarean mother find a comfortable position for breastfeeding. Lying on her side with her baby lying next to her will help to avoid incision pain in the first hours. It also permits breastfeeding even if the mother's head must remain down after spinal anesthesia. She can place pillows behind her back and under her top knee to support her abdomen. Another position is for the mother to lie flat with the baby placed on top of her.

When the mother breastfeeds in a sitting position, she can place a pillow over the surgical incision to cushion it from the pressure of the baby's body. She can use additional pillows placed under her knees for support if she is sitting in bed. Another useful position is with the baby along the side of her body with the arm closest to the breast, tucking her baby under her arm (known as a **clutch hold** or **football hold**). A positive experience with initiating breastfeeding will help to normalize the postpartum experience for mothers who may feel a sense of failure or disappointment that they did not give birth vaginally.

▶ ## CREATING A SUPPORTIVE POSTPARTUM ENVIRONMENT

Treating women as individuals and understanding their lifestyle and previous experiences regarding breastfeeding and parenting will facilitate their learning. Mothers and caregivers must have realistic expectations for the early days of breastfeeding. Both need to understand that, although breastfeeding is instinctive by nature, it often requires learning and practice to accomplish. Especially in the early hours and days, encourage mothers to be flexible and patient. First-time breastfeeding mothers are novices, as are their babies. They need time and patience to adjust to one another's idiosyncrasies as they learn to work together as a team. The mother may feel awkward and clumsy at times. In an accepting atmosphere, her awkwardness will not deter her from continuing. A relaxed and supportive climate will encourage her to seek help, laugh at any missteps, and help her baby learn to breastfeed effectively.

Taking time to instruct the mother and showing a willingness to listen to her concerns demonstrates the importance of breastfeeding. This encourages her to put forth extra effort to continue, ultimately making your role easier and more rewarding. Quality time spent instructing each mother is rewarded tenfold through her assuming responsibility for her baby's care and for her decisions. Your efforts in teaching and supporting the mother will produce long-term health benefits for both mother and baby.

Eliminate Negative and Unnecessary Practices

In order to dispel anxiety of the unknown, pregnant women can learn as much as possible about the hospital's routines and procedures so they will know what to expect during and after delivery. The mother will experience continual interruptions from people entering her room at any hour of the day or night. Her obstetrician will visit her daily to check on her progress. The pediatrician may come to her room to examine her baby or to report to her daily about her baby's progress. The nursing staff will enter her room periodically throughout the day and night to check her baby, monitor her temperature and blood pressure, examine any incisions and IV, check her uterus and breasts, provide medications and snacks, fill her water pitcher, and change her bed linens.

Dietary personnel will bring meals and later pick up empty trays and menus. Housekeeping personnel will clean her bathroom and dust the room. A photographer may stop to take pictures. Someone will come for information for the birth certificate. Other interruptions may occur from members of maintenance, television services, volunteer services, and clergy—not to mention friends and relatives who come for a personal visit. Moreover, these interruptions are doubled if she shares her room with another new mother! Encouraging mothers to request that visitors wait until the family goes home will help mothers get the rest they need. It also allows you time for teaching the mother and assisting her with breastfeeding.

Routines that limit interruptions are a positive contribution to breastfeeding. Routines that inhibit interaction, practices that imply possible failure, and ineffective problem solving can all influence both short-term and long-term breastfeeding. Such questionable practices often stem from tradition and misinformation. With some exceptions, the degree of knowledge regarding breastfeeding care is relatively low among the general population of nurses and physicians (Power, 2003; Arthur, 2003). Breastfeeding advice may derive from personal experience or misconceptions rather than fact-based information. In the absence of sound knowledge of breastfeeding practices, erroneous and incorrect advice can lead to a bumpy start for the mother and baby.

Show Mothers How to Breastfeed

STEP FIVE OF THE TEN STEPS

Show mothers how to breastfeed and how to maintain lactation, even if they should be separated from their infants.

Nurses often cite lack of time as a barrier to providing adequate assistance to mothers (Patton, 1996). However, time taken by the maternity staff for the early initiation of breastfeeding will help the mother establish sound breastfeeding practices. Moreover, it will help avoid difficulties that require additional staff time later spent in problem solving. Every breastfeeding mother should receive basic instruction in day-to-day breast-feeding matters. A knowledgeable caregiver optimally will be present for the first feeding to assist, observe technique, and answer questions. Some mothers may require no help beyond that.

Mothers have an important need for privacy during feedings. Breastfeeding mothers need a place to feed their babies in a quiet, uninterrupted setting. Hospital rooms need to provide privacy and a comfortable chair. Mothers who are separated from their infants need special assistance with establishing milk production. They need to pump 8 to 12 times in a 24-hour period with a hospital-quality pump. Make sure they receive information on pump rental options and milk storage.

The baby may have difficulty in his initial attempts, or he may latch on and begin to suckle immediately. Many newborns sleep most of the time. It is common for a baby born in the hospital to show little interest in nursing the first few times the mother brings him to breast. He may lose up to 7 percent of his birth weight during the first week. Generally, he will regain birth weight by 10 days to 2 weeks. It is important that the mother be aware of this pattern so that his initial weight loss does not worry her. A baby who enjoys unrestricted access to the breast may have little or no weight loss.

Teach Breast Care

Teaching mothers appropriate breast care will help them avoid the discomfort of nipple soreness. Healthy skin contains sufficient moisture to keep it soft and pliable. The nipples require no treatment unless they are tender or sore. A healthy nipple needs no special attention other than observing practices that will preserve the health of the skin. Primary among these practices is making sure the mother positions the baby so he can get a good latch. Some mothers express a drop or two of colostrum and gently rub it into the nipple and areola.

Provide Effective Discharge Planning

Many women will begin breastfeeding with no prior reading or instruction. Some may not even have made the decision to breastfeed until the baby arrives. You may need to guide a new mother in making this decision and help her examine its benefits by answering questions and responding to concerns she may have. Staff cannot assume a mother will automatically know what to do, even if she has previously learned about breastfeeding. Once she is caring for her baby, a review of breastfeeding techniques will help her relate to the information more readily than she did before the baby arrived.

The postpartum period is a time in a mother's parenting experience when she is eager to listen and learn what to do—a teachable moment. Prior to hospital discharge, the postpartum nursing staff must ensure that the mother understands how to breastfeed and how to assess her baby's needs. Learning about typical patterns of feeding and breastfeeding milestones will help her know what to expect. This will help to prevent problems and aid her in continuing to breastfeed for as long as she desires. Mothers also need to learn about risks associated with the use of infant formula and pacifiers and risks of maternal overweight (Dewey, 2003). Observing the mother and baby breastfeed on the third or fourth day postpartum will provide an opportunity to evaluate the mother's understanding of breastfeeding technique.

A mother who is unfamiliar with typical newborn behavior may believe that various infant care matters are associated with breastfeeding. Concerns related to sleep, crying, and sucking needs often are associated with breastfeeding because of its unique nature. Providing anticipatory guidance regarding these normal concerns will help mothers. Because parents receive so much information in the hospital, they will benefit from having someone to call when concerns or questions arise.

Give No Unnecessary Supplements

STEP SIX OF THE TEN STEPS

Give newborn infants no food or drink other than breast-milk, unless medically indicated.

Infants who are given supplements are at increased risk for early termination of breastfeeding (DiGirolamo, 2001). There is clear evidence that breastfeeding infants do not need supplemental water (De Carvalho, 1981). Newborns who breastfeed frequently from birth, every two to three hours or in response to feeding cues, never need water and seldom need an artificial substitute. Routine use of glucose water or formula for breastfeeding babies should be discouraged. Their use may set up long-term allergies and implies to the mother that her milk alone is not sufficient. This undermines her confidence in her ability to provide adequate nourishment for her baby.

Babies often incorrectly receive artificial formula or water to supplement colostrum because of a misconception that colostrum is insufficient for total nourishment. The use of formula supplementation is associated with negative breastfeeding outcomes (Chezem, 2003). The only time breastfeeding babies should receive any type of supplement is in the rare instance of a specific medical need.

Babies should never receive supplements routinely, and a mother should never receive a bottle to give her baby without specific instructions. Staff should never send a mother home with vague instructions regarding supplementation such as "give the baby some formula after every feeding." She needs specific directions, such as "feed the baby one ounce of formula after each time you breastfeed until you come back into the clinic the day after tomorrow." This gives the mother specific guidelines so that she knows that supplementation, although it may be necessary at the moment, will not last long.

Acceptable Medical Reasons for Supplements

In light of the many concerns related to the use of artificial baby milks, it is important to note that on rare occasions some babies will be unable to breastfeed. For the vast majority of babies, human milk is their normal and expected source of nourishment and protection. However, it is crucial that you be aware of situations in which a baby needs a supplement, either expressed mother's milk, donor human milk, or artificial baby milk. There are also rare situations in which breastfeeding must be avoided altogether. The 1997 AAP statement says that untreated active tuberculosis, HIV- positive status of the mother, a small number of drugs (mostly cancer chemotherapy agents), and use of illegal drugs should contraindicate breastfeeding. HTLV-1 is usually a contraindication as well (AAP, 2005).

The debate regarding preterm infants and their nutritional needs, discussed in Chapter 9, may continue for some time. Preterm infants who weigh as much as 1850 grams often receive human milk fortifiers. Babies who experience hypoglycemia that does not improve through increased breastfeeding need to receive additional human milk by an alternate means such as cup, dropper, or spoon until breastfeeding is established. If a baby experiences acute water loss, as with **phototherapy** for jaundice, supplementation of expressed milk may be required if increased breastfeedings do not meet his needs. Babies with certain inborn errors of metabolism, such as phenylketonuria, need supplementation of a low **phenylalanine** formula in addition to breastmilk. Infants with galactosemia are unable to breastfeed, except in the case of a form of galactosemia known as the Duarte variant (Ono, 1999). With Duarte's, it is possible to breastfeed, although the baby's **galactose** levels must be carefully monitored, with some nondairy formula probably provided (Ganesan, 1997).

In rare instances, a baby may be able to breastfeed, but the mother is not. If the mother experiences a severe illness, such as psychosis, eclampsia, or shock, her caregiver may delay breastfeeding or expressing milk. Advice to HIV-positive mothers in countries with sanitary conditions and a safe water supply is to not breastfeed (see Chapter 25). A mother who needs certain medications, such as cytotoxic, radioactive, or some antithyroid (other than propylthiouracil) drugs, will be unable to breastfeed while the drug is at a level that would harm the baby. This may necessitate temporary interruption of breastfeeding while the mother expresses her milk to maintain milk production. The mother might choose to wean and feed her baby donor milk or infant formula (WHO/UNICEF, 1993).

Promote Practices That Support Breastfeeding

A strong set of supportive protocols enables the mother and baby to establish breastfeeding smoothly. Baby-friendly practices encourage the mother to be with her infant. This transmits a belief in her ability to breastfeed and provides sound principles of breastfeeding care. Mothers and babies will remain together from the moment of birth, followed by rooming-in for the remainder of the hospital stay.

Place No Restrictions on Feedings

Baby-friendly healthcare places no rules or restrictions on feedings. Most hospitals will state that they encourage breastfeeding in response to feeding cues. However, babies who remain in the nursery for most of the day customarily feed every three or four hours or when they cry. Feeding a baby on a rigid schedule or ignoring his natural feeding cues does not help the mother learn how to respond to those cues. It often does not allow the baby to begin feeding before he is frantic. Additionally, delaying or rigidly scheduling feedings slows milk production and increases the risk of breast engorgement.

There is an increase in the incidence of jaundice and hypoglycemia in the baby when feedings are limited (ABM, 1999 Varimo, 1986; De Carvalho, 1985;). Clinicians refer to this as "lack of breastfeeding jaundice," indicating that the jaundice is a result of breastfeeding mismanagement. If the mother finds herself governed by a rigid schedule, she may not be breastfeeding often enough to stimulate milk production or satisfy her baby. Prenatal anticipatory guidance includes encouraging expectant parents to determine the hospital's infant feeding policy prior to delivery and negotiate changes if needed. Baby-friendly hospitals place no rules or restrictions on feedings and keep babies with their mothers.

Encourage Rooming-In

STEP SEVEN OF THE TEN STEPS
Practice rooming-in—allow mothers and infants to remain together—24 hours a day.

Rooming-in is a component of family-centered maternity care that is a standard practice or option in most hospitals (see Figure 12.3). Parents often need to make prior arrangements for this accommodation, which may require

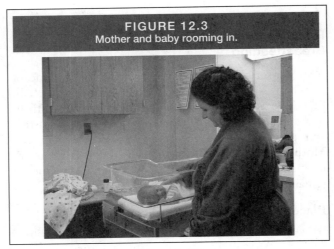

FIGURE 12.3
Mother and baby rooming in.

Printed with permission of Anna Swisher.

a private or semi-private room. Rooming-in provides maximum opportunity for the mother and infant to interact. Keeping the baby with the mother in her room increases the mother's self-confidence in handling her baby. She learns to recognize hunger cues and can feed her baby as frequently as he desires. It is also reassuring for the mother to have her baby close, rather than in the nursery where she cannot see and respond to him. Encourage rooming-in as soon as the mother can care for her baby. If she had a cesarean birth, having a support person stay with her on the postpartum unit facilitates earlier rooming-in.

Variations in Rooming-in Policies

Availability of the various types of rooming-in arrangements will vary from one hospital to another. Expectant parents need to learn what rooming-in options are available to them. They can learn this through childbirth education classes and their prenatal care providers. They can then locate a hospital that will meet their needs. An option of 24-hour rooming-in allows the baby to stay with the mother at all times. Some hospitals allow the baby to remain with the mother during the day except when she is sleeping or showering, and the baby is taken to the nursery at night. Other hospitals require that the baby return to the nursery during visiting hours. Flexible rooming-in permits the mother to have her baby in her room and take him to the nursery if the need arises.

Many mothers find that flexible rooming-in, beginning from the moment of birth, is the most desirable arrangement. It offers new parents the chance to get acquainted with their baby and to learn how to care for him before assuming sole responsibility at home. It also allows the mother with older children an opportunity to get to know her new baby before returning home and dividing her time between her new baby and her other children.

Benefits of Rooming-in to Breastfeeding

Hospital practices alone do not determine how long breastfeeding will continue. However, there is clear evidence for a correlation between rooming-in and longer breastfeeding duration (Lindenberg, 1990; Nylander, 1991). Positive results occur with rooming-in, especially when the mother receives guidance (Perez-Escamilla, 1992). Parents who know their babies' abilities are better able to notice them (Delight, 1991).

Rooming-in offers physical and emotional benefits to the entire family. It allows for bonding and quick relief of fussiness and hunger and incorporates the baby into the family unit immediately after birth. The frequent feedings made possible by this arrangement reduce breast engorgement and encourage early milk production. Mothers who room in with their babies and take no pain or sleep medications sleep just as well as mothers who take medication and leave their babies in the nursery (Keefe, 1988).

Mothers who care for their babies throughout the day and night have babies who are better breastfeeders. The babies have a less disorganized cry, startle less frequently, and feed more often than babies cared for in central nurseries. Optimal feeding occurs when the baby gives cues such as mouthing and hand-to-mouth activity (Anderson, 1989). Rooming-in enables mothers to recognize and respond to their babies' hunger cues.

Babies who room in have more frequent feedings and greater weight gain. Because rooming-in promotes caregiver response, the baby experiences less crying and movement, thereby conserving energy (Yamauchi, 1990). Keeping mothers and babies together during their hospital stay promotes learning and enhances the mother's self-confidence. In this baby-friendly environment, she learns feeding cues and breastfeeding techniques in a setting where she can have her questions answered and her techniques evaluated (Anderson, 1989). Additionally, mothers are able to provide antibodies to the microbes in the vicinity. If a baby remains in a nursery with its set of pathogens, the mother's milk will not reflect this.

When Babies Are Left to Cry in the Nursery

Some hospitals still have centralized nurseries where nursing staff cares for babies most of the 24 hours, particularly at night. It is common for several babies to be crying in the nursery at any given time. "The belief that newborn infants need to cry is not true" (Anderson, 1989). In healthy full-term infants, an adequate functional reserve is present in the lungs after the first breath. The lungs have expanded as fully at 30 minutes postbirth as at 24 hours.

Newborns who self-regulate their care by remaining with their mothers cry less than those whose care is controlled externally by hospital staff. In the first hour after birth, newborns in Anderson's study whose feedings were time-controlled cried for 10 minutes and startled 12 times. They cried for 38 minutes during the first 4 hours. Babies who self-regulated their care cried less than 1 minute in the first hour after birth and did not startle. They cried only 2 minutes during the first 4 hours after birth. Sucking pressures were 4 times as strong and blood pressure averaged 10 mg/Hg lower than babies who were under time-controlled care (Anderson, 1989). Blood glucose levels stay higher when babies do not cry. Crying uses up glycogen stores, which results in a drop in glucose levels (Mazurek, 1999; Aono, 1993).

Teach Mothers Feeding Cues

STEP EIGHT OF THE TEN STEPS
Encourage breastfeeding on demand.

Encouraging breastfeeding on demand means that the mother responds to her baby's feeding cues. There is a clear relationship between a feeding "schedule" and the establishment of sound breastfeeding practices. The ideal "schedule" allows the baby to nurse whenever he demonstrates feeding cues. This enables breastfeeding to get off to a good start. It ensures the early establishment of milk production through frequent breast stimulation and milk removal. Feeding in response to feeding cues encourages bonding between the mother and baby and helps to avoid milk **stasis**, which can lead to problems such as breast engorgement or plugged ducts.

Hospital policies that support responding to the baby will help mothers learn to recognize their baby's hunger cues. Newborns become hungry every 1½ to 3 hours and sometimes sooner. They may feed every 1 to 1½ hours 3 or 4 times in a row and then sleep for 4 or 5 hours. Observing the number of feedings in 24 hours rather than timed intervals between feedings is easier for mothers.

Teach mothers that babies go to the breast and demonstrate feeding cues for many reasons. They may be hungry or thirsty. They may be uncomfortable and need to suckle to relieve the discomfort. They may need to pass gas or have a bowel movement. Breastfeeding is not just another method of feeding a baby; it is a relationship to be nurtured. Mothers may assume that they do not have enough milk if the baby wants to go to the breast frequently. It is important to help them understand how to know their baby is getting enough to eat and that nurturing at the breast is an important component of breastfeeding.

Breastfeeding during the nighttime is essential for establishing milk production. Whenever a baby wakes during the night, he should be breastfed, not offered pacifiers, water, or an artificial substitute. Many nursing mothers make up missed sleep by napping during the day. Frequent feedings day and night encourage early milk production and decrease uncomfortable breast fullness.

Make sure parents understand that cue feeding does not mean feeding the baby only when he cries. Most babies show feeding cues (see Chapter 13) such as mouthing and hand-to-mouth activity for up to 30 minutes prior to sustained crying (Anderson, 1989). Babies who have been crying have difficulty breastfeeding because they are unable to organize themselves to focus on feeding. Crying compromises and disorganizes their suck, and their sucking strength drops. Pediatrician William Sears suggests, "Crying is good for the lungs like bleeding is good for the veins" (Sears, 2003). Mothers need to watch for hunger cues before the baby progresses to crying.

Give No Artificial Teats to Infants

> ### STEP NINE OF THE TEN STEPS
>
> Give no artificial teats or pacifiers (also called dummies or soothers) to breastfeeding infants.

A baby suckles differently on an artificial nipple than on the breast. Thus, the use of bottles and pacifiers can cause considerable confusion for some babies. While some babies may not be confused when given an artificial nipple, they may prefer the smaller, longer, rigid latex or silicone nipple that fits in their mouth like their fingers. Baby-friendly practices avoid the use of bottles unless there is a medical need for supplements. If a medical need for **supplementary feedings** arises, mothers can use a method other than a bottle and artificial nipple to feed her baby (see the discussion on alternate feeding methods in Chapter 21). If the mother is usually not rooming in with her baby, she can ask that the staff bring her baby to her when he is hungry and at frequent intervals. She can also instruct the nursery to bring her baby to her during the night for feedings. This minimizes the possibility of staff feeding the baby when he is not with the mother.

Restrict the Use of Nipple Shields

A nipple shield is an artificial nipple placed over the mother's nipple during breastfeeding. Hospital personnel may give a mother a nipple shield to protect a sore nipple or to help the baby pull out a nipple that is difficult to grasp. Use of a nipple shield is usually not an appropriate intervention for nipple soreness. Sore nipples usually occur due to poor positioning, which the mother can correct. A mother should not receive a nipple shield as a quick fix for a baby who cannot latch.

Nipple shield use can interfere with milk production. It is vital that the mother receive specific guidelines and careful clinical supervision. She should also sign a consent form. See Chapter 21 for guidelines on the use of a nipple shield. A nipple shield can be an effective short-term tool for certain situations (Meier, 2000; Wilson-Clay, 1996). When it is used, appropriate follow-up care by the IBCLC is essential.

Refer Mothers to Support Groups

> ### STEP TEN OF THE TEN STEPS
>
> Foster the establishment of breastfeeding support groups and refer mothers to them on discharge from the hospital or clinic.

A 48-hour hospital stay leaves little time for teaching breastfeeding before the mother is discharged. Legislation passed in 1996 requires health insurance companies in the United States to cover 48-hour maternity hospital stays (Bradley, 1996). However, most hospitals have only a 24-hour stay as the norm for a vaginal delivery unless there are markers for concern, such as the mother testing positive for Group B strep or the baby not voiding or stooling.

Short stays leave little time for assessing breastfeeding knowledge, teaching basic techniques, and evaluating the dyad for effective feeding. Easy-to-read handouts and videos can help to bridge this gap. At discharge, consider what the mother's immediate needs will be when she returns home. Help her plan realistically to meet her needs and her baby's needs. Some mothers will have help at home for several days from relatives, friends, or through a postpartum doula service. However, the majority of mothers will need to manage on their own.

When mothers receive early contact and telephone follow-up from knowledgeable caregivers, the duration of breastfeeding significantly increases (Bernard-Bonnin, 1989). If possible, place a follow-up telephone call at about 2 days after discharge. The baby should optimally have a weight and color check within 48 hours of discharge. Some hospitals provide this only when there are markers for concern at the time of discharge, such as weight loss of over 10 percent or early onset of jaundice.

Mothers can check with their insurance carrier to learn if their insurance plan includes a home health visit. If a mother qualifies, she may be able to arrange a home visit with the public health department or Visiting Nurses Association. Mothers need information on community resources such as local IBCLCs and breastfeeding support groups. The mother may qualify for the local WIC program, so include WIC guidelines and contact numbers in your resource list. One-on-one peer support programs are also helpful (Dennis, 2002). If there are no local breastfeeding support groups, it would be advantageous for a hospital to develop its own. A warm line can also provide support to mothers after they go home. Mothers who need to locate an IBCLC can search for one on the ILCA Web site at www.ilca.org.

▶ **CARE PLAN FOR 48-HOUR HOSPITAL STAY**

In order to provide continuity of care, postpartum staff needs a clear understanding of breastfeeding technique. An informed staff can give breastfeeding mothers the tools that will enable them to establish breastfeeding at home. You can assist the staff in developing a care map that will efficiently utilize their time and talents.

Below are care maps for breastfeeding during a 48-hour hospital stay and a 24-hour hospital stay. They identify for each hospital shift specific responsibilities that will get breastfeeding off to the best possible start. Coordination of care and instruction will ensure that every mother receives the information she needs. This care map covers all areas in which the mother and baby receive care, beginning with labor and delivery and continuing through postpartum care.

Labor and Delivery

After delivery, a mother can learn about positioning her baby for the first feeding. Show the mother the feeding cues her baby is exhibiting at this time. If the baby is not interested in feeding, he can remain with the mother skin to skin. Keep the room quiet, dim the lights, and reduce stimulation. Delay visitors for at least one hour to allow the parents quiet time alone with their baby.

Hours 1–8

Review positioning and the importance of a good latch. Observe a breastfeeding and point out to the mother the difference between **nutritive sucking** and **non-nutritive sucking**. Review feeding cues (see Chapter 13) and put the baby to breast according to cues. Keep the baby with the mother. He may feed only once or several times during the first eight hours. If he has not fed *at all* by ten to twelve hours postbirth (including in labor and delivery), have the mother begin expressing milk by pump or manual expression. Hospitals usually have protocols for the length of time they will allow a baby to go without feeding before supplementing. The Academy of Breastfeeding Medicine's *Model Breastfeeding Policy* describes model protocols (ABM, 2004).

Hours 9–16

Review basic nutrition with the mother, advising her to eat a normal healthy diet and to drink when she is thirsty. The baby should breastfeed two or more times during the next eight hours. If he is not breastfeeding, have the mother feed him expressed milk with an alternative feeding method such as a spoon, **syringe**, or **finger-feeding**. Review risk factors for breastfeeding problems (see Figure 12.4) and take appropriate action.

FIGURE 12.4
Red flags and risk factors for breastfeeding problems.

Maternal Factors

◆ Gained less than 18 pounds during pregnancy
◆ Previous breast surgery or breast trauma
◆ Little or no change in breast size or color during pregnancy
◆ History of low milk supply or breastfeeding "failure" with previous infants
◆ History of hypothyroidism, infertility, polycystic ovarian syndrome (PCOS), or other androgen or endocrine disorder
◆ Hypoplasia of the breasts
◆ Flat or inverted nipples or taut, tight breast tissue
◆ Primipara
◆ Gestational diabetes or diabetic (either oral or insulin dependent)
◆ Epidural in labor
    ◆ In place longer than 3–4 hours before delivery
    ◆ Put in more than one time
    ◆ Received more than 1 bolus of epidural medication
◆ Induction of labor with Pitocin
◆ Received excessive intravenous fluids; on magnesium sulfate; postdelivery edema newly present in ankles
◆ Pain medication for labor more than one hour prior to delivery
◆ Had a cesarean delivery
◆ Breastfeeding initiated more than one hour after delivery
◆ Sore nipples throughout a feeding at time of hospital discharge

Infant Factors

◆ Less than 38 weeks' gestation
◆ Weighs less than 7 pounds
◆ Male infant
◆ Vacuum or forceps used for delivery
◆ Baby has ankyloglossia (tight frenulum) or cleft lip or palate or both
◆ Fetal distress; meconium release during delivery
◆ Insult to the oral cavity (laryngoscope and deep suctioning)
◆ Kept in nursery instead of with mother
◆ SGA (small for gestational age) or LGA (large for gestational age)
◆ Feeding restrictions placed on infant (timed feedings, NPO)
◆ Multiple bottles given during hospitalization
◆ Use of pacifier more than 30 minutes per day
◆ Jaundice
◆ Sleepy, difficult to wake; fails to give clear feeding cues
◆ Difficulty latching on consistently; has not established effective breastfeeding by hospital discharge
◆ 7% or greater weight loss at time of hospital discharge

All factors can contribute to problems with breastfeeding. Some are more significant than others. Multiple factors indicate that the dyad *must* be followed after discharge from hospital. The goal of this list is to identify potential dyads that may have problems establishing either an adequate milk supply or positive milk transfer. The health worker can work with them while they overcome their problems, in a manner that is both safe and supportive of the breastfeeding experience.

Printed with permission of Jan Barger and Linda Kutner.

Hours 17–24

The mother should now be able to demonstrate effective positioning and latch. Observe a feeding and ask the mother to point out nutritive and non-nutritive sucking. The baby should breastfeed two or more times during this period, with at least six feedings in the first 24 hours. If he still is not latching on, the mother should continue to express her milk two or three times during the shift and feed the milk to the baby. The staff should refer her to an IBCLC.

Hours 25–32

Teach the mother the appropriate numbers of feedings, wet diapers, and stools in a 24-hour period. Give her a breastfeeding diary and information on how to know when breastfeeding is going well. Teach her warning signs (see Figure 12.5) that indicate a problem, how to prevent nipple soreness and engorgement, and when to call her board-certified lactation consultant. The baby should breastfeed two or more times during this shift.

Hours 33–40

Make sure the mother can position and latch the baby on by herself. Observe a complete feeding and document the findings. Teach the mother about her nutritional requirements (drink for thirst and eat when hungry), **cluster feedings**, role of the father, avoidance of artificial nipples, and risks of formula use. Discuss cosleeping and provide anticipatory guidance for the first few nights at home.

Hours 41–48

By now, the mother should be able to observe nutritive sucking and swallowing during feedings. Teach her that crying is the last sign of hunger, that feeding cues are in place for 20 to 30 minutes prior to sustained crying, and that crying compromises and disorganizes the baby's suck. The baby should be latching on and feeding well. The mother should appear comfortable holding, dressing, and diapering him.

FIGURE 12.5
Signs that breastfeeding is going well.

Baby's birth date and time _____
Your baby will be 4 days old on _____
Baby's birth weight _____
Baby's discharge weight _____
Baby's first week weight _____
Baby's second week weight _____

Lactation consultant's name

_____

Telephone number

BREASTFEEDING IS GOING WELL IF:

✓ Your baby is breastfeeding at least 8 times in 24 hours.

✓ Your baby has at least 6 wet diapers every 24 hours.

✓ Your baby has at least 3 bowel movements every 24 hours.

✓ You can hear your baby gulping or swallowing at feedings.

✓ Your breasts feel softer after a feeding.

✓ Your nipples are not painful.

✓ Breastfeeding is an enjoyable experience.

Remember! If you go home from the hospital in less than 48 hours, your baby should be seen by a physician 2 or 3 days after discharge and again at 10 days to 2 weeks of age. Generally, these visits are for physical assessments and color and weight checks. It is your responsibility to contact the clinic or doctor to schedule these visits, and to notify them and/or your board-certified lactation consultant if at any time you feel breastfeeding isn't going just right for either you or your baby.

WARNING SIGNS!

CALL YOUR BABY'S DOCTOR OR LACTATION CONSULTANT IF:

✓ Your baby is having fewer than 6 wet diapers a day by the 5th day of age.

✓ Your baby is still having meconium (black, tarry stools) on the 5th day of age or is having fewer than 3 stools by the 5th day of age.

✓ Your breasts feel full but you don't hear your baby gulping or swallowing frequently during breastfeeding.

✓ Your nipples are painful throughout the feeding.

✓ Your baby seems to be breastfeeding "all the time."

✓ You don't feel that your milk supply has become full by the 5th day.

✓ Your baby is gaining less than ½ ounce a day or has not regained his birth weight by 10 days of age.

Printed with permission of Breastfeeding Support Consultants.

Discharge

Make sure the mother understands the signs of adequate milk production as described in Chapter 16. Give her contact information for community resources, including breast pump rental stations if necessary. Notify the pediatric office of any potential problems based on risk factors. Ask the mother to confirm when she will have her baby checked for weight and skin color. Many hospitals schedule this appointment with parents before discharge.

 ## CARE PLAN FOR 24-HOUR HOSPITAL STAY

The AAP has identified milestones for discharging families less than 48 hours after delivery. Their milestones state that the infant must complete at least two successful feedings and be able to coordinate sucking, swallowing, and breathing while feeding. The mother must receive training and demonstrate competency feeding her infant. Trained staff should assess the breastfeeding mother and infant for breastfeeding position, latch-on, and adequacy of swallowing (AAP, 2004). The brevity of 24-hour hospital stays requires abridged teaching. Mothers can be encouraged to see a caregiver at 48 hours to compensate for the early discharge.

Labor and Delivery

After the birth, mothers can learn about positioning and management of the first feeding. Show the mother hunger feeding cues her baby exhibits at this time. If the baby is not interested in feeding, he can remain with the mother skin to skin. Keep the room quiet, dim the lights, and reduce stimulation. Refrain from visitors for at least 1 hour to allow parents quiet time alone with their baby.

Hours 1–8

Review positioning and observe the baby's latch. While observing a breastfeeding, point out to the mother the difference between a nutritive and nonnutritive suck. Review feeding cues, and guide the mother in putting the baby to breast according to cues. Keep the baby with the mother. He may feed only once or several times during the first 8 hours. If he has not fed *at all* by 10 to 12 hours postbirth (including in labor and delivery), initiate expression of milk either by pump or manual expression. Teach the mother the desired number of feedings, wet diapers, and stools in a 24-hour period. Give her a breastfeeding diary and information on how to know when breastfeeding is going well, as well as warning signs (see Figure 12.5) that indicate a problem.

Hours 9–16

The baby should breastfeed two or more times during the next eight hours. If he is not breastfeeding, feed him expressed milk with an alternative feeding method such as a softfeeder, syringe, or finger-feeding. Review risk factors for breastfeeding problems (see Figure 12.5) and take appropriate action.

Hours 17–24

The mother should now be able to demonstrate correct positioning and latch. The baby should breastfeed 2 or more times during this period, with at least 6 feedings in the first 24 hours. If the baby is not latching on by midshift, discharge should be delayed until he has had at least 2 effective feedings. If he still is not latching on, the mother should continue to express her milk 2 or 3 times during the shift and feed the milk to the baby. The staff need to refer the mother to an IBCLC to develop a plan of care.

If the baby is latching on well, teach the mother how to prevent nipple soreness and engorgement and when to call her lactation consultant. Review basic nutrition, and advise her to eat a normal healthy diet and to drink when she is thirsty. Teach parents that crying is the last sign of hunger, that feeding cues are in place for 20 to 30 minutes prior to sustained crying, and that crying compromises and disorganizes the baby's suck. The baby should be latching on and feeding well before leaving the hospital.

Discharge

Make sure the mother understands the signs of adequate milk production as described in Chapter 16. Give her contact information for community resources, including breast pump rental if necessary. Notify the pediatric office of any potential problems based on risk factors. Ask the mother to confirm when she will have her baby checked for weight and skin color. Many hospitals have parents return on the day after discharge for weight and bilirubin checks when families leave within 24 hours.

 ## BABY-FRIENDLY HOSPITAL PRACTICES

You can be most helpful to the mother during her early postpartum days by being alert to the potential for any complications. Make sure she understands the importance of sound breastfeeding practices. Encourage her to view this as a period of learning and adjustment and not to feel discouraged by obstacles. If she receives conflicting advice from you and her other caregivers, you can help her make appropriate compromises and decisions. You can also lead discussions among the postpartum and newborn staff nurses about conflicting advice and the importance of explaining suggestions to mothers. You can support mothers through this transitional time and encourage them to look ahead to the more relaxed atmosphere of their home.

Hospitals undergo evaluation to determine the extent to which they promote and support breastfeeding in order to receive Baby Friendly status. This chapter has explored all *Ten Steps to Successful Breastfeeding* within the context of the mother's hospital experience. Figure 12.6

FIGURE 12.6
Ten steps to successful breastfeeding: self-appraisal tool.

Step 1. Have a written breastfeeding policy that is routinely communicated to all health care staff.

1.1 Does the health facility have an explicit written policy for protecting, promoting, and supporting breastfeeding that addresses all Ten Steps to Successful Breastfeeding in maternity services?

1.2 Does the policy protect breastfeeding by prohibiting all promotion of and group instruction for using breastmilk substitutes, feeding bottles, and teats?

1.3 Is the breastfeeding policy available so all staff who take care of mothers and babies can refer to it?

1.4 Is the breastfeeding policy posted or displayed in all areas of the health facility that serve mothers, infants, and/or children?

1.5 Is there a mechanism for evaluating the effectiveness of the policy?

Step 2. Train all healthcare staff in skills necessary to implement this policy.

2.1 Are all staff aware of the advantages of breastfeeding and acquainted with the facility's policy and services to protect, promote, and support breastfeeding?

2.2 Are all staff caring for women and infants oriented to the breastfeeding policy on the hospital on their arrival?

2.3 Is training on breastfeeding and lactation management given to all staff caring for women and infants within 6 months of their arrival?

2.4 Does the training cover at least eight of the Ten Steps?

2.5 Is the training on breastfeeding and lactation management at least 18 hours in total, including a minimum of 3 hours of supervised clinical experience?

2.6 Has the healthcare facility arranged for specialized training in lactation management of specific staff members?

Step 3. Inform all pregnant women about the benefits and management of breastfeeding.

3.1 Does the hospital include an antenatal care clinic or an antenatal inpatient ward?

3.2 If yes, are most pregnant women attending these antenatal services informed about the benefits and management of breastfeeding?

3.3 Do antenatal records indicate whether breastfeeding has been discussed with the pregnant woman?

3.4 Is a mother's antenatal record available at the time of delivery?

3.5 Are pregnant women protected from oral or written promotion of and group instruction for artificial feeding?

3.6 Does the health care facility take into account a woman's intention to breastfeed when deciding on the use of a sedative, an analgesic, or an anaesthetic (if any) during labor and delivery?

3.7 Are staff familiar with the effects of such medicaments on breastfeeding?

3.8 Does a woman who has never breastfed or who has previously encountered problems with breastfeeding receive special attention and support from the staff of the healthcare facility?

Step 4. Help mothers initiate breastfeeding within a half-hour of birth.

4.1 Are mothers whose deliveries are normal given their babies to hold, with skin contact, within a half-hour of completion of the second stage of labor and allowed to remain with them for at least the first hour?

4.2 Are the mothers offered help by a staff member to initiate breastfeeding during this first hour?

4.3 Are mothers who have had caesarean deliveries given their babies to hold, with skin contact, within a half-hour after they are able to respond to their babies?

4.4 Do the babies born by caesarean delivery stay with their mothers with skin contact at this time, for at least 30 minutes?

Step 5. Show mothers how to breastfeed and how to maintain lactation, even if they should be separated from their infants.

5.1 Does nursing staff offer all mothers further assistance with breastfeeding within 6 hours of delivery?

5.2 Are most breastfeeding mothers able to demonstrate how to position and attach their baby correctly for breastfeeding?

5.3 Are breastfeeding mothers shown how to express their milk or given information on expression or advised of where they can get help, should they need it?

5.4 Are staff members or counselors who have specialized training in breastfeeding and lactation management available full-time to advise mothers during their stay in healthcare facilities and in preparation for discharge?

5.5 Does a woman who has never breastfed or who has previously encountered problems with breastfeeding receive special attention and support from the staff of the healthcare facility?

5.6 Are mothers of babies in special care helped to establish and maintain lactation by frequent expression of milk?

(continued)

FIGURE 12.6
Ten steps to successful breastfeeding self-appraisal tool (continued).

Step 6. Give newborn infants no food or drink other than breastmilk, unless medically indicated.
6.1 Do staff have a clear understanding of what the few acceptable reasons are for prescribing food or drink other than breastmilk for breastfeeding babies?
6.2 Do breastfeeding babies receive no other food or drink (other than breastmilk) unless medically indicated?
6.3 Are any breastmilk substitutes including special formulas that are used in the facility purchased in the same way as any other foods or medicines?
6.4 Do the health facility and all healthcare workers refuse free or low-cost supplies of breastmilk substitutes, paying close to retail market price for any? (Low-cost = below 80% open-market retail cost. Breastmilk substitutes intended for experimental use or "professional evaluation" should also be purchased at 80% or more of retail price.)
6.5 Is all promotion for infant foods or drinks other than breastmilk absent from the facility?

Step 7. Practice rooming-in—allow mothers and infants to remain together—24 hours a day.
7.1 Do mothers and infants remain together (rooming-in 24 hours a day), except for periods of up to an hour for hospital procedures or if separation is medically indicated?
7.2 Does rooming-in start within an hour of a normal birth?
7.3 Does rooming-in start within an hour of when a caesarean mother can respond to her baby?

Step 8. Encourage breastfeeding on demand.
8.1 By placing no restrictions on the frequency or length of breastfeeding, do staff show that they are aware of the importance of breast-feeding on demand?
8.2 Are mothers advised to breastfeed their babies whenever their babies are hungry and as often as their babies want to breastfeed?

Step 9. Give no artificial teats or pacifiers (also called dummies or soothers) to breastfeeding infants.
9.1 Are babies who have started to breastfeed cared for without any bottle feeds?
9.2 Are babies who have started to breastfeed cared for without using pacifiers?
9.3 Do breastfeeding mothers learn that they should not give any bottles or pacifiers to their babies?
9.4 By accepting no free or low-cost feeding bottles, teats, or pacifiers, do the facility and the caregivers demonstrate that these should be avoided?

Step 10. Foster the establishment of breastfeeding support groups, and refer mothers to them on discharge from the hospital or clinic.
10.1 Does the hospital give education to key family members so that they can support the breastfeeding mother at home?
10.2 Are breastfeeding mothers referred to breastfeeding support groups, if any are available?
10.3 Does the hospital have a system of follow-up support for breastfeeding mothers after they are discharged, such as early postnatal or lactation clinic check-ups, home visits, telephone calls?
10.4 Does the facility encourage and facilitate the formation of mother-to-mother or health care worker-to-mother support groups?
10.5 Does the facility allow breastfeeding counseling by trained mother-to-mother support group counselors in its maternity services?

Used with permission of UNICEF/WHO.

---

presents the questions asked under each of the Ten Steps in the self-appraisal process.

SUMMARY

The course of a mother's breastfeeding takes root in her experience during and immediately after her baby's birth. Medications and other interventions in labor and delivery can affect the initiation of breastfeeding. Practices that interfere with breastfeeding need to be replaced with those that promote bonding, encourage breastfeeding within one hour of delivery, offer assistance with the first feeding, and create a climate of acceptance. Such policies will encourage rooming-in, responding to hunger cues, and avoiding use of artificial nipples. It is important that the mother receive information about day-to-day breastfeeding and anticipatory guidance to prepare her for milestones. A sound breast-feeding policy and clear discharge guidelines will provide the framework necessary for preserving and protecting breastfeeding for women and infants.

CHAPTER 12—AT A GLANCE

Facts you learned—

Hospital practices:

◆ Reverse pressure softening (RPS) helps soften the areola and improve latch.

◆ Epidural medications diminish early suckling and increase chances of intrapartum fever.

◆ Putting a baby to breast immediately after deep suctioning can cause breast aversion.

◆ Forceps and vacuum extraction increase the risk of bruising and pain in the infant.

◆ Pitocin and IVs may cause breast and nipple edema and delay milk production.

◆ Kangaroo care is more effective than a radiant warmer in maintaining temperature.

◆ Delaying the first breastfeeding increases the risk that formula will be used.

◆ Bonding is strongest in the first one or two hours after delivery and enhanced with skin-to-skin contact.

◆ Rooting and sucking reflexes are particularly strong in the first one or two hours.

◆ Extended contact between the mother and baby in the first three days promotes behavioral and developmental growth in the infant, more exclusive breastfeeding, and more responsive behavior.

◆ Supplements should not be given routinely and should never be given to a mother without specific instructions.

Applying what you learned—

◆ Develop and communicate breastfeeding policies based on current knowledge.

◆ Teach healthcare staff how to implement breastfeeding policies.

◆ Teach physicians and nurses correct information about breastfeeding.

◆ Promote labor and delivery practices that support early breastfeeding.

◆ Advocate for limiting the use of medications, anesthesia, and other birth interventions.

◆ Promote delaying treating the infant's eyes for one hour to allow bonding.

◆ Teach feeding cues, and encourage mothers to respond to them.

◆ Help with the first breastfeeding in a noninterfering manner, and teach effective positioning and latch.

◆ Help cesarean mothers find a comfortable position for breastfeeding.

◆ Create a relaxed and supportive learning climate that encourages mothers to seek help.

◆ Help mothers limit interruptions and visitors in the hospital.

◆ Teach staff to give supplements only for acceptable medical reasons.

◆ Teach staff to give no artificial nipples to infants and to use nipple shields appropriately.

◆ Encourage rooming-in and place no restrictions on feedings.

◆ Provide effective discharge planning, and refer mothers to support groups.

▶ REFERENCES

Academy of Breastfeeding Medicine (ABM). Clinical protocol number 1: Guidelines for glucose monitoring and treatment of hypoglycemia in term breastfed neonates; 1999. Available at: www.bfmed.org. Accessed October 12, 2004.

Academy of Breastfeeding Medicine (ABM). Clinical protocol number 7: model breastfeeding Policy; February 20, 2004. Available at: www.bfmed.org. Accessed December 15, 2004.

American Academy of Pediatrics (AAP). Breastfeeding and the use of human milk. *Pediatrics* 115:496–506; 2005.

American Academy of Pediatrics (AAP) Committee on Fetus and Newborn. Hospital stay for healthy term newborns. *Pediatrics* 113(5):1434–1436; 2004.

Anderson E, Geden E. Nurses' knowledge of breastfeeding. *JOGNN* 20:58–64; 1991.

Anderson G et al. Early skin-to-skin contact for mothers and their healthy newborn infants. Review. *Cochrane Database Syst Rev* (2):CD003519; 2003.

Anderson G. Risk in mother-infant separation postbirth. *Image* 21:196–199; 1989.

Aono J et al. Alteration in glucose metabolism by crying in children. *N Engl J Med* 329(15):1129; 1993.

Arthur C et al. Breastfeeding education, treatment, and referrals by female physicians. *J Hum Lact* 19(3):303–309; 2003.

Baumgarder D et al. Effect of labor epidural anesthesia on breast-feeding of healthy full-term newborns delivered vaginally. *J Am Board Fam Pract* 16(1):7–13; 2003.

Bernard-Bonnin A et al. Hospital practices and breastfeeding duration: A meta-analysis of controlled trials. *Birth* 16:64–66; 1989.

Bond G, Holloway A. Anaesthesia and breast-feeding: The effect on mother and infant. *Anaesth Intens Care* 20:426–430; 1992.

Bradley W. Newborns' and Mothers' Health Protection Act of 1996. Pub L No. 104–204; 1996.

Buczkowska E, Szirer G. Influence of immediate newborn care on infant adaptation to the environment. *Med Wieku Rozwoj* 3(2):215–224; 1999.

Chezem J et al. Breastfeeding knowledge, breastfeeding confidence, and infant feeding plans: Effects on actual feeding practices. *JOGNN* 32:1;40–47; 2003.

Christensson K et al. Temperature, metabolic adaptation and crying in healthy full-term newborns cared for skin-to-skin or in a cot. *Acta Paediatr* 81:488–493; 1992.

Cotterman KJ. Reverse pressure softening: A simple tool to prepare areola for easier latching during engorgement. *J Hum Lact* 20(2):227–237; 2004.

Crowell K et al. Relationship between obstetric analgesia and time of effective breast feed. *J Nurs Mid* 39(3):150–156; 1994.

De Carvalho M et al. Fecal bilirubin excretion and serum bilirubin concentrations in breastfed and bottle-fed infants. *J Pediatr* 107:786–790; 1985.

De Carvalho M. Effects of water supplementation on physiological jaundice in breastfed babies. *Arch Dis Child* 56:568–569; 1981.

Delight E et al. What do parents expect antenatally and do babies teach them? *Arch Dis Child* 66:1309–1314; 1991.

Dennis C et al. The effect of peer support on breast-feeding duration among primiparous women: A randomized controlled trial. *CMAJ* 166(1):21–28; 2002.

Dewey KG, Nommsen-Rivers LA, Heinig MJ, Cohen RJ. Risk factors for suboptimal infant breastfeeding behavior, delayed onset of lactation, and excess neonatal weight loss. *Pediatrics* 2(3 Pt 1):607–619; 2003.

DiGirolamo A et al. Maternity care practices: Implications for breastfeeding. *Birth* 28(2):94–100; 2001.

Ferber SG, Makhoul IR. The effect of skin-to-skin contact (kangaroo care) shortly after birth on the neurobehavioral responses of the term newborn: A randomized, controlled trial. *Pediatrics* 113(4):858–865; 2004.

Fleming A et al. Testosterone and prolactin are associated with emotional responses to infant cries in new fathers. *Horm Behav* 42(4):399–413; 2002.

Ganesan R. Borderline galactosemia. *New Beginnings* 14(4):123–124; 1997.

Hofmeyer G et al. Companionship to modify the clinical birth environment: Effects on progress and perceptions of labour, and breastfeeding. *Br J Obstet Gynaecol* 98:756–764; 1991.

Johanson R et al. Effect of post-delivery care on neonatal body temperature. *Acta Paediatr* 81:859–863; 1992.

Keefe M. The impact of infant rooming-in on maternal sleep at night. *JOGNN* 122–126; 1988.

Kennell J et al. Continuous emotional support during labor in a US hospital. *JAMA* 265:2197–2201; 1991.

Klaus M et al. Maternal assistance in support in labor: Father, nurse, midwife or doula? *Clinical Consultations in Obstetrics and Gynecology* 4(4):211–217; 1992.

Klaus M et al. *Mothering the Mother.* Menlo Park, CA: Addison-Wesley Publishing Company; 1993.

Klaus M et al. Bonding: *Building the Foundations of Secure Attachment and Independence.* New York: Perseus Publishing; 2000.

Klaus M, Kennell J. *Maternal-Infant Bonding.* St. Louis, MO: CV Mosby Company; 1982.

Kroeger M, Smith L. *Impact of Birthing Practices on Breast-feeding.* Sudbury, MA: Jones and Bartlett; 2004.

Kurinij N, Shiono P. Early formula supplementation of breast-feeding. *Pediatrics* 88:745–750; 1991.

Liberman E et al. Epidural analgesia, intrapartum fever, and neonatal sepsis evaluation. *Pediatrics* 99(3):415–419; 1997.

Lindenberg C et al. The effect of early post-partum mother-infant contact and breast-feeding promotion on the incidence and continuation of breast-feeding. *Int J Nurs Stud* 27:179–186; 1990.

Lucas A et al. Randomized outcome trial of human milk fortification and developmental outcome in preterm infants. *Am J Clin Nutr* 64:142–151; 1996.

Matthews MK. The relationship between maternal labor analgesia and delay in the initiation of breastfeeding in healthy neonates in the early neonatal period. *Midwifery* 5(1):3–10; 1989.

Mazurek T et al. Influence of immediate newborn care on infant adaptation to the environment. *Med Wieku Rozwoj* 3(2):215–224; 1999.

Meier P et al. Nipple shields for preterm infants: Effect on milk transfer and duration of breastfeeding. *J Hum Lact* 16(2):106–113; 2000.

Mizuno K et al. Sucking behavior at breast during the early newborn period affects later breast-feeding rate and duration of breast-feeding. *Pediatr Int* 46(1):15–20; 2004a.

Mizuno K, Mizuno N, Shinohara T, Noda M. Mother-infant skin-to-skin contact after delivery results in early recognition of own mother's milk odour. *Acta Paediatrica* 93:1640–1645; 2004b.

Morton SC et al. Effect of epidural analgesia for labor on cesarean delivery rate. *Obstet Gynecol* 83:1045–1052; 1994.

Nylander G et al. Unsupplemented breastfeeding in the maternity ward: Positive long term effects. *Acta Obstet Gynecol Scand* 71:205–209; 1991.

Ono H et al. Transient galactosemia detected by neonatal mass screening. *Pediatr Int* 41(3):281–284; 1999.

Patton C et al. Nurses' attitudes and behaviors that promote breastfeeding. *J Hum Lact* 12:111–115; 1996.

Perez-Escamilla R et al. Effect of the maternity ward system on the lactation success of low-income urban Mexican women. *Early Hum Dev* 31:25–40; 1992.

Philipp B et al. Sustained breastfeeding rates at a US Baby-Friendly Hospital. *Pediatrics* 112(3):e234–e236; 2003.

Power M et al. The effort to increase breast-feeding: Do obstetricians, in the forefront, need help? *J Reprod Med* 48(2):72–78; 2003.

Righard L, Alade M. Effect of delivery room routines on success of first breastfeed. *Lancet* 336:1105–1107; 1990.

Riordan J et al. The effect of labor pain relief medication on neonatal suckling and breastfeeding duration. *J Hum Lact* 16(1):7–12; 2000.

Sears J et al. *The Baby Book: Everything You Need to Know about Your Baby from Birth to Age Two*. Boston, MA: Little, Brown; 2003.

Sepkoski L et al. The effects of maternal epidural anesthesia on neonatal behavior during the first month. *Dev Med Child Neurol* 32:1072–1080; 1992.

Taveras E et al. Clinician support and psychosocial risk factors associated with breastfeeding discontinuation. *Pediatrics* 112 (1 Pt 1):108–115; 2003.

Varimo P et al. Frequency of breastfeeding and hyperbilirubinemia. *Clin Pediatr* 25:112; 1986.

WHO/UNICEF. Protecting, promoting and supporting breastfeeding: A joint WHO/UNICEF statement. Geneva, Switzerland; 1989.

WHO/UNICEF. Breastfeeding management and promotion in a baby-friendly hospital: An 18-hour course for maternity staff. UNICEF, New York; 1993.

Widstrom AM et al. Gastric suction in healthy newborn infants. *Acta Paediatr Scand* 76:566–572; 1987.

Wilson-Clay B. Clinical use of nipple shields. *J Hum Lact* 12:279–285; 1996.

Yamauchi Y, Yamanouchi I. The relationship between rooming-in/not rooming-in and breastfeeding variables. *Acta Paediatr Scand* 79:1017–1022; 1990.

▶ BIBLIOGRAPHY

Albani A et al. The effect on breastfeeding rate of regional anesthesia technique for cesarean and vaginal childbirth. *Minerva Anestesiol* 65(9):625–630; 1999.

American College of Obstetrics and Gynecology Committee on Obstetric Practice. Induction of labor for vaginal birth after cesarean delivery. *Int J Gynaecol Obstet* 77(3):303–304; 2002.

Anderson GC. Development of sucking in term infants from birth to four hours postbirth. *Res Nurs Health* 5:21–27; 1982.

Ansley-Green A. Glucose: A fuel for thought. *J Paediatr Child Health* 27:21–30; 1991.

Axelsson IG et al. Anaphylaxis and angioedema due to rubber allergy in children. *Acta Paediatr Scand* 77:314–316; 1988.

Barr RG, Elias MF. Nursing interval and maternal responsibility: Effect on early infant crying. *Pediatrics* 81(4):529–536; 1988.

Barros FC et al. Use of pacifiers is associated with decrease of breastfeeding duration. *Pediatrics* 95:497–499; 1995.

Bliss M et al. The effect of discharge pack formula and breast pumps on breastfeeding duration and choice of infant feeding method. *Birth* 24:90–97; 1997.

Blomquist HK et al. Supplementary feeding in the maternity ward shortens the duration of breastfeeding. *Acta Paediatr Scand* 83:1122–1126; 1994.

Brill Y, Windrim R. Vaginal birth after caesarean section: Review of antenatal predictors of success. *J Obstet Gynaecol Can* 25(4):275–286; 2003.

Buton KE, Gielen A et al. Women intending to breastfeed: Predictors of early infant experiences. *Am J Prev Med* 7:101–106; 1991.

Chen D et al. Stress during labor and delivery and early lactation performance. *Am J Clin Nutr* 68:335–344; 1998.

Conrad SC et al. Soy formula complicates management of congenital hypothyroidism. *Arch Dis Child* 89(1):37–40; 2004.

de Jong M et al. Randomised controlled trial of brief neonatal exposure to cows' milk on the development of atopy. *Arch Dis Child* 79:126–130; 1998.

deChateau P, Wiberg B. Long-term effect on mother-infant behaviour of extra contact during the first hour post partum. *Acta Paediatr Scand* 66:145–151; 1997.

Driscoll J. Breastfeeding success and failure: Implications for nurses. Clinical issues in perinatal and women's health nursing: Breastfeeding. *NAACOG* 3(4):565–569; 1992.

Dungy C et al. Effect of discharge samples on duration of breast feeding. *Pediatrics* 90(2):233–237; 1992.

Eidelman A et al. Cognitive deficits in women after childbirth. *Obstet Gyn* 81(5):764–767; 1993.

Eidelman A. Hypoglycemia and the breastfed neonate. *Pediatr Clin North Am* 48(2):377–387; 2001.

Ellis DJ. The impact of agency policies and protocols on breastfeeding. Clinical issues in perinatal and women's health nursing: Breastfeeding. *NAACOG* 3(4):553–559; 1992.

Ertem I et al. The timing and predictors of the early termination of breastfeeding. *Pediatrics* 107(3):543–548; 2001.

Frank D et al. Commercial discharge packs and breastfeeding counseling: Effects on infant feeding practices in a randomized trial. *Pediatrics* 80(6):845–854; 1997.

Gill NE et al. Transitional newborn infants in a hospital nursery: From first oral cue to first sustained cry. *Nurs Res* 33(4):213–217; 1984.

Glover J. Supplementation of breastfeeding newborns: A flow chart for decision making. *J Hum Lact* 11(2):127–131; 1995.

Goldsmith R. Baby's first spring water. *Pediatrics* 90(2 Pt 1):281; 1992.

Gordon N et al. Effects of providing hospital-based doulas in health maintenance organization hospitals. *Obstet Gynecol* 93:422–426; 1999.

Host A. Importance of the first meal in the development of cow's milk allergy and intolerance. *Allergy Proc* 12:227–232; 1991.

Host A. Frequency of cow's milk allergy in childhood. *Ann Allergy Asthma Immunol* 89(6 Suppl 1):33–37; 2002.

Janson S, Rydberg B. Early postpartum discharge and subsequent breastfeeding. *Birth* 25:222–234; 1998.

Laning CI, Touwen BC. Neurological differences between 9-year-old children fed breastmilk or formula as babies. *Lancet* 344:1319–1322; 1994.

Lewinski C. Nurses' knowledge of breastfeeding in a clinical setting. *J Hum Lact* 8(2):143; 1992.

Lie B, Juul J. Effect of epidural vs. general anesthesia on breastfeeding. *Acta Obstet Gynecol Scand* 67:207–209; 1988.

Lifschitz CH et al. Anaphylactic shock due to cow's milk protein hypersensitivity in a breastfed infant. *J Pediatr Gastroenterol Nutr* 7:141–144; 1988.

Maiman L et al. Improving pediatricians' compliance-enhancing practices: A randomized trial. *Am J Dis Child* 142:773–779; 1988.

Mulford C. Swimming upstream: Breastfeeding care in a non-breastfeeding culture. *JOGNN* 24(5):464–474; 1995.

National Center for Health Statistics. Trends in cesarean birth and vaginal birth after previous cesarean, 1991–99. *NVSR* 49(13):1–15; 2001. Available at: www.cdc.gov/nchs/data/nvsr/nvsr49/nvsr49_13.pdf. Accessed December 8, 2004.

Neifert M et al. Nipple confusion: Toward a formal definition. *J Pediatr* 126:S125–S129; 1995.

Newman J. Breastfeeding problems associated with the early introduction of bottles and pacifiers. *J Hum Lact* 6:59–63; 1990.

Nissen E et al. Effects of maternal pethidine on infants' developing breast feeding behavior. *Acta Paediatr* 84:140–145; 1995.

Rajan L. The impact of obstetric procedures and analgesia/anaesthesia during labour and delivery on breastfeeding. *Midwifery* 10:87–103; 1994.

Righard L, Alade M. Sucking technique and its effect on success of breastfeeding. *Birth* 91:185–189; 1992.

Sachdev HPS et al. Water supplementation in exclusively breastfed infants during summer in the tropics. *Lancet* 337:929–933; 1991.

Sankaran K et al. A randomized, controlled evaluation of two commercially available human breast milk fortifiers in healthy preterm neonates. *J Am Diet Assoc* 96:1145–1149; 1996.

Sepkoski C et al. Neonatal effects of maternal epidurals. *Dev Med Child Neurol* 36:375–376; 1994.

Sievers E et al. The impact of peripartum factors on the onset and duration of lactation. *Biol Neonate* 83(4):246–252; 2003.

Snell B et al. The association of formula samples given at hospital discharge with the early duration of breastfeeding. *J Hum Lact* 8:67–72; 1992.

Stickler G et al. Is supplemental water necessary for breast-fed babies? *Clin Pediatr* 29:669; 1990.

Thorp JA et al. Epidural analgesia in labor: An evaluation of risks and benefits. *Birth* 23:63–83; 1996.

Victora CG et al. Pacifier use and short breastfeeding duration: Cause, consequence, or coincidence? *Pediatrics* 99(3): 445–453; 1997.

Waldenstrom U, Nilsson C. No effect of birth centre care on either duration or experience of breast feeding, but more complications: Findings from a randomised controlled trial. *Midwifery* 10:8–17; 1994.

Walker-Smith JA. Cow-milk sensitive enteropathy: Predisposing factors and treatment. *J Pediatr* 121:111–115; 1992.

Williams A. Hypoglycaemia of the newborn: Review of the literature. World Health Organization, Geneva; 1997. Available at: www.who.int/chd/publications/imci/bf/hypoglyc/hypoclyc.htm. Accessed July 23, 2004.

Wolf L, Glass R. *Feeding and Swallowing Disorders in Infancy.* San Antonio, TX: Therapy Skill Builders; 1992.

Zoppi G et al. Respiratory quotient changes in full-term infants within 30 hours from birth before start of milk feeding. *Eur J Clin Nutr* 52:360–362; 1998.

CHAPTER

13

INFANT ASSESSMENT AND DEVELOPMENT

Contributing Authors: Jan Barger and Linda Kutner

When assessing breastfeeding, it is important to be aware of typical newborn reflexes and characteristics. A newborn's behavior is linked closely to breastfeeding. Babies signal to their mothers through feeding cues. In your interactions with mothers, you can point out these behaviors and interpret them for parents. Patterns of behavior, growth, sleeping, crying, and digestion vary from one baby to another. Certain anatomic presentations may require a change in your approach to assisting a mother. Obtaining a complete history of the mother and infant as it pertains to breastfeeding and assessing both of them will help you identify situations that may have an impact on the course of lactation.

KEY TERMS

acrocyanosis	Down syndrome
alveolar ridge	erythema toxicum
anoxia	excoriated
approach behaviors	feeding cues
asymmetry	flexion
average baby	fontanel
avoidance behaviors	food sensitivity
Bauer's response	frenulum
bifurcated	frenum
bovine IgG	gastroesophageal reflux
buccal pads	(GER)
candidiasis	grooming
caput succedaneum	Hirschsprung's disease
cephalhematoma	hunger cues
clavicle	hydration
cleft lip	hypertonic
cleft palate	hypotonic
colic	infant acne
constipation	infant states
cosleeping	intravenous
cow's milk intolerance	lactiferous ducts
cradle hold	lactose overload
Dancer hand position	leaky gut syndrome
diaper rash	leukocytes
diarrhea	macular

molding	spitting up
palate	stooling
perineum	sucking
periosteum	sucking pads
peristalsis	sudden infant death
placid baby	syndrome (SIDS)
projectile vomiting	supine
prone	swaddling
pustule	thrush
pyloric stenosis	turgor
rapid eye movement	uvula
reflexes	ventral
rooting	voiding
sling	yeast infection
soy milk intolerance	

ASSESSMENT OF THE NEWBORN

Generally, any initial contact with a breastfeeding mother should include an assessment of her baby. This applies especially when there is concern about poor weight gain, food intolerance, irritability, lethargy, or sucking difficulties. Perform the assessment with the baby completely undressed and lying on a flat firm surface. Evaluate his posture, skin, head, oral cavity, **clavicle**, reflexes, color, elimination, and feeding cues. Be alert for any areas on his body that cause him pain or discomfort.

Posture

Babies prefer the fetal position, and a healthy, full-term newborn generally holds his arms and legs in moderate **flexion**. His fists are closed and usually held near his face. When awake, the baby will resist having his extremities extended and may cry. Observing the baby's body tone will give you clues about potential problems. As the baby matures, he will remain in the fetal position less often and will spend more time comfortably in semi-extension. When held in the **ventral** position, he will lie on his

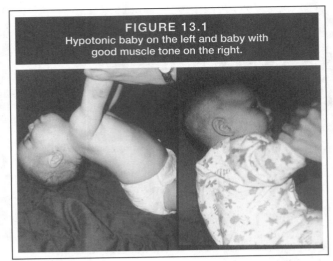

FIGURE 13.1
Hypotonic baby on the left and baby with good muscle tone on the right.

Printed with permission of Kay Hoover.

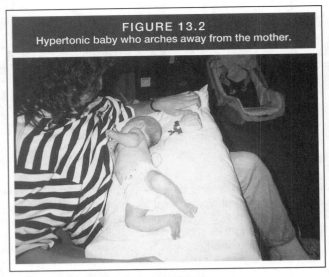

FIGURE 13.2
Hypertonic baby who arches away from the mother.

Printed with permission of Linda Kutner.

abdomen, draped over the examiner's hand, and alternate between trying to bring his head up and putting it down again. At extreme positions, a baby's body tone may be too loose (hypotonic) or too rigid (hypertonic).

Hypotonia

A hypotonic infant has very low body tone and tends to "droop" over the examiner's hand. With **hypotonia**, the baby's posture appears like a wet noodle. His extremities are in extension, and there is little resistance to passive movement. The baby appears floppy, sluggish, and flaccid, as illustrated in Figure 13.1. The hypotonic baby may have difficulty staying latched on to the breast due to a weak suck. He may find it difficult to maintain intraoral negative pressure, even on the examiner's finger. He frequently nurses with his shoulders elevated to just beneath his ears in an effort to support his neck and chin. In the ventral position, the hypotonic baby lays over the examiner's hand with his head hanging down, unable to bring it up. An infant who is preterm or who has **Down syndrome** will show some degree of hypotonia. See Chapter 23 for a discussion on preterm infants and Chapter 25 for a discussion on Down syndrome.

Hypertonia

A hypertonic infant has very rigid body tone. With **hypertonic**, the baby is often in hyperextension, arching away from the breast and away from the mother, as in Figure 13.2. The mother may report that he is difficult to comfort, pulls his head and face away from contact, and does not snuggle into her chest or neck, instead leaning back, away from her. Many hypertonic babies cannot tolerate anyone handling them and prefer to interact from a safe distance. They are often very alert and squirmy, and they will hold their head erect from a

prone position or on the shoulder. When held in the ventral position, the hypertonic baby will be virtually straight, lifting both his head and buttocks, and maintaining them on a horizontal plane. A baby with neurological damage may be hypertonic. See Chapter 25 for a discussion of neurological disorders.

Skin

A healthy newborn's skin is warm and dry, with a pink or ruddy appearance. The ruddiness is a result of increased concentration of red blood cells in the blood vessels, coupled with minimal subcutaneous fat deposits. **Acrocyanosis** (bluish tinge of the hands and feet) may be present after birth due to poor peripheral circulation, especially with exposure to cold. The bluish color should disappear after a few days. Parents often need reassurance that this is normal. It does not mean their baby is cold because of not being dressed warmly enough.

Hydration

Evaluating the **turgor** of the baby's skin is an important part of checking for breastfeeding adequacy. Turgor is the normal strength and tension of the skin, caused by outward pressure of the cells and the fluid that surrounds them. A good area on which to test skin turgor is on the baby's chest, abdomen, or thigh. When gently grasped between your finger and thumb, the skin should spring back to its original shape when you release the tissue. It should not leave an indentation, fold, or wrinkled appearance. Loose skin that slowly returns to a position level with the tissue next to it is a sign of dehydration. The baby's skin may be dry, flaky, or peeling, especially by the end of the first or second week. This is normal, and not a sign of dehydration.

Skin Color

Skin color will vary, depending on the baby's ethnic origin. A significant increase in the newborn's bilirubin level creates a yellowing in his skin color. You can assess for jaundice in natural light by pressing the baby's skin with your index finger and noting the color when you lift your finger. For a quick estimation, some caregivers use a method referred to as the rule of fives to estimate bilirubin levels in the infant.

Jaundice becomes visible in the sclera when the bilirubin level reaches about 5 **mg/dl**. As it continues down the body, the level increases progressively by approximately 5 mg/100 ml from the infant's face to his feet. Jaundice to the level of the shoulders correlates to 5 to 7 mg/dl. Between the shoulders and umbilicus, levels will range between 7 and 10 mg/dl. Between the umbilicus and knees, levels are 10 to 12 mg/dl. Below the knees, bilirubin levels are greater than 15 mg/dl. This progression occurs only when the bilirubin level is rising. When it begins to fall, the skin color fades gradually in all affected areas at the same time (Kramer, 1969). For a complete discussion regarding jaundice and its implications, see Chapter 22.

Erythema Toxicum

Erythema toxicum is a pink to red **macular** area with a yellow or white center. It has no apparent significance and requires no treatment. This is common on the newborn's trunk or limbs and is temporary. It appears one to two days after birth and usually disappears within one week.

Infant Acne

Infant acne resembles adolescent acne. It appears on the face, primarily on the nose, forehead, and cheeks. The appearance changes, depending on whether the baby is hot, cool, crying, or quiet. Infant acne starts at about two weeks of age and disappears at eight to ten weeks. It is a normal response to the maternal hormones of pregnancy.

Diaper Rash

Diaper rash appears as a reddened, small, pimple-like rash. It should respond to careful washing of the buttocks combined with use of a zinc oxide ointment or cream. A diaper rash that does not clear up with appropriate treatment may result from a **yeast infection**. A diaper rash caused by yeast occurs in patches and generally presents as a shiny, red, flat area. It usually occurs on the front of the infant's **perineum** and not around the rectum. If the skin is **excoriated** or has **pustules**, the infant needs to be seen by his caregiver to rule out a bacterial infection.

Head

The newborn's head is large in proportion to the rest of his body, approximately one-fourth of his total body size. The skull bones are soft and pliable. They have not fused before birth, in order to accommodate the infant's descent through the birth canal during second stage labor. After birth, the head may appear **asymmetric** due to the overriding of skull bones, referred to as **molding**. Some infants with severe molding have temporary latching and breastfeeding difficulty.

Caput Succedaneum

Caput succedaneum is a collection of fluid between the skin and cranial bone of the newborn. It usually forms during labor on the presenting area of the head in the cervical opening. The longer the head is engaged during labor, the greater the swelling can be. This condition occurs in 20 to 40 percent of vacuum extractions (Volpe, 2001). There may be red or bruised discoloration, and the baby may be sensitive to pressure on that area. The swelling begins to subside soon after birth. Any bruising increases the risk for jaundice.

Cephalhematoma

A **cephalhematoma**, as shown in Color Plate 14, is a pool of blood between the bones of the head and the **periosteum**, the covering of the bone, which causes swelling. It may begin to form during labor and slowly become larger in the first few days after birth. As the blood reabsorbs, the baby's bilirubin levels may increase. It will take about six weeks to resolve completely. Cephalhematoma is usually a result of trauma, often from **forceps**. Because the baby may be sensitive to touch on that area, the mother will want to avoid touching his head when she positions him at the breast. Again, any bruising increases the risk for jaundice.

Fontanel

The fontanel is a space between the bones of an infant's skull that is covered by tough membranes. The anterior fontanel remains soft until the baby reaches about 18 months. The posterior fontanel closes at about 2 months. Increased brain pressure may cause a fontanel to become tense or to bulge. If the infant is dehydrated, his fontanel may be soft and sunken, especially when he is lying down.

Facial Asymmetry

Facial asymmetry may result from injury to the nerves due to birth trauma and may cause the baby's tongue not to lay centered in his mouth. In this instance, the mother can position her nipple over the center of the baby's tongue rather than the center of his mouth. Facial asymmetry also occurs in utero when the infant's face is wedged against his body or the uterus. The asymmetry usually resolves over several days following birth, depending on the severity.

Eyes

Jaundice, a yellow staining in the white portion of the eye, usually appears when the baby's bilirubin is above 5 mg/dl. Additionally, there may be swelling of the eyelids that will recede in a few days. The baby achieves his final eye color by six to twelve months of age.

Neck

The neck surrounds the infant's esophagus and **trachea**. The **epiglottis** is the cartilage that overhangs the trachea and prevents food from entering the trachea by closing during swallowing. An infant's neck is very short, too weak to provide head support, and needs to be supported at all times. Supporting the baby's neck and shoulders at feedings will avoid the mother pushing on his head, which can be counterproductive.

A baby who keeps his head twisted to the side, usually to the right, may have torticollis, or literally, "twisted neck." Torticollis in infants is a shortening of the muscle that extends from the base of the ear down to the clavicle. The cause may be the baby's position or lack of space in the womb, birth trauma, or low amniotic fluid. Rarely, torticollis can be a marker for serious problems (www.torticolliskids.org, 2001), so the baby needs to be referred to his primary care practitioner. A baby with torticollis may only be comfortable breastfeeding with his head turned to the side. The mother can try nursing in the football hold to provide better control over his neck position. She may also try nursing lying down, with the bed providing postural support. As her baby's range of motion improves through physical therapy, the mother can try other nursing positions.

Oral Cavity

A visual inspection of the mouth is useful. Look for gum lines that are smooth and a palate that is intact and gently arched. The tongue should be able to extend over the lower **alveolar ridge** (gum line) and up to the middle of the baby's mouth when it is open wide. It is not necessary to perform an oral digital exam on all babies, as the newborn's oral cavity is extremely sensitive.

Frenulum

The **frenulum** is the fold of skin under the tongue that checks or controls the tongue's motion. If the baby is unable to extend his tongue over the alveolar ridge, it may be due to **ankyloglossia**—a short frenulum—as shown in Color Plate 15. A short or tight frenulum may cause a heart-shaped appearance to the tip of the tongue when the tongue extends and can interfere with breastfeeding. A short frenulum can make it difficult for the baby to stay attached to the breast during feeding and may result in poor weight gain. Be especially alert to the possibility of a short frenulum as the cause of chronic nipple soreness, slow weight gain, long feedings, low milk production, mastitis or plugged ducts (Ballard, 2002). Clipping the frenulum will enable the baby to extend his tongue adequately (Ramsay, 2004).

Frenum

The labial **frenum** is the fold of skin that anchors the upper lip to the top gum, as shown in Color Plate 16. A large frenum results in a gap between the two top front teeth. A large frenum does not usually interfere with the infant's latch. However, some babies' frenums are so prominent that it is difficult for them to flange the upper lip. Some mothers report compression and discomfort.

Buccal Pads

Buccal pads inside the cheeks (also called fatty pads or **sucking pads**) help decrease the space within the infant's mouth. This feature increases the negative pressure and facilitates milk transfer. If the infant is malnourished or born preterm, the buccal pads may not be present. It may be necessary to position the infant at the breast in such a way that the mother can use her finger against his cheeks to compensate for the lack of fat pads, using the **Dancer hand position**.

Palate

The roof of the mouth divides into the hard palate and soft palate. The hard palate is in the front of the mouth, and the soft palate lies behind it in line with the end of the upper alveolar ridge. The condition and shape of the palate can become an issue in breastfeeding. A high, arched, or bubble palate can cause the mother's nipple to "catch" in the groove and therefore not elongate as it should. This type of palate makes it more difficult for the infant's tongue to compress the breast tissue adequately. Mothers who have infants with such palates often complain of nipple soreness, long feedings, and an unsatisfied infant who needs to nurse frequently.

When an infant has a **cleft lip**, it is immediately obvious to everyone. Frequently, infants with cleft lips also have cleft palates. Occasionally, an infant will have a cleft of the soft palate that escapes initial diagnosis. Infants with a **cleft palate** may choke and gag while nursing. Milk can escape from the baby's nose when milk flow is strong, as when the mother experiences letdown. Changing the infant's position at the breast is often helpful. Infants can have submucosal clefts, where skin covers a cleft of the hard or soft palate. These babies often have a **bifurcated uvula** as well. This can be a marker for genetic disorders. See Chapter 25 for more information on breastfeeding with a cleft of the lip, palate, or both.

Thrush

Thrush is a yeast infection often characterized by white patches that cannot be removed without causing bleeding. It can be located between the baby's gums and lips, on the inside of his cheeks, and on his tongue. Thrush, most frequently caused by the organism *Candida albicans*, is also known as **candidiasis**. The infection may appear on the mother's nipples as well as in the baby's mouth, making it imperative that they both receive treatment at the same time. See the discussion in Chapter 16 on yeast as a cause of nipple soreness.

Clavicle

A fractured clavicle is a common birth trauma, usually identified during the baby's initial examination. However, it may escape detection until later. The baby may restrict the use of his arm and resist breastfeeding in a position that places pressure on the fractured area. For instance, a baby with a fractured left clavicle may be uncomfortable feeding at the right breast in the **cradle hold**. An x-ray will confirm the fracture. Treatment typically consists of immobilizing the arm by pinning it in a t-shirt. A fractured clavicle heals quickly within about three weeks. After healing, there may be a callus on the clavicle, which will disappear as the baby grows.

Reflexes

Reflexes in the newborn are present until his central nervous system has matured. They are a form of communication that tells us much about what the baby needs. Some reflexes are protective, such as blinking or gagging. Other reflexes indicate a need for more or different interaction. The Moro (or startle) reflex results from a loud noise, causing the infant to draw up his legs and fling his arms out. The grasp reflex is initiated by touching the palm of the baby's hand. If left unassisted after birth, it would help the baby find his way to the breast. It is also encouraging to parents, as they see their baby respond to them.

Arching indicates a need for different positioning or a pause from activity. It resembles the positioning of a hypertonic infant (Figure 13.2). If pressure exerted on the back of the baby's head pushes his face into a surface, as against the breast during a feeding, he may arch backward. Pressure on the soles of the baby's feet will elicit spontaneous crawling efforts and extension of the baby's

head, referred to as **Bauer's response**. When positioning the infant, be careful not to press his feet against the back or side of the couch or chair. This could cause him to extend away from the breast. A full-term healthy newborn has many reflexes that aid his breastfeeding. At the forefront of these reflexes are **rooting** and sucking.

Rooting

Stroking the baby's cheek lightly will cause him to turn his head in the direction of the stimulus. His mouth will open, and his tongue will come forward. This is the rooting reflex, as illustrated in Color Plate 17. Gently touching the baby's upper or lower lip causes his mouth to open. The mother can initiate the rooting reflex by brushing her nipple against her baby's cheek, stimulating him to turn toward her breast and search for the nipple.

Sucking

An object placed far enough back into the baby's mouth to reach the juncture between the hard and soft palate will elicit sucking. This may, however, put pressure on the esophageal sphincter and cause regurgitation. The increased definition of newer ultrasound technology suggests that the nipple does not necessarily extend to the juncture of the hard and soft palate, as previously believed. Ultrasound images show the nipple extending only to a few centimeters *before* the hard and soft palatal juncture (Ramsay, 2004).

Babies demonstrate two types of sucking. A high-flow nutritive suck, characterized by a long, deep suck-swallow-breathe pattern, elicits about one suck per second. A low-flow nonnutritive suck, characterized by a light suck, almost a flutter, with short jaw excursions and little or no audible swallowing, elicits about two sucks per second.

▶ DIGESTION

Babies are unique individuals, and each exhibits his own growth and activity patterns. Patterns of digesting food and expelling waste are equally individualized. You can help parents understand these characteristics and encourage them to observe and become familiar with their baby's digestive patterns and particular needs. Patterns of digestion need to take into account the baby's disposition, eating and sleeping patterns, and body temperature. A change in pattern can alert the mother to a problem or illness before it becomes serious. If a mother notices a change, encourage her to look at her baby's overall pattern before contacting her caregiver. This will help her determine whether it is one small change in his habits or a more significant change. The mother also should observe his skin color, changes in breathing, or other signs of illness such as glassy eyes or abdominal cramping. Three functions that occur during digestion—burping, spitting, and stooling—are discussed in the following sections.

Burping

Breastfed babies need to be burped even though they usually do not take in as much air as a bottle-fed baby. Babies who suck vigorously may gulp air. If the mother watches for feeding cues and feeds her baby before he becomes ravenous, the baby will cry less, resulting in less air in his stomach. Burping will make the baby more comfortable because it decreases gas pains and reduces the possibility of spitting up. Air bubbles are interspersed throughout the milk. Gentle patting or rubbing will help them coalesce and rise to the top of the baby's stomach to be expelled. If a baby consistently **spits up** after nursing, the mother may not be taking enough time to burp him and bring up air bubbles.

The mother can sit her baby in her lap, gently rocking him or rubbing his back with her hand. Another method is for the mother to hold her baby against her shoulder and massage or pat him in the middle of his back with a firm pressure from the bottom up. She can also lay her baby on his stomach across her lap, turning his head to one side so that his nose is free, and gently rub his back from the bottom up.

It helps some babies to remain at a 45-degree angle after feedings to bring up air before the mother lays them down for sleep. A baby sling, infant seat, or swing will accomplish this. If the baby has been crying hard, the mother should burp him before putting him to breast. If he is a vigorous feeder, he will need to nurse before he becomes ravenous in order to cut down on the amount of air intake.

Spitting Up

The passage between the baby's stomach and mouth is very short. Additionally, the muscle valve at the upper end of the stomach (the cardiac sphincter, or lower esophageal sphincter) is not as efficient as it will be later in life. As a result, babies may spit up quite often during the early months. Some infants spit up more than others do. Frequent spitting up could be a sign of overfeeding or overactive milk production. If the mother waited too long between feedings, an overabundance of milk may cause the baby to be overanxious and gulp air with the milk. Mucus in the baby's stomach can also cause spitting up. This is more common directly after birth and in the event of an upper respiratory infection.

Although spitting up is messy and inconvenient, it is not usually a cause for serious concern. Because cow's milk protein intolerance and nicotine can cause spitting up, the mother may want to make some adjustments in her lifestyle and diet. Her baby will benefit if she quits smoking or at least cuts down. She can burp her baby more often during a feeding to bring up air bubbles and may even want to burp him before a feeding so any tiny bubbles can coalesce into one big enough to come up. More frequent feeding may also help. Occasionally, if the mother has an oversupply problem, limiting the baby to one breast per feeding is helpful. Make this recommendation only after a complete feeding assessment to ascertain that the mother has oversupply.

Projectile Vomiting

Spitting up differs from vomiting in terms of the force with which the baby expels milk. The baby may dribble milk out with every burp, or he may expel it with some force. A violent expulsion of milk is considered **projectile vomiting** and requires a physician's attention.

If a baby violently expels the contents of his stomach more than once or twice a day, it may indicate a serious medical condition. If he suddenly begins vomiting when he is several weeks old, or if the vomiting gets progressively worse with a decreasing number of wet diapers, he may have **pyloric stenosis**. With pyloric stenosis, the outflow valve of the baby's stomach does not open satisfactorily to permit the contents of the stomach to pass through. It seems to be most common in firstborn white male infants. A sudden onset of vomiting can also indicate an obstruction of the intestines or a strangulated hernia. All of these conditions require careful medical observation and may result in surgery.

Gastroesophageal Reflux (GER)

Some infants spit up only occasionally, and others seem to spit up all the time. Spitting up all the time can be a sign of **gastroesophageal reflux** (GER). GER is a backflow of the contents of the stomach into the esophagus and is often the result of the lower esophageal sphincter failing to close. Gastric juices are acidic and produce burning pain in the esophagus. Infants with reflux may spit up several times after a feeding. Some will spit up even during the feeding.

The constant regurgitation of milk into the esophagus can cause severe irritation or pain for the infant. Some infants with GER learn to limit their intake, having made the association between a full stomach and the pain that accompanies reflux. Regurgitating human milk is not as irritating as regurgitating formula. Because infants digest human milk more quickly than infant formulas, they absorb more milk in the same amount of time. Infants who are breastfed also have a lower pH (measure of the acid level) in their stomach. For these reasons, it is not appropriate to switch a breastfed infant to formula as a treatment for GER.

Frequent spitting up and limited amount of intake may lead to poor weight gain. Infants who experience GER need to be fed in an upright position so that gravity will help the milk stay down. They also benefit from frequent feedings and nursing from only one breast at a feeding, provided the mother has adequate milk production. Both of these actions will help limit the amount of milk the infant takes in at a feeding. It ensures that he gets the heavier hindmilk and allows him to digest and retain more of the milk.

If an infant has more severe reflux, the physician will need to be more involved in his care. Reflux can be severe enough to require medication for the infant. Some medications used for reflux decrease the acid level in the infant's stomach. Others encourage the infant's stomach to pass the mother's milk along more quickly into the infant's intestines.

A physician usually will try medications before resorting to a more invasive test such as a barium swallow, endoscopy, pH probe, or x-ray exam. These tests tend to be done if the baby has poor weight gain or does not respond to medications (Wolf, 1992). In the past, physicians would request that the mother mix her milk with cereal to see if the thicker fluid would stay down better. Another suggestion was for the infant to sleep on an incline and use a pacifier after feedings. These treatments do not appear to have a positive effect on this condition (Carroll, 2002).

The relationship between GER and cow's milk allergy has been examined (Salvatore, 2002). The study showed an association in half the cases of infants with

GER who were less than one year old. In a high proportion of cases, GER not only was associated with cow's milk allergy, but also was induced by it. If a mother tells you her baby has GER or if you see signs consistent with GER, cow's milk allergy may be a factor, either from the mother's diet or from supplemental formula.

GER can be very stressful for parents. It is sometimes like having a baby with colic all day long. Silent reflux may occur, in which the stomach contents fail to come all the way back up. The infant does not spit up but may experience burning and discomfort. Helpful strategies include upright positioning for feeding, holding the baby upright after a feeding, small frequent feedings, and infant massage (Boekel, 2000). You can offer comfort and assurance to the mother that her milk is gentler on the esophagus and digests faster than artificial formula. GER usually subsides by the child's first birthday.

Elimination

Elimination patterns are significant indicators of the baby's intake. Keeping a diary of feedings, voids, and stools for the first week or two postpartum will help parents assess patterns in their new baby's behavior. There is wide variability in stooling and voiding among infants in the early days, especially when there are differences in breastfeeding routine.

Table 13.1 and Table 13.2 show elimination patterns of nine breastfed infants in a suburban North Carolina hospital. As these tables indicate, infants varied as to when they went to the breast for the first time, the

TABLE 13.1
Newborn Birth and Feeding Documentation

Infant	Delivery	Apgar	Comments
1	Vaginal	7–8	Moist lungs; O$_2$ for 2½ hours; all feeds GBF.
2	Vaginal	8–9	Mother told, "Baby smells your milk and that is why he wants to nurse all the time. We could give him some formula." Mother refused.
3	Cesarean	8–9	Circumcision day 2; won't wake to nurse after circumcision.
4	Vaginal	8–9	No problems.
5	Vaginal	8–9	Had 3 poor feeds in first 8 hours with no pumping; first GBF at 15 hours of age.
6	Vaginal	8–9	First 3 feeds PBF; started mother pumping; GBF by 14 hours.
7	Vaginal	8–9	35 weeks' gestation, male infant; isolette for 36 hours; started mother pumping 7 hours after birth.
8	Vaginal	8–9	Night nurse suggested infant could be hungry; cup-fed formula 2 times in nursery.
9	Cesarean	8–9	Breech; cup-fed formula 2 times; no reason stated in nurses' notes; cup-fed 2 times in nursery at mother's request.

GBF—good breastfeed PBF—poor breastfeed
Data gathered at a North Carolina hospital, printed with permission of Linda Kutner, RN, BSN, IBCLC.

						Total Feeds 1st 24 Hours
Infant	**Time of Birth**	**Birth Weight**	**Time of 1st Feed**	**Time of 1st Stool**	**Time of 1st Void**	
1	10:37 pm	8 lb 2 oz	3 hours	3 hours	7 hours	7
2	12:37 pm	7 lb 6 oz	1½ hours	9½ hours	½ hour	8
3	8:18 pm	9 lb	3 hours	7½ hours	7½ hours	7
4	3:30 pm	8 lb 11 oz	¼ hour	1 hour	8 hours	8
5	6:23 pm	8 lb 15 oz	½ hour	2 hours	1 hour	6
6	11:01 am	7 lb 15 oz	1 hour	1 hour	2 hours	9
7	9:14 pm	6 lb 4 oz	1 hour	8 hours	1 hour	8
8	12:35 pm	7 lb 6 oz	1½ hours	9½ hours	½ hour	8
9	1:36 pm	8 lb 8 oz	1½ hours	8 hours	11 hours	8

TABLE 13.2

Newborn Intake and Output Patterns

Data gathered at a North Carolina hospital, printed with permission of Linda Kutner, RN, BSN, IBCLC.

number of feedings they received in a 24-hour period and the frequency with which they stooled and voided. Interestingly, although the number of stools decreased from day one to day two, the number of voids increased.

Clinical observation and bits of information gleaned from unrelated research form the basis for current recommendations regarding output. The problem with such observations and studies is that often they involve infants subjected to birth and postpartum interventions that interfered with exclusive, uninterrupted breastfeeding in the early days of life. Recording intake and output patterns of infants in your practice may shed some light on the relationship of these patterns to breastfeeding. Appendix H contains a Diaper Diary mothers can use to record the baby's output in the first week. (Ordering information is on the form.)

Voiding

Urine should be in the color range of pale yellow to clear. In the first week of life, the baby should have an increasing number of voids daily. Many hospitals correlate the number of voids and stools to the number of days old the baby is, up to day four or five. By the time he is four or five days old, the baby should be voiding at least six times in 24 hours. Pink (copper or "brick dust") stains that appear with urination generally are not significant in the first one to three days of life. However, assessment of the baby's hydration status is necessary, particularly if the stains appear after this time.

Stooling

A breastfed baby's stools differ greatly from those of a formula-fed baby. The newborn's first stools are a black, tarry meconium, usually passed within the first 24 to 36 hours.

Transitional stools are greenish black to greenish brown, as the meconium gives way to brown and then to a golden or mustard yellow color at about 48 to 72 hours of age. The texture may range from watery to seedy yellow to a toothpaste consistency, as illustrated in Color Plate 18. There is no strong odor to the stools of a breastfed infant.

Infants in the first month of life should have at least 3 or more soft, yellow, runny stools a day. An infant who has less than three stools in a 24-hour period may not be getting enough to eat and will need to be weighed, examined, and monitored for adequate intake. Encourage parents to become familiar with their baby's stooling patterns. Every baby's digestive system is different, and each one will exhibit his individual pattern for expelling waste.

Babies' bowel habits change with age. Exclusively breastfed infants will frequently decrease the number of stools they have each day. A mother may find that at around four to six weeks of age, her baby will begin going for longer periods between bowel movements. Frequency in older infants can range from one breastfed baby having several stools every day to only once every three days. Both patterns are acceptable. The characteristics of healthy breastfed stools are described in Table 13.3, along with variations and their possible causes.

Infrequent Stooling

When an infant in the first month of life is not stooling appropriately, the clinician needs to do a complete feeding assessment. Infrequent stooling in the first month of life is usually due to insufficient intake of milk. A baby who is voiding but not stooling or gaining weight may not be receiving enough high-fat hindmilk. Stooling frequency will correct itself with additional feeding or making sure the infant receives more hindmilk at a feeding.

TABLE 13.2 (CONTINUED)
Newborn Intake and Output Patterns

Total Stools 1st 24 Hours	Total Voids 1st 24 Hours	Weight 2nd 24 Hours	Total Feeds 2nd 24 Hours	Total Stools 2nd 24 Hours	Total Voids 2nd 24 Hours	Weight 3rd 24 Hours	
7	1	7 lb 10 oz	Discharged				
5	2	7 lb 1 oz	7	0	2	Discharged	
3	4	8 lb 11 oz	5	4	6	Discharged	
8	3	8 lb 6 oz	8	5	5	Discharged	
3	7	8 lb 12 oz	Discharged				
4	5	7 lb 10 oz	8	3	7	Discharged	
6	7	6 lb 1 oz	10	6	3	5 lb 13 oz	Discharged
5	2	7 lb 3 oz	5	0	3	7 lb 11 oz	Discharged
4	1	8 lb 5 oz	9	3	3	8 lb 2 oz	Discharged

If the mother has good milk production and the infant is gaining at least one ounce per day and has established a good pattern of weight gain, **Hirschsprung's disease** may be the cause of infrequent stooling. In Hirschsprung's disease, a part of the infant's intestines lacks proper nerve innervation and the stool cannot pass easily beyond that point. These infants frequently have large, bloated abdomens from the collection of stool and gas. Breastfed infants with this condition may escape detection until the parents add solid foods to their diet and their stools become more bulky and solid. Although this is a rare condition, any exclusively breastfed infant who is gaining adequately but not stooling frequently needs careful monitoring.

Constipation

Constipation is rare in breastfed infants. Lack of a daily bowel movement or straining at stooling does not indicate constipation. These are normal aspects of toileting. Constipation is diagnosed by the consistency of the stool, not by frequency. As long as the infant's stool is soft, he is not constipated. Constipated stools are molded and firm to the touch like pellets or marbles. In young infants, nursing more frequently will resolve most infrequent stooling problems. Iron supplements may contribute to an infant's constipation; if this is the case, discontinuing them for a few days will allow his system to return to normal.

Constipation sometimes occurs when parents add solid foods to the baby's diet. If the mother is giving large amounts of cereal, she can stop or decrease the cereal for several days until normal stooling is reestablished. She can then reintroduce the cereal in smaller amounts less frequently. She might also add more fruits and vegetables. If the baby is old enough to receive them, yogurt, oatmeal, or prune juice may help. The mother should not treat her infant with suppositories unless the caregiver prescribes them.

Diarrhea

Teach mothers to distinguish between diarrhea and the typically loose stool of a breastfed baby. A mother who has been supplementing with formula and then returns to exclusive breastfeeding may mistakenly believe her baby has diarrhea because of the typically loose stool consistency of exclusively breastfed babies. A mother whose other children were not breastfed might also need to recognize the difference. Grandmothers who did not breastfeed may worry that a normal breastmilk stool is diarrhea.

With diarrhea, the stool is much looser than normal, is very watery, may be greenish, and may be very foul smelling. It may indicate the beginning of an illness or a reaction to antibiotics taken by either the mother or the baby. If diarrhea is suspected, advise the mother to continue breastfeeding. Diarrhea removes valuable intestinal bacteria that aid in the digestion of food, and such bacteria can build back up with human milk. If the infant's diarrhea does not improve quickly or if he appears sick or dehydrated, the mother should contact his caregiver.

▶ INFANT COMMUNICATION

According to one study, infants are more positive socially when their mothers understand how to respond sensitively to infant signals. At twelve months of age, babies in that study demonstrated more secure attachments (Vanden Boom, 1994). In another study, parents who were better at recognizing cues were more empathetic when their babies were three months old (Graham, 1993). You can

TABLE 13.3

Stool Patterns of a Breastfed Baby

Characteristics	Normal Stool	Variations	Possible Causes
Color	A newborn's stool is black, brown, or green in the first 3 days. This is meconium. Later, color ranges from brown or green to mustard yellow.	Unexplained color changes. Black, brown, or red spots.	Mother's or baby's diet. Mother's cracked nipples (possible bleeding—there is no harm to the baby). Bleeding from baby's rectum. If no known cause, the mother should consult the physician.
Consistency	Ranges from a toothpaste-like texture to a liquid with curds.	Very watery.	Foods in diet other than mother's milk, antibiotics, or illness.
		Hard pellets.	Foods in diet other than mother's milk, insufficient fluids, or baby tense or ill.
		Mucous.	Newborn mucus, cold, congestion, or allergy to mother's or baby's diet.
		Fibrous.	Bananas and cereal present in the baby's diet.
Odor	Very little, not unpleasant.	Unpleasant.	New foods in addition to mother's milk, antibiotics, or illness.
Frequency	Ranges from one with every feed to four a day under one month of age. Decrease in frequency after the first month of life.	Sudden change in frequency. Watch carefully and look for other symptoms.	Foods, maturity, or illness.
Volume	Varies with frequency. More frequent stools mean less volume per diaper.	Any sudden change. Watch carefully and be alert to other symptoms.	Foods, maturity, or illness.
Ease of expulsion	Easy and semicontrolled with some straining by the baby.	Flows out continually.	Foods other than mother's milk, illness, or antibiotics.
		Very difficult with extreme straining.	Foods other than mother's milk or insufficient fluids.

play an important role by teaching parents to recognize infant signals and praising them when they respond appropriately to their babies' cues.

Approach and Avoidance Behaviors

Infants exhibit specific behavior that indicates a willingness to be approached. Approach behavior is integrated, stable, balanced, exploratory, and self-regulated. These signals, shown in Figure 13.3, are characteristic of a more mature infant. Likewise, infants also display avoidance behavior

that indicates a desire to withdraw, as shown in Figure 13.4 and Figure 13.5. Recognizing these behaviors will help parents know how to respond to their baby. See Table 13.4 and Table 13.5 for descriptions of infant approach and avoidance behaviors.

Feeding Cues and Stages of Alertness

Many infant approach behaviors signal an interest to breastfeed. The baby may demonstrate feeding cues when he is hungry or thirsty or when he needs to be

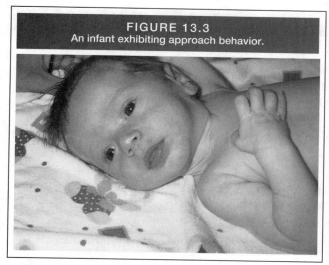

FIGURE 13.3
An infant exhibiting approach behavior.

Printed with permission of Linda Kutner.

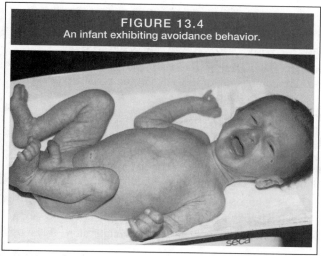

FIGURE 13.4
An infant exhibiting avoidance behavior.

Printed with permission of Kay Hoover.

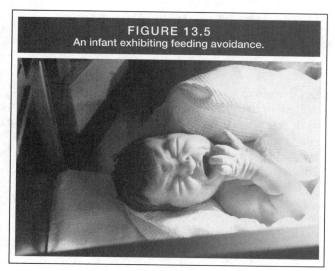

FIGURE 13.5
An infant exhibiting feeding avoidance.

Printed with permission of Carole Peterson.

comforted at the breast. He will give cues the same way, regardless of the reason. His interest in feeding depends on his level of alertness, as described in Table 13.6. Teaching hunger cues to parents will help them know when their baby is ready to go to breast. If parents wait until their baby cries, he will already be exhibiting the final sign of hunger. Pointing out feeding cues during a breastfeeding assessment will help the mother recognize what to look for.

Knowing When to Initiate a Feeding

Hunger cues may be evident during the light sleep, drowsy, and quiet alert states. The baby will begin to wriggle his body, and his closed eyes will exhibit rapid eye movement (REM). He will pass one or both of his hands over his head and bring his hand to his mouth (Figure 13.6). He will make sucking motions, and if his cheek or mouth is touched at this stage, he will begin to root. Soon, more vigorous sucking begins. He then will settle back into a less active state.

The baby may exhibit feeding cues several times in the span of 20 to 30 minutes. If his signals remain unheeded, he could become frustrated and cry. Conversely, he could become exhausted and fall back asleep without having received any nourishment. The missed feeding opportunity can have consequences for the next feed. This is common in preterm or compromised infants or infants who remain in a hospital nursery and are fed by the clock or ignored in an attempt to establish a schedule.

Crying can easily cause a newborn to appear disorganized in his motor functions. It may take several minutes for him to settle enough to breastfeed. He may be unable to breastfeed at all until he has slept again for a

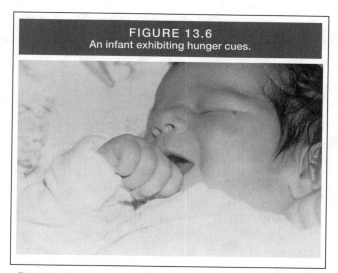

FIGURE 13.6
An infant exhibiting hunger cues.

Printed with permission of Kay Hoover.

TABLE 13.4

Infant Approach Behaviors

Behavior	Description
Tongue extension	The infant's tongue either is extended toward a stimulus or it repeatedly extends and relaxes.
Hand on face	The infant's hand or hands are placed onto his face or over his ears, and are maintained there for a brief period.
Sounds	The infant emits undifferentiated sounds. At times, it may sound like a whimper.
Hand clasp	The infant grasps his own hands or clutches his hands to his own body. His hands each may be closed and touch each other.
Foot clasp	The infant positions his feet against each other, foot sole to foot sole. Or he folds his legs in a crossed position with his feet grasping his legs or resting on them.
Finger fold	The infant interweaves one or more fingers of each hand.
Tuck	The infant curls or turns his trunk or shoulders, pulls up his legs, and tucks his arms. He uses the examiner's hands or body to attain tuck flexion.
Body movement	The infant adjusts his body, his extremities, or his head into a more flexed position. He may turn to the side or attempt to attain a tonic neck response.
Hand to mouth	The infant attempts to bring his hand or fingers to his mouth. He does not have to be successful.
Grasping	The infant makes grasping movements with his hands. He may grasp either toward his own face or body, in midair, toward the examiner's hands or body, or toward the side of the bassinet.
Leg and foot brace	The infant extends his legs and/or feet toward an object in order to stabilize himself. He may push against the examiner's body or hands, the surface he is on, or the sides of the bassinet. Once touching, he may flex his legs or he may restart the bracing.
Mouthing	The infant makes mouthing movements with his lips or jaws.
Suck search	The infant extends his lips forward or opens his mouth in a searching fashion, usually moving his head at the same time.
Sucking	The infant sucks on his own hands or fingers, clothing, the examiner's fingers, a pacifier, or other object that he has either obtained himself or that the examiner has inserted into his mouth.
Hand holding	The infant holds onto the examiner's hand or finger with his own hands. He may have placed them there himself, or the examiner may have positioned them there. The infant then actively holds on.
"Ooh" face	The infant rounds his mouth and purses his lips or extends them in an "ooh" configuration. This may be with his eyes open or closed.
Locking visually and/or auditorily	The infant locks onto the examiner's face or an object or sight in the environment. He may lock on above or to the side of the examiner's face and maintains his gaze in one direction for observable periods. The sound component of an environmental stimulus may contribute to his locking.

The behaviors described are adapted and printed with permission of Sarah Coulter Danner.

while. In either case, the mother has missed a feeding opportunity. If a mother needs to wake her baby for a feeding, she should wait until he is in a light sleep or a drowsy state. Most babies will move from deep to light sleep in approximately 20- to 30-minute cycles.

▶ INFANT BEHAVIOR PATTERNS

The first few weeks of a baby's life are a series of adjustments and readjustments for everyone. For parents, it is a period when love, patience, and understanding for their infant are most important. Because her baby totally relies on her to meet all his needs, a mother may spend nearly all of her time and energies during the first month caring for her baby. At times, she may feel physically drained and emotionally frustrated by his helplessness, while at the same time she enjoys the closeness and warmth of their growing relationship.

A baby's disposition and his patterns of sleeping and eating can affect his nourishment. First-time mothers sometimes become concerned about their babies' dispositions. It helps them to know that babies experience a variety of behavior patterns, ranging from easygoing and undemanding to active and fussy. Studies show that an infant's temperament is inborn. Your specific advice to a

TABLE 13.5

Infant Withdrawal or Avoidance Behaviors

Behavior	Description
Spit up	The infant spits up, with more than a passive drool. However, the amount of vomit may be quite minimal.
Gag	The infant appears to choke momentarily or to gulp or gag. Swallowing and respiration patterns are not synchronized. This is often accompanied by at least mild mouth opening.
Hiccough	The infant hiccoughs.
Bowel movement grunting or straining	The infant's face and body display the straining often associated with bowel movements. He emits the grunting sounds often associated with bowel movements.
Grimace, lip retraction	The infant's lips retract noticeably. His face is distorted in a retracting direction.
Trunkal arching	The infant arches his trunk away from the bed or the mother's body.
Finger splay	The infant's hands open strongly, and the fingers are extended and separated from each other.
Airplane	The infant's arms either are fully extended out to the side at approximately shoulder level or the upper and lower arm are at an angle to each other and are extended out at the shoulder.
Salute	The infant's arms are fully extended into midair, either singly or simultaneously.
Sitting on air	The infant's legs are extended into midair, either singly or simultaneously. This may occur when the infant is lying flat on his back or upright.
Sneezing, yawning, sighing, or coughing	The infant sneezes, yawns, sighs, or coughs.
Averting	The infant actively averts his eyes. He may momentarily close them.
Frowning	The infant knits his brows or darkens his eyes by contracting his muscles.
Startle	The infant's limbs jerk once, occasionally followed briefly by a slight amount of jitteriness and possibly crying.

The behaviors described are adapted and printed with permission of Sarah Coulter Danner.

TABLE 13.6

The Six Infant States

Infant State	Description
Deep sleep	Characterized by limp extremities, a placid face, quiet breathing, no body movement, and no rapid eye movement (REM). The baby lies very still, with an occasional twitch or sucking movement. He cannot easily be aroused.
Light or active sleep	Resistance in the extremities when moved, mouthing or sucking motions, body movement, and facial grimaces. The baby is awakened more easily and is likely to remain awake if disturbed. Most of the baby's sleep is spent in this state, with less regular breathing and rapid eye movement (his eyes flutter beneath the eyelids). Although he may stir and move about, he can return to sleep if left undisturbed.
Drowsy	The baby is aroused easily and may drift back to sleep. His eyes may open and close intermittently, and he may murmur, whisper, yawn, and stretch.
Quiet alert	The baby looks around and interacts with others. This is an excellent time to breastfeed. The baby is extremely responsive. His body is still and watchful, his eyes are bright, and his breathing is even and regular.
Active alert	The baby moves his extremities and plays. He is even more attentive, being wide-eyed, with rapid and irregular breathing. He may become fussy and is more sensitive to the discomfort of a wet diaper or excessive stimulation.
Crying	The baby is agitated and needs comforting.

mother concerning breastfeeding may depend on the type of baby she has. Understanding the various behavior patterns, dispositions, and sleeping and eating patterns will help you offer appropriate suggestions. It may take some time for parents to discover all the variations and subtle nuances.

Average Baby

The average newborn who is exclusively breastfed will nurse anywhere between 8 and 12 times in 24 hours. Nursing more frequently is very normal, especially during times of cluster feeding. He sleeps from 12 to 20 hours a day, with one or two longer periods of sleep balanced by one or two fussy periods. The fussy period typically occurs in the early evening. Usually responsive when handled, he is generally quiet, alert, and listening when he is awake. He soon may learn to soothe himself by sucking on his fist or displaying some other type of comfort measure.

Easy Baby

The breastfeeding pattern of an easy baby is the same as that of an average baby, about eight to twelve feedings per day. However, he will have longer sleep periods and will be less demanding, with relatively little or no fussiness. The mother may need to make a conscious effort to give her baby the tactile stimulation and attention he needs for his emotional growth and physical development. Having an undemanding baby may allow her more free time, and she will want to take care not to overexert herself physically as a result. She can make good use of her free time by devoting some of it to her baby, even though he does not make many bids for attention.

Placid Baby

A placid baby may request as few as four to six feedings a day. The mother will need to monitor him to guard against his becoming undernourished. Because he is sleeping as much as 18 to 20 hours a day, he is usually quietly alert and tranquil when awake. Although he makes few demands for attention, the infrequent feedings do not indicate a lack of hunger. He may wake, feel hungry, and need to nurse. However, he will not cry or demonstrate specific feeding cues to let his mother know he is awake and hungry. Rather, he soon falls back asleep until he awakes again and repeats the same pattern. The result can be an undernourished baby.

A lack of attention and stimuli for a placid baby can lead to poor emotional nourishment as well. Unlike the easy baby, the mother does not meet his needs for nourishment because he does not know how to give the necessary cues. With such vital physical and emotional needs going unfulfilled, he may become withdrawn and lethargic. Mothers often describe a placid baby as being "such a good baby" who does not cry and sleeps through the night. You can discreetly ask the mother of a "good" baby about his breastfeeding and elimination patterns. These babies are typically slow weight gainers.

The mother of a placid baby must take care to meet his needs without receiving many cues from him. She can place a noise device in his crib, such as a rattle, bell, or squeaky toy, which will alert her when he awakes and moves about. The mother can set an alarm clock for herself and check on her baby every two to three hours. When she finds him awake, she can pick him up, stimulate him, and encourage him to nurse. Parents of a placid baby should avoid any pacifying techniques such as pacifiers, cradles, or swings. If the baby sucks his thumb, the mother can encourage him to satisfy his sucking needs at the breast instead of his thumb.

Active and Fussy Baby

An active, fussy baby may nurse more frequently than the average baby, perhaps because of a greater need to calm or comfort himself. He may seem insatiable at the breast and impatient for the milk to let down. He will sleep fewer hours than average and, when awake, will be active and frequently unable to calm himself. He may have several periods during the day when he cries and cannot easily be quieted. He may overreact to freedom and stimulation, and he will need gentle, slow, and soothing movements. The mother can keep him warm and **swaddle** him to keep him from startling himself. She and other family members can hold him often, close to their bodies.

An active, fussy baby may respond well to nursing, dozing, and playing at the breast for generous periods. His greater need to calm and comfort himself at the breast, combined with increased milk intake, may cause him to spit up often from being overly full. The mother might try limiting him to one breast at a feeding, so that he can nurse at his leisure on an empty breast and not take in more milk than he can handle. The mother may need to burp him often as his overeagerness at feedings can cause him to swallow more air. Some of these babies do well when the parents carry them in a sling and hold them upright after nursing.

▶ INFANT GROWTH

When assessing infant growth, note the infant's weight gain since his last weight check. Also look at the overall pattern of gain since the lowest weight he experienced. Record his growth in length and his increase in head circumference. Monitor signs of adequate intake in relation to weight gain, including alertness, skin turgor, moist mucous membranes, and adequate output.

Caloric Intake

Ample evidence indicates that infants are able to control their intakes of food, provided there is no arbitrary scheduling or limit imposed on feeding duration. Giving breastfed babies water can affect their caloric intake. Sterile water has no calories, and sugar water (D5W) has 6 kcal/oz. Until 4 months, mature milk contains 20 kcal/oz, and after 4 months caloric content is typically about 26 kcal/oz. Every ounce of dextrose water the baby consumes can thus reduce his caloric intake by two-thirds.

Breastfed babies utilize breastmilk very efficiently and have a leaner body mass (Heinig, 1993). These lower caloric (energy) intakes by breastfed infants explain their lower percent body fat beginning at five months (Dewey, 1993a). Compared to formula-fed infants, breastfed infants' energy intake is lower throughout the first 12 months (Heinig, 1993). At one month of age, formula-fed infants were found to take an average of 118 kcal/kg/d versus 101 kcal/kg/d for breastfed infants. This discrepancy persisted at four months: 87 kcal/kg/d on average for formula-fed infants versus 72 kcal/kg/d for breastfed infants (Butte, 1990a). Energy needs per day decrease as the baby gets older (Whitehead, 1995). Breastfed infants have lower sleeping metabolic rates, rectal temperature, and heart rates. This may account for the differences in energy intake and expenditure (Butte, 1991; Garza, 1990). A study of infants at 12 and 24 months revealed no difference in intake at these ages, suggesting that the different rates of growth and body composition do not persist into the second year of life (Butte, 2000).

Weight Gain

The baby initially may lose up to seven percent of his birth weight due to a loss of fluids and the passage of meconium. If the mother receives excessive **intravenous** fluids, there can be a fluid shift to the infant, which artificially increases the baby's birth weight. These infants typically void large amounts of urine in the first 24 hours of life and can lose more weight than the average infant. Exposure to medications during labor can depress the baby's central nervous system, and lead to fewer feedings in the first days of life.

A weight loss of more than seven percent indicates the need for evaluation and perhaps assistance with breastfeeding. By day three, the full-term infant should not lose any more weight, and the baby's weight should stabilize

TABLE 13.7
Typical Infant Weight Gain

Baby's Age	Baby's Weight
First month	5–10 oz/week
1–3 months	5–8 oz/week
3–6 months	2.5–4.5 oz/week
6–12 months	1–3 oz/week

Source: Dewey, 1993b.

by the end of the first week. The baby should have regained his birth weight by 10 to 14 days. Infants who are not back to birth weight by this time require evaluation. Table 13.7 presents a typical weight gain pattern for a breastfeeding baby. It is important to recognize that this pattern may vary from one baby to the next.

The 1977 growth charts from the U.S. National Center for Health Statistics (NCHS) were based on one demographic group of primarily formula-fed infants and are not reliable for charting "normal" growth in breastfed babies. The 2000 U.S. CDC growth charts are useful for plotting breastfed infant growth if used with caution.

Growth charts published by the Centers for Disease Control and Prevention (CDC) for standardized length and weight appear in Appendix I. Spanish- and French-language versions of these charts are available at www.cdc.gov/growthcharts. There are notable differences between the growth pattern of breastfed infants and the expected growth pattern on the CDC charts. From birth to about three months, breastfed infants tend to gain weight at similar or greater rates than artificially fed infants. Some studies show that breastfed infants gain weight faster during this time (Fawzi, 1997). Others reveal similar rates (Motil, 1997), statistically insignificant differences (Butte, 1990b), or even slower weight gain (Butte, 1990a). After three or four months, breastfed infants tend to gain more slowly than formula-fed infants. From six to twelve months, breastfed infants tend to weigh less than formula-fed infants do.

A chart based on healthy breastfed infants is required to correctly assess if a baby's growth pattern follows international feeding recommendations (de Onis, 2003). The 2000 CDC growth chart reference population includes data for both formula-fed and breastfed infants in approximately the same proportion of representation. A working group of the World Health Organization is collecting data at seven international study centers to develop a new set of international growth charts for infants and children through five years old. These charts will be based on the growth of exclusively or predominantly breastfed children (CDC, 2002). WHO expects to have new charts based on breastfed infants worldwide in 2005.

▶ SLEEPING PATTERNS

Although the specific amount of sleep each baby needs varies, all babies require a great amount of sleep. Some babies sleep as few as 8 hours in a 24-hour period. Some sleep as many as 20 hours a day. Understanding her baby's typical sleep patterns will help a mother adapt to his needs. The factors that cause variations among babies' sleep patterns may be developmental, environmental, or nutritional. Overtiredness or overstimulation can cause fretfulness before and during sleep. Sounds, lights, the temperature of the room and bedding, and low humidity, which causes difficulty in breathing, can interfere with sleep.

Babies who sleep separated from their mothers may wake at night to seek nourishment and physical contact. The absence of the mother's body warmth and skin contact with her may make it more difficult for the infant to fall asleep and sleep undisturbed. A baby may also have trouble sleeping if the mother consumes too much caffeine, which passes to the baby through her milk. See Chapter 17 for a discussion of developmental factors that affect sleep.

Encouraging Baby to Sleep

Many parents voice concerns about their babies' sleep habits. You can help a mother determine whether she has realistic expectations. Perhaps she can keep a written record for several days of her baby's sleep patterns over a 24-hour period, including even 5-minute naps. Gaining a better understanding of her baby's behavior may help her relax and not allow sleep to be such an important goal of hers for her baby. If she finds that her baby's sleep habits are robbing her of her own sleep, she could make it a practice to sleep when her baby does, taking several daytime naps. She could go to bed early in the evening and take her baby to bed with her. Or, during the night, the baby's father can bring the baby to bed for nursing, allowing her to stay in bed.

Establishing a bedtime ritual can be enjoyable for both parents and baby. A routine will help teach the baby to go to sleep easily at an established time every night. Quiet, soothing activities directly before bedtime such as a bath, story, rocking, and nursing will be effective in preparing the baby for sleep. The mother can warm his sleeping area with a heating pad or hot water bottle before putting him down. Flannel sheets may help keep him from waking because of the initial coolness of cotton sheets.

A baby may sleep for longer periods during the day than at night. Parents can reverse the baby's schedule by waking him every two to three hours during the day to discourage him from sleeping for longer periods. This will enable the mother to nurse him more frequently and let the baby know that nighttime is for undisturbed sleep, not daytime.

Breastfeeding Issues with Sleep

An older baby who is well nourished will usually be able to sleep for longer periods at night. Therefore, the mother will want to nurse her baby frequently during the day. Nursing him right before bedtime will help soothe him and will give him a full stomach. If she nurses him while lying down in the middle of the bed, she can leave him there when he falls asleep. She can later move him to his crib when he is in a deeper sleep, or keep him in her bed until morning or until after the next feeding.

When the baby wakes in the middle of the night to nurse, the mother will want to avoid stimulating him any more than necessary. Placing a night light in the room where the baby sleeps will avoid the need to turn on a bright light. If the baby's diaper needs to be changed, the mother can do it before she puts him to the second breast. He then will be able to nurse on the second breast and fall back to sleep without being disturbed for a diaper change. Keeping the baby and mother warm will help both of them return to sleep more easily.

Cosleeping

In most non-Western cultures and among many subgroups within Western cultures, an infant stays with his mother continually, both day and night. The warmth and familiar smell of his mother comforts the infant when he sleeps in his parents' bed (referred to as cosleeping). He can nuzzle at her breast and nurse whenever he wishes. The mother is not required to leave her bed to nurse her hungry infant. Thus, the mother is able to both get the sleep she needs and meet her infant's needs. The AAP recommends that mothers and babies should sleep in proximity to one another to facilitate breastfeeding (AAP, 2005).

Cosleeping infants arouse more often and in greater synchrony with their mothers than do separate sleepers (McKenna, 1994). This suggests that cosleeping may reduce the risk of Sudden Infant Death syndrome (SIDS) (Stuart-Macadam, 1995). The more frequent arousal also promotes nighttime breastfeeding (Pollard, 1999). Mothers who cosleep with their babies nurse them three times more frequently than do mothers whose babies sleep in a separate room (McKenna, 1997). Contrary to popular thinking, breastfeeding mothers who routinely sleep with their infants receive more total sleep than do those who routinely sleep separately. Moreover, the routine bedsharing mothers evaluate their sleep more positively than do the solitary sleeping mothers (Mosko, 1997).

Cosleeping is a component of responsive parenting that is becoming a more common and accepted practice. A family bed shared by mother, father, and baby may be an effective alternative for parents whose baby has difficulty falling asleep or falls asleep in their arms and cries out when placed in his bed (Figure 13.7). It will also be helpful with a baby who wakes frequently during the night. As an alternative, parents can use a crib that attaches to their bed. See the discussion of attachment parenting in Chapter 19.

Some parents worry that it is emotionally unhealthy for an infant to share a bed with his parents or that once he forms the habit it may be difficult to break. Some fear the mother could harm her baby by inadvertently rolling over onto him while she is asleep. Most mothers, however, instinctively recognize their babies' presence and respond accordingly. The baby would most likely cry out and awaken the mother if she were to roll too close to him. You can reassure parents that most infants worldwide sleep with their parents. It is a *cultural* norm in the U.S. for infants to sleep separated from their parents, not a *biological* norm.

Parents who choose to bedshare with their infant must evaluate their sleep environment and make it as safe as possible for their baby. Both parents should feel comfortable with the decision to cosleep with their baby and be committed to following appropriate safety precautions. No one sleep environment is guaranteed to be risk free, but there are ways of reducing risk in both cribs and adult beds (Donohue-Carey, 2002). Figure 13.8 contains precautions for cosleeping as well as creating a safe sleep environment in a crib.

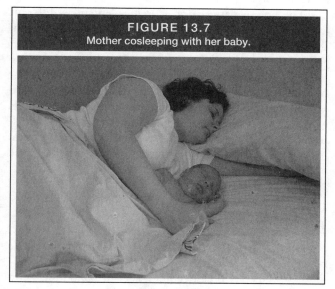

FIGURE 13.7
Mother cosleeping with her baby.

Printed with permission of Anna Swisher.

FIGURE 13.8
Creating a safe infant sleep environment.

Adapted from Infant Sleep Environment Safety Checklist by Patricia Donohue-Carey, BS, LCCE, CLE. Solitary or Shared Sleep: What's Safe? *Mothering*; 44–47 September/October 2002. Printed with permission.

Precautions for cribs and adult beds:

◆ Use a firm mattress to avoid suffocation.
◆ Have no gaps between the mattress and the frame.
◆ Keep bedding tight around the mattress.
◆ Avoid strings or ties on baby's and parents' nightclothes.
◆ Avoid soft items such as comforters, pillows, featherbeds, stuffed animals, lamb skins, and bean bags.
◆ Keep the baby's face uncovered to allow ventilation.
◆ Put the baby on his back to sleep.
◆ Do not overheat the room or overdress baby.
◆ Do not place a crib near window cords or sashes.

Additional precautions for cribs:

◆ When baby learns to sit, lower the mattress level to avoid falling or climbing out.
◆ When baby learns to stand, set the mattress level at its lowest point and remove crib bumpers.
◆ When baby reaches a height of 35 inches or the side rail is less than three-quarters of his height, move the baby to another bed.
◆ Crib bumpers should have at least six ties, no longer than six inches.
◆ Hang crib mobiles well out of reach and remove when baby can sit or reach.
◆ Remove crib gyms when baby can get up on all fours.

Additional precautions for cosleeping:

◆ Parents pull back and fasten long hair.
◆ Do not use alcohol or other drugs, including over-the-counter or prescription medications.
◆ Have no head/foot board railings with spaces wider than allowed in safety-approved cribs.
◆ Use no bed rails with infants less than one year.
◆ Do not allow siblings in bed with a baby less than one year old.
◆ Do not cosleep in a waterbed.
◆ Avoid placing bed directly alongside furniture or a wall.

Additional precautions regarding infant sleep:

◆ Do not sleep with baby on sofas or overstuffed chairs.
◆ Do not put baby to sleep alone in an adult bed.
◆ Do not place baby to sleep in car or infant seats.

Sources: American Academy of Pediatrics policy statement, *Changing Concepts of Sudden Infant Death Syndrome: Implications for Infant Sleeping Environments and Sleep Position* (RE9946); March 2000. Available at: www.aap.org/policyrRe9946.html.

American Academy of Pediatrics. *Caring for Your Baby and Young Child, Birth to Age 5* (New York: Bantam Books, 1998), 16–17.

SIDS Alliance. *Safe Infant Bedding Practices.* Available at: www.sidsalliance.org/Healthcare/default.asp.

Sudden Infant Death Syndrome (SIDS)

SIDS is the sudden death of an infant under one year of age which remains unexplained after an autopsy, examination of the death scene, and review of the clinical history (Willinger, 1991). Typically, parents find their seemingly healthy infant lifeless in his bed. Most SIDS deaths occur between the ages of two and six months. The occurrence peaks at about ten weeks of age. A baby who is not breastfed may be at greater risk for SIDS, presumably because of an immunological protection in human milk that he does not receive. The greater risk also may be related to differences in mothering styles between mothers who breastfeed and those who formula feed (Bernshaw, 1991).

The position in which the mother places her baby for sleep is a major factor in the risk of SIDS. Placing the baby in a **supine** position (on his back), rather than in a prone position (on his stomach) substantially reduces the incidence of SIDS (Irgens, 1995; Guntheroth, 1992). Breastfeeding mothers who cosleep predominantly put their infant on his back to facilitate reaching the breast.

Breastfed infants are more easily aroused from active sleep at two to three months of age than are formula-fed infants. This age coincides with the peak incidence of SIDS, and may be another protective mechanism of breastfeeding. "Arousal from sleep is believed to be an important survival mechanism that may be impaired in victims of SIDS" (Horne, 2004). Some researchers believe that infants' immature control mechanisms can be aggravated by environmental factors (Kahn, 2003).

There are increased risks for SIDS when parents smoke in conjunction with bedsharing, put the baby to sleep in the prone position, and do not breastfeed (Gilbert, 1995). Several studies reveal that two of the most significant risk factors for SIDS are sleeping prone and maternal smoking (Daltveit, 2003; Kahn, 2003; L'Hoir, 1998). Another risk factor is the baby's inhalation of passive smoke, even if parents co-sleep (Blair, 1996; Klonoff-Cohen, 1995). Parents who smoke around their baby need to be educated about the dangers to their baby. Blair found "no evidence that bed sharing is hazardous for infants of parents who do not smoke" (Blair, 1999), although the study did warn against bedsharing under certain conditions. The study showed an increased risk of SIDS when the baby sleeps in a separate room versus sleeping in the same room with his parents. Another study found 36 percent of 745 deaths attributable to the baby sleeping in a separate room (Carpenter, 2004).

▶ CRYING AND COLIC

New parents envision a smiling baby who smiles, coos, and snuggles; not one who is fussy and cries a lot. Parents of a fussy baby may worry that crying is a reflection of their ability to parent. You can help parents recognize that babies fuss and cry because of their needs, not because of their parenting. Encourage them to focus on positive elements, such as, "You have a high-need baby . . . your baby is fortunate to have parents who are so tuned into his needs" (Sears, 1996). Table 13.8 describes several combinations of temperament that can affect a baby's disposition.

People stare at the parents of a crying baby, and the parents may feel out of control. During pregnancy, the mother was in control and was the center of attention. Now it may seem that the baby has both the attention and the control. Mothers are vulnerable to the negative reaction to their colicky baby. Many times the problem lies in the parents' expectation of what parenting will be like.

Parents are often advised not to pick up their crying infant and are encouraged to let him cry it out. See Chapter 19 for a discussion on such "baby training" and its impact on breastfeeding. Infant crying is a powerful communicator used by the baby to interact with his environment. In a cause-and-effect relationship, the baby learns that he has the ability to make things happen through crying. By crying and eliciting his parents' response, he learns they will meet his needs. He forms a greater attachment to his parents, develops trust more readily, and cries less. A baby repeatedly left to cry alone ultimately learns that his needs will not be met and stops asking (crying).

Mothers may perceive infant fussiness as dissatisfaction with breastfeeding and conclude that supplementing with infant formula or cereal will provide a solution. It is important that parents understand that crying is a baby's method of communicating with his world. It is meant to get attention. The decibel level of a baby's cry is actually higher than street noise and can be 20 decibels louder than normal speech.

The crying pattern for a preterm infant is different from that of a full-term infant (Robb, 2003; Goberman, 1999). The preterm infant has a different rhythm, pause, and inhalation-exhalation pattern. His cry is a full octave higher, signaling a greater urgency. In response to her baby's cry, the mother's heart beats louder, her blood pressure increases, and the temperature in her breasts increases. A crying infant, shown in Figure 13.9, is disturbing and aggravating. Perhaps this is nature's design to ensure that the newborn receives the attention he needs.

The Effect of Crying on the Infant

Sears (2003) suggests, "Crying is good for the lungs like bleeding is good for the veins." Babies who have been crying have difficulty breastfeeding. They are often unable to organize themselves and their behavior for a period after

TABLE 13.8
Influences on Baby's Disposition

Baby's Disposition	Mother's Disposition	Probable Outcome
Easy baby	Responsive mother	This is a predictable and cuddly baby whose mother is in tune with him. The mother feels good about her parenting based on the positive interactions with her baby.
Easy baby	Restrained mother	This baby is not very demanding, and such behavior may lead the mother to feel somewhat unnecessary. The mother initially may not develop comfort skills, believing they are unnecessary. She may divert her energies elsewhere, and her baby may, in time, exhibit more fussy behavior.
High-need baby with good attachment-promoting behaviors	Responsive mother	The mother cannot ignore the needs of her baby and responds to him. She is rewarded with occasional satisfied responses from her baby. She will continue to explore alternative responses until she finds one that reaches her baby. Because of his mother's responsiveness, the baby will also fine-tune his attachment-promoting skills, resulting in a parent-child relationship of mutual sensitivity.
High-need baby with poor attachment-promoting skills	Responsive mother	This type of baby often is referred to as slow to warm up. He shows little or no effort to respond to or be comforted by his mother's efforts. The mother's nurturing responses are fine-tuned by her baby's responses. When the baby's responsiveness is lacking, this may seriously jeopardize the mother-baby relationship. In some situations, it is helpful for the mother to seek assistance from a professional who is trained in interaction counseling.
High-need baby	Restrained mother	This situation places the mother-baby relationship at risk. Often, the mother has been advised to let the baby cry it out or to not spoil him. Continued lack of response to his needs will lead this baby to one of two outcomes. He will intensify his high-need behaviors, or he will give up. The baby who gives up essentially shuts down his communication and withdraws into himself. He is prone to attach to objects rather than persons.

Adapted from Sears W., Sears M. *The Fussy Baby Book: Parenting Your High-Need Child from Birth to Age Five.* New York: Little Brown & Company; 1996.

the crying spell. When an infant cries or startles during the first four to five days of life, there is an increase in blood pressure, which, in turn, increases intracranial pressure. Poorly oxygenated blood flows back into circulation rather than into the lungs. Large fluctuations in blood flow increase cerebral blood volume and decrease cerebral oxygenation. A fluctuating pattern of cerebral blood flow is associated with intracranial hemorrhage (Anderson, 1989).

Crying decreases cerebral oxygenation in infants with respiratory problems (Brazy, 1988). Crying significantly raises the baby's heart rate and blood pressure (Dinwiddie, 1979). Crying decreases the absorption of inhalant medications, which frequently are given to preterm babies (Iles, 1999). Because of the extreme pressure caused by crying, some question whether it puts the baby at risk for a **pneumothorax**—a collection of air or gas in the chest that causes the lung to collapse (Theilade, 1978).

Metabolically, crying leads to increased glucose expenditure. In the immediate postpartum period, this could result in hypoglycemia. Crying also increases gastric distention and may result in a very discontented baby due to gas pain. Crying increases levels of cortisol, a stress hormone (Ahnert, 2004). Current neurological research focuses on the effects of early life events on neurobiological stress systems (Pruessner, 2004). Clinical data suggest a correlation between traumatic attachments and adult mental illness, presumably through

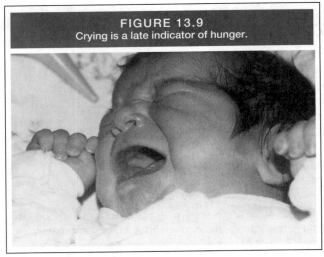

FIGURE 13.9
Crying is a late indicator of hunger.

Printed with permission of Kay Hoover.

organizing brain development (Sullivan, 2003). In one study, the quality of infants' attachment moderated the relation between cognitive level and cortisol reactivity. Infants with low security scores had higher cortisol responses to the test stressors (confrontation with a stranger and a scary robot). The researchers believe these findings may have implications for the development of self-regulation (van Bakel, 2004).

Identifying the Cause of Crying

Although some babies may cry periodically as a way to release tension, a baby's cry usually indicates some form of physical discomfort. As parents become accustomed to their baby, they will learn to distinguish among different types of cries. An infant's cry may indicate hunger, pain, or a reaction to his environment. Too often, a mother immediately assumes that hunger is the cause and may blame low milk production or poor quality milk for her baby's fussy disposition. You can encourage mothers to investigate other causes for crying, especially if the baby has nursed recently and does not appear to be hungry. As parents become better acquainted with their baby's particular communication, they will learn to distinguish the cause for his crying.

Crying from Hunger

In the early weeks, it is common for the baby to require frequent feedings and to sleep for short, frequent periods. As the mother tunes into her baby's pattern of sleeping and waking, she will learn to recognize a hunger cry. She will want to consider how long it has been since the last feeding and how much he nursed at that time. Other factors are his general disposition,

whether he can easily be soothed, and the feeding cues he demonstrates.

A newborn usually cries from hunger about one and a half to two hours or more after a feeding. A hunger cry is more prevalent in the evening hours when the mother's milk production seems lowest and the environment feels harried. As a result, cluster feeding is common in the early evening. Mothers who respond to hunger cries by nursing their babies will most likely have a more contented baby. He will cry less frequently than one whose mother maintains a strict feeding schedule regardless of her baby's cries. You can teach mothers to recognize hunger cues so that they feed on cue rather than waiting until the baby cries.

Crying from Body Discomfort

Wet or soiled diapers themselves are not usually sufficient to cause crying. However, when the diaper cools, the drop in temperature is a potential cause of discomfort. Cooling may actually make the baby more responsive to stimulation and more likely to cry for other reasons. Babies also may cry from too much heat. First-time mothers tend to overdress a new baby even on the hottest summer day, fearing he may become chilled. In warm weather and cold weather alike, babies can be dressed in the same type of clothing that an adult would wear.

Even when temperature is controlled, babies may cry when they are undressed and lose the warm secure feeling of clothing and blankets. A baby who is especially sensitive to this may benefit from swaddling. The texture of the cloth that touches his body is important. Plastic or rubber is more irritating than soft toweling or blanketing. Other skin irritations such as heat rash or diaper rash can be a cause of a baby's cries. In addition to comfortable body temperature, swaddling, and avoidance of skin irritants, a baby may find comfort in close skin-to-skin contact with his parents. The mother can take her baby into the bathtub with her or lie in bed with him.

A baby may cry from an internal discomfort such as gas or overfullness. If the mother finds her baby is constantly fussy during feedings, and she is confident that breastfeeding management is not the cause, she may need to burp him more often to help him bring up a bubble of air. Gas in the intestines can cause discomfort. The mother can help her baby pass his gas by using the techniques for comforting a colicky baby described later in this chapter. Some babies take in more milk than they are able to handle. Such overfullness causes pressure, which, in turn, can produce discomfort. Mothers can encourage the baby to nurse long enough on one breast before offering the other one. When parents have tended to the physical needs of their baby and he continues to cry, they will want to look for an external cause for the crying.

External Stimuli That Cause Crying

Babies may startle and cry in reaction to sudden movement, touch, smell, light, noise, and excessive handling. This often accounts for the initial fussiness when the baby makes the transition from hospital to home. Constant, soft, soothing noise can be an effective comfort measure. The steady movement of being rocked is comforting, as is the motion of a car ride.

Swaddling and being held by a parent are the most effective sources of comfort to a newborn. Swaddling provides a baby with constant touch stimulation. It reduces the amount of movement he can make and thus the amount of stimulation he experiences from his movements. Confining his arms and legs will prevent him from startling himself and provide him with a feeling of warmth and security. Although this may increase the time a baby sleeps and decrease time spent crying, it does not necessarily do so at the expense of time spent quietly awake.

Pediatrician Harvey Karp popularized the concept of a "fourth trimester," in which re-creating the sounds and feeling of the womb comforts a baby. He is a proponent of swaddling newborns (Karp, 2004, 2003). Figure 13.10 shows another comforting technique of "wearing" the baby in a sling. This provides him with the secure feeling of swaddling, with the added benefit of closeness to the person who "wears" him.

Some babies do not like being swaddled. They will cry or squirm when they are wrapped too tightly or held too close. Such a baby may push away from the breast when held too closely. He may need to nurse in such a way that he has no constraints on his movements. For a young baby, the mother can lie on her side to nurse. She can either lightly support the baby from behind or put a pillow behind him for support. She could also lean above a reclining baby and put him to breast.

Through touch, a baby gets important information about the world around him. A mother whose touch is tentative and light may have an irritable baby who cries frequently. With a firm touch, a mother communicates to her baby that she is confident and that he can relax and trust her to care for him. Gently stroking an infant's body during a feeding—called **grooming**—increases the mother's prolactin level. Such quiet, gentle touching does not usually interfere with feedings. However, if a mother distracts her baby during nursing by poking or jiggling him, it could be difficult for him to relax and he may react by crying.

Overhandling by well-meaning adults can cause a baby to cry in an attempt to tell them, "Please leave me alone!" Babies at times may prefer to lie quietly in their cribs and will react unhappily when picked up. Some become very agitated when they are tired and might cry themselves to sleep. If parents have ruled out hunger or discomfort, their baby may settle on his own after a few minutes. They need to be encouraged to focus on the cues their baby gives in response to their parenting approach. If their baby is responding positively to a technique, it can be encouraged. If their baby exhibits withdrawal or avoidance behaviors, they will want to try a new approach.

Distinguishing Crying from Colic

Much of the fussiness that practitioners see and parents describe is actually colic-like behavior and not true colic. The accepted research definition of colic is "inconsolable crying for which no physical cause can be found, which lasts more than three hours a day, occurs at least three days a week and continues for at least three weeks; spasmodic contractions of smooth muscle, causing pain and discomfort" (Wessel, 1954). This is quite different from the pattern of one or two fussy periods a day experienced by most infants. Duration is more important than frequency in defining colic (Barr, 1992).

The term "colic" derives from the Greek word *kolikos*, an adjective derived from *kolon*, meaning "large colon." It is estimated that as many as 16 to 30 percent of all infants experience colic-like symptoms. These symptoms subside by 16 weeks of age in the majority of infants (Pinyerd, 1992). There seems to be little distinction in the occurrence of colic between bottle-feeding and breastfeeding infants. Colic does seem to be more common when infants begin solid foods younger than three months of age.

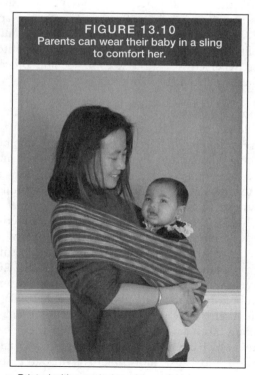

FIGURE 13.10
Parents can wear their baby in a sling to comfort her.

Printed with permission of Anna Swisher.

A colicky baby exhibits unexplained fussiness, fretfulness, and irritability. He appears to suffer from severe discomfort during the colicky period. His cries are piercing, explosive attacks. A rumbling sound may be audible in the baby's gut. Excessive flatulence (gas) and apparent abdominal pain may cause the baby to draw his legs up sharply into his abdomen. He may clench his fists and appear intense, energetic, excitable, and easily startled. He may grimace, stiffen, and twist his body, and may awaken easily and frequently. Continuous crying may cause him to swallow air and further aggravate the discomfort.

Causes of Colic

The exact cause of colic has not been determined medically. Not everyone even agrees about the incidence of colic. Some theories relate colic to stress and tension in the mother and child during pregnancy and lactation. Others believe the cause to be an immature digestive and intestinal system or allergies. Pregnancies with **hyperemesis** (pregnancy marked by long-term vomiting, weight loss, and fluid and electrolyte imbalance), pelvic pain, and distress often correlate to infants with colic. A similar relationship exists for second-born infants and those with a family history of colic (Hogsdall, 1991).

Immature Gastrointestinal and/or Neurological Systems

Compared with other young mammals, a human baby is born in an extremely immature state. He is essentially neurologically incomplete. At one month, the infant's stomach capacity is one-tenth the size of an adult stomach. He has only four percent of the gastric glands that secrete digestive enzymes. The muscle layers surrounding the stomach and intestines are thin and weak, and his intestines lack the ridges and hair-like filaments that help process food.

Colicky infants transmit more macromolecules across the epithelium (lining) of the gut than those without colic symptoms (Lothe, 1990). Peristalsis (wavelike rhythmic contraction of smooth muscle) can be irregular, faint, forceful, or spasmodic. Additionally, lack of muscle tone can cause food to move up out of the stomach as well as down into the intestines. The colons of colicky infants may contract violently during feedings. Whereas the colon in normal infants takes several hours to empty, the colon may empty in less than one minute for some colicky infants. Interestingly, one recent study found a correlation between colic and feeding disorders, including reflux (Miller-Loncar, 2004).

Hormones

At birth, babies have high levels of progesterone, which helps relax the muscles of the intestines. The progesterone level drops after one to two weeks and may account for the increase in colic symptoms at that time. Infants with colic-like behavior have high levels of motilin from the first day of life. Motilin is a digestive hormone that stimulates muscle contractions. Human milk has high levels of many enzymes that are necessary for digestion and thus may aid in reducing the intensity of colic in some infants.

Intrauterine and Birth-Related Problems

Increased crying occurs in infants who were born prematurely, who were small for gestational age (SGA), or who experienced birth trauma or **anoxia** (lack of oxygen). Increased excitability and fussiness are seen in infants whose mothers were hypertensive (had high blood pressure). Mothers who received epidural anesthesia may be at higher risk for a colicky baby (Murray, 1981; Thomas, 1981). By the fifth day of life, these babies cried more and, at one month, were less adaptable, more intense, and difficult to manage. Maternal distress during pregnancy results in a threefold increased risk of infant colic (Sondergaard, 2003). The passage of time seems to be the most effective course for colic-like behavior caused by birth interventions. Some parents seek help from a chiropractor or craniosacral therapist. One study found that osteopathic treatment offered symptom relief (Colli, 2003).

Prenatal Intake of Street Drugs

Prenatal maternal abuse of heroin, marijuana, barbiturates, or cocaine can result in colic-like behavior in the infant. Infants of a substance abuser often exhibit signs of nervous system instabilities. Symptoms may not appear until a week or more after birth. Symptoms include excitability, trembling, restlessness, ravenous appetite, jitteriness, hyperactivity, shrill scream, feeding problems, and either hypertonia or hypotonia.

Smoking Parent

A clear correlation exists between infant fussiness and parental intake of nicotine. The infants of smokers are more excitable and hypertonic than other infants. They require more careful handling, and show more stress/abstinence signs, specifically in the central nervous system (CNS), gastrointestinal, and visual areas (Law, 2003). Only about 20 percent of women who smoke will initiate breastfeeding. There is a two-fold increase in colic among infants whose mothers smoked during pregnancy or postpartum (Sondergaard, 2001). However, this incidence is lower among smoking mothers who breastfeed their infants (Reijneveld, 2000).

The levels of the peptide somatostatin are increased in smoking mothers. This peptide inhibits the release of prolactin, which can lead to a decrease in maternal milk production and cause more infant crying and fussing. Smoking 15 or more cigarettes per day significantly lowers basal prolactin levels (Anderson, 1982). No difference is apparent in milk production between women who smoke or who use a nicotine patch (Ilett, 2003).

Encourage a mother to stop smoking or to decrease the amount of cigarettes she smokes. She can also discuss the possible use of nicotine gum or patches with her physician. Acquaint yourself with smoking cessation programs available in your area. Discuss with both parents the need to refrain from smoking in the same room or car as the baby. The mother may need help establishing and maintaining adequate milk production. If smoking lowers her milk supply and she is unwilling to quit smoking, she may benefit from the use of galactogogues (see Chapter 18).

Food Sensitivity

A typical infant who reacts to something in his mother's diet is calm at the start of a feeding and then begins to pull off the breast, stiffens his body, cries, and then reattaches. He may repeat this many times during the feeding. Symptoms can be continuous or can start after a feeding. It is rare for symptoms of a food sensitivity to show up before three weeks. Signs of food sensitivity are:

- A stuffy or drippy nose without any other sign of having a cold
- Frequently pulling off the breast and arching and crying while feeding
- An itchy nose
- A red, scaly, oily rash on the forehead or eyebrows, in the hair, or behind the ears
- Eczema
- A red rectal ring
- Fretful sleeping or persistent sleeplessness
- Frequent spitting up or vomiting
- Diarrhea or green stools, perhaps with blood in them
- Wheezing
- Typical colic-like symptoms and behaviors

Cow and Soy Milk Intolerances

Cow's milk protein is a common cause of intolerance in infants. The mean level of bovine immunoglobulin G (IgG) in colicky babies' mothers' milk is higher than levels for non-colicky babies. Almost all mammal milks contain some IgG (Clyne, 1991). In this study, bovine IgG levels in the milk of colicky babies reached 0.42 mg/ml, compared to 0.32 mg/ml among babies who did not have colic. The range in human milk was from 0.1 to 8.5 mg/ml, compared to 0.6 to 128 mg/ml in cow's-milk formulas. Highest levels occurred in powdered formula, with lowest levels in formula concentrate. Bovine IgG levels can be so high or the half-life so long that trials of two to seven days on a diet free of cow's milk may not be long enough to see results. A 14-day trial may be necessary. There is no bovine IgG in soy or hydrolysate formulas.

About 30 percent of colic-like behavior in breastfed infants is due to cow's milk protein intolerances. Some researchers have found a decrease in colic in breastfed babies when the mother omits dairy products (Host, 2002; Lindberg, 1999). A mother who suspects that her baby is intolerant to cow's milk can try eliminating dairy foods from her diet for two weeks. If cow's milk was the cause of her infant's colic-like behavior, she may see some improvement in 48 hours, although it may take several days. The mother can reintroduce dairy slowly into her diet after two weeks of a dairy-free diet. She can start with hard cheeses or yogurt the first week, add soft cheeses the second week, butter and ice cream the third week, and cow's milk in small quantities the fourth week. Any time the infant becomes fussy or other symptoms return, the mother can once again reduce her intake of dairy products. A true milk-free diet means the mother takes in no milk, whey, casinate, or sodium casinate. Lactose is acceptable since it is a sugar and not a cow's milk protein. Caution mothers using a dairy elimination diet to read food labels. Casein is used as a binder in many processed foods.

Mother's and Infant's Diets

Removal of possible sources of intolerance may provide relief to a colicky baby. The mother should feed him nothing but her milk. Even vitamins, fluoride, and iron supplements may be a source of discomfort. Babies who receive antibiotics may be at a greater risk for developing food allergies. Antibiotics are linked to **leaky gut syndrome**, a condition in which the intestinal lining first becomes inflamed, and then thin and porous. Proteins that do not completely digest may cross from the intestines into the bloodstream. **Leukocytes** attack such proteins and lead to an antigen-antibody reaction, which manifests itself as an allergic reaction with subsequent exposure to that protein.

Babies are usually not bothered by foods in their mothers' diets. If the mother has a very sensitive baby, she may want to monitor her food intake, because some of what she consumes may pass through her milk. Medications, vitamin supplements, caffeine, high-protein foods, milk, wheat, chocolate, eggs, and nuts are all potential sources of discomfort to an intolerant baby. Many mothers report that foods that make them gassy (e.g., cabbage, beans, and broccoli) also make their babies gassy, especially in the early days. Because many colicky babies become food-intolerant children, there may be some validity to the theory of allergy as a cause of colic-like behavior.

Lactose Overload

Colic-like symptoms may occur when a baby consumes an unbalanced amount of milk, receiving too much lactose and too little fat. The amount of lactose in human milk is the same in both foremilk and hindmilk, but the amount of fat is low in foremilk and high in hindmilk. If the infant receives an unbalanced feeding, he will get a higher percentage of lactose in comparison to the percentage of fat. This results in the lactose fermenting in the baby's gut, which can lead to gassiness and fussiness.

Lactose overload can result from an overactive letdown, overabundant milk production, or insufficient hindmilk intake (Woolridge, 1988). When a mother places limits on her baby's time at the breast, she may remove him from one breast before letdown has occurred or before he has been able to obtain the amount of hindmilk he needs. This results in the baby ingesting a large quantity of foremilk. He then nurses on the other breast and fills up on foremilk again. Computer imaging research has found that fat intake varies between feedings, and that the emptier the breast, the higher the fat content (Daly, 1993).

In addition to typical colic-like symptoms, the infant's stools may be green, frothy, loose, and frequent. He may have poor weight gain, a bloated abdomen, and a great deal of gas. Lactose overload can be a temporary problem when either the mother or the infant has been on prolonged antibiotic therapy. To avoid lactose overload, it is important that the mother allow her baby to nurse from the first breast until he has received the fatty hindmilk. Some babies may need to nurse repeatedly on the same breast before they switch to the other breast. If the mother has documented overabundant milk production, she may try nursing on one breast for several feedings before switching. Although some caregivers prescribe simethicone (Mylicon) drops for colic due to gas, these aids have not proved to be effective. The symptoms of lactose overload are very similar to those of food intolerance. Never suggest to a mother that she only feed on one side or reduce her supply without a full feeding assessment that includes AC/PC weights (weight before and after feeding) on a digital scale and pumping for residual milk.

Treatment of Colic-Like Symptoms

One theory holds that colic indicates an overreactive nervous system. This causes the baby to become tense easily and to react with discomfort to most stimuli, including parental handling. He may appear to reject his mother by crying and pushing her away when she picks him up. The mother needs to learn that these reactions do not indicate he dislikes her but that he needs to be soothed.

Some parents find massage effective for soothing an infant with colic-like symptoms. Touch has relaxing effects on both the baby and parent. The mother can hold her naked baby on her lap, supine, with his head on her knees. She gently massages his stomach, shoulders, head, hands, and feet, and then turns him over to massage his back. Then she holds him against her shoulder and soothes him until he is calm. Sometimes the baby will cry throughout the massage but be calm by the end. Other infants may respond immediately.

One study found both infant massage and a crib vibrator useful in reducing crying in colicky babies (Huhtala, 2000). The use of reflexology treatment (massage corresponding to specific organs) gave a "significantly better outcome" to a group of colicky babies compared to the observation group in one study (Bennedbaek, 2001). Massage on preterm babies in the NICU is linked to greater weight gain, earlier discharge, and increased developmental scores (Vickers, 2004; Beachy, 2003).

Many cultures promote home remedies such as chamomile, catnip, fennel, dill, and anise for colic symptoms (Humphrey, 2003). One study found that fennel oil emulsion eliminated colic in 65 percent of the treatment group (Alexandrovich, 2003). However, you should caution parents to discuss options with their baby's caregiver before they use any over-the-counter, herbal, or folk remedy. A blend of Chinese and Japanese types of anise resulted in two infant poisoning cases when used for treatment of colicky pain (Minodier, 2003).

Time seems to be the actual cure for colic-like behavior. Parkin (1993) found in a randomized controlled trial that none of three interventions was better than the others in the management of persistent crying. When crying stops temporarily, parents cannot necessarily assume the cause is clear (Pinyerd, 1992). Table 13.9 identifies some interventions parents may wish to try. One of the techniques, shown in Figure 13.11, is for the mother to place her baby across her lap. If all measures used to comfort the baby fail, the parents should consult their baby's caregiver to rule out illness. Resources on infant massage include *Infant Massage—Revised Edition: A Handbook for Loving Parents* (McClure, 2000); *Loving Hands: The Traditional Art of Baby Massage* (Leboyer, 1997); and *Baby Massage: The Calming Power of Touch* (Heath, 2000).

Supporting the Parents of a Colicky Baby

When a baby experiences colic-like symptoms, parental stress and concern increase. Colic seems severe enough to some parents that they visit the hospital emergency room. Crying accounted for 19 percent of emergency room visits in one study (Perez, 2003). Beebe (1993) reported that 10 to 30 percent of infants cry for three hours or more a day in the first three months, and stress was higher for the mothers of these babies.

TABLE 13.9
Measures for Comforting a Colicky Baby

Holding techniques	"Wear" the baby around the house in a cloth baby sling, walking and dancing in a soothing manner. Hold the baby upright against the parent's shoulder near the neck. Place the baby on his stomach across the parent's lap or knees. Carry the baby against the parent's hip. Lay the baby face down on the parent's chest. Lay the baby face down on the inside of the parent's forearm with the baby's head held in the crook of the parent's arm. The pressure on the stomach feels good and the parent can use the free hand to pat and rub the baby's back. Pick up the baby as soon as he starts to fuss. This will decrease the length of time he is fussy and prevent it from escalating.
Sounds and motion	Provide a steady noise from a vacuum, clothes dryer, music, humming, or tapes of the mother's heartbeat. Play a recording of the baby's own cry. Parents speak closely and softly in whispers. Baby look at the mother's and father's face. Provide an unexpected distraction to startle the baby to cease crying. Take the baby for a car ride to provide soothing, rhythmic motion. Bounce, swing, rock, and walk in slow, rhythmical movements.
Security and warmth	Place the baby in a warm bath. Check for any rashes that could indicate reaction to the fiber or detergent in clothing or blankets. Swaddle the baby to provide closeness and security, or unswaddle him if the blanket seems too constricting. Check the diaper for dampness and keep the baby warm with sweaters or blankets. Place a warmed hot water bottle against the baby's stomach area to help him release tension and thereby encourage the passing of gas. Fold his legs up to his stomach in a bicycle motion to help him eliminate gas.

Parents of a colicky baby will need support, frequent contact, and reassurance. Depending on their reading level and desire, you can suggest appropriate reading material. *The Fussy Baby Book* (William and Martha Sears, 1996); *The Baby Book: Everything You Need to Know About Your Baby from Birth to Age Two* (Revised and Updated Edition) (James Sears et al., 2003); *Crying Baby, Sleepless Nights* (Jones 1992); and *The Happiest Baby on the Block* (Karp, 2003) are all helpful resources.

The mother of a colicky baby may experience frustration, and guilt for resenting him. Physical exhaustion is common from constantly trying to soothe and comfort a crying baby. A baby may react to his mother's emotional state when she is holding him. She may find that her baby is comforted immediately when another person picks him up, which can further add to her feelings of guilt. She may believe that her baby is rejecting her and that she is the cause of her baby's colic-like behavior. The mother will need a great deal of emotional support and frequent close contact.

One study suggests an emotional component to colic, reporting that both parents of colicky infants had worse parent-child interaction compared with control parents. Interaction problems were most pronounced between fathers and infants in the severe colic group. Severely colicky infants did not interact as well as the controls. Interaction between the parents was more often dysfunctional in the severe colic group (Raiha, 2002).

Tension can aggravate a baby's colicky condition. The mother will need an avenue for venting her anger and frustration. She will benefit from the support of someone who is receptive, caring, and reassuring. Parents may also need to take a break and spend some time away from the baby when necessary in order to keep their perspective.

Encourage parents to get help if they feel they cannot cope with their baby's crying. Shaking the baby to stop his crying, or shaking him too roughly in play, can cause shaken baby syndrome. Make sure both parents and caregivers know the causes of shaken baby syndrome, and that they know to never shake their baby or handle him roughly. Shaking can cause brain damage, blindness, and death. Although it is difficult to estimate how many children die from being shaken, one study found that

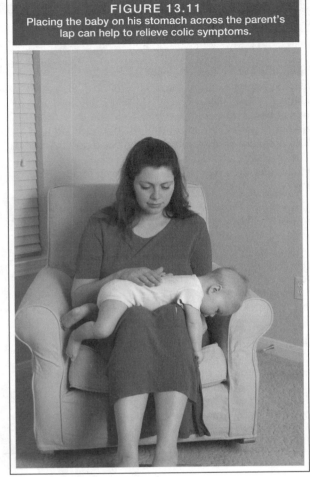

FIGURE 13.11
Placing the baby on his stomach across the parent's lap can help to relieve colic symptoms.

Printed with permission of Nelia Box.

53 percent of traumatic brain injuries were inflicted (Keenan, 2003). The study also found that relative to the general population, children who incurred an increased risk of inflicted injury were born to young mothers (under 21 years), non-European American, or products of multiple births. The National Center on Shaken Baby Syndrome has helpful information on recognizing and preventing this form of child abuse. Its Web site is www.dontshake.com.

You have the opportunity to educate parents about normal baby behavior. Many parents have never held a baby until they hold their child. One study concluded that some babies with normal irritability are wrongly diagnosed with medical conditions. The results are unnecessary medication and the potential for "lifelong problems for these infants and their families" (Armstrong, 2000). Your experience with many healthy babies at different developmental stages will help you familiarize parents with what is normal.

▶ SUMMARY

Infant assessment is a significant part of your role with breastfeeding mothers. Recognizing deviations from normal in the infant's posture, skin, head, and reflexes will provide important clues to his condition. An assessment of the infant's oral cavity and patterns of voiding and stooling will assist you in determining any need for changes in approach. Teaching parents how to recognize and interpret infant signals will help them tune into their baby's needs. Understanding typical patterns of behavior, growth, sleeping, crying, and digestion will be a source of comfort to parents as they learn to interpret their baby's patterns.

▶ CHAPTER 13—AT A GLANCE

Applying what you learned—

Teach the mother:

- How to help her hypotonic baby stay latched.
- How to find a position for feeding her hypertonic baby.
- Dancer hand position for a baby who lacks sufficient buccal pads.
- Rooting and other reflexes.
- How to recognize nutritive and nonnutritive sucking.
- What to do for frequent spitting up.
- Appropriate number of voids and stools.
- Approach and avoidance behaviors.
- Feeding cues.
- How to stimulate a sleepy baby and comfort a fussy baby.
- Expected weight patterns.
- Cosleeping and responsive parenting.
- How to distinguish among different types of cries.

Evaluate the baby for:

- Skin turgor for breastfeeding adequacy.
- Body tone for clues about potential problems.
- Ability to extend his tongue over the alveolar ridge.
- Short frenulum or frenum.
- Fractured clavicle or sensitivity from forceps or cephalhematoma.

▶ REFERENCES

Ahnert L et al. Transition to child care: Associations with infant-mother attachment, infant negative emotion, and cortisol elevations. *Child Dev* 75(3):639–650; 2004.

Alexandrovich I et al. The effect of fennel (Foeniculum Vulgare) seed oil emulsion in infantile colic: A randomized, placebo-controlled study. *Altern Ther Health Med* 9(4):58–61; 2003.

American Academy of Pediatrics (AAP). Policy Statement on Breastfeeding and the Use of Human Milk. *Pediatrics* 115(2):496–506; 2005.

Anderson A et al. Suppressed prolactin but normal neurophysin levels in cigarette smoking breastfeeding women. *Clin Endocrinol* 17:363; 1982.

Anderson G. Risk in mother-infant separation postbirth. *Image* 21:196–199; 1989.

Armstrong K et al. Medicalizing normality? Management of irritability in babies. *J Paediatr Child Health* 36(4):301–305; 2000.

Ballard JL et al. Ankyloglossia: Assessment, incidence, and effect of frenuloplasty on the breastfeeding dyad. *Pediatrics* 110(5); 2002.

Barr CS, Newman TK, Shannon C et al. Rearing condition and rh5-HTTLPR interact to influence limbic-hypothalamic-pituitary-adrenal axis response to stress in infant macaques. *Biol Psychiatry* 55(7):733–738; 2004.

Barr RG, Rotman A, Yaremko J, Leduc D, Francoeur TE. The crying of infants with colic: A controlled empirical description. *Pediatrics* 90:14–21; 1992.

Beebe S et al. Association of reported infant crying and maternal parenting stress. *Clin Pediatr* 32:15–19; 1993.

Beachy J. Premature infant massage in the NICU. *Neonatal Netw* 22(3):39–45. Review; 2003.

Bennedbaek O et al. Infants with colic. A heterogeneous group possible to cure? Treatment by pediatric consultation followed by a study of the effect of zone therapy on incurable colic. *Ugeskr Laeger* 163(27):3773–3778; 2001.

Bernshaw NJ. Does breastfeeding protect against sudden infant death syndrome? *J Hum Lact* 7:73–79; 1991.

Blair P et al. Babies sleeping with parents: Case-control study of factors influencing the risk of the sudden infant death syndrome. CESDI SUDI research group. *BMJ* 319(7223):1457–1461; 1999.

Blair P et al. Smoking and the sudden infant death syndrome: Results from 1993–5 case-control study for confidential inquiry into stillbirths and deaths in infancy. Confidential enquiry into stillbirths and deaths regional coordinators and researchers. *BMJ* 313(7051):195–198; 1996.

Boekel S. *Gastroesophageal Reflux: The Breastfeeding Family's Nightmare.* Presentation at ILCA International Conference, Washington, DC; July 27, 2000.

Brazy J. Effects of crying on cerebral blood volume and cytochrome aa3. *J Pediatr* 112(3):457–461; 1988.

Butte N et al. Infant feeding mode affects early growth and body composition. *Pediatrics* 106(6):1355–1366; 2000.

Butte N et al. Sleep organization and energy expenditure of breast-fed and formula-fed infants. *Pediatr Res* 32:514–519; 1992.

Butte N, Smith E, Garza C. Heart rates of breast-fed and formula-fed infants. *J Pediatr Gastroenterol Nutr* 13(4):391–396; 1991.

Butte N et al. Energy expenditure and deposition of breast-fed and formula-fed infants during early infancy. *Pediatr Res* 28(6): 631–640; 1990a.

Butte NF, Smith EO, Garza C. Energy utilization of breast-fed and formula-fed infants. *Am J Clin Nutr* 51(3):350–358; 1990b.

Carpenter R et al. Sudden unexplained infant death in 20 regions in Europe: Case control study. *Lancet* 363(9404): 185–191; 2004.

Carroll A et al. A systematic review of nonpharmacological and nonsurgical therapies for gastroesophageal reflux in infants. *Arch Pediatr Adolesc Med Review* 156(2):109–113; 2002.

Centers for Disease Control and Prevention (CDC), National Center for Health Statistics. CDC growth charts: United States; May 30, 2000. Page updated on June 7, 2002. Available at: www.cdc.gov/growthcharts. Accessed August 12, 2003.

Clyne P, Kulczycki A. Human breast milk contains bovine IgG. Relationship to infant colic? *Pediatrics* 87:439–444; 1991.

Colli R et al. Osteopathy in neonatology. *Pediatr Med Chir* 25(2):101–105; 2003.

Daltveit A et al. Circadian variations in sudden infant death syndrome: Associations with maternal smoking, sleeping position and infections. The Nordic Epidemiological SIDS Study. *Acta Paediatr* 92(9):991–993; 2003.

Daly S et al. Degree of breast emptying explains changes in the fat content but not fatty acid composition of human milk. *Exp Physiol* 78:741–755; 1993.

de Onis M, Onyango AW. The Centers for Disease Control and Prevention 2000 growth charts and the growth of breast-fed infants. *Acta Paediatr* 92(4):413–419; 2003.

Dewey K et al. Adequacy of energy intake among breast-fed infants in the DARLING study: Relationships to growth velocity, morbidity, and activity levels. *J Pediatr* 119:538–547; 1991.

Dewey K et al. Breast-fed infants are leaner than formula-fed infants at 1 year of age: The DARLING study. *Am J Clin Nutr* 57:140–145; 1993a.

Dewey K et al. Growth of breast-fed and formula-fed infants from 0 to 18 months: The DARLING study. *Pediatrics* 89: 1035–1041; 1993b.

Dinwiddie R et al. Cardiopulmonary changes in the crying neonate. *Pediatr Res* 13:900–903; 1979.

Donohue-Carey, P. Solitary or shared sleep: What's safe? *Mothering* 39–43; September/October 2002.

Garza C, Butte N. Energy intakes of human milk-fed infants during the first year. *J Pediatr* 117(Suppl):S124–S131; 1990.

Gilbert RE. Bottle-feeding and the sudden infant death syndrome. *Br Med J* 310:88–90; 1995.

Goberman A, Robb M. Acoustic examination of preterm and full-term infant cries: The long-time average spectrum. *J Speech Lang Hear Res* 42(4):850–861; 1999.

Graham M. Parental sensitivity to infant cues: Similarities and differences between mothers and fathers. *J Pediatr Nurs* 8:376–384; 1993.

Guntheroth WG, Spiers PS. Sleeping prone and the risk of sudden infant death syndrome. *JAMA* 267:2359–2362; 1992.

Heath A et al. *Baby Massage: The Calming Power of Touch.* New York: DK Publishing; 2000.

Heinig MJ et al. Energy and protein intakes of breast-fed and formula-fed infants during the first year of life and their association with growth velocity: The DARLING study. *Am J Clin Nutr* 58:152–161; 1993.

Hogsdall C et al. The significance of pregnancy, delivery and postpartum factors for the development of infantile colic. *J Perinat Med* 19:251–257; 1991.

Horne R et al. Comparison of evoked arousability in breast and formula fed infants. *Arch Dis Child* 89(1):22–25; 2004.

Host A. Frequency of cow's milk allergy in childhood. *Ann Allergy Asthma Immunol* 89(6 Suppl 1):33–37; 2002.

Huhtala V et al. Infant massage compared with crib vibrator in the treatment of colicky infants. *Pediatrics* 105(6):E84; 2000.

Humphrey S. *The Nursing Mother's Herbal.* Minneapolis, MN: Fairview Press; 2003.

Iles R et al. Crying significantly reduces absorption of aerosolised drug in infants. *Arch Dis Child* 81(2):163–165; 1999.

Ilett K et al. Use of nicotine patches in breast-feeding mothers: Transfer of nicotine and cotinine into human milk. *Clin Pharmacol Ther* 74(6):516–524; 2003.

Irgens LM et al. Sleeping position and sudden infant death syndrome in Norway 1967–91. *Arch Dis Child* 72:478–482; 1995.

Jones S. *Crying Baby, Sleepless Nights.* Boston, MA: Harvard Common Press; 1992.

Kahn A et al. Sudden infant deaths: Stress, arousal and SIDS. *Early Hum Dev* 75 S147–166; 2003.

Karp H. *The Happiest Baby on the Block: The New Way To Calm Crying and Help Your Newborn Baby Sleep Longer.* Bantam: New York; 2003.

Karp H. The "fourth trimester": A framework and strategy for understanding and resolving colic. *Contemporary Pediatrics* 21:94; 2004.

Keenan HT et al. A population-based study of inflicted traumatic brain injury in young children. *JAMA*; 290:621–626; 2003.

Klonoff-Cohen HS et al. The effect of passive smoking and tobacco exposure through breast milk on sudden infant death syndrome. *JAMA* 273:795–798; 1995.

Kramer LI. Advancement of dermal icterus in the jaundiced newborn. *Am J Dis Child* 118:454–458; 1969.

Law K et al. Smoking during pregnancy and newborn neurobehavior. *Pediatrics* 111(6 Pt 1):1318–1323; 2003.

Leboyer F. *Loving Hands: The Traditional Art of Baby Massage.* New York: Newmarket Press; 1997.

L'Hoir M et al. Sudden unexpected death in infancy: Epidemiologically determined risk factors related to pathological classification. *Acta Paediatr* 87(12):1279–1287; 1998.

Lindberg T. Infantile colic and small intestinal function: A nutritional problem? *Acta Paediatr Suppl* 88(430):58–60; 1999.

Lothe L et al. Macromolecular absorption in infants with infantile colic. *Acta Paediatr Scand* 70:417–521; 1990.

Malloy M et al. Sudden infant death syndrome and maternal smoking. *Am J Public Health* 82:1380–1382; 1992.

Matheson I, Rivrud GN. The effect of smoking on lactation and infantile colic. *JAMA* 261:42; 1989.

McClure V. *Infant Massage: A Handbook for Loving Parents.* New York: Bantam; 2000.

McKenna J et al. Bedsharing promotes breastfeeding. *Pediatrics* 100:214–219; 1997.

McKenna J, Mosko S. Sleep and arousal, synchrony and independence among mothers and infants sleeping apart and together (same bed): An experiment in evolutionary medicine. *Acta Paeidatr Suppl* 397:94–102; 1994.

Miller-Loncar C et al. Infant colic and feeding difficulties. *Arch Dis Child* 89(10):908–912; 2004.

Minodier P et al. Star anise poisoning in infants. *Arch Pediatr* 10(7):619–621; 2003.

Mosko S et al. Maternal sleep and arousals during bedsharing with infants. *Sleep* 201(2):142–150; 1997.

Motil K et al. Human milk protein does not limit growth of breast-fed infants. *J Pediatr Gastroenterol Nutr* 24(1):10–17; 1997.

Murray AD et al. Effects of epidural anesthesia on newborns and their mothers. *Child Dev* 52:71–82; 1981.

Nacey K. Infant colic. *J Emerg Nurs* 19:65–66; 1993.

Parkin P et al. Randomized controlled trial of three interventions in the management of persistent crying of infancy. *Pediatrics* 92:197–201; 1993.

Perez Solis D et al. Neonatal visits to a pediatric emergency service. *An Pediatr (Barc)* 59(1):54–58; 2003.

Pinyerd B. Strategies for consoling the infant with colic: Fact or fiction. *J Pediatr Nurs* 7:403–411; 1992.

Pollard K et al. Night-time nonnutritive sucking in infants aged 1 to 5 months: Relationship with infant state, breastfeeding, and bed-sharing versus room-sharing. *Early Hum Dev* 56(2–3):185–204; 1999.

Pruessner J et al. Dopamine release in response to a psychological stress in humans and its relationship to early life maternal care: A positron emission tomography study using [11C] raclopride. *J Neurosci* 24(11):2825–2831; 2004.

Raiha H et al. Excessively crying infant in the family: Mother-infant, father-infant and mother-father interaction. *Child Care Health Dev* 28(5):419–429; 2002.

Ramsay D. Ultrasound Imaging of the Sucking Mechanics of the Term Infant. Presentation at *Human Lactation: Current Research & Clinical Implications*. Amarillo, TX; October 22, 2004.

Reijneveld S et al. Infantile colic: Maternal smoking as potential risk factor. *Arch Dis Child* 83(4):302–303; 2000.

Robb M. Bifurcations and chaos in the cries of full-term and preterm infants. *Folia Phoniatr Logop* 55(5):233–240; 2003.

Salvatore S, Vandenplas Y. Gastroesophageal reflux and cow milk allergy: Is there a link? *Pediatrics* 110(5):972–984; 2002.

Sears J et al. *The Baby Book: Everything You Need to Know about Your Baby from Birth to Age Two.* Boston, MA: Little, Brown; 2003.

Sears W, Sears M. *The Fussy Baby Book: Parenting Your High-Need Child from Birth to Age Five.* Boston, MA: Little, Brown; 1996.

Small M. *Our Babies, Ourselves: How Biology and Culture Shape the Way We Parent.* New York: Anchor Books; 1998.

Sondergaard C et al. Psychosocial distress during pregnancy and the risk of infantile colic: A follow-up study. *Acta Paediatr* 92(7):811–816; 2003.

Sondergaard C et al. Smoking during pregnancy and infantile colic. *Pediatrics* 108(2):342–346; 2001.

Stuart-Macadam P, Dettwyler K (eds). *Breastfeeding: Biocultural Perspectives.* New York: Aldine de Gruyter; 1995.

Sullivan R. Developing a sense of safety: The neurobiology of neonatal attachment. *Ann N Y Acad Sci* 1008:122–131; 2003.

Theilade D. Nasal CPAP employing a jet device for creating positive pressure. *Intensive Care Med* 4(3):145–148; 1978.

Thomas D. Aetiological associations in infantile colic: An hypothesis. *Aust Paediatr J* 17(4):292–295; 1981.

van Bakel H, Riksen-Walraven J. Stress reactivity in 15-month-old infants: Links with infant temperament, cognitive competence, and attachment security. *Dev Psychobiol* 44(3):157–167; 2004.

Vanden Boom D. The influence of temperament and mothering on attachment and exploration: An experimental manipulation of sensitive responsiveness among lower-class mothers with irritable infants. *Child Dev* 65:1457–1477; 1994.

Vickers A et al. Massage for promoting growth and development of preterm and/or low birth-weight infants. *Cochrane Database Syst Rev*(2):CD000390. Review; 2004.

Volpe J. *Neurology of the Newborn.* 4th ed. Philadelphia: WB Saunders; 2001.

Wessel M et al. Paroxysmal fussing in infancy, sometimes called "colic." *Pediatrics* 114:421–434; 1954.

Whitehead R. For how long is exclusive breastfeeding adequate to satisfy the dietary energy needs of the average young baby? *Pediat Res* 37(2): 239–243; 1995.

Willinger M et al. Defining the sudden infant death syndrome (SIDS): Deliberations of an expert panel convened by the National Institute of Child Health and Human Development. *Pediatric Pathology* (11):677–684; 1991.

Wolf L, Glass R. *Feeding and Swallowing Disorders in Infancy: Assessment and Management.* San Antonio, TX: Therapy Skill Builders; 1992.

Woolridge M. Colic, "overfeeding," and symptoms of lactose malabsorption in the breast-fed baby: A possible artifact of feed management? *Lancet* 2:382–384; 1988.

www.torticolliskids.org. Information Web site for parents of children with torticollis; 2001. Accessed June 12, 2004.

 ## BIBLIOGRAPHY

American Academy of Pediatrics (AAP) Work Group. Infant feeding practices and their possible relationship to the etiology of diabetes mellitus. *Pediatrics* 94:752–754; 1994.

Barr RG et al. Nursing interval and maternal responsivity: Effect on early infant crying. *Pediatrics* 81:529–536; 1988.

Behrman R, Kliegman R, Jenson H. *Nelson Textbook of Pediatrics*, 17th ed. Philadelphia, PA: WB Saunders; 2003.

Bick D et al. What influences the uptake and early cessation of breast feeding? *Midwifery* 14(4):242–247; 1991.

Fanaroff A, Martin R. *Neonatal-Perinatal Medicine: Diseases of the Fetus and Infant*, 7th ed. St. Louis, MO: Mosby; 2001.

Gurry D. Infantile colic. *Aust Fam Phys* 23:337–346; 1994.

Lothe L et al. Motilin and infantile colic: A prospective study. *Acta Pediatr Scand* 79(2):410–416; 1990.

MacArthur C et al. Investigation of long term problems after obstetric epidural anaesthesia. *BMJ* 304(6837):1279–1282; 1992.

Matheny R et al. Control of intake by human-milk-fed infants: Relationships between feeding size and interval. *Dev Psychobiol* 23:511–518; 1990.

Minchin M. *Food for Thought.* Sydney, Australia: Unwin Paperbacks; 1986.

Mohrbacher N, Stock J. *The Breastfeeding Answer Book.* Schaumburg, IL: La Leche League International; 2003.

Montagu A. *Touching: The Human Significance of the Skin*, 3rd ed. New York: HarperCollins; 1986.

National Center on Shaken Baby Syndrome. Ogden, UT. Available at: www.dontshake.com. Accessed November 12, 2004.

Rapp D. *Is This Your Child?* New York: William Morrow and Company; 1992.

Riordan J. *Breastfeeding and Human Lactation*, 3rd ed. Sudbury, MA: Jones and Bartlett Publishers; 2005.

CHAPTER
14

GETTING BREASTFEEDING STARTED

▶ Most mothers and babies are capable of easily mastering breastfeeding. Breastfeeding is a combination of instinct and learned skill for both mother and baby. Mothers have the desire to snuggle and cuddle with their newborns. Often they hold their babies in positions that are very close to breastfeeding during nonfeeding times. The baby may have difficulty in his initial attempts at breastfeeding, or he may be a natural pro. Both mother and baby will learn the art of breastfeeding with time, patience, and gentle guidance as they learn to coordinate their natural behaviors with one another. Mothers who give birth to more than one baby require ingenuity and resourcefulness in managing breastfeeding. You also may encounter mothers who have a nursing child at home when they give birth to a new infant. You can assist these mothers as they balance the needs of both children.

KEY TERMS

baby-led feeding	fussy baby
calming techniques	latch-on
C-hold	lying down position
clutch hold	motility
cradle hold	posture feeding
cross-cradle hold	prone position
Dancer hand position	rooting reflex
dominant hand hold	rousing techniques
flanged	tandem nursing
football hold	

▶ GETTING READY TO NURSE

Mothers typically look forward to their first breastfeeding session with anticipation and excitement. Ideally, a mother will nurse her baby directly after birth on the same bed in which she birthed him. The earlier she begins to breastfeed, the earlier her baby will receive colostrum, and the sooner he will begin stooling. This early suckling begins milk production sooner than for a woman whose first breastfeeding is delayed. Mothers and babies should be kept together and not subjected to unnecessary separation that interferes with this process.

Delays in initiating breastfeeding can contribute to engorgement and low milk production. There is also evidence that a delay can affect the duration of breastfeeding. "A study was done . . . with two groups of mothers who had expressed a desire to breastfeed. One group received their babies to suckle shortly after birth. The other group did not have contact with their babies until 16 hours later. No mother in either group had to stop breastfeeding for physical reasons. Two months later, the mothers who had had their infants to suckle right after birth were all still breastfeeding. In the other group, five out of six had stopped" (MacFarlane, 1997).

Establish a Breastfeeding Routine

Mothers who are breastfeeding for the first time may feel an initial awkwardness in trying to get comfortable while the baby settles onto the breast. Assure mothers that this feeling of awkwardness is common and to be expected. Breastfeeding is a new venture for the mother, and she needs time to learn it. These first sessions are ideal practice times for the mother and her baby as they both learn how to nurse.

By establishing a regular routine for every feeding, the mother will develop self-confidence, increase the ease with which she breastfeeds, and ensure effective breastfeeding. The mother can attend to her physical needs before settling down for a feeding. She can use the bathroom, wash her hands, and gather whatever she will need during the feeding. This may include pillows to help position herself and her baby, a beverage, a cloth for burping her baby, reading material, breast pads, diapers, wipes, and a change of clothes for her baby. A mother may find it helpful to gather a basket of the items she will want so she can carry it anywhere in her house. She may choose not to answer the telephone so that she and her baby will be undisturbed. Other suggestions for relaxing and creating an optimal climate for feedings appear in Table 14.1.

TABLE 14.1	
Creating a Relaxing and Effective Climate for Nursing	
Issue	**Suggestions for the Mother**
Relaxation techniques	◆ Spend a few minutes before going to sleep to analyze your own relaxation techniques, e.g., movements, positions, and room darkness. Repeat these techniques at other times for relaxation.
	◆ Remove distractions, e.g., find a quiet spot and take the phone off the hook.
	◆ Get comfortable, e.g., empty your bladder; find a cozy chair or bed; get pillows for support; remove eyeglasses, shoes, or tight clothing; adjust room temperature.
	◆ Listen to relaxing music.
	◆ Take a deep breath and let it out slowly. Repeat this several times.
	◆ Breathe steadily and rhythmically, noting the faint movement of your body, and breathe slowly to relax further.
	◆ Tense your entire body and relax the tension slowly. Concentrate on one muscle at a time, starting from your toes, and progress up to the facial muscles, until your limbs, eyelids and all body parts feel heavy.
	◆ Use massage or warm compresses on tense parts of your body.
	◆ Take a warm shower or bath.
	◆ Close your eyes and move them back and forth or up and down. Then rest your eyes and feel the release of tension. Relax your eyes by thinking about a ship sailing away from you and disappearing over the horizon.
	◆ Allow your mind to drift into a sleepy state and think pleasant thoughts, e.g., enjoyable moments, pleasures, or dreams.
	◆ Think about your baby, of milk flowing, or of water rushing.
	◆ Think about, write down or talk with someone about your fears, stresses, tensions, and what you feel causes them. Then let your mind drift or think of pleasant thoughts and feel the release of tension.
	◆ Visualize some strenuous or precarious activity, such as walking across thin ice, and then pretend it has ended and you are at ease.
	◆ Pray.
	◆ Meditate on a passage of a text from a favorite author.
Creating an optimal climate	◆ Nurse in a quiet spot away from distractions.
	◆ Avoid embarrassing or stressful situations for feeding.
	◆ Drink juice, water, or noncaffeinated tea before and during feeding.
	◆ Set up a routine for beginning a feeding.
Recharging your batteries	◆ Nap or rest when the baby rests.
	◆ Simplify daily chores and establish priorities around the baby.
	◆ Get help with household, child care, and other responsibilities.
	◆ Take a break from the daily routine with an evening out, shopping, a walk, or lunch with a friend.
Feeding-related techniques	◆ Use warm compresses before feeding.
	◆ Express a little milk and gently stimulate the nipple.
	◆ Use breast compression while the baby is nursing.
	◆ Lie down to nurse.
	◆ Nurse the baby in bed at night.
	◆ Hold the baby skin to skin during feeding.

Encourage Baby-Led Feedings

Newborns have an amazing ability to tell their parents when they need to eat and when they are finished. The feeding cues described in Chapter 13 tell the mother when her baby is ready for a feeding. The baby is equally able to let her know when he has fed long enough and wishes to end the feeding.

Babies have the ability to self-regulate their feedings to meet their individual needs for optimal growth (Cregan, 1999; Daly, 1993; Woolridge, 1990). Encourage mothers to allow the baby to begin the feeding on the side that received the least stimulation at the previous feeding and to allow him to continue nursing on that breast until he removes himself. If it has been only a short time and he unlatches for burping or discomfort, the mother may address the cause and resume nursing on that breast again. If he has been on one breast for some time, the mother may watch for further feeding cues and then switch him to the other breast. Mothers do not need to use both breasts at every feeding. However, in the early days of nursing, most mothers will want to stimulate both breasts equally, to assure optimal milk production in both breasts.

Each baby will pace his feeding himself in his own unique way. Confusing a mother and baby with exact times for feeding and length of feedings will lead to frustration for both. No adult eats a meal in exactly the same amount of time as all other adults. Nor do adults enjoy having their meals regulated by a clock. The same is true with babies. Imposing time restrictions will alter a baby's natural regulation of his intake of foremilk and hindmilk. Switching breasts without cues from the baby overrides his natural ability to self-regulate his feedings. Such overriding of a baby's freedom can set up negative reactions and behaviors in the newborn that may lead to breast refusal.

Interference with the intake of foremilk and hindmilk can lead to colic-like symptoms in babies, as discussed in Chapter 13. Limiting a baby's time on one breast in order for him to nurse on the other breast can result in less hindmilk intake. The increased foremilk intake coupled with less hindmilk may result in lactose dumping into the small intestine (Woolridge, 1988). Lactose overload in the small intestine causes fermentation and consequently increased gas and gut **motility** in the gastrointestinal tract. This can lead to a very uncomfortable, fussy baby.

Imposing time-related rules for breastfeeding is a frustrating and unnecessary burden at a period when the mother is becoming acquainted with her new baby. Such restrictions on feedings can lead to frustration and physical symptoms in the baby. Mothers need to be encouraged to watch their babies, not the clock. Their babies cannot tell time. They only know that they are unhappy when they are hungry and content when they are full.

When a mother learns how to recognize hunger in her baby, she is able to let him lead the way. Help mothers learn how to observe their baby's feeding readiness. A baby who is often placed in a position for feeding at times when he is not ready to feed can become frustrated and wary of the whole process. Only the baby knows when it is time to nurse, and he will exhibit a progression of signs that indicate a desire to feed. See Chapter 13 for a description of infant feeding cues.

Exceptions to Baby-Led Feedings

There are two caveats to watching the baby and not the clock. The first is in the case of a medicated birth, discussed in Chapter 12. Many babies born after long medicated labors have a depressed central nervous system (CNS), latching problems, and sleepiness (Kroeger, 2004). The other babies to watch carefully are the near-term, 36–38 weekers who go home without competent breastfeeding skills (Wight, 2003).

Babies in both of these categories are sleepy, difficult to rouse, ineffective at the breast, and often appear "content to starve." They frequently develop jaundice, which increases the sleepiness. These babies need a lot of stimulation to nurse, frequent feedings, and often supplementation with alternative feeding methods (see Chapter 23). Mothers of these babies do need to "watch the clock" temporarily and be vigilant about getting calories into them.

Very early preterm babies are usually discharged at about the age of a near-term infant, and the same feeding concerns apply to them. In addition, they often have significant health problems, such as cardiac or respiratory issues, that require continual monitoring and care by the parents. See Chapter 23 for more discussion on very preterm babies.

The mother of a near-term infant can focus on three goals: feeding the baby, protecting the mother's milk supply, and transitioning the baby to the breast. Usually, when the baby reaches his due date, he suddenly wakes up to nurse. Encourage the mother of a sleepy, medicated baby that the sleepiness will pass and that the baby will soon exchange sleepiness for fussiness, probably in the evening hours!

▶ BEGINNING THE FEEDING

The manner in which the mother brings her infant to breast determines in large part the quality of the feeding. When discussing positioning, it is convenient to consider four zones within which the mother and baby interact. These zones include the mother's body, the mother's breast, the baby's body, and the baby's mouth (Kutner, 1996). A mother must be in a comfortable position to support her baby during a feeding, and the baby's position needs to enable him to latch onto the breast and keep it in his mouth. The mother can respond to verbal communication and thus is easier to work with. The baby can usually be positioned easily to accommodate breastfeeding. In most cases, the baby's mouth will work correctly if the mother's and baby's body positions do not interfere.

The Mother's Body: Zone One

The mother needs to find a comfortable position, with her back and arms supported by pillows where necessary, as illustrated in Color Plate 19. When the mother is positioned well, her posture will be relaxed, with her shoulders resting comfortably against the back support. If she is sitting, her feet will rest comfortably on the floor or a footstool, so that her knees are higher than her hips. This encourages the baby to remain close to the mother's chest rather than away from her. Placing her knees higher than her hips also helps prevent the mother from leaning over her baby to breastfeed.

A mother who delivers by cesarean birth may want to place a pillow on her lap to protect her abdominal incision. Alternately, she can position the baby at her side with pillows to raise him to a level near the breast and protect her abdomen. Typical postpartum discomforts need to be addressed, particularly in the perineal and incision areas. Positioning should place the least stress on any sore areas. If the mother is in pain, you may see her toes curled, facial grimacing, or hunched shoulders. She may also become uncomfortable if she remains in the same position for a long time. When the mother is positioned comfortably, she is ready to bring her baby to breast.

The Mother's Breast: Zone Two

For the first several weeks, it is often helpful for the mother to support her breast, especially if she is large-breasted. The weight of the breast may cause it to pull slightly from the baby's mouth, preventing him from getting a good latch. The mother can cup her free hand to form the letter C—referred to as the **C-hold**—with her thumb on top and her fingers curved below the breast, well behind the areola, as in Color Plate 20. She can then gently guide her baby to the breast and center the nipple in his mouth.

Some babies latch on better with the nipple angled up toward the hard palate. This helps trigger the baby's suck reflex and encourages him to take in more of the areola below the nipple. After the mother and baby have mastered the technique and the baby is older, it will not be necessary for the mother to support her breast. In the early weeks, however, some sort of support is often helpful in preventing nipple soreness and encouraging positive milk transfer.

A slight variation of the C-hold works well with premature infants and other babies who have weak muscle development and find it difficult to hold the jaw steady while they suck. This position, the Dancer hand position, begins in the C-hold position. The mother then brings her hand forward to support her breast with the first three fingers. She supports the baby's chin by resting it in the area of her hand between her thumb and index finger, as illustrated in Color Plate 21. The mother bends her index finger slightly so that it gently holds the baby's cheek on one side, with her thumb holding the other cheek. This hold helps decrease the available space in the baby's mouth and increases negative pressure. When the mother uses steady, equal pressure while holding her baby's cheeks, she avoids interfering with the rooting reflex. As his muscle tone begins to improve, she can place her thumb back on top of the breast, leaving the index finger to support the baby's chin.

The Baby's Body: Zone Three

Improper positioning of the baby at the breast is the major cause of nipple soreness. When the baby's positioning avoids pulling on the nipple, the potential for pain is lessened. That is not to say that mothers will not react with surprise at the sensation of the first latch, as evidenced in Figure 14.1. It is common for mothers to feel a certain amount of discomfort when they first begin breastfeeding. However, it should subside after time and should not escalate to prolonged pain.

Properly positioned, the baby will be well supported and cuddled around the mother. The mother holds him chest-to-chest, level with her breast. His ear, shoulder, and hip are all in alignment, and his body is in a flexed posture. The baby's cheeks are both the same distance from the breast. The mother holds him closely enough so his chin presses deeply in the breast. If the mother's breast obstructs his breathing, she can pull his back and shoulders in toward her body. This will angle his head slightly away from the breast and allow him to breathe freely.

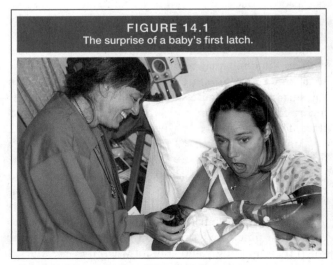

FIGURE 14.1
The surprise of a baby's first latch.

Printed with permission of Tammy Arbeter.

The Baby's Mouth: Zone Four

With her baby positioned as described in zone three, the mother is ready to begin the feeding. Either gently stroking his cheek with her nipple or tickling his upper lip with it will provide the signal for him to open his mouth. The mother needs her baby to open his mouth wide to get a large mouthful of breast tissue. She should position his mouth slightly below the center of the breast so that he reaches up to it. Lining up the baby's nose with the mother's nipple is often a helpful reference. This will result in his lower lip covering more of the areola than his upper lip. His tongue will extend over his lower gum (alveolar ridge), many times far enough to extend out to the lower lip. If her baby turns his head away from the breast, she can entice him to turn back toward the breast and open his mouth by stimulating his rooting reflex.

Rooting Reflex

When eliciting the rooting reflex, the mother will want to take care not to touch any other part of her baby's face. He will instinctively root toward the source of the stimulation and may become confused and frustrated. A 1993 study by Widstrom looked at the placement of infants' tongues during rooting and prior to the first suckle. The infants were between one and two hours old. When they showed an interest in feeding, the mother elicited the rooting reflex by touching the cheek with her nipple. In ten of the eleven infants, as the infant turned his head toward the stimulus, his mouth opened wide and his tongue extended out of his mouth. Licking movements preceded rooting when the infant was in an alert state.

A baby who is crying will place his tongue up toward the palate. If forced to the breast (even with gentle force), he may remember the forced situation and defend himself by placing his tongue in the palate at subsequent feedings. This may also occur if a mother forces her baby to the breast when he is not hungry. Forcing the baby to the breast can disturb the rooting-tongue-reflex system. Color Plate 22 shows the baby beginning to open his mouth. If the mother were to attempt to latch him on at this point, he would fail to get far enough back on the breast. In Color Plate 23, he has opened his mouth wide enough for the mother to pull him onto the breast for a good latch. Chapter 15 discusses latch in detail.

▶ USING A VARIETY OF BREASTFEEDING POSITIONS

Mothers can use a variety of positions for holding the baby at the breast. The most common positions are the cradle hold, football hold, cross-cradle hold, and lying down. **Posture feeding** and some other unique variations are also useful in particular circumstances. The following breastfeeding positions describe a mother nursing her baby at her right breast.

Cradle Hold

The cradle hold is the traditional sitting position in which the mother sits with her baby's body across her abdomen. With her baby at the right breast, she places his head in the crook of her right arm and supports his body with her right hand, as in Color Plate 24. This position may not be optimal if the mother and baby are experiencing any problems with latch or milk transfer. When using this hold, the mother has limited control over the movement of her baby's head. Thus, she cannot assist or guide him to a better latch. However, the cradle hold is the position most mothers instinctively use, and you should not interfere with it unless it is clearly ineffective. Avoid saying anything negative when the mother first positions her baby, to avoid undermining her confidence or increasing her anxiety.

Football (Clutch) Hold

In the football or clutch hold, the mother holds her baby under her arm much in the same way she clutches a purse to her side or a football player holds the ball while running. She places her baby so his body is along her right side and his feet are toward her back. Pillows help support the baby and the mother's arm. Holding the baby's head in her right hand, she supports his body with her right forearm and raises his head to breast level, as in Color Plate 25.

Such positioning is especially effective for nursing a preterm baby, who fits snugly under the mother's arm. It is also useful for full-term infants who have difficulty latching on. The mother is able to hold her baby's entire body on her arm and can control his body movements better. She can hold and form her breast with the other hand and can also perform **breast massage** easily. This hold is helpful in tricking a baby into nursing on a breast that he refuses in the traditional sitting position. It helps with babies who have a short tongue or ankyloglossia and for nursing multiples or for mothers with very large breasts.

Cross-Cradle (Dominant Hand) Positions

The cross-cradle hold combines the football hold and cradle hold, with the mother resting her baby's head in her hand. It is sometimes referred to as the **dominant hand**

position, though the mother can use either her dominant or less dominant hand for the cross-cradle hold. In the dominant hand position, the right-handed mother rests the baby's head in her right hand and supports his body with her forearm. She then moves her arm with the baby across her body to the opposite breast, as in Color Plate 26. This makes it possible to begin the feeding at one breast in the football hold and end it with the cross-cradle hold on the opposite breast without repositioning her hold on the baby. Holding the baby with the dominant hand is especially helpful in early feedings, because it allows the mother better control over her baby's movements. Feedings are easier to manage, which increases the mother's self-confidence.

Lying Down Position

Lying down to nurse will help the mother get needed rest. To use this position, the mother lies on her side, with her knees slightly bent. Pillows placed under her head, between her legs and behind her back will help her get into a comfortable position. She can position her lower arm under her head and use her top arm to support the baby's head and back. Alternatively, she can place her lower arm under the baby's head or along the back of his body, using that arm to support him. She can put her baby to breast first and then raise or lower the breast by rolling her body. To nurse on the top breast, she can roll toward the baby so that her top breast is level with his mouth. She may need to rearrange the pillows to provide necessary support. Another method for changing breasts is for the mother to hug her baby against her chest and roll together with him to the opposite side, shown in Color Plate 27.

Prone Position (Posture Feedings)

If the mother has an overabundant milk supply that causes excessive amounts of milk to gush into her baby's mouth, the prone position, also called posture feeding, may be useful. Posture feeding is a term popularized in Australia, where women tend to have copious milk production (ABA, 1995). In this position, the mother places her baby above the breast in order to achieve better control over milk flow. The mother lies on her back with her baby lying tummy to tummy on top of her (see Color Plate 28). To get into this position easily, the mother can begin in a sitting position, put her baby to breast, and then lean back. The heel of her hand can support his forehead to help him hold his head up and away from the breast.

Prone feeding may be useful at times when letdown seems strongest, as in the early morning. It also is useful for babies who bite or retract their tongue, as it encourages the jaw to fall forward by gravity. Caution mothers not to use the posture feeding position excessively. Because gravity does not aid milk flow, there is a danger of incomplete milk removal if used too often. In addition, the baby can become accustomed to nursing in this position and refuse to nurse in any other position.

Other Creative Breastfeeding Positions

Women have devised some unusual breastfeeding positions to meet their needs. Conventional nursing positions may aggravate a sore spot on the nipple, or the mother may not be able to clear a plugged duct by using such positions. She might place her baby on the bed, as in Color Plate 29, and lean over him on her hands and knees. She can then position the breast in his mouth by rotating his body. To avoid back strain, she can raise the baby by placing pillows or blankets under him. This position is useful for babies who are in traction or have had surgery. As an alternative, the mother can lie on her back and place the baby on his stomach with his feet over her shoulder, as in Color Plate 30. Such variations demonstrate that there is no one correct position for nursing. As long as the baby is able to manage an effective latch, mothers can continue to be creative in their approach.

▶ BREASTFEEDING MULTIPLES

Mothers of multiples can attain the same breastfeeding outcomes as the mother of a single baby. Although there may be more demands on her time and some special challenges, the mother will find that breastfeeding brings a calming element to an otherwise hectic life. It is certainly a more pleasurable expenditure of time than preparing formula and heating bottles while listening to the cries of hungry babies! It also saves parents the expense of buying double or triple the amount of infant formula and the increased medical expense of more frequent illness.

When a woman learns she is expecting more than one baby, she may be told that she cannot breastfeed or that she will have to feed her babies on a schedule. You can help her sort through conflicting advice and find what arrangement will work best for her. The greatest gift you can give her is reassurance that she can make enough milk for her babies. Records from 1900 reveal that wet nurses in France were able to furnish 2230 grams of milk per day. One woman yielded as much as 2840 grams (Budin, 1907), over 100 ounces!

The few possible exceptions to an ample milk supply include a woman with hormonal problems or one with true insufficient glandular development. IBCLCs have noted that some infertile women who conceive through reproduction technology have difficulty with milk production. See the discussion on insufficient milk supply in Chapter 25.

As many as 60 percent of triplets and 90 percent of quadruplets may be conceived through reproduction technology. In 2002, there were 31 sets of twins out of every 1000 births, an increase of 38 percent since 1990 and 65 percent since 1980. Triplets and other higher-order multiple births dropped to 184 sets per 100,000 births in 2002, the third decline in 4 years, after an increase of more than 400 percent between 1980 and 1998 (CDC, 2003).

Breastfeeding encourages the mother to regard each baby's needs individually. The mother of multiples may need to pay closer attention to her breastfeeding schedule than is usually the case with the mother of a single baby. With creative planning and flexibility, she will find a routine that works best for her. Breastfeeding encourages the mother to spend more time in close physical contact with her babies, enabling her to provide a maximum amount of skin contact with each one. Encourage her to breast-feed her babies separately at least once every day and to spend other time alone with each baby as well. Bonding is important to the emergence of individuality in each baby. Breastfeeding enhances this attachment (Noble, 2003).

Breastfeeding Routine

A mother of multiples will benefit from special help with feedings. While in the hospital, it is important that she have all of her babies together for feedings. If one baby must remain in a special care nursery, she can nurse the baby who is able to be with her and express her milk for the other one. Some hospitals find that keeping multiples together in the same bassinet or **isolette**, referred to as "cobedding," is beneficial to the babies. Having the babies together for feedings will enable the mother to learn the practical aspects of feeding them. The mother will need plenty of pillows to help her position more than one baby during a feeding. She may require the help of another person to keep one baby positioned at the breast while she helps the second baby latch onto the other breast. If she has more than two babies, she can feed the other baby with an alternative method while two are nursing. Rotating babies at each feeding will give all of them equal time at the breast.

Positioning the Babies

Many mothers prefer to nurse their twins simultaneously rather than separately. The mother can enjoy nursing times more if she does not hear the hunger cries of her other baby. Otherwise, she may rush through the feeding and find it less relaxing. She may also have less opportunity to interact in a meaningful way with her babies. Figure 14.2 illustrates three positions for nursing both babies simultaneously.

Feeding Pattern

There are a variety of options for managing simultaneous feedings. The mother may confine each baby to one breast only and always reserve the same breast for the same baby. One drawback to this is that one baby may have a stronger suck, which can cause the mother to develop a larger breast on that side because of greater stimulation and milk production. Another drawback is the baby's visual development. Feeding a baby from two different sides stimulates different parts of their bodies and provides equal vision stimulation to both eyes. Alternating babies between breasts at each feeding or every few feedings will ensure equal stimulation of both breasts and coordinated visual development. Alternatively, each baby may nurse on one breast each day and switch to the other breast the next day.

One baby may exhibit hunger cues at a time when the other baby is not interested in nursing. The mother might choose to delay feeding the hungry baby until the other one is willing to nurse so that she can economize on the time she spends feeding them. It is important that you not add to the mother's dilemma by causing her to feel guilty about doing this. Each mother must work out her own routine and will appreciate your support in her decision. At another time, you can discuss with her each baby's individual needs and the importance of responding to them. Perhaps she can breastfeed the hungry baby and keep the second one close by, in hopes that letdown and proximity will stimulate his interest in feeding. She can also waken the second baby to feed.

Breastfeeding more than two multiples requires even more creativity than breastfeeding twins. In the early days, the mother will most likely need the help of another person at feedings. It is not possible for a mother to nurse all babies at one time, and it would be very time-consuming to nurse each baby separately. She can nurse two babies at one time while she or someone else feeds the other baby with an alternative feeding method. Alternatively, she can nurse the first two babies simultaneously and the other or others on both breasts afterward. The mother will eventually be adept at managing feedings on her own. As with twins, she will want to be sure that all babies receive the same amount of time at the breast and that both of her breasts receive equal stimulation. The mother should be sure to offer the breast to all three babies throughout the day so that

---

FIGURE 14.2
Positions for nursing multiples.

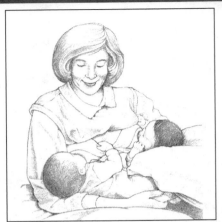
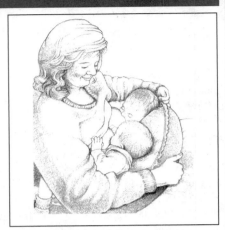

Babies are crisscrossed, with each one in the cradle hold, with support from the mother's hands under their buttocks and pillows placed under the mother's elbows.

Babies are placed with one in the cradle position and one in the football (clutch) position, with pillows supporting the mother's arms. A pillow on her lap may also help.

Both babies are placed on a pillow in the football (clutch) position. A footstool can add to the mother's comfort.

Illustrations by Marcia Smith.

---

they all receive milk from the breast. It may be helpful to keep a log for each baby's diapers and feeds.

Parenting Challanges with Multiples

Initial bonding may be complicated with multiples. It may be even more complex when one baby remains hospitalized longer than the other one. The mother will have bonded with one baby and may find it difficult to establish the same attachment with the other(s) after the delay in coming home. She may need to actively work at developing a close relationship with both or all of her babies. When the later baby arrives home, she can make arrangements that will allow her to spend more time getting to know the new arrival. Sometimes this dilemma is never resolved.

The mother's reaction to parenting multiples can range from delight to dismay. The quality of the parents' support system is a large factor in the mother's coping abilities. Her emotions are likely to fluctuate, depending on how each day goes for her. She may feel stressed by the constant demands on her time and energy. Household priorities will need to accommodate the demands of more than one baby. Timesaving techniques will help the mother manage her daily routine, and simple, nutritious meals will safeguard her health and sense of well-being.

Mothers who can afford to may hire part- or full-time help or use shopping and cleaning services. Other mothers will not have these options. You can compile a resource list for area food banks, resale or charity clothing stores, and appropriate governmental assistance. Many seasoned mothers of older multiples are happy to be resources for new mothers. As you work with mothers, you can ask them if they would like to help other mothers and give their permission to be contacted.

Mastitis may be more common for mothers of multiples, partially because of fatigue and the mother's abundant milk supply. A missed feeding by one or all babies can result in engorged breasts more quickly than in the case of a mother with one baby. Because of this, the mother with multiples will need to be accessible to her babies for feedings. When she is away, she must be sure to express milk to avoid engorgement and the possibility of plugged ducts.

Multiples will develop and grow at varying rates, just as with other siblings. Although growth spurts may occur simultaneously, it is more likely that they will come at slightly different times for each baby. The babies may be ready for solid foods and weaning at different times as well. Mothers of multiples are more likely to supplement their babies early. They may feel pressured by well-meaning friends and family to begin supplemental foods earlier than usual or to wean at an earlier age.

Some mothers of multiples may breastfeed exclusively for several months, whereas others may elect to supplement every day. Occasional supplements given by another person will allow the mother to have some time alone for a few hours if she wishes. This will help her keep a perspective on her mothering and can provide a workable compromise. It may be the only way for some mothers to manage breastfeeding their multiples. You can provide support to these mothers by affirming that any breastmilk is better than no breastmilk. Although exclusive breastfeeding is optimal, breastfeeding does not have to be "all or nothing" for these mothers. Breastfeeding is a rewarding and comforting element in the lives of babies whose individual personalities are emerging. It enables babies to bond with their mother. There is a tendency to regard multiples as a single entity, a group. Nurturing at the breast and feeling the close special attention of his mother is reassuring to each individual baby (Gromada, 1999).

Most mothers know before birth that they are carrying multiples, especially when the pregnancy results from infertility treatment. Anticipatory guidance and information are especially helpful. One resource that encourages breastfeeding multiples is the Web site for Breastfeeding and Attachment Parenting Twins (Breastfeeding and Attachment, 2004). Stories from mothers who have breastfed triplets and quadruplets are very empowering and can help reassure expectant mothers about their abilities. This site may be helpful for breastfeeding mothers of singletons as well, regardless of their parenting philosophy. See Table 14.2 for counseling suggestions with mothers of multiples.

Support from you and other significant people in her life will be important in helping the mother accommodate breastfeeding to the busy routine of parenting multiples. Mothers of Multiples clubs, which offer excellent support and advice about caring for multiples, are available in many communities. However, the purpose of Mothers of Multiples clubs is not to provide breastfeeding support, and many mothers in these groups have chosen to bottle-feed. Help in this area can occur simultaneously with support from a lactation consultant or breastfeeding support group, preferably one with other mothers nursing multiples.

TABLE 14.2
Counseling Mothers with Multiples

Mother's Concern	Suggestions for Mother
Lack of time for all tasks	◆ Plan nursing schedule. ◆ Carefully evaluate priorities. ◆ Use time-saving methods for household chores. ◆ Prepare simple nutritious meals. ◆ Enlist help from others.
Bonding with more than one baby	◆ Breastfeed separately at least one time every day. ◆ Spend time alone with each baby every day.
Bonding with a baby who has a delayed homecoming	◆ Regard babies as individuals and meet their separate needs. ◆ Obtain help with babies who are already settled in, and spend more time with the new arrival.
Nursing two babies at the same time	◆ Let each baby nurse exclusively on one breast. ◆ Put babies on alternate breasts at each feeding. ◆ Let each baby nurse on one breast for the entire day and alternate breasts daily.
Spending too much time nursing babies separately	◆ Whenever one baby is hungry, nurse both.
Nursing three or more babies	◆ Nurse two at a time and get help from another person to feed the other baby. ◆ Alternate babies so a different one is fed with alternate means at each feeding. ◆ Nurse two babies simultaneously and the other baby on both breasts afterward.
Greater susceptibility to mastitis	◆ Avoid long periods away from the babies. ◆ Remove milk from your breasts when feedings are missed.

▶ TANDEM NURSING

Tandem nursing describes the breastfeeding of two or more children of different ages. A mother may still be breastfeeding when she begins another pregnancy. She may choose to continue nursing throughout the pregnancy and to nurse both babies when the new baby arrives. A child who had previously weaned may show a renewed interest in breastfeeding when he sees the new baby at his mother's breast. A very warm relationship can develop between nursing siblings and their mother. Breastfeeding can provide a good lesson in sharing and touching and encourages affection and close friendships between siblings.

Breastfeeding During Pregnancy

A mother who becomes pregnant while still nursing a previous child may be reluctant to give up the special relationship she and her nursing child enjoy. Additionally, her child may be reluctant to give up nursing and may resist attempts at weaning. The American Academy of Family Physicians has voiced strong support for "extended" breastfeeding. They recommend that breastfeeding continue beyond infancy and that women receive ongoing support and encouragement. They also acknowledge that it is common for women to continue nursing when they are pregnant with another child (AAFP, 2001).

One concern about tandem nursing is that the developing baby may be undernourished. One study found no significant differences in fetal growth, although mothers had reduced maternal fat stores when less than 6 months had elapsed between pregnancies (Merchant, 1990). In another study, 17 percent of children were weaned during a new pregnancy, which resulted in higher mortality rates for the weaned child in non-industrialized countries (Jakobsen, 2003). Other studies have found a correlation between the mother breastfeeding during pregnancy and lower weight gains for the new baby (Marquis, 2002).

One study found that lactating women gained less weight during the first trimester of pregnancy than non-lactating women did. While they gained more during the third trimester, suggesting a rebound effect, weight for the total pregnancy was still less. The authors recommended that the mothers consume more energy and nutrients to meet the demands of pregnancy and breast-feeding (Siega-Riz, 1993). This nutritional recommendation seems appropriate for all pregnant breastfeeding mothers. If the mother continues to nurse during a pregnancy, she will want to be sure that she is eating nutritiously. Encourage her to consume enough nutrients to meet her nutritional needs as well as those of her fetus and her nursing child. Although her child will receive additional nourishment from supplemental foods, he will still be depleting the mother's nutritional stores.

The exception to breastfeeding during pregnancy may be a woman who has experienced a preterm birth or who is at risk for premature labor. The concern is that the oxytocin released during breastfeeding might trigger preterm labor. It thus may be necessary to wean her child to avoid the possibility of miscarriage. Mothers in this situation may need to abstain from sexual relations as well. Encourage the mother to discuss her situation with her caregiver, and be available to help the mother with weaning.

Nipple tenderness is common in early pregnancy. The mother may experience discomfort when the child touches her breasts. Some pregnant women feel nauseated when the older child nurses. These discomforts may discourage some women from nursing when they are pregnant. The older child may react as well. Hormones of pregnancy alter the composition and taste of the mother's milk. This difference in taste and consistency causes some children to self-wean. Some mothers experience a decrease in milk yield about the fourth or fifth month of pregnancy. This causes some children to lose interest in breastfeeding and wean themselves. One study reported that 57 percent of children weaned during pregnancy (Moscone, 1993). In another study of 503 pregnant nursing mothers, 69 percent of the nurslings weaned during pregnancy (Newton, 1979).

If the woman's baby is under one year old when she conceives, frequent weight checks can monitor adequate intake. If her milk supply decreases to the point that it does not meet his needs, supplements may be necessary. Remind the mother that children under one year of age should not receive whole cow's milk. They should not have goat's milk either, despite the perception in some circles that goat's milk is "closer" to human milk than bovine milk is.

Breastfeeding Siblings

Mothers may worry that they will not have sufficient milk to sustain both an older child and a new infant. Adequate milk production is usually not an issue in tandem nursing. The increased suckling will continue to increase the mother's milk production. The important factors are the emotional needs of her older child and the mother's own comfort. If she believes that her older child will benefit from the emotional nurturing of breastfeeding, she may choose to continue nursing. If she is uncomfortable with her child nursing, it may be better to wean the older child rather than feel resentment when he nurses.

If the mother weans her older child, she will want to do so gradually, as in any other weaning situation. It can be more difficult when she is still nursing her young baby because the older child may want to nurse whenever he sees the baby at the breast. The mother can try to nurse her baby at times when the older child is not around or when he is happily occupied with other things. Substituting other special activities and snacks in place of breastfeeding may help her older child move easily toward total weaning. The father can take over evening rituals such as baths and reading bedtime stories. Encourage the mother to substitute an ample amount of hugs, cuddles, and touching to help the older child feel included.

The toddler who continues to nurse can position himself at the breast, making simultaneous feedings manageable. He may be old enough to understand the need to wait to nurse and the concept of taking turns. This can facilitate separate feedings. Each child will indicate a preference to nurse at a particular time of day. The mother may want to nurse each of them separately at this special time in order to give them each close individual attention.

Because the older child is receiving additional nutrients from other foods, the mother needs to put her younger baby to breast first, when milk production and release is greatest. The older child can then nurse on the less full breast, thereby obtaining less milk. Another option is to reserve a particular breast for each child and to alternate breasts daily to equalize nipple stimulation. Because the toddler is a more efficient nurser and will increase the mother's milk production, the mother may find that she produces so much milk that her younger baby receives too strong a flow of milk and chokes when attempting to nurse. In this event, she can allow her older child to briefly nurse first before putting her baby to breast. A resource for pregnant nursing mothers is *Adventures in Tandem Nursing: Breastfeeding during Pregnancy and Beyond* (Flower, 2003).

▶ ASSISTING AT A FEEDING

During the early postpartum weeks, the most important adjustment for parents is becoming acquainted with their baby. Parents learn to become sensitive to their baby's physical needs, his disposition, and his behavior at the breast. He may prefer quiet at one time and stimulation at another time. During these early weeks, parents learn the many things that make their baby unique.

Acquainting parents with typical infant patterns will help them adapt their routines to meet the needs of their baby. Learning these patterns of behavior may be challenging in the early days. Help parents understand that it will become more natural and easier with time. Let them know, too, that learning to interpret their baby's signals may occur more slowly with babies who demonstrate ambiguous signals than babies whose signals are clear. You can explore with the mother ways to modify her baby's patterns, when necessary, and adapt to her baby's nuances. Being available to assist her at

early feedings will help build her confidence and put the parents on the road to long-term enjoyment.

Observing the Feeding

After the baby has latched on is an ideal opportunity for you to sit back and watch the mother and baby. Observe the mother's posture, noting whether she is comfortable and has her back supported. Watch how she holds the baby, and whether she needs to hold her breast to assist with latch. Note the position of the baby's body, the position of his mouth on the breast, the placement of his tongue, and the position of his head and hands. He should appear comfortable, with his body in good alignment. His lips should **flange** out, and his cheeks should be smooth, with each an equal distance from the breast.

The baby should settle into long, deep sucks, with about one suck per second. You should be able to hear swallowing, with an absence of clicking sounds. Listen for a suck-swallow-breathe pattern. When a large quantity of milk is flowing, a baby suckles about once per second. He suckles about twice per second when there is little milk flow. This may signal the time between milk ejection reflexes or the end of the feeding on that breast. If he exhibits the latter pattern throughout an entire feeding, he may not have a good latch or little milk may be available.

Assisting a Reluctant Nurser

In the early days of breastfeeding, a baby's reluctance to nurse is frequently a result of something unrelated to feeding. The mother and baby may simply need time to learn how to respond to one another. Observe the mother and baby at a feeding to consider what is happening. Learn from the mother and baby, and trust that they will work it out. Do not be in a hurry to do or say anything until you have determined that they need help. If the baby's reluctance continues for several hours or days, the mother will need to express milk to maintain production and prevent engorgement.

It is common in the early days for the baby to seem unresponsive to the mother's attempts to breastfeed. He may be sleepy or medicated from the delivery or from the mother's pain medication during her postpartum recovery. He simply may not be hungry at the time the mother attempted to feed him. He often can be encouraged to nurse by expressing milk onto his lips.

There may be times during the early days that a baby will not be ready to breastfeed when the mother wants or needs to nurse. When this occurs, the mother can stimulate the baby to nurse by using the rousing techniques listed in the following section. She can use these techniques both before and during a feeding when necessary. If the mother notices that her baby develops a pattern of being reluctant to nurse at a particular time of day, he may simply not want to nurse at that time. Watching her baby for feeding cues will help her determine the times when he is most receptive for feeding.

The Baby Who Is Sleepy

There may be times when a mother needs to wake her baby in order to feed him. This often happens in the early days because the baby may be sleepy from labor medications, or simply because of his immature system. The mother needs to nurse frequently enough to establish milk production. It may be necessary to wake her baby at times to establish a pattern of good feedings. Many newborns sleep for longer periods during the day and nurse more at night. Waking these babies periodically during the day will help turn the schedule around and encourage longer sleep periods at night. Parents will need to be patient, because it may take several weeks to reverse the baby's rhythm.

Possible Causes of the Baby's Sleepiness

You can help the mother explore possible causes for her baby's sleepiness. The cause may be:

◆   The mother received medications during labor.

◆   A traumatic birth resulted from a long labor or long second stage labor.

◆   The baby was born prematurely.

◆   It is the baby's usual sleepy period.

◆   The first feeding was delayed.

◆   The mother overlooked feeding cues.

◆   The baby has sensory overload, as in a loud nursery.

◆   Crying is in response to interventions, particularly circumcision.

◆   The baby is jaundiced.

◆   A schedule was imposed on feedings.

◆   The mother had a cesarean delivery.

◆   The baby is experiencing hypothermia.

Plan of Care for a Sleepy Baby

After exploring causes for the baby's sleepiness, you and the mother can determine a plan of care. In the hospital, you can encourage 24-hour rooming-in with skin-to-skin contact. Help parents learn to distinguish between deep sleep and light sleep. Teach feeding cues to the parents so they learn how to respond to their baby. The mother can attempt to put her baby to breast every half hour to hour, when he shows signs of a light sleep state.

Until feedings are established, the mother will need to pump or hand express her milk to feed to her baby. Using an alternative feeding method will avoid the potential for the nipple preference that would result if the baby received a bottle. If her milk or donor milk is not available, she will need to feed the baby artificial baby milk. It is important that the mother monitor her baby's output and watch for symptoms of dehydration or hypoglycemia (Maccagno-Smith, 1993). The Academy of Breastfeeding Medicine has developed a protocol for appropriate supplementation of healthy, full-term breastfed infants, available at www.bfmed.org.

There are a number of rousing techniques parents can try when attempting to interest their baby in feeding. Attempting a feeding when the baby demonstrates feeding cues will achieve better results than attempting to feed a baby who is in a deep sleep. The first step, on picking him up, is to loosen his blankets to expose him to the air. Because he will likely be in need of a diaper change anyway, this can be the next step.

Skin-to-skin contact often facilitates an interest in nursing. Therefore, the mother can unclothe her baby and cuddle him upright between her bare breasts. If he still does not awaken, the mother can hold him in an upright position and talk to him. Dimming the lights will encourage the baby to open his eyes. If he does not waken, the mother can allow him to sleep for another half to one hour and then try again.

Rousing Techniques

◆   Talk to the baby and try to make eye contact.

◆   Loosen or remove blankets.

◆   Hold the baby upright in a sitting or standing position.

◆   Partially or fully undress the baby.

◆   Change the baby's diaper.

◆   Stimulate the baby through increased skin contact, such as massage or gently rubbing his hands and feet.

◆   Stimulate the baby's rooting reflex.

◆   Stimulate the baby's sense of smell by bringing him close to the breast so that he can detect the scent of the mother's skin.

◆   Stimulate the baby's sense of taste by expressing milk onto the nipple or into his mouth.

◆   Wipe the baby's forehead and cheeks with a cool moist cloth.

◆   Manipulate the baby's arms and legs by playing pat-a-cake, doing baby exercises, and so on.

◆   Give the baby a bath or, better yet, take a bath with the baby to provide increased skin-to-skin contact.

◆   If the baby takes the breast but does not maintain a rhythmic suck-swallow-pause pattern, try stroking under his chin from front to back. Also, compress the breast, as with manual expression.

The Baby Who Cries and Resists Going to Breast

At times, a baby may seem to resist when his mother puts him to breast. When moved toward the breast, he cries loudly instead of starting to suckle. The longer the mother tries, the more the baby cries and fights against it. Some babies seem to be more fussy and irritable during the first month of life. These babies may cry frequently and require continuous attention during their waking hours. They are easily stimulated and excited. They may be especially sensitive to being handled or become frightened by their flailing arms and legs. Swaddling the baby to restrict startling and movement may help (Karp, 2004).

The mother will need to soothe her fussy baby before putting him to breast. A crying baby will have difficulty coordinating breathing and swallowing, and may choke or swallow air. Similarly, a baby who is overly hungry may choke and gag due to his overeagerness to nurse. The mother can prevent this by carefully observing her baby and beginning the feeding before he becomes too upset or overly hungry. The mother may not always be able to anticipate hunger or fussiness, however, and will benefit from suggestions for calming a fussy baby. She can try these suggestions before and during the feeding, as well as at other times during the day.

When a sensitive baby is fussy, the mother may become tense and frustrated by his behavior. The baby could notice this tension, causing him to cry even more. When this happens, the mother needs to break the cycle by changing her behavior in some way. She can leave the room for several minutes and use relaxation and breathing techniques to calm herself. She can get relief away from the baby for longer periods by enlisting the help of the father, another relative, or a friend to care for the baby. Talking with you or someone close to her about her feelings of anger, frustration, and inadequacy will help relieve her tension. She may also benefit from a walk outdoors or a soothing bath or massage.

A mother can improve her outlook by keeping her body in good condition and eating nutritious foods. Advise her to plan easy meals and snacks that include sufficient protein to ensure a feeling of well-being and adequate B vitamins for calm nerves. She will want to rest whenever possible, nurse while lying down, and enlist the help of others to care for the baby while she naps. See Chapter 13 for further discussion on crying and care of a fussy or colicky baby.

Possible Causes of Fussiness

- Caregivers have handled the baby too much.
- The baby is in pain or has experienced pain.
- The mother received medication during labor or postpartum that passed to the baby.
- The baby has discomfort from forceps, vacuum extraction, internal monitor lead, or cephalhematoma.
- The baby has oral aversion because of deep suctioning or other invasive procedures.
- The baby is irritable.
- The baby received an artificial nipple or pacifier, which resulted in nipple preference.
- The mother's lack of confidence causes her to hold her baby tentatively.
- The baby needs to be swaddled to provide boundaries or to be soothed by being cuddled skin-to-skin with the parent.
- The baby has shut down from too much intervention, such as someone attempting to push him on the breast.
- The mother and baby were separated, resulting in missed feeding cues and missed imprinting.
- Rarely, fussiness in a baby can be a sign of serious problems, such as neurological disorders.

Plan of Care for a Fussy Baby

Encourage the mother to hold her baby calmly and to cuddle him skin-to-skin at the breast. Limit attempts to attach him to no more than a few minutes at a time. If he starts to cry or fight the breast, stop and try again about 10 or 15 minutes later, after he is calm. Avoid placing pressure on a potentially painful site. Also avoid holding the baby in a feeding position when administering medical treatment. As with a sleepy baby, it is important for the mother to express or pump her milk and feed it to the baby until feedings are established. He should receive no unnecessary bottles or pacifiers. The baby's caregiver may prescribe medication to calm the baby. Encourage the mother to ask questions about its possible side effects.

Calming Techniques

- Limit invasive procedures to minimize crying.
- Provide skin-to-skin contact.
- Cuddle without pushing the baby to breastfeed.
- Work with the baby for short periods.
- Be sensitive to and respect the baby's cues.
- Build the mother's confidence.
- Use slow, calm, deliberate movements in caring for the baby.
- Cuddle, hold, and walk with the baby.
- Talk or sing to the baby in a soft voice.
- Swaddle the baby.

◆ Nurse in a dark, quiet room.

◆ Rock in a rocking chair to relax both the mother and baby.

◆ Burp the baby often (unless burping seems to upset him). Burp before switching to the other breast at a feeding.

◆ Carry the baby in a position that puts gentle and firm pressure on his abdomen, for example, on the mother's hip or shoulder.

◆ Play music, create a monotonous noise by running a vacuum cleaner or dishwasher, or play a recording of such sounds.

◆ Change the baby's diaper when it becomes damp or soiled.

◆ Mother and baby sleep or nap together so the baby is comforted by her body warmth and heartbeat.

◆ Massage the baby for 10 to 15 minutes (the baby may fuss during the massage and then become quiet afterward).

◆ Use a sling to carry the baby close to the mother's body.

◆ Use a baby swing for times when individual attention is not possible.

◆ If the baby is full-term and has established good temperature control, remove his clothes and expose him to the air for limited amounts of time.

◆ Lay the baby on his stomach on the mother's lap while she gently bounces her knees or moves them back and forth.

◆ Have the mother and baby take a bath together.

◆ Provide monotonous movement with a stroller or car ride.

◆ Remove allergens from the mother's diet.

Ending the Feeding

A baby who nurses robustly and effectively will gently release the breast when he is finished. If the mother needs to remove her baby from the breast before this occurs (i.e., to achieve a better latch), she can break the suction by inserting her finger gently into the corner of his mouth between his gums. Color Plate 31 demonstrates this. In addition, she can press a finger against her breast near the corner of the baby's mouth. Her breast can then slip easily out of his mouth.

The baby should not chew or tug on the end of the nipple. If the mother notices her baby chewing on her nipple toward the end of a feeding to the extent that it causes discomfort, she may need to remove him from the breast. When the mother's finger touches the baby's lips to begin breaking suction, the baby will automatically

begin to suck faster. This is a reflexive response to having his lip touched while at the breast. The mother can continue her efforts to remove her baby from the breast.

Generally, however, advise the mother to continue a feeding until the baby releases the breast spontaneously. She can put him to breast on the other side after he has finished the first breast and continue to nurse at both breasts, one after the other, for as long as the baby wants. There is always milk in the breast unless there are maternal problems, as discussed in Chapter 20. Unless the mother feels pain or discomfort, encourage her to allow her baby to stay at the breast as long as he is still suckling and swallowing.

▶ **SUMMARY**

Learning to recognize their baby's instincts, reflexes, and responses will guide parents in meeting their baby's needs. The mother's early days with her baby are important in the establishment of a strong foundation for breastfeeding. Establishing a routine for feedings will help the mother become comfortable with the process. Teach mothers how to recognize feeding cues and to trust their instincts in nurturing their babies. Ensure that mothers understand the principles of positioning and attachment, and make it a goal to observe every mother and baby at a breastfeeding to assess technique and offer any necessary assistance. Be available to assist with babies who have difficulty latching on. Provide support for mothers whose babies are sleepy or fussy, and offer suggestions for rousing or calming the baby. The time spent by caregivers assisting mothers in these early feedings will influence the course of the mother's long-term breastfeeding. Assure the mother that the learning process passes quickly.

▶ **CHAPTER 14—AT A GLANCE**

Applying what you learned—

◆ Create a relaxing and effective climate for mothers.

◆ Enable a mother to nurse her baby directly after birth and offer help.

◆ Keep mothers and babies together.

◆ Limit unnecessary interventions.

◆ Protect the mother's milk production.

◆ Allow the baby to pace his feedings.

◆ Make sure no time-related rules are imposed on feedings.

◆ Observe an entire breastfeeding for effective technique.

Teach mothers:

- Exclusive breastfeeding in response to feeding cues.
- Positioning of the baby's body for feedings.
- Common nursing positions.
- C-hold for early feedings when necessary.
- Typical infant patterns.
- How to stimulate a sleepy baby to nurse.
- How to comfort a fussy baby for an effective feeding.
- How to watch her baby for signs that he wants to end a feeding.
- Signs of good attachment
  - The baby's mouth is open wide.
  - The baby's chin is touching the breast.
  - The baby's lower lip is curled outward.
  - The baby suckles, pauses, and suckles again—in slow, deep sucks.
  - The mother hears the baby swallowing.
- Signs of poor attachment
  - The nipple looks flattened or striped as it leaves the baby's mouth at the end of the feeding.
  - The mother experiences nipple soreness during and after feedings.
  - The mother's breasts are engorged.
  - There is inefficient removal of milk from the breast.

Teach mothers of multiples:

- Breastfeed babies separately at least once every day.
- Spend non-feeding time alone with each baby.
- Co-bedding.
- Options for positioning, scheduling, and simultaneous feedings.
- Responsive parenting and support groups.

If nursing during pregnancy:

- Ensure adequate nutrition.
- Consult caregiver in pregnancies at risk for preterm labor.
- If weaning older child, do so gradually.
- Delay cow's milk until one year of age.
- Ways to substitute nursing and include older child.
- If tandem nursing, put younger baby to breast first.

▶ REFERENCES

American Academy of Family Physicians (AAFP). *AAFP Policy Statement on Breastfeeding.* Breastfeeding: Position Paper; 2001.

Australian Breastfeeding Association (ABA). *Too Much, Coping with an Over-Abundant Milk Supply.* Nunawading: ABA; 1995.

Breastfeeding and Attachment Parenting Twins. Available at: http://members.tripod.com/~breastfeedingtwins/. Accessed June 19, 2004.

Budin P. *The Nursling: The Feeding and Hygiene of Premature and Full-Term Infants.* Paris 1907. Lecture 3, Authorized translation by Malony WJ. London: Caxton Publishing Co. Available at: www.neonatology.org/classics/nursling/nursling.html. Accessed January 7, 2005.

Centers for Disease Control (CDC). Births: Final data for 2002. *National Vital Statistics Report* 52(10); 2003.

Cregan M, Hartmann P. Computerized breast measurement from conception to weaning: Clinical implications. *J Hum Lact* 15(2):89–96; 1999.

Daly S et al. The short-term synthesis and infant-regulated removal of milk in lactating women. *Exp Physiol* 78:209–220; 1993.

De Carvalho M. Effects of frequent breastfeeding on early milk production and infant weight gain. *Pediatrics* 72:307–311; 1983.

Flower H. *Adventures in Tandem Nursing: Breastfeeding During Pregnancy and Beyond.* Schaumburg, IL: La Leche League, International; 2003.

Fox-Bacon C et al. Maternal PKU and breastfeeding: Case report of identical twin mothers. *Clin Pediatr* 36:539–542; 1997.

Gromada K. *Mothering Multiples: Breastfeeding and Caring for Twins or More.* Rev ed. Schaumburg, IL: La Leche League, International; 1999.

Jakobsen M et al. Termination of breastfeeding after 12 months of age due to a new pregnancy and other causes is associated with increased mortality in Guinea-Bissau. *Int J Epidemiol* 32(1):92–96; 2003.

Karp H. The "fourth trimester:" A framework and strategy for understanding and resolving colic. *Contemporary Pediatrics* 21:94; 2004.

Kroeger M, Smith, L. *Impact of Birthing Practices on Breastfeeding.* Sudbury, MA: Jones and Bartlett; 2004.

Kutner L. *Lactation Management Course.* Chalfont, PA: Breastfeeding Support Consultants Center for Lactation Education; 1996.

Maccagno-Smith R, Young M. Breastfeeding the sleepy infant. *Can Nurse* 89:20–22; 1993.

MacFarlane A. *The Psychology of Childbirth.* Boston, MA: Harvard University Press; 1997.

Marquis G et al. Postpartum consequences of an overlap of breastfeeding and pregnancy: Reduced breast milk intake and growth during early infancy. *Pediatrics* 109(4):e56; 2002.

Mead L et al. Breastfeeding success with preterm quadruplets. *JOGNN* 21(3):221–227; 1992.

Merchant K et al. Maternal and fetal responses to the stresses of lactation concurrent with pregnancy and of short recuperative intervals. *Am J Clin Nutr* 52(2):280–288; 1990.

Moscone S, Moore MJ. Breastfeeding during pregnancy. *J Hum Lact* 9(2):83–88; 1993.

Neifert M, Thrope J. Twins: Family adjustment, parenting, and infant feeding in the fourth trimester. *Clin Obstet Gynecol* 33:102–112; 1990.

Newton N, Theotokatos M: Breast-feeding during pregnancy in 503 women: Does psychobiological weaning mechanism exist in humans? *Emotion Reprod* 20B:845; 1979.

Noble E, Sorger L. *Having Twins and More: A Parent's Guide to Multiple Pregnancy, Birth, and Early Childhood*, 3rd ed. New York: Mariner Books; 2003.

Siega-Riz A, Adair L. Biological determinants of pregnancy weight gain in a Filipino population. *Am J Clin Nutr* 57(3): 365–372; 1993.

Sollid D et al. Breastfeeding multiples. *J Pernat Neonat Nurs* 3:46–65; 1989.

Widstrom AM et al. The position of the tongue during rooting reflexes elicited in newborn infants before the first suckle. *Acta Paediatr* 82:281–283; 1993.

Wight N. Breastfeeding the borderline (near-term) preterm infant. *Pediatric Ann* 32(5):329–336; 2003.

Williams R, Medalie J. Twins: Double pleasure or double trouble? *Am Fam Phys* 49:869–873; 1994.

Woerner J. The joy of multiples. *Int J Childbirth Education* 8:35–36; 1993.

Woolridge M, Fisher C. Colic, overfeeding, and symptoms of lactose malabsorption in the breast-fed baby: A possible artifact of feed management? *Lancet* ii:382–384; 1988.

Woolridge MW et al. Do changes in pattern of breast usage alter the baby's nutrient intake? *Lancet* 336:395–397; 1990.

▶ BIBLIOGRAPHY

Dewey K. Growth patterns of breastfed infants and the current status of growth charts for infants. *J Hum Lact* 14:89–92; 1998.

La Leche League, International. *The Womanly Art of Breastfeeding*, 7th ed. Schaumburg, IL: La Leche League International; 2004.

Lang S. *Breastfeeding Special Care Babies*, 2nd ed. London: WB Saunders; 2002.

Levindon P et al. Randomised controlled trial of sucrose by mouth for the relief of infant crying after immunisation. *Arch Dis Child* 78:453–456; 1998.

Lobo M et al. Current beliefs and management strategies for treating infant colic. *J Pediatr Health Care* 18(3):115–122; 2004.

Lucassen P et al. Effectiveness of treatments for infantile colic: Systematic review. *Br Med J* 316:1563–1569; 1998.

Matthews M. Mothers' satisfaction with their neonates' breastfeeding behaviors. *JOGNN* 20(1):49–55; 1991.

Skadberg B et al. Abandoning prone sleeping: Effect on the risk of sudden infant death syndrome. *J Pediatr* 132:340–343; 1998.

Walker M. Breastfeeding the sleepy baby. *J Hum Lact* 13(2): 151–153; 1997.

Wilson-Clay B, Hoover K. *The Breastfeeding Atlas*, 2nd ed. Austin, TX: Lactnews Press; 2002.

Wolke D et al. An epidemiologic longitudinal study of sleeping problems and feeding experience of preterms and term children in southern Finland: Comparison with a southern German population sample. *J Pediatr* 133:224–231; 1998.

15

INFANT ATTACHMENT AND SUCKING

Contributing Authors: Linda Kutner and Jan Barger

Although there may be an occasional baby who needs assistance in initiating effective suckling, the majority need no help. Caregivers need to trust in the innate abilities, reflexes, and instincts of both the mother and baby. Always remain aware that there should be a good reason for putting anything in the baby's mouth other than the breast. A sound understanding of infant sucking will help in evaluating the appropriateness of any intervention. This chapter explores the baby's sucking and suckling as they relate to breast attachment and milk transfer.

KEY TERMS

bolus	orbicularis oris muscles
carpal tunnel	peristalsis
craniosacral therapist	pharynx
intervention levels	SGA
intubation	soft palate
latch	suck training
masseter muscle	sucking
milk transfer	sucking needs
neuromotor	sucking pattern
dysfunction	suckling
nutritive sucking	syringe feeding
oral cavity	trough

SUCKING AND SUCKLING

Sucking is a baby's means of comfort and nourishment. It is pleasurable, both physically and emotionally. The sucking associated with nursing stimulates saliva, which contains enzymes that help predigest food before it reaches the stomach enzymes. Farther down in the gut, sucking stimulates gastrointestinal secretions, hormones, and motility. The release of certain hormones, including cholecystokinin (CCK) in the gut, also promotes satiety and sleepiness in the baby.

Sucking can have a calming effect on the baby and helps him pass gas and stool. It activates prolactin release in the mother, thus stimulating milk production and

feelings of yearning for her baby. As sucking continues, oxytocin is released, which causes cuddly and warm feelings in the mother. This triggers her milk to let down and helps her uterus return to its prepregnant size.

Sucking needs vary from one baby to another. Many babies are born with red marks or blisters on their hands or wrists, an indication that they were sucking in utero. Babies use their thumbs, fingers, and hands as a means of soothing and calming themselves. The need for sucking is usually greater in the first three months than at any other time. Encourage mothers to be sensitive to this important aspect of their babies' health. Satisfying a baby's sucking needs will enhance his emotional well-being and growth.

The Infant's Sucking Pattern

A breastfeeding baby sucks in a rhythm that corresponds inversely to the amount of milk that is available. High rates of milk flow result in slower sucking rates of about one suck per second. As the baby obtains milk, his sucking rate increases until he reaches about two sucks per second, when milk removal is minimal (Mathew, 1989; Bowen-Jones, 1982). A newer study showed that infant suck rates increase from 55/minute in the immediate postnatal period to 70/minute by the end of the first month, and swallow rates increase from about 46 to 50/minute. Feeding efficiency almost doubled over the first month (Quereshi, 2002). These rates of sucking, termed nutritive and nonnutritive respectively, have two distinctly different patterns. There is also a distinction between sucking and suckling. *Sucking* describes the act of the baby drawing the breast into his mouth and maintaining negative pressure to keep it there. He then actively *suckles* the milk out with his tongue.

Suckling and feeding develop in a predictable and organized way after birth (Widstrom, 1987). Several investigators have found that drugs given to the mother in labor that depress the central nervous system adversely affect nutritive sucking (Baumgarder, 2003; Riordan, 2000; Crowell, 1994; Righard, 1990). Letting the baby cry can compromise his innate sucking behavior and result in a disorganized suck. See the discussion on the effect of crying on the infant in Chapter 13.

Changes in sucking rate during breastfeeding are gradual. At the beginning of a feeding, the baby suckles rapidly to initiate milk flow. When letdown occurs and he swallows, his sucking pace slows. He returns to more rapid suckling to stimulate further milk flow and then slower sucking as he obtains milk. He will continue to alternate between nutritive and nonnutritive sucking throughout the feeding.

Multiple milk ejections are common during breastfeeding. Mothers typically only notice the first one, and many mothers do not feel their letdown at all. The number of milk ejections is related to the amount of milk ingested by the baby (Ramsay, 2004a). When the baby switches to the other breast, he resumes the same pattern. Full-term neonates younger than 24 hours old exhibit less rhythmic sucking than older term infants.

During the first two or three days, the baby sucks with several short, fast bursts per swallow. This pattern is an indication that volume of colostrum is relatively small. Around the third or fourth day, a regular feeding rhythm becomes established. This indicates that the mother is producing transitional milk with increased volume. At around four to five days, the full-term infant typically swallows with every suck, which indicates milk flow following letdown.

Babies who exhibit short suckling bursts and shorter overall suckling times have more feeding difficulties at 6 weeks of age compared to babies who have longer, continuous suckling bursts and longer suckling times (Ramsay, 1996). For this reason, it is important that you thoroughly assess the baby's early suckling pattern and work with the mother to help her baby continue at feedings rather than stop after short efforts.

Physiology of Suckling

The baby uses his tongue to draw the nipple and areola into his mouth and forms a cone-shaped extension of the breast that conforms to the shape of his mouth, as shown in Figure 15.1. It is important to recognize that when the baby draws sufficient breast tissue into his mouth, his tongue is free from frictional movement against the breast. There is no in-and-out movement—only a one-way exchange of milk from the breast to the baby.

Ultrasound studies from the 1980s suggest that the baby's tongue moves in a peristaltic motion from the front of the mouth toward the back. It appeared the nipple was drawn back completely to the juncture of the **hard** and **soft palate** (Woolridge, 1986; Weber, 1986; Bosma, 1990). Smith described more of a piston-like movement (Smith, 1988). More recent studies combining ultrasound,

video, and intra-oral pressure measurement suggest new findings (Ramsay, 2004b). The areola and nipple press upward against the upper gum and the hard palate as described previously. However, the nipple does not appear to reach completely to the juncture of the hard and soft palates. It appears that it is the negative pressure of the baby's suck that transfers milk, with much greater milk flow when the tongue is down than when the tongue is up (Ramsay, 2004b). The negative pressure, along with the alternate compression and release of the gums, moves the milk through the milk ducts and out the nipple. When the baby's jaw drops, the increased negative pressure allows the milk to move from the nipple to the baby's mouth. Multiple letdowns also facilitate milk transfer. Ramsay's research found that mothers may have one to nine milk ejections per feeding, with an average of 2.5.

Suckling increases the mother's prolactin level and releases oxytocin in a pulsatile manner (Yokoyama, 1994). The newborn is capable of adjusting his sucking rate, suggesting an ability to cope with letdown (Al-Sayed, 1994). One study demonstrated that bottle-feeders breathe less often than breastfeeders, with two of the 15 bottle-feeders experiencing decreased heart rates during feeding. The number of sucks per minute was also higher in breastfeeders (Mathew, 1989). A more recent study found that preterm babies were more stable, with lower heart rates, higher oxygen saturations, and less desaturations during cup feedings than during bottle-feedings (Marinelli, 2001). Preterm babies that are cup-fed have fewer desaturations and higher breastfeeding rates at three months than do preterm bottle-feeders (Rocha, 2002).

In functional suck/swallow/breathe sequencing, swallowing does not occur simultaneously with breathing.

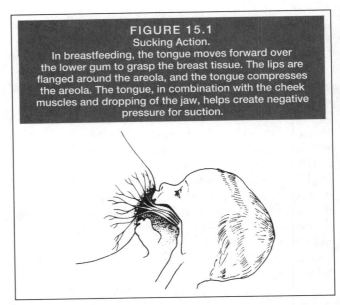

FIGURE 15.1
Sucking Action.
In breastfeeding, the tongue moves forward over the lower gum to grasp the breast tissue. The lips are flanged around the areola, and the tongue compresses the areola. The tongue, in combination with the cheek muscles and dropping of the jaw, helps create negative pressure for suction.

Source: King FS. *Helping Mothers to Breastfeed*, Revised Edition, p. 14. Nairobi, Kenya: AMREF. Reprinted with permission.

Swallowing while breathing results in aspiration, taking foreign matter into the lungs. A pattern of more sucks per minute is associated with fewer swallows. Therefore, a higher sucking frequency correlates with more breaths and higher oxygen saturations. Babies pause between bursts of suckling and are able to regulate their breathing. Suckling develops on a continuum with fewer sucks per burst and longer pauses in preterm infants.

▶ SUCKLING AT THE BREAST VERSUS SUCKING ON A BOTTLE

Suckling action in breastfeeding involves the baby's entire mouth—his lips, gums, tongue, cheeks, and his hard and soft palates. The soft breast molds to the baby's mouth, and the baby actively suckles the breast in order to receive milk. This is quite different from the sucking motion used for extracting milk from a bottle, as shown in Figure 15.2. In bottle-feeding, the baby draws the nipple into his mouth and must alter his mouth to accommodate the shape of the artificial nipple. He must generate suction pressure so that the milk flows freely from the bottle. New ultrasound studies show that the baby's tongue pushes against the nipple, with compression of the nipple and a hook-like lift of the posterior tongue (Ramsay, 2004b).

What may appear to be dysfunctional on a bottle, that is, wide jaw excursions, is not dysfunctional in breastfeeding. Wide jaw excursions are indicative of nutritive suckling in a breastfeeding baby. This belies the argument that preterm infants must "prove" themselves on a bottle before they are allowed to go to breast (Meier, 1994). Further, high flow rates from artificial nipples cause preterm infants to swallow continuously, thus limiting their chances to breathe. Preterm infants can

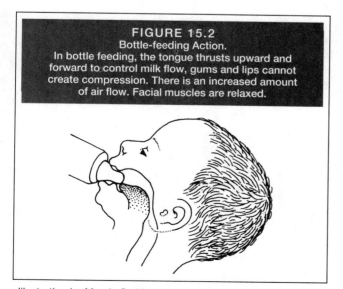

FIGURE 15.2
Bottle-feeding Action.
In bottle feeding, the tongue thrusts upward and forward to control milk flow, gums and lips cannot create compression. There is an increased amount of air flow. Facial muscles are relaxed.

Illustration by Marcia Smith.

coordinate suck-swallow-breathing as early when breastfeeding as when bottle-feeding. Moreover, the baby is better able to maintain stable body temperature and higher oxygen saturation at the breast (Morton, 2003).

Because of the very different way in which babies suck on a bottle and the breast, alternating between the two can create problems. This is especially true in the early weeks when the baby is mastering his technique. Artificial teats—both bottle nipples and pacifiers—can cause the baby to develop a preference for the teat over the breast. Milk flows more readily and quickly from a bottle nipple. When he returns to the breast, he must suckle actively to receive milk. Healthy, full-term breastfed babies should not routinely be given an artificial nipple. DiGirolamo (2001) found the strongest risk factors for early breastfeeding termination were late breastfeeding initiation and supplementing the infant. Compared with mothers experiencing all five baby-friendly practices, mothers experiencing no baby-friendly practices were approximately eight times more likely to stop breastfeeding early.

If parents consider other alternative feeding methods too stressful, time-consuming, or impractical, you can teach them paced bottle-feeding (Wilson-Clay, 2002; Kassing, 2002), as described in Chapter 21. Feeding specialists have noted that babies who cannot breastfeed well usually cannot bottle-feed well either. When you encounter a baby who cannot breastfeed, carefully observing him being bottle-fed will be an important part of your evaluation. For an infant who cannot breastfeed, bottle-feeding can be a helpful tool when used judiciously (Noble, 1997).

Consequences of Extended Bottle or Pacifier Use

The use of bottles and artificial nipples during infancy may have far-reaching health consequences. Babies who suck for extended periods on a bottle or pacifier may compromise proper development of the oral cavity and swallowing pattern. The greatest development of the craniofacial structure takes place within the first four years of life (Shepard, 1991). Extended use of artificial devices in the infant's mouth may contribute to abnormal craniofacial development during a very sensitive period.

Bottle-feeding may alter proper development of swallowing, which can extend into adulthood (Palmer, 2004b, 1999). A proper adult swallowing pattern mirrors that of a breastfeeding baby, with a peristaltic motion from the tip of the tongue to the soft palate. The tongue should not exert any pressure on any teeth and should rest against the hard palate until the next swallow. In bottle-feeding, the baby draws his tongue inside his mouth to protect the bottom of the tongue from the trauma of being compressed between the nipple and his gum pad. He also places his tongue at the back of the throat in a protective posture to prevent too much liquid from going down his throat.

To limit the flow of formula, the baby may use his tongue in a thrusting motion against the bottle nipple. This tongue thrusting can continue into adulthood, causing the adult to push against his teeth and create spaces. Tongue thrusting may be the greatest contributor to the development of a malocclusion (improper alignment of the teeth). Research shows a greater incidence of malocclusion among infants who are not breastfed (Labbok, 1987). Bottle feeding and non-nutritive sucking activity (pacifier use) more than doubles the risk of posterior cross-bite (Viggiano, 2004). In 1996, the American Academy of Pediatric Dentistry reported that 89 percent of youths aged 12 to 17 had some degree of malocclusion (AAPD, 1996). A study in the 1930s evaluated the teeth, facial contours, and mouths of thousands of people in nonindustrialized cultures and skulls from burial sites. Nearly all had ideal occlusions and dental arches and minimal decay (Price, 1997). This population had no access to artificial formula, bottles, or pacifiers.

As the baby removes formula from the bottle, a vacuum may form in the bottle, causing him to suck excessively in order to increase flow. The greater the sucking action needed within the mouth, the greater the potential for collapse of the oral cavity. It can narrow the dental arch to a V-shape rather than the normally wide U-shape. It also contributes to a high palate, which can infringe on the nasal cavity and increase resistance to air flow. This may lead to increased risk for obstructive sleep apnea in adulthood (Palmer, 2004b).

Bottle-feeding weakens the baby's suck. This, in turn, reduces the strength of the **masseter muscle** and increases the strength of the **orbicularis oris muscles**. Facial muscles develop in the exact opposite pattern from which they were intended (Legovic, 1991). Palmer (2004a) explains that a "key point about breastfeeding is that all the perioral musculature gets involved. Breastfeeding is a complex process needing coordinated efforts by all the muscles of the mouth and jaw. Infants have to 'work' all the muscles during breastfeeding . . . . Farmers who milk cows by hand have strong hands, arms and shoulders. Those who use milking machines don't."

▶ LATCHING THE BABY ON

The moment of contact of the baby's mouth on the mother's breast is referred to as *latching on* or *attachment*. A good latch enables the baby to take a large amount of breast tissue into his mouth. He needs to get as much of the areola as possible into his mouth and to have his lips positioned well behind the nipple. This enables him to release milk from the underlying ducts. With good position accomplished, the baby is then able to suckle and

obtain milk. Removal of milk, in turn, relieves milk pressure in the breast and maintains milk production.

When a baby latches on well, the mother observes audible swallows or long, drawing, nutritive, high-flow sucks. In the first 24 to 48 hours, the swallows often sound like little puffs of air after 3 to 4 high-flow, nutritive sucks. The mother may report a tugging or pulling sensation with a good latch. However, she should be free of pain, both during and after the feeding. If she experiences pain, she needs to adjust her baby's position. Figure 15.3 and Figure 15.4 show the differences between a baby who has a good latch and one who does not.

Principles of an Effective Latch

Principles of a good latch are just that—general principles. There is no rule that a baby must latch on in one particular way. That said, babies will have more effective

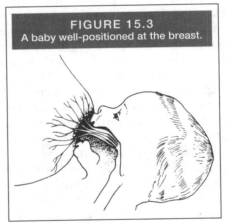

FIGURE 15.3
A baby well-positioned at the breast.

Source: King FS. *Helping Mothers to Breastfeed*, Revised Edition, p. 14. Nairobi, Kenya: AMREF. Reprinted with permission.

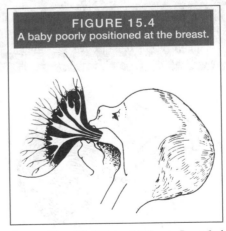

FIGURE 15.4
A baby poorly positioned at the breast.

Source: King FS. *Helping Mothers to Breastfeed*, Revised Edition, p. 14. Nairobi, Kenya: AMREF. Reprinted with permission.

milk transfer and mothers will have less discomfort in the technique described here. In order to achieve a good latch, the baby first needs to be in a receptive state in which he can settle and organize himself. He will turn his head toward the mother's breast and open his mouth wide. The position for optimal suckling is for the breast to be slightly above the center of the baby's open mouth. His lips flange out and open wide at an angle of about 140 degrees. His bottom lip will cover most of the areola and his top lip will cover somewhat less of the areola in an asymmetrical, or off-center, latch. This ensures adequate compression of the ducts underneath the areola.

With a good latch, the mother's breast tissue completely fills the baby's oral cavity, as depicted in Figure 15.5. In order for the baby to take a large enough amount of breast tissue into his mouth, he must be close to and facing the mother's breast. If the baby does not take enough breast tissue into his mouth, he will have difficulty extracting milk and fail to gain weight. He will compensate by increasing suction and compressing his lips to hold the nipple securely. This could result in nipple soreness. A change in positioning can improve the baby's suckling (Morton, 1992).

With a good latch, the baby's tongue is under the breast and extends outward far enough to cover the alveolar ridge (bottom gum line). With his mouth open wide and his lips flanged, he will take in a large mouthful of breast tissue. His tongue will form a **trough** through which the milk will flow. He will then draw the nipple into the center of his mouth or tongue. His jaws are well behind the nipple and compress the milk ducts rhythmically. He will continue to hold the breast in his mouth as he establishes a pattern of repeated bursts of suck/swallow/pause . . . suck/swallow/pause. A good latch usually means that the mother feels no pain (Kutner, 1996).

The Baby's Latch in the First Few Days

In the early days of breastfeeding, it is common for a baby to have some difficulty latching on to the breast. This is particularly true if the mother's labor and birth involved interventions and medications (Kroeger, 2004; Baumgarder, 2003). If the baby misses the nipple when he roots toward it, the mother can wait a few seconds and stroke his cheek again. If his rooting reflex appears to be weak, she can express milk onto his lips to lead him to the breast. If the baby still does not latch on to the nipple, the mother can withdraw her breast, relax, reposition the baby, and repeat the rooting reflex stimulus. Establishing this routine will help the baby develop a pattern for getting onto the breast. Encourage the mother to think of the early days as a learning period and not to become discouraged if she and her baby have difficulty getting started.

▶ MILK TRANSFER

Before addressing possible problems with suckling and attachment, it is first helpful to understand how the baby receives milk, and how interaction between the baby and the breast can affect milk transfer. Two essential elements for efficient milk transfer are a functioning letdown in the breast and appropriate suckling by the infant. It is important that everyone involved in the mother's and baby's care understand that milk transfer is an interaction between the mother and her baby. They each exert influence over the other. The manner in which the baby's mouth physically meets and then stimulates the breast is crucial to effective milk transfer.

The Transfer Process

Milk transfer occurs when the baby's suckling delivers a **bolus** of food to the **nasopharynx** and is swallowed. Earlier studies describe a peristaltic wave of contraction in the tongue muscle that progresses backward along the teat from an anterior to a posterior direction (Woolridge, 1986; see Table 15.1). More recent ultrasound research reveals little tongue movement other than up (compression) and down (negative pressure), with more milk delivered when the tongue is down than when it is up (Ramsay, 2004b).

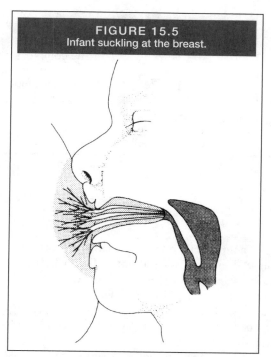

FIGURE 15.5
Infant suckling at the breast.

Source: Woolridge MW. The anatomy of infant sucking. *Midwifery* 2:164–171; 1986. Reprinted with permission.

TABLE 15.1

Peristaltic Wave Theory of Milk Transfer

Step		Description
1	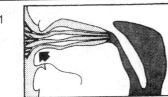	The baby takes breast tissue into his mouth and forms a teat from the mother's nipple, areola, and breast tissue. It is important to note that the teat formed by the breast and nipple fills the baby's mouth, leaving no room for movement of the breast within the mouth. As he draws the teat far into his mouth, his tongue cups around the teat to form a trough for the milk. The baby's tongue stays cupped along the sides of the breast and nipple teat, and covers the alveolar ridge throughout the suckling cycle.
2	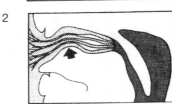	The suck cycle begins. The end of the nipple is drawn back to the soft palate by a combination of suction and compression. When it is fully extended, the nipple is approximately three times as long as it is at rest. This suggests that the baby cannot traumatize the breast tissue if he has a good mouthful of breast. It is compressed for only a fraction of a second and will not look flattened or compressed when the feed ends if the baby was attached correctly. When the nipple touches the soft palate at the back of the oral cavity, it elicits the baby's suck reflex. The baby then raises his lower jaw to pinch off milk that collects in the lactiferous sinuses. At the same time, the anterior tip of his tongue begins to push upward against the breast tissue.
3	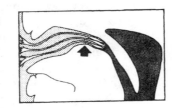	The baby strips milk from the breast. A peristaltic wave of compression moves along the underside of the teat. The baby's tongue pushes against his hard palate, thus compressing the sinuses. A bolus of milk is then squeezed from the teat. Note that when the sinuses are compressed, milk flows from the breast. The baby does not get milk from the breast by suction.
4	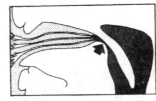	The wave of compression continues to the back of the tongue, which pushes against the soft palate and rises to seal the nasal cavity. The trachea and vocal chords are closed off by the **epiglottis**, and milk is propelled into the esophagus. This, in turn, initiates the baby's swallow reflex.
5	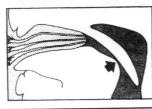	The compression ends at the posterior base of the tongue. The back of the tongue depresses, which creates negative pressure. The breast is then drawn back into the baby's mouth to begin another cycle.

Source: Woolridge MW. The anatomy of infant sucking. *Midwifery* 2:164–171; 1986. Reprinted with permission.

The mother's nipple, areola, and breast tissue form a teat within the baby's mouth. The baby's tongue cups along the sides of the teat and forms a trough. The baby alternately compresses the nipple and swallows when the back of his mouth fills with milk. Suckling typically occurs in a continuous cycle of suck/swallow/breathe (Mathew, 1989).

The baby's tongue covers the alveolar ridge throughout the suckling cycle. The baby draws the end of the nipple back to within a few centimeters of the soft palate. His lower jaw and tongue rise to compress the breast. The combination of positive pressure in the alveoli created by the letdown reflex and suction caused by the jaw lowering causes milk to enter the teat. Some milk is released when the breast is compressed, but more is released when the compression ends and the baby's jaw opens (Ramsay, 2004b).

Milk reaching the back of the baby's mouth stimulates him to swallow. Negative pressure retains the breast in the baby's mouth and may help milk move down the ducts. Thus, the amount of breast tissue the baby takes into his mouth plays a role in how easily he can extract the milk. Watching the baby's sucking action and jaw movement in relation to the frequency of swallowing can give clues to the amount of milk that is being transferred to him. Pre-feed and post-feed weights on a digital scale will measure the amount precisely if necessary, as in the case of a low weight gain or preterm baby.

Signs of Effective Milk Transfer

After observing that the baby has latched on effectively, you can evaluate the transfer of milk to her baby. The vast majority of babies will accomplish milk transfer remarkably well when the mother uses sound breastfeeding practices. There are some babies, however, who may have difficulty and require assistance. Signs of good milk transfer include:

- The baby moves from short rapid sucks to slow deep sucks early in the feeding.
- The mother notices signs of the milk ejection reflex.
- No dimpling or puckering of the baby's cheeks is noted.
- Breast tissue does not slide in and out of the baby's mouth when the baby sucks or pauses.
- No smacking or clicking sounds are evident with sucking.
- Swallowing is evident after every one to two sucks.
- The baby is able to maintain his latch throughout the feeding.
- The mother's breast softens as the feeding progresses (noted after Stage II lactogenesis).
- The baby spontaneously unlatches and is satiated.
- The mother's nipple does not blanch or compress when the baby unlatches.
- The baby is content between most feedings.
- The baby's voiding and stooling are appropriate for his age.

▶ PROBLEMS WITH LATCH

It is common for a baby to have some difficulty latching on to the breast in early attempts. Help mothers approach early feedings in a calm manner and with a sense of humor. This will decrease potential frustration in both the mother and the baby. When there are difficulties, encourage mothers to keep the attempts to breastfeed very short. Depending on the baby's tolerance, the mother may be able to work with him for as long as ten minutes.

As soon as the baby cries, pushes away, or demonstrates other withdrawal or avoidance behaviors such as hic-coughing, coughing, gagging, or sneezing, she should stop that attempt, calm the baby, and try again later.

The mother may also try feeding on the other breast or try holding her baby in a different position. (See Chapter 14 for discussion of positioning.) If the baby rejects the breast after a few such attempts, advise that she stop all efforts for that feeding. She can snuggle skin to skin with her baby and watch for the return of approach behaviors such as tongue extension, bringing his hand to his mouth, or rooting. She can then gently bring him to breast again.

The mother will need to express milk from her breasts to maintain milk production if the baby continually refuses to nurse. Until the baby achieves an effective latch, he can receive expressed milk with an alternative feeding method. Occasionally, latch problems are due to oral intrusion such as vigorous oral suctioning (Wiswell, 2000; Widstrom, 1987) or unnecessary digital exams. The first thing placed into a baby's mouth should be the mother's breast. The information in Table 15.2 will help you explore the possible causes for problems with latch so that you can determine appropriate measures.

Possible Signs of a Poor Latch

- The baby is unable to stay on the breast for more than several sucks.
- The mother has pain during or after feedings.
- Dimpling or puckering of the baby's cheeks is noted.
- The breast slides in and out of the baby's mouth throughout sucking.
- Clicking or smacking noises are heard when the baby suckles.
- Little or no swallowing is evident during a feeding.
- The baby is fussy during or after feedings.
- The mother's nipple appears flattened, creased, or blanched after the baby unlatches.
- Little or no breast changes occur from the beginning to the end of a feeding after Stage II lactogenesis.
- The baby has inadequate voiding, stooling, or both.

Feeding Adjustments to Improve Latch

When a baby continues to have difficulty with latch the mother can explore alternative ways to manage feedings. Suggest that she provide lots of skin-to-skin contact without attempting to put the baby to breast. She can lie on her back with the baby between her breasts, just as she would immediately after birth. If the baby begins

TABLE 15.2	
The Baby Who Cannot Get Attached	
Cause	**Suggestions for Management**
The baby is being held in a position that requires him to twist his neck in order to breastfeed.	Help the mother hold her baby close, directly facing and slightly lower than the center of the breast.
The baby does not open his mouth wide enough.	Tease the baby with the nipple, by gently touching his upper lip, until he opens his mouth wide before attaching.
The baby has been given an artificial nipple and has a sucking preference. He may thrust or hump his tongue when he tries to attach and suckle	Give no artificial nipples to the baby; allow him only to suckle at the breast. If supplementation is necessary, use a small spoon, cup, or a tube at the breast.
The mother's nipples are flat because of engorgement.	Be sure the mother's breasts do not become too full because of limited feedings. If the breasts are engorged, express milk to help the nipple protrude and soften the areola. Try reverse pressure softening.
The mother's nipples are inverted to the point that the baby cannot get attached.	Draw out an inverted nipple with mild suction before the feeding, using an everter, inverted syringe or pump. Note that inverted nipples do not necessarily interfere with breastfeeding. Babies attach to the breast, not to the nipple.

to root around for the breast, she can help guide him to the breast, making sure not to push him on.

The mother may have more success getting her baby attached if she holds him in a position where her dominant hand is in control. A right-handed mother could use the football hold on the right breast or the cross-cradle hold with the left hand supporting the left breast. This reverses for a left-handed mother. Such positions will give the mother control over the baby's head movement and help her hug him to the breast as soon as his mouth is opened wide enough.

If her baby tends to approach the breast without opening his mouth, the parents can encourage him to open his mouth wider. When the baby is content, awake, and happy, they can tickle his upper lip with a finger, talking to him all the time, saying slowly, "o..p..e..n..w..i..d..e." When he responds, they can gently put a finger into his mouth, pad side up, to suck on as a reward. Dipping the finger into the mother's expressed colostrum or milk or sweetened water may be an added incentive. In addition, babies often imitate facial expressions. Parents can demonstrate a wide mouth by opening their mouths wide so that the baby will mirror the action.

The Baby Who Cannot Stay Attached

Some babies initially may achieve a good latch and then form a pattern of popping on and off the breast during a feeding. The baby attaches and begins to nurse, and after a short time, falls away from the breast and cries or chokes. This may happen several times during a breastfeeding. Table 15.3 will help you explore the causes and then determine the appropriate measures. It sometimes happens in the early days postpartum before the mother's milk has come in; or it could occur when her mature milk is in.

First rule out an overactive supply resulting from a strong milk ejection reflex (MER). Any of these situations can cause the baby to have trouble latching on and generating enough suckling pressure to hold onto the breast. The mother may have very large breasts, and the baby may be near-term (37–38 weeks) or small for gestational age (SGA). In situations like this, the mother can learn how to help her baby stay with the analogy of a "breast taco" or a "breast sandwich" (Wiessinger, 1998). You can describe how she holds a taco or sandwich horizontally, not vertically, to eat it. She can use the same principle to help her baby get a substantial part of her breast in his mouth by flattening her breast so that it "fits" the plane of his mouth.

Figure 15.6 shows a mother using the taco hold. The mother first uses the C-hold and then provides additional support for her baby's cheek and chin. Her thumb and index finger help to flatten her breast into a "breast taco" so her baby can take in a mouthful of breast tissue. Her thumb is on the outer part of her areola. Mothers are usually advised to put their fingers behind the areola; if this mother did so, she would be too far back for her baby to achieve a good latch. Her breasts and areola are so large that her breast would round back out, and the baby would slide down on her nipple as before. This is an example of the uniqueness of

TABLE 15.3
The Baby Who Cannot Stay Attached

Cause	Suggestions for Management
The baby must reach or twist his neck to keep the breast in his mouth.	Be sure the mother is holding her baby close, directly facing and slightly lower than the breast, with his nose and chin touching the breast and the baby's ear, shoulder, and hip in alignment.
The baby is unable to breathe when he is at the breast.	Avoid flexing the baby's head forward in such a way that his nose is pushed against the breast. His head needs to be slightly extended so that his chin and nose are just touching the breast. Pull his bottom in more, and his head will angle out.
The mother is moving either her breast or her baby, or not supporting the baby enough so that the breast falls away.	Hold the baby in a side-sitting position with his head cradled in the mother's hand for greater head control (avoiding pushing at the back of his head). Help the mother identify a good attachment and focus on what it feels like so she can recognize the baby's gradual slipping off the breast. Put pillows or blankets under her arm so a fatigued arm muscle will not let the baby slip. Help her check during the feeding for good attachment and learn trauma-free unlatching and relatching so that both she and the baby develop the habits of a wide-open, mouth-full attachment. If you can see the problem and the mother cannot, she will continue doing the wrong thing.
The mother's milk is flowing too forcefully.	Be sure the mother's breasts do not become too full because of limited feedings. If the breasts are engorged, expressing milk will help the nipple to protrude. Suggest that the mother express milk before a feeding so that the flow is less forceful. Allow the baby to feed on only one breast per feeding, with no time limitations, until the initial oversupply has diminished. The mother may need to express milk from the other breast for comfort. If she has an overabundance of milk, she may want to nurse the baby on the same side two or three times before changing to the other breast.

each mother and baby pair. Flexibility and creativity are two of your most important tools. Mothers usually only need this type of assistance in the early days or until the near-term baby reaches his due date. You can reassure the mother of this, and encourage her that very soon her baby will be able to latch on well by himself.

Consequences of a Poor Latch

A mother whose baby cannot latch on effectively will very likely experience nipple soreness. Incorrect latch is the primary cause of nipple soreness. In turn, the pain—or anticipation of pain—when the baby latches on may inhibit the mother's milk ejection reflex and prevent sufficient milk from reaching her baby. Because a poorly latched baby is unable to remove milk from the mother's breasts adequately, the mother is at risk for engorgement, plugged ducts, and mastitis. Milk production will diminish, and lactation failure is likely to result in the absence of any intervention. It is important that the mother pump or express her milk if the baby is not latching on and breastfeeding effectively.

Consequences of a poor latch are inevitable for the baby as well. Because of the mother's decreased milk ejection reflex, he receives primarily foremilk. This results in increased hunger, fussiness, and perhaps colic-like symptoms. His urine and stool output may be low, and he may develop jaundice. The baby may be unable

FIGURE 15.6
The "Breast Taco" or "Breast Sandwich" hold.
Printed with permission of Anna Swisher.

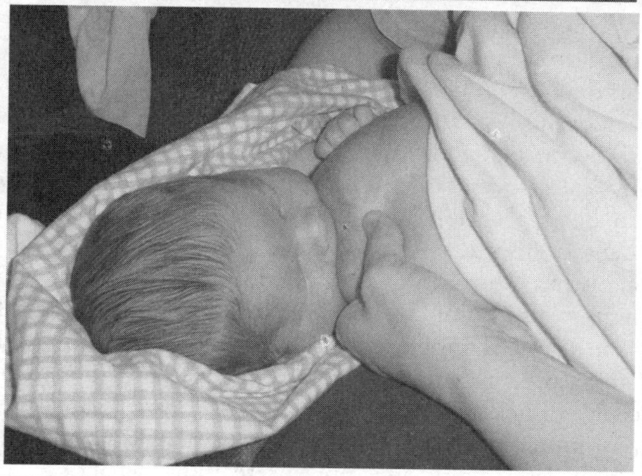

to obtain enough high-fat hindmilk, resulting in failure to gain adequate weight or even in weight loss. To preserve the baby's health, he may need formula supplements. This could mark the end to breastfeeding, unless the plan of care includes suggestions on ways to increase the mother's milk production. Making adjustments in the baby's latch can prevent the situation from progressing to this point.

Physical Pathologies That Can Affect Latch

In some cases, difficulty with latch may be a result of breast or nipple abnormalities. It could also result from acute or chronic physical conditions such as low back pain, carpal tunnel syndrome, or pain related to delivery, particularly perineal or cesarean incision pain. It may be a result of the infant having a cleft lip or palate, neurological or orthopedic problems, Down syndrome, a fractured clavicle, ankyloglossia (tight frenulum), or a high palate. If comfort measures have not resulted in improvement, these factors need to be explored as possible causes for the baby's difficulty with attachment.

Some babies engage in rapid side-to-side head movements, making it impossible to achieve a good latch. You can use a dropper of the mother's milk or water to touch the midline of the baby's upper lip. When the baby stops his head movement, the mother can lead him to the breast, placing a couple of drops of fluid on his tongue as he opens his mouth. You can also do this with tubing and a syringe.

Devices to Help with Latch

The mother can feed her baby her expressed milk while she continues to put him to breast at every feeding. A nipple shield may help her baby latch on at the beginning of the feeding. It is important that she attempt to remove it after a few minutes and place her baby directly on the breast to suckle. The mother will need to continue to express milk from her breasts to maintain milk production until the baby weans from the shield. Remain flexible in your approach with mothers. Do only what a particular mother can tolerate. This may require providing more alternatives in some cases than in others.

Some practitioners use periodontal syringes for finger feeding or for supplementing at the breast. Use care when syringe-feeding babies. It removes control from the baby and places it in the hands of the mother or caregiver. Care must be taken not to accidentally poke the baby if he moves suddenly. The syringe should deliver only a few drops at a time, which allows the baby to set the pace of swallowing. See the discussion of feeding alternatives in Chapter 21.

▶ PROBLEMS WITH SUCKLING

Most feeding difficulties result from incorrect attachment or faulty positioning of the baby at the breast. In many cases, patience, practice, and repositioning of the baby's body and his mouth on the breast will alleviate these suckling difficulties. Righard and Alade (1992) demonstrated the importance of correcting early sucking problems. Their study revealed that uncorrected babies stopped nursing sooner. Hence, suggesting that the baby will figure it out when the milk comes in is not always adequate. When the mother adjusts positioning to achieve a good latch, the baby's suckling will usually improve (Morton, 1992).

A thorough assessment of both the mother and baby will help determine if the problem is one of attachment or if the baby has a truly **dysfunctional suck**. Most attachment or sucking difficulties are short-lived. They usually resolve with the passage of time, as long as the baby receives sufficient calories. A baby may have a weak or ineffective suck because he is actually weak from insufficient nourishment. Many times, a baby's suckling will improve simply by getting more calories into him. **Intubation** is another factor to consider when evaluating an infant's suck, especially with preterm infants. One study showed intubated babies took longer to develop a normal nutritive suck. Both breastfeeders and bottle-feeders were included in this study, however, and they were not analyzed separately (Bier, 1993).

The Baby Who Attaches and Is Not Suckling Nutritively

An occasional baby may achieve a good latch and yet make no effort to establish a nutritive suck. It is possible that he is sleepy and not hungry at the moment. For these babies, you need to determine whether they are receiving any artificial feedings of water or infant formula, or are using a pacifier. These are simple factors to correct by elimination, and the baby will probably be back exclusively at the breast easily.

Some babies have difficulty initially mastering the physical process of suckling. **Disorganized suckling** can be due to illness, prematurity, drugs given to the infant or mother, or a delay in the first breastfeeding at birth. Neuromotor dysfunction, variations in oral anatomy, and nipple preference due to the introduction of an artificial nipple all affect suckling ability as well. Table 15.4 presents a summary of the causes of a baby having difficulty suckling and suggests possible measures the mother can take. A careful assessment is an integral part of determining the appropriate course of action.

TABLE 15.4
Causes of Latch or Sucking Problems

Cause	Suggestions for Management
Medication received by the mother during labor	Encourage childbirth educators to focus on labor support issues and to educate couples about the effects of epidurals and cesareans.
Forceps delivery or vacuum extraction	Watch positioning of the baby to avoid pressure on his head.
Post-birth interventions such as deep laryngeal suctioning or circumcision	Avoid putting the baby to breast immediately following deep suctioning or other oral insult until the baby demonstrates readiness. Avoid circumcision until the baby has fed well at the breast at least three times.
Prolonged crying, especially due to interventions	Prevent prolonged crying by helping the mother with her baby. Comfort the baby before putting him to breast. Teach the mother and staff the importance of feeding on cue rather than when the baby cries. Keep the mother and baby together rather than having the baby in the nursery.
Baby has a fractured clavicle or cephalhematoma	Position the baby in a manner that prevents pressure on the affected area.
Mother has tight, taut breast tissue with flat or inverted nipples	Massage breasts before the feeding. Use a hold that enables the mother to maintain control over her baby's head movement (clutch hold or cross-cradle hold). Use an inverted syringe to form the nipple (see Chapter 21). The mother may need to use a nipple shield (see Chapter 21).
Incorrect positioning at the breast	Correct any positioning problems. Make sure both mother and baby are comfortable.
Mother's lack of confidence in handling baby and putting baby to breast	Give encouragement to the mother and help her see that she and her baby will become more comfortable with one another with practice and time. Show the mother how to handle her baby and put him to breast. Avoid doing it for her.
High-arched or bubble palate	Use the clutch hold. Take the baby off the breast after 30–60 seconds and reattach. The second latch helps draw more tissue farther back into the baby's mouth.
Short or tight frenulum	Contact the pediatrician, dentist, oral surgeon, or ear-nose-throat specialist for evaluation and possible clipping of the frenulum.
Cleft lip	The lip usually molds around the breast to form suction. If this is not the case, the mother can cover the cleft area with her breast or finger. Massage the breasts before and during the feeding.
Cleft palate	Nurse in a semiupright position. Hold the breast in the baby's mouth during feedings. Interrupt feeding as necessary to allow the baby to burp or breathe. Supplement with the best device for the individual baby. An obturator (a feeding plate placed over the cleft) may be helpful. The mother will need a referral to a cleft palate team.
Hypoglycemia in the baby	Feed the baby expressed colostrum via cup, spoon, or syringe. Use an artificial baby milk if expressed mother's milk is not sufficient for the baby's needs. Make sure that the baby is fed at regular intervals. Wake him to feed if necessary.
Hypotonia or hypertonia in the baby	Positioning is the key. Some hypertonic babies may need to find their own position of comfort. A hypotonic baby will need to be supported well. The mother may need to supplement if the baby does not feed well. These babies respond well to tube-feeding at the breast. Decrease external stimulation for the hypertonic baby. Use rousing techniques for the hypotonic baby, starting with infant massage. Use gentle massage to calm the hypertonic baby. Short, very frequent feeding (every 1½ to 2 hours) will be more effective than longer feedings at longer intervals. Condition the baby by establishing a routine for getting on the breast, especially if the baby's rooting reflex is not well developed. Supplement with expressed milk in a cup or bottle after nursing if the baby is unable to obtain enough through use of a tube-feeding device at the breast. Express milk and supplement the baby until the condition improves.

(continued)

TABLE 15.4 (CONTINUED)	
Causes of Latch or Sucking Problems	
Cause	**Suggestions for Management**
Baby engages in tongue sucking or tongue thrust	A baby who consistently sucks his tongue may have been doing so in utero for months. Have the baby learn to suck progressively on the mother's small finger, middle finger, and then thumb to gradually increase the baby's comfort level with larger sizes of objects in his mouth. Use finger feeding until the baby can latch on.
Baby has received bottles and prefers an artificial nipple	Because babies suck differently on an artificial nipple than they do on the breast, it is important to avoid using a rubber/silicone nipple as much as possible. The long, firm object stimulates his palate and initiates a suck almost immediately. He does not have to draw it into his mouth. Any kind of sucking stimulus on the bottle nipple will cause fluid to flow into his mouth; hence, he will be unable to suck non-nutritively on the bottle as he can on the breast. He will have to hump his tongue at the front of the nipple to control milk flow. When the breast is drawn into the baby's mouth, it conforms to the shape of his mouth, whereas the bottle nipple not only does not fill the baby's mouth, but he must alter his mouth shape to work with the artificial nipple. Discontinue the bottle and supplement with a cup, spoon, syringe, or medicine dropper.
Baby has a stuffy nose due to a cold or allergies	Nurse the baby in an upright position. Saline nose drops or a drop of the mother's milk in the baby's nostrils helps clear a stuffy nose. Using a bulb syringe to clear the nose may irritate the delicate mucous membranes and cause swelling.
Mother is taking medication that affects the baby through her milk	Ask the physician about switching to a drug that will have less effect on the baby. Alter feeding times and drug administration so that the baby nurses when the amount of drug in the mother's milk is lowest. If possible, delay drug use until the baby is older. If reactions are serious (i.e., extreme colic-like behavior or lethargy) and the drug cannot be discontinued, do not breastfeed. Pump and dump to maintain lactation.

Plan of Care for Sucking Problems

A plan of care for sucking problems must focus on the assessed problem, not on an assumption of dysfunctional suck. The goal is to resolve the cause of the sucking problem instead of just the symptoms. In other words, you need to resolve why the baby has poor weight gain. Do not just feed formula to the baby. Take the mother's situation and emotional state into account, and include her in the planning. Be cautious not to overwhelm parents with too many things to do.

Consider the long-term consequences of your plan of care. Will using a bottle cause nipple preference? Might a nipple shield lower the mother's milk production? Will a bottle or nipple shield be a useful tool that saves breastfeeding for this mother? Will feeding become a chore for the mother and a difficult procedure for the baby? You need to develop a practical plan that the mother is likely to take ownership of and use.

Most breastfeeding problems relate to poor latch rather than dysfunctional sucking. There is a difference between a disorganized suck and a dysfunctional suck. Babies may exhibit an uncoordinated suck in the first few days of life because of sucking habits in utero, birth interventions, or early artificial nipple feedings. In some cases, the cause is unexplained. Most uncoordinated sucking is resolved with the passage of time and with increasing the baby's caloric intake.

The initiation of any intervention in the hospital for a healthy term infant can result in poor or ineffective feeding behaviors. The baby's oral cavity is extremely sensitive and has many complex innervations. Excessive or inappropriate manipulation can result in an aversion to anything going into his mouth, including the breast. You should put your finger into the baby's mouth only if you have received appropriate training.

Barger (1998) identifies five levels of intervention for babies who have difficulty suckling. When there is a true need for assistance, the clinician should always start with the least complex and intrusive method. Progressing to the highest degree of intervention is rarely necessary and should occur only when there is a clear need. Whenever possible, follow a course that places the baby in control of the feeding rather than special devices or techniques. Refer to Chapter 21 for further details on the techniques described below.

Noninterventive Techniques

The least invasive approach is to determine the probable cause of the suckling difficulty and consider whether the situation is one that will improve with time. If poor positioning is the cause, help the mother correct the positioning. Then wait for the "golden moment," the time before crying begins when the baby is rooting, hungry, and opens his mouth wide. The mother can express colostrum onto her nipple to entice the baby. Alternatively, she may drip some glucose water on the nipple to stimulate sucking. The sweeter the solution, the more vigorously the baby may suck. Make sure mothers do not use honey, which can cause botulism in infants.

Minimal Level of Intervention

If enticing the baby has been unsuccessful, you or the parent can place an index finger in the baby's mouth to pacify him or to initiate rhythmic sucking. Using a supplemental feeding device at the breast will help get calories into the baby and stimulate sucking at the same time. The baby can receive either expressed mother's milk or formula through the device, depending on the availability of mother's milk. If the baby is not latching on to the breast, a feeding tube at the breast will not be helpful. However, a feeding tube is helpful for a baby who attaches and does not suckle adequately.

Low-Level Intervention

If less invasive techniques have failed to achieve a good suck, you can insert your index finger into the baby's mouth to evaluate his oral cavity and his suck. It is not routinely necessary to assess infant oral structure other than visually. Oral examination is an invasion of the baby's mouth, done only if the clinician suspects a problem. If a short frenulum is causing difficulty, you can help the mother find someone to clip the frenulum. A baby who is not breastfeeding effectively will need to receive nourishment by an alternative feeding method until the issue is resolved.

Moderate-Level Intervention

If other measures have been unsuccessful, you can place your index finger in the baby's mouth, with the pad side up, to organize his sucking. This technique involves placing light pressure on the midline of the baby's tongue, pulling the finger out slowly to encourage the baby to suck it back in. The baby receives verbal reinforcement when he sucks correctly. In the minimal level and low-level interventions, the baby was in control. This intervention involves more control by the caregiver through manipulation of the finger in the baby's mouth. Its use is appropriate only after other measures have failed to elicit effective suckling.

Some babies respond well to finger feeding with a supplemental nursing system. Parents can use this tool to help a baby who is having trouble suckling. The feel of a parent's finger resembles the mother's breast more than a silicone or latex nipple does. See Chapter 21 for a discussion on finger feeding. If the mother has flat or inverted nipples or edema that does not respond to reverse pressure softening or if the baby has a high bubble palate or thin buccal pads, a nipple shield may be

a successful bridge to direct breastfeeding (Meier, 2000; Wilson-Clay, 1996).

High-Level Intervention

Suck training is the highest degree of sucking intervention. This level of intervention is beyond the scope of most nurses and IBCLCs. If there is a need for suck training, other neurological problems, such as cerebral palsy, may be present. The suck may be the first area in which the problem presents. Suck training involves placing the index finger in the baby's mouth to stimulate certain portions of his oral anatomy in order to train him to suck. Suck training is not an appropriate technique for an untrained clinician to attempt. The baby must be referred to a professional who is trained and skilled in this field, such as a physical, occupational, or speech therapist experienced in working with breastfeeding babies.

Some parents find improvement with chiropractic help or with a branch of massage therapy known as **craniosacral therapy** (see Figure 15.7). Developing a list of reliable allied health professionals will enable you to refer parents appropriately. You will need to work in concert with the baby's caregiver and other specialists as a part of the healthcare team. A referral to an organization that assists the neurologically impaired child and his family may be necessary. Refer to Appendix A for a list of national organizations that may be helpful for intervention referrals.

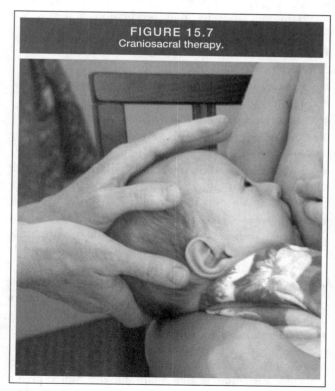

FIGURE 15.7
Craniosacral therapy.

Printed with permission of Anna Swisher.

▶ SUMMARY

An awareness of the mechanics of infant sucking will help caregivers understand the transfer of milk from the breast to the baby. The fact that the studies on milk transfer lead to different descriptions of infant sucking illustrates the continual evolution of insights into the intricacies of breastfeeding. Simply because certain views go against each other does not mean that either is incorrect. It is not the differences in descriptions that are important; it is the fact that the mechanics of breastfeeding are substantially different from those of bottle-feeding. The manner in which a baby suckles the breast, his sucking needs, and the pattern he establishes will affect this transfer. Although some infants may have difficulty suckling, most causes of attachment or suckling difficulties are reversible without direct intervention by the caregiver. When it becomes necessary to intervene, clinicians must begin with the least invasive method. High-level interventions are appropriate only after exhausting less intrusive alternatives. Many suckling difficulties will be resolved by time and by making sure the baby is receiving sufficient calories.

▶ CHAPTER 15—AT A GLANCE

Facts you learned about—

Sucking:

- Sucking stimulates saliva, gastrointestinal secretions, hormones, motility, milk production, and maternal yearning.
- Cholecystokinin (CCK) promotes satiety and sleepiness.
- Sucking rhythm corresponds inversely to the amount of milk available.
- Nutritive sucking is affected by CNS depressants.
- Suckling at the breast is very different from sucking on a bottle.
- Ineffective suckling places the mother at risk for engorgement, plugged ducts, mastitis, and compromised milk production.
- Ineffective suckling places the baby at risk for increased hunger, fussiness, colic-like symptoms, low urine and stool output, jaundice, inadequate weight gain, or weight loss.
- Latch difficulties may result from breast or nipple abnormalities, pain, cleft lip or palate, neurological or orthopedic problems, ankyloglossia, or high palate.
- Suckling can be disorganized due to illness, prematurity, drugs given to the infant or mother, delay in the first breastfeeding at birth, neuromotor dysfunction, variations in oral anatomy, and nipple preference due to the introduction of an artificial nipple.

- Too much inappropriate intervention can result in oral aversion.
- When possible, the feeding should be controlled by the baby rather than by special devices or techniques.
- Extensive suck training is beyond the scope of most nurses and IBCLCs.

Applying what you learned—

Teach mothers that:

- Wide jaw excursions indicate nutritive suckling.
- Alternating between breast and bottle can compromise breastfeeding.
- Extended bottle or pacifier use may cause malocclusion and sleep apnea in adulthood.
- Audible swallows or long, drawing, nutritive, high flow sucks indicate a good latch.
- The early days of breastfeeding are a learning period.
- With a good latch, the breast is slightly above the center of the baby's open mouth, lips are flanged, bottom lip covers most of the areola off-center, and tongue is under the breast and over the alveolar ridge, forming a trough.
- Efficient milk transfer requires a functioning letdown and appropriate suckling.
- A nipple shield may help a baby latch on at the beginning of a feeding.
- Most feeding difficulties are caused by incorrect attachment or faulty positioning.
- Most uncoordinated sucking is resolved with the passage of time and with increasing the baby's caloric intake.
- A baby who is sleepy or not hungry may not suckle nutritively.

Teach the mother how to:

- Observe her baby for signs of a good latch and good milk transfer.
- Handle problems with the baby's latch and assist a baby who cannot stay attached.
- Maintain milk production when her baby is unable to nurse effectively.
- Preserve her baby's health with supplements when necessary.

▶ REFERENCES

Al-Sayed L et al. Ventilatory sparing strategies and swallowing pattern during bottle-feeding in human infants. *J Appl Physiol* 77:78–83; 1994.

American Academy of Pediatric Dentistry (AAPD). Special issue: Reference manual. *Pediatr Dent* 17(6); 1995–1996.

Anderson G. Risk in mother-infant separation postbirth. *Image Journal of Nursing Scholarship* 21:196–199; 1989.

Barger J. *Lactation Management Course.* Breastfeeding Support Consultants Center for Lactation Education, Chalfont, PA; 1998.

Baumgarder D et al. Effect of labor epidural anesthesia on breast-feeding of healthy full-term newborns delivered vaginally. *J Am Board Fam Pract* 16(1):7–13; 2003.

Bier J et al. The oral motor development of low-birth-weight infants who underwent orotracheal intubation during the neonatal period. *Am J Dis Child* 147:858–862; 1993.

Bosma J et al. Ultrasound demonstration of tongue motions during suckle feeding. *Dev Med Child Neurol* 32(3):223–229; 1990.

Bowen-Jones A et al. Milk flow and sucking rates during breast-feeding. *Devel Med Child Neurol* 24:626–633; 1982.

Crowell MK et al. Relationship between obstetric analgesia and time of effective breastfeed. *J Nurse Midwifery* 39(3):150–156; 1994.

DiGirolamo A et al. Maternity care practices: Implications for breastfeeding. *Birth* 28(2):94–100; 2001.

Kassing D. Bottle-feeding as a tool to reinforce breastfeeding. *J Hum Lact* 18(1):56–60; 2002.

Kroeger M, Smith L. *Impact of Birthing Practices on Breastfeeding.* Sudbury, MA: Jones and Bartlett; 2004.

Kutner L. *Lactation Management Course.* Breastfeeding Support Consultants Center for Lactation Education, Chalfont, PA; 1996.

Labbok M, Hendershot G. Does breastfeeding protect against malocclusion? *Am J Prev Med* 3:227–232; 1987.

Legovic M, Ostric L. The effects of feeding methods on the growth of the jaws in infants. *J Dent Children* 58(3):253–255; 1991.

Marinelli, K et al. A comparison of the safety of cupfeedings and bottlefeedings in premature infants whose mothers intend to breastfeed. *J Perinatol* 21(6):350–355; 2001.

Mathew O, Bhatia J. Sucking and breathing patterns during breast- and bottle-feeding in term neonates. *Am J Dis Child* 143:588–592; 1989.

Medoff-Cooper B et al. Neonatal sucking as a clinical assessment tool: Preliminary findings. *Nurs Res* 38:161–165; 1989.

Meier P et al. Nipple shields for preterm infants: Effect on milk transfer and duration of breastfeeding. *J Hum Lact* 16(2):106–114; 2000.

Meier P. Transitional suck patterns in premature infants. *J Perinat Neonat Nurs* 80:vii–viii; 1994.

Morton J. Ineffective suckling: A possible consequence of obstructive positioning. *J Hum Lact* 8:83–85; 1992.

Morton J. The role of the pediatrician in extended breastfeeding of the preterm infant. *Pediatric Ann* 32(5):308–316; 2003.

Noble R, Bovey A. Therapeutic teat use for babies who breastfeed poorly. *Breastfeed Rev* 5(2):37–42; 1997.

Palmer B. Breastfeeding: Reducing the risk for obstructive sleep apnea. *Breastfeeding Abstracts* 18(3):19–20; 1999.

Palmer B. The importance of breastfeeding to total health, 2004a. Available at: www.brianpalmerdds.com. Accessed May 21, 2004.

Palmer B. Sleep apnea from an anatomical, anthropologic and developmental perspective, 2004b. Presentation to the Academy of Dental Sleep Medicine, June 4, 2004. Available at: www.brianpalmerdds.com.

Price WA. *Nutrition and Physical Degeneration*, 6th ed. New Canaan, CT: Keats Publishing; 1997.

Quereshi M et al. Changes in rhythmic suckle feeding patterns in term infants in the first month of life. *Dev Med Child Neurol* 44(1):34–39; 2002.

Ramsay D et al. Ultrasound imaging of milk ejection in the breast of lactating women. *Pediatrics* 113(2):361–367; 2004a.

Ramsay D. *Ultrasound imaging of the sucking mechanics of the term infant.* Presentation, Human Lactation: Current Research and Clinical Implications, Amarillo, TX; October 22, 2004b.

Ramsay M, Gisel E. Neonatal sucking and maternal feeding practices. *Dev Med Child Neurol* 38:34–47; 1996.

Righard L, Alade M. Effect of delivery room routines on success of first breastfeed. *Lancet* 336:1105–1107; 1990.

Righard L, Alade M. Sucking technique and its effect on success of breastfeeding. *Birth* 19:185–189; 1992.

Riordan J et al. The effect of labor pain relief medication on neonatal suckling and breastfeeding duration. *J Hum Lact* 16(1):7–12; 2000.

Rocha N et al. Cup or bottle for preterm infants: Effects on oxygen saturation, weight gain, and breastfeeding. *J Hum Lact* 18(2):132–138; 2002.

Shepard JWJ, Gefter WB, Guilleminault C et al. Evaluation of the upper airway in patients with OSA/SDB. *Sleep* 14:361–371; 1991.

Smith W, Erenberg A, Nowak A. Imaging evaluation of the human nipple during breast-feeding. *Am J Dis Child* 142(1):76–78; 1988.

Viggiano D et al. Breast feeding, bottle feeding, and non-nutritive sucking; effects on occlusion in deciduous dentition. *Arch Dist Child* 89(2):1121–1123; 2004.

Weber F et al. An ultrasonographic study of the organization of sucking and swallowing by newborn infants. *Dev Med Child Neurol* 28:19–24; 1986.

Weber F, Woolridge M, Baum J. An ultrasonographic study of the organisation of sucking and swallowing by newborn infants. *Dev Med Child Neurol* 28(1):19–24; 1986.

Widstrom AM. Gastric suction in healthy newborn infants. *Acta Pediatr Scand* 76:566–572; 1987.

Wiessinger D. A breastfeeding tool using a sandwich analogy for latch-on. *J Hum Lact* 14(1):51–56; 1998.

Wilson-Clay B. Clinical use of silicone nipple shields. *J Hum Lact* 12(4):279–285; 1996.

Wilson-Clay B, Hoover K. *The Breastfeeding Atlas.* 2nd ed. Austin, TX: Lactnews Press; 2002.

Wiswell T et al. Delivery room management of the apparently vigorous meconium-stained neonate: Results of the multicenter, international collaborative trial. *Pediatrics* 105(1 Pt 1):1–7; 2000.

Wolf L, Glass R. *Feeding and Swallowing Disorders in Infancy.* San Antonio, TX: Therapy Skill Builders; 1992.

Woolridge M. Anatomy of infant suckling. *Midwifery* 2:164–171; 1986.

Yokoyama U et al. Releases of oxytocin and prolactin during breast massage and suckling in puerperal women. *Eur J Obstet Gynecol Reprod Biol* 53:17–20; 1994.

▶ **BIBLIOGRAPHY**

Ardran G, Kemp M, Lind J. A cineradiographic study of breast feeding. *Br J Radiol* 31(363):156–62; 1958.

Ardran G, Kemp M, Lind J. A cineradiographic study of bottle feeding. *Br J Radiol* 31(361):11–22; 1958.

Cox D et al. Studies on human lactation: The development of the computerized breast measurement system; 1998. Available at: www.biochem.uwa.edu.au/PEH/PEHRes.html. Accessed June 30, 2004.

Daly S et al. Degree of breast emptying explains changes in the fat content but not fatty acid composition of human milk. *Exp Physiol* 78:741–755; 1993.

Daly S et al. The short-term synthesis and infant-regulated removal of milk in lactating women. *Exp Physiol* 78:209–220; 1993.

Matthews MK. Developing an instrument to assess infant breastfeeding behaviour in the early neonatal period. *Midwifery* 4:154–165; 1988.

Morris SE. Overview of the anatomy and physiology of the oral pharyngeal mechanism. In Palmer MM (ed). *The Normal Acquisition of Oral Feeding Skills: Implication for Assessment and Treatment* (pp. 19–32). New York: Therapeutic Media; 1982.

Narayanan I et al. Sucking on the "emptied" breast: Nonnutritive sucking with a difference. *Arch Dis Child* 66(2):241–244; 1991.

Prieto C et al. Sucking pressure and its relationship to milk transfer during breastfeeding in humans. *J Reprod Fertil* 108:69–94; 1996.

Ramsay M et al. Infant sucking ability, non-organic failure to thrive, maternal characteristics, and feeding practices: A prospective cohort study. *Dev Med Child Neurol* 44(6): 405–414; 2002.

Smith W et al. Imaging evaluation of the human nipple during breast-feeding. *Am J Dis Child* 142:76–78; 1988.

Stevenson RD, Allaire JH. The development of normal feeding and swallowing. *Pediatr Clin N Am* 38(6):1439–1453; 1991.

BREASTFEEDING
IN THE EARLY WEEKS

The early weeks with a new baby are a time of great adjustment for families. Some mothers seem to sail through this time with little difficulty. Others encounter situations that require extra assistance. Providing anticipatory guidance at key times will help the mother manage any difficulties with minimal disruption. During the early weeks of breastfeeding, the mother will be establishing milk production and refining her technique. She will benefit from your guidance and support as she learns how to respond to the needs of her baby. Your assistance at this critical time can help her avoid problems with sore nipples, engorgement, plugged ducts, and mastitis.

KEY TERMS

abscessed breast	mastitis
alternate massage	milk bleb
ankyloglossia	milk blister
autocrine control	milk stasis
breast compression	palliative care
Candida albicans	phytoestrogens
candidiasis	plugged duct
cholecystokinin (CCK)	postmature babies
colostrum	Raynaud's phenomenon
edema	recurrent mastitis
engorgement	spontaneous lactation
feedback inhibitor of	sublingual
lactation (FIL)	suppressor peptides
galactorrhea	thrush
hyperprolactinemia	transient nipple soreness
labial frenum	vasospasm
lingual frenulum	

► COMMITMENT TO BREASTFEED

Why do some women breastfeed for months and years, whereas others wean after a few days or weeks? In the industrialized world, there is a clear perception that, although breastfeeding is best, alternatives are acceptable. Generally, mothers who breastfeed do so out of choice, not because of perceived necessity or tradition. This has a significant impact on duration. When an acceptable alternative exists, confidence and commitment may wane in the absence of support and encouragement.

Reasons Women Continue to Breastfeed

Bottorff (1990) examined why women continue to breastfeed beyond the early days. She noted that it may be influenced by the baby's responsiveness, the mother's satisfaction, and the compatibility of breastfeeding with her lifestyle. Bottorff also identified the key role a mother's persistence and commitment play in the decision. A woman saying, "I will try to breastfeed," is quite different from one who says, "I will breastfeed." When a woman commits herself to breastfeeding, she is able to do so despite most difficulties that may arise. Breastfeeding is a journey into the unknown and the unpredictable. It involves ongoing learning. Part of a mother's persistence is recognizing the need for help and then finding that help.

A more recent study of women in Hong Kong breastfeeding for more than six months found the same qualities. "Despite family opposition, frequently from their mother-in-law, and lack of societal acceptance, difficulties were overcome by what the Chinese people call *hung-sum* or determination" (Tarrant, 2004). An Australian study found that maternal confidence, or "breastfeeding self-efficacy," was a "significant predictor of breastfeeding duration and level" (Blythe, 2002).

Early contact and early breastfeeding contribute to how long a woman breastfeeds. Leff (1994) identified areas that are important in evaluating the overall breastfeeding experience. Mothers who see their babies grow, gain weight, rarely become ill, settle with breastfeeding, and fall asleep during or after breastfeeding are likely to view breastfeeding as successful. Satisfaction is higher when breastfeeding is comfortable and when any painful phases are short lived. Mothers in the Leff study identified breastfeeding as an important part of the maternal role. They spoke of a harmonized relationship between themselves and their babies that made breastfeeding feel successful. In other words, breastfeeding worked for both the mothers and their babies.

Women in the Leff study rated their breastfeeding success relatively low if they perceived their baby as not being satisfied. If the baby was satisfied, high levels of success also depended on maternal enjoyment, attainment of the desired maternal role, and lifestyle compatibility. The baby's satisfaction is not totally the mother's responsibility. His sucking competence, alertness, stamina, and abilities to self-regulate and to respond to soothing also influence his satisfaction. It takes time for mothers to find ways to work with the individual characteristics of their babies (Lothian, 1995).

Your role in encouraging the continuation of breastfeeding involves helping the mother prioritize her baby's needs. Boosting a mother's confidence empowers her to continue breastfeeding. Her confidence will soar when you point out positive things about her baby, such as, "He is growing so fast," or "He looks so healthy." Point out her abilities as well, as in, "You're such a good mom," or "You pick up on your baby's cues really well." Help the mother recognize and respond to her baby's language and cues. Acknowledge that she knows her baby better than anyone else. Validate her concerns and her wide range of emotions as a normal part of mothering.

Misconceptions That Interfere with Breastfeeding

There are numerous unfounded beliefs about breastfeeding that confuse parents and interfere with sound medical advice. Parents and caregivers alike are subject to these beliefs. You can assist both parents and caregivers in understanding these misconceptions and recognizing factors in sound breastfeeding practices. Some of the more common misconceptions are cited below.

Common Misconceptions

◆ **Bottles and artificial baby milk given to breastfeeding babies do not interfere with breastfeeding.** Any artificial nipple given to an infant in the early weeks of establishing breastfeeding has the potential to create a preference for the artificial nipple (see Chapter 21). Additionally, formula exposes the infant to a greater risk of disease and sensitizes him to cow's milk protein (see Chapter 9). It is not necessary to feed breastfeeding babies with a bottle in the early days postpartum in order to train them to accept a bottle later.

◆ **Time at the breast needs to be limited in the early days to prevent nipple soreness.** Poor positioning is the major cause of sore nipples, not the amount of time a baby nurses. Babies need unlimited access to the breast. Early, frequent feedings increase the mother's milk production and avoid complications (see the discussion in this chapter). Enforced time limits increase the incidence of jaundice and inadequate weight gain in the baby and engorgement and low milk production in the mother.

◆ **Even with time limits, most breastfeeding women will experience nipple soreness.** The vast majority of sore nipples are a result of poor positioning of the baby at the breast. Women typically experience brief moments of latch-on tenderness or initial **transient nipple soreness** that disappears within a few days to a week. This transient pain does not interfere with breastfeeding. Breastfeeding should be pain free through the whole feeding and after.

◆ **Newborn babies typically need to eat every four hours.** Breastfeeding babies may want to nurse as frequently as every one to two hours in the early days. Enforced scheduling of feedings ignores hunger cues and interferes with mothering. By learning how to read hunger cues, mothers can trust their babies to determine the timing of feedings. See Chapter 13 regarding infant feeding cues, and see the discussion of feeding frequency later in this chapter.

◆ **Water supplementation will help prevent or reduce jaundice in breastfeeding infants.** A jaundiced baby needs the increased stooling facilitated by receiving colostrum. The correct response is to increase the number and effectiveness of feedings. Water supplementation can decrease the amount of human milk the baby consumes, increasing bilirubin levels and resulting in weight loss (see Chapter 22). Water supplementation does not coat the gut as human milk does. It does not have the laxative effect of colostrum to help with the excretion of meconium. Giving water to the baby can reduce effective suckling at the breast, increase the incidence of engorgement, and cause nipple preference when given by bottle. It also reduces the baby's caloric intake and his ability to self-regulate his intake.

◆ **Formula supplementation is necessary when the mother has low milk production.** Initial remedies for low milk production are to increase the frequency of feedings and ensure correct positioning and attachment (see Chapter 18). **Alternate massage** during a feeding will help increase the volume of milk transferred. Supplementing with artificial baby milk by bottle can result in nipple preference, difficulty with attachment, less time at the breast, inadequate milk removal, and allergies. It can also cause the mother to doubt her competence or ability to breastfeed. Breastfeeding babies should receive no artificial baby milk unless medically indicated. If the problem lies with the baby and not with the mother's milk supply, the first choice for supplementation is her own pumped milk. If formula supplementation is medically necessary, as in the rare case of PKU, it should be given by a method that will interfere least with breastfeeding (see Chapter 21).

◆ **Weaning is recommended when mothers are taking most medications.** The American Academy of Pediatrics advises that most maternal use of medications does not require weaning (see Chapter 10). Refer to the latest edition of the Hale (2004) text *Medications and Mother's Milk* for information about specific drugs. Also visit Hale's Web site at www.ibreastfeeding.com.

◆ **Breastfeeding mothers and babies take more of the caregiver's time than do those who bottle-feed.** Mothers who room in with their babies in the hospital assume more care of their babies, freeing hospital staff for other tasks (see Chapter 12). Mothers who receive anticipatory guidance and appropriate teaching make fewer phone calls and visits to the pediatrician (see Chapter 2).

◆ **The best time to start breastfeeding is after the mother's milk "comes in."** Colostrum is present from about the fourth month of pregnancy onward. Delaying the start of breastfeeding can lead to engorgement, a delay or decrease in milk production, and interference with the mother's instincts (see Chapter 12). Mothers should be given the opportunity to breastfeed within 1 hour of birth.

◆ **The best way to tell that a baby is getting enough of his mother's milk is that he sleeps for several hours after each feeding.** Sleeping is not an indication of the baby receiving enough milk. The more calorically deprived a baby is, the more he will sleep. Mothers need to watch for the number of wet diapers and bowel movements, the baby's disposition during and between feedings, and other growth indicators (see Chapter 13).

◆ **After the mother's milk production is established, the baby will usually take most of the milk in the first five to seven minutes.** Each baby's breastfeeding pattern is different. As babies become older, they are able to remove milk more quickly from the breast. However, they still should determine the end of the feeding rather than having arbitrary time limits imposed (see Chapter 14).

◆ **Mothers need to nurse from both breasts at every feeding; therefore, the mother should limit sucking time on the first breast so the baby will take the second breast.** The amount of time it takes a baby to remove both foremilk and hindmilk from a breast varies. If the mother removes her baby from the breast before he receives hindmilk, he will ingest large amounts of foremilk. This could result in colic-like behavior or poor weight gain (see Chapter 16). Some babies nurse from only one breast at a feeding and will follow this pattern for all feedings, whereas others may nurse from one breast until late afternoon or evening and then nurse from both. Others will always nurse from both breasts. Initially, encouraging the baby to take the second breast after he comes off the first on his own will stimulate milk production in both breasts.

◆ **Artificial baby milk is just as healthy as human milk.** There are profound differences between artificial baby milk and human milk. See Chapter 9 for a detailed discussion about the properties and health benefits of human milk and a comparison to infant formula health risks.

◆ **Breastfeeding is essentially an alternative to infant formula.** Breastfeeding is much more than human milk. It is a dynamic bonding process, a biological relationship between a mother and her baby. Breastfeeding involves people, not simply infant food (see Chapter 3). This is an especially important reminder for adoptive mothers or mothers with low milk production.

◆ **It is important to wait at least two to three hours between feedings so the breast can refill and the baby does not use the mother as a pacifier.** The breast is never empty. As the baby removes milk, the breast produces more milk. The shorter the period between feedings, the higher the fat content of the milk (Daly, 1993). Waiting a specified period between feedings can decrease milk production and the amount of fat the baby receives (see Chapter 7). Additionally, sucking is soothing to the baby. He should be pacified at the breast rather than on a rubber nipple. The breast is for nurture, not just nutrition.

◆ **A mother cannot make enough milk for more than one baby.** Most women can make far more milk than their baby requires and, in fact, regulate their supply to their singleton's needs. Wet nurses once nursed up to five babies and produced up to 2230 ml of milk per day (Budin, 1907). One of Budin's wet nurses produced as much as 2840 ml per day! Exclusive breastfeeding of twins is common in breastfeeding support circles. Exclusive breastfeeding of triplets or a higher order of multiples, while a time and energy management challenge, is biologically feasible (Noble, 2003; Gromada, 1999).

▶ ESTABLISHING MILK PRODUCTION

Milk, in the form of colostrum, is present from about the fourth month of pregnancy onward. At birth, the delivery of the placenta triggers a reduction in the woman's progesterone levels that removes the inhibition of milk production and allows the elevated levels of prolactin to function. Increased amounts of blood and lymph in the breast form the nutrients for milk production. These fluids cause the breasts to become fuller, heavier, and sometimes tender. As regular, frequent breastfeedings progress, this normal fullness diminishes. By about two weeks postpartum, when lactation is well established, the breasts become comfortably soft and pliable, even when they are full with milk. Regular, frequent feedings will maintain this condition.

A woman's production of milk requires a functioning letdown response and adequate milk removal on a regular basis. The process of milk production is believed to occur through local autocrine control after the initial postpartum period (DeCoopman, 1993). Removal of milk is just as important as nipple stimulation and letdown. When a baby nurses frequently, there is greater nipple stimulation and greater removal of milk, and consequently, increased milk production. Thus, to ensure good milk production, the mother will want to avoid missed feedings, especially in the early days when she is still establishing milk production.

Generally, mothers should allow the baby to remain at the breast until he spontaneously releases the breast on his own. If the baby tends to "linger" at the breast, the mother can watch for a change from nutritive to nonnutritive sucking. Nonnutritive sucking does not provide the stimulation necessary for increasing milk production. If the mother removes him from the breast at this time, it should not significantly affect milk quantity. However, mothers should be encouraged to gauge their baby's needs. Some babies need more comfort sucking at the breast than others need.

During the first month of life, the baby establishes patterns of milk intake that will continue through the next twelve months (Mitoulas, 2002). Parents need to avoid strict schedules and allow the baby to lead his feedings. This supports the individual nature of infant needs and the importance of baby-led feedings. Each baby's own rhythm will reflect his feeding patterns.

One Breast or Two

In the first few days, feedings may be shorter, lasting only about 10 to 15 minutes, than after the mother has established milk production. The baby may nurse on only one breast at each feeding and then drift off to sleep. When he is put to the other breast he may be too drowsy or too full to nurse. His drowsiness is due in part to the release of cholecystokinin (CCK) in his system during suckling. CCK is a gastrointestinal hormone that enhances digestion and sedation and induces a feeling of satiation and well-being. The baby's suckling releases CCK in both the baby and mother. The baby's CCK level peaks immediately after a feeding and again about 30 to 60 minutes later (Uvnas-Moberg, 1989). If, during the time between the two peaks, the mother puts the baby to breast on the side that has not yet been nursed, he may arouse enough to nurse.

As the days pass and the baby becomes more alert, feeding times will increase and he will be more likely to feed at both breasts at a session. Encourage mothers to remain flexible, especially in the early days while the mother and her baby are both establishing themselves in this new venture. Let the baby be the guide. If milk production is plentiful and the baby is gaining weight, a mother need not be concerned about her baby's refusal of the second breast. This is common in the early days and may persist for many months. One-breast feedings can be adequate (Righard, 1993). Some babies never nurse on both breasts at a feeding. If the mother experiences uncomfortable fullness of the second breast, she can encourage her baby to nurse on that side to relieve the fullness and prevent engorgement. She can then begin the next feeding on the side that is fuller. Some mothers, especially those returning to work, may choose to pump the full breast and save the milk for feedings during separation.

Duration of Feedings

In general, the baby's needs should determine feeding length. When the flow of milk diminishes from one breast, the sucking rate will move from the long, drawing nutritive suck to a faster, gentler suck. The baby's eyes will close, his fists will relax, and his hands will come away from his face. He may release the breast and let it slide out of his mouth. Allowing the baby to remove himself from the breast will ensure that he has received the high-fat hindmilk needed for optimal growth. The mother can then nurse him from the other breast until he self-detaches.

Hospital procedures and other practices that restrict feeding frequency and duration are detrimental to the initiation of breastfeeding. Limiting the time spent on a breast may result in the baby's receiving foremilk from both breasts and becoming too full to obtain a significant amount of hindmilk from either breast. This type of high-volume, low-fat feeding can result in poor weight gain and colic-like symptoms. As the baby matures, he will become more efficient at extracting milk, and the time spent at the breast will usually decrease. Flexibility on the mother's part will allow for variations in the baby's nursing style, hunger, and daily temperament.

Unlimited suckling time beginning directly after birth improves breastfeeding (Philippe, 2003). One group of women studied was on a timed regimen that began with three minutes on each breast and increased gradually to ten minutes over the next four days. The other group of women nursed for any length of time they wished. When interviewed at six weeks, 80 percent of the second group was still breastfeeding, compared with only

57 percent of the timed group. There were ten percent fewer cases of breast engorgement in the untimed group and no significant differences in the incidence of nipple problems between the groups (Slavein, 1981).

Until breast tissue becomes accustomed to suckling, mothers may experience some initial nipple discomfort that usually peaks between the third and sixth day postpartum. Decreasing the time or frequency of feedings will not prevent this tenderness. Nipple soreness results primarily from improper positioning of the baby at the breast. The best insurance against soreness is holding the baby with his body facing the mother and bringing him to the breast in a position that does not stress the end of the nipple. Using these techniques, the mother can be comfortable nursing for as long as her baby requires.

Frequency of Feedings

During the first month, feeding frequency for a healthy, fully developed baby may range from 8 to 14 feedings daily. Most babies require at least 8 to 10 feedings. The baby who nurses more frequently may nurse as often as every one to two hours, with nighttime feedings spaced farther apart. The AAP states, "In the early weeks after birth, nondemanding babies should be aroused to feed if four hours have elapsed since the beginning of the last feeding" (AAP, 2005). When it is clear that the baby is gaining weight well and breastfeeding more than eight times during a 24-hour period, the mother need not wake her baby at night.

It is common for a baby to feed as often as every hour or hour and a half during the day or several times during the night. Every baby's needs are different. Encourage mothers to remain flexible to meet their babies' requirements. You can reassure parents by having them look at their baby's feeding pattern over the course of a day. For example, a mother whose baby has gained well, has breastfed ten times during the daytime, had six clear, heavy wet diapers, and three to five ample stools can relax if he sleeps longer that night and can enjoy her extra rest! Help mothers learn to watch their babies rather than clocks.

By eight to twelve weeks of age, a baby has usually developed a pattern of feeding every two to three hours, sometimes less often during the night. The longer nighttime stretch may alternate with a period of almost constant wakefulness and suckling at some other time of the day, generally the early evening. These are referred to as clustered or bunched feedings. As the baby matures and becomes a more efficient breastfeeder, he will obtain more milk in a shorter period and will begin to space his feedings farther apart.

Increases in Feeding Frequency

A mother may periodically notice an increase in the frequency with which her baby wishes to feed. All babies experience periods of sudden growth during their early months. They react to these growth spurts by feeding more frequently. Such periods of increased feedings usually last only a few days. Growth spurts can occur at any time, although there are predictable ages. Mothers who have established a robust supply of milk through frequent breastfeeding in the early postpartum days easily carry through during these times of feeding frequency until the growth spurt has passed (Dewey, 1991).

First Days at Home

A baby whose feedings were restricted during the hospital stay may nurse more frequently when allowed to establish his own routine. At home, he may feel overstimulated by eager parents or siblings and turn to nursing for comfort. He may react to the dramatic difference between the hospital environment (his first extrauterine experience) and his home, particularly at night. Although home births have better health and breastfeeding outcomes for infants, babies can still feel overstimulated by excited family members.

10 to 14 Days

At about 10 to 14 days, the baby experiences his first growth spurt and he will want to nurse more often. It is around this time that the mother also loses the initial fullness in her breasts. She may worry that increased feedings and smaller breasts indicate that her milk production is dwindling. Anticipatory guidance will help avoid concerns that would cause her to question her ability to nourish her baby. Teaching parents to expect increased frequency in the baby's hunger around this time will help forestall concerns of low milk production. In the United States, samples of artificial baby milk will predictably arrive on parents' doorsteps. Formula manufacturers obtain expectant and new parent information from direct marketing firms and mailing lists sold to them by retail stores, parent magazines, and other sources (Walker, 2001). They aggressively target mailing of "free" formula to coincide with the two-week growth spurt to take advantage of mothers' concerns at this stage.

Three to Six Weeks

In addition to a second growth spurt that occurs at around three to six weeks, the baby may nurse more often in response to an increase in his mother's activity level. By six weeks, mothers often resume many or all of their prepregnant activities, including a return to work or school. The increase in activity may lead to a drop in milk production. The baby's response is to nurse more frequently to rebuild the supply. He may go to the breast more frequently to reassure himself that his mother is still available to him.

Three and Six Months

As the baby continues to grow, he will periodically nurse more frequently to increase milk production to meet his needs. These growth spurts typically occur at about three and six months. The mother may incorrectly interpret these increased feedings as a sign of her baby's readiness to begin solid foods. Again, anticipatory guidance will prevent mothers from misinterpreting this increase in feeding frequency.

Other Times of Increased Feedings

Times of illness, overstimulation, emotional upset, or physical discomfort may cause a baby to turn to the breast for security and comfort. You can help the mother through these times by reminding her that babies nurse for comfort as well as for nutrition. Remind her that when a baby is sick she produces antibodies to the virus and passes these antibodies back to the baby. Breastfeeding is the only time in a mother's life when she will be able to protect her baby in this unique way. Being able to comfort her baby at the breast is one of the marvelous benefits of breastfeeding.

Mothers who nurse in response to their babies' cues may not even notice growth spurts. Often, however, mothers are aware of fussiness in a previously contented baby, a baby who wants to nurse more frequently than usual, or a baby who has suddenly begun to nurse more vigorously. You can prepare the mother for these events before they occur, so that such incidents do not undermine her confidence or cause her to consider early weaning. Reassurance, support, and a listening ear can be pivotal to a mother who finds herself with a fussy baby who requires a lot of attention. Encourage her to respond to her baby's needs during this growing time.

Decreases in Feeding Frequency

A mother often becomes concerned when her baby begins dropping feedings, especially if she has not yet begun giving him solid foods or other supplements. She may worry that he is not being nourished sufficiently if he had been nursing eight or nine times in 24 hours and suddenly drops to six or seven feedings. This schedule change is common when the baby reaches about three months of age. It is usually a result of his having become a more efficient nurser. He is able to obtain a greater amount of milk in a shorter period and can go longer between feedings. He may decrease the time he remains on the breast at a feeding as well, because he is able to obtain the milk he needs more quickly.

Encourage the mother to observe her baby's overall disposition and health. If he appears content, is voiding and stooling appropriately, is increasing his weight and body length, and has good skin tone, she will know he is well nourished and that there is no cause for worry. If, however, decreased feedings occur when the baby is unhealthy or has inadequate growth, advise the mother to consult her baby's caregiver immediately. You will need to assess her breastfeeding practices to help her make necessary adjustments.

Signs of Sufficient Milk

Mothers can watch for a number of signs that the baby is receiving enough milk. Sufficient urine output to soak at least six or more regular diapers by day four indicates adequate milk volume. This is in the absence of supplemental fluids. If super-absorbent diapers are used, the number of diapers may be less. After day four or five stooling also indicates adequate milk transfer. In the first month, the baby should stool three or more times daily. Parents should call their baby's practitioner any time in the first month when their baby does not have at least three yellow, seedy stools larger than a quarter per day.

As long as a baby is not typically placid or fussy, a pleasant disposition generally is a sign of adequate nourishment. A mother needs to understand that crying does not necessarily mean that her baby is hungry. She should be alert to other indications of adequate nourishment. Regular intervals of wakefulness, sleep, and feeding will reassure a mother that she is providing her baby with enough milk. Healthy skin tone and color, periods of alertness and engagement, and eye contact are other signs of proper nourishment.

An infant's growth pattern also is evidence that he is thriving on his mother's milk. The most obvious signs are fat creases in his arms and legs, and the baby filling out his clothing. The mother should look for increases in length and head size, as well as regular weight gain. It is common for a breastfed baby to experience an initial weight loss of up to seven percent of his birth weight during the first week of life. If feedings are restricted in the early days, this weight loss could be as high as ten or twelve percent. More frequent breastfeedings will help the baby regain his birth weight by day ten. This pattern is less pronounced in babies who nurse frequently from birth. These babies have less initial weight loss and more rapid weight gain. Assure a mother that her baby's removal of her milk will create the supply he needs.

▶ LEAKING

It is common for some women to experience milk leaking from their breasts during the first few weeks of breastfeeding. In most cases, leaking results from fullness in the breast or the mother's milk letting down. Leaking is a normal part of the process of breastfeeding. It may occur during a feeding from the opposite breast, directly before a feeding when the breasts are full, or if the mother misses a feeding entirely. The range of leaking is extremely variable from one woman to another.

For many women, milk leaking from the breast is an encouraging sign that their milk supply is plentiful and that their letdown reflex is functioning well. In most cases, leaking will subside as harmony develops between the baby's needs and the mother's milk production, usually by six weeks postpartum. Failure to leak milk is not an indication that milk production is low. Many women never experience leaking. An absence of leaking may indicate that the sphincter muscles within the nipple function well to close off the nipple pores. It is possible that a mother who does not leak is feeding more frequently and is therefore less prone leak.

Causes of Leaking

Leaking can be caused by overfull breasts, stimulation during lovemaking, overuse of breast shells, frequent milk expression, clothing that rubs against the nipples, overproduction of milk, or hormone imbalances. It may be a result of psychological conditioning of letdown. A woman may leak in response to hearing a baby cry, picking up her baby to nurse, or simply thinking about breastfeeding or her baby. Many women's breasts leak during sexual intercourse. Oxytocin releases during orgasm, which triggers the letdown reflex.

Controlling Leaking

Although women generally consider leaking to be a nuisance, they usually accept it as a part of breastfeeding and use appropriate measures to control it. Assure mothers that this phase of lactation passes quickly. Suggestions for controlling leaking are to:

◆ Wear breast shells between feedings or on the opposite breast during a feeding.

◆ Press the heel of her hand over the breast or cross her arms and press.

◆ Wear absorbent breast pads and change them often.

◆ Feed the baby before lovemaking and use absorbent towels over bedding.

◆ Decrease pressure on the breast and elastic in the bra cup; loosen the bra or wear a larger size.

◆ Discontinue practices that stimulate nerves in the nipple, such as clothing rubbing on the nipple, or holding or cuddling the baby in a particular manner.

◆ Express or pump milk when it is necessary to miss or delay a feeding.

◆ Wear dark, patterned clothing or a sweater to conceal moist spots.

◆ Check for the use of medications or herbs that stimulate milk production, and discontinue their use.

Excessive or Inappropriate Leaking

Occasionally, a woman's leaking is excessive, or she may experience leaking past the early weeks of establishing breastfeeding. Excessive leaking may be a sign of an imbalance in other body functions. In some women, milk production greatly exceeds the baby's needs. In others, leaking continues after the baby weans or occurs at times unrelated to birth or breastfeeding. Such milk production post-weaning is termed galactorrhea, also referred to as **spontaneous lactation**.

Inappropriate milk production in a nonlactating breast may be due to the use of medications such as thyrotropin-releasing hormones, theophyllines, amphetamines, or tranquilizers (MacFarlane, 1977). Chest or breast surgery, a fibrocystic breast, or herpes zoster may stimulate nerves enough to induce milk production significantly. In some cases, a woman's body may be especially sensitive to normal levels of prolactin. If no underlying disorder is found through medical examination, special efforts should be made to decrease breast stimulation.

Galactorrhea is a symptom, not a disease. It may indicate an underlying health problem that causes elevated prolactin levels (**hyperprolactinemia**). Possible causes of hyperprolactinemia are hypothyroidism, hyperthyroidism, psychosis and anxiety medications, chronic renal failure, pituitary tumors, and uterine and ovarian tumors. Abnormal lactation can occur in connection with surgery and stress related to such tumors.

Any unexplainable excessive milk flow during lactation, or milk production that continues beyond three to six months after the baby weans, is not normal. The woman should be encouraged to undergo a general physical examination. Infrequently, mothers may use medications to suppress lactation, but these medications are often only temporary measures. Generally, treatment of galactorrhea requires treating the underlying cause (Lawrence, 1999).

▶ NIPPLE SORENESS

Although sore nipples occur with relative frequency, they are not a normal part of breastfeeding. Initial tenderness, or transient nipple soreness, is part of the typical postpartum course for the majority of mothers. Women often describe it as tenderness with the initial latch and first few sucks (Cable, 1997). The peak periods of nipple tenderness occurs in the first week postpartum, particularly between the third and sixth days (Ziemer, 1990). It is possible that this period of tenderness is associated with the breast adjusting to the frequency of use in breastfeeding or to hormonal changes postpartum. It is common for mothers to experience nipple tenderness during their menstrual cycles and with new pregnancies.

Pain is a sign that something is not right within the body. This applies to nipple pain during breastfeeding as well. Nipple pain requires investigation if it occurs beyond the transient soreness of the first week or lasts after the first few sucks following attachment. It can constitute a breastfeeding emergency because it is a common reason for early weaning (Sheehan, 2001). Nursing on a sore nipple is similar to painful friction on a scraped knee or knuckle. Untreated, nipple pain can progress to the development of a crack. The crack offers a portal of entry for bacteria and yeast that are present on the skin surface and may lead to infection. The increased severity of pain when untreated may decrease a woman's desire to put her baby to breast. This, in turn, may lead to engorgement, reduced milk production, and premature weaning.

Causes and Prevention of Nipple Soreness

Myths abound regarding the cause of nipple soreness. A long-held belief that a baby left too long on the breast would cause soreness led to time restrictions for early feedings. Quite to the contrary, restriction of feedings only prolongs the onset of soreness. Such restrictions also interfere with the baby's regulation of milk production (Renfrew, 2000). Women previously learned to toughen their nipples prenatally with the hope of avoiding soreness, an unpleasant and unnecessary practice that damages nipple skin (Woolridge, 1986). There was also a theory that fair-skinned women are prone to nipple soreness. However, they do not experience soreness at greater rates than other women (Hewat, 1987). You can give mothers correct information if they receive any of this outdated advice (often from older relatives or older healthcare providers).

Positioning and Attachment

Two of the most common causes of nipple soreness are poor position and attachment at the breast. Prenatal education needs to emphasize correct positioning and attachment. Postpartum caregivers need correct information regarding assessment of latch and positioning. Maternity policies need to reflect this as well. Prevention should focus on proper positioning of both mother and baby. Blair (2003) found that more optimal latching, including rooting, gaping, sealing, and sucking behavior, were slightly related to lower levels of reported pain, although a more defined study is needed.

The baby needs a deep, slightly off-center or asymmetrical latch, with a mouthful of breast tissue rather than just the nipple. Positioning presents a problem when the baby's body is not in alignment with his head or when his head is not facing the breast. "Nipple to nose" is a great catch phrase to aid a mother in optimal alignment. This refers to aligning the nipple with the baby's nose so the mother can brush his upper lip with her nipple and the baby will aim up and not down. Nursing is difficult for the baby when he does not face the breast and must swallow with his head turned to the side or tipped too far back. (You can alert mothers to this misalignment by asking them to imagine swallowing water with their head turned to one side.) The mother's breast undergoes extra tension and negative pressure exerted by a poor position.

Poor latch is frequently evident after the introduction of an artificial nipple from a bottle or pacifier. The mechanism of suck on a bottle nipple is very different from suckling at the breast. The rate of flow is much faster, even with "slow flow" nipples. The baby's suckling controls milk flow unless the mother's letdown is strong. Conversely, milk flows from the bottle until the baby stops it. When mothers combine breastfeeding and bottle-feeding, it often produces an unenthusiastic and incorrect suck when the baby returns to the breast. Artificial nipples should be avoided in the early days of breastfeeding unless used therapeutically (Kassing, 2002; Wilson-Clay, 2002) or unless a bottle is the only alternative feeding device parents will accept.

Other Factors

Nipple pain can result from nipple shape, engorgement, and improper use of breast pumps or nipple shields. Breast and nipple skin can be tender from thrush (see Color Plate 33), impetigo, or eczema (ILCA, 2002). Psoriasis (see Color Plate 34), herpes (see Color Plate 35), and poison ivy (see Color Plate 36) can damage the skin. Bacterial infection is common (Livingstone, 1996), and sensitivity to topical ointments can occur.

Nipple pain can result from anomalies in the infant's oral structure, such as ankyloglossia, a short tongue, or a high or bubble palate. These anatomical differences can create difficulty with suckling. Clenching and compressing the nipple is common with near-term, SGA, LBW, and **postmature** babies, due to thin cheeks and sparse buccal fat pads. A very eager nurser combined with minimal milk flow in the first day or two may lead to pain, as can a mother pulling her baby off the breast without first breaking suction.

Strong pain due to sucking pressure beyond the first four or five days when mature milk should be in might indicate the mother has low milk flow. The baby is working with all his might, but there is no meal there! The center of the mother's nipple will often appear to have a "hickey" when this has happened. Another infant response is to clamp down if the mother has a strong letdown. The baby may compress the nipple and areola to try to stop the overwhelming gush of milk. Sometimes the baby will slide down onto the nipple, or come off the breast, choking or sputtering.

Assessment of Sore Nipples

The assessment of nipple soreness requires an in-person visit to determine the cause and suggest appropriate measures. As with any other condition, it is important to note the age of the baby and when the soreness began. The mother's description of how the pain feels and at what times it feels a certain way can yield clues to the cause. Ask open-ended questions to elicit descriptive adjectives from the mother. "Burning" pain may indicate thrush. "Throbbing" may indicate mastitis. Pain upon exposure to cold may indicate **Raynaud's phenomenon.** Note any chronic conditions of the mother, as well as medication usage. Ask about the use of soaps, creams, lotions, laundry products, and perfumes, especially in terms of recent product changes. Nipple soreness may also develop when the baby begins teething, or when the mother begins menstruating or becomes pregnant. Your assessment should address these milestones.

Level of Soreness

Descriptors many lactation professionals use for nipple soreness include such terms as *cracked*, *macerated*, and *abraded*. Mohrbacher (2004) proposes a grading scale for identifying the severity of nipple trauma, similar to terms used in the medical field for other types of anomalies. Table 16.1 presents four stages of nipple trauma, ranging from a superficial and intact nipple to one that has deep damage throughout the dermis. These descriptors may help lactation professionals quantify the severity of nipple damage in much the same way they use descriptors to evaluate a breastfeeding. The descriptors will clarify whether the skin is broken and, if so, how deep the damage occurs.

Note the appearance of the nipple before the feeding. If you observe signs of infection (angry red streaks, swelling, pus), refer the mother to her caregiver right away. Have the mother attach the baby and nurse briefly. It is essential to see the baby's attachment and positioning during a feeding. You need to observe the baby's alignment and closeness to the breast, the mother's position, and the mouth-breast connection, as described in Chapter 14. After the baby has suckled for a few minutes, ask the mother to remove him from the breast and examine the nipple. Blanching and/or flattening of the nipple are clues to poor latch, as are the nipple looking like an "orthodontic" nipple, with the top rounded, but the bottom flattened.

If the mother reports that she ends feedings, rather than allowing the baby to self-detach, observe her technique. Pulling her baby off the breast without breaking suction can cause nipple pain and damage the skin. Visually assess the baby's oral cavity, paying close attention to the tongue, palate, and frenulum. If no obvious cause can be found by observing the feeding, a digital exam of the baby's oral structure should be done. Explaining to the parents what you are assessing is reassuring (see Chapter 21). Also explain the reasons for allowing the baby to end feedings.

Treatment and Plan of Care

If positioning appears to be the cause of nipple soreness, help the mother make the necessary adjustments. The baby should be level with and facing the breast, and his body should be aligned with his head. If the mother

TABLE 16.1

Scale of Nipple Pain and Trauma

Stage	Type of Wound	Description	Could Include
Stage I	Superficial intact (see Color Plate 37)	Pain or irritation with no skin breakdown noted	Redness, bruising, red spots, or edema
State II	Superficial with tissue breakdown (see Color Plate 38)	Pain with some tissue breakdown noted	Abrasion, shallow crack or fissure, compression stripe, blister, hematoma, or shallow ulceration
State III	Partial thickness erosion (see Color Plate 39)	Skin breakdown with destruction of the epidermis to the lower layers of the dermis	Deep fissure or deep ulceration with more advanced erosion
Stage IV	Full thickness erosion (see Color Plate 40)	Deeper damage throughout the dermis	Could include full erosion of some parts of the nipple

Printed by permission of Nancy Mohrbacher, IBCLC, *Nipple Pain and Trauma: Causes and Treatment*, June, 2004.

has been using only one position and has developed soreness, using another position can provide relief to the sore area. The mother's body position is also important. If she does not adequately support her baby's head, he may bite down reflexively. If her arms tire during a feeding, the baby may not remain level with the breast and slip down. He may then exert more pressure on the nipple or slide to the nipple base.

Correcting Latch

The baby's latch must consistently be correct in order for him to transfer milk, as well as for the mother's comfort. The baby's mouth should open wide and optimally should be slightly off-center from the nipple. Since only the lower jaw moves, positioning his mouth so that he takes in more of the underside of the nipple will help compress the ducts most effectively. To encourage the baby to open wide, the mother can hold him in a position that allows gravity to aid him, such as the football hold. Babies mimic facial expressions of others, so the mother can demonstrate a wide-open mouth for him and repeatedly say "o . . . p . . . e . . . n" as he works to latch on. This is useful for a baby who "chews" his way onto the nipple. His lips should flange outward, and his mouth should have a wide angle when he begins sucking. The mother needs to watch for correct lip placement and help her baby flange either or both lips when needed.

Babies who bite at the breast often respond well to prone positioning, chin support, or **sublingual** pressure (gentle pressure under the chin). Jaw clenching can cause nipple **vasospasms** (constriction of blood vessels within the nipple), identified by pain and blanching of the nipple. The mother can work with her baby to establish a good latch to avoid this. There are now helpful video clips demonstrating correct latch techniques at breastfeeding Web sites (see partial list in Appendix A).

Vasospasms

Vasospasms of the nipple during breastfeeding create a Raynaud-like phenomenon. Mothers describe the pain as stinging, tingling, burning, very painful, and persisting after the feeding. This phenomenon is characterized by a triphasic color change: the nipple turns white (blanches), then turns blue (cyanotic), and then turns red (rubor) (Anderson, 2004; Lawlor-Smith, 1997). Raynaud's is a common condition that affects up to 22 percent of women 21–50 years of age (Olsen, 1978). Some mothers with nipple vasospasms report the pain also occurs when exposed to cold. Pain in the extremities when exposed to cold is a marker for Raynaud's phenomenon.

Treatment for vasospasm includes avoiding cold and applying heat to the nipples after a feeding. Caffeine and nicotine constrict blood vessels and have been shown to increase the severity of Raynaud's. Therefore, removing caffeine from her diet may bring relief. Increasing the mother's intake of vitamin B_6 has helped some mothers. However, high doses, such as 600 mg, can lower milk production. Additionally, B_6 passes readily into mother's milk, and too much can harm an infant's liver (Hale, 2004). Hale suggests not consuming more than 25 mg/day. Calcium channel blockers, such as nifedipine, have been helpful for some mothers (Hale, 2002). The Hale text also contains dosing protocols for the caregiver. For some mothers, your validation that their nipple pain is abnormal and has a cause is a big relief. See Chapter 25 for further discussion of Raynaud's.

Ankyloglossia

Ankyloglossia, or tongue-tie, is a common cause of breastfeeding pain (see Color Plate 15). If the **lingual** frenulum is too tight and the tongue is unable to extend over the lower lip, the frenulum may need to be clipped (Messner, 2003, 2000; Ballard, 2002). The labial frenum on the upper lip (see Color Plate 16) could also be tight and cause problems (Zeretzke, 2004; Wiessinger, 1995). Refer the mother to the baby's caregiver for further assessment and treatment.

Treating Other Causes of Soreness

If the cause of nipple pain is dried milk sticking to the mother's bra or breast pads, she can moisten the fabric before removing them. If the mother has been pulling her baby off the breast without releasing suction, she can learn to break suction with her finger between the baby's gums before removing him. When her soreness is relieved, she needs to understand the importance of allowing her baby to determine when to end the feeding. Pain connected to a retracted or inverted nipple may find relief from techniques that gently encourage eversion of the nipple, as described in Chapter 7.

Plan of Care

After identifying the cause of nipple pain, it is important to institute a plan for **palliative care** (care that provides a measure of pain relief). The mother needs suggestions for immediate physical comfort. She can place ice in a wet cloth and apply the cloth to her nipples prior to a feeding. (Make sure she does not place the ice directly on her skin.) Starting a feeding with the least sore breast first, initiating the milk ejection reflex before putting the baby to breast, and eliminating prolonged nonnutritive (comfort) sucking at the breast are other measures to relieve the mother's discomfort. For the duration of nipple soreness, the mother can gently remove her baby from the breast when she notices he is no longer actively feeding and has not yet released the breast.

Alternate massage will help sustain sucking and swallowing and relieve long periods of negative pressure. In alternate massage, the mother massages and compresses the breast each time the baby pauses during a feeding. If the mother is unable to tolerate any sucking at all, she can pump her milk with a quality electric breast pump while she heals and provide her milk to her baby with an alternative feeding method. Some mothers find an anti-inflammatory such as ibuprofen helpful, if it is approved for use by the mother's caregiver.

Alternating Breastfeeding Positions

Teaching the mother various nursing positions can help alleviate nipple soreness. In order to avoid further irritation to a sore spot, she can keep the baby's chin, and thus his tongue, away from that area. Thinking of her breast as a clock can help the mother describe the location of the soreness. In turn, you can suggest nursing positions to minimize further irritation. Figure 16.1 illustrates the relationship between the most common nursing positions and the resulting sore spots. Other positions, such as with the mother and baby lying down with the baby's feet pointing above the mother's head, will also provide relief for the mother and distribute stress more evenly. (See Chapter 15 for discussion of various nursing positions.)

Topical Creams and Ointments

Research is mixed on the results of using topical agents on sore nipples. Many practitioners recommend that the mother apply her expressed milk to the sore area and allow for air-drying of the areola. Mothers should first consider whether they need to adjust their positioning and latch technique before using topical creams. Additionally, they should avoid any topical

agents that need to be removed before a feeding. A mother sometimes will need to remove dead tissue from the skin, referred to as *debriding* (Wilson-Clay, 2002). Unnecessarily removing topical agents can further aggravate any existing nipple damage.

It is important to read research with a critical eye before recommending any clinical practice. Some topical agents that are suggested for sore nipples actually delay healing time, cause possible irritations or allergies (ILCA, 2002), and contain harmful substances such as the pesticides found in regular lanolin. Oils, including vitamin E, do not facilitate moist wound healing. The oil stays on the surface of the skin and does not provide moisture for healing (Huml, 1994). Increased serum concentrations of vitamin E were present in breastfed babies 6 days after ingesting milk from their mothers who were using topical vitamin E on their nipples (Marx, 1985). This is a cause for concern because high doses of Vitamin E can cause liver damage (Hale, 2004).

Hypoallergenic, medical-grade anhydrous, or modified, lanolin has been encouraged for use on sore nipples for many years. The allergens and impurities of regular lanolin are removed, and modified lanolin has been found to "provide a semi-occlusive moisture barrier that slows down internal moisture loss without clogging the pores, thus acting as a moist wound healer" (Huml, 1994). However, modified lanolin has been found to have an insignificant effect on nipple pain or damage during days one to five postpartum (Spangler, 1993).

Brent (1998) found lanolin and breast shells were more effective and had a lower rate of infection than hydrogel pad use. One study analyzed the use of 3 comfort measures in alleviating nipple pain: USP-modified lanolin, warm water compresses, and the mother's expressed milk with air-drying. It found no significant

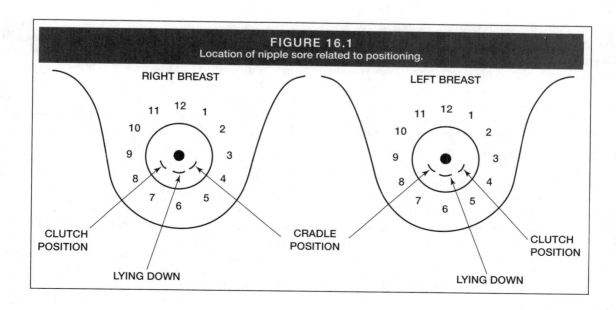

FIGURE 16.1
Location of nipple sore related to positioning.

RIGHT BREAST

LEFT BREAST

CLUTCH POSITION

CRADLE POSITION

CLUTCH POSITION

LYING DOWN

LYING DOWN

differences in pain intensity, pain affect, or duration of breastfeeding (Pugh, 1996). While modified lanolin may not be appropriate for routine use in all mothers, it may be a perceived benefit to some mothers.

In the 1990s and early 2000s, studies emerged suggesting that hydrogel dressings helped mothers with sore nipples by providing "moist wound healing" (Cable, 1997; Ziemer, 1995). Brent's study (1998) had found such high rates of infection with gel pads that their use was discontinued. A newer study comparing the use of lanolin and hydrogel pads found that 8 mothers in the lanolin group had breast infections, with no infections reported in the hydrogel group. There was no difference in the duration of breastfeeding between the two groups (Dodd, 2003).

The advent of any new technology or product can be tempting to view as a "quick fix." There is no substitute for your time, clinical judgment, and education of the mother on the basics of optimal latch-on and positioning for comfortable nursing. If pain persists, validate the mother's concerns and do not minimize her perceptions of pain. Some mothers may find an ointment or pad comforting, while others will prefer not to use them. Your experience will help you become proficient at discerning the difference. Table 16.2 summarizes the treatment options for sore nipples.

Interruption of Breastfeeding

When treatment fails to provide relief, some mothers prefer to stop breastfeeding for several feedings or even a few days in order to preserve long-term breastfeeding. When a mother experiences an interruption in breastfeeding, she will need to use a hospital-grade electric breast pump to maintain milk production. She can double pump for about 15 minutes every 2 to 3 hours, closely matching her baby's feeding frequency. Some mothers find a small amount of olive oil dabbed on the flange before pumping can lessen the pulling on the areola within the flange and make pumping more comfortable. The pump should be on the lowest suction at the beginning to avoid pain. As her condition improves, she can increase the suction setting, although stronger suction does not necessarily produce better results. See Chapter 21 for further discussion of breast pumps.

To avoid nipple preference during this time, the mother can feed her baby by a method that does not involve bottles. When resuming breastfeeding, the baby should nurse at the breast when the mother feels ready. Depending on how quickly her nipples heal and on how well the latch and suckle have been improved, she can put the baby to breast for every second or third feeding. She can then increase the frequency of feedings at the breast as tolerated. Encourage the mother to maintain a lot of skin-to-skin contact during this time. This will ensure that the baby continues to associate her smell and skin with nurture and nourishment.

Cracked Nipples

When soreness persists, a crack or fissure may develop, appearing either crosswise or lengthwise along the nipple (see Color Plate 41). Infrequently a woman's nipple may fold over, causing a stress point at the fold. Bleeding may result during nursing when the baby stretches the nipple to 2 times its resting length. If the baby receives a significant amount of blood, he may vomit or have black stools. The baby's caregiver may want to interrupt breastfeeding for a short time to rule out internal bleeding. If the baby has black stools or vomits blood because of the cracked nipples, the symptoms will cease when he stops nursing.

When the integrity of the nipple skin has been compromised, the open wound is a pathway for bacteria. It is important for the mother to cleanse her nipples. She may benefit from an antibacterial ointment such as mupirocin or polysporin, just as she would for a scraped knee or other open sore. Encourage the mother to ask her caregiver for a recommended topical ointment. Figure 16.2 presents a compounded ointment for nipples that has found wide acceptance in Canada and the United States. Most compounding pharmacies have become proficient in preparing this ointment, available by prescription. The combination presented here gives a total volume of approximately 30 grams. Clotrimazole powder to a final concentration of 2 percent may be substituted if miconazole powder is unavailable (Newman, 2003a). If other methods of healing are ineffective, the mother may wish to interrupt breastfeeding for a couple of days until her nipples heal. She needs to express her milk during that time. Table 16.3 summarizes the treatment options for cracked nipples.

▶ CANDIDIASIS

A yeast infection usually develops from *Candida albicans*, a fungal organism commonly found in the mouth, gastrointestinal tract, and vagina of healthy persons. Under normal conditions, the body's flora keeps *candida's* growth in check. Predisposing factors that may disturb the normal flora and lead to yeast infection include diabetes, illness, pregnancy, oral contraceptive use, poor diet, antibiotic therapy, steroid therapy, and immunosuppression. In addition, local factors such as obesity or excessive sweating provide consistently warm, moist areas in which *Candida* can thrive (Amir, 1995).

While *Candida* does not normally appear on skin such as the nipple, it may be present during lactation. Yeast on the nipples has been associated with nipple damage early in lactation, mastitis, recent use of antibiotics in the postpartum period, long-term antibiotic use before pregnancy, and vaginal yeast infection (Amir, 1991). In one study, nearly two-thirds of mothers with

TABLE 16.2
Causes and Treatment of Sore Nipples

Causes	Actions for the Mother
Soreness from newborn suckling	◆ Check to ensure that baby is put on and comes off breast properly. ◆ Check to ensure that nipple is back far enough in baby's mouth. ◆ Hold baby closely during nursing so nipple is not being pulled. ◆ Use pure anhydrous lanolin or hydrogel pad as a temporary comfort measure.
Dried colostrum or milk causing nipple to stick to bra or breast pads Poor positioning	◆ Moisten bra or pads before taking off so as not to remove keratin. ◆ Bring baby close to nurse, so he does not pull on breast. ◆ Bring baby to breast so that he has a big mouthful of breast tissue.
Baby chewing or nuzzling onto nipple	◆ Form nipple for baby. ◆ Set up pattern of getting baby onto breast, using rooting reflex.
Baby nursing on end of nipple	◆ Ensure that baby is positioned properly at breast. ◆ Check for tight frenulum. ◆ Check for inverted nipple. ◆ Check for engorgement.
Baby chewing his way off nipple or nipple being pulled out of baby's mouth at end of feeding	◆ Remove baby from breast by placing a finger between baby's gums to ensure suction is broken. ◆ End feeding when baby's sucking slows, before he begins to chew on nipple.
Baby overly eager to nurse	◆ Respond to feeding cues promptly. ◆ Pre-express milk to hasten letdown and avoid vigorous sucking.
Inadequate letdown	◆ Use massage and relaxation before feedings. ◆ Condition letdown by setting up routine for getting baby onto breast.
Nipples not allowed to dry	◆ Check for leaking milk. ◆ Check that there are no plastic liners in breast pads. ◆ Eliminate synthetic fabrics in bra and clothing; wear cotton or cotton blends. ◆ Air dry breasts after feedings. ◆ Change breast pads frequently.
Improper use of nipple shield	◆ Use shield only to draw nipple out, then have baby nurse on breast. ◆ Avoid shields with inner ridges that irritate nipples.
Inadequate milk supply; baby tugging or sucking on empty breast	◆ Nurse more frequently (every 1 to 1½ hours). ◆ Nurse long enough to facilitate good milk production.

(continued)

TABLE 16.2 (CONTINUED)

Causes and Treatment of Sore Nipples

Causes	Actions for the Mother
Nipple skin not resistant to stress	◆ Improve diet, especially adding fresh fruits and vegetables and vitamin supplements. ◆ Eliminate or decrease use of sugary foods, alcohol, caffeine, and cigarettes. ◆ Check for use of cleansing or drying agents.
Natural oils being removed or keratin layers broken down by drying agents such as soap, alcohol, shampoo, or deodorant	◆ Eliminate irritants. ◆ Wash breasts with water only. ◆ Use lanolin or hydrogel pads after air drying.
Nipple irritated by going braless under rough clothing or by rubbing against bra during vigorous exercise	◆ Wear a bra or change to one with more support (sports bra). ◆ Wear softer fabric blouse.
Residue of laundry products present on clothing	◆ Use less detergent, and rinse wash loads twice. ◆ Try different laundry products.
Teething causes increased feedings, chomping down on nipple, irritation by a change in baby's saliva or medication used for baby's gums	◆ Wash breast after every feeding in plain warm water to remove baby's saliva or other irritants. ◆ Breastfeed before giving solid foods rather than after. ◆ Use soothing techniques instead of nursing to comfort baby. ◆ Stop feeding after the first incident of biting and resume when baby is more hungry. ◆ Keep finger ready to break suction and stop feeding when sucking pattern changes.
Baby falls asleep and clamps down on breast	◆ Remove baby before he falls asleep.
Teeth marks on breast (not usually cause for soreness but mother may say baby is biting)	◆ Alternate nursing positions.
Irritation from food particles in toddler's mouth	◆ Check toddler's mouth before feedings. ◆ Offer toddler a sip of water or wipe his mouth with clean moist cloth before nursing. ◆ Breastfeed before offering solid foods.
Mother menstruating or pregnant	◆ If menstruating, discomfort will last only a few days. ◆ If pregnant, discuss plans for continued nursing or weaning.
Thrush (a yeastlike infection; see discussion thrush)	◆ Have physician check and prescribe medication for both of mother and baby. ◆ Discard or boil any items that baby puts in his mouth.

TABLE 16.3
Cracked Nipples

Causes	Actions for the Mother
All causes of sore nipples carried to extreme	◆ Consult physician about using ibuprofen, acetaminophen, or other painkiller. ◆ Improve nutritional status, increasing protein, vitamin C, and zinc. ◆ Refer to actions for sore nipples.
Nipple folds over (crack may appear at fold)	◆ Air dry breasts after feeding.
Local infection (baby with staph or other organism may have infected mother's nipples)	◆ Have physician check nipples, culture baby's throat and mother's nipples, and treat accordingly.
Baby overly eager at feedings	◆ Respond to feeding cues promptly. ◆ Limit nursing times to 10 minutes per breast until nipple heals. ◆ Pre-express milk to hasten letdown. ◆ Nurse in a position that does not aggravate crack.

FIGURE 16.2
Jack Newman's all-purpose nipple ointment.

Mupirocin 2 percent ointment (not cream): 15 grams
Betamethasone 0.1 percent ointment (not cream): 15 grams
To which is added miconazole powder so that the final
   concentration is 2 percent miconazole
Sometimes it is helpful to add ibuprofen powder as well, so that
   the final concentration of ibuprofen is 2 percent.

vaginal yeast infections transmitted the infection to their infants (von Maillot, 1978). The baby contracts oral yeast as he passes through the birth canal and, in turn, transfers the infection to the mother's nipple when he breastfeeds. Preterm infants or infants in the NICU for other physical problems are prone to *Candida* infection (Kaufman, 2004; Chapman, 2003; Benjamin, 2000). For this population *Candida* can be fatal.

A yeast infection that occurs in the baby's mouth is thrush. Thrush presents as white patches that look like milk curds, as illustrated in Color Plate 42. The mother will not be able to wipe the patches off, which is how she can distinguish it from milk in her baby's mouth. In the diaper area, yeast may present as a raised, very red area with a sharply defined border. Babies with a yeast infection often seem to be gassy and fussy. Symptoms of vaginal yeast are usually difficult to miss. The vaginal area and vulva are tender and very red, with intense itching. There may also be a cheesy, white vaginal discharge.

Yeast on the nipple does not always present with visual symptoms. It is unusual to see white patches or redness on the nipple, although it is possible (see Color Plate 33). The most obvious symptom is usually breast and nipple pain. When a mother presents with severely sore nipples after a period of pain-free breastfeeding, a yeast infection may be the cause. Mothers often describe the pain as intense and burning, radiating through the breast during or after feedings. Lawrence (1999) describes it as "feeling like hot cords burning in their chest wall".

Mothers may not be able to tolerate the feel of clothing on the nipple or the spray of water during a shower. They may feel a stinging sensation deep within the breast ducts and may have pain between feedings. Sometimes the areola will have a very shiny, pinkish cast, easily detected with a small flashlight or other focused beam of light. Clinicians have observed a break in the skin similar to a positional compression stripe at the base of the nipple shank where the nipple joins the areola. There may also be some very slight edema noted in the areola (Berens, 2004).

One study comparing yeast in breastfed and artificially fed infants found that *Candida* species were much less frequent in infants who were predominantly breastfed than in those who were bottle-fed. However, yeast was much more frequent on the breasts of lactating women (Zollner, 2003). The lower incidence of yeast among breastfed babies in spite of the mothers' cultures may be because human milk is fungistatic (Andersson, 2000).

Treatment of a Yeast Infection

When a mother has yeast on her nipples, her baby often has oral thrush. The reverse is also true. It is imperative that both the mother and the baby receive treatment simultaneously, even if only one of them exhibits visible symptoms. In addition to the baby's mouth and mother's nipples, any other sites of infection need treatment as well. This includes the diaper area and vagina, as well as other family members who harbor the infection. It is important to follow the full course of treatment even after symptoms subside. A yeast infection recurs very easily. In one case, six weeks of treatment were necessary (Bodley, 1997).

Treatment Options

The strain of yeast on the mother's nipples and the baby's mouth can be different from that found in a diaper rash. Many strains of yeast are resistant to the common medications. Various treatment regimens exist for both oral and nipple yeast. Antifungal topical agents used to treat yeast include nystatin, clotrimazole at one percent, miconazole nitrate at two percent, ketoconazole at two percent, ciclopirox at one percent, and naftifine hydrochloride. Although nystatin is often the first treatment suggested, the other topicals are more effective (Huggins, 1993; Lawrence, 1999). Clotrimazole and miconazole are available over the counter, and the others require a medical prescription.

The usual treatment of oral yeast infection in the baby is to rinse his mouth with water after breastfeeding, shake and pour nystatin into a cup, and apply it to all surfaces of the baby's mouth with a cotton swab. The swab should never be dipped back into the original vial of nystatin. The mother can rinse her nipples with a solution of one cup of plain, tepid water and one tablespoon of vinegar, and air-dry them. She can then apply the antifungal cream sparingly so it soaks in by the time she is ready to feed again. It does not need to be washed off the nipple. She should change breast pads at every feeding (Amir, 1995). Air drying and brief exposure of the breasts to sunlight or artificial light may be helpful, since yeast thrives in dark, moist environments.

Gentian violet is a very effective treatment for both oral and nipple yeast infection. It is available over the counter and should be 0.5 percent solution (Huggins, 1993). The mother dips a cotton swab in the gentian violet and swabs the baby's mouth. When the baby latches onto the breast, the mother's nipple is treated by direct contact. Some clinicians advise that the mother swab both of her breasts once a day as well. Newman recommends applying gentian violet to the mother's breasts once daily for several days. The mother should discontinue use of gentian violet when the pain subsides. If her pain continues, she can use it for up to a total of seven days (Newman, 2003b). Caution mothers that

ulceration of the mucous membranes in the baby's mouth may result with excessive use or with strengths higher than 0.5 percent (Huggins, 1993).

Exercise caution in how you discuss treatment options with mothers unless you have a medical license that includes prescriptive privileges. It is helpful to describe the treatments for yeast as a continuum. The lowest level of treatment includes home remedies such as rinsing the mother's nipples and exposing them to sunlight. The next level includes over-the-counter options such as topical antifungals and gentian violet. Farther along on the continuum are the powerful, systemic antifungals such as fluconazole and ketoconazole, which require a prescription.

The mother should be encouraged to discuss treatment options with her own and her baby's caregivers, particularly with persistent cases that do not respond to conventional topical medications. The protocol for breastfeeding candidiasis outlined in *Clinical Therapy in Breastfeeding Patients* (Hale, 2002) may be helpful for the mother's healthcare provider. If the nipple soreness persists, referral to a dermatologist may be appropriate. Although culturing the breast for yeast has been difficult in the past, a new technique offers promise for more precise measurement (Morrill, 2003).

Stopping the Spread of Yeast

Further considerations during the course of yeast treatment focus on family hygiene. Good hand washing before and after diapering, using the toilet, or breastfeeding will help stop the spread of yeast. Anything that comes in contact with the mother's breast, such as a bra, breast shells, or breast pump parts, needs to be boiled once a day for at least 20 minutes. These items are vehicles for reinfection, and boiling kills the *Candida*. The same is true for anything that has contacted the baby's mouth, such as a pacifier, bottle nipple, or teething ring. The mother should discard bottle nipples, pacifiers, and teethers after one week. Toys should be cleaned thoroughly with hot soapy water, and all of the family's clothing should be laundered in very hot water (Zeretzke, 1998).

The mother's diet can also be a factor in a persistent yeast infection. She may need to decrease dairy products and sugars while increasing her intake of acidophilus, garlic, zinc, and B vitamins (Baumslag, 1992). If the mother is pumping, she can feed her fresh milk to her baby but not frozen milk, since freezing will not kill *Candida* (Rosa, 1990). There is debate among lactation specialists as to whether giving previously frozen milk with *Candida* in it will reinfect a healthy baby. Lawrence states, "Freezing pumped breastmilk while infected with *Candida* does not kill the fungus. The milk must be pasteurized or discarded" (Lawrence, 1999). To pasteurize, the mother can heat the frozen milk for about 20 minutes at a slow boil in a double boiler or steamer so there is no direct contact with the water.

ENGORGEMENT

At birth, delivery of the placenta triggers a reduction in the woman's progesterone levels that helps stimulate the production of mature milk. Increased amounts of blood and lymph circulate in the breast and are the source of nutrients for milk production. Enlarged blood vessels are often visible beneath the skin of the lactating breast. These fluids cause the breasts to become fuller, heavier, and sometimes tender. Color Plate 43 shows a normally full breast. With unlimited, exclusive breastfeeding, this normal fullness diminishes. By about 10 days postpartum, when lactation is fully established, the breasts become comfortably soft and pliable, even when they are full of milk.

Engorgement, on the other hand, is a serious condition. It is important to distinguish between it and the normal postpartum fullness. Engorgement is essentially *over*fullness that occurs when the mother fails to remove milk adequately or frequently enough from the breast. Engorgement is **iatrogenic**, caused by medical interference with the natural process in the form of regulations, schedules, and poor management of lactation. Sometimes engorgement results from the mother having received IV fluids in the hospital, which can create edema in her feet and ankles as well (see Figure 12.2 in Chapter 12). If the duct system does not clear of colostrum sufficiently before milk begins to accumulate after delivery, pressure produces breasts that feel firm, hard, tender, and warm or hot to the touch. The skin may appear shiny and transparent, as in Color Plate 44. The nipples may flatten and, in extreme cases, can be indistinguishable from the rest of the breast. Table 16.4 characterizes four stages of breast fullness when describing engorgement (Kutner, 1996).

A mother can experience engorgement at any time during lactation when milk is not removed regularly. The most common time for engorgement to occur is in the early days, when breastfeeding is beginning and feeding patterns are irregular. Engorgement can develop when the baby begins sleeping through the night and whenever the mother and baby miss feedings because of separation. It is a risk during the weaning process, especially if rapid weaning is necessary. Encourage mothers to remove milk from their breasts whenever they have a feeling of fullness, before they become uncomfortable. Figure 16.3 illustrates the causes and results of engorgement.

Consequences of Engorgement

Engorgement creates serious problems with milk production. Breast tissue elasticity allows milk storage for up to 48 hours before the rate of milk production and secretion begins to decrease rapidly. When milk remains longer, the pressure on alveoli and ducts increases. This, in turn, decreases the flow of blood and lymph within the breast. Consequently, fewer nutrients become available to make milk. The possibility of infection increases because the lymphatic system does not remove bacteria at a normal rate.

Engorgement presents a danger of permanently harming breast tissue. The increased milk pressure can cause some alveolar cells and myoepithelial cells to shrink and die off. This atrophy of milk-producing cells can permanently compromise the milk-producing ability of the breast for that particular breastfeeding experience. The **suppressor peptide**—feedback inhibitor of lactation (FIL)—in human milk has a negative effect on milk production if the milk remains in the breast for extended periods. Suppressor peptides are inhibiting peptides in human milk that bring about the cessation of milk secretion during milk stasis and engorgement. Unrelieved severe engorgement can cause insufficient milk production (Knight, 1998; Wilde, 1998). These mothers and babies need close follow-up.

Engorgement adversely affects the mother's letdown mechanism. The flattened nipple of the engorged breast becomes difficult for the baby to grasp. He therefore may not stimulate the nerves within the nipple and areola sufficiently, and letdown may not occur. Without letdown, the baby cannot remove milk from the breast efficiently. Pressure then increases in the ducts even more. When engorgement causes flattening of the nipples, the baby can grasp only the ends of the nipples. This often results in sore, cracked nipples, which can further inhibit letdown.

TABLE 16.4	

Four Stages of Breast Fullness

Stage	Definition
+1	Breasts are soft. Milk flows freely.
+2	Breasts are firm and nontender. Milk flows freely.
+3	Breasts are firm and tender. Milk release is slow and relief is obtained quickly.
+4	Breasts are hard and painful. Milk release is slow and relief is not obtained quickly.

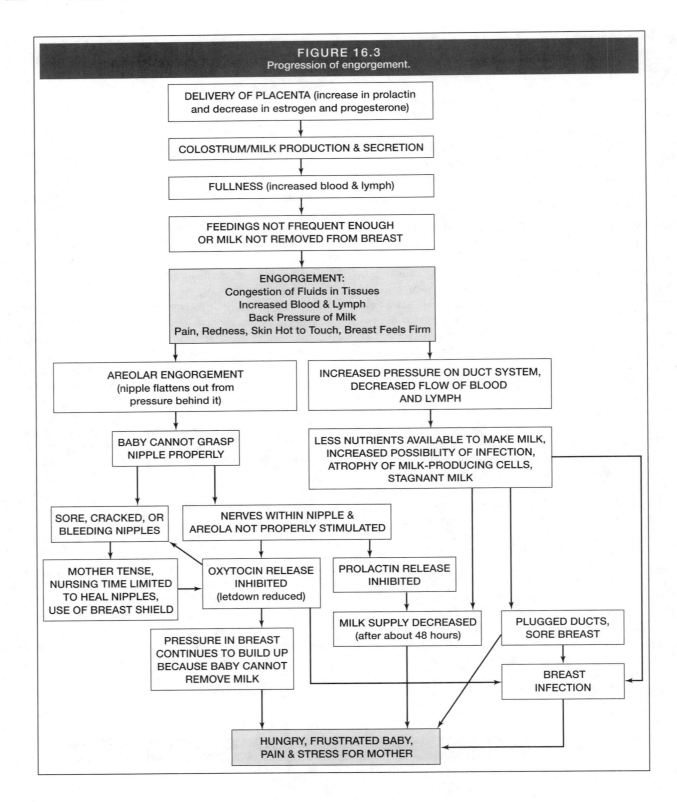

FIGURE 16.3
Progression of engorgement.

Preventing Engorgement

The practices promoted in Chapter 12 offer preventive measures for engorgement. Initiating breastfeeding within the first hour of life sets the stage for the prevention of problems. When mothers and babies remain together 24 hours a day, the mother becomes familiar with her baby's feeding cues and learns to act on them. Breastfeeding in response to baby cues for as long as the baby needs must be encouraged as the norm. Eight or more feedings in 24 hours, including night feedings, will keep milk flow paced with production. If breast fullness increases, the mother can be encouraged to wake her baby and put him to breast for relief. For times when the baby is very sleepy and not nursing adequately, mothers need to know how to express their milk. Each mother and baby must be assessed for correct latch and positioning. If latch and positioning are not correct, it may lead to decreased milk removal. Parents should avoid the use of artificial nipples, which do not promote efficient suckling and may confuse the baby when he returns to the breast. Education of maternity staff, midwives, and doulas must focus on these key areas for the postpartum period. Minimizing interference with breastfeeding is often the best prevention of engorgement.

Helping Mothers Relieve Engorgement

Treating engorgement involves a combination of identifying and correcting the cause and offering palliative measures. Engorgement can be a frightening experience for a mother. It is helpful for her to know it is temporary, and that engorgement usually is resolved within 24 to 48 hours with proper treatment. If the mother has been limiting feedings with respect to either frequency or duration, encourage her to breastfeed at least every two hours or sooner if her baby desires and to allow him to nurse as long as he needs. After the engorgement is resolved, advise the mother to nurse her baby at least eight times in every 24-hour period. Gentle **breast compression** helps the mother drain the breast more completely (Newman, 2000). If breastfeeding alone does not reduce the engorgement, she may need to express milk between feedings. (See the following guidelines for pumping.)

If engorgement has progressed to the degree that the baby is unable to latch onto the breast, the mother can express milk before a feeding to soften the areola. Suggest that she express milk in the shower, as water spraying on the mother's back and shoulders will help to relax her. Reverse pressure softening, described in Chapter 21, has been helpful for some mothers in softening the areola and enabling the baby to latch on (Cotterman, 2004). Cold compresses applied between feedings will help decrease the mother's discomfort. A frozen pack of vegetables such as peas or corn works well because it conforms to the shape of the breast. The mother can refreeze them for reuse, making this an easy and affordable compress. The mother may also lie flat on her back to elevate the breasts and help reduce swelling. Cabbage leaves worn inside the bra provide a simple remedy that many mothers use.

Guidelines for Pumping When Engorged

With appropriate guidelines, pumping or hand expressing for engorgement will preserve the mother's milk production. Pumping for engorgement is usually necessary for only 24 to 48 hours. Continuing to pump beyond that time could maintain the mother's milk production at a level that is higher than needed. A double pump will pump both breasts at the same time, which is especially important if the breasts feel hard and there is poor milk release.

If engorgement occurs in only one breast, the mother does not need to pump the other one. Single pumping is appropriate when there is +2 or +3 engorgement and the baby is still able to nurse (see Table 16.4 for definitions). If the areola is firm or hard, the mother will need to pump before nursing. She should pump only long enough to soften the areola so that the baby can latch on easily and not cause nipple trauma. The mother should then put her baby to breast to nurse. Following the feeding, she can pump her breast again if needed. If milk removal was easy and the mother heard her baby gulping, she need only pump until the milk stops flowing quickly. If she heard only periodic swallowing, she should pump for at least ten minutes after the feeding. If the milk continues to flow quickly at the end of ten minutes, she should continue to pump until it slows.

If the mother pumps only one breast at a time, she can use her other hand to massage the breast while she is pumping. She can apply cabbage leaves or ice packs to her breasts between feeding and pumping sessions. She will want to stop the pre-feed pumping as soon as possible. She can then pump after nursing only when necessary. Reassure the mother that very soon she will be able to discontinue pumping, relax, and enjoy her baby.

The Use of Cabbage for Engorgement

The use of fresh green cabbage leaves to treat engorgement is not a new phenomenon. *The Glory of Woman*, published in 1896, describes the application of fresh, young cabbage leaves to the "gathered" breast. An article in 1988 was instrumental in reviving the practice (Rosier, 1988). It may be that **phytoestrogens** present in cabbage contribute to reducing swelling in the tissues. Cabbage is effective on other parts of the body for swelling caused by sprains and strains. Many mothers have had positive results from the use of cabbage for reducing edema in breast engorgement and inflammation caused by plugged ducts and mastitis. Some mothers use prolonged applications of cabbage to wean or to suppress lactation. Folklore has it that farmers were careful to keep their cows out of the cabbage patch because consumption of cabbage decreased milk production.

Roberts (1995b) found that mothers reported significantly less pain with using cabbage, either chilled or room temperature, than before treatment. There may be a psychological value for the mother who uses alternative treatments such as cabbage (Ayers, 2000). A large Cochrane review states, however, that three different studies using cabbage leaves or cabbage leaf extracts found no overall benefit (Snowden, 2001). The review concluded that prevention of engorgement should

TABLE 16.5

Treatment Options for Engorgement

Causes	Actions for the Mother
Missed or infrequent feedings	◆ Room in with baby in the hospital. ◆ Breastfeed baby 10 to 12 times each 24 hours, or more if he is willing, around the clock. ◆ Watch baby for feeding cues, and respond to them. ◆ Use rousing techniques for sleepy baby. ◆ Increase skin-to-skin contact to encourage baby to nurse. The mother can remove her shirt and bra, and hold her baby with only a diaper on. ◆ Pump breasts or hand express any time baby is unwilling or unable to nurse.
Milk removal not adequate at feedings	◆ Check that baby's latch and position are appropriate. ◆ Stop the use of all artificial nipples. ◆ Increase skin-to-skin contact during feedings. The mother can remove her shirt and bra and hold baby with only a diaper on. ◆ Do breast compression during feedings to encourage baby to suckle. ◆ Pump breasts or hand express *after* the feeding with a hospital-grade electric breast pump only to remove the milk that flows quickly and easily. ◆ Pump breasts *between* feedings for comfort, if necessary, only as long as the milk flows quickly and easily.
Inadequate letdown due to edema and pain	◆ Relax in warm shower with water running over back, avoiding the breasts, and hand express to relieve fullness. ◆ Breastfeed *after* the breast has softened enough to allow baby to latch on. ◆ Use relaxation techniques and gentle breast massage during feedings. ◆ Lie flat on back between feedings to elevate breasts. ◆ Apply cool packs to the breasts and under arms. ◆ Apply green cabbage leaves to breasts.

remain the key priority. Anecdotally, at least, cabbage helps many women, and mothers will benefit from knowing how to use it.

Application of Cabbage to the Breast

To use cabbage for the relief of engorgement, the mother places cabbage leaves on her breasts and holds them in place with her brassiere (see Color Plate 45). The procedure for applying cabbage is simple. After discarding the outer leaves, pull off several leaves, wash them, pat them dry, and crush them slightly to break up the veins. Place the leaves on the engorged breasts and hold them in place with a bra. The remainder of the cabbage can be stored in the refrigerator and remain chilled for later use.

After a short period, women will sometimes report that their breast feels "different"—sometimes described as tingly and cool. When the mother feels this sensation, when milk begins to leak, or when there is evidence of softening of the tissues, she can remove the cabbage. She can then put her baby to breast, or pump if the baby still cannot latch on. With severe engorgement, the cabbage will actually wilt because of the heat of the breast. The mother can apply fresh leaves about every 2 hours for about 20 minutes. As soon as the baby or pumping provides the needed relief, the mother should discontinue the use of cabbage. To dry up the milk completely, as in sudden weaning or suppressing lactation, the mother leaves cabbage on her breasts around the clock, changing it as needed until milk production ceases.

The amount of relief experienced by women varies. Some will get relief in as little as 20 to 30 minutes. Others may need to apply the cabbage over a period of 24 hours. In some cases, the decrease of edema is so pronounced that the milk ducts will stand out in bold relief on the breast after the cabbage is removed. Cabbage helps women with plugged ducts and mastitis as well. The mother washes and crushes it and applies it to the plug or the area where the mastitis inflammation is evident. She leaves it on the breast until she obtains relief. There are no reports of untoward effects from the cabbage (Roberts, 1995a, 1995b). Table 16.5 presents treatment options for engorgement.

PLUGGED DUCT

Sometimes a plug forms in a duct, consisting of cells and other milk components shed within the ducts. A plugged duct causes localized soreness, swelling, lumpiness, or slight pain. The localized pain is not accompanied by a symptom in any other part of the body, such as fever or flu-like symptoms (which could indicate a breast infection).

Plugs may be absorbed quickly by the body and not appear in the milk. A plug that releases and comes out with the milk may be brownish or greenish in color, as well as thick and stringy (see Color Plate 46). The mother can remove it manually with no ill effects. Although the baby may reject the milk with the plug due to the taste or texture, most babies easily return to nursing afterward. There is no known danger to the baby.

Causes of Plugged Ducts

The cause of a plugged duct is incomplete milk removal or outside pressure on specific areas of the breast. Any practice that inhibits free flow of milk in the ducts can create pressure. The source could be a tight or underwire bra, bunched-up clothing under the arm, or a baby sling. It may be from consistently holding, carrying, or rocking the baby in the same position. Sleeping in a position that puts pressure on the breast or pressure from a breast pump flange can also lead to a plugged duct.

Treatment of Plugged Ducts

Plugs can be broken up and worked down the ducts by regular frequent feedings and hand massage in the direction of the plug toward the nipple. Moist heat over the area of the plug may help move it along the duct. Plugs can also be encouraged to move by rotating the baby's position for feedings so that his tongue stimulates more milk flow in the area of the plug. Beginning a feeding on the breast with the plug will help with removal by taking advantage of the baby's more vigorous suck early in the feeding.

Lawrence (1999) found that consuming lecithin and reducing saturated fats in their diets helped women prevent recurring plugged ducts. The recommended dosage of lecithin, an emulsifier, is one tablespoon three or four times a day, or one to two capsules (1200 milligrams each) three or four times a day. The measures listed earlier for releasing a plug are helpful, as well as the techniques in Table 16.6. Encourage the mother to make every effort to remove the plug quickly. A plugged duct can develop into a larger blocked-off area referred to as a *caked breast*. Left untreated, it could also develop into mastitis. Advise the mother to call her caregiver if a plug does not respond to treatment.

MILK BLISTER

Occasionally, milk clogs a nipple pore and causes a **milk blister**—also called a **milk bleb** or blocked nipple pore (see Color Plate 47). It is referred to as a bleb or blocked nipple pore when it is open. When the skin closes over the pore and forms a blister, it is referred to as a nipple blister or milk blister. Many healthcare providers use the terms interchangeably.

Milk blisters and blebs are intensely painful, because milk cannot flow from the duct and stays in the breast. This type of blister or bleb is very different from the sucking blisters some mothers experience in the early days. Some specialists believe that nipple blisters lead to plugged ducts; others believe that plugged ducts actually cause the blisters (Newman, 2000). Either way, they are terribly painful for most mothers who have them, and they can lead to mastitis because of milk stasis.

One method for removing a blister is for the mother to soak her nipple with a warm wet compress or in a comfortably hot bowl of water. Sometimes very gentle rubbing with a washcloth will remove the pore covering. The mother may even see the hardened plug of dried or crystallized milk come out. The mother can then nurse her baby, who may remove the plug through his suckling. If this works, the mother usually feels instant relief as the backed-up milk is removed (Watson-Genna, 2004). Soreness may remain for a few days.

The mother can use a topical antibiotic ointment to prevent infection of the blister. If the baby's suckling does not remove the plug, the mother's practitioner may open The blister or bleb with a sterile needle. The best time for this to be done is immediately after breastfeeding the baby. When the blister is opened in this manner, the backed-up milk will often stream out. Again, the mother usually feels immediate relief. Gentle breast compression will aid in draining the breast. Encourage the mother to breastfeed her baby very frequently and thoroughly on the affected breast to prevent recurrence.

	TABLE 16.6
	Treatment Options for a Plugged Duct
Causes	**Actions for the Mother**
Poor positioning	◆ Try a variety of positions for better milk removal. ◆ Nurse baby with his chin pointed toward the plugged duct.
Breasts overfull due to missed feedings, irregular nursing patterns, engorgement	◆ If prone to plugged ducts, avoid missed feedings or pump to remove milk. ◆ If baby does not adequately remove milk from the breasts, pump or express milk after feedings.
Incomplete removal of milk from the breast	◆ Nurse long enough on each breast for the baby to remove sufficient milk. ◆ If baby does not remove milk, pump or express milk after feedings. ◆ While nursing on affected side, use massage and heat to encourage drainage. ◆ Nurse more frequently on affected breast. ◆ Gently roll, pull, and rub plug down while in warm shower. ◆ Use moisture to remove any dried secretions blocking nipple pores.
External pressure on the breast	◆ Avoid positions that put pressure on one spot for long periods, e.g., always sleeping on one side, always holding the baby one way, or baby sleeping on mother's chest. ◆ Use larger nursing bra or a bra extender. ◆ Avoid bunching up sweater or nightgown under arm during a feeding. ◆ Use nursing bra instead of pulling up conventional bra to nurse in order to avoid pressure on ducts.

▶ MASTITIS

Mastitis is inflammation of the breast, usually (although not always) from bacterial infection. Infection can develop from a crack in the nipple skin that provides a pathway into the breast for *Staphylococcus* and other organisms. It is associated with milk stasis and engorgement and can result from a plugged duct that went unnoticed or untreated, or that failed to respond to treatment. The inflamed area of the breast becomes red, hot, and tender to the touch (see Color Plate 48). More than just a localized soreness, a breast infection usually produces fever and flu-like symptoms in the woman. Any time a breastfeeding mother feels flu-like symptoms, she needs to rule out the possibility of mastitis. If she has mastitis, she will want to begin treatment immediately in order to reduce the severity and protect her milk production.

The occurrence of mastitis varies considerably, according to the literature. In one study, mastitis developed in 12 to 35 percent of mothers with sore nipples who were not treated with systemic antibiotics, compared to 5 percent of mothers who were treated with systemic antibiotics (p < .005) (Livingstone, 1999). Another study found 9.5 percent out of 946 mothers had reported cases of mastitis (Foxman, 2002). Up to 20 percent of breastfeeding mothers experience mastitis in the first 6 months

of breastfeeding, with most incidents in the 2- to 3-week postpartum period (Hale, 2002). Many mothers may self-treat an infection and not seek medical treatment. A separate study, using the same cohort of 946 mothers, associated mastitis, breast or nipple pain, bottle use, and milk expression (pumping) in the first 3 weeks with weaning (Schwartz, 2002). Any mother who contacts you with symptoms of mastitis is at risk for weaning and needs immediate assistance.

Causes of Mastitis

The anticipatory guidance you give to mothers will alert them to times when breast infections are most likely to occur. Mastitis can occur during the newborn period, when the mother is more likely to be tired and her immunity lowered by pregnancy. While she establishes breastfeeding, any interruption in breastfeeding or change in nursing pattern can cause milk to remain in the ducts. An infection can also develop when the mother's time and energy become overextended, as with holidays, vacations, houseguests, family crises, or when the baby is ill.

Riordan (1990) noted that mothers ranked fatigue and stress as the most common conditions that preceded a bout of mastitis. Other factors identified in her survey include plugged ducts, change in feeding frequency, milk stasis (lack of flow), engorgement, sore or cracked nipples, an infection in the family, and trauma to the breast. The most frequent site of inflammation was the upper outer quadrant of the breast unilaterally, with near-equal distribution in the right and left breasts.

Breast infections most often result from bacteria in the baby's mouth or in the home environment. The Vancouver Breastfeeding Centre showed that when pain was moderate or severe and when cracks were present, mothers had a 54 percent chance of having an infection caused by *Staphylococcus aureus*, an easily transmitted bacterium of moderate virulence (Livingstone, 1996).

Because the infection probably came from the baby's mouth or her home, the mother is likely to have produced antibodies in her milk already. Most breast infections are located outside the ducts in surrounding breast tissue and do not enter the milk. Therefore, it is reasonably safe for the baby to nurse through an infection. The mother will need to continue nursing in order to remove milk. The baby's suckling removes milk much more effectively than a pump or hand expression does. Additionally, frequent feedings provide a cleansing effect on the breast, which can prevent milk stasis from developing (Melnikow, 1994). Some mothers report their baby rejects the infected breast, possibly because of a salty taste resulting from increased sodium and chloride levels (Lawrence, 1999). If the baby will not nurse on that breast, the mother needs to pump the affected breast to prevent stasis.

Treatment of Mastitis

Treatments for mastitis include efficient milk removal, warm moist compresses to the site of inflammation, anti-inflammatory medication, and antibiotics. Some clinicians have found relief from the application of cabbage leaves. Cabbage may work because it contains rapine, which some herbalists regard as an antifungal antibiotic (Lawrence, 1999). The mother needs total rest to help her body fight the infection. If she works outside the home, she might need to ask for a short sick leave.

When mastitis develops, an assessment of a feeding will ensure that the baby's latch provides adequate milk removal. Advise the mother to breastfeed as frequently as her baby desires and to express milk from the affected breast after every feeding. Soaking the affected breast in warm water for short periods facilitates blood flow and drainage. Having her baby begin a feeding on the affected breast will allow the baby's more vigorous suck to drain the milk better.

When it has been determined that a mother has a breast infection, advise her to contact her primary healthcare provider immediately. If she is running a temperature higher than 100 degrees and symptoms have not resolved within 24 hours, her caregiver will probably place her on antibiotic therapy for 10 to 14 days. In the absence of a fever, the caregiver may be willing to wait a few days to determine whether other measures are effective. Table 16.7 provides treatment suggestions relative to specific causes. The basic measures for treating a breast infection are:

◆ Heat—apply warm, moist compresses to the inflamed area before and during the feeding.

◆ Rest—get as much bed rest as possible.

◆ Remove milk from the breast—nurse the baby with his chin pointed toward the inflamed area.

◆ Breastfeed as often as possible—use of breast compression and massage may help drain the breast more effectively.

◆ Call the caregiver for an antibiotic—follow through on the entire regimen, even if the infection seems to clear quickly.

Recurrent Mastitis

Some mothers seem to be prone to mastitis. After a mother has recovered from a breast infection, advise her to be watchful for signs of recurring infection. She will want to be especially careful to remove milk regularly from her breasts. If she must miss a feeding, she will need to express her milk. Caution her against becoming overly tired or overworked. At the first sign of an infection or plugged duct, warm compresses, more frequent feedings, and bed rest will help to shorten the length of the infection.

If infection recurs within two months, the mother will need to see her caregiver. Many caregivers will prescribe over the telephone without seeing the woman. Over the past 50 years, staph has become more resistant to antibiotics, especially those that are penicillin-based. Methicillin-resistant *staphylococcus aureus* (MRSA) occurs more frequently now and requires much stronger antibiotics than those usually used to treat staph infection. MRSA occurs more commonly among people in hospitals and other healthcare facilities. It can also occur in the community and is associated with recent antibiotic use, sharing contaminated items, having active skin diseases, and living in crowded settings (CDC, 2003).

A culture of the mother's milk and nipple and the baby's throat will determine the appropriate antibiotic. This may be especially important if outbreaks of MRSA are common in your community. Two of the antibiotics used to treat MRSA, vancomycin and teicoplanin, are expensive. They may be toxic to patients and must be administered to the mother by intravenous infusion. Patients infected with MRSA require hospital treatment (AMM, 1995). Adding the oral antibiotic rifampin to

TABLE 16.7

Treatment Options for Mastitis

Causes	Actions for the Mother
Milk stasis: Poor milk removal from the breast	◆ Nurse as long as the baby desires. If breast is full after he is finished, express milk for relief.
Milk stasis: Breasts overfull due to missed feedings, irregular nursing pattern, or engorgement	◆ Avoid missed or delayed feedings. ◆ When feedings are delayed, pump or hand express to remove milk from breasts.
Overwork	◆ Rearrange priorities and daily schedule. ◆ Get help with tasks.
Low resistance to infection due to anemia, poor diet	◆ Improve diet. ◆ Exercise. ◆ Reduce stress.
Lack of adequate sleep; fatigue	◆ Take daytime naps or rest periods (sleep rebuilds the immune system). ◆ Nurse lying down. ◆ Take baby to bed at night.
Failure to clear a plugged duct	◆ Work plug down manually, if it is not too painful. ◆ Have baby nurse with chin pointed toward plug.
Infection via cracked nipple	◆ Eliminate non-nutritive sucking. ◆ Briefly soak breasts in saline solution (¼ tsp salt in 8 oz water) after feeding and air dry.
Infection passed from baby or other family member	◆ Treat primary infection in conjunction with mother's infection.

vancomycin treatment increases its efficacy (Hale, 2002). Table 16.7 describes some of the possible causes of mastitis and actions that will alleviate the infection.

Anemia or other deficiencies predispose some women to recurrent mastitis. Recurring episodes also can occur when the mother fails to respond to a particular antibiotic or does not follow the entire course of treatment. Sometimes a woman will stop taking an antibiotic after several days because she no longer has symptoms of an infection. However, without the complete regimen of antibiotic, the infection may not fully clear and instead recur as soon as her resistance lowers again. The bacteria may be resistant to the antibiotic she took. As discussed previously, the caregiver may need to culture the milk to determine the type of bacteria. Broader spectrum antibiotics may be necessary.

Mothers who experience recurrent mastitis should check for poor hygiene when handling of the breast as a possible source. The mother may want to evaluate her hygiene and overall health in terms of diet, rest, and exercise. She may need to reduce daily activities and commitments such as work, volunteer activities, and chauffeuring older children. She can work toward a more healthful and less stressed lifestyle, at least while she is breastfeeding. It is important for her family members to help.

If the mother lacks a support system among family or friends, help her find community resources. Many church groups offer meals for postpartum mothers and support groups for single parents. Neighborhood preteens may be available to assist with simple household chores for less money than an older teen would charge. Check around to find what private and government resources are available in your community so you are able to refer mothers who need help. Lack of support is a risk factor for postpartum depression. As a caregiver, you can do your part to form a safety net around mothers like these.

Abscessed Breast

An **abscess** is a localized collection of pus that forms from an infection that has no opening for drainage. In the breast, an abscess forms from an untreated breast infection or one that did not respond to treatment. The indications of an abscess are the same as for mastitis—fever, flu-like symptoms, nausea, extreme fatigue, and aching muscles. However, symptoms are less severe than with mastitis because the abscess is isolated from the rest of the breast. The infection site becomes red, swollen, and tender (see Color Plate 49). Occasionally, an abscess can occur in the absence of any systemic symptoms. If treatment does not resolve what seems to be a plugged duct within 48 hours, the mother needs to see her physician.

An abscess improperly treated with hydrogen peroxide resulted in an oxygen embolism in one woman (Agostini, 2004). Abscesses have also been associated with polyarthritis postpartum (Demetriadi, 2004). An abscess can be a serious health hazard that requires the mother to see her physician immediately for treatment.

The abscess usually is lanced and drained (see Color Plate 50). At the same time, the mother receives medication for the infection. She may be able to continue to nurse on one or both breasts. This will depend on the location of the abscess, the pain associated with it, and the medication her physician prescribed. If the mother is unable to nurse, she will need to express milk from the affected breast, or she may choose to wean from that breast.

If the mother wishes to continue breastfeeding on the affected breast, she can implement the suggestions in Table 16.7 for treating a breast infection. If she chooses to wean, let her know that many mothers practice one-sided nursing and produce sufficient milk for their baby. Whether she weans from the affected breast only or totally weans her baby, she will need to do it slowly to avoid another infection. Abscesses occur in about five to ten percent of mastitis cases (Hale, 2002). Mothers can prevent them with appropriate breastfeeding management and immediate treatment of mastitis. Abscesses can occur in non-lactating women as well (Berna-Serna, 2004).

▶ SUMMARY

You can provide much reassurance and assistance to breastfeeding women in the early weeks. Discussing common breastfeeding expectations can ease the mother through this time of great change. By being available to her when difficulties arise and providing support and guidance, you can be the catalyst for her reaching her breastfeeding goals. The anticipatory guidance you provide for early breastfeedings, care of the breast, and leaking will avoid unnecessary concern for her. Educating her about prevention and treatment of nipple soreness, engorgement, thrush, plugged ducts, and mastitis will make it less likely that these problems will arise. If they

do occur, giving mothers appropriate treatment options will help to prevent a prolonged occurrence or recurrence. You can help achieve consistency among caregivers in their approach to these events by educating them and being available as a resource.

▶ CHAPTER 16—AT A GLANCE

Applying what you learned—

Counseling the mother:

◆ Help her prioritize her baby's needs.

◆ Boost her confidence.

◆ Point out positive things about her baby.

Teach mothers that:

◆ Limiting time at the breast does not prevent nipple soreness.

◆ Use of artificial nipples can create nipple preference.

◆ Poor positioning is the major cause of sore nipples.

◆ Babies may breastfeed every 1–2 hours (8–14 feedings) in the early days.

◆ Water supplementation should not be given to breastfeeding infants.

◆ Formula supplementation is appropriate only if medically indicated.

◆ Most medications are safe for breastfeeding, but check with caregiver first.

◆ The baby needs sufficient time at each breast to remove both foremilk and hindmilk.

◆ Regular frequent feedings will maintain milk production.

◆ The baby should determine when a feeding ends.

◆ Tight frenulum, tight frenum, short tongue, and palate shape may affect suckle.

Teach mothers about:

◆ Risk factors of infant formula.

◆ Key times for increases and decreases in feeding frequency.

◆ Signs of sufficient milk transfer.

◆ Correct positioning and attachment.

◆ Importance of alternating breastfeeding positions.

◆ Causes and treatment of recurrent mastitis.

Teach mothers how to:

◆ Count wet and dirty diapers; note the baby's disposition during and between feedings, and other growth indicators.

◆ Control leaking.

◆ Prevent and treat nipple soreness.

◆ Apply topical creams and ointments.

◆ Handle an interruption in breastfeeding due to soreness.

◆ Check for and treat thrush in the baby and yeast on the nipples.

◆ Stop the spread of yeast.

◆ Identify, avoid, and treat engorgement, plugged ducts, and mastitis.

◆ Use gentle breast compression to drain the breast.

◆ Prevent a breast abscess.

▶ **REFERENCES**

Agostini A. Oxygen embolism after hydrogen peroxide irrigation of a breast abscess. *Gynecol Obstet Fertil* 32(5):414–415; 2004.

American Academy of Pediatrics (AAP). Policy Statement on Breastfeeding and the Use of Human Milk. *Pediatrics* 115(2):496–506; 2005.

Amir L, Hoover K, Mulford C. Candidiasis and breastfeeding. *LLLI Lactation Consultant Series, Unit 18*. Garden City Park, NY: Avery Publishing; 1995.

Amir L. Candida and the lactating breast: Predisposing factors. *J Hum Lact* 7:177–181; 1991.

Anderson J et al. Raynaud's phenomenon of the nipple: A treatable cause of painful breastfeeding. *Pediatrics* 113(4):e360–e364; 2004.

Andersson Y et al. Lactoferrin is responsible for the fungistatic effect of human milk. *Early Hum Dev* 59(2):95–105; 2000.

Association of Medical Microbiologists (AMM). *The Facts about MRSA*. London; 1995. Available at www.amm.co.uk/newamm/files/factsabout/fa_mrsa.htm. Accessed December 12, 2004.

Ayers J. The use of alternative therapies in the support of breastfeeding. *J Hum Lact* 16(1):52–56; 2000.

Ballard J et al. Ankyloglossia: Assessment, incidence, and effect of frenuloplasty on the breastfeeding dyad. *Pediatrics* 110(5):e63; 2002.

Baumslag N, Michels D. *A Woman's Guide to Yeast Infections*. New York: Pocket Books; 1992.

Benjamin D et al. When to suspect fungal infection in neonates: A clinical comparison of *Candida albicans* and Candida parapsilosis fungemia with coagulase-negative staphylococcal bacteremia. *Pediatrics* 106(4):712–718; 2000.

Berens P. *Breast Complications While Breastfeeding*. La Leche League of Texas Area Conference, San Antonio, TX; June 12, 2004.

Berna-Serna J, Madrigal M, Berna-Serna J. Percutaneous management of breast abscesses: An experience of 39 cases. *Ultrasound Med Biol* 30(1):1–6; 2004.

Blair A et al. The relationship between positioning, the breastfeeding dynamic, the latching process and pain in breastfeeding mothers with sore nipples. *Breastfeed Rev* 11(2):5–10; 2003.

Blythe R et al. Effect of maternal confidence on breastfeeding duration: An application of breastfeeding self-efficacy theory. *Birth* 29(4):278–284; 2002.

Bodley V, Powers D. Long term treatment of a breastfeeding mother with fluconazole-resolved nipple pain caused by yeast: A case study. *J Hum Lact* 13:307–311; 1997.

Bottorff J. Persistence in breastfeeding: A phenomenological investigation. *J Adv Nurs* 15:201–209; 1990.

Brent N et al. Sore nipples in breast-feeding women: A clinical trial of wound dressings vs. conventional care. *Arch Pediatr Adolesc Med* 152(11):1077–1082; 1998.

Budin P. Le Nourisson, Paris: Octave Doin; 1900 (Malony WJ, transl): *The Nursling: The Feeding and Hygiene of Premature and Full-Term Infants*, Lecture 3. London: Caxton Publishing Co; 1907. Available at: www.neonatology.org/classics/nursling/nursling.html.

Cable B et al. Nipple wound care: A new approach to an old problem. *J Hum Lact* 13:313–318; 1997.

Centers for Disease Control and Prevention (CDC). *MRSA–Methicillin Resistant Staphylococcus Aureus Fact Sheet*; March 7, 2003. Available at: www.cdc.gov/ncidod/hip/Aresist/mrsafaq.htm. Accessed May 30, 2004.

Chapman R. Candida infections in the neonate. *Curr Opin Pediatr* 15(1):97–102; 2003.

Cotterman K. Reverse pressure softening: A simple tool to prepare areola for easier latching during engorgement. *J Hum Lact* 20(2):227–237; 2004.

Daly S et al. Degree of breast emptying explains changes in the fat content but not fatty acid composition of human milk. *Exp Physiol* 78:741–755; 1993.

DeCoopman J. Breastfeeding after pituitary resection: Support for a theory of autocrine control of milk supply? *J Hum Lact* 9:35–40; 1993.

Demetriadi F, Steuer A, Hall A. Post-partum polyarthritis associated with a staphylococcal breast abscess. *Rheumatology* (Oxford) 43(6):810–811; 2004.

Dewey K et al. Maternal versus infant factors related to breast milk intake and residual milk volume: The DARLING study. *Pediatrics* 87:829–837; 1991.

Dodd V, Chalmers C. Comparing the use of hydrogel dressings to lanolin ointment with lactating mothers. *JOGNN* 32(4): 486–494; 2003.

Fawzi W et al. Maternal anthropometry and infant feeding practices in Israel in relation to growth in infancy: The North African Infant Feeding Study. *Am J Clin Nutr* 65(6): 1731–1737, 1997.

Foxman B et al. Lactation mastitis: Occurrence and medical management among 946 breastfeeding women in the United States. *Am J Epidemiol* 155(2):103–114; 2002.

Gromada K. *Mothering Multiples: Breastfeeding & Caring for Twins or More.* Schaumburg, IL: La Leche League International; 1999.

Hale T, Berens P. *Clinical Therapy in Breastfeeding Patients.* Amarillo, TX: Pharmasoft Publishing; 2002.

Hale T. *Medications and Mothers' Milk.* Amarillo, TX: Pharmasoft Publishing; 2004.

Hewat R, Ellis D. A comparison of the effectiveness of two methods of nipple care. *Birth* 14:41–45; 1987.

Huggins K, Billon S. Twenty cases of persistent sore nipples: Collaboration between lactation consultant and dermatologist. *J Hum Lact* 9(3):155–160; 1993.

Huml S. Moist wound healing for cracked nipples in the breastfeeding mother. *Leaven* 29(1):2–6; 1994.

International Lactation Consultant Association (ILCA) (Walker M ed). *Core Curriculum for Lactation Consultant Practice.* Sudbury, MA: Jones and Bartlett; 2002.

Kassing D. Bottle-feeding as a tool to reinforce breastfeeding. *J Hum Lact* 18(1):56–60; 2002.

Kaufman D. Fungal infection in the very low birthweight infant. *Curr Opin Infect Dis* 17(3):253–259; 2004.

Knight C, Peaker M, Wilde C. Local control of mammary development and function. *Rev Reprod* 3(2):104–112; 1998.

Kroeger M, Smith L. *Impact of Birthing Practices on Breastfeeding.* Sudbury, MA: Jones and Bartlett; 2004.

Kutner L. *Lactation Management Course.* Chalfont, PA: Breastfeeding Support Consultants Center for Lactation Education; 1996.

Lawlor-Smith L, Lawlor-Smith C. Vasopasm of the nipple: A manifestation of Raynaud's phenomenon. *BMJ* 314:644–645; 1997.

Lawrence R. *Breastfeeding: A Guide for the Medical Profession.* Philadelphia, PA: CV Mosby; 1999.

Leff E et al., Maternal perceptions of successful breastfeeding. *J Hum Lact* 10(2):99–104; 1994.

Livingstone V et al. Staphylococcus aureus and sore nipples. *Can Fam Physician* 42:654–659; 1996.

Livingstone V, Stringer J. The treatment of Staphyloccocus aureus infected sore nipples: A randomized comparative study. *J Hum Lact* 15(3):241–246; 1999.

Lothian J. It takes two to breastfeed: The baby's role in successful breastfeeding. *J Nurse Midwife* 40:328–334; 1995.

MacFarlane A. *The Psychology of Childbirth.* Boston, MA: Harvard University Press; 1977.

Marx CM et al. Vitamin E concentrations in serum of newborn infants after topical use of vitamin E in nursing mothers. *Am J Obstet Gynecol* 152:668–670; 1985.

Melnikow J, Bedinghaus J. Management of common breastfeeding problems. *J Fam Pract* 39:56–64; 1994.

Messner A et al. Ankyloglossia: Incidence and associated feeding difficulties. *Arch Otolaryngol Head Neck Surg* 126(1): 36–39; 2000.

Messner A et al. Ankyloglossia: Does it matter? *Pediatr Clin North Am* 50(2):381–397; 2003.

Mitoulas L et al. Variation in fat, lactose and protein in human milk over 24 h and throughout the first year of lactation. *Br J Nutr* 88(1):29–37; 2002.

Mohrbacher N. *Nipple Pain and Trauma Algorithm.* Libertyville, IL: Hollister; 2004.

Morrill J et al. Detecting *Candida albicans* in human milk. *J Clin Microbiol* 41(1):475–478; 2003.

Newman J, Pitman T. *The Ultimate Breastfeeding Book of Answers.* Roseville, CA: Prima Publishing; 2000.

Newman J. Handout #3b. *Treatments for Sore Nipples and Sore Breasts.* January 2003a. Available at: www.breastfeedingonline. com. Accessed June 23, 2004.

Newman J. Handout #6. *Using Gentian Violet.* Revised January 2003b. Available at: www.breastfeedingonline.com. Accessed December 29, 2004.

Noble E, Sorger L. *Having Twins and More: A Parent's Guide to Multiple Pregnancy, Birth, and Early Childhood,* 3rd ed. Boston, MA: Houghton Mifflin; 2003.

Olsen N, Nielson S. Prevalence of primary Raynaud's phenomenon in young females. *Scand J Clin Lab Invest* 37:761–776; 1978.

Philippe B et al. Sustained breastfeeding rates at a US baby-friendly hospital. *Pediatrics* 112(3 Pt 1):e234–e236; 2003.

Pugh L et al. A comparison of topical agents to relieve nipple pain and enhance breastfeeding. *Birth* 23(2):88–93; 1996.

Renfrew M et al. Feeding schedules in hospitals for newborn infants. *Cochrane Database Syst Rev* (2):CD000090; 2000.

Righard L et al. Breastfeeding patterns: Comparing the effects on infant behavior and maternal satisfaction of using one or two breasts. *Birth* 20:182–185; 1993.

Riordan J, Nichols F. A descriptive study of lactation mastitis in long-term breastfeeding women. *J Hum Lact* 6(2):53–58; 1990.

Riordan J. *Breastfeeding and Human Lactation,* 3rd ed. Sudbury, MA: Jones and Bartlett Publishers; 2004.

Roberts K et al. A comparison of chilled cabbage leaves and chilled gel paks in reducing breast engorgement. *J Hum Lact* 11(1):17–20; 1995a.

Roberts K et al. A comparison of chilled and room temperature cabbage leaves in treating breast engorgement. *J Hum Lact* 11(3):191–194; 1995b.

Rosa C et al. Yeasts from human milk collected in Rio de Janeiro, Brazil. *Rev Microbiol* 21(4):361–363; 1990.

Rosier W. Cool cabbage compresses. *Breastfeed Rev* 1(12):28–31; 1988.

Schwartz K et al. Factors associated with weaning in the first 3 months postpartum. *J Fam Pract* 51(5):439–444; 2002.

Sheehan D et al. The Ontario mother and infant survey: Breastfeeding outcomes. *J Hum Lact* 17(3):211–219; 2001.

Slaven S, Harvey D. Unlimited suckling time improves breastfeeding. *Lancet* 1(8210):392–393; 1981.

Snowden HM, Renfrew MJ, Woolridge MW. *Treatments for Breast Engorgement during Lactation* (review). Cochrane Database of Systematic Reviews, The Cochrane Library. Oxford: Update Software. MIRU No: 2001.29; 2001.

Spangler A, Hildebrandt E. The effect of modified lanolin on nipple pain/damage during the first ten days of breastfeeding. *Int J Childbirth Ed* 8(3):15–18; 1993.

Tarrant M et al. Becoming a role model: The breastfeeding trajectory of Hong Kong women breastfeeding longer than 6 months. *Int J Nurs Stud* 41(5):535–546; 2004.

Uvnas-Moberg, K. The gastrointestinal tract in growth and reproduction. *Scientific American* 261:78–83; 1989.

von Maillot K et al. Candida mycosis in pregnant women and related risks to the newborn. *Mykosen* 1:246–251; 1978.

Walker M. *Selling Out Mothers and Babies: Marketing Breast-Milk Substitutes in the USA.* Weston, MA: NABA REAL; 2001.

Watson-Genna C. *Nipple Blebs/Blisters.* Medela Breastfeeding Fact Sheet. McHenry, IL: Medela; 2004.

Wiessinger D, Miller M. Breastfeeding difficulties as a result of tight lingual and labial frena: A case report. *J Hum Lact* 11(4):313–316; 1995.

Wilde C et al. Autocrine regulation of milk secretion. *Biochem Soc Symp* 63:81–90; 1998.

Wilson-Clay B, Hoover K. *The Breastfeeding Atlas,* 2nd ed. Austin, TX: Lactnews Press; 2002.

Woolridge M. Aetiology of sore nipples. *Midwifery* 2: 172–176; 1986.

Zeretzke K. Yeast infections and the breastfeeding family: Helping mothers find relief for symptoms and treatment for the infection preserves the breastfeeding relationship. *Leaven* 34(5):91–96; 1998.

Zeretzke K. Personal email correspondence; April 19, 2004.

Ziemer M et al. Methods to prevent and manage nipple pain in breastfeeding women. *West J Nurs Res* 12(6):732–744; 1990.

Ziemer M et al. Evaluation of a dressing to reduce nipple pain and improve nipple skin condition in breastfeeding women. *Nurs Res* 44:347–351; 1995.

Zollner M, Jorge A. Candida spp. occurrence in oral cavities of breastfeeding infants and in their mothers' mouths and breasts. *Pesqui Odontol Bras* 17(2):151–155. Epub; 2003.

▶ **BIBLIOGRAPHY**

Amir L. Candida albicans: Is it associated with nipple pain in lactating women? *Gynecol Obstet Invest* 41:30–34; 1990.

Amir LH, Pakula S. Nipple pain, mastalgia and candidiasis in the lactating breast. *Aust N Z J Obstet Gynecol* 31:378–380; 1991.

Amir L et al. Candida Albicans: Is it associated with nipple pain in lactating women? *Gynecol Obstet Invest* 41(1):30–34; 1996.

Barros F et al. Use of pacifiers is associated with decreased breast-feeding duration. *Pediatrics* 95:497–499; 1995.

Brooten D et al. A comparison of four treatments to prevent and control breast pain and engorgement in nonnursing mothers. *Nurs Res* 32(4):225–229; 1983.

Daly S et al. The short-term synthesis and infant-regulated removal of milk in lactating women. *Exp Physiol* 78:209–220; 1993.

Dewey K et al. Growth of breast-fed and formula-fed infants from 0 to 18 months: The DARLING Study. *Pediatrics* 89 (6 Pt 1):1035–1041; 1992.

Dewey K. Effects of exclusive breastfeeding for four versus six months on maternal nutritional status and infant motor development: Results of two randomized trials in Honduras. *J Nutr* 131(2):262–267; 2001.

Dewey K. Maternal and fetal stress are associated with impaired lactogenesis in humans. Review. *J Nutr* 131(11):3012S–3015S; 2001.

Fetherston C. Risk factors for lactation mastitis. *J Hum Lact* 14:101–109; 1998.

Horowitz BJ et al. Sexual transmission of candida. *Am J Obstet Gynecol* 69(6):883–886; 1987.

Johnstone HA: Candidiasis in the breastfeeding mother and infant. *JOGNN* 19(2):171–173; 1990.

Kaufmann R, Foxman B. Mastitis among lactating women: Occurrence and risk factors. *Soc Sci Med* 33:701–705; 1991.

Matheny R et al. Control of intake by human-milk-fed infants: Relationships between feeding size and interval. *Dev Psychobiol* 23:511–518; 1990.

Milsom I, Forsman L. Repeated candidiasis: Reinfection or recrudescence, a review, part 2. *Am J Obstet Gynecol* 152(7): 956–959; 1985.

Moon S, Humenick S. Breast engorgement: Contributing variables and variables amenable to nursing intervention. *JOGNN* 18(4):309–315; 1989.

Perez Escamilla R et al. Infant feeding policies in maternity wards and their effect on breast-feeding success: An analytical overview. *Am J Public Health* 84:89–97; 1994.

Pugh L et al. A comparison of topical agents to relieve nipple pain and enhance breastfeeding. *Birth* 23:88–93; 1996.

Riordan J. Mastitis: A new look at an old problem. *Breastfeeding Abstracts* 10:1; 1990.

Rippon JW. *Medical Mycology*, 2nd ed. Philadelphia, PA: WB Saunders; 1992.

Roberts K et al. Effects of cabbage leaf extract on breast engorgement. *J Hum Lact* 14:231–236; 1998.

Sharp DA. Moist wound healing for sore or cracked nipples. *Breastfeeding Abstracts* 12(2); 1992.

Shrago L. Engorgement revisited. *Breastfeeding Abstracts* 11(1); 1991.

Simkin P. Intermittent brachial plexus neuropathy secondary to breast engorgement. *Birth* 15(2):102–103; 1988.

Utter AR. Gentian violet treatment for thrush: Can its use cause breastfeeding problems? *J Hum Lact* 6(4):178–180; 1990.

Ziemer M, Pigeon J. Skin changes and pain in the nipple during the first week of lactation. *JOGNN* 22:247–256; 1993.

BREASTFEEDING BEYOND THE FIRST MONTH

Contributing Author: Carole Peterson

As babies mature beyond their first month, some aspects of breastfeeding change in response to their increased age and development. Babies are awake for longer periods, expanding their world in the direction of physical and social development. Parents learn to adjust their child care practices to accommodate breastfeeding to these changed patterns. New challenges will present themselves in the form of breastfeeding in public, traveling with a nursing baby, returning to work, and adjusting breastfeeding practices as the baby grows.

Over time, parents will learn to recognize their baby's unique means of communication. Waking and sleeping patterns, crying and cooing, and smiling and frowning will elicit responses and readjustments in routine. The baby progresses from an awareness of his mother as a satisfier of his needs through the development of motor skills for self-amusement and an awareness of his environment. He experiences teething, crawling, standing, separation anxiety, experimenting with vocabulary sounds, feeding himself, and drinking from a cup. Mothers face the challenges of nursing a toddler and, ultimately, weaning. You can help parents appreciate these developmental milestones and recognize ways to adjust their parenting to accommodate them.

KEY TERMS

allergens	mother-led weaning
baby-led weaning	nursing strike
Bauer's response	Palmer grasp
body length	Pincer grasp
food intolerance	prone position
gradual weaning	reflexes
head circumference	REM sleep
minimal breastfeeding	soporific
Moro reflex	tonic neck reflex

PATTERNS OF GROWTH IN A BREASTFED BABY

During the first 3 months, babies usually gain 5 to 10 oz/week. In the next 3 months, their gain is about 2.5 to 4.5 oz/week (Dewey, 1992). Breastfed infants typically double their birth weight by five to six months and triple it by one year. In the first few months, breastfed infants generally grow at about the same rate as their formula-fed counterparts. After this time, formula-fed infants typically begin to exceed breastfeeding infants in weight, while breastfed infants tend to gain more length. Formula-fed infants are less energy efficient, taking in more milk and using nutrients less efficiently than infants who are breastfed (Dewey, 1992). Head circumference is similar.

Body length and head circumference are indicators of appropriate growth. At one year of age, a baby's length should be approximately one and one half his length at birth. Brain growth is quite rapid in the first year of life. Head circumference should increase approximately 7.6 cm (3 inches) by one year of age. Dewey's study on infant growth found length and head circumference to be similar in breastfed and formula-fed infants until after four months of age. Infants breastfed for twelve or more months are leaner than formula-fed infants because of their lower energy intake (Dewey, 1993).

INFANT DEVELOPMENT

In the first hours and days after birth, a mother becomes acutely aware that her baby has a distinct personality. As she becomes familiar with his waking and sleeping patterns, his crying and cooing, and his smiling and frowning, she will learn how to adapt her responses and her mothering to suit his specific needs. Despite each baby's individuality, there are many characteristics and patterns that all babies exhibit as they develop mentally, emotionally, and physically. Caregivers who have experience with a large number of infants are able to identify ones who do not exhibit age-appropriate reflexes and developmental milestones. Babies develop as individuals within certain parameters. Parents need to be aware of developmental milestones and talk with their healthcare provider if their baby appears not to develop as expected.

Infant Development in the First Year

There are wide variations of normal, and each baby progresses at his or her own rate. Humans develop progressively: from head to foot and from the center of the body or torso out to the extremities. This progression aids us in attaining mobility. Parents often look forward to their baby's new abilities as he develops. A mother who is aware of these developmental stages in advance is better prepared to respond appropriately to the changes in her baby as he grows. She will learn to alter her nursing patterns and other caregiving to meet her baby's ever-changing needs.

Reflexes

Reflexes that were present at birth will remain in place until the baby develops finer skills to replace them. These reflexes are necessary for survival. Reflexes such as rooting, suckling, grasping, and swallowing enable the baby to obtain food. A gag reflex protects him from choking as he learns to take in food. He will continue to exhibit the **Moro reflex**, startling in response to sudden noise. The Palmer grasp will enable him to grasp his parents' fingers. He will exhibit the **tonic neck reflex** until three or four months of age. It is a normal body reflex, also referred to as the "fencer position." When the baby lies on his back, he extends the arm and leg on the side of his body opposite to the direction his head is turned. This prevents him from rolling over until adequate neurologic and motor development occurs. Pressure on the soles of his feet will continue to elicit Bauer's response, with the baby making movements similar to crawling or kicking. Of these reflexes, Moro, **Palmer grasp**, and tonic neck will disappear at about four months. Bauer's response and the rooting and suckling reflexes will continue to about nine months.

Head and Body Control

At about three months, the baby will begin to raise his head from a prone position. By four to five months, as he gains head and neck strength, he can raise his head higher and hold it for longer periods. He becomes alert and turns his head toward a voice or movement. He will begin to rest on his forearms as his torso becomes stronger. By six months, large motor development has advanced to allow the baby to roll over. The torso is strengthening to allow the baby to prepare for crawling. By seven months, he can roll over in either direction. Babies need to spend time on their tummies to encourage these developmental stages.

Hand Movement

At four to five months, the baby is able to control hand movements and begins to play with his fingers. He will wave and bat at objects, fascinated by movement. By six months, he will master visually directed reaching so that he can grasp desired items and pull them toward his mouth. Tongue movement now allows him to take solid foods and begin to learn the social art of eating. Many babies at this age begin reaching for foods when they join the family for meals. By seven months, the baby's hands and arms are more developed. He learns to wave bye-bye and can transfer objects from hand to hand. He begins to use his thumb and forefinger to pick up objects, called the **pincer grasp**, at about eight to nine months of age.

Sitting

At four months, the baby's back is rounded and his head erect when held in a sitting position. By five months, his body will be erect when supported. At six months, increased head and neck control make it possible to pull him to a sitting position. By this age, most babies can sit if they are propped. By seven months, they can sit without being propped. By nine months, they can sit well in a chair and pull themselves into a sitting position.

Crawling and Walking

Babies become very active by seven months, a time when they expand their world through physical movements (Figure 17.1). Many babies begin the early stages of crawling at about six to eight months, raising themselves onto their hands and knees and rocking back and forth. By ten to twelve months, the beginning of locomotion has arrived. This is an expansive age for the baby as he vigorously and enthusiastically practices many new motor skills while he avidly explores his environment. He learns to cruise by using tables and chairs to balance himself as he begins to learn to walk (Figure 17.2). By one year, babies are interested in everything and show their pleasure and displeasure easily.

A mother can help satisfy her baby's strong desire to explore by giving him freedom to move within safe limits at home. Babies are able to reach many items that can pose a danger to them. Therefore, parents need to examine their house for potential hazards. As early as ten months, babies can crawl up stairs but they cannot crawl down them. Parents may want to place a baby gate at both ends of the stairs for safety.

Many parents lived in one- or two-child households when they were young. They may not have been around babies or toddlers or know common-sense safety precautions. If you visit their home, be alert to potential hazards and gently point them out. Explain why something is dangerous so parents understand. You also can

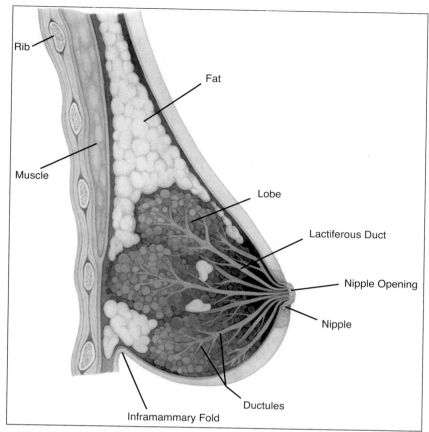

COLOR PLATE 1. Anatomy of a lactating breast.

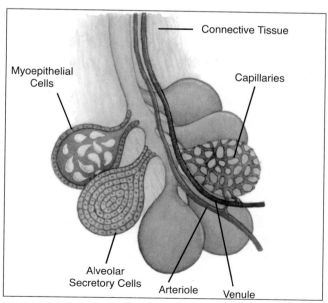

COLOR PLATE 2. Myoepithelial cells.

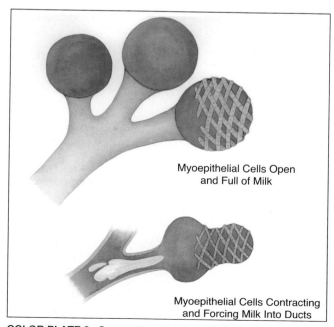

Myoepithelial Cells Open
and Full of Milk

Myoepithelial Cells Contracting
and Forcing Milk Into Ducts

COLOR PLATE 3. Contraction of myoepithelial cells.

Common Types of Breasts

COLOR PLATE 4. Type 1: Round breasts, normal lower medial and lateral quadrants. (Printed with permission of Anna Swisher.) See page 117.

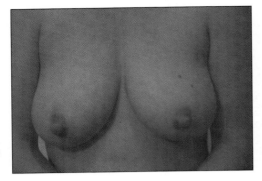

COLOR PLATE 5. Type 2: Hypoplasia of the lower medial quadrant. (Printed with permission of Anna Swisher.) See page 117.

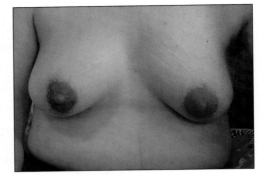

COLOR PLATE 6. Type 3: Hypoplasia of the lower medial and lateral quadrants. (Printed with permission of Anna Swisher.) See page 117.

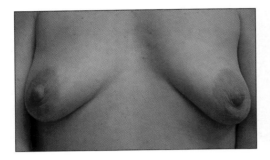

COLOR PLATE 7. Type 4: Severe constrictions, minimal breast base, areolae may be very bulbous. Breasts may be 'udder' shaped, with significant asymmetry. (Printed with permission of Anna Swisher.) See page 117.

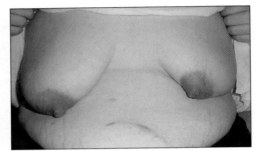

COLOR PLATE 8. Scar from breast surgery can be a marker for severed ducts. (Printed with permission of Chele Marmet.) See page 125.

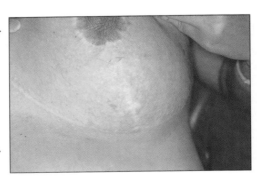

COLOR PLATE 9. Nipple appears normal. (Printed with permission of Kay Hoover.) See page 126.

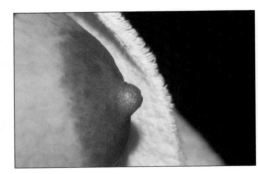

COLOR PLATE 10. Nipple from Color Plate 9 inverts when stimulated. (Printed with permission of Kay Hoover.) See page 126.

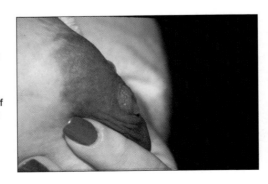

COLOR PLATE 11. Nipple appears dimpled. (Printed with permission of Kay Hoover.) See page 126.

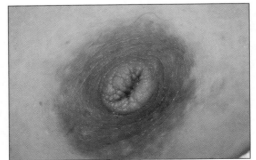

COLOR PLATE 12. Nipple in Color Plate 11 everts after pumping to release adhesions. (Printed with permission of Kay Hoover.) See page 126.

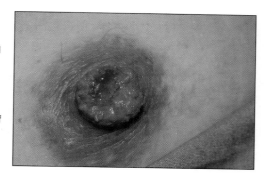

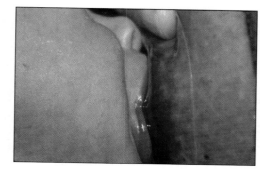

COLOR PLATE 13. Baby latching onto the breast with the aid of a nipple shield. (Printed with permission of Kay Hoover.) See page 126.

COLOR PLATE 14. Baby with a cephalhema-toma. (Printed with permission of Anna Swisher.) See page 245.

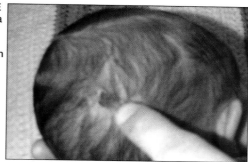

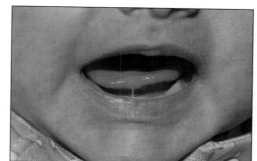

COLOR PLATE 15. A tight frenulum can interfere with the baby's ability to open his mouth wide enough for a good latch. (Printed with permission of Kay Hoover.) See page 246.

COLOR PLATE 16. A tight frenum can sometimes cause difficulty with latch. (Printed with permission of Anna Swisher.) See page 246.

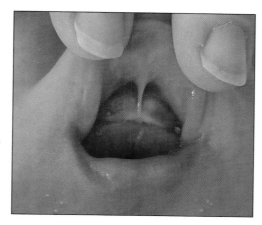

Positioning and Latch

COLOR PLATE 17. Rooting for the nipple is a feeding readiness signal from the baby. (Printed with permission of Debbie Shinskie.) See page 247.

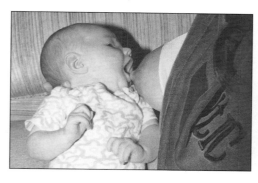

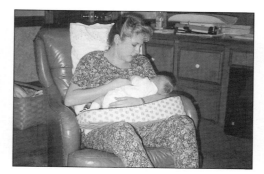

COLOR PLATE 19. A mother positioned with pillows to help with positioning and comfort. (Printed with permission of Linda Kutner.) See page 276.

COLOR PLATE 20. Using the C-hold to support the breast during a feeding. (Printed wih permission of Kay Hoover.) See page 276.

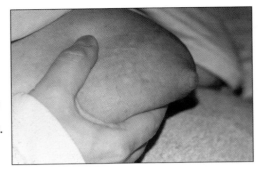

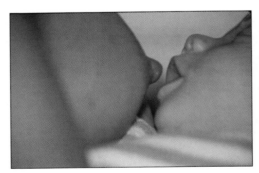

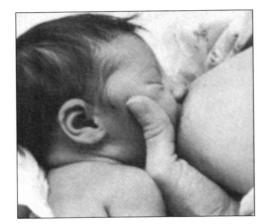

COLOR PLATE 21. Dancer hand position supports the baby's mouth and gently compresses his cheeks. (Printed wih permission of Sarah Coulter Danner.) See page 276.

COLOR PLATE 22. The baby begins to open his mouth; if the mother were to put him to breast at this point he would not get a good mouthful of breast tissue. (Printed with permission of Kay Hoover.) See page 277.

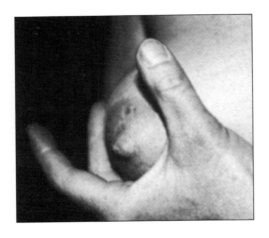

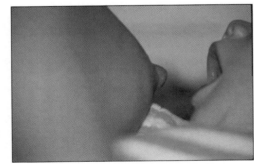

COLOR PLATE 23. The baby has continued to open his mouth wide and is now ready to be put to the breast. (Printed with permission of Kay Hoover.) See page 277.

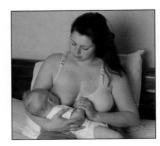

COLOR PLATE 24. Cradle hold nursing position. (Printed with permission of Nelia Box.) See page 277.

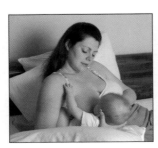

COLOR PLATE 25. Football (clutch) nursing position. (Printed with permission of Nelia Box.) See page 277.

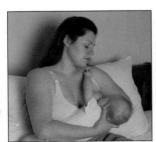

COLOR PLATE 26. Cross cradle (dominant hand) nursing position. (Printed with permission of Nelia Box.) See page 278.

Diapers of the Breastfed Baby

Looking at a baby's poop and pee can help you tell if your baby is getting enough to eat.

The baby's poop should change color from black to yellow during the first 5 days after birth.

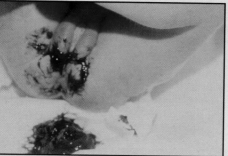

The baby's first poop is black and sticky.

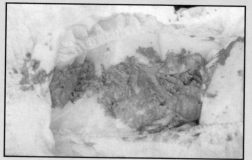

The poop turns green by Day 3 or 4.

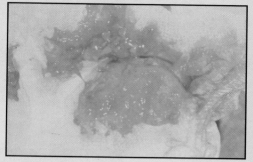

The poop should turn yellow by Day 4 or 5.

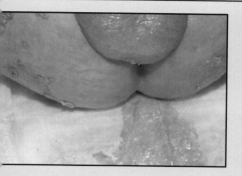

Poop can look seedy.

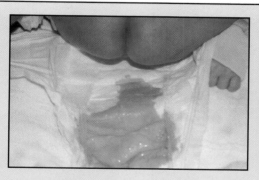

Poop can look watery.

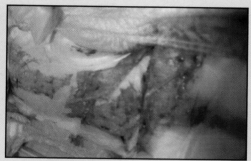

Illness, injury, or allergies can cause blood in poop. Call Doctor.

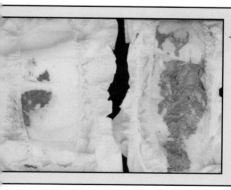

Babies make some large and some small poops every day.

Only count poops larger than this. ▶

By Day 4, most breastfed babies make 3 or 4 poopy diapers every day.

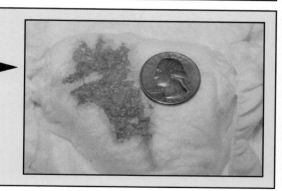

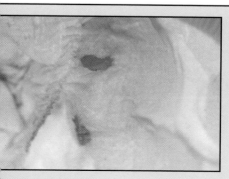

◀ On Day 1 or 2 some babies have orange or red pee.

By Day 3 or 4, breastfed babies should make 3 or 4 wet diapers with pee that looks like <u>clear water</u>.

A wet diaper is as heavy as 3 tablespoons of water. ▶

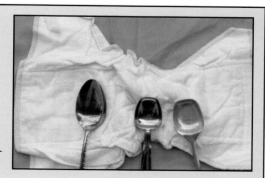

COLOR PLATE 18. Variations in stools. (Printed with permission of Kay Hoover and Barbara Wilson-Clay.) See page 250 and Appendix H on page 665

COLOR PLATE 27. Lying down nursing position. (Printed with permission of Nelia Box.) See page 278.

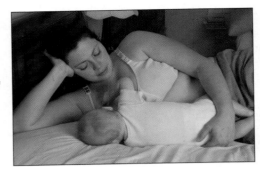

COLOR PLATE 28. Posture feeding position. (Printed with permission of Nelia Box.) See page 278.

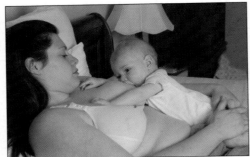

COLOR PLATE 29. Leaning over the baby. (Printed with permission of Nelia Box.) See page 278.

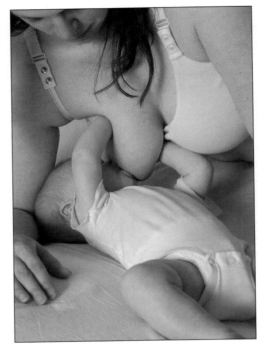

COLOR PLATE 30. Baby lying over the mother's shoulder. (Printed with permission of Nelia Box.) See page 278.

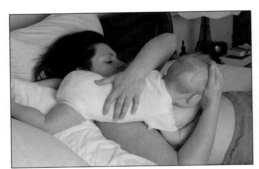

COLOR PLATE 31. A finger placed in the corner of the baby's mouth helps break suction so the breast can be removed gently. (Printed with permission of Kay Hoover.) See page 286.

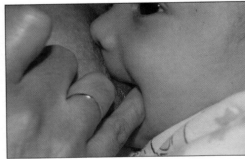

Breast Conditions

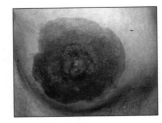

COLOR PLATE 32. Paget's disease on the nipple. (Printed with permission of S. J. Parker.) See page 128.

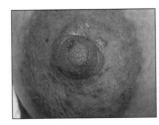

COLOR PLATE 33. Thrush on the nipple. (Printed with permission of Kay Hoover.) See page 312 and 319.

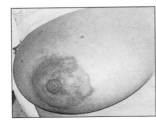

COLOR PLATE 34. Psoriasis on the nipple. (Printed with permission of Karen Ford.) See page 312.

COLOR PLATE 35. Herpes on the nipple. (Printed with permission of Chele Marmet.) See page 312.

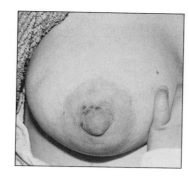

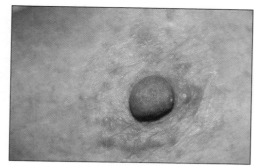

COLOR PLATE 36. Poison ivy on the nipple. (Printed with permission of Kay Hoover.) See page 312.

COLOR PLATE 37. Stage I nipple trauma—superficial intact. (Printed with permission of Kay Hoover and Barbara Wilson-Clay.) See page 313.

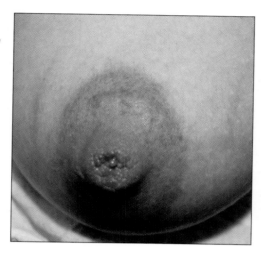

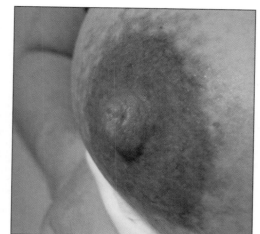

COLOR PLATE 38. Stage II nipple trauma—superficial with tissue breakdown. (Printed with permission of Anna Swisher.) See page 313.

COLOR PLATE 39. Stage III nipple trauma—partial thickness erosion. (Printed with permission of Anna Swisher.) See page 313.

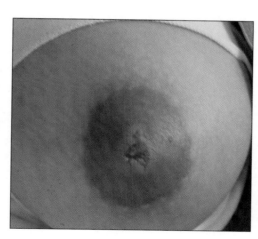

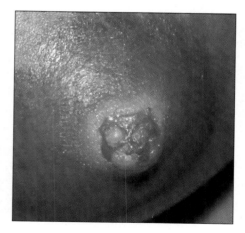

COLOR PLATE 40. Stage IV nipple trauma—full thickness erosion. (Printed with permission of Kay Hoover and Barbara Wilson-Clay.) See page 313.

COLOR PLATE 41. Cracked nipple. (Printed with permission of Kay Hoover.) See page 316.

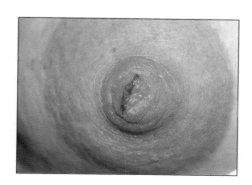

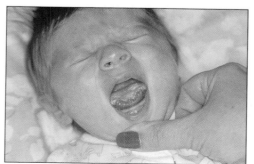

COLOR PLATE 42. Baby with thrush in his mouth. (Printed with permission of Chele Marmet.) See page 319.

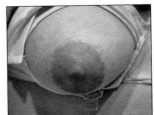

COLOR PLATE 43. A normal full breast. (Printed with permission of Linda Kutner.) See page 321.

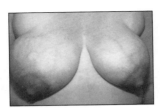

COLOR PLATE 44. An engorged breast. (Printed with permission of Debi Bocar.) See page 321.

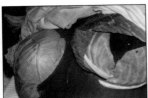

COLOR PLATE 45. Mother with cabbage on her breasts to relieve engorgement. (Printed with permission of Kay Hoover.) See page 324.

COLOR PLATE 46. Milk released from a breast infection. (Printed with permission of Kay Hoover and Barbara Wilson-Clay.) See page 325.

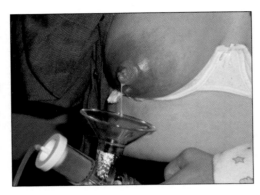

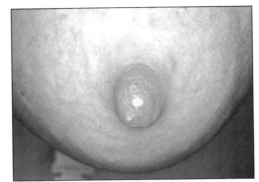

COLOR PLATE 47. Milk blister on the nipple. (Printed with permission of Jan Riordan.) See page 325.

COLOR PLATE 48. Mother with mastitis. (Printed with permission of Sarah Coulter Danner.) See page 326.

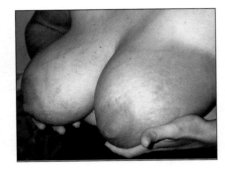

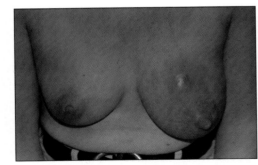

COLOR PLATE 49. Breast abscess before surgery. (Printed with permission of Kay Hoover.) See page 329.

COLOR PLATE 50. Breast abscess after surgery. (Printed with permission of Donna Corrieri.) See page 329.

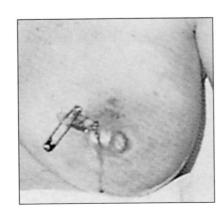

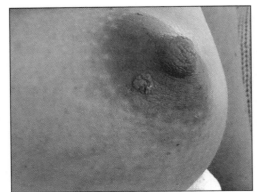

COLOR PLATE 51. Scar on breast from childhood injury. (Printed with permission of Anna Swisher.) See page 365.

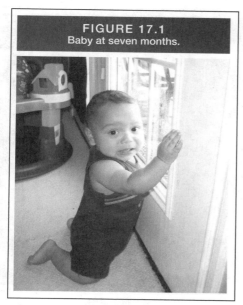

FIGURE 17.1
Baby at seven months.

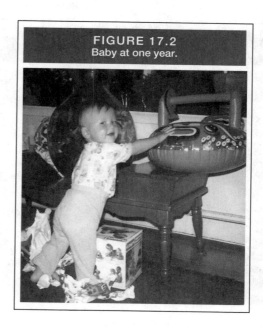

FIGURE 17.2
Baby at one year.

Printed with permission of Anna Swisher.

give parents a brochure on baby-proofing their home. Child safety information is available from many sources, including the Home Safety Council. The Web site is www.homesafetycouncil.org. Many businesses provide child safety assessments and child-proofing services. Providing a list of those in your area may be helpful.

Sleep Pattern

Each baby's physical development determines when he will be able to sleep through the night. The ability to sleep for longer periods will increase as the central nervous system develops. Differences in sleep organization and energy expenditure between breastfed and formula-fed infants may indicate that breastfeeding enhances maturation of the central nervous system (Butte, 1992).

Newborns spend 50 percent of their time in REM sleep, which is essential for brain growth and maturation. By six to twelve months of age, this decreases to 30 percent. Adults spend only 20 percent of sleep time in REM sleep. As the baby approaches three months, his sleeping pattern usually shifts to at least one longer rest period and several naps each day. A baby's personality may determine which part of the 24-hour cycle he sleeps for a longer period. The mother can adjust his cycle by initiating feedings more frequently during the day. When changes in the baby's sleep pattern occur, the mother may awaken with more fullness in her breasts than previously. Nursing her baby directly before she retires for the evening will help him sleep for the longest period at night and provide her with five or six hours of uninterrupted sleep.

At around eight months of age, a baby may experience separation anxiety if he awakes during the night and realizes that his mother is not nearby. Even after he has developed the ability to sleep for longer periods, a baby may find his sleep disturbed by dreams. The need to nurse can also cause disturbed sleep. This is common during periods of rapid physical and mental growth, increased activity during the day, and teething. In a child's second year, he may still need close physical contact in order to fall asleep (Montagu, 1986).

Social Development

The baby's world broadens as he develops an awareness of his mother as the person who responds to his needs. By three months (Figure 17.3) he regards himself and his mother as a single entity, and his need for her is absolute. The mother may have ambivalent feelings about such constant demands on her time and presence. She may enjoy the dependency because it helps her feel important and useful. At the same time, she may wish she had more time to herself for relaxation and recreation. She will continue to make adjustments as she defines her new role, enabling her to establish priorities in baby care while learning to postpone her own needs.

Interaction

By three months, the baby responds to stimuli and becomes very social. He begins to focus on objects around him and interacts with his environment. Visual acuity is clearer, and he will bat at objects in an attempt to touch and move them. He will respond more readily to high-pitched voices and may show interest in children while ignoring adults. This interest encourages siblings to entertain and interact with him.

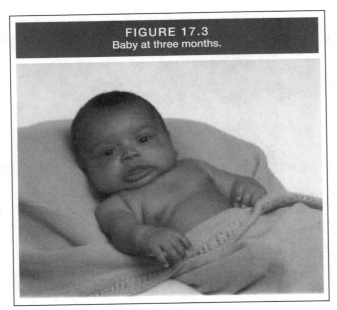

FIGURE 17.3
Baby at three months.

Printed with permission of Anna Swisher.

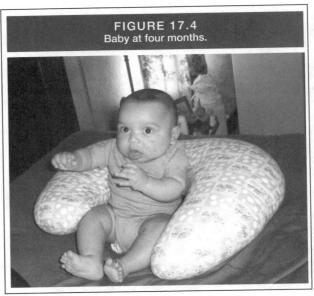

FIGURE 17.4
Baby at four months.

Printed with permission of Anna Swisher.

At three months, the baby will be awake for more hours each day and will be much more alert and responsive. The mother will interact with him in ways other than breastfeeding, exposing him to everyday household sounds and providing bright, colorful toys and decorations. Varying his positions and environment during the day will help provide the stimulation he needs for physical and mental growth. Parents will enjoy playing with their baby. Allowing him to play on his tummy will promote muscle development and prevent his head from flattening by being on his back the majority of the day.

At ten to twelve months, the baby is eager to participate in family activities and will especially want to take part in mealtimes. Parents can give him finger foods that he can study, touch, turn over, and taste. Mealtime becomes a time of discovery and interaction. By participating in his feeding, he experiences the independence he craves. As his mobility increases, he discriminates further between himself and his mother. He freely moves away from her to explore his environment, while continually checking back for assurance that she will be there when he returns.

Disposition

Big smiles are evident by three months, and the baby recognizes voices of his caregivers. He learns to express unhappiness, delight, and excitement during this time. The baby may show a preference for his parents, especially the mother, and may fuss when others care for him. At three months, he is able to sense tension in his caregiver. He will respond with tension and fussiness, quieting down only when held in a calm and relaxed manner. His eating and sleeping take on a more definite pattern, which may integrate easily into the family schedule.

By four months, babies have mastered the art of laughing aloud, to the delight of everyone around them (Figure 17.4). At this time, most parents have adapted their lives to the needs of their new baby and feel more confident in their ability to care for him. Their hours of patience, understanding, and love are rewarded by his responsiveness and the development of elementary skills. Their baby begins to gain independence through use of motor skills for self-amusement, and his demands on his parents will decrease accordingly.

At about nine months, the baby's awareness of his mother's ability to be apart from him may bring on separation anxiety, or dismay when a loved one leaves the room. As a result, he may cry in anticipation of her leaving or while she is away. He may wake during the night and cry out for reassurance that his parents are nearby. The baby has learned that his parents are important but does not have the awareness that they will return. Parents need to recognize this as a natural stage in their baby's development.

At nine months, it is common for babies to prefer their mothers to their fathers. The baby's increased awareness of differences in people may cause him to react fearfully to a stranger. He may continue his need for contact with his mother for reassurance. Parents do not need to protect him from exposure to new people. Observing strangers will enhance the baby's awareness of his mother as a special person in his life. The baby's fearful reactions to strangers are normal behavior at this age.

At ten to twelve months, the baby becomes so involved in physical achievements that he may feel overwhelmed by outside stresses such as contact with strangers, separation from his mother, and changes in schedule. He may react with shyness or fear, or begin clinging to his mother like a much younger baby. He may climb into her lap to escape stresses as well as for emotional refueling. Although he may not appear tired, he needs several periods of rest from active exploration each day in order to renew his energy.

Vocalization

By four to five months, the baby begins to imitate sounds. By six months, babbling, cooing, and squealing mark the beginning of language. Babbling is the vocalization of vowel-consonant combinations. As he experiments with language, he interacts with those around him. Responding to the baby's language efforts is essential for his development. This is a very active and social period for babies. At ten to twelve months, the baby's recognition vocabulary (words that he understands and responds to) increases noticeably, and he begins experimenting with vocabulary sounds. He expands his sociability, often seeming to interact with others in a negative manner by repeatedly saying, "No!"

Breastfeeding Behavior

Baby-friendly practices encourage a mother to nurse her baby immediately after birth. However, many babies do not actively feed at this time. They may be sleepy following delivery or simply need time to explore how to suckle and grasp the breast. Breastfeeding patterns will settle in over the first several weeks postpartum.

One Month

By one month, the baby is efficient at suckling and will actively nurse for 15 minutes or more at a feeding. He establishes a pattern ranging between 8 and 16 feedings per day. Periods of increased appetite and growth can occur at any time. Babies typically experience appetite spurts at about two weeks, six weeks, three months, and six months of age. During this time, the baby nurses much more frequently, in spurts that last two to three days. Encourage mothers to respond with frequent feedings and lots of snuggling.

Two to Three Months

By two to three months, the baby will typically spend less time at each feeding. His suckling becomes more efficient as he matures, and he may use methods other than nursing for self-comforting. A mother may perceive this as her baby's decreased interest in breastfeeding. In addition, hormonal changes during this period cause the mother's breasts to be less firm. The mother may worry that she has lost her milk, which can increase her apprehension. You can help mothers anticipate these as normal events in breastfeeding. Focusing on her baby's disposition, appearance, number of wet diapers and stools, weight gain, and

general health and vigor will be reassuring to her. This will encourage her to continue breastfeeding and help her feel secure in the knowledge that she and her baby are working in harmony to provide him with the precise amount of milk that will support his optimal growth.

At three months, the mother may need to leave her baby regularly. Many mothers must return to work, some as early as six weeks after birth. Make sure the mother knows how to express milk for her absences. You can suggest alternative feeding options other than a bottle. Breastfed babies often find the transition to a cup easier than to a bottle. See Chapter 21 for a discussion of expressing and feeding milk to the baby.

Four to Six Months

By four months, most babies become noticeably more efficient at suckling. Feedings will be shorter in length and will occur less frequently. The baby becomes very interested in his surroundings and may shorten or miss some feedings because he is so curious about everything. Mothers need to watch the baby's output and weight gain during this time. Because he requires less time at the breast to satisfy his hunger needs, the mother may consider feeding solid foods to him. You can remind her that her baby's swallowing mechanism and gastrointestinal tract will not mature enough to handle solid foods until six months of age or later. Assure her that her milk is still the ideal food to support his growth. The AAP recommends exclusive breastfeeding for the first six months of life.

At four months, the baby will continue to need his mother's attention and expand his world beyond breastfeeding. The mother can share in his growth by providing opportunities for him to develop to his full potential. Breastfeeding will continue to serve as a quiet, secure retreat from the stimulation of learning about the world apart from his mother.

By four to five months, the baby may pat or stroke the breast and strain his body away from his mother to have a better look at her or to scan his environment. Mothers may regard this as a sign of the baby's desire to separate himself from exclusive breastfeeding or even as a rejection of them as mothers. Some babies may go through what is referred to by some as a **nursing strike**. A nursing strike occurs when a baby who has previously been breastfeeding well becomes unhappy and fussy at the breast. The mother knows he is hungry, but he resists going to the breast, pulls off, and starts crying. In some instances, the baby may not cry but still pushes away. See Chapter 22 for further discussion of nursing strikes.

The apparent loss of interest or tendency toward distraction is actually a positive step forward in the baby's growth and development. It shows that he is reaching out to learn more about the world around him. Breastfeeding continues easily during this expansive time as the baby internalizes his new knowledge and gains confidence.

By six months, the frequency of feedings usually will continue to diminish. The longest nursing usually will take place before being put to bed for the night. Solid foods will begin around this time, and the baby may wake more often during the night to nurse. Teething will begin soon, which can result in increased feedings for comfort and reassurance. The baby may drool, suck on his fingers, or chew on objects. Suckling can induce pain in the baby's tender gums and may cause him to pull off the breast abruptly. These fluctuations in the nursing pattern, coupled with those caused by the baby's distractibility at this age, may result in less milk removal and the potential for engorgement, plugged ducts, and mastitis. Wiping the nipples with clear water after feedings will help prevent skin irritation. Regular milk removal will keep milk ducts open and prevent the development of plugs and infections.

Somewhere between four and six months, babies who have been sleeping through the night commonly begin waking at night to nurse. Developmentally, the baby is doing more during the day. Nursing at night enables him to receive the calories he may have missed during the day. It also allows him to reconnect with his mother. Cosleeping enables the baby to nurse frequently, maintains milk production, and provides the baby with a sense of security (Pryor, 1997).

Seven to Twelve Months

Most babies will have begun teething by seven to nine months. During this period, they will actively seek to nurse any time and anywhere, pulling at the mother's clothing or attempting to unbutton her blouse. The baby may hold the breast with one or both hands when he nurses. Over the next couple of months, he may distract easily, and the mother will need to find quiet locations for uninterrupted feedings.

By ten to twelve months, newly found freedom can result in further changes in nursing patterns. Some babies increase the frequency and duration of their feedings as the many new events and experiences in the baby's life prompt a need for reassurance that there are safe and familiar aspects in his world. The constant need for reassurance and closeness, as well as increased feedings, may upset a mother who thought her baby was on the verge of weaning. She may feel discouraged by his apparent lack of progress toward independence. You can assure her that satisfaction of his emotional needs now will lead to emotional growth and subsequent independence later.

By ten to twelve months, the baby has mastered motor skills and established regular meal patterns. He may turn to his mother more frequently for comfort and reassurance, increasing the number of feedings. A mother may interpret this as a sign that her baby is becoming overly dependent on her or on breastfeeding. The apparent dependence can be her baby's way of expressing his need for the reassurance of the safe, comfortable part of his world. It may indicate that he needs more time to adapt to his new experiences. You can let the mother know that her baby's current need for closeness will eventually lead to more independence. What may seem like a step away from independence may actually provide the security that will give him confidence to move toward self-reliance.

By twelve months, outside pressure may lead a mother to consider weaning. Her baby is now capable of obtaining his nourishment away from the breast, and it may appear that he is outgrowing breastfeeding. However, you can assure the mother that he still needs the security and comfort of nursing as a stabilizing factor in his life. Solid foods do not usually contain the special fatty acids present in human milk needed for continued brain growth. Only mother's milk contains the immunities and antibodies specific to the baby's environment. Remind the mother that the American Academy of Pediatrics recommends breastfeeding for the first year and beyond (AAP, 1997). WHO recommends breastfeeding for the first two years of life (WHO, 1989). The American Academy of Family Physicians recommends breastfeeding beyond infancy (AAFP, 2001).

There is a prevalent belief in U.S. culture that a mother's milk is no longer beneficial after the first year. You can educate parents about the continuing nutrition and protection given by human milk in the second year of life. If a mother chooses to wean at this time, your role is to support and validate her decision. Help her replace her usual nursing periods with other types of close interaction. A mother who breastfeeds an older baby will benefit from support and encouragement. It is difficult to breastfeed in a bottle-feeding culture. Praise her for overcoming any obstacles, and validate the pride she feels in nourishing her child.

Overfeeding a Breastfed Baby

Sometimes a mother may worry that her baby is nursing too frequently and for too long at a feeding. This worry could stem from a baby who seems to be overweight or who spits up milk. A baby is considered overweight if he is about two categories above the weight for his height, as determined by standard height and weight charts. A normal weight gain is one to two pounds per month for the first four or five months. This rapid weight gain should not continue into the second half of the first year.

Some families have heavier babies who thin down in the second year, regardless of whether they are breastfed or bottle-fed. If the baby is significantly heavier than other family members were, he may be getting too much milk. An older baby who often spits up or vomits from an overly distended stomach may be overfed. The mother can shorten or decrease feedings and substitute other activities for breastfeeding until the spitting up diminishes.

Overfeeding can occur when a baby nurses frequently for comfort or has a great sucking need. You can suggest to the mother alternate ways of comforting her baby so that she does not use feeding as a response to every cue. Encourage her to see the total picture of the developing mother-child relationship and to refine her parenting skills to meet her child's needs. As the months go by, the mother needs to interact with her baby with activities other than nursing in order to expand his world in the direction of optimal physical and social development.

Actions to avoid overfeeding:

- Let the baby suck on his thumb or finger.

- Nurse at one breast per feeding and allow the baby to continue sucking on the less full breast.

- Learn other ways to interact with the baby—rock, carry, keep him within view of the mother, talk to him, change his position, play with him, sing to him, etc.

- Interest the baby in other activities—a stroll, toys, baby exercises, and so on.

Infant Development After One Year

As a baby advances into toddlerhood, the changes in his social, emotional, and physical development are reflected in his breastfeeding. Many babies will continue to nurse far beyond one year. Others will wean themselves and never seem to miss breastfeeding. Providing anticipatory guidance to parents will relieve concerns and help them enjoy this exciting and entertaining stage of their children's lives.

Social and Emotional Development

Sometime between 12 and 15 months, the baby may again demonstrate a fear of strangers and a dislike for separation from his mother. He may regress to earlier behaviors in order to adjust to such incidents. A mother who works outside the home may be especially aware of these regressions. She will want to make certain that her baby's caretaker provides the attention and caring he needs to develop emotional stability.

Overstimulation during the day or separation anxiety may cause a baby to wake at night. He may especially appreciate the closeness of breastfeeding to soothe him back to sleep. Love and reassurance freely given are likely to be the best cure for insecurity. Recognizing this may appease the mother of a baby who clings and nurses more frequently than she may wish. Many mothers separated

from their babies during the day treasure their evenings and nights together. The baby's outside interests soon will become more important than breastfeeding. The mother's love, patience, and understanding are rewarded when she sees her child as a secure and independent individual.

As the baby grows older, communication and play become increasingly important. He primarily extends his world to increase his interaction with his father, who presents the novelty of another personality with different ideas and responses. A mother who returns home at the end of the day may offer this same type of diversion. When the baby begins to develop a close relationship with another person, the mother may worry that her role is diminishing. In reality, her baby needs her in new ways as he reaches out to others. This positive step in his development will eventually lead to the beginnings of his ability to identify and understand the separate interests of his parents. Eventually, he will learn that absent parents will return, which minimizes emotional upset over temporary separations. Allowing the baby opportunities to become self-reliant and to proceed at his own pace will encourage his growth and independence.

Breastfeeding Behavior

The expansion of the baby's world carries over to mealtimes. The mother can provide opportunities to breastfeed as she perceives her baby needs it. He will enjoy using a spoon to feed himself and will practice picking up and drinking from a cup. As with all other tasks that the baby attempts, the mother will want to encourage exploration and practice. Accepting mistakes and spills as a part of learning is a helpful approach for parents to adopt concerning their child's eating habits.

In his second year of life, a child no longer requires as much food as he did previously, and his interest focuses on other things. This shift in focus contributes to a decrease in his appetite. He may have gained as much as 16 pounds in the first year and may double his weight after another three years. Food preferences become better defined, and a low-key approach to food selection may be the most effective method of ensuring an adequate diet. The mother can be satisfied if her one-year-old eats one balanced meal a day plus two other partial meals and nutritious snacks.

The mother's milk will continue to supply significant calories, vitamins, and minerals and immunity to illness (Slusser, 1997). Breastfeeding is encouraged throughout the second year and beyond. The composition of milk changes as the baby's nursing pattern changes. The "weaning" milk of a toddler has a higher concentration of secretory IgA, which helps protect a toddler who puts his hands into his mouth as he explores an unsanitary world.

As his needs change during this expansive age, the baby's breastfeeding patterns will fluctuate. He may nurse less frequently when he is busy experimenting with new skills, or more frequently because of an increased need for security or attention. He may also seek to nurse when he is getting ill. Testing other possibilities before putting the baby to breast helps the mother ensure that she does not initiate breastfeeding as the sole solution to his bids for attention. This will ease the transition to a more comfortable pattern for the mother and child. Setting aside several special times during each day for total interaction with her baby will result in fewer interruptions at other times. These times will help a mother fulfill her baby's need for attention and social interaction in a positive manner.

▶ BREASTFEEDING AN OLDER BABY

As the baby grows and breastfeeding progresses, many events occur that require a mother to expand her child care and parenting techniques. You can help her identify ways that breastfeeding fits into these events. The mother may need to make choices about how she will nurse in front of others or in public places. She may require suggestions for comforting her baby when he is teething or ways of coping with his biting. At some point, her baby may lose interest in nursing or develop a preference for one breast over the other. If she finds that she is still nursing her baby beyond the point at which she had planned to stop, you can help her reevaluate her goals. Anticipatory guidance will help the mother progress through breastfeeding in a rewarding and positive way.

Breastfeeding in Public

Each individual mother makes her breastfeeding experience unique according to her attitudes and philosophies. Some mothers prefer to nurse only in the privacy of their homes. Others are comfortable breastfeeding in the homes of friends and family. Many women enjoy taking their babies along with them for shopping and dining out and are comfortable breastfeeding in public places. Some may be uncomfortable breastfeeding in the presence of other people, worrying that they are the center of attention and that others will disapprove. Several U.S. states have passed legislation protecting a mother's and baby's right to breastfeed anywhere. Pointing this out may provide reassurance to mothers who question the acceptance of public breastfeeding. When a mother learns techniques that eliminate awkwardness and obscure her body from public view, she will often become more comfortable nursing in public.

A mother can gain confidence by watching other women nurse their babies, observing practical methods and other people's reactions. She will also feel more self-assured after she practices discreet nursing in front of a mirror or another person. The baby's father is often a great "mirror" for the mother, as he may be more likely to give candid comments of what others might see. Another excellent place to try discreet nursing is within breastfeeding support groups, where other mothers can learn from one another.

If a mother knows she will be away from home, she can prepare for discreet nursing by selecting appropriate clothing. Loose-fitting clothes allow easy access to the breast, and a sweater, jacket, or other such garment worn over her shoulders can conceal her breast from those who may view her from the side. A baby sling will provide support and extra cover, as well as ease in mobility. To avoid attracting attention, she can feed her baby before he is overly hungry and starts to fuss. She will need to allow time for this feeding in her schedule.

A mother can also allow time to look for a comfortable place to nurse if she is unfamiliar with her location. A spot that is out of the way of aisles and walkways will be more comfortable for the mother and less distracting for the baby. Such places include a corner table or booth in a restaurant, a bench next to a wall, sitting next to her partner or friends, a department store dressing room or lounge, or a parked car. Mothers should never breastfeed in a restroom or other highly unsanitary environment. A restroom is not an appropriate place for any type of eating!

With forethought and planning, a mother can choose a time and location for nursing in which she can be relaxed and comfortable. Most women grow in confidence as they learn they can breastfeed in public and that few people even notice. Breastfeeding in public will gain acceptance as more people recognize the importance of breastfeeding for lifelong health. Many facilities now offer nursing lounges for mothers.

Traveling with a Breastfeeding Baby

Sometime after her baby is about six weeks old, the mother's physical recovery is nearly complete. She may be ready to leave home with her baby for extended periods. A baby between the ages of six weeks and six months is usually an ideal traveler. His routine is predictable, he does not yet eat solid foods, and he is not very mobile. Babies at this age often sleep through the monotony of an automobile, train, bus, or airplane ride, making the trip that much easier for parents. Traveling with a baby decreases the worry a mother might experience about being apart from her baby.

Planning for the Trip

Although traveling with a baby is more cumbersome than traveling alone, careful planning and preparation can help make it both convenient and enjoyable. In order not to be overburdened, parents can confine baby care items to those that are essential. Breastfeeding eliminates the need for supplemental foods or artificial baby milk, as well as the equipment necessary to prepare and transport them. It also eliminates the worry about the possibility of using contaminated water to reconstitute formula.

A lightweight diaper bag can double as a purse, and using disposable diapers will further decrease baggage. Parents can purchase them conveniently along the way, so only a few need to be packed. Several changes of baby clothing in the diaper bag, as well as plastic pants worn over diapers to contain potentially messy stools, will decrease the need to open suitcases in search of clothing while en route. For long trips, parents can take along a few items to keep the baby amused. Colorful pictures, rattles, and toys tied onto a string will capture the baby's attention temporarily.

Traveling by Foot

A baby sling is convenient for walking with a baby. It is more versatile than a stroller, especially in crowded shops, on stairways, on hiking trails, and in the sand. Wearing the baby in a sling also helps prevent the baby from touching things in stores. The comfortable position and motion often lulls him to sleep. A lightweight cloth sling will fit easily into the mother's bag, ready to use at any time. For added protection in cold weather, parents can place the baby in the sling under their coat.

Traveling by Automobile

For safety, a baby should be strapped securely into an approved infant car seat when traveling by automobile. Infant car seats are also effective for other modes of travel and are more comfortable for the baby than adult seats. Parents should never hold their baby in a moving automobile. A sudden stop could result in the parent losing hold and hurling the baby from the car or against the car's interior. Likewise, caution parents against carrying their baby in a sling or baby carrier while they are riding in the car. The force of the parent's body could cause serious injury to the baby in the event of a sudden stop.

A mother should be discouraged from breastfeeding during an automobile ride unless she is able to nurse her baby while he remains in his rear-facing car seat and she has her seat belt securely fastened. A bottle of expressed milk may help stretch out nursing times and parents can stop every two or three hours to allow for nursing and for the baby to move around freely. While this will mean a longer trip, ultimately it will be more enjoyable when everyone arrives safely and comfortably at their destination. Allowing extra time for these accommodations is part of families meeting everyone's needs.

At times, parents may need to endure the baby's crying if they cannot find a suitable distraction. This is probably the most difficult part of traveling with a child. It usually occurs near the end of the trip, when the parents are pushing to arrive at their destination. You can help parents understand that babies are not able to tolerate very long periods of travel. Encourage them to relax their schedule to accommodate their baby.

Traveling by Air

When planning a trip by air, a mother can request the roomier seat behind the bulkhead. Babies should be in their car seats strapped into a regular seat. Strollers and other baby equipment can be well marked and checked with the luggage, leaving the mother free to carry her baby and only those items she will need during the flight. Airlines usually allow parents with small children to board the plane before other passengers so they can get settled and avoid waiting in line. Mothers need to be aware that changes in cabin pressure may affect the baby's ears. Breastfeeding during takeoff and descent can help minimize this discomfort.

Teething and Biting

Babies typically cut their first tooth between six and eight months of age, although teething can occur anywhere between 4 and 14 months. As a tooth erupts, it causes swelling and irritation in the gums. When the baby sucks, blood rushes to his gums, which adds to the swelling that is already present and causes immediate discomfort. Thus, when the baby begins to nurse, he may quickly pull away from the breast and cry out with pain. The mother may notice additional clues that her baby is teething. He may become irritable, have a slight fever, begin drooling more than usual, and occasionally spit up or develop loose stools for no apparent reason. He may also begin waking during the night to seek comfort.

Overcoming Teething Pain

The baby soon discovers that chewing and rubbing his gums reduces teething pain. A teething baby may rub his jaw or pull on his ear to relieve discomfort. The same nerves to the teeth branch out to the face, cheek, and outer ear. If the baby cries out when the mother rubs his gums, he may be teething. Continued rubbing on the gums should comfort him and help him to settle down. Providing the baby with a cooled teething ring or rubbing ice or a cold cloth on his gums before breastfeeding can relieve the soreness long enough for him to nurse. Providing suitable objects and hard foods such as toast for the baby to chew on helps relieve the pain and promote tooth eruption. Parents can soothe their baby's teething pain with over-the-counter pain relievers or locally acting over-the-counter preparations that temporarily numb gum tissue. The mother will want to consult her baby's caregiver before using such medications.

Discouraging Biting

Teething may cause the baby to clamp down on the breast during feeding. The mother can be especially observant at this time and watch for signs that the feeding is ending. When there is a slowing of the suck-swallow rhythm, she can remove the baby from her breast. If biting occurs in the middle of a feeding, the mother can remove her baby immediately, say "No", and wait a few minutes before resuming the feeding. If the baby bites again, she can end the feeding promptly and gently give another verbal reprimand.

Because of the sucking mechanics involved during breastfeeding, it is impossible for the baby to suckle and bite at the same time. Clamping down tightly will interfere with the tongue compressing the nipple. If the baby is biting, he probably is not hungry enough to nurse at that time. The mother can end the feeding and try again later when his hunger returns. If she suspects teething pain to be the cause of biting, she can try some comfort measures and then resume nursing.

Biting may occur at the end of a feeding as the baby falls asleep and closes his jaw. The mother can prevent such clamping down on her nipple by inserting her finger in the baby's mouth between his gums and removing her breast when she perceives he is nearly finished. Withdrawing her finger slowly will break suction and avoid discomfort. When a baby bites for the first time, the mother may react with an outcry and a startled jerk away from her baby. Let her know that this is a common reaction. She can be cautious not to respond so strongly in the future so that the baby does not interpret this as a sign of rejection and discontinue nursing because of it. Assure her that she can overcome biting and that it need not be a reason to wean.

▶ SUSTAINING BREASTFEEDING BEYOND ONE YEAR

There are a number of techniques you can suggest to mothers to help them continue breastfeeding for two years and beyond as is recommended by WHO and UNICEF. As the baby becomes more alert and more easily distracted, she can breastfeed in a quiet place to limit distractions and interruptions. When the mother adds supplemental foods to her baby's diet, she can breastfeed first and then offer the complementary food. A baby who has begun eating other foods may wish to breastfeed less frequently. He will continue to diminish the frequency and duration of breastfeedings as he receives more foods in his diet. The mother can continue to put her baby to breast and respond to his wishes. As she approaches weaning, she will want to allow him to lessen the number of feedings gradually and be sure he receives plenty of other foods each day.

Breastfeeding a Toddler

Breastfeeding patterns in other cultures show that with loving patience from their parents, children outgrow their need to nurse in their second, third, or even fourth year of life. Most often, cultural practices set the standards for weaning times in a society, without regard for the baby's biologic need. Within social groups where early weaning is common, a mother who chooses **baby-led weaning** is often pressured by lack of acceptance and misinformation about breastfeeding her older baby.

Misinformation about breastfeeding a toddler takes several forms. Some people believe that breastfeeding a baby beyond infancy will make him more dependent on his mother. However, in cultures where mothers typically breastfeed beyond twelve months, babies walk and crawl earlier than those that are primarily bottle-fed (Dewey, 2001). Many studies have shown that satisfying a baby's emotional needs will encourage his self-reliance. Normal sucking needs can last for several years, and babies may require a substitute for sucking if weaning occurs before sucking needs subside. Some people believe that nighttime feedings cause the baby to continue waking during the night. However, sleep patterns most often are the result of neurological development and environmental factors, not the availability of breastfeeding.

One study found that women who breastfed longer than twelve months were older, better educated, and had exclusively breastfed longer. About a third of the mothers slept with their babies (Hills-Bonczyk, 1994). Mothers who want to breastfeed into the toddler stage need reassurance that it is perfectly natural and normal to do so. The support of others within their social structure will validate their choice. They will be empowered further by informed professionals who can answer their questions. These mothers will benefit from the emotional support and practical suggestions of other mothers who understand their circumstances and are willing to listen to them.

Gradually presenting the concept of breastfeeding a baby beyond infancy enables mothers to consider this parenting option objectively. Each society defines the term "older baby" differently when used in the context of breastfeeding. Many American women will describe an older baby as 18, 15, or even 9 months of age, and most do not expect to continue breastfeeding their infants into the toddler years. They simply respond to their babies' breastfeeding needs on a daily basis as a natural part of mothering. Describing breastfeeding a toddler as an extension of the warm infant-mother relationship will help women view it positively.

Rewards of Breastfeeding a Toddler

Breastfeeding a toddler is rewarding and satisfying for the mother who recognizes that she is meeting her child's needs (Figure 17.5). It can be a source of great comfort and stability to the child, especially when he feels stressed, is injured, has his feelings hurt, is feeling shy, or is in a new and strange environment (Wrigley, 1990). Breastfeeding provides a comforting way for the active child to connect with his mother between explorations. Particularly during the toddler period, breastfeeding offers the mother a reassuring way to communicate her love even though she and her child may be at odds over his behavior. A child who is able to communicate verbally can bring his mother great joy by expressing his feelings about breastfeeding. There can be love and humor in this relationship, with both mother and child being the giver and receiver. These aspects of breastfeeding serve as a transitional parenting technique from infancy to childhood.

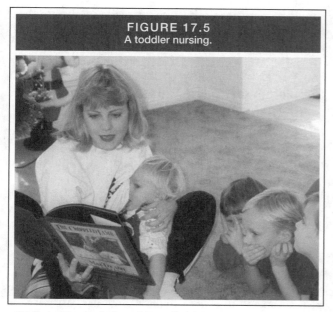

FIGURE 17.5
A toddler nursing.

Printed with permission of Anna Swisher.

Challenges to Breastfeeding a Toddler

Although breastfeeding a toddler can be very rewarding, it may also cause inconveniences and conflicts that rival those of the newborn period and that often cause mothers to consider weaning. The physical act of nursing a toddler can be quite different from breastfeeding an infant. The older baby may not wish to be held and will assume a position that allows him to conveniently view the room, including standing or straddling (Figure 17.6). For a time, his developing teeth may leave pressure marks on the areola until he learns to hold the breast with his lips. Crumbs or food particles left in the child's mouth may irritate the mother's nipples during feedings.

Some women may consider weaning because they feel they have lost control of their bodies or that their babies are manipulating them. The child may insist on nursing at inconvenient or embarrassing moments. He may tug at the mother's clothing, even partially disrobing her. He may enjoy fondling her body, which embarrasses her when others notice. She may feel trapped and controlled by her child and resent that she did not expect this phase of breastfeeding.

The mother can prevent such potential negative feelings by guiding her child in his breastfeeding, just as she guides him in other aspects of his life, such as eating, sleeping, and playing. She can limit breastfeeding to certain times and eliminate overindulging him. Feedings can be limited to coincide with the mother's needs so that breastfeeding continues to be a source of pleasure for both of them. If touching the other breast while breastfeeding is unpleasant, the mother can tell the toddler, "No." Help her adopt a balanced view of breastfeeding as an integral part of parenting so she can continue to enjoy this special relationship with her baby as he matures.

A mother can work out with her baby some signals and times for breastfeeding that are reasonably acceptable to both. The family may adopt a special name for nursing, so that when the toddler asks to breastfeed while out in public the mother can avoid embarrassment. Rather than arguing with him at every request, she can try to stretch the intervals between feedings. He may, for example, be satisfied with a drink or treat just before the usual time for nursing. The mother can suggest other activities to take his mind off breastfeeding. Encourage her to remain flexible enough to adjust her approach if it causes stress in the child. The concept of time is often difficult for a child to comprehend, and nursing can be linked to a special location instead. For instance, he will understand if she says, "Let's nurse when we get home in Mommy's chair." Being consistent in restricting breastfeeding to a particular place is the key to making this mutually satisfying for both mother and toddler.

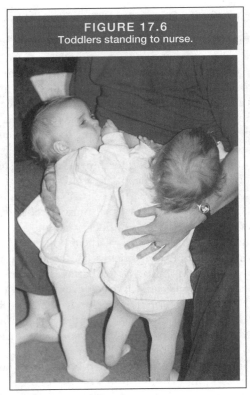

FIGURE 17.6
Toddlers standing to nurse.

Printed with permission of Kay Hoover.

Opposition from Others

Sometimes the baby's father will object to his older baby continuing to nurse. He may believe that the child appears too dependent while nursing, or he may worry about the social and sexual implications of breastfeeding an older baby. If the mother complains about breastfeeding, the father may wonder why she continues. Help the mother learn what the father's precise objections are and develop a breastfeeding plan to resolve the issue. She can discuss with him the baby's physical and emotional needs at this stage in his development, as well as her desire to continue breastfeeding. If he continues to object, she can avoid nursing in his presence. He may accept the situation better if he does not actually see the toddler nurse, or he may benefit from seeing other children continue to nurse, as in a support group. He can also read books such as *Becoming a Father* (Sears, 2003). The mother will benefit from your support if she continues breastfeeding despite the father's objection.

People other than the baby's father are often uncomfortable seeing a woman breastfeed a toddler. To avoid this, mothers can be encouraged to breastfeed discreetly. A mother can also refrain from breastfeeding in front of people who she knows are critical, in order to defray reactions and avoid feeling intimidated by them.

She will need to remain firm in her conviction that she is doing what is best for her child. Chapter 20 presents suggestions on helping the mother handle criticism about breastfeeding her toddler.

Siblings may appear to resent the special attention the breastfeeding child receives from his mother. Reevaluating her children's needs and setting aside special time with each child may eliminate such reactions. The mother may inadvertently be responsible for prolonging breastfeeding by nursing her toddler in order to keep him from disturbing her older children's toys or disrupting their play. Providing storage places and play areas that are inaccessible to the baby can prevent him from interfering with siblings, so that the mother does not resort to breastfeeding to keep him occupied.

You can listen to the mother's concerns with a sympathetic ear and help her work out solutions that fit her situation. She may not know another person who will praise her for her efforts and reassure her that she has chosen the right action for her child and family. Whether she chooses to wean or to continue breastfeeding, she needs an accepting listener who will support her in her decision. Attending a breastfeeding support group will also be helpful to her.

▶ NOURISHMENT AWAY FROM THE BREAST

Mothers need to understand that any nourishment the baby receives away from the breast may alter his breastfeeding pattern. The greater the frequency and amount of other food, the greater the impact will be on breastfeeding. The lactation community distinguishes between supplementary feeding—food in place of the mother's milk—and complementary feeding—necessary nourishment that cannot be provided by the mother's milk.

Supplementary Feedings

The most common definition of a supplementary feeding is a food other than human milk fed to the infant following or in place of a breastfeeding. Some refer to it as "topping off" the breastfed infant with liquids other than mother's milk, such as water or infant formula. While some sources refer to these substitutes as complementary foods, complementary foods differ significantly, as described later in this chapter.

Some consider the mother's expressed milk to be a supplementary feeding because the baby does not obtain it directly at the breast. The mother's milk is certainly preferred over water or formula. Encourage the mother to plan ahead and to express milk on a regular basis for these feedings. If she wishes to use formula for supplementary feeding she needs to consider the WHO, UNICEF, and

AAP recommendations for exclusive breastmilk to age six months. She also needs to check that there is no history of allergies in the family and discuss with her baby's caregiver which type of formula to use.

Many mothers take their babies with them or plan activities around the baby's feeding times and never have a need for supplementary feedings. Others wish to have time away from their babies without the worry of delayed feedings or needing to rush back in time for the next feeding. Mothers may experience an accident, illness, or other unforeseen happening, such as getting stuck in traffic or having an automobile breakdown. A substitute feeding can eliminate the worry of an unhappy and hungry baby.

Feeding Method for Supplementary Feedings

Mothers need to introduce supplementary feedings in such a way that the amount of supplement does not interfere with the baby's breastfeeding pattern. Therefore, it is best to delay any supplementary feedings until the baby is at least three weeks old and has firmly established good nursing habits. Parents should initiate a supplementary feeding when the baby is not fussy or too hungry.

Because of the potential for nipple preference, parents may want to avoid bottles when other feeding methods are possible. Most babies will accept feeding by a cup, which avoids the nipple preference associated with a bottle. Learning to drink from a cup is often easier for breastfeeding babies than for those fed exclusively with a bottle. If a mother prefers to use a bottle, the baby's acceptance of feeding from a bottle may require several attempts. A baby sometimes will accept a bottle, reject it the next few times, and then accept it again later. The mother can continue to offer the bottle until her baby accepts it. Encourage her to use paced feeding techniques to slow the feeding rate, as described in Chapter 21.

Many fathers and grandparents enjoy feeding their baby. They can be relied on not to overfeed him when they understand the relationship between the amount of milk the mother produces and the amount the baby needs. They or someone else can feed the baby about one ounce of fluid in a cup or bottle once or twice a week. The baby may refuse the alternative feeding method if the mother is even in the same room. The couple can plan for her to enjoy some time away from home while the father does this.

If supplementary feeding results in a missed breastfeeding, the mother's breasts may become full. She can nurse or express milk just before she departs, or she can express her milk while she is away. If she prefers that her baby nurse immediately when she returns, wearing a larger bra may help to avoid pressure on her full breasts that could cause blockage of her milk ducts. Mothers

who work outside the home or return to school or an active social life soon learn how to manage such absences without experiencing discomfort from full breasts. Having prepared supplementary feedings ahead of time, they feel secure in their babies' willingness to accept substitute nourishment.

Complementary Feeding

A complementary feeding refers to new foods added to the growing breastfed infant's diet that are intended to meet the energy and nutrient needs that are not met by the mother's milk alone. Some use this term interchangeably with supplemental feeding and interpret it as "topping off" the breastfed infant with liquids other than the mother's milk (i.e., water or infant formula). The most common definition of complementary foods refers to solid foods added to the child's diet.

Mothers need to understand that when a baby receives his first complementary food, the weaning process has begun. The introduction of solid foods begins to establish eating patterns that will last a lifetime. Parents recognize this as a giant step in their baby's development that requires many decisions on their part. They wonder when to begin solid foods, what types of food are best, how to offer the food, and how to make sure their baby receives adequate nutrition. You can give parents the information that will help them make responsible decisions about foods for their baby.

Pressure to Begin Complementary Foods

New parents receive a deluge of messages from baby food manufacturers proclaiming the many advantages of commercially processed foods. They often receive an overabundance of advice from family and friends on when and how to introduce these foods. Books, magazines, and newspapers advocate various methods and times for starting solid foods. Parents must evaluate this assortment of facts and opinions in the context of their baby's needs. This may be one of the parents' first forays into advocating for their child as informed consumers, searching out and evaluating information available to them.

Counseling Implications for Complementary Feeding

You can be a valuable source of information for parents about introducing solid foods to their baby. Provide them with clear, accurate, well-documented facts to eliminate their possible confusion from contradictory advice. A mother needs encouragement and a high level of self-esteem to continue exclusive breastfeeding despite pressure to start solid foods. Reassure her that her baby looks and acts healthy and is well nourished from her milk alone. Assure her that she has an adequate milk supply and the capacity to increase milk production to meet her child's increased needs. You can be an active force in helping her delay solid foods until an appropriate age by giving her the support that will build her confidence in her mothering skills.

Sometimes the baby's caregiver will suggest that a mother start her baby on solid foods when it does not seem appropriate or when the mother does not feel ready. Encourage her to ask the caregiver to clarify the reason for suggesting solid foods. Did the caregiver say that she *may* begin solid foods if she wishes? Did the caregiver recommend solid foods for a specific reason? It may be that the caregiver is not familiar with the recommendation by the American Academy of Pediatrics that babies receive nothing but breastmilk before six months of age. The mother can reinforce her breastfeeding goals and discuss such pertinent aspects of her baby's health as weight gain, family weight patterns, allergies, and anemia.

Sleeping through the Night

The suggestion for complementary feeding often occurs in relation to sleep issues. There is no conclusive evidence that a particular feeding method promotes longer nighttime sleep. Because human milk is digested more quickly than cow's milk, it seems reasonable that a breastfed baby would wake up hungry in the middle of the night. A baby who is exclusively breastfed at five months may sleep eight hours at night. That same baby may have been up every three or four hours during the night at one month old. It seems more likely, then, that the reason for longer sleep at five months is due to a more fully developed nervous system and is unrelated to nutritional factors.

Some people will tell parents that a baby needs cereal just before going to bed in order to "fill him up." However, sleeping through the night is a developmental event that parents cannot change by feeding the baby cereal (Macknin, 1989). When adults experience restless sleep, having a light snack such as warm milk before they retire often helps. They do not choose a heavy meal that could cause indigestion and further encourage wakefulness. Warm milk contains a **soporific** (sleep-inducing) agent that helps people fall asleep. In that case, human milk is the ideal food for encouraging a baby to sleep.

Choosing the Appropriate Time to Introduce Complementary Foods

The introduction of solid foods expands a baby's dietary choices and serves as a complement to the mother's milk during weaning. There are many factors to consider in deciding when to add solid foods to a baby's diet. In general, the ideal time falls somewhere between when the baby's system is mature enough to handle solid foods and when he needs more nutrients than he can obtain solely

from his mother's milk. Beginning solid foods before six months or in response to growth spurts seriously compromises milk production and may precipitate food allergies.

Babies of average birth weight with adequate fetal stores of fat and iron do well on mother's milk alone until about six months of age. This is why the AAP recommends that exclusive breastfeeding is ideal nutrition and is sufficient to support optimal growth and development for the first six months after birth. Human milk provides all the calories, vitamins, and minerals in the proper proportions needed by the baby. In addition, its protective factors help prevent allergies and illness. Introducing other foods before the baby's body is ready can lead to frequent digestive upsets, increased upper respiratory infections, poor nutrient absorption, and excessive weight gain due to increased calorie consumption.

Early introduction of solid foods correlates with higher weight at 8, 13, and 26 weeks of age. At 14 to 26 weeks of age, early solid foods correlate with increased respiratory illness (Forsyth, 1993). Excessive weight gain in infancy can lead to lifelong obesity. Not all babies will be able to wait until six months of age to start solid foods, however. Some babies who begin nursing constantly at four or five months and never seem to be satisfied may need further nourishment from solid foods. Every baby will be ready for solid foods at a slightly different age. Parents can watch their baby for signs of readiness.

Signs of the Baby's Readiness for Complementary Foods

The baby displays obvious outward signs that he is ready for solid foods when his internal functions have developed to the point where they can efficiently handle a more diverse diet. At around six months of age, neuromuscular development allows for proper chewing and swallowing of non-liquid foods. Intestinal maturation promotes more complete digestion and absorption of a variety of foods. This enables the baby's body to handle the waste products from solid foods. His immunologic system has also begun to function, so that he no longer must depend on the protection provided by his mother's milk.

Other signs of a baby's readiness for additional foods include the eruption of teeth, the ability to sit up, the disappearance of the tongue extrusion reflex, improved eye-hand coordination, and the ability to grasp objects with his thumb and forefinger (Figure 17.7). The most obvious sign is the baby's behavior when others are eating. He may watch them intently, imitate their chewing, and reach for food while loudly vocalizing his desire for it. An intensified demand to nurse that is not satisfied after several days of increased breastfeedings may be an additional clue to the mother that it is time to begin solid foods.

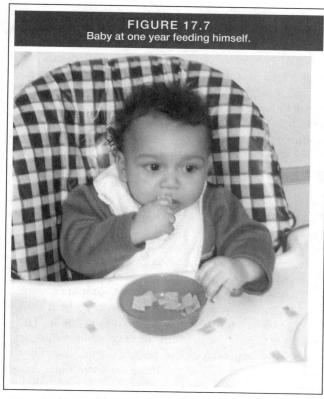

FIGURE 17.7
Baby at one year feeding himself.

Printed with permission of Anna Swisher.

Parents sometimes consider starting solid foods in order to solve an unrelated problem. Misconceptions about breastfeeding or about the baby's behavior patterns may cause parents to believe that some aspects of their relationship with their baby are feeding-related. Such misconceptions may involve frequency of feedings, milk production, richness of the mother's milk, sleep, crying, and infant development. By correcting these misconceptions, you can help parents avoid starting solid foods prematurely. In the DARLING study (Davis Area Research on Lactation, Infant Nutrition and Growth), the age of starting solid foods was unrelated to the frequency of night feedings. Early solid feeders had lower intake of their mother's milk at ages six and nine months (Heinig, 1993).

Supplementing to Provide Iron

Parents may consider starting solid foods to supply their baby with iron. In a healthy full-term baby, this is not usually necessary. The mother's milk typically supplies sufficient iron for her baby until he triples his birth weight. Her milk contains lactoferrin, an iron-binding protein that increases the absorption of the normal amounts of iron that are available in the milk. Outside sources of iron disrupt this process. Adding iron too soon interferes with the disease-protection qualities of lactofer-

rin. Lactoferrin binds iron and increases its absorption. This robs some microorganisms of the iron they require in order to grow and multiply. Premature infants and infants of anemic mothers will need iron supplementation whenever a **hematocrit** (hemoglobin blood test) determines that iron stores are low.

How to Introduce Complementary Foods

The introduction of solid foods should be a pleasant experience for a mother and her baby. Slow and gradual introduction of foods will prevent the baby from feeling overwhelmed by this new way of eating. His digestive system will have a chance to get used to each new change in diet. Offering complementary foods to the baby after he has nursed will maintain the mother's milk production. It allows the mother and baby to rely on breastfeeding as a means of relaxation and comfort during this time of change. With breastfeeding as a stabilizing factor in his life, a baby will be better able to adapt to the new experience.

Parents can begin at a slow pace, with one complementary feeding every one or two days. The best time to initiate this is at times when the baby is still hungry after a breastfeeding. Often, the afternoon and early evening hours are times when the baby will accept additional foods more readily. This usually coincides with the time when the mother is most tired and busy with other tasks. It provides an opportunity for the father or other family member to interact with the child and offer her a break from baby care.

Age of the Baby

Breastfeeding should be allowed to diminish slowly as solid foods increase to the point that they are the primary source of nutrition for the child. The mother's milk can still meet three-fourths of her baby's nutrient needs during the second six months of life. Even during the baby's second year, her milk continues to be nutritionally valuable (Slusser, 1997).

By the age of seven to nine months, one or two complementary feedings a day with regular breastfeeding will satisfy the baby's nutritional needs. By around nine to twelve months, as he becomes an active participant at family meals, he will have a schedule of three meals a day. He will still require nutritious snacks several times a day, as well as several separate nursing times. Breastfeeding will gradually decrease as he learns to eat balanced meals and drink from a cup.

Texture of Complementary Foods

Foods initially will be highly puréed and diluted with liquid. As the baby becomes accustomed to eating solid foods, liquid content can give way to a coarser texture. This will eventually transition to chunky foods, finger foods, and finally table foods. Delaying solid foods until eight or nine months avoids the need to prepare puréed foods. The baby can start with finger foods and chunky foods.

The texture of foods needs to be compatible with the baby's ability to chew and swallow. Table 17.1 provides guidelines for a child's ability to feed himself as he develops and matures. As illustrated in the table, the average baby will begin eating small chunky finger foods by nine months. By one year of age, he will be eating regular table food, cut up to sizes appropriate for his age and capabilities, along with the rest of the family.

Types of Foods Given

The types of food the baby receives depends on his age, preferences of the parents or pediatrician, and his willingness to accept them. The baby will need to begin with foods relatively high in protein (AAP, 2003) because the protein requirement in the baby's diet begins to exceed what he receives from his mother's milk. Single-grain infant cereals, such as rice or barley, will provide additional energy and iron. Therefore, these cereals are often the pediatrician's choice for the first complementary food. The mother can express some of her milk or use warm water to mix with the cereal.

Typically, rice cereal is first, followed by vegetables, fruits, and meats, in that order. Babies do not require juice and parents should limit its use. When solid foods begin after five or six months of age, the order of introduced foods seems to be of little importance. Babies require no desserts and no sweeteners added to their foods. Sweet foods are a poor substitute for foods with greater nutritional value. They cause tooth decay and promote poor eating habits.

Single-ingredient foods are the best choice, started one at a time at weekly intervals to allow an opportunity to identify potential food sensitivity and avert development of potential food intolerance or allergies. If the baby receives several foods together, the mother is unable to identify one that causes a reaction. If food sensitivity occurs, the mother can discontinue the food and reintroduce it later. She may find that small amounts of a food can be tolerated, whereas larger amounts will cause reactions. See the discussion that follows on allergy considerations.

If the baby objects to a particular food, the mother can withhold it for several weeks before offering it again. The experience of trying new foods should be pleasant for the baby. Parents should not force him to eat something he finds unpleasant. They should avoid starting new foods when he is ill or has recently had an inoculation.

Giving the baby water with his solid food enables him to meet his fluid needs without taking in extra calories. Additional water is often necessary to help rid the baby's body of the waste products in solid foods. This is especially the case with meats and egg yolks. Fruits, fruit juices, and vegetables pose less of a problem for the baby. In the second year of life, a child no longer needs a special infant diet. At that time, he can begin sharing modified family meals, prepared without excessive salt or spices, cut into appropriate-sized pieces, and served at a moderate temperature.

Extremely restrictive vegetarian diets such as fruitarian and raw food diets are not appropriate for infants. However, when vegetarian infants receive adequate breastmilk and their diets contain goods sources of energy, iron, vitamin B_{12}, and vitamin D, growth is normal. Guidelines for the introduction of solid foods are

TABLE 17.1	
Child's Ability to Self Feed	
Age	**Characteristics**
6 to 9 months	Holds, sucks, and bites finger foods.
9 months to 1 year	Enjoys finger foods, eats most table foods, drinks from cup with help, will hold and lick spoon after it is dipped into food.
15 months	Begins to use spoon, turns it before it reaches mouth; may no longer need bottle; may hold cup; likely to tilt cup rather than head, spilling contents.
1 to 2 years	Eats with spoon, often spilling; turns spoon in mouth; requires assistance; holds glass with both hands, size of glass is important.
2 years	Puts spoon in mouth correctly, occasionally spilling; holds glass with one hand; distinguishes between food and inedible materials.
2 to 3 years	Feeds self entirely, with occasional spilling; uses fork; pours from pitcher; can obtain drink of water from faucet without assistance.

Excerpted from *Child Health Encyclopedia: The Complete Guide for Parents* by The Children's Hospital Medical Center and Richard Feinbloom, M.D. Reprinted by permission of Delacorte Press/Seymour Lawrence.

the same as for nonvegetarian infants. Protein-rich foods include tofu, legumes, soy or dairy yogurt, cooked egg yolks, and cottage cheese. Foods rich in energy and nutrients such as legumes, tofu, and avocado should be used when the infant is being weaned (ADA, 2003).

Amount of Food Given

Mothers often wonder how much complementary food they should feed to their babies. When first presenting a food, the mother will frequently prepare a small dishful, only to find that her baby scarcely tastes it. She can begin with a teaspoon or so of creamy consistency food and then work up to a few tablespoons at a rate determined by the baby's appetite. Too often, babies are overfed because parents expect them to consume an entire jar of commercially prepared baby food in one sitting. Parents need to be aware of their baby's signals that he has had enough.

At first, the mother can expect to see more food running down the sides of her baby's mouth than getting into his stomach. This will change as he learns to use his newly developed swallowing mechanism. Messiness is a normal and sometimes amusing part of this new experience. It will be evident again when the baby starts feeding himself. Some babies are not very interested in solid foods until they can handle the food themselves. Others love to eat right from the start. Caution the mother not to overfeed an eager baby. Solid foods contain more calories per volume than milk. A young baby's mechanism for determining hunger is by volume of food. Overfeeding can manifest itself as constipation, spitting up, excessive weight gain, or a rapid decrease in the number of breastfeedings.

Allergy Considerations

When babies are breastfed exclusively, components in the mother's milk coat the intestinal tract to prevent foreign proteins from entering the baby's system and causing allergic reactions. Eventually the baby's body develops the ability to protect itself without the mother's milk. However, children of parents with a history of allergy appear to have a more prolonged dependence on the protective factors in human milk. These children have an increased susceptibility to ingested food proteins. The hereditary risk of food allergy seems lower when the baby is breastfed exclusively for several months (Saarinen, 1995). Avoidance of the most potent allergenic foods during the first year is effective in reducing allergic reactions in children.

The degree of response to foreign proteins varies widely from one baby to another. Some babies exhibit sudden and clear-cut allergic reactions. Others may be slightly fussy or irritable. The signs of food reactions that may help a mother to recognize intolerance in her baby appear in the following section. Food reactions may be mistaken for signs of illness or drug reactions and vice versa. If symptoms persist, parents should contact the physician, since these symptoms may also indicate illness in the baby.

Signs of Food Intolerance

- Runny nose, stuffiness, and constant cold-type symptoms
- Skin rashes, eczema, hives, and sore bottom
- Asthma
- Ear infections
- Intestinal upset, gas, diarrhea, spitting up, and vomiting
- Fussiness, irritability, and colic-like behavior
- Poor weight gain due to malabsorption of food
- Red itchy eyes, swollen eyelids, dark circles under the eyes, constant tearing, and gelatin-like fluid in the eyes

Family History of Allergies

Parents with a family history of allergies should notify the physician whenever they suspect an allergic response in their baby. The physician can help them pinpoint the offending allergen and may provide medication to relieve the symptoms. The mother should limit her consumption of milk and eggs, especially during the last month of pregnancy. She can substitute other foods to ensure a balanced, nutritious diet. When the mother eats an excessive amount of a particular food, it may cause an allergic reaction in her baby. She can avoid this by eating a variety of foods in moderation. To eliminate a reaction entirely, she may need to exclude a food from her diet. By experimenting with known allergens, the mother can identify and eliminate the offending foods. If she eats a particular food and notices repeated symptoms with that food after she breastfeeds her baby, that food may be the cause.

If a mother eliminates a food from her diet, especially one such as cow's milk, which is high in protein and calcium, she will need to substitute another food or supplement to obtain the necessary nutrients to support lactation. Mothers do not need to eliminate foods from their diets unless they suspect that a particular food is causing problems. They can continue to consume in moderation any foods they have been accustomed to eating.

When the potentially allergic baby begins consuming complementary foods, parents need to be especially cautious about introducing one food at a time and waiting at least one week for a possible reaction. Foods to avoid in the first year include cow's milk and milk products, citrus fruits and fruit juices, eggs, tomatoes, chocolate, fish, pork, peanuts and other nuts, and wheat. A baby younger than one year of age should never receive honey because of its potential to cause infant botulism. The baby's skin should not be in contact with wool clothing and blankets or with lanolin products. There should be no smoking near the baby and preferably nowhere in the home.

▶ WEANING

It is far too impersonal and arbitrary for a mother to allow cultural influences to dictate how long she will nurse her baby. The suitable time for weaning will define itself when the mother is knowledgeable about breastfeeding and weaning. With the appropriate information, she will be confident that she is basing her decision on her baby's physical and emotional needs. She will then be less likely to allow misconceptions or pressure from others to cause her to initiate weaning before her baby is ready.

Baby-Led Weaning

The biologically normal and desired method for weaning is to allow the baby to wean himself at his own pace. When a mother is relaxed about breastfeeding and has no pressures or problems that lead her to wean, she can allow her baby to establish his own nursing pattern and weaning time. Through baby-led weaning, the baby will drop feedings gradually and the mother will nurse only when he indicates a need for it.

Signs a Baby Is Ready to Wean

When weaning takes place buffered from societal pressures, natural times for ending breastfeeding seem to fall between the periods of the baby's greatest developmental activity. Globally, the normal range for weaning is somewhere between 2½ and 7 years of age (Stuart-MacAdam, 1995), around when the first molars erupt. Common ages for weaning in Western Culture are 12 to 14 months, 18 months, 2 years, and 3 years.

The mother can follow her baby's feeding cues and subsequent pattern for weaning by neither denying nor initiating breastfeeding. The baby may become more self-reliant and go for long stretches without nursing, perhaps accepting a drink or snack as a substitute. He may show his disinterest in breastfeeding by being easily distracted at the breast, spending less time at feedings, frequently refusing the breast, and showing a greater interest in solid foods. These signs indicate to the mother that her baby

may be ready to wean. The mother can view it as a natural step toward her baby's maturity.

A baby may start to wean when his mother does not want or expect it, and she may respond by trying to entice him to nurse more frequently. You can help her learn to appreciate his maturity by stressing his new achievements and showing her new ways to interact with him and continue their close relationship.

A mother may overlook her baby's signs of readiness to wean and initiate feedings she could have eliminated. She may put her baby to breast as soon as he awakens instead of preparing breakfast for him. She may nurse to keep him quiet while she talks on the telephone or engages in other activities. If the mother wishes to change these patterns, she can read stories to her baby, offer him a snack, or provide him with toys and activities to occupy his time. Rocking, cuddling, singing, and holding can effectively replace the coziness and comfort of breastfeeding. Two resources that have been helpful to many mothers nursing beyond U.S. cultural norms are *Mothering Your Nursing Toddler* (Bumgarner, 2000) and *How Weaning Happens* (Bengson, 2000).

Mother-Led Weaning

Mother-led weaning describes a mother's attempt to end breastfeeding without having received cues from her baby. Your use of guiding skills will help her explore her goals and her baby's needs. Some mothers become impatient for their baby to wean. If a mother has begun to resent breastfeeding, it may be time for her to wean. She may be feeling pressure from others or may have received poor information or advice. She may be planning to return to work and believes that she must wean in order to do this. She may feel that her baby is no longer satisfied with breastfeeding.

Help the mother determine what is best for her and her baby. Weaning is a transitional period that mothers need to manage with appreciation for the baby's needs. Many mothers delay weaning so they can avoid bottles and progress directly to a cup. When a mother brings up the topic of weaning, she may actually be unsure whether she wishes to wean at that time. If she does want to wean, she may approach the subject with hesitation because she knows you advocate extended breastfeeding. Be sensitive to her cues and let her know that you will help her whether she chooses to wean or to continue breastfeeding. Your nonjudgmental approach will encourage her to express her concerns freely and to define her questions clearly, so that she can understand the nature of weaning.

Most mothers in the United States wean before nine months. Ending breastfeeding between three and six months is largely a matter of physical management. Mother-led weaning of a three-year-old may involve a greater challenge, perhaps including bargaining with the child to establish acceptable substitute activities. It is important that you adopt a nonjudgmental attitude and support a mother's decision to wean. Your role is to educate and advise her about weaning. Once she has made the decision, your role is to support that decision and help her through the weaning process.

Gradual Weaning

If the mother wishes to initiate weaning, she can eliminate the least preferred feeding first, allowing at least two days for her baby and her breasts to adjust to the dropped feeding. In its place, the mother can substitute a drink, snack, cuddling, or a favorite activity. When she drops an early morning feeding, she can have breakfast ready when the baby awakens. When she drops a late night feed, she can consider alternate ways of getting him to sleep. As she and the baby adjust to each new substitution, she can proceed to drop another feeding, continuing in this manner for several weeks or months. The child may wish to continue one preferred feeding and may decrease his frequency to once every few days until he stops breastfeeding entirely.

If weaning proceeds too quickly, the baby may react by demanding more attention, wanting to nurse more frequently, or exhibiting physical changes such as allergic reactions, stomach upsets, or constipation. Weaning too quickly may cause the mother's breasts to become uncomfortable. She can express her milk to relieve the discomfort, while being careful not to express so much that she actually increases production. She will want to watch for any symptoms of plugged ducts or mastitis and can wear a supportive bra that is not binding. She may want to consider comfort measures such as a pain reliever, ice packs, or cabbage leaves. The mother and baby both adjust better when weaning is gradual and tailored to their needs. By allowing several months for weaning, any physical and emotional discomforts are minimal.

Miscues That Cause Mothers to Consider Weaning

Weaning ideally occurs when both the mother and baby are ready. If the baby no longer desires to nurse, encourage the mother to accept this sign of his maturity and to discontinue putting him to breast. When the mother decides to end breastfeeding, she can find other ways of satisfying her baby's needs. In both of these situations, the mother usually learns to accept weaning without guilt or resentment. Unfortunately, weaning sometimes results from misconceptions, outside pressure, or a change in personal circumstances. When this happens, the mother can react with anger, resentment, or guilt because she was unable to continue breastfeeding. Miscues that lead to untimely weaning are described below.

Crying

A mother may have a baby who cries a lot, which causes her to doubt that she is satisfying his hunger. His behavior may be stressful, and she may decide to wean to avoid further stress. You can help her explore the reason for his crying which may be due to allergies, pain, distress, or hunger. Teach her comforting techniques and explain how she can increase milk production, if necessary. Teaching her about feeding cues and normal output may help to reassure her that her baby is getting enough milk. Feeling successful about her mothering skills will help her continue to breastfeed with confidence.

Teething, Biting, or Illness

When teething, biting, or illness occur, the mother may become frustrated and fatigued with trying to manage breastfeeding and comforting her baby. She may decide to wean in an effort to decrease tension or so that someone else can feed the baby while she rests. You can help her understand that this is a temporary stage. Further, bottle-feeding is not likely to improve the situation if a baby is ill. Weaning at this time can produce the additional discomfort of engorgement and the inconvenience of trying to decrease milk production. In times of stress, a baby needs the closeness and reassurance of breastfeeding.

Nighttime Feedings

Continued nighttime feedings may cause a mother to be so fatigued from lack of sleep that she does not function well during the day. If her baby is older, weaning may be the answer. It may be possible simply to drop night feedings. Help her explore the reasons for her baby's wakefulness. It may be from separation anxiety, habit, insufficient daytime feedings to satisfy his hunger, or a need for attention. Perhaps she can respond to night feedings if she gets into the habit of napping during the day or cosleeping with her baby at night.

Changes in the Family

A family's life becomes complicated with moving, job changes, illness, emotional upsets, or other stressful situations. It might appear that weaning would make life simpler for the mother at such a time. However, her baby's needs for security and continuity are even greater when there are significant changes in his life. Ending breastfeeding at this time could lead to fussiness, increased illness, and increased demands for attention. You can guide the mother in developing ways to integrate breastfeeding into her lifestyle so that she feels less stressed. If she does wean, she needs to do so gradually, so that her baby has time to adjust to his new environment.

The mother may consider weaning because she fears pregnancy and wants to start or resume taking oral contraceptives. You can give her some information about other methods of contraception (see Chapter 19) that are compatible with breastfeeding. Encourage her to discuss them with her caregiver. Ideally, she will find one that is acceptable to both her and her partner.

Sadly, there are cases in which breastfeeding babies have become emotional "footballs" between parents who are involved in divorce. In one case, a mother breastfeeding her older child was accused of child abuse by the child's father. Other mothers have felt pressured to wean in order to allow extended visitation between the father and child. However, visitation can take place in a way that accommodates breastfeeding. Information on breastfeeding in the context of family law and the best interests of the child is available at www.lalecheleague.org.

Societal Pressure

Pressure or comments from family members or friends can prompt a mother to consider weaning. Suggestions that her baby is becoming too dependent because of breastfeeding may cause her to worry that this is actually the case. She can examine her breastfeeding pattern to determine whether she initiates nursing in response to all of her baby's bids for attention. In some instances, she may need to find other ways to respond. Her baby becomes self-reliant when he can depend on his mother for comfort and security. She can continue to breastfeed knowing that it provides emotional benefits to her baby.

The baby's father may suggest weaning because he feels left out when he sees the mother and baby constantly together. Perhaps he misses evenings out together or simply would like more of her attention. She can explore his reasons for wanting her to terminate breastfeeding and try to find a suitable compromise. Special times together for the couple or fewer feedings when he is home may satisfy the father. Ultimately, the mother may decide to wean to maintain harmony in the home. Your role is to support her in her decision.

A mother may be criticized for breastfeeding an older baby and begin to wonder if breastfeeding is still beneficial. Let mothers know that their milk has nutritional advantages for a toddler and is dose-dependent. In other words, the more breastmilk he receives, the greater the nutritional benefits. Furthermore, the emotional security of breastfeeding can be a stabilizing factor in a child's life. In order to decrease criticism, she can avoid nursing in front of those who disapprove and keep a toy or snack ready as a distraction to postpone feedings. She can also avoid taking her child places when she anticipates he will be hungry or tired and wish to nurse.

If the mother senses others are receptive, she can attempt to educate them about the continuing benefits of breastfeeding. She may simply need to indicate her determination to continue nursing by standing firm and nursing discreetly. She will benefit from your encouragement and support to offset the negative influences around her. Contact with other women who are breastfeeding older babies will help build her confidence and maintain her perspective.

Untimely Weaning

Mothers must sometimes wean their babies abruptly, with no time for preparation or forethought. If **emergency weaning** is unavoidable, the mother must put aside her ideal vision of gradual, comfortable weaning. If she is able to take several days to wean, she can drop every other feeding the first day. In place of those feedings, she can express just enough milk to relieve discomfort but not so much that she stimulates further production. She can then eliminate the remainder of the feedings, making sure she includes extra nurturing and attention for her baby.

Emergency Weaning

If a mother must wean immediately, she may experience about 24–48 hours of painful engorgement. This will subside gradually. She can wrap her breasts in cabbage leaves to reduce swelling. (See Chapter 16 for guidelines in applying cabbage to engorged breasts.) Ibuprofen can relieve her pain and help reduce swelling. In addition, she can place ice wrapped in a towel on her breasts to reduce swelling and pain. She will want to avoid heat because it increases blood flow and swelling and can promote milk flow. Plugged ducts or mastitis could occur because of the lack of milk flow. Your attention and availability will be critical to her as she experiences this period of stress. Some outdated medical literature and older relatives may recommend breast binding, a practice that can lead to plugged ducts and mastitis, and intensify the mother's pain or illness. Mothers should never bind their breasts!

Unintentional Weaning

Sometimes a mother inadvertently weans her young baby while actually wanting to continue nursing. Perhaps she started giving occasional bottles of formula and before she realized the consequences, her milk production had diminished. She may feel breastfeeding has slipped away from her to the extent that she is unable or unwilling to turn back. She will especially need your acceptance and support at this time to help her through her disappointment.

Should the mother express a desire to **relactate**, you can refer to the discussion of relactation in Chapter 24. Untimely weaning can shake a woman's confidence in her competence as a mother. Encourage her to continue giving her baby the same nurturing and attention she gave him when she was breastfeeding, holding him close and providing eye contact during feedings.

Unavoidable Weaning

Some circumstances outside the mother's control may lead to weaning. The mother may develop a serious illness or require medication that would pass through her milk and harm her baby. She may return to work or school and find it difficult to continue to breastfeed. Her baby may suddenly refuse to nurse and fail to resume breastfeeding. She may become pregnant, and her history of miscarriage or premature birth may preclude breastfeeding. The discomfort of sore nipples during pregnancy coupled with a decrease in milk production may suppress her desire to continue nursing.

After such forced weaning, the mother may grieve over the loss of breastfeeding. She may feel guilty or incompetent because she could not continue this part of her mothering role. Listening to and accepting her feelings will help her work through this personal loss. You can stress the benefits she provided her baby during the time she breastfed and teach her other mothering skills to substitute for the closeness of breastfeeding.

Minimal Breastfeeding

Many women find that **minimal breastfeeding** provides an attractive compromise to total weaning. Minimal breastfeeding describes a pattern of breastfeeding one to three times a day, with complementary foods providing the remaining nourishment. This may be an option when the mother and baby are separated for regular periods, as when the mother returns to work or school. Breastfeeding two to three times a day can help a mother continue to experience the special connection to her baby that accompanies breastfeeding. One study showed that 49 percent of mothers used minimal breastfeeding (feeding one to two times per day) for an extended period as a comfortable transition to weaning (Williams, 1989).

After Weaning

It is common for mothers to feel some regret or sadness when breastfeeding ends, even if they had wanted to wean. Every woman will benefit from support and understanding by those close to her in order to overcome these feelings. Help the mother recognize that new skills for comforting her baby will replace breastfeeding. Help her regard weaning as another step in her child's development, and encourage her to look forward to new stages.

Physical Changes with Weaning

The mother may experience several physical adjustments after weaning. Anticipatory guidance will help her expect these changes. To avoid gaining weight, most women will need to adjust their diets to eliminate calories they used during lactation. Some are pleased to find a sudden weight loss of a few pounds resulting from a loss of fluid and fat from the body's fat stores. If menstruation did not resume until after weaning, menstrual cycles may be somewhat irregular for a few months, with intermittent bleeding, light flow, or spotting.

The breasts may become soft, flat, or droopy for a few months. Some women find that their breasts gradually return to their prepregnancy size, while other women's breasts remain larger than they were before they became pregnant. Some observe that their breasts never fully regain the fatty layer that was present before conception. The Montgomery glands recede, and the areola may remain darker than before pregnancy. Stretch marks may be apparent on the mother's breasts.

Continued Milk Secretion

Some mothers continue to secrete milk for several months after weaning. This will gradually diminish and turn to a colostrum-like consistency. If the mother is still spontaneously secreting milk six months after weaning, she can evaluate any circumstances that may be stimulating milk production. Perhaps she is holding her baby against her chest, wears clothing that rubs against her nipples, or is sensitive to sexual foreplay that involves her breasts.

The total cessation of milk secretion varies greatly from one woman to the next. It may last several weeks or as long as one year after weaning. After milk secretion has stopped completely, if the mother notices the appearance of a discharge, she will want to consult her caregiver to determine the cause. Sometimes old milk works its way out. Other times, fluid may result from an infection or growth. Review the discussion in Chapter 16 to investigate whether there is an underlying medical reason for her continued milk secretion.

▶ SUMMARY

Anticipatory guidance will help parents recognize the normal events to expect as their babies develop throughout their first year and beyond. Adjustments in routines and practices will help to accommodate breastfeeding to these developmental stages. The baby will expand his world and develop both physically and socially. He will learn that certain cues elicit responses from his parents. He will cry, coo, smile, or frown depending on his needs. Whereas his mother first represents his entire world, he soon expands to an awareness of others and to his environment. Motor skills will develop further as he begins to crawl and walk. Teething, shorter feedings, separation anxiety, experimenting with vocabulary sounds, feeding himself, and drinking from a cup all will evolve gradually. Mothers will find creative ways to nurse their toddler and eventually manage weaning. This expansive time can be both exhilarating and challenging for parents. They will appreciate your advice and support as they make the necessary adjustments to meet their baby's needs.

◆ CHAPTER 17—AT A GLANCE

Applying what you learned—

Teach mothers about:

◆ What to expect with each of the baby's developmental stages.

◆ Her baby's innate reflexes of rooting, sucking, grasping, swallowing, and gagging.

◆ When her baby will be able to sleep through the night.

◆ Appetite spurts and decreased time at feedings because of efficiency in suckling.

◆ Adjusting breastfeeding when her baby begins teething.

◆ Typical weight gain.

◆ Her breasts becoming less firm being unrelated to milk supply.

◆ Delaying solid foods until six months or later.

◆ The value of her milk throughout the second year and beyond.

◆ Signs that her baby is ready for complementary foods.

◆ Resisting pressure to begin complementary foods too early.

◆ Cow's milk food allergy and signs of food intolerance.

◆ Role of family history in allergies.

◆ Signs a baby is ready to wean.

◆ Importance of baby-led weaning or gradual mother-led weaning.

◆ Miscues that cause mothers to consider weaning.

◆ Minimal breastfeeding as an alternative to weaning.

◆ Physical changes to expect after weaning.

Teach mothers how to:

◆ Adapt breastfeeding to each developmental stage.

◆ Adapt to changes in eating and sleeping patterns.

◆ Fit breastfeeding into resuming social activities.

◆ Help her baby overcome teething pain and discourage biting.

◆ Sustain breastfeeding beyond one year.

◆ Manage supplementary and complementary feedings.

◆ REFERENCES

American Academy of Family Physicians (AAFP). *AAFP Policy Statement on Breastfeeding*. Breastfeeding Position Paper; 2001.

American Academy of Pediatrics (AAP). Policy Statement on Breastfeeding and the Use of Human Milk. *Pediatrics* 115(2):496–506; 2005.

American Academy of Pediatrics (AAP). *Pediatric Nutrition Handbook*, 5th ed. Elk Grove Village, IL: AAP; 2003.

American Dietetic Association and Dietitians of Canada. Position of the American Dietetic Association and Dietitians of Canada: Vegetarian diets. *J Am Diet Assoc* 103(6):748–765; 2003.

Bengson D. *How Weaning Happens*. Schaumburg, IL: La Leche League International; 2000.

Bumgarner N. *Mothering Your Nursing Toddler*. Schaumburg, IL: La Leche League International; 2000.

Butte N et al. Sleep organization and energy expenditure of breast-fed and formula-fed infants. *Pediatr Res* 32:514–519; 1992.

Dewey K et al. Growth of breastfed and formula-fed infants from 0 to 18 months: The DARLING study. *Pediatrics* 89:1035–1041; 1992.

Dewey K et al. Breast-fed infants are leaner than formula-fed infants at 1 y of age: The DARLING study. *Am J Clin Nutr* 57(2):140–145; 1993.

Dewey K. Effects of exclusive breastfeeding for four versus six months on maternal nutritional status and infant motor development: Results of two randomized trials in Honduras. *J Nutr* 131(2):262–267; 2001.

Forsyth J et al. Relation between early introduction of solid food to infants and their weight and illness during the first two years of life. *Br Med J* 306:1572–1576; 1993.

Heinig M et al. Intake and growth of breast-fed and formula-fed infants in relation to the timing of introduction of complementary foods: The DARLING study. *Acta Paediatr* 82:999–1006; 1993.

Hills-Bonczyk S et al. Women's experiences with breastfeeding longer than 12 months. *Birth* 21:206–212; 1994.

Macknin M et al. Infant sleep and bedtime cereal. *Am J Dis Child* 143:1066–1068; 1989.

Montagu A. *Touching: The Human Significance of the Skin*. New York: Harper Row; 1986.

Pryor G. *Nursing Mother, Working Mother: The Essential Guide for Breastfeeding and Staying Close to Your Baby After You Return to Work*. Boston, MA: Harvard Common Press; 1997.

Saarinen U, Kajosaari M. Breastfeeding as prophylaxis against atopic disease: Prospective follow-up study until 17 years old. *Lancet* 346(8982):1065–1069; 1995.

Slusser W, Powers NG. Breastfeeding update I: Immunology, nutrition and advocacy. *Pediatri Rev* 18(4):111–119; 1997.

Stuart-MacAdam P, Dettwyler K eds. *Breastfeeding: Biocultural Perspectives (Foundations of Human Behavior).* New York: Aldine de Gruyter; 1995.

Williams K, Morse J. Weaning patterns of first-time mothers. *American Journal of Maternal Child Nursing* 14L:188–192; 1989.

World Health Organization (WHO). *Protecting, Promoting, and Supporting Breastfeeding: A Joint WHO/UNICEF Statement.* Geneva, Switzerland; WHO: 1989.

Worthington H et al. Interventions for preventing oral candidiasis for patients with cancer receiving treatment. Review. *Cochrane Database Syst Rev* (3):CD003807; 2002.

Wrigley E, Hutchinson S. Long-term breastfeeding: The secret bond. *J Nurse Midwife* 35:35–41; 1990.

▶ **BIBLIOGRAPHY**

Allen K, Marotz L. *By the Ages: Behavior and Development of Children Pre-birth through Eight.* Albany, NY: Delmar Thompson Learning; 2000.

Beatty J. *Observing Development in the Young Child.* Columbus, OH: Charles Merrill; 1990.

Bee H. *The Developing Child.* New York: Harper and Row; 1989.

Buschbach D, Schaub Bordeaux M. *Newborn Physiologic and Developmental Transitions: Integrating Key Components of Perinatal and Neonatal Assessment.* Washington, DC: AWHONN; 2002.

de Bruin, N et al. Energy utilization and growth in breast-fed and formula-fed infants measured prospectively during the first year of life. *Am J Clin Nutr* 67:1256–1264; 1998.

Dewey K. Effect of age of introduction of complementary foods on iron status of breast fed infants in Honduras. *Am J Clin Nutr* 67:878–884; 1998.

Goldman A. Association of atopic diseases with breast-feeding: Food allergens, fatty acids, and evolution. *J Pediatr* 134:5–7; 1999.

Hendricks K, Badruddin S. Weaning recommendations: The scientific basis. *Nutr Rev* 50:125–133; 1992.

Hill P et al. Effects of parity and weaning practices on breastfeeding duration. *Public Health Nursing* 14:227–234; 1997.

Hughes FP et al. *Child Development.* St. Paul, MN: West Publishing; 1988.

Isolauri E et al. Breast-feeding of allergic infants. *J Pediatr* 134:27–32; 1999.

Jiang Z et al. Energy expenditure of Chinese infants in Guangdong Province, south China, determined with use of the doubly labeled water method. *Am J Clin Nutr* 67:1256–1264; 1998.

Keener M et al. Infant temperament, sleep organization, and nighttime parental interventions. *Pediatrics* 81:762–771; 1988.

Kendall-Tackett K, Sugarman M. The social consequences of long-term breastfeeding. *J Hum Lact* 11(3):179–184; 1995.

Kendall-Tackett K, Sugarman M. Weaning ages in a sample of American women who practice extended breastfeeding. *Clin Pediatr (Phila)* 34(12):642–647; 1995.

Lloyd B et al. Formula tolerance in postbreastfed and exclusively formula-fed infants. *Pediatrics* 103(1):E7; 1999.

Lorick G. Untimely weaning: Assisting the mother who may grieve. *Int J Childbirth Education* 8:41; 1993.

Maekawa K et al. Developmental change of sucking response to taste in infants. *Biol Neonate* 60(supp 1):62; 1991.

Rowe L et al. A comparison of two methods of breastfeeding management. *Aust Fam Phys* 21:288–294; 1992.

Sears W et al. Becoming a Father, 2nd ed. Schaumburg, IL: La Leche League International; 2003.

Victora C et al. Breast-feeding and growth in Brazilian infants. *Am J Clin Nutr* 67:452–458; 1998.

Winchell K. Nursing strike: Misunderstood feelings. *J Hum Lact* 8(4):217–219; 1992.

PROBLEMS WITH MILK PRODUCTION AND TRANSFER

Contributing Author: Linda Kutner

The most common reason women give for stopping breastfeeding is that they believe they do not have enough milk. Studies from around the world reveal that this is a universal belief, transcending nationalities and cultures (Simic, 2004; Al-Jazzir, 2003; Borges, 2003; Shani, 2003; Blythe, 2002; Colin, 2002). This is also why most women give their babies supplements. The information presented in this chapter will assist you in helping a mother recognize when her milk production truly is low. You will learn to recognize when a newborn is receiving sufficient amounts of his mother's milk, and when he is not. Measures for increasing milk production and for efficient transfer are presented as well. With appropriate teaching and follow-up, you and the mother can maximize the chances of an adequate milk supply and a baby who thrives on his mother's milk.

KEY TERMS

augmentation
breastfeeding after
    reduction (BFAR)
digital baby scale
donor milk
failure-to-thrive

Human Milk Banking
    Association of North
    America (HMBANA)
insufficient milk supply
poor weight gain
slow weight gain

INSUFFICIENT MILK SUPPLY: PERCEIVED OR REAL?

A mother might perceive a problem with her milk for a number of reasons. She may believe it is not rich enough or satisfying enough. She may worry that her milk is causing an allergic response or excessive gas in her baby. By far the most common concern for mothers is that they have an inadequate amount of milk. When a mother says she does not have enough milk for her baby, you first need to determine why she says this. While it is possible that she has low milk production, the comment may actually result from a lack of confidence or a lack of knowledge about typical newborn behavior. Helping the mother identify whether she actually has a problem, and reassuring her when you have determined that her

production is fine, will have a tremendous influence on breastfeeding duration among your clients.

Reasons for a Perceived Low Milk Supply

There are differences between women who perceive they have insufficient milk and those who do not. IBCLCs need to be aware of some of these differences and view them as red flags so that mothers receive special help or information. Mothers who perceive their milk production to be insufficient worry that the baby does not seem satisfied and is fussy after feedings. They are also concerned about too frequent feedings and poor infant weight gain.

Some women lack confidence in their bodies' ability to function as nature intended. The medical profession's use of negative terminology in women's health could be a contributing factor. Such terms as *lactation failure*, *failure to progress*, and *incompetent cervix* can undermine a woman's self-confidence and self-esteem. Messages such as these can compromise a mother's confidence at a time when she is extremely vulnerable to negativism.

Because many new parents do not live near their nuclear family, they may lack a strong support system and positive role models for birthing and parenting. Women who choose to breastfeed in a culture that is saturated with bottle-feeding messages face many societal challenges. Female friends and relatives often have bottle-fed their babies. The expectations of society and the media are that babies are fed by bottles. One mother, when asked if she were still breastfeeding her twins, replied, "No, I'm feeding them the regular way." Often, caregivers either have a lack of correct information regarding breastfeeding care (Power, 2003; Akuse, 2002) or are noncommittal to avoid making mothers "feel guilty" if they choose not to breastfeed (Dettwyler, 1999).

The stress of becoming a new mother can feed into a woman's worries about competence. Most families in industrialized countries are small and many parents have had little or no experience in caring for small infants.

Parents want to know they are doing the best for their baby. A mother's misconceptions about the realities of motherhood can cause her to question her choices and doubt her mothering abilities. Her preconceived notion of babies may not match the reality of her baby or her baby's needs. Misconceptions of normal behavior can create anxieties in inexperienced parents, and they may incorrectly blame breastfeeding as the cause for fussiness, wakefulness, or other newborn behaviors. One study measuring parental self-efficacy found a significant correlation between levels of maternal self-confidence and perceived insufficient milk (McCarter-Spaulding, 2001).

Recognizing Sufficient Milk Production

Mothers have fewer worries about inadequate milk production when they understand that milk removal triggers further milk production and what to expect in normal newborn behavior. Knowing how to tell that their baby receives sufficient milk will prevent the unnecessary early weaning caused by a mother's perception that she does not have enough milk for her baby. The signs below indicate that breastfeeding is going well.

Signs That Breastfeeding Is Going Well

◆ By day four, the baby has at least six wet diapers in each 24-hour period.

◆ The baby has pale, dilute urine.

◆ By day four, the baby has three or more ample stools that are yellow or at least are turning yellow.

◆ The baby continues to have at least three stools in each 24-hour period until he is about five to six weeks old.

◆ The baby routinely breastfeeds at least 8 to 12 times in each 24-hour period.

◆ The mother's breasts feel softer after a feeding (although some women have no dramatic change).

◆ The mother's nipples are not painful during or after feedings.

◆ The baby regains his birth weight by 10 to 14 days.

◆ The baby gains four to eight ounces a week.

◆ During a feeding, the baby's sucking rhythm changes and slows as he obtains milk, and the mother hears swallowing or gulping.

◆ The baby is alert and active.

◆ The baby is content between feedings and usually rests for one to two hours, wakes on his own, and signals to breastfeed again (although well-fed infants may be fussy for other reasons).

It is important that the mother feel secure in her ability to breastfeed her baby. Help her to feel confident that she can produce the milk her baby will need. If she and her baby went home in 48 hours or less, the baby's primary caregiver needs to see him within two to four days (AAP, 2004). The mother will typically have a second visit at around two weeks for a physical assessment and another weight check. It should be sooner if the baby's condition warrants it. These safeguards will help to assure a healthy baby and a confident mother.

Identifying Mothers at Risk

Your role in the case of low milk production or transfer involves helping the mother explore the possible causes. There usually are multiple factors that cause a baby not to gain adequate weight, some more significant than others. Factors may relate to the mother, to the baby, or to breastfeeding practices. When multiple factors exist at birth, it is important that the mother and baby receive follow-up. Figure 12.4 in Chapter 12 identifies potential problems for establishing either adequate milk production or effective milk transfer.

Poor breastfeeding technique may be the cause of slow or poor weight gain. Some feeding-related causes are the baby's inability to suck well, improper positioning, or inadequate time at each breast. Mothers also find that their milk supply diminishes after they begin supplemental or complementary feedings (Hill, 1991). Prolactin inhibitors and an inhibited or unstable letdown can cause problems with weight gain. A specific cause may not always be apparent. When the mother and baby are both more proficient at nursing, problems that cause low milk production often diminish. See Chapter 25 for a discussion of maternal factors for true insufficient milk supply.

Measures to Increase Milk Production

You can work with the mother and baby while they increase milk production in a manner that is both safe and supportive of breastfeeding. A need to increase milk production may occur at any time during in the early days of lactation, at times of growth spurts, or whenever the baby nurses less often. The baby may have poor weight gain that requires the mother to increase her milk production. The mother may have started giving supplements to her baby too early and wish to reduce or eliminate the amount of supplement her baby receives.

The degree to which a mother is able to increase milk production will depend on the age of her baby, his willingness to nurse, and the degree of breast involution. It will also depend on the condition of the baby and any corresponding medical factors. Whether the baby is currently taking a supplement and the amount taken will

TABLE 18.1	
Measures to Increase Milk Production	
Actions for the mother	◆ Rest as much as possible, and relax during breastfeedings to help the milk flow.
	◆ Spend 100 percent of her time with the baby for 48 hours, concentrating on increasing feedings and resting. Get help with all other tasks.
	◆ Take special precautions to prevent sore nipples.
	◆ Use local galactogogues (foods, drinks, or herbs believed to increase milk production).
	◆ Keep a record of feedings (both breastfeedings and any supplements). This can show how quickly the milk production is increasing and help the mother find a workable feeding pattern.
	◆ Use a hospital-grade electric breast pump to provide additional stimulation to the breasts.
	◆ Improve diet by eating more protein, fresh fruits and vegetables, and B vitamins.
Management of feedings	◆ Encourage letdown by relaxation techniques and following a daily feeding routine.
	◆ Prepare the baby so he is alert and ready to nurse by rousing or soothing him as needed.
	◆ Make sure the baby is attached for effective suckling.
	◆ Put the baby to both breasts at a feeding, several times each, to increase stimulation.
	◆ Encourage the baby to feed more frequently and longer, both day and night.
	◆ Nurse long enough for the baby to receive hindmilk. This will vary from one baby to another.
	◆ Nurse for comfort if the baby is fussy.
	◆ Get into bed with the baby for feedings to increase skin contact.
	◆ Resume night feedings if they had been dropped.

influence the length of time it takes to increase production. A mother's motivation to give her time and energies fully to breastfeeding her baby will determine her success. Her baby needs to breastfeed at least 10–12 times in 24 hours. Mothers least at risk for insufficiency are those who breastfeed more frequently and longer at each feeding (Hill, 1993).

You can help the mother increase milk production by offering some of the suggestions presented in Table 18.1. As with other aspects of breastfeeding, several measures can be considered when developing a plan with the mother to increase her milk production. Be careful not to overwhelm her with too many suggestions or with measures that do not appeal to her. Each mother's needs are different. The mother will need close contact and support from you. This is especially the case in the first few days when she is trying to sort out the methods that work most effectively for her.

Galactogogues

Many mothers are able to increase milk production simply by altering their pattern of feedings. Some respond well to galactogogues—foods, drinks, medications, or herbs believed to increase milk production. Some women use fenugreek, blessed thistle, and other herbs as galactogogues. *The Nursing Mother's Herbal* (Humphrey,

2003) may be helpful for mothers seeking an herbal approach.

Domperidone

Many women use domperidone to increase milk production, because a side effect of the medication is an increase in prolactin levels. Before domperidone became available, women used metoclopramide, which also raises prolactin levels. However, because of metoclopramide's other side effects of fatigue, irritability, and depression, domperidone is now preferred.

In 2004, the U.S. Federal Drug Administration issued a warning against the use of domperidone by breastfeeding women. Responses from breastfeeding experts underscored the long history of safe use of domperidone for increasing milk production in breastfeeding women. Domperidone is available in many countries, even as a non-prescription medication in some. It is not available in the United States except by compounding—combining drugs to create a new substance. In addition to warning the public about use of domperidone, the FDA issued an Import Alert asking FDA personnel to be on the lookout for the drug being imported into the United States (FDA, 2004). These warnings occurred at a time when the pharmaceutical industry was fighting against importation of drugs into the United States. The FDA issued the warning on the same day as the largest breastfeeding promotion campaign in U.S. history was launched by the Department of Health and Human Services.

Newman points out that domperidone should not be the first approach to correcting breastfeeding difficulties. Its use is appropriate only after exploring all other factors that may result in insufficient milk supply and responding appropriately. Problem solving should include correcting the baby's latch, correcting sucking problems, and using breast compression during feedings and milk expression after feedings to increase milk production (Newman, 2003b).

▶ CONCERNS ABOUT INFANT GROWTH

Several factors contribute to the total picture of a baby's adequate growth. Birth weight should have doubled by four months and tripled by twelve months (Lawrence, 1999). Body length is a significant indicator of growth. The baby should have increased in length by 50 percent at twelve months. Head circumference, which indicates brain growth, should have increased by 7.6 cm (3 inches) at one year. Other signs of healthy growth are sufficient voids and stools, which will be frequent in the first month and less frequent thereafter. Bright eyes, an alert manner, and good muscle and skin tone also indicate a healthy baby. If there is a family history of small stature or slow weight gain, the parents' children will most likely exhibit a similar pattern. All of these factors need consideration before you determine that a problem may exist.

To ensure the health of every infant in your care, be alert to weight gain and to the factors that could contribute to low milk production. Understand each mother's and baby's feeding pattern to help you assess adequate growth. Consider all growth indicators and possible causes of poor growth as you and the mother develop a care plan for improvement.

Few mothers actually have insufficient milk production, although their numbers are increasing (Marasco, 2000). Most cases of insufficient milk result from ineffective breastfeeding, which the mother can correct. Be careful not to confuse the maternal inability to produce adequate amounts of milk with the lack of *opportunity* to produce the milk.

Newborn Dehydration

When a baby does not receive a sufficient amount of fluids, he can become dehydrated. This can occur when a breastfed baby is not receiving an adequate amount of his mother's milk. Many mothers and babies leave the hospital before someone who is knowledgeable about breastfeeding has evaluated their breastfeeding technique. Consequently, some mothers will not have had a good breastfeeding before they go home. Because of short hospital stays, very few mothers will have established milk production (Lactogenesis II) prior to discharge. There is evidence that high milk sodium levels, rather than *causing* dehydration, seem to occur after milk production slows (Scott, 2003; Sofer, 1993).

It is imperative that mothers and babies who go home early receive some form of follow-up shortly after discharge. Mothers need to know how to assess adequate breastfeeding, stools, and wet diapers. There is never any reason for a healthy newborn to progress to the point of dehydration. Hospital staff needs to teach the mother how to recognize when her baby achieves an effective latch, signs that breastfeeding is going well, and warning signs of potential problems (see Chapter 12). Just because a baby's jaw moves up and down does not mean he is taking in milk.

Giving the mother a diary to document feedings, stools, and voids will help her monitor her baby's output. If she has not established effective breastfeeding at the time of discharge, the mother and baby need a follow-up visit to the physician's office or lactation clinic within one to two days post-discharge. The office staff must recognize the impact of the number of feedings, stools, and voids. Recognizing the symptoms of dehydration will help you identify infants at risk.

Symptoms of Dehydration

- ◆ Few or no stools
- ◆ Scant urinary output
- ◆ Infant sleeps at the breast
- ◆ Infrequent feedings
- ◆ Weight loss greater than 10–15 percent of birth weight
- ◆ Lethargy
- ◆ Weak cry
- ◆ Dry mucous membranes
- ◆ Lack of tearing
- ◆ Poor skin turgor
- ◆ Sunken fontanels

Problems with Infant Weight Gain

Concerns about the baby's weight usually surface within the first month. Weight gain problems that start after the first month are more likely to have organic causes (Lukefahr, 1990). As discussed in Chapter 13, weight loss beyond 10 to 15 percent in the first week warrants an evaluation and assistance with breastfeeding. There should be no further weight loss after the third day for full-term infants, and weight gain should begin by day four. By 10 to 14 days, the baby should be back to birth weight (Merlob, 1994). If he has not regained his birth weight by 14 days, you need to explore the mother's breastfeeding practices to rule out inadequate milk intake. This encompasses both the infant not taking enough milk and the mother not producing enough milk.

In order to assess milk transfer, weigh the baby before and after feedings. Test weighing on a digital electronic scale will assure accuracy (Meier, 1994). Reserve this assessment for problems associated with milk intake. Occasionally, some parents have serious doubts that their baby is taking in enough milk. Weighing him before and after a feeding can give them reassurance.

Breastfed and formula-fed infants consume dramatically different amounts of calories. By eight months a formula-fed infant consumes about 30,000 more Kcal than a breastfed infant (Garza, 1987). By four months of age, gross energy intakes by exclusively breastfed infants are significantly less than current recommendations, which are based on artificial feeding. Furthermore, breastfed infants have normal growth rates that differ from the growth rates of formula-fed infants. They also have lower total daily energy expenditure, sleeping metabolic rates, rates of energy expenditure, rectal temperature, and heart rates (Garza, 1990).

In unfavorable environments, babies may have higher-than-usual energy requirements. Rather than low milk production or intake, the baby's environment could explain the growth differences. This may be an issue for babies who live in high-poverty areas. Babies who lack restful sleep or who have multiple care providers may also have increased caloric needs (Butte, 1993). Although breastfed infants develop leaner body mass, the pattern does not continue into the second year (Butte, 2000). Because of the difference in growth in exclusively breastfed infants and those fed artificial baby milk, there is a need for growth charts for breastfed infants. World Health Organization growth charts should be available in 2005.

Infant with Slow Weight Gain

Every child develops at his own rate. Some adolescents experience a growth spurt and grow six inches in one year. The same is true for babies. Some babies naturally gain weight more slowly than others. It is important to distinguish between a baby who is not gaining weight *adequately* and one who is simply gaining weight *slowly*. A slow-gaining infant will demonstrate a slow and steady growth over time; will grow proportionally for weight, length, and head circumference; and will develop appropriately for his age.

In the absence of other risk factors, minimal intervention, if any, is required. You can observe a breastfeeding to evaluate the mother's technique. Ask about her baby's feeding pattern and suggest any necessary changes. Some mothers believe they should nurse on only one breast at a feeding. Simply changing to two breasts can have a significant improvement in weight gain. Make sure the baby receives no pacifiers or bottles that would limit his sucking time at the breast. Confirm that the mother is not trying to schedule or restrict feedings or is limiting her baby's time at the breast (see Chapter 19 for cautions about "baby training"). Review feeding cues with the mother to be sure she responds to her baby at appropriate times. Suggest that she have her baby weighed weekly and record his weights to monitor his growth. These measures may be all that is necessary for a slow-gaining infant.

Infant with Poor Weight Gain

A newborn who remains below birth weight by several ounces at day 14 may need more direct intervention. The same is true of an older baby who is not gaining or who is gaining less than three ounces per week. Make sure the infant receives a minimum of eight to twelve feedings per day around the clock and an appropriate number of complementary foods in the case of older babies. Feedings should last 20 to 40 minutes with a lot of swallowing observed.

If you are concerned that a baby may be an inefficient feeder, obtain pre- and post-feeding weights on a digital scale and have the mother pump after the feeding. This will help you determine whether the baby is ineffective in removing milk or the mother has low milk production. The pumped milk can be fed to the baby at the next feeding. Teach the parents paced feeding to slow the flow rate if they choose to supplement with a bottle (Kassing, 2002; Wilson-Clay, 2002). (See Chapter 21 for information about paced feeding.) Caution against the use of pacifiers for a baby with poor weight gain. Emphasize to parents that all sucking needs to be nutritive to increase caloric intake.

Suggest that the baby be weighed at least twice a week, and record his weights to monitor his gain. If the baby is an inefficient feeder, the mother will need to use a breast pump to remove any milk left in the breast at the end of the feeding and provide quality nipple stimulation to maintain milk production. This will be necessary until the baby is more effective at transferring milk.

In the event of poor weight gain, the goal is twofold. First, the baby needs to receive calories. Increasing his weight is essential. If the mother's milk production is low, the baby will need to receive supplemental donor milk or formula. If the baby is preterm or has other health problems, his physician can prescribe donor milk. Some insurance companies and Medicaid will cover the use of donor milk for these babies. Compile a list of the human milk banks, and become familiar with the **Human Milk Banking Association of North America's** (HMBANA) guidelines. Those who live outside Canada, the United States, or Mexico can check with their health ministry or department. HMBANA's Web site is www.hmbana.org.

The second goal is to increase the mother's milk production to the level that it can sustain her infant. Only then can the mother discontinue supplements. Supplementing the baby through a tube at the breast will accomplish both goals at the same time. The baby receives the nourishment he needs and the mother's breasts receive the stimulation necessary for milk production. Pumping with a hospital-grade electric breast pump immediately after feedings will further help to increase milk production.

Make sure the baby's physician is aware of the plan of care you and the mother develop. The mother's primary caregiver also needs to be involved if the mother has an impaired milk supply. Send a report of your consultation to both caregivers, or call them with your evaluation and suggestions. Encourage the mother to stay in close contact with you and her caregivers until the baby's weight gain has been resolved. As the baby begins to gain weight, the mother can slowly decrease the amount of supplement he is receiving, after she is confident he is transferring more from the breast. Caregivers should become concerned when growth deviates downward by 2 major percentiles on the growth chart. When this occurs, the baby is diagnosed as failure to thrive.

Signs of Inadequate Weight Gain

The above factors will help you to identify mothers and babies who are at risk for low milk production or transfer. Unfortunately, you may not always have the opportunity to see these mothers and infants before a problem develops. You need to recognize signs that will alert you to problems. Babies who are not gaining adequately will frequently sleep for long periods to conserve energy. They may fuss when removed from the breast and then go back to sleep as soon as they return to the breast. A mother may tell you that she is nursing "all the time" because she cannot put her baby down without him fussing. Another mother may tell you she has a "good" baby who nurses infrequently. These infants usually sleep through the night and have few periods of quiet alert time.

A baby with poor weight gain often looks worried or anxious. He holds his body in a flexed fetal position to help maintain his temperature. If a baby has lost a large amount of weight, he will have hanging folds of skin on his thighs and buttocks. His cry may be a high-pitched sound like the "mew" of a cat. Urinary output may be decreased, or the baby may pass concentrated urine. In an older baby, urine may smell strongly of ammonia. A baby less than 5 to 6 weeks of age will pass few stools. In a young infant, parents frequently report that he is still passing meconium after the fourth day of life.

Failure-to-Thrive

Lawrence defines a failure-to-thrive (FTT) infant as one who continues to lose weight after 10 days of life, does not regain his birth weight by 3 weeks of age, or has a weight gain below the tenth percentile beyond 1 month of age (Lawrence, 1999). In older infants, a weight that is 2 standard deviations or more below where it should be on a standard growth chart is an indication of FTT. A growth chart that shows normal weight for each age is a tool for determining whether growth is within established guidelines. Plotting the baby's predictable growth curve on a chart will help assess his progress.

A baby who fails to thrive may be lethargic, hypertonic, irritable, and difficult to soothe (Figure 18.1). He may sleep excessively or be continuously fussy. His compromised status could relate to his physical condition or that of his mother. Table 18.2 identifies causes related to the mother and infant. In many cases, failure to thrive is a consequence of ineffective breastfeeding. It is important to realize that even a baby who appears to be satisfied can fail to thrive. An easy, placid baby is vulnerable to failure to thrive because he does not display appropriate hunger cues. An interesting phenomenon occurs when the mother corrects her breastfeeding technique. These babies have a tendency toward obesity, perhaps due to inactivity or a defect in appetite control (Habbick, 1984).

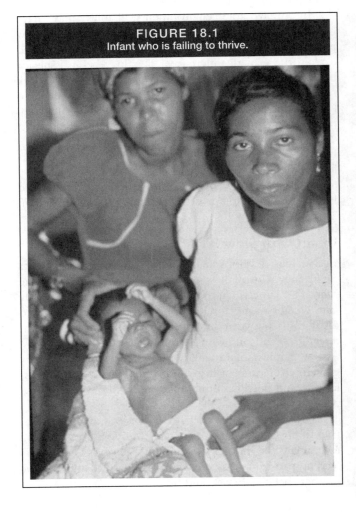

FIGURE 18.1
Infant who is failing to thrive.

TABLE 18.2
Causes of Failure-to-Thrive

Maternal causes

◆ Previous breast surgery, either reduction or augmentation, or breast trauma

◆ Back or thoracic surgery

◆ Polycystic ovarian syndrome or history of infertility

◆ Hypoprolactinemia

◆ Anatomic position of the ducts

◆ Insufficient mammary tissue

◆ Hormonal disorders, including untreated hypothyroidism

◆ Sheehan's syndrome

◆ Disrupted neurohormonal pathways

◆ Inappropriate use of a nipple shield

◆ Retained placental fragments

◆ Poor breastfeeding practices, such as scheduling or restricting feedings

Infant causes

◆ Neuromotor problems

◆ Preterm or SGA infant

◆ Tight frenulum

◆ Systemic illness

◆ Sleepy infant

◆ Inability to compress breast adequately

◆ Mother's anatomy versus infant's oral cavity

◆ Disorganized suck

◆ "Good" baby who does not exhibit hunger cues

Issues to Address with the Mother

Identifying the causes of failure to thrive can require detective work on your part. The mother whose breast is depicted in Color Plate 51 answered, "No," when asked if she had ever had a breast injury. Upon examination, the IBCLC could clearly see a two-and-a-half-inch scar across the areola. With further questioning, the mother recalled that when she was nine years old she ran into the propeller on her family's boat! Her milk supply did not seem impaired by the injury, although this breast did produce less milk than the right breast. Below are issues you can address with the mother.

◆ *How much weight did you gain during pregnancy?* This may give you a clue to low fat in the mother's milk or the possibility of an eating disorder.

◆ *Describe the changes that occurred in your breasts during pregnancy.* This may help you determine if she has sufficient mammary tissue.

◆ *Do you have a history of infertility or miscarriages?* Miscarriage is a marker for thyroid disorders.

◆ *Are you aware of having any thyroid dysfunction?* (Know the markers for hypothyroidism and hyperthyroidism.)

◆ *Have you had any breast procedure, such as a biopsy, cyst removal, augmentation, or reduction? Have you ever had a breast injury?*

◆ *During delivery, was there excessive blood loss or the use of Pitocin or IV fluids?* Hemorrhage or edema may delay onset of milk production.

◆ *Are you using oral contraceptives?* Estrogen can reduce milk production.

◆ *Describe your diet.* While this is rarely a factor, this information will help to paint a total picture.

◆ *Do you smoke cigarettes? How many per day?* Smoking has been associated with low supply (Hale, 2004).

◆ *Do you drink alcohol? How much and how often?* Alcohol has been associated with a reduction in milk production (Mennella, 2001, 1998).

◆ *Have you experienced any breast engorgement or mastitis?* Pathologic engorgement may lead to loss of milk producing cells.

◆ *Describe your breastfeeding routine.* How often does the baby feed in a 24-hour period and for how long, and on both breasts or one.

◆ *How many voids and stools has your baby had in the last 24 hours? What color and size were they?* Scant or no stooling indicates inadequate intake. Green stools may mark imbalance in foremilk and hindmilk.

◆ *How often does your baby use a pacifier?* Pacifier use has been associated with reduced breastfeeding (Adair, 2003; Ullah, 2003; Benis, 2002).

◆ *How much time does your baby spend in a swing?* Use of devices to delay or avoid feedings can contribute to underfeeding your baby.

◆ *Is there a particular parenting program or schedule that you are trying to follow?* "Baby training" programs are associated with low weight gain and maternal loss of milk supply (Aney, 1998; Marasco, 1998). See Chapter 19 for further discussion.

Reversing the Trend of Failure-to-Thrive

If failure-to-thrive is suspected, measures must begin immediately to reverse the pattern of weight loss. The actions taken will depend on whether the issues affecting lactation lie with the baby, the mother, or both. Your assistance and support can be pivotal in helping a mother reverse her baby's weight pattern. Interventions may be required for a long time, so help her form realistic expectations. It is very common for the mother of a failure-to-thrive infant to feel highly stressed. As her baby's condition begins to improve, caution the mother to proceed slowly with decreasing the amount of supplement and frequency of milk expression. Sometimes interventions, as described below, are required for the entire time the baby is breastfed.

Interventions for an Infant Who Fails To Thrive

◆ Assess the baby's latch, sucking technique, and positioning at the breast. If oral anomalies are noted, refer to the baby's caregiver for referral to an appropriate specialist. For example, babies with ankyloglossia are often referred to ear, nose, and throat specialists or to pediatric dentists for frenotomies (clipping the frenulum).

◆ Perform pre- and post-feeding weights on a digital baby scale to assess milk transfer.
  ◆ If the baby does not transfer a significant amount of milk (two ounces or more), and the mother is able to pump two ounces or more, refer her to the baby's physician for assessment.
  ◆ If the baby is able to transfer two ounces, increasing frequency and duration of feedings may be appropriate.

◆ Breastfeed the baby 10–12 times in 24 hours around the clock until he has three stools per 24 hours for three days in a row.

◆ Switch breasts when the baby's suckling pattern changes and swallowing ceases.

◆ Use alternate breast compression to increase milk flow (Newman, 2003a).

◆ Limit feedings to 40 minutes per session no matter which combination of feeding methods are used.

◆ Supplement after every feeding until the baby is gaining well, per the physician's guidelines.

◆ Pump immediately after nursing. Using a hospital-grade electric breast pump, double pump for 10–15 minutes or until milk stops flowing to help stimulate milk production. She can then massage her breasts and pump a few minutes more.

◆ Meet the baby's caloric needs with frequent feedings and supplements as recommended by the baby's physician.

◆ Ensure that the baby visits his physician frequently.

◆ Weigh the baby frequently and record weight changes.

◆ Advise the mother to stay in close contact with you and her baby's physician.

◆ As things improve, discuss with the mother what intervention stresses her the most, and try to eliminate or decrease that aspect of the feeding plan. The mother frequently will ask to discontinue nighttime supplements when things improve. Encourage her to continue to breastfeed at least once during the night to take advantage of higher prolactin levels.

Supplementing the FTT Baby

It is crucial that the baby receive adequate nourishment while the mother is increasing her milk production. If milk production is too low to give sufficient calories, she will need to supplement her baby with formula or donor milk until her milk production increases. The baby should receive no pacifiers, to ensure that all sucking is nutritive.

Encourage the mother to breastfeed first and follow with the supplement. Pumping after feedings will provide further stimulation. She can feed her baby any residual milk that remains in the breast at the end of a feeding. When her milk production improves, she can reduce supplements slowly and continue with the increased number of breastfeedings.

Amount to Supplement

Mothers must regulate supplements and give them in measured amounts. This will ensure that the baby does not receive too much supplement and consequently becomes disinterested in nursing. Suggest that the mother plan the number of ounces to feed her baby during a 24-hour period. A standard physician order of "Nurse first and supplement afterward" may be misleading. Some babies nurse as few as six times a day, while others nurse as many as twelve times. The baby could consume so much formula this way that nursing may never resume.

The mother can ask her baby's caregiver how much supplement per day her baby must receive. The recommended number of ounces can be divided into two, three, or four feedings, depending on the amount. The baby can receive supplements at predetermined times through a tube at the breast. If he does not finish it at one feeding, he may not require as much supplement in his daily diet. On the other hand, he may need those few ounces sometime later within that 24-hour period. Advise the mother to watch her baby carefully for signs of hunger and to respond accordingly.

A feeding assessment will help determine the amount of supplementation the baby needs. He should not have nursed for about two hours prior to the assessment, and the mother should delay expressing her milk until after the feeding assessment. Weighing the baby on a digital scale before and after a feeding will establish how much

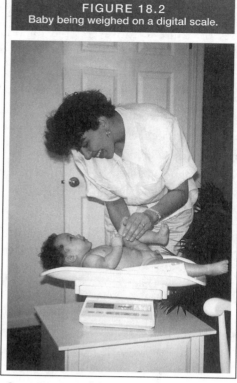

FIGURE 18.2
Baby being weighed on a digital scale.

Courtesy of Medela, Inc.

he consumes during the feeding (see Figure 18.2). The mother then pumps her breasts to measure the amount of residual milk left in the breast. The amount of milk the infant consumed, added to the amount of residual milk, gives a good indication of the mother's milk production over the preceding two or three hours.

The calculations in Table 18.3 will help you determine the baby's total daily requirements. Divide it by the number of feedings he takes or should take during a 24-hour period. Knowing what he consumed compared to what he should have consumed will give you and the mother an accurate measurement of the amount of supplement her baby will require. A convenient reference

list for determining feeding requirements appears in Appendix G.

Explain clearly to the parents that feeding charts are guidelines. Although charts can be helpful tools when a baby is not gaining, they are not ironclad rules. Babies differ in the amounts of milk they consume. Breastfed babies typically consume 26–32 ounces during a 24-hour period. However, averages are just that—average—and no baby is "average."

Weaning from the Supplement

Encourage the mother to keep a record of how much supplement her baby is getting, as well as the number of feedings, wet diapers, and stools. The mother needs to give her baby enough supplement to provide adequate infant growth. At the same time, she must make sure her breasts receive enough quality stimulation to increase milk production. Caution her to decrease the amount of supplement slowly, with frequent weight checks to make sure her baby continues to gain.

A mother should *never* dilute formula in an attempt to cut back on supplements, as this may lead to insufficient caloric intake for the baby. The process of eliminating formula and increasing her milk production to replace it may take several weeks of concentrated effort. Following a consistent pattern of nursing while offering supplements and watching for small daily successes will aid her in reaching her goal of exclusive breastfeeding. Your close contact with her will give her the support and objectivity she needs to succeed.

Counseling Issues with FTT

A baby who fails to thrive plays into a mother's fears and insecurities about her parenting and her ability to breastfeed. It is important that you approach the mother with sensitivity, offering validation and reassurance. She may cry frequently and may need to express her fears and feelings of guilt. Lack of familiarity with infant development and a lack of follow-up support from the healthcare system are factors in most cases of failure-to-thrive. See

TABLE 18.3	
Determining the Number of Ounces an Infant Needs	
Example for an infant weighing 4 pounds and 2 ounces	
Convert infant's weight to ounces.	4 lb + 2 oz = 66 oz
Divide total ounces by 6 to determine amount required for a 24-hour intake.	66 oz ÷ 6 = 11 oz
Divide the 24-hour requirements by the number of feedings per 24-hour period to determine how much is required per feeding.	11 oz ÷ 8 feedings = 1.37 oz per feeding
	11 oz ÷ 6 feedings = 1.83 oz per feeding

Chapter 25 for a discussion of biological insufficient milk supply (IMS) and ways to counsel and help those mothers optimize their breastfeeding.

In a case of breast trauma, especially augmentation or reduction surgeries, the mother will need to come to terms with impaired milk production. She may feel anger at herself for having an elective procedure performed or at the surgeon for minimizing or failing to explain the risk of surgery on lactation. She may feel guilt for not being able to provide her baby's entire nutrition. You can help her recognize the difference between regret and guilt. She may want to channel her anger into productive ways of coping, such as lobbying for consumer healthcare education and protection.

The mother may benefit from the long-term support of a breastfeeding group such as Breastfeeding After Reduction. Their Web site is www.bfar.org. Another resource for mothers with impaired milk production due to surgery is *Defining Your Own Success: Breastfeeding After Breast Reduction Surgery* (West, 2001). Be alert to recognizing when a mother's emotional needs are beyond your scope of practice or ability to help her. Referral to a counselor specializing in women's issues may be appropriate.

▶ SUMMARY

Caregivers have a responsibility to give mothers the information and support they need in order to feel confident in their ability to provide sufficient milk to their baby. A mother who is physically unable to establish milk production or an infant who is physically unable to achieve milk transfer is uncommon in the general population. IBCLCs in private practice often receive referrals for such occurrences. Problems with milk production and transfer usually result from inappropriate breastfeeding technique. Identifying the cause and taking appropriate action will prevent serious consequences for the baby. No breastfed baby should reach the point of dehydration or failure-to-thrive. Be alert to significant barriers to milk production or positive milk transfer. Understanding the issues presented in this chapter will help you, as a practitioner, avoid such serious consequences.

▶ CHAPTER 18—AT A GLANCE

Applying what you learned—

Teach the mother about:

◆ When to consult a healthcare practitioner.

◆ Signs her baby's weight needs to be monitored with a baby scale.

◆ Signs of a healthy slow weight gain.

◆ Signs that a baby is not gaining adequate weight.

◆ Causes of failure-to-thrive and the importance of supplementing the baby.

Teach the mother how to:

◆ Recognize sufficient milk production.

◆ Avoid practices that compromise milk production.

◆ Avoid newborn dehydration.

◆ Increase milk production.

◆ Recognize signs of adequate growth in her baby.

◆ Recognize and manage failure-to-thrive.

▶ REFERENCES

Adair S. Pacifier use in children: A review of recent literature. *Pediatr Dent* 25(5):449–458; 2003.

Akuse R, Obinya E. Why health care workers give prelacteal feeds. *Eur J Clin Nutr* 56(8):729–734; 2002.

Al-Jazzir M et al. A review of some statistics on breastfeeding in Saudi Arabia. *Nutr Health* 17(2):123–130; 2003.

American Academy of Pediatrics (AAP) Committee on Fetus and Newborn. Hospital stay for healthy term newborns. *Pediatrics* 113:1434–1436; 2004.

American Academy of Pediatrics (AAP) Work Group on Breastfeeding. Breastfeeding and the use of human milk. *Pediatrics* 100:1035–1039; 1997.

Aney M. Babywise advice linked to dehydration, failure to thrive. AAP News; April 1998. Article available at: www.ezzo.info/Aney/aneyaap.htm. Accessed January 10, 2005.

Benis M. Are pacifiers associated with early weaning from breastfeeding? *Adv Neonatal Care* 2(5):259–266; 2002.

Blythe R et al. Effect of maternal confidence on breastfeeding duration: An application of breastfeeding self-efficacy theory. *Birth* 29(4):278–284; 2002.

Borges A, Philippi T. Opinion of women from a family health unit about the quantity of mother milk produced. *Rev Lat Am Enfermagem* 11(3):287–292, Epub; 2003.

Butte N et al. Higher energy expenditure contributes to growth faltering in breast-fed infants living in rural Mexico. *J Nutr* 123:1028–1035; 1993.

Butte N et al. Infant feeding mode affects early growth and body composition. *Pediatrics* 106(6):1355–1366; 2000.

Colin W, Scott J. Breastfeeding: Reasons for starting, reasons for stopping and problems along the way. *Breastfeed Rev* 10(2):13–19; 2002.

Dettwyler K. *Promoting Breastfeeding or Promoting Guilt.* La Leche League International Conference. Orlando, FL; 1999.

FDA Talk Paper. FDA warns against women using unapproved drug, domperidone, to increase milk production; June 7, 2004. Available at: www.fda.gov/bbs/topics/ANSWERS/2004/ANS01292.html. Accessed November 2, 2004.

Garza C et al. Growth of the breastfed infant. In Goldman A, et al. *Human Lactation #3*:109–121. New York: Plennum Press; 1987.

Garza C, Butte N. Energy intakes of human milk-fed infants during the first year. *J Pediatr* 117:S124–S131; 1990.

Habbick B, Gerrard J. Failure to thrive in the contented breast-fed baby. *Can Med Assoc J* 131(7):765–768; 1984.

Hale T. *Medications and Mothers' Milk*. Amarillo, TX: Pharmasoft Publishing; 2004.

Hill P, Aldag J. Insufficient milk supply among Black and White breast-feeding mothers. *Res Nurs Health* 16:203–211; 1993.

Hill P. The enigma of insufficient milk supply. *Maternal Child Nursing* 16:312–316; 1991.

Kassing D. Bottle-feeding as a tool to reinforce breastfeeding, *J Hum Lact* 18(1):56–60; 2002.

Lawrence R. *Breastfeeding: A Guide for the Medical Profession*. 5th ed. St. Louis, MO: Mosby; 1999.

Lukefahr JL: Underlying illness associated with FTT in breast-fed infants. *Clin in Perinatology (Phil)* 29(8):468–470; 1990.

Marasco L, Barger J. Cue vs. scheduled feeding: Revisiting the controversy. *Mother Baby Journal* 3(4):38–42; 1998.

Marasco L et al. Polycystic ovary syndrome: A connection to insufficient milk supply? *J Hum Lact* 16(2):43–48; 2000.

McCarter-Spaulding D, Kearney M. Parenting self-efficacy and perception of insufficient breast milk. *JOGNN* 30(5):515–522; 2001.

Meier P et al. A new scale for in-home test-weighing for mothers of preterm and high risk infants. *J Hum Lact* 10:163–168; 1994.

Mennella J. Short-term effects of maternal alcohol consumption on lactational performance. *Alcohol Clin Exp Res* 22(7):1389–1392; 1998.

Mennella J. Alcohol's effect on lactation. Review. *Alcohol Res Health* 25(3):230–234; 2001.

Merlob P et al. Continued weight loss in the newborn during the third day of life as an indicator of early weaning. *Israeli J Med Sci* 30:646–648; 1994.

Newman J. Breast compression; January 2003a. Available at: www.breastfeedingonline.com. Accessed May 13, 2004.

Newman, J. Domperidone is a prescription drug that can help women increase their milk supplies; January 2003b. Available at: http://www.breastfeedingonline.com/domperidone.shtml. Accessed July 4, 2004.

Power M et al. The effort to increase breast-feeding: Do obstetricians, in the forefront, need help? *J Reprod Med* 48(2):72–78; 2003.

Scott J et al. Neonatal hypernatraemic dehydration and malnutrition associated with inadequate breastfeeding and elevated breast milk sodium. *J Indian Med Assoc* 101(5):318, 321; 2003.

Shani M, Shinwell E. Breastfeeding characteristics and reasons to stop breastfeeding. *Harefuah* 142(6):426–428, 486; 2003.

Simic T et al. Breastfeeding practices in Mostar, Bosnia and Herzegovina: Cross-sectional self-report study. *Croat Med J* 45(1):38–43; 2004.

Sofer S et al. Early severe dehydration in young breast-fed newborn infants. *Isr J Med Sci* 29:85–89; 1993.

Ullah S, Griffiths P. Does the use of pacifiers shorten breast-feeding duration in infants? *Br J Community Nurs* 8(10):458–463; 2003.

West D. *Defining Your Own Success: Breastfeeding After Breast Reduction Surgery*. Schaumburg, IL: La Leche League International; 2001.

Wilson-Clay B, Hoover K. *The Breastfeeding Atlas*, 2nd ed. Austin, TX: Lactnews Press; 2002.

 ## BIBLIOGRAPHY

American Academy of Pediatrics (AAP) Work Group on Breastfeeding. Breastfeeding and the use of human milk. *Pediatrics* 100:1035–1039; 1997.

Cadwell K et al. *Maternal and Infant Assessment for Breastfeeding and Human Lactation: A Practitioner's Guide*. Sudbury, MA: Jones and Bartlett Publishers; 2002.

Edwards A et al. Recognizing failure to thrive in early childhood. *Arch Dis Child* 65:1263–1265; 1990.

Frantz K. The slow-gaining breastfeeding infant: Clinical issues in perinatal and women's health nursing. *Breastfeeding NAACOG* 3(4):647–655; 1992.

Grossman L et al. The effect of postpartum lactation counseling on the duration of breastfeeding in low-income women. *Am J Dis Child* 144:471–474; 1990.

Hill PD. Insufficient milk supply syndrome: Clinical issues in perinatal and women's health nursing. *NAACOG* 3(4):605–612; 1992.

Human Milk Banking Association of North America (HMBANA). The value of human milk: Position paper on donor milk banking; 2003. Available at: www.hmbana.org. Accessed December 23, 2004.

Kaplan J et al. Fatal hypernatremic dehydration in exclusively breast-fed newborn infants due to maternal lactation failure. *Am J Forensic Med Pathol* 19:19–22; 1998.

Parents Anonymous Inc. Available at: www.parentsanonymous.org. Accessed October 12, 2004.

SPECIAL CARE

CHANGES IN THE FAMILY

One who bears her children is a mother in part,
But she who nurses her children is a mother at heart.
–Jacob Cats (1577–1660)

Family dynamics, roles, and relationships all take on new dimensions when a baby enters the picture. As a couple merge into new roles as parents, both the mother and father undergo adjustments with one another and with their baby. If other children are at home, their adjustments to the new baby will present further challenges. You can provide assistance and support as the family settles into newly defined roles and relationships.

KEY TERMS

amenorrhea	lochia
anovulatory	menses
anticipatory stage	natural family planning
attachment	oral contraceptives
baby blues	patches
baby training	perineum
barrier methods	personal stage
contraception	post-traumatic stress
Edinburgh postnatal	disorder
depression scale	postpartum depression
fertility	postpartum psychosis
formal stage	sexual abuse
implants	sterilization
informal stage	tubal ligation
injectables	urethra
intrauterine device (IUD)	uterus
Kegel exercises	vaginal ring
lactational amenorrhea	
method (LAM)	

ACQUIRING THE PARENTAL ROLE

One role common to most people is that of parent. Although we receive special instruction to qualify us for driving an automobile, for employment, and for other life skills, society does little to formally prepare us for the important job of parenting. At the same time, fewer and fewer couples live near their extended families, and many have no family support system for everyday parenting. Couples increasingly are on their own as they use trial and error to establish themselves as parents.

Bonding to the baby by both the mother and father in the first hours and days of life seems to encourage the acceptance of their roles as parents and ensure their attachment to the baby (see Figure 19.1). The mother's physical recovery and the development of realistic expectations can help her maintain a positive perspective. This enables her to make a smooth transition to the role of mother, just as her partner redefines his role as a new father. The couple will learn to support one another through this transition by helping each other adjust to the changes occurring in their lives.

Learning about Parenting

No amount of preparation can totally predict a couple's parenting style and interactions with their unique children. However, parents typically progress through predictable stages as they prepare for and care for their first

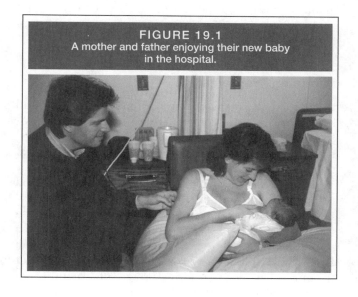

FIGURE 19.1
A mother and father enjoying their new baby in the hospital.

child. The four stages of role acquisition are anticipatory, formal, informal, and personal (Bocar, 1987; Mercer, 1981).

Anticipatory Stage

The **anticipatory stage** is when parents begin to learn about their new roles. They may take classes, read books, and subscribe to parenting and child care magazines. They often begin asking questions of their own parents and of other family or friends who already have children.

Formal Stage

After taking in and considering new information, parents move into the **formal stage**. During this time, they begin to view their roles as parents more personally. They often strive for "parenting perfection" with a goal of doing it "just right."

Informal Stage

The frustration of trying to achieve perfection and the realization that "just right" is very individual leads parents into the **informal stage**. This stage is a time of modifying, blending, and individualizing their roles to fit their unique family.

Personal Stage

As parents become more comfortable in their parenting role, they move into the **personal stage**. Their style of parenting evolves to be consistent with their personalities—parenting that fits them like an old glove. The roles of the mother and father evolve in response to the needs of their baby, their family backgrounds, and the couple's interaction. Both parents define their roles gradually through experience, which is enhanced and made more enjoyable through open communication between them.

Parenting Programs

While there are many effective parenting programs and books, others cause concern within the healthcare profession. Parent Effectiveness Training (PET) and Systematic Training for Effective Parenting (STEP) are two programs that have been around for several decades. They focus on consistency, treating children with respect, and teaching children logical and natural consequences. Other programs based on a rigidly structured approach to child rearing are so worrisome that the AAP passed a resolution in 1998 to investigate and monitor them. Parents who follow these rigid programs find it difficult to move beyond the formal stage of parenting to develop a personal style. There are concerns not only about the potential physical problems that can ensue from parents following such strict rules, but also about

the psychological outcome of children left to "cry it out" (Francis, 1998; Hunter, 1998; CAPCOC, 1996).

Baby Training Programs

Several books and parenting programs teach parents to schedule feedings in order for the baby to sleep through the night from an early age. These teachings contradict the AAP's guidelines on infant feeding and baby care. They promote their parenting method as the "right" way to raise a child, with no scientific basis for any of their teachings. Such books and programs unfortunately are very popular among young parents. Table 19.1 contrasts the feeding advice in six of these books with the AAP infant feeding policy (AAP, 2005) and the AAP Media Alert on scheduled feedings (AAP, 1998).

Parents Drawn to These Programs

The generation in western cultures who are having babies today reached adulthood during a time of economic prosperity. They may begin their lives together as two upwardly mobile, career-minded professionals. The parenting approaches of baby training programs pander to couples in this lifestyle. They direct parents not to allow their baby to be "the center of the family universe" (Ezzo, 2001) and stress the importance of the parents establishing time for themselves (Hogg, 2001).

A baby's grandparents may give a book like this to their children. It affirms the rigid scheduling of their own parenting practices and validates the way they raised their children. However, lack of knowledge about infant physiology and the day-to-day care of a baby can set parents up for unrealistic expectations of what to expect with their new baby.

Parents who ascribe to these programs may be in a peer group with other first-time parents who are using them. Religiously based programs such as Growing Families International (GFI) invest families spiritually in its teachings. They teach parents to form a "like-minded . . . moral community" within a social sphere that can become a closed loop (Gordon, 1999; Terner, 1998). Because parents rely on the program for parenting details, it is difficult for them to move beyond the formal stage of learning and to mature in their parenting style. Of greater concern to medical and mental health professionals are the behaviors observed in some infants subjected to these teachings. These infants can demonstrate detachment, depression, eating issues, and self-stimulating and self-soothing behaviors (Webb, 2003; Williams, 1999, 1998).

Effect on Breastfeeding

Baby training programs blame demand feeding for sleep deprivation, maternal depression, low milk production or quitting breastfeeding, failure to thrive, and selfish

TABLE 19.1

Advice from American Academy of Pediatrics versus Baby Training Books

Source	Feeding Frequency	Longest Interval Between Feedings	Who Should Design Feeding Schedule	Most Reliable Way to Know If Baby Needs Feeding
American Academy of Pediatrics (AAP) www. aap.org	On demand: "8–12 feedings at the breast every 24 hours"—Breastfeeding Policy Statement, 2/05	4 hours—Breastfeeding Policy Statement, 2/05	Babies, because those "designed by parents may put babies at risk for poor weight gain and dehydration" (AAP Media Alert, 4/98)	An infant's feeding cues: "increased mouthing, or rooting. Crying is a late indicator of hunger." (AAP Media Alert, 4/98)
On Becoming Babywise and Let the Children Come Along the Infant Way (formerly *Preparation for Parenting*)	◆ Parent-Directed Feeding (PDF) Routine: "approximately every 2½–3 hr" (p. 74) ◆ Translates to 8–9.6 feeds per day (1998 and 2001 eds; 2002 AIW)	◆ 5 hours for breastfeeding baby ◆ No limits given for formula-fed infant (pp. 112, 119; 1998 ed) (p. 112; 2001 ed)	Parents, because babies are "not capable of regulating their hunger patterns" (p. 47) (1998 and 2001 eds)	Acknowledges infant feeding cues, but repeatedly insists they be interpreted through the lens of the PDF schedule or the baby's routine will be so altered as to represent a new routine (1998 and 2001 eds)
Secrets of the Baby Whisperer	◆ Approximately every 2½–3 hr ◆ Author "never advocates demand feeding" (pp. 43, 100) ◆ Translates to 8–9.6 feeds per day	◆ No limits given for babies being fed by either method ◆ Author recommends against waking a baby who has slept through a feeding, even in the early days, unless baby weighs less than 5.5 lbs (p. 104)	Parents, because following baby's cues alone will result in a demanding, insecure, less healthy baby; an exhausted mother; and a chaotic household (pp. 42, 49, 51, 83, 100)	Acknowledges infant feeding cues, but repeatedly states that referring to the author's E.A.S.Y. routine is the best way in which to interpret what baby needs (pp. 81, 87, 100, 115, 117)
The Contented Little Baby Book	◆ 2 wk: 3–4 hr/daytime (max 7); 4–5 hr at night (p. 77) ◆ 2–6 wk: 6 feeds, 1x night if waking (pp. 90–96) ◆ 6–12 wk: 5 feeds, water at night (pp. 104–110) ◆ 3–5 mo: 5 feeds, 0 at night (pp. 116–118); add 1–2 solids by 4 mo (pp. 144–146) ◆ 5–6 mo: 4 feeds, 0 at night, 1–3 solids (pp. 126–128; pp. 144–146) ◆ 6–9 mo: 3 feeds, 3 solids (pp. 133–138) ◆ Table on p. 79 outlines feeds	◆ No longer than 3 hr during day and 4–5 hr at night (pp. 63, 77) ◆ Every 3 hr during day, 1 feeding at night (p. 82); 12.5 hr by 5 mo (p. 79)	Parents, to avoid "months of sleepless nights, colic, feeding difficulties and many of the other problems that the experts convince us are a normal part of parenting" (p. xiv)	Clock (pp. 88–89)

(Continued)

TABLE 19.1 (CONTINUED)

Advice from American Academy of Pediatrics versus Baby Training Books

Source	Feeding Frequency	Longest Interval Between Feedings	Who Should Design Feeding Schedule	Most Reliable Way to Know If Baby Needs Feeding
My First 300 Babies	◆ Birth to 4 mo: 5 feedings in 24 hr (p. 12) (conflicts with schedule in "publisher's note," p. xix, which allows 7 feeds from birth to 2 mo) ◆ 4 mo: 3 bf, 1 cup feeding (juice or cow's milk), 3 solids (meats, veggies, fruit) (p. 13) ◆ 9–12 mo: 2 bottles, 2 juices, 3 solids (p. 14)	◆ Birth to 2 mo: 4 hr (p. 12) ◆ 4 mo: 5 hr, 12 hr at night (p. 13) ◆ 9 mo: 13 hr at night (p. 14)	Author used this exact schedule for all of her "300" babies, "no exceptions" (p. 3); makes analogy that while all people are unique, they must all obey same traffic laws, so while all babies are different, they must "be individually obedient to what denotes order and proper procedure" (p. 3)	Author's schedule (pp. 12–14)
Parenting Principles: From the Heart of a Pediatrician	◆ Birth to 2 mo: every 4 hr; never awaken at night (pp. 152–153, 160) ◆ 2 wks: start solid food with 2 solid feedings (pp. 157, 160) ◆ 2 mo: 4 feedings (5 oz), 2 solid feeds; add fruit (pp. 158, 160) ◆ 3–4 mo: 4 feeds (5 oz) + 3 solids; add vegetables (pp. 158, 160) ◆ 5 mo: 4 feeds (5 oz) + 3 solids with added desserts, juice (pp. 159, 161) ◆ 6 mo: 4 feeds (5 oz) + 3 solids; intro cup & use 2% cow's milk, not formula (pp. 159, 161) ◆ 6–12 mo: 3 meals/day (pp. 160, 161)	◆ From birth, at least 4 hr ◆ Goal is to have 2-week baby sleep through the night (8 hr) without feedings ◆ Allow regular crying for 15–20 min (pp. 153–154)	Parents "must bring this child home . . . with the attitude and determination that you are going to be in authority and you are going to be in control" (p. 152)	Does not address

Comparison compiled by Patricia Donohue-Carey, BS, LCCE, CLE; Anh Gordon, MD; and Anna Swisher, MBA, IBCLC. Printed with permission.

children. Parents are encouraged to let their babies cry from 15 minutes to an hour at a time. Anticipatory guidance will be especially important for these parents, preferably prenatally during childbirth or breastfeeding classes. Mothers who use baby-training techniques frequently experience low milk supply, low infant weight gain, or the baby rejecting the breast. Infrequent feedings postpartum will down regulate milk production. Many of these mothers lose their milk supply at three to four months postpartum (Moody, 2002; Aney, 1998).

Mothers who schedule feeding as part of a broader parenting philosophy are sometimes told that lactation consultants have a bias towards "attachment parenting." They are urged not to follow recommendations to cosleep, use a baby sling, or feed frequently (Ezzo, 2002, 2001). You can help these parents understand the reasons behind your recommendations. Staying up-to-date on lactation research will enable you to discuss the scientific reasons behind the variance in each mother's milk storage capacity and synthesis rate (Cox, 1998; Daly, 1995a, 1995b).

Baby training books and programs dismiss the idea that crying is harmful to babies. Teaching parents about the effects of stress and extended crying on infants will be helpful (Anderson, 2003, 1989; Mazurek, 1999; Aono, 1993; Yamauchi, 1990). One important claim to address with parents is that non-scheduled babies will miss feedings. Parents of a preterm or sleepy baby who does not demonstrate feeding cues do need to temporarily "watch the clock" and rouse the baby to feed frequently, not allowing more than four hours without feeding (AAP, 2005). However, this is not necessary for other babies.

Parents who follow baby training for religious reasons may be responsive to theological arguments. Christian leaders reject the materials (MacArthur, 2000; Dobson, 1999; Hanegraaf, 1998–1999) and several articles argue against the teachings on theological grounds (Webb, 2003; Cox, 2001; Terner, 1998). Use of reflective listening will enable you to be accepting of these parents without implying endorsement of their practices. A nonjudgmental approach is important to creating a climate in which parents can question the information. While you may have strong feelings about these parenting techniques, it is important for you to share information objectively and to give current and relevant resources.

You have a unique opportunity to empower parents who find it difficult to move beyond the formal stage of acquiring their parental role. After you address scheduled feedings and present information from reliable medical sources, you need to step back from the situation and the parents' practices. Document any concerns you have regarding the baby's health or mother's milk supply. Stay in close communication with the parents' physicians or other caregivers. Be sure the baby's care-giver is aware that the mother is using scheduled feedings so the baby's weight gain can be monitored.

▶ BECOMING A MOTHER

All women respond in their own ways to motherhood. Most new mothers have one characteristic in common, however: They have little or no idea of what to expect in their babies' behavior and development! They may have formed opinions on child care but find that these ideas do not work with their baby. They may have had preconceived ideas about types of babies but find that theirs is another type entirely. Mothers eventually realize they need to develop their own parenting skills and that their competence and confidence will grow with practice, experimentation, observation, and self-education.

Every mother has some adjustments to make after her baby is born. This is a wonderful phase in a family's life. At the same time, it can be frustrating. A mother may not feel prepared for the fact that caring for her baby is a round-the-clock job. She cannot return to her life as she knew it.

One of the pitfalls of counseling an experienced mother is to assume that she does not need your support. She is constantly making adjustments, and although her questions and concerns will be different from those of a first-time mother, they are just as significant. She often must help others in the family, such as siblings and grandparents, make their own adjustments. Having a supportive person with whom she can share her concerns can be especially important to her.

Emotional Adjustments

Emotions during the postpartum period rival those of the adolescent years. Hormonal shifts are dramatic within the first 24 hours after giving birth. Suddenly, the mother has a baby who is entirely dependent on her. At the same time, she is coping with extraordinary body changes and her emotions are subject to biochemical, psychological, and societal influences. Her birth experience may have been exhilarating, confusing, exhausting, or devastating. Her ideas about parenting and her expectations of herself, her baby, and her family may not reflect the reality of her situation.

The Lactation Consultant's Role with Mothers

Help mothers see that their reactions are normal and that the blissful image of a perfect mother is far from reality. Encourage each mother to develop realistic expectations about her baby and about motherhood. Help her see that not all problems with her baby are associated with breastfeeding. If she is considering weaning, help her understand that weaning may not solve her other problems. Her baby will still cry, and she will still feel tired and tied down at times. Bottle-feeding mothers have these challenges, too!

Normal Postpartum Adjustments

There is a tendency to assume that a highly educated woman is comfortable with and adequately prepared for parenting (Pridham, 1991). However, women often feel unprepared for their new role as mother. They may lack personal experience in caring for a baby and may not have family close by to support them in the early weeks. A mother's uncertainty may show up as a specific concern or worry, such as handling a fussy baby or insufficient milk production (Bottorff, 1990). If she quit working, she will experience a loss of additional income. Additionally, decreased contact with adults can create feelings of isolation and loneliness.

Motherhood is a new, constant job, and the stress of the new expectations may seem overwhelming at times. The mother may have a baby who is continually fussy and rarely sleeps, who fails to live up to her expectations of a happy, responsive baby. She may have had a disappointing or unpleasant birth or may have experienced an unwanted pregnancy. Poor nutrition and lack of rest can also cause emotional distress in the new mother, especially when coupled with the many adjustments to a new baby.

Women's emotional adjustments to motherhood vary greatly during the postpartum period. Some women need do no more than make room for the new baby. Many women, however, will have a few rough days balanced by high moments. This brief despondency, referred to as **baby blues**, frequently appears around the third day postpartum and could last for a couple of weeks. The mother may have bouts of tearfulness and sadness, mingled with happiness and excitement. These emotions are more common in women who have their first baby. A positive birth experience and an abundance of emotional support and practical help following the birth help to minimize baby blues.

Postpartum Depression

Some women become clinically depressed for weeks or months after giving birth. They will require professional help that is beyond your role as lactation consultant. Typically, this mother will be depressed from one to six weeks postpartum. **Postpartum depression** creates mood changes, loss of pleasure, poor concentration, low self-esteem, guilt at failing as a mother and wife, sleep disturbances, fatigue, and a flat affect in voice tone.

A mother in the throes of postpartum depression may lack confidence in her ability to breastfeed and can experience a sudden dramatic drop in milk production. She may say she is lonely, has no visitors, and has no place to go. She may not answer her telephone, or she may stay away from home in an attempt to keep busy. She may demonstrate a lack of tolerance for other family members and feel detached from her baby, evidenced by a failure to refer to her baby by name. Premature weaning occurs more frequently among depressed women (Cooper, 1993).

A woman suffering from postpartum depression generally feels unable to cope with life and worries that something is not "right." She may even entertain occasional thoughts of harming herself. This requires urgent evaluation by a psychiatrist (Kendall-Tackett, 2001), preferably one who has a special interest in antenatal and postpartum women. These psychiatrists are more likely to support breastfeeding and try to treat the mother without interfering with breastfeeding. Loss of control is a significant emotion experienced after the birth of a baby and is not an identifying symptom of postpartum depression.

Effective education will help the mother understand the difference between baby blues and postpartum depression. Help her understand that postpartum depression is a common illness and is treatable, like any other biological illness. When the mother and her partner understand this, there is less likely to be obstacles around diagnosis and treatment, and the mother is likely to recover more quickly.

Postpartum depression occurs in an estimated 10 to 20 percent of U.S. mothers, with a higher incidence in women who have a personal or family history of depression (Misri, 2002). A careful history will reveal if there is a family background of depression. The current view is that the physiological changes that accompany birth can trigger major depression in women with a preexisting predisposition (Wisner, 1997).

You should never attempt to counsel an emotionally distressed mother alone. Gently urge the mother to contact her caregiver for a referral to a psychiatrist. In addition to counseling, treatment may involve medications, most of which are compatible with breastfeeding. You can be a source of information for the mother by citing current medication information and providing her with resources.

Edinburgh Postnatal Depression Scale

Depression makes it difficult, if not impossible, to experience real pleasure and joy. The **Edinburgh Postnatal Depression Scale** (Figure 19.2) was developed to help primary care health professionals detect mothers suffering from postnatal depression. These mothers may cope with their baby and with household tasks, but their enjoyment of life is seriously affected and it is possible that there are long-term effects on the family. The Edinburgh Scale (Cox, 1987) is an easy self-rating depression

FIGURE 19.2
Edinburgh Postnatal Depression Scale (EPDS)

Instructions for users:

The mother is asked to underline the response which comes closest to how she has been feeling in the previous 7 days. All ten items must be completed. Care should be taken to avoid the possibility of the mother discussing her answers with others. The mother should complete the scale herself, unless she has limited English or has difficulty with reading. The EPDS may be used at 6–8 weeks to screen postnatal women. The child health clinic, postnatal check-up or a home visit may provide suitable opportunities for its completion.

Name: _____   Baby's Age: _____

Address: _____

As you have recently had a baby, we would like to know how you are feeling. Please UNDERLINE the answer which comes closest to how you have felt IN THE PAST 7 DAYS, not just how you feel today.

1. I have been able to laugh and see the funny side of things.
   a. As much as I always could – 0
   b. Not quite so much now – 1
   c. Definitely not so much now – 2
   d. Not at all – 3
2. I have looked forward with enjoyment to things.
   a. As much as I ever did – 0
   b. Rather less than I used to – 1
   c. Definitely less than I used to – 2
   d. Hardly at all – 3
*3. I have blamed myself unnecessarily when things went wrong.
   a. Yes, most of the time – 3
   b. Yes, some of the time – 2
   c. Not very often – 1
   d. No, never – 0
4. I have been anxious or worried for no good reason.
   a. No, not at all – 0
   b. Hardly ever – 1
   c. Yes, sometimes – 2
   d. Yes, very often – 3
*5. I have felt scared or panicky for not very good reason.
   a. Yes, quite a lot – 3
   b. Yes, sometimes – 2
   c. No, not much – 1
   d. No, not at all – 0

*6. Things have been getting on top of me.
   a. Yes, most of the time I haven't been able to cope at all – 3
   b. Yes, sometimes I haven't been coping as well as usual – 2
   c. No, most of the time I have coped quite well – 1
   d. No, I have been coping as well as ever – 0
*7. I have been so unhappy that I have had difficulty sleeping.
   a. Yes, most of the time – 3
   b. Yes, sometimes – 2
   c. Not very often – 1
   d. No, not at all – 0
*8. I have felt sad or miserable.
   a. Yes, most of the time – 3
   b. Yes, quite often – 2
   c. Not very often – 1
   d. No, not at all – 0
*9. I have been so unhappy that I have been crying.
   a. Yes, most of the time – 3
   b. Yes, quite often – 2
   c. Only occasionally – 1
   d. No, never – 0
*10. The thought of harming myself has occurred to me.
   a. Yes, quite often – 3
   b. Sometimes – 2
   c. Hardly ever – 1
   d. Never – 0

Response categories are scored 0, 1, 2, and 3 according to increased severity of the symptoms. Items marked with an asterisk are reverse scored (i.e., 3, 2, 1, and 0). The total score is calculated by adding together the scores for each of the ten items. Users may reproduce the scale without further permission providing they respect copyright by quoting the names of the authors, the title and the source of the paper in all reproduced copies.

Cox LL, Holden JM, Sogovsky R. *British Journal of Psychiatry*.

scale that indicates the normal range of postpartum emotions and degree of danger for depression.

Developed at health centers in Livingston and Edinburgh, it consists of ten short statements. The mother underlines one of four possible responses that describe how she has been feeling during the past week. The validation study showed that mothers who scored above the threshold of 92.3 percent were likely to be suffering from a depressive illness. The EPDS score should not override clinical judgment or careful clinical assessment to confirm diagnosis. The scale will not detect mothers with anxiety neuroses, phobias, or personality disorder.

Postpartum Psychosis

An estimated 1 to 2 out of 1000 postpartum women develop psychosis. This involves symptoms far more serious than those of baby blues or depression (Gale, 2003; Gold, 1995). The mother's symptoms may progress beyond insomnia, fatigue, and depression. **Postpartum psychosis** occurs on a much more intense level than postpartum depression. It can lead to a loss of control, rational thought, and social functioning. The mother experiences overwhelming delusions and hallucinations.

Due to the severity of depression, the mother may attempt suicide. This illness is a medical emergency. A

British review found that psychiatric disorder, specifically suicide, is the leading cause of maternal death. Suicide accounted for 28 percent of maternal deaths from 1997 to 1999. Women also died from other complications of psychiatric disorders, and a significant minority died from substance misuse (Oates, 2003).

The mother may be at risk for harming her child or children. The priority for this mother is to keep her and her child safe and to get her into effective treatment immediately. The world was horrified in 2001 by the multiple murders by a mother with a history of severe postpartum depression and two suicide attempts. She methodically drowned each of her five children, including her baby, whom she had breastfed for four months (O'Malley, 2004). The mother had breastfed all her children (Yates, 2004).

Survivors of Sexual Abuse

As many as one in three women has reported being sexually assaulted in their lifetime, often in childhood (Bass, 1994). The estimated incidence ranges from 7 to 36 percent of all women and 3 to 29 percent of all men (Finkelhor, 1994). Past sexual abuse affects the functioning of at least 20 percent of adult survivors, predisposing women to major depression or post-traumatic stress disorder (PTSD) (Briere, 1991).

Pregnancy and childbirth are common times for a sexual abuse survivor to remember her past abuse. Because of the intimate nature of breastfeeding, past sexual abuse may cause a disruption or disturbance in breastfeeding. Memories, flashbacks, and feelings from the abuse may interfere with the mother's ability to breastfeed. Flashbacks are a sign of PTSD and require professional help. Memories may be triggered by the sounds or feelings of giving birth, the sensation of the baby at the breast, the loss of control felt in the early days of parenting, or even the sight of milk during letdown. Any of these events can trigger a flashback that causes the woman to feel uncomfortable with breastfeeding (Kendall-Tackett, 1998).

Identifying a Sexual Abuse Survivor

In some instances, a woman may feel comfortable telling you about her sexual abuse because you take the time to listen to her concerns. Assisting the mother with such an intimate topic draws on your ability to listen intently with warmth and caring and to regard the woman with openness and acceptance. A suspicion of abuse may stem from the way the mother positions herself for feedings or from an apparent discomfort with holding her baby while discussing breastfeeding. Some warning signs that may indicate a history of sexual abuse are late prenatal care, substance abuse, mental health concerns, eating disorders, poor compliance with self-care,

or sexual dysfunction. She may feed expressed milk to her baby with a bottle and not put him to breast (Kendall-Tackett, 1998). Although these signals do not necessarily indicate a history of sexual abuse, they are signs that can alert you to the possibility.

Breastfeeding Implications for the Survivor

The most stressful time in breastfeeding for a survivor will be during the early postpartum period, when the new mother feels stressed, tired, and vulnerable. Although all new mothers experience fluctuations in their emotions at this time, abuse survivors may be more emotionally fragile due to memories of abuse or depression. Because sexual assault tends to occur at night or at bedtime, nighttime breastfeeding can be especially difficult. Having someone feed her milk to the baby for nighttime feedings may help this situation. When the baby gets older and becomes more playful, the mother may seem reluctant to continue breastfeeding. Assuring the mother that her infant needs and desires her milk may help her breastfeed longer.

Be prepared to meet the mother's needs, and to support her. Her choices in breastfeeding may include expressing her milk and feeding it to her baby by bottle. They may not be what you would choose. Remember that those choices are best for her. Each mother's reactions to a situation may vary widely, and you must meet the mother on her own terms. Some mothers find breastfeeding too uncomfortable to continue. Others find breastfeeding to be quite healing. Be alert to the mother's feelings and provide support when possible, including support for weaning if that is her choice.

A lactation consultant is not qualified to treat or investigate sexual abuse situations. Refer the mother to a licensed therapist or counselor who specializes in sexual abuse, preferably one who is familiar with breastfeeding mothers. You can meet with counselors in your community to provide appropriate breastfeeding information. A helpful book for mothers dealing with depression or past abuse is *The Hidden Feelings of Motherhood: Coping with Stress, Depression and Burnout* (Kendall-Tackett, 2001). See Appendix A for additional resources for sexual abuse survivors.

Physical Recovery Following Birth

After a woman gives birth, many changes take place within her body to return it to its prepregnant state. Having just completed nine months of pregnancy, she may feel disappointed that her abdomen still protrudes because of stretched muscles. Her walk may seem more of a waddle because of loosened pelvic ligaments and stitches or pads. The fullness in her breasts may be slightly uncomfortable, and she may have little energy left to cope with her appearance and the stresses of daily life.

Assure mothers that these physical responses are normal. For the first six weeks, new mothers need rest for physical recovery. A mother who receives insufficient rest may develop excessive bleeding, exhaustion, dizziness, or weak pelvic floor muscles. Add breastfeeding to the mix, and she may experience sore nipples or a breast infection.

Encourage mothers to get as much bed rest as possible. Staying in her bathrobe for the first few weeks will discourage a new mother's visitors from staying too long. She can nap when her baby naps and nurse lying down to catch up on needed rest. A reminder of the need for moderation is especially helpful in the early weeks following delivery. By this time, the mother will begin to feel energetic and restless at home and could be more apt to overexert herself. Caution her to minimize household tasks and not to resume strenuous activities too quickly. Her family can help by limiting visitors during that time.

Familiarize the mother with normal physical changes that occur during the weeks following delivery. In addition to the usual postpartum recovery involving the uterus and perineum, she may experience variations in body functions or minor physical irritations. The resumption of menstruation and the possibility of another pregnancy are a concern for many new mothers. Breastfeeding speeds uterine recovery, encourages the mother to rest while nursing, relieves breast fullness, and delays the return of fertility and menses.

Uterus

The uterus, which attained a weight of about 2.5 pounds by delivery, begins to diminish in size soon after the baby's birth. By one week postpartum, it has decreased to about 1 pound, and at 6 weeks, it is usually reduced to approximately 2 ounces. This time of involution is accompanied by a discharge of blood, mucus, and tissue called **lochia**, which is the gradual sloughing off of the extra tissue lining the uterus. Its color transforms from red to pink and then to white in about three to four weeks. A change in color from pink to white and back to red may indicate that the mother's level of physical exertion is too high. She will need to report this to her caregiver and cut back on her activity level.

There is often an increase in lochia flow during feedings because of uterine contractions caused by the release of oxytocin. The contractions may cause what is commonly referred to as afterpains, which usually last for only a few days to one week. Multiparous women may find these contractions more severe. The mother can reduce afterbirth pains by emptying her bladder before breastfeeding and by doing deep breathing. Ibuprofen can alleviate the pain, if approved for use by her caregiver. Reassure her that the pains are nature's way of limiting blood loss and returning her body to its prepregnant state.

Perineum

A vaginal delivery causes swelling and tenderness in the perineum, the region between the vagina and rectum. An episiotomy, a surgical incision between these two points, enlarges the vaginal opening during delivery. It may increase postpartum swelling and cause a pulling sensation. Ice packs, sitz baths, sprays, cooling cotton pads, and medications can provide comfort for the mother.

Perineal floor exercises, known as **Kegel exercises**, will help the mother regain muscle tone in the pelvic floor, where stretching is most pronounced during labor. If these muscles remain weak, the uterus may tip or sink down into the vagina and the mother may have difficulty controlling urination. To perform Kegel exercises, the woman inhales and then tightens the muscles surrounding her vagina, **urethra**, and rectum as she exhales. You can help mothers visualize this by telling them these are the same muscles used to stop the flow of urine. Performing Kegel exercises regularly throughout the day will help return muscle tone and enable the mother to control urination.

Body Functions

In the first few days postpartum, the mother may notice changes in her body functions. She may need to urinate frequently as she loses extra fluids accumulated during pregnancy. Some women have difficulty urinating, especially if they had a **catheter** inserted in the bladder to keep it empty during labor and delivery. A mother might not have a bowel movement until two or three days postpartum.

Initially, a woman who delivered vaginally may find it unsettling to assume a position that is similar to the position in which she had recently delivered her baby. She may fear expelling her uterus, rupturing her episiotomy, or increasing her pain. A mother who had a cesarean delivery may have difficulty with bowel movements until her intestines resume normal functioning. The manipulation of the intestines during cesarean delivery causes gas and temporary bowel dysfunction. Deep breathing exercises, rocking back and forth in a rocking chair, and alternating between abdominal tightening and relaxing will help. She will need bulk and fluids in her diet, and may require a stool softener if other methods fail. Medication used by some hospitals to reduce gas have not been shown to cause problems for breastfeeding babies.

Minor Irritations

Among other minor irritations, some women experience backaches in the early weeks because of the hormones that softened or loosened the sacroiliac ligaments and allowed more flexibility of the pelvic structure for birth. Backaches are also associated with the use of epidural anesthesia (Kroeger, 2004; MacArthur, 1993). Heat, massage, pelvic rocking exercises, and correct lifting and breast-feeding positions will help. Heavy perspiration, particularly at night, results from the body removing surplus fluid from pregnancy. The mother can wear cool, loose clothing and take frequent showers to help her feel better. The extra-large sanitary pads used postnatally may be irritating. As the lochia discharge subsides, the mother may be more comfortable with a minipad.

Changing Priorities

Caution mothers that when they overexert physically, their baby may be fussy the next day. An overactive lifestyle can lead to a breast infection. Each mother makes her own decision about the importance of a task. She may need to relax her standards and priorities concerning household chores. If she has responsibilities such as an outside job, volunteer work, or transporting older children to activities, perhaps she can make some compromises or trade-offs that will allow her the time she needs for herself and her baby. Encourage her to resume obligations slowly, to watch her baby and other family members for signs of distress, and to cut back when necessary. Help her realize that the intense amount of time her baby now consumes will diminish rapidly. As the baby becomes efficient in expressing and meeting his needs, the mother's schedule will become more relaxed, and time will steadily increase for other responsibilities and relaxation.

The mother can be imaginative in developing arrangements to return to her previous obligations. She could explore telecommuting, working at home, employing a teenager, or trading favors with another mother. She might participate in only those activities where her baby is welcome, arrange to take her baby with her, or work out some other method to suit her needs. There are organizations of mothers who have made a variety of lifestyle decisions, such as the National Association of At Home Mothers. Searching the Internet may lead to connections with other mothers who find it hard to leave home for adult conversation. La Leche League has online meetings for breastfeeding women (www.lalecheleague.org).

The mother's ability to adapt her lifestyle to motherhood will depend on her emotional state, her physical recovery, her maturity, and the support she receives from family and friends. She can hasten her recovery and her return to a workable schedule by resting during the early weeks. Help her form realistic expectations, and point out options she may have with household chores, child care, and obligations outside the home.

▶ BECOMING A FATHER

Men experience social, emotional, and behavioral adjustments as they redefine themselves as fathers. A new father will adapt to a changed relationship with his partner, now a mother. He will embrace changes brought about by a new family member—a newborn baby who poses a very serious responsibility. His role expands to one of supporter and helpmate to his wife and protector and provider for his newborn infant. This represents an awesome responsibility to many men, and each will adjust in his own way. It is important that the mother accept her partner's definition of his new role. Encourage couples to share their feelings with one another, both positive and negative, openly and honestly.

The father learns his role through society's definitions, experience with his own father, and peer pressure from other men. Pressure or encouragement from within his family is also a factor in his growth as a father. Each father will choose his own level of involvement in the care and nurturing of his baby. Being actively involved in the pregnancy and the birth will enhance his level of participation.

Fathers and Common Parenting Issues

Anticipatory guidance can help fathers ease into the parenting role. Even before the childbearing years, boys and girls alike deserve exposure to discussions of infant feeding and the importance of breastfeeding. Often, you have an opportunity to provide such education through school, hospital, and community outreach programs. Planting the seed for future generations will empower them to make knowledgeable choices regarding infant feeding. Such early education results in breastfeeding becoming more acceptable and, therefore, the norm.

When a couple discovers that they are expecting, they frequently seek out prenatal classes to prepare for parenting. Learning what to expect and how to cope will help both parents ease into their roles. Much focus in prenatal breastfeeding education is on the mother. However, researchers have identified a need for also educating fathers regarding the realities of breastfeeding. This will strengthen their involvement and validate their reactions in the early postpartum period (Freed, 1992; Gamble, 1992; Jordan, 1990). Fathers often cite concerns related to breastfeeding, such as limited initial opportunity to develop a relationship with their children, feeling inadequate, and feeling separated from their partners (Jordan, 1990). Incorporate sensitivity to these concerns and appropriate guidance into classes.

Prenatal classes need to address issues related to the mother and father as a couple. The father often feels as though he has lost his partner, who seems immersed in the care of their new baby. Early parenting is both physically and emotionally intense, whether the baby is breastfed or not. Fortunately, breastfeeding simplifies some aspects of these early days. Nighttime feedings are easier for both the mother and father, as there is no special preparation required for feeding and the baby's food is always available.

Other aspects of life with a new baby, such as physical recovery from childbirth and changes in roles of the couple as new parents, will benefit from anticipatory guidance. Although breastfeeding enhances a woman's physical recovery from childbirth, the mother will still experience fatigue, discomfort, and breast changes in the early days. Parenting expands the couple's relationship to a wonderfully new dimension. This change is not without periods of stress and uncertainty. You can acknowledge these points when educating couples and emphasize that they are normal. Encourage them to communicate with one another regarding their feelings and to keep a focus on their relationship as a couple through this time of great change.

Fathers experience a hormonal response to their babies' cries, with a rise in prolactin and testosterone levels. They are more responsive to infant cues than are non-fathers (Fleming, 2002). The father can bond with his baby through infant care tasks, such as bathing, burping, and diapering. He can help the mother with positioning to breastfeed, carry the baby in a sling, and provide skin-to-skin contact. Fathers benefit from learning about infant cues and responsiveness in order to recognize what is normal and how to interact with their young infants (Delight, 1991).

The baby initially may show a preference for the mother, so the father needs time alone with the baby in order to develop his own parenting style and bond with his child. Although he will have different methods from the mother, his methods are no less important or effective. He needs encouragement in his new role (Eidelman, 1994; Graham, 1993; Jordan, 1993). Fathers may be further encouraged by the fact that they are the first person in their baby's life who teaches him that food and love must not always come from the same person! Books that are helpful in assisting the father in his personal parenting journey include *Becoming a Father: How to Nurture and Enjoy Your Family* (Sears, 2003) and *Fathering Right from the Start: Straight Talk about Pregnancy, Birth and Beyond* (Heinowitz, 2001).

Learning about breastfeeding will enable fathers to provide their partners with practical help. A father who attends prenatal classes may be better able to assist his partner in tangible ways, such as helping her get comfortable. He can fill in pieces of information the mother may have forgotten and provide encouragement when she is having a bad day. Prenatal classes expose fathers to the normalcy of breastfeeding and the reasons why breastfeeding is important for babies. They learn practicalities of breastfeeding, such as the economics, the ease of nighttime feedings, health issues, and overall convenience. These influences may further cement their support of their partner's decisions to breastfeed.

Support Person for the Mother

A breastfeeding mother benefits from an abundance of emotional support from those close to her. Ideally, a major portion of this support will come from the baby's father. Discussing plans for breastfeeding will enable couples to share their opinions and concerns and arrive at mutual decisions. The breastfeeding experience is much more rewarding and fulfilling when shared by the entire family in a positive and accepting atmosphere.

Support by the father takes many forms. It can range from physical care of the baby to helping with household chores to a strong philosophical support. A lack of sharing of tasks often becomes a source of the mother's complaints. She may wish that her mate would take more initiative in helping or that he were more competent with baby care and household chores. You can help her understand that learning these tasks is like learning a new job. Her partner needs time and encouragement to develop confidence and competence. Because mothers typically spend more time with the baby than fathers do, they tend to learn quickly how to interact with and care for their baby. A mother needs to be patient and give her mate the same opportunity to learn what works for him and how he fits in. When the mother encourages the father in his new role, she often finds that he becomes her best supporter and an outspoken advocate of breastfeeding.

Father's Interaction with the Baby

Each father will choose his own manner and level of involvement with his baby. Ideally, a father will participate in the birth process and begin to bond with his baby immediately after birth. This father is likely to respond more openly and readily to the baby than one whose first interaction occurs after the baby comes home. Devoting the first hours and days to becoming acquainted with his newborn child will enable the father to learn the skills necessary to care for him. Mothers and fathers both need to learn these parenting skills, which do not come naturally, as some parents expect.

A father can be invaluable in helping to soothe a fussy baby through walking, rocking, singing, and cooing. He can share in his baby's care and provide the mother some free time alone. He can bathe, burp, diaper, and play with his baby. Bringing the baby to the mother for nighttime feedings will help her get needed sleep.

Many mothers find that their mates' involvement increases as the baby gets older and responds to his attentions. Whatever type of interaction the father chooses, the mother should be careful not to discourage his efforts by criticizing the way he does things to the point that he limits his involvement. She can offer instructive guidance, particularly when a certain practice might be harmful to the baby (e.g., she can point out the need to support the baby's head when carrying or holding him). Encourage the mother to avoid unwarranted criticism. Although the father may do things differently from the mother, his way may be very satisfying for him and his baby.

Babies whose fathers interact with them continually and consistently show an eagerness for learning. They may have a more positive self-image and show more confidence in relating to males. These babies are more likely to have a sense of humor and a longer attention span. Fathers benefit as well by interacting with their babies. They can learn how to care for the baby, can read to him, and can be supportive in easing the intensity of motherhood.

▶ CHANGES IN FAMILY RELATIONSHIPS

The responsibility of being parents presents a major adjustment to many couples. At times, some new parents may resent their baby for disrupting their lives and interfering with their freedom. Help them understand that such ambivalence is normal and often is balanced by deep feelings of affection and love for their infant. Parents need not feel guilty about their reactions. Encourage them to share their feelings honestly and openly with one another.

The need for open and honest communication is especially great during the first few months of parenthood. Both partners will feel inadequacies and a need for support in establishing their new roles as father and mother. They may react strongly to the ways in which the other performs his or her role. They may resent the fact that the baby now receives a lot of the affection and intimacy previously monopolized by the other partner. Remaining sensitive to one another's needs will help them make compromises and adjustments.

Sexual Adjustments

Open communication between the couple and the passage of time will be major factors in reestablishing enjoyable sexual relations. By reassuring the mother that the need for sexual adjustment is common to most new parents, you can make it easier for her to discuss her feelings with her partner. New babies consume a great deal of time and energy, and at the end of a tiring day, lovemaking may seem like just one more chore. As the mother settles into her new role, she may be encouraged to look for ways to boost her energy level. She can nap when her baby naps, nurse lying down, and sleep with her baby at night. You can help the mother look at her dietary practices and offer her suggestions for improvement through quick and healthy food choices (see Chapter 8). The

mother can also explore ways to prioritize her household tasks and ask for help to maximize her efficiency.

As a result, she will have more time and energy to enjoy companionship, conversation, and lovemaking with her partner. New fathers, as well as new mothers, need to be reassured that they are good parents. Fatherhood is a part of manhood, and a confident man is more likely to inspire an enthusiastic sexual response from his partner. He will need to be understanding about the physical demands of motherhood and, at times, compromise his own needs.

Resuming Sexual Intercourse

The recovery period following birth may take several months. Many caregivers advise women that they may resume sexual intercourse after the six-week checkup, while some suggest waiting until the mother's lochia discharge has completely stopped. The six-week checkup indicates how the mother's recovery is progressing and whether any complications exist. Some couples resume sexual relations before this checkup. The mother will want to listen to her body before resuming intercourse.

Emotional Adjustments

In the early weeks or months after giving birth, some women have little or no desire for lovemaking or other forms of intimacy. It may take several months for a new mother to regain her desire or for her responses to return to normal. This may be due in part to the fact that her baby provides her with sufficient affection and emotional gratification, and she does not feel a need for further intimacy. You can assure the mother that this response is normal and that it usually subsides as she adjusts to her maternal role.

A woman's breasts may be overly sensitive during foreplay or, at the other extreme, she may experience no sensual response to her partner's touch. Her responses usually will return to normal within several months after delivery, although for some women this change continues throughout lactation. Some women describe themselves as becoming sexually aroused or experience an increased sensuality when nursing the baby. The sensation is a result of the hormone oxytocin released during both lactation and orgasm. Women need reassurance that nothing is wrong or inappropriate and that they can enjoy this aspect of breastfeeding.

Either partner may be reluctant to engage in foreplay that involves the woman's breasts for fear of passing on germs. If the skin of the breast is healthy and unbroken, chances of transmitting an infection are minimal. The mother produces antibodies to her partner's germs, which pass to her baby through her milk and protect him from infection. She can shower or wash her breasts before nursing the baby, if she so desires.

Physical Adjustments

A new mother may experience some physical discomfort when she first resumes sexual intercourse. The hormones involved with lactation cause a decrease in vaginal lubrication, which may result in discomfort. The mother can relieve this discomfort with an artificial lubricant such as K-Y jelly. Interventions the mother experienced during birth can interfere with her desire for intimacy in the postpartum period. Intercourse may be painful because of an episiotomy, abdominal incision, or internal injury from the use of forceps. If either partner does not experience physical sensations during intercourse, it may be the result of stretched pelvic floor muscles. Kegel exercises will help with general toning and facilitate entrance in intercourse.

Overfull or leaking breasts may be a source of discomfort for the mother. Sexual orgasm releases the hormone oxytocin, which also facilitates the letdown of the mother's milk. For this reason, leaking during intercourse is very common and indicates a positive hormonal response. If the couple is uncomfortable with the dampness that results, a towel can protect bed linens. An adjustment in positioning can alleviate pressure on the woman's breasts. Nursing the baby before intercourse will decrease fullness as well as leakage.

Adjusting Sexual Routine

Adjustments in positioning can help alleviate physical discomfort caused by painful incisions or full breasts. A change in the couple's timing for lovemaking can also help. They may be tense if lovemaking begins at a time when the baby usually wishes to nurse, or even if the baby is pleasantly awake. Nursing the baby immediately before bedtime and taking advantage of moments alone during nap time can provide parents an opportunity for intimacy.

The stresses of discomfort and demands of the baby are easier to cope with when there is tenderness between partners. Often it is effective for couples to have a period of rekindling their tenderness for each other by spending time just holding and cuddling. It is important for a couple to understand that their need for sexual adjustment is normal and common to new parents regardless of whether the mother is lactating. Variations in technique or routine may enhance lovemaking. If the mother experiences discomfort or lack of response in her breasts during foreplay, developing new patterns of foreplay can be an enjoyable solution. It is reassuring to both parents to learn that what they are experiencing is normal and that coping requires simply a little understanding and willingness to adapt.

Menstruation and Fertility

Menstruation and fertility are delayed for varying periods during lactation. The delay occurs as part of the mother's physiologic response to her baby's suckling and other stimuli. This changes the release of brain hormones and reproductive hormones, thus disrupting the cycle of ovulation and menstruation. The single most important factor in suppressing ovulation during lactation is the early establishment of frequent and strong suckling (Tay, 1996; McNeilly, 1993). Prolactin was previously thought to play a major role in this suppression. However, research now suggests that a variety of hormones are involved, with a link between levels of growth hormone, leutinizing hormone, follicle-stimulating hormone, and estrogen (McNeilly, 1993).

Return of Menses

In the initial postpartum period and for several months thereafter, a breastfeeding mother experiences a phase of amenorrhea (lack of menstruation). The menstrual cycle can be delayed for several months, followed by a period of resumed menstrual cycles that may be **anovulatory** (producing an inadequate ovum). The length of amenorrhea and infertility is linked to breastfeeding frequency, short intervals between feedings (Gray, 1993), duration of feedings (Diaz, 1991; Gellen, 1992; McNeilly, 1994; Vestermark, 1994), the presence of nighttime feedings, (Vestermark, 1994), and the absence of supplemental foods in the baby's diet (Diaz, 1992).

Menstruation may resume at any time during lactation and is greatly dependent on overall breastfeeding patterns. The rate of return of menses is between 19 and 53 percent by 6 months postpartum in women who breastfeed exclusively (Lawrence, 1999). Although a very small percentage of women resume menstruation as early as 6 to 12 weeks, others may not menstruate until breastfeeding has ceased totally. Some women produce a scanty show before their full menstrual cycles resume. The onset of menstruation should not be confused with any normal or abnormal postpartum bleeding. If the mother suspects abnormal bleeding, she should consult her caregiver.

Some women report bleeding around days 42 to 56. This may signal an end to lochial discharge, or it may reflect a change in the mothers' activity level (Visness, 1997). Other bleeding, or bleeding with breastfeeding difficulties, is a sign to seek immediate healthcare advice. Menstruation causes no significant changes in the composition of the mother's milk, and mothers can continue nursing during menstrual cycling. Hormonal changes may alter the taste of her milk, however, which can prompt the baby to be fussy during a feeding or even refuse to nurse. The baby's reaction may also result from heightened tension in the mother or to swelling in the breast caused by menstrual edema and hormones. Any of these factors can affect letdown.

Contraception

During the postpartum period, parents face important decisions about birth control. They may gather information about various contraceptive devices through reading, talking with friends, and consulting their caregiver. Often, a woman may ask about birth control methods that are compatible with breastfeeding. Some women fear another close pregnancy and will not breastfeed if it precludes using a method that provides full protection. These women may not be receptive to a family planning method that relies on breastfeeding and their body's signals. You are not responsible for a mother's final choice; you are responsible only for ensuring that your counseling is based on scientific evidence and that it supports her goals. Referral to other providers may help the mother find the solution that is best for her.

Lactational Amenorrhea Method (LAM)

The absence of ovulation and menstruation during lactation is not merely a convenience to the mother. Research has demonstrated that lactation can delay the return of fertility during the postpartum period. Women who are breastfeeding fully (that is, frequently, day and night), and are experiencing **lactational amenorrhea** are more than 98 percent protected from pregnancy for 6 months after birth (Hight-Laukaran, 1997; Kennedy, 1998; Labbok, 1997, 1994). This protection has given rise to the lactational amenorrhea method (LAM) of contraception (Figure 19.3).

Three conditions are necessary for the mother to rely on the lactational amenorrhea method to prevent pregnancy. First, the mother's menses must not have returned. Second, she must breastfeed around the clock, without significant amounts of other foods in her baby's diet. Third, the baby must be younger than six months of age. If any one of these conditions is not met, the mother will be at increased risk of pregnancy and should supplement with another method to ensure adequate

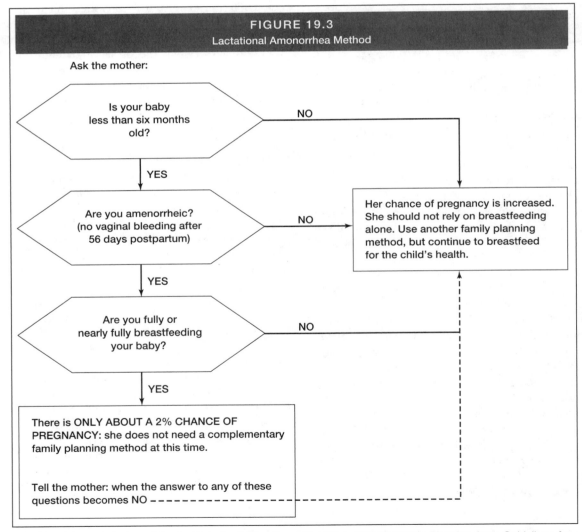

FIGURE 19.3
Lactational Amonorrhea Method

Ask the mother:

Is your baby less than six months old?

NO → Her chance of pregnancy is increased. She should not rely on breastfeeding alone. Use another family planning method, but continue to breastfeed for the child's health.

YES ↓

Are you amenorrheic? (no vaginal bleeding after 56 days postpartum)

NO →

YES ↓

Are you fully or nearly fully breastfeeding your baby?

NO →

YES ↓

There is ONLY ABOUT A 2% CHANCE OF PREGNANCY: she does not need a complementary family planning method at this time.

Tell the mother: when the answer to any of these questions becomes NO - - - - - -

Reprinted by permission of the Institute for International Studies in Natural Family Planning from *Guidelines for Breastfeeding in Family Planning and Child Survival Programs,* Washington, DC, Georgetown University, Labbok M, Koniz-Booher P, Cooney K, Shelton J, and Krasovac K (eds); January, 1990.

protection. For LAM to be most effective, it is recommended that the baby breastfeed beginning soon after birth and continue to breastfeed exclusively, day and night, for six months. The use of artificial nipples, such as a bottle or pacifier, interferes with frequency and duration of suckling at the breast, and the mother should avoid them.

LAM offers a method of protection from pregnancy at a vulnerable time in the mother's life—the first 6 months postpartum. It does so with no side effects to either the mother or child. Many mothers find this an excellent opportunity to be in tune with their bodies' natural rhythms. LAM requires only that the mother learn the three conditions and that she breastfeed her child in an optimal manner. Such a method, which allows a mother to meet both her needs and her baby's needs in a safe manner, deserves to be included in prenatal and postpartum education. Mothers need to understand that as soon as there is a decline in breastfeeding, either because the baby begins solid foods or supplements or because he is nursing less often, contraceptive protection decreases.

Natural Family Planning

Periodic abstinence, or natural family planning, involves charting the basal body temperature (temperature taken on waking, at around the same time each day) or checking vaginal secretions. It requires keeping a careful calendar record of menstrual periods to predict fertile days. This method is more reliable than the rhythm method, which estimates the woman's fertile period from the calendar records of menstrual periods alone.

In total natural family planning, changes in cervical mucus before ovulation help signal the beginning of the fertile days. Women who are familiar with natural family planning will probably have more success with it postpartum than new users, because the signs can be quite different during lactation. Cervical mucus patterns in the first few breastfeeding months postpartum may be less clearly defined than after regular cycles have resumed. Mucus changes from a scant semisolid white or yellowish matter to an abundant thin, clear, watery, and slippery fluid that allows the sperm to penetrate the canal of the cervix easily.

Fluctuations in the woman's basal body temperature aid the couple in determining fertile periods. During menses and up to ovulation, basal body temperature is at its lowest. After ovulation, the temperature will rise, leveling off until just before the onset of menses. Monitoring mucous and temperature changes will identify the five to seven days per month when pregnancy may occur. Clients interested in using natural family planning can read *Breastfeeding and Natural Child Spacing: How Ecological Breastfeeding Spaces Babies* (Kippley, 1999) or visit the Web site for the Couple to Couple League at www.ccli.org.

Oral Contraceptives

Combination oral contraceptives contain the hormones estrogen and progesterone. They appear to cause the most difficulty in lactating women, especially in the early postpartum period before lactation is well established. Estrogen can lower milk production (IPPF, 2002; WHO, 2000, 1998; Koetsawang, 1987). Additionally, the long-term effects of oral contraceptive use on babies are not known. There are concerns related to milk composition as well (Erwin, 1994).

Women have used birth control pills for over 40 years with no reports of adverse effects on their children. Research into the long-term effects of oral contraceptives is limited, however, reaching only to the age of puberty for the exposed children (Pardthaisong, 1992). The effects this hormonal exposure will have on the reproductive potential of these children needs consideration.

Generally, advice to breastfeeding women is that they use non-estrogen contraceptive methods. Progestin-only oral contraceptives (the mini-pill) do not appear to interfere with milk production and therefore are acceptable during lactation (Bjarnadottir, 2001; Kelsey, 1996; Dunson, 1993; Speroff, 1992–1993). However, the long-term effects remain unknown. Bjarnadottir noted slight adverse effects in some mothers and children but concluded that the mini-pill appeared to be safe for lactating women. Generally, women should not use this method before six weeks postpartum. Practitioners have received numerous anecdotal reports of mothers experiencing drops in milk production after starting the progesterone-only pill. Milk production recovers when mothers cease taking the pill.

Intrauterine Devices (IUD)

The IUD is a copper or hormonal device placed into the uterus. The copper affects the lining of the uterus and prevents a fertilized egg from implanting (Williams, 2003). The non-hormonal IUD does not seem to have any effect on lactation (Koetsawang, 1987). Hormonal IUDs prevent pregnancy by releasing the hormone progesterone. This causes a thickening in the cervical mucus and acts as a barrier to prevent sperm from entering the uterus, thereby preventing implantation of a fertilized egg. Hormonal IUDs need replacement within one year (Williams, 2003). Use of a progesterone-releasing IUD was associated with a slight decrease in milk volume, compared to use of a copper IUD (Kelsey, 1996).

Vaginal Ring

The vaginal ring is a hormone-releasing ring a woman can self-insert. One study found similar effectiveness rates between the efficacy of a progesterone-releasing vaginal ring and a copper IUD in lactating mothers. Milk production and infant growth were within normal limits for women who used a vaginal ring and those who used an IUD (Sivin, 1997). At least one vaginal ring on the U.S. market contains both progesterone and estrogen. Although the company Web site says that it contains "half the estrogen of a commonly used oral contraceptive," a mother might be prudent to consider non-estrogen alternatives (Organon, 2004).

Implants

Levonorgestrel is a progestin implant made of small plastic rods, which is inserted surgically under the skin of the upper arm. The rods slowly release progesterone into the body for up to five years. About half of women using levonorgestrel continue to ovulate, and about half have the implants surgically removed before the third year due to unpleasant side effects (Hatcher, 1995). Neurovascular injury can occur with removal (Sarma, 1995).

Injectables

Depo-Provera is a progestin injection given every three months. Infertility may last up to one year. Although many lactation consultants have noted a connection between the administration of Depo-Provera immediately postpartum and an impaired milk supply, one clinical study showed no impact on lactation (Danli, 2000). Mothers should delay use of Depo-Provera until lactation is well established, since it is the precipitous drop in progesterone postpartum that initiates stage II lactogenesis (Kennedy, 1997).

Patches

The "patch" is a birth control system that delivers hormones directly through the skin into the bloodstream via a thin patch. It is a combination contraceptive, containing both estrogen and progesterone. The patch is a newer form of birth control with no proven safety record in lactating mothers. It is about as effective as combination oral contraceptives.

Barrier Methods

Barrier methods include condoms, diaphragms, cervical caps, and the use of a spermicide, with or without physical barriers. Spermicides prevent pregnancy by destroying sperm before it can reach and fertilize an egg. Studies of spermicides show variable failure rates averaging 21–26 percent for typical users. A male condom is a thin latex or silicone sheath that covers the penis. A female condom is a thin polyurethane sheath with two soft rings at each end. One ring, covered with the polyurethane, fits over the cervix and acts as an anchor. The larger, open ring stays outside the vagina, covering part of the perineum and labia during intercourse. Male condoms have about a 14 percent failure rate (Williams, 2003). Diaphragms and cervical caps have a higher failure rate among women who have had vaginal births (Williams, 2003).

Sterilization

Some mothers choose sterilization through bilateral **tubal ligation**, a procedure that ties the mother's fallopian tubes to prevent conception. Most mothers in the United States who choose tubal ligation have the procedure almost immediately postpartum. Although there is no evidence that tubal ligation hampers milk production, the operation immediately postpartum can potentially affect the mother's pain level. The IV fluids she receives can increase edema and make it difficult for her baby to latch on in the early days.

Some fathers choose sterilization by vasectomy, in which the vas deferens (the main duct through which sperm travel during ejaculation) is snipped. Sterilization is a permanent decision (Hatcher, 2005). Parents considering this option may want to let time lapse before deciding to end their family size.

Points for Parents to Consider

Most caregivers' offices provide information on family planning, sex education, parenting, and sterilization. Literature on each of the individual birth control methods is available free of charge. Prenatal classes can encourage couples to discuss contraception with their providers during pregnancy to provide sufficient time for careful consideration. The obstetric provider knows the woman's general medical history, family history, and other needs that may influence her options.

The choice of contraceptive method is the parent's responsibility. Restrict your help to that of suggesting options that are compatible with breastfeeding, rather than giving advice. The following considerations may be helpful to parents in selecting a form of contraceptive:

◆ Religious and ethical feelings about birth control

◆ Concerns regarding contraceptive effectiveness and the possibility of another pregnancy

◆ Choice of who will take responsibility for contraception

◆ Convenience in terms of remembering to use it and wishing to use it every time

◆ Association between the method and intercourse

◆ Expense, inconvenience, use of foreign objects, messiness, and loss of spontaneity

▶ SIBLING REACTIONS AND ADJUSTMENTS

Homecoming for parents and their new baby can range from a very smooth adjustment to a distant or demanding attitude by siblings. Reactions will depend on many

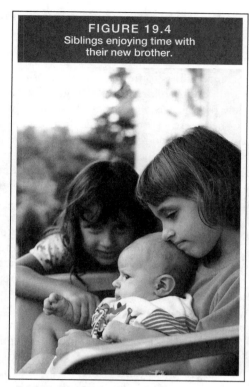

FIGURE 19.4
Siblings enjoying time with their new brother.

Printed with permission of Debbie Shinskie.

factors, including the age of the child and the length of his separation from his mother. Prepare the mother for possible changes in her older children, and let her know that these reactions are common. She may be engrossed with the baby and feel less close to her other children for a while. This can cause the children to display jealousy and perhaps develop a closer relationship with their father or other relative in the early weeks, while appearing distant with the mother. Relationships will mend as all family members learn to bond with the baby in their own way (Figure 19.4).

Helping Siblings Prepare for the New Baby

Parents can begin preparing their children for the baby's arrival by sharing the events of pregnancy with them. They can explain how a baby develops, visits their mother will make to her caregiver, and what she will do in the hospital. They can read books to their children that show a new baby in the family. Children can participate in preparing for the baby by helping with baby clothes and equipment and packing the mother's suitcase. If the child's sleeping arrangements will change, it should be done early and in a way that the older child does not feel crowded out by the new baby.

The mother can make a construction paper booklet with magazine pictures about what it is like in the hospital (physicians, nurses, nursery pictures), coming home, at

home with the baby (bathing, sleeping, nursing, crying), and the new family. Looking at their family's current baby pictures can be fun, too. She can prepare the child for what new babies do, such as nursing, sleeping, and crying, and the fact that they are not yet able to play. There are many children's books that show breastfeeding as a normal, routine part of infant care and family life. A list is available at the La Leche League Web site at www.lalecheleague.org/cbi/bfbookshort.htm.

Parents can explain any changes that will take place in usual family activities and the reasons for the changes. The mother can involve her child in caring for the new baby, assuring him she needs his help with such things as bringing diapers and clothes to her, holding the baby, talking to him, and getting him to smile. Siblings can visit a family with a new baby to see what a baby looks and sounds like and how it has changed their family.

Preparing for a Home Birth

Many families prefer the option of home birthing as the natural, low-intervention way to welcome their child into the world. It is the parents' decision whether their other children will attend the labor and birth. Some mothers worry that the intensity of labor could frighten a young child. The level of participation parents are comfortable with probably depends on the age, maturity, and personality of the children.

Regardless of whether the child is present for the labor and birth, the continuous presence of his mother in the home eliminates the concern about the child's reaction to her absence. Other siblings are able to see the baby during or immediately after birth. They can welcome the new baby to their home, free from hospital interventions and interruptions. A caregiver for the children can tend to their needs during and after labor.

Preparing for the Mother's Absence

If the mother plans to give birth in a hospital, it is important that the older child be prepared for his mother's absence during her hospital stay. He will want to understand where the mother is going, why, for how long, and what she will do while she is there. Visiting the hospital with him during the pregnancy will help him understand what will take place. Many hospitals offer sibling classes and tours, and sibling visitation during the mother's postpartum stay can be worked out at that time. The mother can plan to maintain contact with her family through telephone calls and visits. Because of the brevity of U.S. hospital stays, the mother will usually be away only one or two nights.

Some parents wish to have siblings present at the baby's birth. Such a choice requires preparation about what birth is like and how the mother will act. When siblings are present at the birth, a caregiver needs to be present to meet the needs of the children during the experience. The sibling can decide whether he is comfortable being present at the actual time of delivery. Many hospitals with family-centered care allow siblings to stay with their parents at the hospital after the delivery.

Adjusting to the New Baby

Whenever a new baby joins a family, the role of each family member is redefined and expanded. An older child who previously had been the "baby of the family" loses his position as the center of attention. He may need to assume responsibility for tasks previously performed by his parents. Parents may expect him to dress himself, help with household chores, and generally fend for himself instead of always relying on someone to help him. The ease with which he can do this will depend on his age at the time of his sibling's birth, his personality, and his sense of security.

Each child needs time and understanding in assuming his new role. The parents can help him adjust by making him feel special in new ways. The mother can begin fostering her older child's emotional growth by giving him her undivided attention the first time she sees him following the birth of the baby. She can have another adult hold the baby while she renews contact with her older child and expresses her love for him. After the family is settled, the parents can create situations where each child can look at, touch, or hold the baby. Setting aside special moments each day for the other children individually will let each one know how she appreciates his unique qualities.

Sibling's Behavior During Feedings

During feedings, a sibling may want to be included in the closeness and interaction he observes between his mother and the new baby. The mother can accommodate this by nursing her baby where there is ample room for all family members, such as the bed, couch, or floor. She can plan activities to share with her toddler during nursing times, such as reading books, playing simple games ("I spy something red"), and activities (paper and crayons, tea party, puzzles, or playing music).

A toddler who had weaned may ask to nurse again. If the mother gives him the opportunity to do so, his mother's awareness of his needs and her willingness to respond favorably will be reassuring to him. He may want only to taste the milk, in which case the mother can put some of her milk in a cup to satisfy his curiosity. This renewed interest in breastfeeding is usually temporary. A toddler occasionally resumes nursing on a regular basis,

and the mother may need your support in tandem nursing (see Chapter 14).

Adjustment Challenges

Despite parents' efforts toward a smooth transition, some toddlers and young children exhibit regressive behaviors when a new baby arrives. Reactions can include whining, baby talk, bed-wetting or accidents from a previously toilet-trained child, waking during the night, clinging to the mother, or hitting the baby. Such behavior may be the child's way of seeking attention. A child often will develop mixed feelings. He may enjoy cuddling and talking to the baby but at the same time may find it difficult to share his mother's attention with him.

The mother can reassure her child that she understands and accepts his feelings and him. She can read to him about new babies and emphasize his importance as an older child in protecting and amusing their baby. She can help him find his new position in the family by giving him special opportunities to demonstrate his capabilities in caring for the baby. She can point out the many benefits and privileges of being more independent and self-reliant. Spending focused time with each parent—especially the mother—can help alleviate the older child's feelings of displacement and help the adjustment to being the new older brother or sister.

▶ SUMMARY

Your availability and support to couples will help them as they evolve into the parental role. Understanding typical postpartum adjustments and the aspects of physical recovery will help mothers avoid needless worry. Fathers have their own unique adjustments as they provide support to the mother and learn how to interact with their new baby. The mother and father will experience adjustments in their sex life and consider contraceptive options that are compatible with breastfeeding. Siblings will benefit from preparation for the birth, as well as patience and understanding as they adjust to the new baby. This is an exciting time for the family as they welcome a new baby into their home and learn to respond to one another in new ways.

▶ CHAPTER 19 — AT A GLANCE

Applying what you learned—

Counseling the mother:

◆ Encourage mothers to express their feelings.

◆ Encourage women to develop friendships with other new mothers.

◆ Encourage realistic expectations about the baby and motherhood.

- Help mothers see that not all problems with the baby are related to breastfeeding.
- Help mothers cope with baby blues.
- Recognize when baby blues progresses to depression or psychosis.
- Recognize your limitations and when to refer.
- Recognize characteristics of survivors of sexual abuse.

Teach parents about:

- Dangers of baby training programs.
- Physical recovery and emotional adjustments following birth.
- Changes in priorities with a new baby.
- Importance of the father's support to the mother.
- The father's interaction with the baby.
- Sexual adjustments and physical discomfort.
- Lactational amenorrhea method and other contraceptives.
- How to respond to their baby's needs.
- Helping siblings prepare for and adjust to the new baby.

REFERENCES

American Academy of Pediatrics (AAP). *Media Alert: AAP Addresses Scheduled Feedings vs. Demand Feedings.* Chicago, IL; April 20, 1998. Available at: www.ezzo.info/Aney/aapmediaalert.pdf. Accessed January 26, 2005.

American Academy of Pediatrics (AAP). Policy Statement on Breastfeeding and the Use of Human Milk. *Pediatrics* 115(2):496–506; 2005.

Anderson G et al. Early skin-to-skin contact for mothers and their healthy newborn infants. Review. *Cochrane Database Syst Rev* (2):CD003519; 2003.

Anderson G. Risk in mother-infant separation postbirth. *Image* 21:196–199; 1989.

Aney M. Babywise linked to dehydration, failure to thrive. *AAP News*; April 1998.

Aono J et al. Alteration in glucose metabolism by crying in children. *N Engl J Med* 329(15):1129; 1993.

Bass E, Davis L. *The Courage to Heal.* New York: Harper Collins; 1994.

Bjarnadottir R et al. Comparative study of the effects of a progestogen-only pill containing desogestrel and an intrauterine contraceptive device in lactating women. *BJOG* 108(11):1174–1180; 2001.

Bocar DL, Moore K. *Acquiring the Parental Role.* Lactation Consultant Series #16. New York: Avery Publishing Group; 1987.

Bottorff J, Morse J. Mothers' perceptions of breast milk. *JOGNN* 19:518–526; 1990.

Briere J, Runtz M. The long-term effects of sexual abuse: A review and synthesis. *New Dir Ment Health Serv* (51):3–13; 1991.

Child Abuse Prevention Council of Orange County (CAPCOC). *Religious Parenting Programs: Their Relationship to Child Abuse Prevention. Parenting Program Review Committee*; May 14, 1996. Available at: www.geocities.com/thetruthaboutgfi/. Accessed February 24, 2005.

Cooper P et al. Psychosocial factors associated with the early termination of breastfeeding. *J Psychosom Res* 37:171–176; 1993.

Cox DB, Owens RA, Hartmann PE. Studies on human lactation: The development of the computerized breast measurement system. 1998. Available at: www.biochem.uwa.edu.au/PEH/PEHRes. html. Accessed September 15, 2004.

Cox J. Utah Chapter, American Academy of Pediatrics. (UCAAP). *Got time? The Growing Times.* September/October 2001. Available at: www.ips-aap.org/newsIndexDetail.asp?articleId=39. Accessed August 10, 2004.

Cox LL, Holden JM, Sagovsky R. Edinburgh postnatal depression scale (EPDS). *British Journal of Psychiatry* 150:782–786; June 1987.

Daly S, Hartmann PE. Infant demand and milk supply, Part 1: Infant demand and milk production in lactating women. *J Hum Lact* 11:21–26; 1995a.

Daly S, Hartmann P. Infant demand and milk supply, Part 2: The short-term control of milk synthesis in lactating women. *J Hum Lact* 11:27–37; 1995b.

Danli S et al. A multicentered clinical trial of the long-acting injectable contraceptive Depo Provera in Chinese women. *Contraception* 62(1):15–18; 2000.

Delight E et al. What do parents expect antenatally and do babies teach them? *Arch Dis Child* 66:1309–1314; 1991.

Diaz S et al. Early difference in the endocrine profile of long and short lactational amenorrhea. *J Clin Endocrinol Metab* 72:196–201; 1991.

Diaz S et al. Relative contributions of anovulation and luteal phase defect to the reduced pregnancy rate of breastfeeding women. *Fertil Steril* 58:498–503; 1992.

Dobson J. Focus on the family. Radio Broadcast August 25, 1999: In response to on-air question. Available at: www.ezzo.info/Focus/dobsontranscript.htm. Accessed May 24, 2004.

Dunson T et al. A multicenter clinical trial of a progestin-only oral contraceptive in lactating women. *Contraception* 47:23–35; 1993.

Eidelman A et al. Comparative tactile behavior of mothers and fathers with their newborn infants. *Isr J Med Sci* 30:79–82; 1994.

Erwin P. To use or not use combined hormonal oral contraceptives during lactation. *Fam Plann Perspect* 26:26–30; 1994.

Ezzo G, Bucknam R. *On Becoming Babywise.* Simi Valley, CA: Parent-wise Solutions; 2001.

Ezzo G, Ezzo A. *Let the Children Come Along the Infant Way.* Louisiana, MD: Growing Families International; 2002.

Finkelhor D. The international epidemiology of child sexual abuse. *Child Abuse Negl* 18(5):409–417; 1994.

Fleming A et al. Testosterone and prolactin are associated with emotional responses to infant cries in new fathers. *Horm Behav* 42(4):399–413; 2002.

Francis B. Growing Families International: An extreme response to attachment parenting. *Christian Association for Psychological Studies West Newsletter* 25(3):2,7; August 1998.

Freed G, et al. Attitudes of expectant fathers regarding breastfeeding. *Pediatrics* 89:224–227; 1992.

Gale S, Harlow B. Postpartum mood disorders: A review of clinical and epidemiological factors. Review. *J Psychosom Obstet Gynaecol* 24(4):257–266; 2003.

Gamble D, Morse J. Fathers of breastfed infants: Postponing and types of involvement. *JOGNN* 22:358–365; 1992.

Gellen J. The feasibility of suppressing ovarian activity following the end of amenorrhea by increasing the frequency of suckling. *Int J Gynecol Obstet* 39:321–325; 1992.

Gold M. *The Good News about Depression: Cures and Treatments in the New Age of Psychiatry*. Rev ed. New York: Bantam; 1995.

Gordon A. *Differing Parenting Philosophies*. La Leche League International Texas Area Conference; Dallas, TX; June, 1999.

Graham M. Parental sensitivity to infant cues: Similarities and differences between mothers and fathers. *J Pediatr Nurs* 8: 376–384; 1993.

Gray R et al. The return of ovarian function during lactation: Results of studies from the US and the Philippines. In Gray R (ed). *Biomedical and Demographic Determinants of Reproduction*. Oxford, UK: Oxford University Press, 428–445; 1993.

Hanegraaf H. Christian Research Institute: Commentary on radio broadcast of The Bible Answer Man, July 28, 1998, October 6, 1998, October 8–9, 1998, October 26, 1998, October 27, 1998, March 25–26, 1999. Available at: www.equip.org. Accessed March 15, 2003.

Hatcher R et al. *Contraceptive Technology*, 18th ed. New York: Ardent Media Inc; 2005.

Hatcher R, Sarma S. How we can save Norplant contraceptive implants. Trouble in paradise? *Contracept Technol Update* 16(1): 14–15; 1995.

Heinowitz J. *Fathering Right from the Start: Straight Talk about Pregnancy, Birth and Beyond*. Novato, CA: New World Library; 2001.

Hight-Laukaran V et al. Multicenter study of the lactational amenorrhea method (LAM) II: Acceptability, utility, and policy implications. *Contraception* 55:337–346; 1997.

Hogg T. *Secrets of the Baby Whisperer*. New York: Ballantine Books; 2001.

Hunter B. *The Power of Mother Love* (chapter on attachment). New York: Waterbrook Press; 1998.

International Planned Parenthood Federation (IPPF). IMAP statement on hormonal methods of contraception. *IPPF Med Bull* 36(5):1–8; 2002.

Jordan P, Wall V. Breastfeeding and fathers: Illuminating the darker side. *Birth* 17:210–213; 1990.

Jordan P, Wall V. Supporting the father when the infant is breastfed. *J Hum Lact* 9:31–34; 1993.

Kelsey J. Hormonal contraception and lactation. *J Hum Lact* 12(4):315–318; 1996.

Kendall-Tackett K. Breastfeeding and the sexual abuse survivor. *J Hum Lact* 14(2):125–130; 1998.

Kendall-Tackett K. *The Hidden Feelings of Motherhood: Coping with Stress, Depression and Burnout*. Oakland, CA: New Harbinger; 2001.

Kennedy K et al. Premature introduction of progestin-only contraceptive methods during lactation. *Contraception* 55:347–350; 1997.

Kennedy K et al. Users' understanding of the lactational amenorrhea method and the occurrence of pregnancy. *J Hum Lact* 14: 209–218; 1998.

Kippley S. *Breastfeeding and Natural Child Spacing: How Ecological Breastfeeding Spaces Babies*. Reprint ed. Cincinnati, OH: Couple to Couple League International; 1999.

Koetsawang S. The effects of contraceptive methods on the quality and quantity of breast milk. *Int J Gynaecol Obstet* 25 Suppl:115–127; 1987.

Kroeger M, Smith, L. *Impact of Birthing Practices on Breastfeeding*. Sudbury, MA: Jones and Bartlett; 2004.

Labbok M et al. The Lactational Amenorrhea Method (LAM): A postpartum introductory family planning method with policy and program implications. *Adv Contracept* 10(2):93–109; 1994.

Labbok M et al. Multicenter study of the lactational amenorrhea method (LAM) I: Efficacy, duration, and implications for clinical application. *Contraception* 55:327–336; 1997.

Lawrence R. *Breastfeeding: A Guide for the Medical Profession*. New York: Mosby; 1999.

MacArthur C, Knox G. Association with backache is real. *Br Med J* 307:64; 1993.

MacArthur J. Grace Community Church: Public Statement, July 25, 2000. Available at: www.ezzo.info/GCC/macarthur.htm. Accessed May 12, 2004.

Mazurek T et al. Influence of immediate newborn care on infant adaptation to the environment. *Med Wieku Rozwoj* 3(2):215–224; 1999.

McNeilly A et al. Physiological mechanisms underlying lactational amenorrhea. *Ann NY Acad Sci* 709:145–155; 1994.

McNeilly A. Lactational amenorrhea. *Endocrinol Metab Clin North Am* 22:59–73; 1993.

Mercer R. A theoretical framework for studying factors that impact on the maternal role. *Nurs Res* 30:73–77; 1981.

Misri S. *Shouldn't I Be Happy? Emotional Problems of Pregnant and Postpartum Women*. New York: Free Press; 2002.

Moody L. Case studies of moms who had problems using Babywise or Preparation for Parenting, 2002. Available at: www.angelfire.com/md2/moodyfamily/casestudies.html. Accessed June 3, 2004.

O'Malley S. *Are You There Alone? The Unspeakable Crime of Andrea Yates*. New York: Simon & Schuster; 2004.

Oates M. Perinatal psychiatric disorders: A leading cause of maternal morbidity and mortality. *Br Med Bull* 67(1): 219–229; 2003.

Organon USA Inc. Nuvaring consumer information. Available at: www.nuvaring.com. Accessed June 23, 2004.

Pardthaisong T et al. The long term growth and development of children exposed to Depo-Provera during pregnancy or lactation. *Contraception* 45:313–324; 1992.

Pridham K et al. Early postpartum transition: Progress in maternal identity and role attainment. *Res Nurs Health* 14: 21–31; 1991.

Sarma S, Hatcher R. Neurovascular injury during removal of levonorgestrel implants. *Am J Obstet Gynecol* 172(1 Pt 1):120–121; January, 1995.

Sears W et al. *Becoming a Father*, 2nd ed. Schaumburg, IL: La Leche League International; 2003.

Sivin I et al. Contraceptives for lactating women: A comparative trial of a progesterone-releasing vaginal ring and the copper T 380A IUD. *Contraception* 55(4):225–232; 1997.

Speroff L. Postpartum contraception: Issues and choices. *Dialogues in Contraception* 3:1–3, 67; 1992–1993.

Tay C et al. Twenty-four hour patterns of prolactin secretion during lactation and the relationship to suckling and the resumption of fertility in breast-feeding women. *Human Reprod* 11:950–955; 1996.

Terner K, Miller E. More than a parenting ministry: The cultic characteristics of Growing Families International. *Christian Research Journal* 20(4); 1998. Available at: www.equip.org/free/DG233.htm. Accessed June 23, 2004.

Vestermark V et al. Postpartum amenorrhoea and breastfeeding in a Danish sample. *J Biosoc Sci* 26:1–7; 1994.

Visness C et al. The duration and character of postpartum bleeding among breastfeeding women. *Obstet Gynecol* 89:159–163; 1997.

Webb C. Is the Babywise method right for you? What you should know about Babywise and Growing Kids God's Way. *Tulsa Kids*; July 2003.

Williams M. Epigee Birth Control Guide. August 2003. Available at: www.epigee.org. Accessed February 8, 2004.

Williams N. Counseling challenges: Helping mothers handle conflicting information. *Leaven* 34(2):19–20; April–May 1998.

Williams N. Dancing with differences: Helping mothers handle conflicting information, including scheduled feeding and sleep training. La Leche League International 1999 Conference, Orlando, FL; July 5, 1999.

Wisner KL, Stowe ZN. Psychobiology of postpartum mood disorders. *Semin Reprod Endocrinol* 15(1):77–89; 1997.

World Health Organization (WHO). Effects of hormonal contraceptives on breast milk composition and infant growth. *Stud Fam Plann* 19:36–69; 1988.

Yamauchi Y, Yamanouchi I. The relationship between rooming-in/not rooming-in and breastfeeding variables. *Acta Paediatr Scand* 79:1017–1022; 1990.

Yates R. Review of *Are You There Alone? The Unspeakable Crime of Andrea Yates*. January 18, 2004. Available at: www.yateskids.org/are_you_there_alone.php. Accessed April 12, 2004.

▶ **BIBLIOGRAPHY**

Beck C. A checklist to identify women at risk for developing postpartum depression. *JOGNN* 27:39–46; 1998.

Beck C. Teetering on the edge: A substantive theory of postpartum depression. *Nurs Res* 42:42–48; 1993.

Blume ES. *Secret Survivors: Uncovering Incest and Its After-Effects in Women*. New York: John Wiley & Sons; 1990.

Bohn DK. Domestic violence and pregnancy: Implications for practice. *J Nurse-Midwife* 35(2):86–98; 1990.

Cox DB, Owens RA, Hartmann PE. Blood and milk prolactin and the rate of milk synthesis in women. *Experimental Physiology* 81:1007–1020; 1996.

Ezzo G, Ezzo AM. *Preparation for Parenting*, 6th ed. Simi Valley, CA: Growing Families International; 1998.

Focus on the Family. Letter of concern regarding GFI. Original letter 1993; current revision dated January 13, 1999. Available at: www.ezzo.info/Focus/FOTFstatement.htm. Accessed May 5, 2004.

Ford G. *The Contented Little Baby Book*. New York: New American Library; 2001.

Ford G. The mumsnet session. Q&A; 2003. Available at: www.mumsnet.com/onlinechats/livechat03.html. Accessed May 10, 2004.

Growing Families International (GFI). Available at: www.gfi.org. Accessed May 10, 2004.

Hendrick G. *My First 300 Babies*. Goleta, CA: Hurst Publications; 1999.

Holz KA. A practical approach to clients who are survivors of childhood sexual abuse. *J Nurse-Midwife* 39(1):13–18; 1994.

Huysman A. *The Postpartum Effect: Deadly Depression in Mothers*. New York: Seven Stories Press; 2003.

Kennedy K et al. Consensus statement on the use of breast-feeding as a family planning method. *Contraception* 39: 477–496; 1989.

Kennedy KI, Labbok MH, VanLook PFA. Consensus statement: Lactational amenorrhea method for family planning. *Int J Gynecol Obstet* 54(1):55–57; 1996.

Marasco L. *Common Breastfeeding Myths*. Schaumburg, IL: La Leche League International; 1999.

Mullen PE et al. Impact of sexual and physical abuse on women's mental health. *Lancet* 16:841–845; 1988.

Murphy S. Siblings and the new baby: Changing perspective. *J Pediatr Nurs* 8:277–288; 1993.

Newton N. Psychologic differences between breast and bottle-feeding. *Am J Clin Nutr* 24:993–1004; 1971.

Parenting Principles. Available at www.parentingprinciples. org. Accessed May 10, 2004.

Rein, S. A collection of resources and concerns about Growing Families International (GFI). Available at: www.ezzo.info. Accessed January 16, 2005.

Richards L. January Interview; March 2001. Available at: www. januarymagazine.com/profiles/thogg.html. Accessed May 10, 2004.

Shelov S. ed. The American Academy of Pediatrics. *Caring for Your Baby and Young Child Birth to Age 5*. New York: Bantam Books; 1998.

Sherar C. Background information for leaders. *Leaven* 34(2): 20–21; April–May 1998.

Simkin P. Memories that really matter. *Childbirth Instructor* 4(1):20–23, 39; 1994.

Slonecker W. *Parenting Principles: From the Heart of a Pediatrician*. Nashville, TN: Broadman and Holman; 2003.

Tyre P. Cries and whispers. *Newsweek,* 54; February 26, 2001.

20

SPECIAL COUNSELING CIRCUMSTANCES

Contributing Author: Carole Peterson

Lactation consultants meet women with a rich variety of lifestyles. At times, circumstances may affect a mother's options and decisions. Tailoring your approach and counseling to women's circumstances will give them the support they need to overcome challenges. When a woman encounters negative reactions from significant people in her life, she may question her decision to breastfeed. Single parents or those who live on a limited income often have special challenges, as do teenage mothers. Meeting the needs of women from cultures other than your own will require sensitivity to their traditions and beliefs. These issues are all explored in this chapter, as well as the important role of support groups for breastfeeding women.

KEY TERMS

acculturated
anticipatory guidance
lifestyle
mother-to-mother support
   group

opposition to breastfeeding
outreach counseling
respiratory distress
   syndrome

MOTHER'S LIFESTYLE

Some women have factors in their lives that detract from breastfeeding and interfere with building understanding and rapport with you. Mothers who live in the city differ in their frame of reference from those who live in suburbia or a more rural setting. Low-income families and those from other cultures may have values and health practices that differ from your own. It is important that you not make unfounded assumptions about others' lifestyle choices. You cannot presume that a mother is married or that the baby's father is living with the mother and baby, or even that there is enough food for the family to eat. Single-parent households are common, and a breastfeeding woman who is solely responsible for her baby's care may have many challenges in her life. A woman in the United States with an unwanted pregnancy is less likely to initiate or continue breastfeeding

than is a woman with an intended pregnancy (Taylor, 2002). A teenage mother may be coping with single parenthood as well as the usual adjustments of adolescence. All of these circumstances present special counseling challenges. Your approach and availability to the mother can greatly influence her mastery of the situation.

Having realistic expectations for each mother and her goals for breastfeeding is important. Beliefs and practices vary widely among cultural groups. Breastfeeding, especially exclusive breastfeeding, may be more than some mothers can handle or even desire. Learn about cultural differences and trends in your community so that you can respond to the individual needs of each mother. Remaining flexible and objective in your approach will help mothers fit breastfeeding into their lifestyles. By working in partnership with the mother, you can develop innovative approaches for providing accurate information and support to all women.

OPPOSITION TO BREASTFEEDING

Despite the strong endorsement of breastfeeding by the American Academy of Pediatrics (AAP, 2005), the World Health Organization (WHO, 1989), and other major health organizations, mothers often receive questions and comments that prompt them to explain and defend their decision to breastfeed. Such remarks can undermine a mother's confidence and cause her to doubt her decision or her capability to breastfeed. Most of the people commenting do not truly oppose breastfeeding; they simply do not understand it. When the mother is confident in her decision to breastfeed, she may be able to educate some of these people and familiarize them with the feeding patterns of a breastfed baby.

Opposition to breastfeeding often manifests itself as subtle undermining of the mother's efforts rather than blatant remarks. Professionals and laypersons alike, quick to state that breastfeeding is "the best" infant food, often point to breastfeeding as the cause when the baby cries or the mother expresses a concern. The mother is encouraged to "rest" and feed her baby with a bottle, implying that breastfeeding and bottle-feeding are interchangeable. Mothers will benefit from your education and support to get them through challenging times when doubts surface that undermine their confidence.

Unsupportive questions or remarks mothers may receive:

◆ How long do you plan to nurse?

◆ Are you still breastfeeding?

◆ Isn't he getting a little old to nurse?

◆ Does he want to nurse again so soon?

◆ He seems hungry all the time; maybe your milk isn't rich enough, or maybe you don't have enough milk.

◆ How long are you going to do *that*?

A mother may receive opposition from strangers, friends, her employer, colleagues, coworkers, her caregiver, the baby's grandparents and other relatives, and even the baby's father. Objections from people close to the mother are more difficult for her to cope with. It is no surprise that mothers who have a strong support system for breastfeeding have better outcomes (Rose, 2004; Ekstrom, 2003; Sikorski, 2003). You can help a mother identify the various breastfeeding supporters within her network of friends and family. Their support will help the mother through the challenges she may face when others oppose or question her choice to breastfeed. You can also provide positive support, suggest ways for her to cope with the opposition, and personally make an extra effort to boost her morale and self-confidence.

Opposition from Strangers

When a mother is confident and knowledgeable about her decision to breastfeed, she is less likely to yield to the opinions or rude remarks of a stranger. In order to minimize the potential for such comments, she can ensure that she is discreet when she breastfeeds in public. She can wear clothing that allows easy access to her breast while still providing coverage. Practicing discreet breastfeeding in front of a mirror will help her become confident with techniques that work for her. Breastfeeding in public normalizes breastfeeding and helps increase cultural acceptance.

Opposition from Friends

Opposition from friends may prove more difficult for the mother to handle. Depending on the nature of the friendship, a mother may attempt to educate a friend who opposes breastfeeding. She needs to find a comfort level with such a friend in order to maintain both their relationship and her breastfeeding. Developing friendships and relationships with people who are supportive of breastfeeding or who are breastfeeding mothers themselves can help her become more confident with breastfeeding (Dykes, 2003).

Opposition from an Employer

Some women who return to work while they are breastfeeding experience negative reactions from their employers. A mother can avoid the stress and tension of an unsupportive work environment by speaking frankly with her employer about her plans to breastfeed. She can discuss any special needs she will have, such as breastfeeding her baby at work or expressing milk for her baby, as well as her desire to combine breastfeeding with working.

The mother may need to convince her employer that any needs related to breastfeeding will not interfere with her job performance. She can point out that the health benefits of breastfeeding result in less time off and less use of health benefits. Employers who have had previous experience with breastfeeding employees often react more positively to combining employment with breastfeeding (Dunn, 2004). Negative attitudes tend to result from lack of understanding and experience, rather than outright opposition (Bridges, 1997). You can educate employers in your community about breastfeeding's contribution to infant and maternal health and their implications for employment.

Employers are more responsive when they recognize breastfeeding's importance and the cost savings to the company. The monograph *Advancing Women's Health: Health Plans' Innovative Programs in Breastfeeding Promotion* describes model programs and promotion within the insurance industry. It explores eight organizations that promote breastfeeding coverage and provide benefits to breastfeeding employees (AAHP, 2001).

Some women are uncomfortable approaching their employer, especially if they work in a male-dominated profession or have little job security. They may worry that they are jeopardizing their position with such a "feminine" request. These mothers need to consider which aspects of the job are compatible with breastfeeding. They may find books, articles, and Web sites for employed breastfeeding mothers helpful, such as the book *Nursing Mother, Working Mother* (Pryor, 1999). They can learn their legal rights and consider how to approach their employer before the baby arrives. Be sure to address employment issues in prenatal education classes as part of your anticipatory guidance.

In some cases, a woman may be unable to resolve her employer's lack of support. If the situation undermines her breastfeeding, she may need to reevaluate her priorities and motives regarding working and breastfeeding. She can refer unreasonable and unfair treatment by an employer to her human resources department, local labor relations board, or, in the United States, the Equal Employment Opportunity Commission (EEOC). Some work environments are not compatible with breastfeeding. You can assist the mother in developing a plan within the parameters of her employment. See Chapter 24 for further discussion of combining breastfeeding with employment.

Opposition from a Physician

It is often difficult for a mother when her physician does not support breastfeeding. Women value their physicians' opinions and trust their judgments about their family's healthcare. A physician who does not seem committed to breastfeeding may be unsupportive and unintentionally give misinformation. If the mother has a good rapport with her physician, she may be able to resolve differences about breastfeeding. If the mother does not have a good rapport with her physician, she may need to consider whether this relationship is in the best interests of her and her baby.

Well-meaning physicians may not realize that their remarks to a woman can undermine her confidence. A mother with an unsupportive physician needs a lot of extra contact and confidence building. Anticipatory guidance will help this mother through times of change and uncertainty. A perceived lack of support by a physician may actually stem from lack of knowledge and experience with breastfeeding. Giving her research articles to share with her physician can reinforce her efforts, and raise the physicians level of appreciation for the importance of breastfeeding and understanding of breastfeeding care. Chapter 2 has further discussion of the relationship between physicians and mothers with respect to breastfeeding.

Opposition from Grandparents and Other Relatives

In many cultures, the baby's grandmother has a pivotal role in a mother's breastfeeding experience (Ekstrom, 2003). A new mother often will turn to her own mother for encouragement and wisdom as she merges into her parenting role. This is particularly true if she is a first-time mother. Breastfeeding is a part of feminine identity. Women from the 1940s on were discouraged from breastfeeding for a multitude of poor reasons, which remain part of many grandmothers' understanding of the childbearing continuum. It is often difficult for their daughters to disregard these beliefs without feeling guilty.

A grandmother may see the choice to breastfeed by her daughter as a reflection on her own parenting decisions. Grandparents often sympathize with the strains of early parenting, such as lack of sleep, coping with crying, and physical recovery from birth. They may perceive that breastfeeding increases those strains and may therefore encourage the mother to reduce stress by supplementing breastfeeding or weaning. A mother who receives negative comments from her mother or mother-in-law needs to understand the grandmother's concern for both the mother and baby. She may not want her daughter to experience the same disappointment and failure that she did. On the other hand, she may be envious that her daughter can do something she was not able to do.

You can help the mother recognize that her own mother did the best she could at the time with the information and support that was available to her. She can gently explain that she understands that her mother did her best and that she is now doing the same today for her child with current information. The grandmother may not understand the typical feeding pattern of a breastfed baby. She may worry that his frequent feedings indicate inadequate nourishment. She may not know that loose stools are normal for breastfeeding babies and may worry that her grandchild has diarrhea. Remarking about her concerns can undermine the new mother's confidence and come through as lack of support.

You can encourage the mother to be patient and understanding of any relative, especially a grandparent, whose opposition stems from a genuine concern for her and her baby. She can attempt to educate the grandparents and enlist their support by giving them literature. She can ask the grandmother to accompany her to a breastfeeding support group meeting. At times, a mother may simply need to accept the grandmother's point of view and not allow it to affect her breastfeeding. She will need to stay firm in her resolve while remaining kind and considerate.

Some health and breastfeeding organizations have information geared directly to grandparents (TDH, 2002). You can direct mothers to this literature or develop a small handout with current recommendations that address past beliefs or practices. It may include the following recommendations:

- Babies should be breastfed for at least one year or longer.
- Putting a baby to bed with a bottle is unsafe and causes tooth decay.
- Feeding cereal through the bottle can cause the baby to choke.
- Feeding solid foods to babies before they are four to six months old can cause health problems.
- Placing the baby on his back to sleep helps prevent SIDS.
- Babies should not be exposed to secondhand smoke.

Occasionally, a grandmother may be overly helpful or overly controlling. She may pressure the mother to breastfeed. If you encounter an overbearing grandmother in the hospital, you can encourage nurses to limit visitors. If you are visiting the mother in her home and the grandmother is dominating the conversation, you might ask her to help with the baby or with other children. You may need to simply state that you and the mother need to meet privately. HIPAA does not permit you to discuss the mother's situation with her in front of others unless she gives verbal permission.

Opposition from the Baby's Father

It is especially difficult for a mother to encounter opposition from the baby's father. A father's preference typically is significant in the mother's choice for infant feeding. Thus, his opposition will weigh greatly on her decision to initiate or continue breastfeeding (Kong, 2004; Rose, 2004; Chang, 2003). A father may seem unsupportive of breastfeeding because he wants his child to be independent and worries that breastfeeding will make the baby too dependent on the mother. It can be helpful for him to learn that meeting a child's present needs will actually make him less dependent in the future. Sharing information with the baby's father about the importance of breastfeeding provides a springboard for discussing the mother's need for his support.

If the father believes breastfeeding interferes with the couple's sex life, help him see that having a baby interferes with all parents' sex lives, no matter how they feed their baby! If he seems jealous, you can suggest that the mother plan some special time alone with him. The father's opposition may stem from the same concerns as those of grandparents and other relatives—the health and well-being of his partner and baby. You can point out the positive aspects of this concern and suggest ways for the mother to reassure and educate the father that breastfeeding is beneficial to the entire family and that *not* breastfeeding increases health risks for both the mother and baby.

The mother can point out how breastfeeding enhances their baby's pleasant disposition and contributes to family harmony. The father will recognize the nutritional value of human milk when he sees evidence of health benefits in his baby's growth and development. If he feels left out of his baby's care because he is not able to feed him, the mother can suggest ways for him to be involved other than with feedings. She can remind the father that most babies start solid food at 6 months and he can feed the baby then. See Chapter 19 for more discussion of the father's interactions.

Western culture promotes women's breasts in a sexual manner in all forms of media (Stuart-Mccadam, 1995). As a man's role changes from mate to father, it may be difficult for him to regard his partner's breasts as something other than sexual. The father may subconsciously believe that the baby is invading his territory. The biological purpose of the female breast has always been to nurture babies. Encourage the couple to discuss these issues with sensitivity and understanding.

As the baby grows older, a previously supportive father may question the need or appropriateness of continuing to breastfeed. He may worry about a loss of masculinity due to an overdependence on the mother. The mother can remind the father about the benefits of breastfeeding for their baby at any age, both nutritionally and developmentally. Breastfeeding is dose-dependent, with longer duration providing greater protection against diseases such as diabetes (Sadauskaite-Kuehne, 2004), and promotes higher IQ development (Anderson, 1999).

The mother can help him understand the baby's needs and her desire to continue breastfeeding. Networking with families of older nursing babies and children will enable the father to meet breastfeeding families and find it more acceptable. See Chapter 19 for further discussion of the father's role in supporting breastfeeding.

A mother who cannot resolve the father's opposition to breastfeeding will need a great deal of support and will benefit from frequent contacts. If she decides to wean her baby because of the father's opposition, you need to accept this decision and help her wean gradually and with love. Help the father understand the need for her to wean slowly to avoid mastitis.

Avoid placing yourself in the middle of a conflict between a mother and an unsupportive partner. You can listen, suggest reading material for the father, and offer extra support and encouragement. A referral to a mother-to-mother support group will provide the additional support the mother needs at this time. It is important that you accept the father's position and help the mother cope without judging or becoming involved in any conflicts that arise.

Because of the intimate nature of your role with mothers, you are in a unique position to witness a couple's interaction. If you see bruises or unexplained injuries, suspect domestic violence, or witness the father verbally ridiculing or abusing the mother, you can mention this privately to the mother. Provide her with hotline numbers and local community resources, such as battered women's shelters or safehouses (see the resources in Appendix A). If she denies the situation or makes excuses, you can gently reflect what you see to her and encourage her to talk with her caregiver or a counselor about what is occurring. If you suspect the baby or other children are being abused, you must report it to the appropriate authorities.

Mother's Confidence

Breastfeeding is a confidence game! Maternal confidence is a significant predictor of the duration and level of breastfeeding. A mother who is confident in herself and in her commitment to breastfeed will continue despite setbacks or problems. Likewise, there is a correlation between low parental confidence and a high perception of milk insufficiency (McCarter-Spaulding, 2001). Enhancing a mother's feelings of self-efficacy and increasing her confidence in her ability to breastfeed will help her persevere if she does encounter difficulties (Blythe, 2002).

A mother's self-esteem increases with a positive breastfeeding experience (Locklin, 1993). Prenatal and postnatal care needs to go beyond education to encompass enhancing the mother's confidence regarding breastfeeding (Ertim, 2001). You can build the mother's confidence by pointing out her baby's positive aspects and showing her how well he is growing. Positive feedback helps the mother recognize that she is doing well and validates her choice to breastfeed.

▶ LOW-INCOME MOTHER

The income level of some mothers in your care may be near or below the poverty level. Poverty is often associated with lower self-esteem, limited expectations, and lower educational and occupational levels. Low-income women may live in an area in which many unfavorable conditions exist. They may face the challenge of overcrowding, run-down housing, crime, and inadequate community services. They may experience physical and mental health problems, broken families, relocation problems, isolation, alienation, or language differences.

Low-income women may avoid childbirth classes because of cost, availability, or lack of interest. In one study, attendance at childbirth classes was associated with a 75 percent increase in the odds that a child would be breastfed. It also cited significant sociodemographic disparities in attendance at childbirth classes (Lu, 2003).

The mother may have received prenatal care in one place and delivered her baby in another. She may seek attention for her sick children from a clinic or emergency room and for her well children from a child health station. You can inform her of local health services and suggest that she take advantage of programs that assist low-income populations with supplemental foods. In the United States, the Women, Infants, and Children (WIC) program provides these services. See Chapter 2 for further discussion about the U.S. WIC program and the Canada Prenatal Nutrition Program (CPNP).

Psychosocial Issues

Other barriers can impede a low-income mother's commitment to initiate or continue breastfeeding. She may lack support and accurate information (Rose, 2004). She may face challenges related to survival (England, 2003). Low-income mothers often hold two jobs and have little discretionary time or money. Life can be a series of crises. Statistically, substance abuse and alcoholism are high among this population. One study showed that 25 percent of the at-risk women did not breastfeed or quit breastfeeding because of the fear of passing "dangerous things" to their infants through their milk (England, 2003). In a survey of low-income formula feeders, 84 percent knew that breastmilk was better for their babies but chose not to breastfeed due to concerns about pain, smoking, and work (Noble, 2003).

Family and community support for breastfeeding can be lacking in a low-income community (McIntyre, 2001). Low-income mothers often feel they cannot control their lives and surroundings, and may feel detached from society. A sense of despair or stress can prevail. The mother may feel that her immediate circle of relationships is not comfortable or supportive. She might distrust you because her life is insecure and you represent the "system" that has been unkind to her. She may consider breastfeeding as one more stress in her life and may worry that breastfeeding will be one more failure in her life. She also may be unaware of the many community resources available to low-income women.

The Decision to Breastfeed

Research has shown that a low-income woman is more likely to choose breastfeeding if she has a higher level of education (Sharp, 2003; MacGowan, 1991; Michaelsen, 1994), is married (Sharp, 2003; MacGowan, 1991), or has greater ego maturity and is thus more able to deviate from community norms (Jacobson, 1991). The greatest motivator seems to be a support person she respects who had a positive breastfeeding experience. Access to support and accurate information play vital roles in her breastfeeding experience. Her perception of family and peer support, particularly from another woman with whom she is close, is another factor (Locklin, 1993).

Medical personnel, respected for their expertise, can be instrumental in encouraging low-income women to continue breastfeeding. You can help these women recognize that babies are healthier, and therefore happier, when their mothers breastfeed. Let the mother know that more women breastfeed now, so that she will not feel as different. Praise her for making an intelligent decision based on sound medical fact rather than fads or advertising claims.

Introduction of artificial baby milk, particularly through the hospital, undermines the mother's confidence in her ability to breastfeed (Michaelsen, 1994). She may believe that a substitute is equally good, or perhaps better because it is more "scientific." There may be little family or community support for breastfeeding compared to bottle-feeding. The use of infant formula is implicitly advocated when it is given by postpartum hospital staff in gift packs (Donnelly, 2000). Receiving free formula negatively affects breastfeeding rates (Fooladi, 2001).

Your support during the mother's hospital stay and the first week postpartum can be critical to her breastfeeding. As breastfeeding continues, you can capitalize on the mother's achievements. More than in other populations, a low-income woman may find that breastfeeding builds her self-confidence and self-esteem. Realizing that breastfeeding contributes to her child's well-being and that she accomplished it through her own resources enhances her self-image. This can improve her parenting skills and encourage her to share her success with others. Some women report that childrearing was the experience that enabled them to become active learners, as they became advocates for their children's health.

Peer Support

Several studies show an increase in breastfeeding rates among low-income women when their local healthcare clinics increase breastfeeding support to include classes, one-on-one instruction, and peer counselors. Women who receive community-health intervention breastfeed for a longer time, and their babies have fewer sick visits and less medication (Pugh, 2002). In a **pilot study**, low-income women received visits in the hospital and at home by a community health nurse and peer counselor, followed by telephone support. By five months, women who received intervention had the highest breastfeeding rate. They reported less nipple discomfort in the first month; significantly less fatigue in the fourth month; and less fatigue, depression, and anxiety in the third and fifth months (Pugh, 2001).

Grossman (1988) found that only 17 percent of women who received no extra education or support chose to breastfeed at delivery. Those who received classes, one-on-one education, and peer counselor support chose to breastfeed at a rate of 66 percent at delivery. Peer counselor support has a positive effect on breastfeeding initiation and duration, as does the mother's choice to breastfeed exclusively (Kistin, 1994, 1990). The Rush Mothers' Milk Club, a NICU support group for mothers of preterm infants, has had outstanding success at helping primarily low-income women pump for their preterm babies. Many have gone on to breastfeed directly (Meier, 2004).

Although breastfeeding discussion groups can serve as an effective teaching arena, attendance may be minimal for low-income women. Many women feel overwhelmed with work, child care, and obtaining the necessities of life. Adding a class to the mother's routine may be more than she can handle. Those who are receptive are more likely to attend meetings in surroundings they find comfortable such as a private residence, church, or community center. When participants have a major role in planning and organizing such meetings, they feel part of the process. They can also determine the day, time, and topics that are most relevant to them.

A low-income woman may be very isolated, with no support system and no acquaintances who breastfed. Discussion groups with other mothers who face the same challenges can provide the peer support she needs to succeed and help build trust in your services. In order to make the meetings enjoyable, keep presentations short and to the point. Address issues that are relevant to the mother's needs, using a casual, informal approach that encourages discussion.

Teaching and Support Strategies

When a mother is in crisis, you will need to put aside theoretical and background information for the moment and first concentrate on the problem at hand (Hardy, 1989). Adopt an approach that accounts for unchangeable factors such as personality or the limitations of her lifestyle. Suggestions need to be practical rather than general. Simply advising that she nurse her baby more often will not be as useful as helping her figure out times and ways she can do it. Help her with practical solutions to improve nutrition for herself and her family. Refer her to a local WIC clinic or food bank for nutritious foods to supplement her diet.

A low-income mother's literacy level could impede her ability to absorb information. Offer attractive, simply written brochures with illustrations that cover only the essential points she needs to know. Make sure the reading level of the material is appropriate, being sensitive to visual images and the amount of words on each page. If too many words make a brochure overwhelming, she may not read or absorb the information.

When teaching the mother about breastfeeding techniques, reinforce verbal explanations with visual aids. Provide her with a checklist of the suggestions you discussed as a reminder. If you are assisting her over the telephone, reinforce the basic points of your conversation. Try to get some feedback from the mother to indicate that she has understood your message and will act on your suggestions. Make sure she understands the consequences of her practices, and be patient and persevering in areas of importance. The mother and baby will both benefit from your sincerity and concern.

Make sure women know when you are available and how to contact you. Reach out to them in their neighborhoods through community bulletin boards, clinics, and other public places. If you make home visits, it is important that you be conscious of safety issues. Low-income homes are often in high-risk areas. Plan visits during daylight hours. Leave behind information with a colleague or family member that includes where you will visit, times you expect to arrive and leave, and the route you will take. A map and cellular telephone are essential when visiting a client's home. Recognize that circumstances may make it unsafe for you to visit a mother's home alone. In this case, arrange to have someone accompany you on the visit, or meet with the mother in a different location. Be sensitive and tactful when you discuss these arrangements with the mother to avoid offending her.

▶ SINGLE MOTHER

A mother may have sole responsibility for her baby because of divorce, separation, death of her partner, a choice to remain unmarried, or a situation that requires the baby's father to be away from home for extended periods. The number of single mothers has increased dramatically over the past two decades. In 2003, 34 percent of births in the United States were to unmarried women (NCHS, 2004a). U.S. Census Bureau statistics in 2002 showed that over 4 million mothers were never married and 23 percent of children were living with only their mother.

A single mother may live alone or may reside with her parents or a friend. Each situation presents unique challenges. Over 7.5 million single mothers in the United States maintain a household alone. These women juggle one or more jobs, schooling or training, household responsibilities, and parenting. Work affords opportunities for adult companionship, instills a sense of independence, and furnishes necessary income. Yet, when she returns home from a long day of work, she faces all the other household routines waiting for her.

A mother who lives with her parents can benefit from their support and security. At the same time, she may struggle to maintain her identity as an adult and a mother, and to preserve an identity as a family unit for herself and her baby. It can be difficult for two family units to live harmoniously in the same home. The mother may receive criticism about her parenting, and other family members may discipline her child. Lack of privacy can interfere with her breastfeeding. Many mothers view their return home as a temporary situation until they secure other living arrangements.

When a mother's single status has resulted from divorce or the death of a spouse, emotional stress and other demands of the aftermath may result in missed feedings and lowered milk supply. Her baby may tune in to her emotional state and want to nurse more frequently. Breastfeeding can provide comfort to both the mother and baby in times of stress. Any increase in frequency will help maintain milk production as well.

A single mother will benefit from your support. She may have little or no support system among friends and family, and no one with whom she can share concerns or parenting responsibilities. She may attempt to be a "supermom" in order to meet her baby's needs as well as those of everyday life. This leaves little time for herself. She can meet her own and her baby's needs at the same time by taking a walk with her baby in a backpack or stroller or enrolling in a baby swim class or exercise class with other mothers and babies. Her nutritional status may be compromised because of a lack of desire or time to prepare well-balanced meals for just herself. Single mothers are likely to appreciate your care and concern. They can also contact a local Parents Without Partners or other support group. Many churches have single parent ministries that offer food assistance, free automobile care, parenting classes, and babysitting services.

▶ TEENAGE MOTHER

Globally, teenage birth rates have declined, but U.S. rates exceed those in most developed countries (NCHS, 2001). In 2002, 10 percent of U.S. births were to teens aged 15 to 19 (CDC, 2003). Many pregnant teenagers elect to keep their babies, and about 17 percent go on to have a second child within 3 years (NCHS, 2004b). Some will breastfeed, although rates are lower for teen mothers than adults, partly because of lack of knowledge (Dewan, 2002). Many of the young people becoming parents today lack active guidance from parents and other adults. It is important to understand teen mothers and fathers against this backdrop (Parker, 2000). Figure 20.1 identifies common reasons teens become pregnant.

FIGURE 20.1
Reasons teens become pregnant.

- ◆ It will never happen to me. (denial and invulnerability)
- ◆ Everyone else has a baby. (power, social status, peer pressure)
- ◆ I thought he'd marry me. (seeking permanence)
- ◆ I didn't mean to. (date-rape, substance abuse, impulsivity)
- ◆ I wanted out of the house. (physical, emotional, sexual, substance abuse)
- ◆ It's not fair—I used birth control. (ignorance, inconsistent or improper use)

Source: Denise Parker and Nancy Williams, 2000

Most pregnant teens do not marry the father of their baby. They do not feel pressured socially to have a mate or a father for their babies. They may not complete high school because of the demands on their time, and they may be unable to care for their babies because they lack the skill or income. They often have no job skills and are dependent financially on their families and society. Young mothers wish to be treated as adults and do not respond well to lecturing, advice, or a patronizing manner that suggests an adult-child relationship. They need you to listen to their concerns and respond as you would with an older mother.

Learning how to approach a teen mother sensitively and respectfully will enable you to be a positive influence in her life. You can empower her to form her own individuality, take ownership of her life, and learn to advocate for her baby. Because she is in the process of learning to think abstractly, it is normal for her adolescent focus to be self-centered. Talking to a teen mother about the benefits of breastfeeding for her (or the risks of *not* breastfeeding for her) may carry more weight than a litany of information about the baby's health.

Prenatal Issues

There is a frequent pattern of inadequate prenatal care and poor nutrition among pregnant teens. Some young mothers attempt to hide or deny their pregnancy in the early months. Consequently, they begin prenatal care much later than usual, many times as late as the end of the second trimester. Teens, therefore, have a higher incidence of prematurity, low-birth-weight infants, stillbirths, and neonatal death than do postadolescent mothers (March of Dimes, 2002).

A pregnant teenager may be fearful and unhappy about the physical changes that occur with her body during pregnancy. She may feel apprehensive about the impending labor and delivery. She may be concerned about the reactions of family, friends, teachers, and her baby's father. Depending on the degree of her emotional adjustment to pregnancy, she might doubt her self-worth and have a poor self-image.

Many teenagers have poor eating habits. Pregnant teenagers need to understand the importance of good nutrition to the developing fetus and to the mother's body. Pregnancy compromises the health of a young mother, whose growth needs compete with the growth needs of her baby. She will be reluctant to gain weight and can be encouraged and praised for the weight she gains and its benefit for her baby. She may need to consume more food than older mothers do and will benefit from ongoing individualized advice regarding her diet. The adolescent who recently experienced puberty may require even more calories to support the rapid growth that follows. If she lives with her parents, she may

FIGURE 20.2
How a teen mother's health affects her baby.

◆ Low weight gain increases the risk of having a low weight baby. Low birth weight babies may have undeveloped organs. This can lead to lung problems, respiratory distress syndrome, brain bleeding, vision loss and serious intestinal problems. Low birth weight babies are more than 20 times as likely to die in their first year of life than normal weight babies.

◆ More teens smoke than adults. Smoking doubles a woman's risk of having a low birth weight baby, and also increases the risk of miscarriage, pregnancy complications, premature birth and stillbirth.

◆ Pregnant teens are least likely to get early and regular prenatal care.

◆ A teen mother is at greater risk than women over 20 for pregnancy complications such as premature labor, anemia and high blood pressure.

◆ Three million teens are affected by sexually transmitted diseases (STDs) per year. These include chlamydia (which can cause sterility), syphilis (which can cause blindness and maternal and infant death) and HIV, which may be fatal to both mother and baby.

Source: March of Dimes, *Facts You Should Know About Teenage Pregnancy*, March 2002

have limited influence on meal planning. Nutrition education is a primary achievement for all pregnant teenagers. Figure 20.2 shows how a teen mother's health can affect her baby.

After the Baby Is Born

Adolescent mothers often feel threatened and overwhelmed by the hospital environment and will be reluctant to ask for anything from the nursing staff. Consequently, they may be less likely to arrange for immediate or prolonged contact with their babies following birth. Teens may not understand the importance of early contact for bonding, and are inclined to consider the social aspect of visitors to be more important. Hospital personnel can be sensitive to this and invite interaction between the mother and her baby, rather than relying on the mother to ask that someone bring her baby to her. Childbirth is a time of vulnerability for all new mothers. For a teen mother, whose confidence is very fragile, it may be the first realization of the responsibility ahead of her.

After she is at home with her baby, a young mother may question her adequacy as a parent and have difficulty coping with the daily responsibilities of parenthood. In some cases, her own mother raises the baby, with the baby's mother having little to do with his care. The mother's maturity and attitude are determining factors in how she copes with parenthood and breastfeeding. The less mature teenager may have difficulty devoting love and attention to her baby at a time when her own needs for such nurturing are so great. However, other young mothers are ready to accept the responsibilities of motherhood and respond in much the same way as an older mother.

Some teens are engaged in a power struggle with their mothers over the care of the baby. The teen may want to assert herself as a parent, but her mother may believe she is too young to care for a baby. Providing the teen mother with accurate information on baby care may help the teen allay her mother's misgivings. The teen's mother may feel threatened by her daughter's desire to breastfeed. Perhaps she did not breastfeed her daughter and may worry that her grandchild will not receive proper nutrition. She may worry that her daughter's choice to breastfeed reflects negatively on her own child-rearing techniques (see the discussion on grandparents earlier in this chapter). Some teens breastfeed in order to establish control, seeing breastfeeding as the one thing that only they can do for their baby. They may also breastfeed to limit the biological father's involvement in the baby's care for as long as possible.

Breastfeeding Decision

Not surprisingly, breastfeeding rates among teenage mothers are much lower than among adult mothers. Yet the babies of teens are the ones who most need to receive the health benefits of breastfeeding. Teens tend to deliver earlier, have lower-birth-weight babies, and have more delivery complications. They typically live in less healthful environments, and their children are more at risk for cognitive and behavioral problems (McAnarney, 1993). Breastfeeding and its associated health benefits is especially important to this population.

As with adult mothers who choose not to breastfeed, teens are less likely to be married and more likely to have low educational and income levels. Generally, teens have issues about their sexuality and body image that may interfere with the desire to breastfeed (Peterson, 1992). Older teens who are married and no longer in school during their pregnancy are the most likely to breastfeed (Lizarraga, 1992). Teens who see other women breastfeed and who were breastfed as babies are more inclined to breastfeed (Lefler, 2000). Younger, single teens who are enrolled in school and have little exposure to breastfeeding need the most outreach and encouragement. Studies have found these factors consistently across countries and cultures, including Canadian Native Ojibwas (Martens, 2001), Quebecois (Ross, 2002), Brazilians (Nakamura, 2003), and Nigerians (Ojofeitimi, 2001).

Neifert (1988) looked at the motivating factors for teen mothers who breastfeed. She found that, similar to the adult population, 83 percent of the teens in her study decided whether to breastfeed before the third trimester of pregnancy. This demonstrates the need to reach teens in early pregnancy regarding infant feeding and to capitalize on opportunities to incorporate breastfeeding into school curricula for all students. Neifert found that 65 percent of breastfeeding teen mothers "chose breastfeeding because it was 'good for the baby,' and 67 percent identified the 'closeness' of the nursing relationship as the most enjoyable part of breastfeeding." Obstacles to breastfeeding included concern about modesty and the need to return to school within 2 months postpartum. One prenatal program resulted in 97.6 percent of pregnant teens wanting to breastfeed and 82.8 percent breastfeeding at discharge (Greenwood, 2002). While duration was lower than for older women, there was evidence of improved attitudes and knowledge.

Breastfeeding Management

Teens who encounter difficulties are less likely than adults to overcome them and continue breastfeeding. It was believed in the past that adolescent mothers have difficulty producing sufficient amounts of milk (Stout, 1992). However, the greatest proliferation of mammary ducts occurs during pregnancy, and teens thus have the same potential for milk production as other women do. They may not breastfeed often enough to produce a robust supply. Asking open-ended questions will help a teen mother learn to quantify her breastfeeding pattern. Ask questions such as:

- How many times did your baby breastfeed over the past 24 hours?
- How many minutes did your baby nurse on each side?
- How many times does your baby pee and poop each day?
- How many bottles of formula do you give your baby each day?
- How much formula is in each bottle?

Teens are inclined toward exaggeration. Therefore, when a teen tells you that her baby cries "all day long," help her measure what that means. Help her learn that she can reduce her baby's crying by using a sling or snuggly carrier. Teach her infant feeding cues so she can learn to feed her baby before he starts crying. If she says he "never sleeps," suggest that she keep a notepad handy to record his naps. Whereas this might be tedious for a more mature mother with a better grasp of time, it may help a young mother learn to modulate, analyze, and describe her baby's behaviors more observantly.

Teens may feel overwhelmed by parenting responsibilities and a need for support for breastfeeding among family and friends. They may lack futuristic thinking, failing to anticipate the consequences of their actions and not understanding that a problem can be resolved "in the moment." That said, some teens have an excellent support system and will breastfeed for the same amount of time as the average breastfeeding mother.

Interactions with Teenage Mothers

A teenage mother usually has a great need for a one-to-one relationship with someone who cares about her and understands her needs. She wants consistency and personal involvement in this relationship. It is important to get to know her as an individual and not just as the baby's mother. An adolescent mother needs a trusting relationship with her mother, grandmother, partner, or pregnancy coordinator (Dykes, 2003). Ask her about herself—how she is adjusting, how the birth went, how she feels, and what her needs are. Demonstrating interest in her as a person will help build rapport and develop trust in the relationship. Help her see how she will benefit from breastfeeding her baby.

Classroom Teaching

Interaction with teens often takes place in a class setting. To meet their needs effectively, find out what the teens already know about breastfeeding and what they would like to learn. This can be a challenge, because teen mothers will often not volunteer information and may not ask questions, fearing peer ridicule. Asking teens to write out their questions or concerns anonymously encourages them to think about the situation and protects their privacy.

Because teens may not attend every educational offering or appointment, you will need to cover breastfeeding basics whenever possible. New information needs to be in simple, clear terms that do not overwhelm them. After 15 minutes of new information, teens typically lose interest, so you need to make the time together both humorous and informative. Allow for nonthreatening participation, and plan meaningful interaction. To demonstrate the importance of positioning the baby, for example, teens can be asked to swallow some water looking straight ahead and then to repeat it turning their head to the side. This demonstrates how difficult it is for a baby to swallow if he must turn his head to latch on. A doll will help you demonstrate how to hold their baby. A golf ball can illustrate the size of a newborn's stomach. Use audiovisual aids and handouts that depict other teens, rather than adults, in breastfeeding and parenting situations. When teaching teens in a group setting, make yourself available for individual time.

Encourage teens to bring family or friends with them to classes to help build a support system. Giving information to friends and family about breastfeeding can help them learn how to support the mother. Recognize that the teen may not have help or support for breastfeeding at home. Her mother may not have breastfed, and her peers are much less likely to have breastfed. Interactions between the teen and her mother may or may not be positive. She may be in disfavor with her family because of her pregnancy. Her mother also may have unresolved issues about her own breastfeeding experience or lack of it. Convey your support to the teen and be accepting of her situation.

Become familiar with organizations that assist teen mothers. Agencies that reach out to teenage mothers in the United States include WIC, the March of Dimes, and the United States Government Department of Health and Human Services (DHHS). See Appendix A for source information for these organizations.

▶ Mothers with Cultural Differences

Families who leave their native country have several characteristics in common when they work toward becoming part of a new culture. They share a sense of loss of their own culture, an environment in which they developed a set of beliefs and attitudes that are central to their lives. A person's degree of **acculturation** (integration into a new culture) depends on how firmly they cling to traditional values. Members of succeeding generations replace old values with new ones as cultural differences become more diffuse.

Other factors that influence behavior are age, educational and social exposure, the intent to return to their country of origin, economic status, contact with older relatives, and the part of the country in which they reside. The lower classes tend to hold onto traditional values, whereas the middle and upper classes generally incorporate new practices into their value system. Practically speaking, this means that women from other cultures exhibit a wide range of value systems, family support, and interest in breastfeeding.

Family Dynamics

In many Western cultures, the individual is the basic social entity and the building block of all social relations and institutions. In other cultures, the family is the dominant unit, and decision making is the responsibility of the family rather than the individual member. Decisions may be the responsibility of the eldest male or other male figure in the family group. Extended family often provides a support system for raising children. In order to counsel effectively, you must take care not to interfere with support from family and peers. Instead, you can strengthen family support by providing clear, accurate information in a climate of acceptance. A woman's cultural beliefs are more important to her than you are.

Health and Illness Behaviors

Cultural beliefs may create health and illness behaviors that vary significantly from your own. Understanding these differences will avoid alienating a mother with recommendations that are irrelevant or ignored. A mother's culture affects the way she regards health and the measures she will take to prevent or treat illness. She may place considerable reliance on cultural patterns as a method of coping. Cultural and religious practices can be therapeutic and foster social support from her community. In order to counsel a woman from another culture effectively, you will need to understand her values and cultural practices and learn how they can influence her breastfeeding.

Cultural Beliefs Regarding Breastfeeding

Your approach in helping these mothers will need to be flexible. Learn about their beliefs and adapt your suggestions to meet their needs. Inappropriate advice can upset or confuse a mother and cause friction with other family members. You risk losing credibility and rapport with the mother if you discredit beliefs she has held her entire life. Do not try to change culturally based practices unless they are detrimental to her health or the baby's health.

Each mother's cultural heritage and economic standing will have a direct bearing on how long she breastfeeds and her ability to deal with reactions from her partner, family, or friends. Values and priorities will vary greatly among women of different cultural backgrounds. Some regard healthcare providers and the scientific community with great respect. Others place more faith in self-care or folk medicine. Some cultures regard colostrum as valueless or undesirable and do not encourage breastfeeding until the second or third postpartum day. You can inform these mothers about the medical value of colostrum, realizing at the same time that their cultural beliefs may predominate.

You can seek ways to work around culturally based practices so they benefit rather than harm breastfeeding. For example, some women of Mexican heritage who work outside in the heat believe their milk will spoil in their breasts during the day, and so they wean before returning to work. One caregiver used this belief as a motivating factor to continue to breastfeed by instructing the women to express out the "bad" milk and throw it away, and then to nurse their babies when they returned home. The mothers were able to continue breastfeeding, with formula supplements given to the babies during the daytime, similar to the way some other working mothers manage breastfeeding.

Some cultures discourage new mothers from consuming cold foods and beverages for several weeks or months. Hot teas and soups will help these mothers meet their fluid requirements. Some cultural beliefs place limitations on activity for the postpartum mother that an uninformed caregiver may interpret as a lack of compliance. By recognizing this, you can encourage the involvement of extended family in the mother's care. Cultural restrictions may carry over to how others relate to the baby as well. Certain ways of touching the baby or referring to the baby may be taboo. Always ask permission when you wish to touch the baby. Gentle, honest inquiries about the mother's customs will help you learn appropriate responses.

Language and Communication

Cultural barriers may seem greater when accompanied by a language difference. A sensitive understanding of the woman's culture and language is essential to establishing effective communication. Speak slowly and clearly, and provide simple explanations. Maximizing communication is especially important if the mother has a breastfeeding problem she needs to discuss. A woman with a limited understanding of English can usually converse well enough about breastfeeding in general. When she has a specific problem, however, she may need to converse in her native language in order to be understood and to comprehend your advice.

Bilingual Aids

If you are not bilingual, you can learn common phrases used in breastfeeding in the languages used by mothers in your community (see the Spanish glossary in Appendix J). Many communities offer classes in conversational medical terminology, called *meducation*. It would be helpful to have the services of a colleague who can speak comfortably in a second language. If you practice in a hospital, a translator should be on staff. Spanish is the second most common language in the United States, and French is the second most common language in Canada.

If there is no one available in your practice who speaks the language of a particular mother, you can ask her if she has a bilingual friend or relative who can assist. You can also contact a local high school or university to request a volunteer to serve as interpreter. It is important that the interpreter be another woman, because the mother may be reluctant to share intimate information with a male other than her partner. Try to ensure that the interpreter is communicating accurately and not adding opinions or values that differ from what you are attempting to convey to the mother.

Women who have difficulty reading English cannot take advantage of lengthy books on breastfeeding. Brief pamphlets with simple themes and illustrations written at an appropriate reading level can help these mothers. You might also arrange to have some of your literature translated so that the mothers can benefit even more. Demonstrations with visual aids and the use of flash cards with translations may be helpful. Bilingual teaching aids are available through La Leche League International and other sources (see Appendix A). Local social services and library materials may be useful as well.

Body Language and Customs

Because body language is an important communication tool, personal contact is preferable to telephone contact. Be alert to differences in body language. In some cultures, nodding and smiling do not denote understanding as they do in Western society. You cannot assume that a mother comprehends what you are saying because of these gestures. Watch for nonverbal cues and messages through facial and body expressions. A nod of the head accompanied by a bland or puzzled look can imply confusion. To ensure that a woman understands your instructions, you can ask her to repeat them. You can also demonstrate a technique and summarize the important points at the end of your conversation. Use of listening skills is critical in determining motivation to breastfeed and cultural factors that may be involved.

Visiting a woman in her home will help you obtain a more complete picture of her physical and emotional environment. Families may be reluctant to invite strangers into their homes or may feel embarrassed by their living arrangements. They may respond to a friendly and sincere interest in their welfare. Learn cultural customs of greeting and inclusion of others before you make this visit. Become familiar with the cultural practices of the ethnic groups in your community. For example, it is customary to remove one's shoes upon entering the home in many Asian countries. Americans tend to be very businesslike and customarily do not accept offers of tea and food on a home visit, considering it a professional call. However, offers of tea or food are important rituals in some cultures, and it can be considered rude to refuse.

Taking cues from your clients will help you respond appropriately and show your interest and respect for the woman and her culture. If you are unsure about the etiquette in a particular situation, ask your client what the correct practice is. Most immigrants are pleased to share their customs. Remember that the Western way is not the best or only way. Most other countries and cultures have higher breastfeeding rates than the United States. Western culture has much to learn. Open yourself up to learn the ideas and choices that work in other places.

Promoting Breastfeeding to Women of Other Cultures

In addition to learning to function within a woman's culture, you may face the challenge of promoting breastfeeding among an ethnic group that favors formula feeding. A woman from that culture who breastfed her own baby can help your promotion efforts. She can help you learn beliefs and child-rearing practices that are predominant in her culture. She can also help you understand the most effective measures for supporting and educating mothers.

One study found that Hispanic women intending to breastfeed in the United States had more education, were bilingual, had been born and educated in one country, and had received prenatal care. Single women with less education and no prenatal care were less likely to breastfeed. Multiparous women born in Mexico, primiparous women educated in Mexico were more likely to intend to breastfeed (Byrd, 2001). Another survey reported that Hispanic women who intended to breastfeed felt supported by significant people in their lives (Libbus, 2000).

Among mothers immigrating to the United States, breastfeeding rates and duration decrease for children who are U.S.-born (Ghaemi-Ahmadi, 1992). This decrease inversely correlates with the mother's need to return to work or school and the availability of free infant formula. Breastfeeding education needs to address the feasibility and practicality of breastfeeding when the mother works or attends school.

James (1994) noted a correlation between free formula and decreased breastfeeding rates among women living in the United States who were originally from other countries. Receiving free formula samples in the hospital undermines a mother's confidence in her ability to produce milk. It sends a message that her caregivers do not take her decision to breastfeed seriously and implies that formula feeding is the "American" way (Donnelly, 2000). Another study found that immigrant mothers were more likely to experience hospital practices detrimental to breastfeeding than non-immigrant mothers were. However, they were more likely to receive professional breastfeeding support in the community (Loiselle, 2001). This underscores the importance of connecting mothers to strong community resources.

A mother who wishes to acculturate in her new home country may believe that formula feeding is one way to achieve it. Family support for breastfeeding is an integral part of breastfeeding education. In the absence of an extended family, a mother tends to rely heavily on the father's infant feeding preference. Prenatal education should actively seek to include the father and members of the extended family.

Women generally wish to do what is best for their babies and will be more likely to follow your suggestions

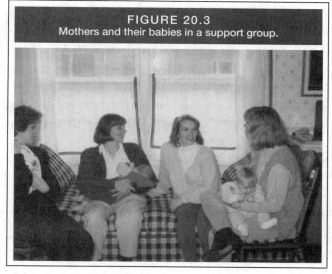

FIGURE 20.3
Mothers and their babies in a support group.

Printed by permission of La Leche League International Schaumburg, Illinois.

when they fully understand the reasons behind your advice. While learning about a woman's culture and her unique beliefs, you may become more attuned to your own beliefs. You need to leave your beliefs and assumptions behind when counseling women from cultures different than your own. Intercultural experiences provide an opportunity for personal growth by enabling you to view yourself and others more objectively.

▶ MOTHER-TO-MOTHER SUPPORT GROUPS

As breastfeeding rates continue to rise, a majority of babies leave the hospital being breastfed, either partially or exclusively. However, many of these mothers fail to continue because they lack the necessary support and information. Mother-to-mother support groups provide support through written materials, counseling services, regular discussion groups, and special programs (Figure 20.3). It is important to become aware of and involved in all lactation services and support available within your community.

Support groups reinforce women's traditional patterns of seeking and receiving advice from relatives and friends. A mother can seek help at any time, day or night, and help usually is available in her own community. Experienced mothers lead discussion groups and offer support to new mothers, helping them gain a feeling of self-reliance and reassurance. Starting a mother-to-mother support group can provide a needed service to women in your community and further the promotion of breastfeeding. See the discussion in Chapter 2 regarding your relationship to mother-to-mother support groups.

The goal of a mother-to-mother support group is to educate women about options and to help them make informed choices. The group should accommodate the style and needs of the women and the community it serves. Contact between a counselor and mother is encouraged from the baby's birth through weaning. These groups usually emphasize exclusive breastfeeding for at least six months, baby-led weaning, and limited separation of mother and baby. Helping mothers manage breastfeeding and working, supporting early weaning, and other variations in breastfeeding styles that require compromises will reflect the group's flexibility and acceptance.

The positive working relationship you develop with peer counselors, the mothers they counsel, and their caregivers will be essential to meeting women's needs. Be careful not to place yourself, counselors, or mothers in opposition to other members of the medical community. This will discourage healthcare providers from referring mothers to you and will diminish your credibility in the community. Open communication and cooperation between the medical community and other breastfeeding counselors is essential, with the mother making decisions based on information from both.

Outreach Counseling

A mother-to-mother support group provides anticipatory guidance to help mothers learn what to expect, avoid potential problems, and resolve issues before they become obstacles. Inviting women to group meetings and contacting them by telephone are effective forms of outreach. Other ways to actively reach out to women include speaking at childbirth classes and clinics, sharing information with professionals, and visiting high school health classes.

Regular meetings for breastfeeding mothers in the community provide a valuable counseling opportunity. Meeting formats should encourage friendly and informal discussion and provide a supportive environment for a mother who lacks contact with other breastfeeding women. The primary factors influencing meetings should be the needs of the women who will be attending. The goal should be to involve mothers as much as possible and help them feel comfortable in taking part, with questions, demonstrations, small group discussions, and book reviews.

If a support group is not available in your community, you can provide ongoing support and appropriate written materials. In the absence of community support, it is especially important that you provide follow-up to mothers after hospital discharge and after they have experienced a difficulty. You might also help develop a mother-to-mother support group, train group leaders, or be available as a resource to the group.

▶ SUMMARY

You can provide valuable support and guidance to mothers navigating through special circumstances. When a mother experiences opposition to her choice to breastfeed, she will greatly value a listening ear, praise, and practical suggestions, particularly if the opposition is from someone close to her. You can also be a valuable resource to a mother who is experiencing challenges such as low income, single parenthood, or teen parenthood. Such mothers often bear burdens that go well beyond the scope of breastfeeding. They benefit from thoughtful suggestions and referrals tailored to their special needs. A mother whose culture or nationality differs from your own will need you to remain open and flexible so that you can gauge suggestions accordingly. Mother-to-mother support groups provide valuable support to mothers and will benefit from your support as well.

▶ CHAPTER 20 — AT A GLANCE

Applying what you learned—

Counseling the mother:

- Help her cope with opposition to breastfeeding.
- Educate an unsupportive father about health risks associated with not breastfeeding.
- Avoid placing yourself in the middle of conflicts with an unsupportive family member.
- Build the mother's confidence with positive feedback.
- Adapt your counseling to each woman's income level, educational level, lifestyle, and support system.
- Give practical suggestions rather than general advice.
- Use visual aids to reinforce verbal explanations.
- Provide reading materials at an appropriate literacy level.
- Reach out to mothers in their own neighborhoods.
- Help mothers access supplemental food programs.
- Recognize the needs of single mothers.
- Refer women to a breastfeeding support group.

Recognize special needs of a teenage mother:

- Need for sound prenatal care and nutrition.
- Ability to feel adequate as a parent.
- May be engaged in a power struggle with her mother.
- Tendency not to breastfeed often enough to produce a robust supply of milk.
- Need for a one-to-one relationship.
- Need to be treated as an adult.

- Need for concrete suggestions and simple, clear information.

Tailor counseling and expectations to cultural differences:

- Accept health and illness behaviors that do not compromise breastfeeding.
- Ask permission before touching the mother or baby.
- Learn customs and body language to help you respond appropriately.
- Learn phrases in common languages within your community.
- Teach with visual aids and return demonstrations.
- Enlist help from other women in the culture to promote breastfeeding.

▶ REFERENCES

American Academy of Pediatrics (AAP). Policy Statement on Breastfeeding and the Use of Human Milk. *Pediatrics* 115(2):496–506; 2005.

American Association of Health Plans (AAHP). Health Plans' Innovative Programs in Breastfeeding Promotion. August 2001. Available at: www.aahp.org. Accessed December 8, 2003.

Anderson J et al. Breast-feeding and cognitive development: A meta-analysis. *Am J Clin Nutr* 70(4):525–535; 1999.

Blythe R et al. Effect of maternal confidence on breastfeeding duration: An application of breastfeeding self-efficacy theory. *Birth* 29(4):278–284; 2002.

Bridges C et al. Employer attitudes toward breastfeeding in the workplace. *J Hum Lact* 13:215–219; 1997.

Byrd T et al. Acculturation and breast-feeding intention and practice in Hispanic women on the US-Mexico border. *Ethn Dis* 11(1):72–79; 2001.

Centers for Disease Control (CDC). Births: Final data for 2002. *National Vital Statistics Report* 52(10); 2003.

Chang JH, Chan WT. Analysis of factors associated with initiation and duration of breast-feeding: A study in Taitung Taiwan. *Acta Paediatr Taiwan* 44(1):29–34; 2003.

Cohen R et al. Comparison of maternal absenteeism and infant illness rates among breast-feeding and formula-feeding women in two corporations. *Am J Health Promot* 10(2):148–153; 1995.

Dewan N et al. Breast-feeding knowledge and attitudes of teenage mothers in Liverpool. *J Hum Nutr Diet* 15(1):33–37; 2002.

Donnelly A et al. Commercial hospital discharge packs for breastfeeding women. *Cochrane Database Syst Rev* (2):CD002075; 2000.

Dunn B et al. Breastfeeding practices in Colorado businesses. *J Hum Lact* 20(2):170–177; 2004.

Dykes F et al. Adolescent mothers and breastfeeding: Experiences and support needs: An exploratory study. *J Hum Lact* 19(4):391–401; 2003.

Ekstrom A et al. Breastfeeding support from partners and grandmothers: Perceptions of Swedish women. *Birth* 30(4): 261–266; 2003.

England L et al. Breastfeeding practices in a cohort of inner-city women: The role of contraindications. *BMC Public Health* 3(1):28; 2003.

Ertim I et al. The timing and predictors of the early termination of breastfeeding. *Pediatrics* 107(3):543–548; 2001.

Fooladi M. A comparison of perspectives on breastfeeding between two generations of Black American women. *J Am Acad Nurse Pract* 13(1):34–38; 2001.

Ghaemi-Ahmadi S. Attitudes toward breastfeeding and infant feeding among Iranian, Afghan, and Southeast Asian immigrant women in the United States: Implications for health and nutrition education. *J Am Diet Assoc* 92:354–355; 1992.

Greenwood K, Littlejohn P. Breastfeeding intentions and outcomes of adolescent mothers in the Starting Out program. *Breastfeed Rev* 10(3):19–23; 2002.

Grossman L et al. Prenatal interventions increase breastfeeding among low-income women. *Am J Dis Child* 142:404; 1988.

Hardy J, Streett R. Family support and parenting education in the home: An effective extension of clinic-based preventive health care services for poor children. *J Pediatr* 115:927–931; 1989.

Jacobson S et al. Incidence and correlates of breastfeeding in socioeconomically disadvantaged women. *Pediatr* 88:728–736; 1991.

James D et al. Factors associated with breastfeeding prevalence and duration among international students. *J Am Diet Assoc* 94:194–196; 1994.

Kistin N et al. Breastfeeding rates among Black urban low-income women: Effect of prenatal education. *Pediatr* 86: 741–746; 1990.

Kistin N et al. Effect of peer counselors on breastfeeding initiation, exclusivity and duration among low-income urban women. *J Hum Lact* 10:11–15; 1994.

Kong S, Lee D. Factors influencing decision to breastfeed. *J Adv Nurs* 46(4):369–379; 2004.

Lefler D. U.S. high school age girls may be receptive to breastfeeding promotion. *J Hum Lact* 16(1):36–40; 2000.

Libbus M. Breastfeeding attitudes in a sample of Spanish-speaking Hispanic American women. *J Hum Lact* 16(3):216–220; 2000.

Lizarraga J et al. Psychosocial and economic factors associated with infant feeding intentions of adolescent mothers. *J Adolesc Health* 13:676–681; 1992.

Locklin M, Naber S. Does breastfeeding empower women? Insights from a select group of educated, low-income, minority women. *Birth* 20:30–35; 1993.

Loiselle C. Impressions of breastfeeding information and support among first-time mothers within a multiethnic community. *Can J Nurs Res* 33(3):31–46; 2001.

Lu M et al. Childbirth education classes: Sociodemographic disparities in attendance and the association of attendance with breastfeeding initiation. *Matern Child Health J* 7(2):87–93; 2003.

Luddington-Hoe S et al. Breastfeeding in African-American women. *J Natl Black Nurses Assoc* 13(1):56–64; 2002.

MacGowan R et al. Breastfeeding among women attending Women, Infants, and Children clinics in Georgia, 1987. *Pediatrics* 87:361–366; 1991.

March of Dimes National Foundation. *Facts You Should Know about Teen Pregnancy.* White Plains, NY: March of Dimes; 2002.

Martens P. The effect of breastfeeding education on adolescent beliefs and attitudes: A randomized school intervention in the Canadian Ojibwa community of Sagkeeng. *J Hum Lact* 17(3):245–255; 2001.

McAnarney E, Lawrence R. Day care and teenage mothers: Nurturing the mother-child dyad. *Pediatrics* 91:202–205; 1993.

McCarter-Spaulding D, Kearney M. Parenting self-efficacy and perception of insufficient breast milk. *JOGNN* 30(5):515–522; 2001.

McIntyre E et al. Attitudes towards infant feeding among adults in a low socioeconomic community: What social support is there for breastfeeding? *Breastfeed Rev* 9(1):13–24; 2001.

Meier P et al. The Rush Mothers' Milk Club: Breastfeeding interventions for mothers with very-low-birth-weight infants. *JOGNN* 33(2):164–174; 2004.

Michaelsen K et al. The Copenhagen cohort study on infant nutrition and growth: Duration of breastfeeding and influencing factors. *Acta Paediatr* 83:565–571; 1994.

Nakamura S et al. School girls' perception and knowledge about breastfeeding (Portuguese). *J Pediatr (Rio J)* 79(2): 181–188; 2003.

National Center for Health Statistics (NCHS). Births to teenagers in the United States, 1940–2000. NVSR; Hyattsville, MD: NCHS; September 25, 2001.

National Center for Health Statistics (NCHS). *Births: Preliminary Data for 2003.* NVSR 53:9, Hyattsville, MD: NCHS; 2004a.

National Center for Health Statistics (NCHS). *Trends in Characteristics of Births by State: US 1990, 1995 & 2000–2002.* NVSR 52:29, Hyattsville, MD: NCHS; 2004b.

Neifert M et al. Factors influencing breastfeeding among adolescents. *J Adolesc Health Care* 9:470–473; 1988.

Newman J, Pitman T. *The Ultimate Breastfeeding Book of Answers.* Roseville, CA: Prima; 2000.

Noble L et al. Factors influencing initiation of breast-feeding among urban women. *Am J Perinatol* 20(8):477–483; 2003.

Ojofeitimi E et al. Promotion of exclusive breastfeeding (EBF): The need to focus on the adolescents. *Nutr Health* 15(1): 55–62; 2001.

Parker D, Williams N. *Lactation Consultant Series Two: Teens and Breastfeeding.* Schaumburg, IL: La Leche League International; 2000.

Peterson C, DaVanzo J. Why are teenagers in the United States less likely to breastfeed than older women? *Demography* 29: 431–450; 1992.

Pryor G. *Nursing Mother, Working Mother.* Schaumburg, IL: La Leche League International; 1999.

Pugh L et al. The breastfeeding support team for low-income, predominantly-minority women: A pilot intervention study. *Health Care Women Int* 22(5):501–515; 2001.

Pugh L et al. Breastfeeding duration, costs, and benefits of a support program for low-income breastfeeding women. *Birth* 29(2):95–100; 2002.

Rose V et al. Factors influencing infant feeding method in an urban community. *J Natl Med Assoc* 96(3):325–331; 2004.

Ross L, Goulet C. Attitudes and subjective norms of Quebecian adolescent mothers towards breastfeeding (French). *Can J Public Health* 93(3):198–202; 2002.

Sadauskaite-Kuehne V et al. Longer breastfeeding is an independent protective factor against development of type 1 diabetes mellitus in childhood. *Diabetes Metab Res Rev* 20(2): 150–157; 2004.

Sharp P et al. Health beliefs and parenting attitudes influence breastfeeding patterns among low-income African-American women. *J Perinatol* 23(5):414–419; 2003.

Sikorski J et al. Support for breastfeeding mothers: A systematic review. *Paediatr Perinat Epidemiol* 17(4):407–417; 2003.

Stout R. Composition of milk in adolescents. *J Adolesc Health* 13:261; 1992.

Stuart-Mccadam P, Dettwyler K. *Breastfeeding: Biocultural Perspectives.* New York: Aldine de Gruyter; 1995.

Taylor J, Cabral H. Are women with an unintended pregnancy less likely to breastfeed? *J Fam Pract* 51(5):431–436; 2002.

Texas Department of Health (TDH), Bureau of Nutrition Services. *Just for Grandparents.* #13-06-11288; 2002.

U.S. Census Bureau. Available at: www.census.gov. Accessed June 23, 2004.

World Health Organization. *Protecting, Promoting, and Supporting Breastfeeding: A Joint WHO/UNICEF Statement.* Geneva: WHO; 1989.

▶ **BIBLIOGRAPHY**

Abramson R. Cultural sensitivity in the promotion of breastfeeding. *NAACOG's Clin Issues* 3(4):717–722; 1992.

Bocar D. Combining breastfeeding and employment: Increasing success. *J Perinat Neonat Nurs* 11:23–42; 1997.

Brent N et al. Breast feeding in a low-income population. *Arch Pediatr Adolesc Med* 149:798–803; 1995.

Bryant CA, Coreil J, D'Angelo SL, Bailey DFC, Lazarov M. A strategy for promoting breastfeeding among economically disadvantaged women and adolescents. *NAACOG's Clin Issues* 3:723–730; 1992.

Buckner E, Matsubara M. Support network utilization by breastfeeding mothers. *J Hum Lact* 9:231–235; 1993.

Clark AL (ed.). *Culture and Childbearing.* Philadelphia, PA: FA Davis; 1981.

Corbett-Dick P, Bezek S. Breastfeeding promotion for the unemployed mother. *J Pediatr Health Care* 11:12–19; 1997.

D'Avanzo C. Bridging the cultural gap with Southeast Asians. *MCN* 17:204–208, 1992.

Editorial. A warm chain for breastfeeding. *Lancet* 344: 1239–1241; 1994.

Ellis J. Southeast Asian refugees and maternity care: The Oakland experience. *Birth* 9(3):191–194; 1982.

Faught P. Special people, special needs: The adolescent challenge. *Int J Childbirth Ed* 10:15–17; 1995.

Gunnlaugsson G, Einarsdottir J. Colostrum and ideas about bad milk: A case study from Guinea-Bissau. *Soc Sci Med* 36:283–288; 1993.

Hoddinott P, Pill R. Qualitative study of decisions about infant feeding among women in east end of London. *Br Med J* 318:30–34; 1999.

Humphreys A et al. Intention to breastfeed in low-income pregnant women: The role of social support and previous experience. *Birth* 25:169–174; 1998.

Ibrahim M et al. Breastfeeding and the dietary habits of children in rural Somalia. *Acta Paediatr* 81:480–483; 1992.

Julion B. Letter. *J Nurse Midwife* 38:179–180; 1993.

Kanashiro H et al. Consumption of food and nutrients by infants in Huascar (Lima), Peru. *Am J Clin Nutr* 52:995–1004; 1990.

Kannan S et al. Cultural influence on infant feeding beliefs of mothers. *J Am Diet Assoc* 99:88–90; 1999.

Kavanaugh KH, Kennedy P. *Promoting Cultural Diversity: Strategies for Health Care Professionals.* Thousand Oaks, CA: Sage; 1992.

Kendall-Tackett K. Breastfeeding and the sexual abuse survivor. *J Hum Lact* 14:125–133; 1998.

Kyenkya-Isabirye M, Magalheas R. The mothers' support group role in the health care system. *Int J Gynecol Obstet* 31 (Suppl 1):85–90; 1990.

Levitt M et al. Social support and relationship change after childbirth: An expectancy model. *Health Care Women Int* 14: 503–512; 1993.

Locklin M. Telling the world: Low income women and their breastfeeding experiences. *J Hum Lact* 11:285–291; 1995.

Lynch EW, Hansen MJ. *Developing Cross-Cultural Competence.* Baltimore, MD: Paul H Brookes; 1992.

McNatt M, Freston M. Social support and lactation outcomes in postpartum women. *J Hum Lact* 8:73–77; 1992.

Morse J et al. Initiating breastfeeding: A world survey of the timing of postpartum breastfeeding. *Int J Nurs Stud* 27:303–313; 1990.

Motil K et al. Lactational performance of adolescent mothers shows preliminary differences from that of adult women. *J Adolesc Health* 20:442–449; 1997.

Naeye PIL. Teenaged and pre-teenaged pregnancies: Consequences of the fetal-maternal competition for nutrients. *Pediatrics* 67(1):146–150; 1981.

Riordan J. *Breastfeeding and Human Lactation*. Sudbury, MA: Jones and Bartlett; 2004.

Romero GE, Carias L. Breastfeeding intentions and practices among Hispanic mothers in southern California. *Pediatrics* 84:626–632; 1989.

Romero GE. Breastfeeding pattern among Indochinese immigrants in Northern California. *Am J Dis Child* 143:804–808; 1989.

Sciacca J et al. Influences on breast-feeding by lower income women: An incentive based partner-supported educational program. *J Am Diet Assoc* 95:323–328; 1995.

Serdula M et al. Correlates of breastfeeding in a low-income population of whites, Blacks and Southeast Asians. *J Am Diet Assoc* 91:41–45; 1991.

Spector R. *Cultural Diversity in Health and Illness*. Stamford, CT: Appleton and Lange; 1996.

Thomas RG, Tumminia PA. Maternity care for Vietnamese in America. *Birth* 9(3):187–190; 1982.

Tyler VL. *Intercultural Interacting*. Provo, UT: Brigham Young University Publications; 1987.

Waxler-Morrison et al. *Cross-Cultural Caring: A Handbook for Health Professionals*. Vancouver, BC: UBC Press; 1990.

Williams E, Pan E. Breastfeeding initiation among a low-income multiethnic population in Northern California: An exploratory study. *J Hum Lact* 10:245–251; 1994.

CHAPTER
21

BREASTFEEDING TECHNIQUES AND DEVICES

The United States and other developed countries seem to be fascinated with gadgets and gizmos. Breastfeeding is no exception, with a variety of devices intended to facilitate feedings. In such a climate, it is important for caregivers and parents alike to ask themselves what a woman truly needs in order to breastfeed. Moreover, what do parents truly need in order to care for an infant? Advertisements for baby care items often focus on separation of the mother and baby and seem to imply that separation is the desired norm. This trend is evident in breastfeeding devices as well, with use of a breast pump often reflecting an assumption that the mother and baby will be apart. Suggesting appropriate and conservative uses of breastfeeding devices will increase your effectiveness with mothers. Overuse of devices can overwhelm a new mother and make breastfeeding seem like a lot of work. Teaching them techniques to assist with feedings will help them become self-sufficient.

KEY TERMS

alternate feeding method
breast massage
breast pump
breast shells
C-hold
cup feeding
Dancer hand position
digital techniques
disorganized suck
drip milk
dysfunctional suck
flat nipple
HMBANA
Holder pasteurization
human milk bank
hydrogel dressing
inverted nipple

inverted syringe
manual expression
nipple shield
nursing supplementer
olfactory senses
oral aversion
paced feeding
pacifiers
paladai
pinch test
pooled milk
reverse pressure softening
spoon feeding
suck reorganization
tube feeding
uncoordinated suck
universal precautions

BREASTFEEDING TECHNIQUES

Some simple techniques are helpful to women prenatally and in the early weeks of breastfeeding. Performing a pinch test, for instance, will help the mother determine whether her nipple will evert for feedings. Learning how to massage her breasts will help her with early feedings and facilitate removing milk from her breasts through pumping or hand expression. Supporting her breast during feedings can help the baby maintain a good latch during the early days of nursing.

Pinch Test

The pinch test can be used prenatally to assess a mother's nipples for protrusion. When a mother learns she has retracted or inverted nipples near the end of her pregnancy, she can begin manipulating her nipples to help increase protraction. Figure 21.1 shows a mother's breast before performing the pinch test. To test the protractility of the nipple, the mother grasps the base of the nipple with her forefinger and thumb, as in Figure 21.2. She then presses the thumb and forefinger together several times around the base.

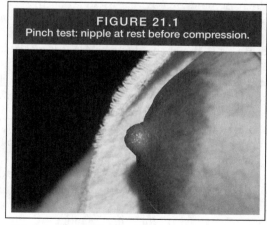

FIGURE 21.1
Pinch test: nipple at rest before compression.

Printed with permission of Kay Hoover.

411

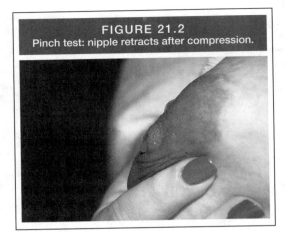

FIGURE 21.2
Pinch test: nipple retracts after compression.

Printed with permission of Kay Hoover.

If the nipple moves forward, it is a normal, protracting nipple and needs no special intervention. A retracting nipple moves inward rather than outward, as depicted in Figure 21.2. It may benefit from the use of a nipple eversion device or a breast pump after the baby is born. A nipple may appear inverted on visual inspection and then evert when pinched. Although this type of nipple may need shaping before latching the baby on, it will most likely not interfere with breastfeeding. A completely inverted nipple appears inverted on visual inspection and does not respond to stimulation. This type of nipple may improve with manipulation. See Chapter 7 for a discussion on differences in nipples.

Breast Massage

Breast massage, or breast compression, can be helpful at various times and for a variety of reasons. Any form of massage encourages the mother to relax. Because touch causes myoepithelial cells to contract, breast massage helps stimulate letdown. During breast massage, oxytocin levels increase, and they remain high while the massage continues (Yokoyama, 1994). Working in combination with oxytocin and the myoepithelial cells, massage helps "push" the milk down the ducts where it is available for the baby to remove or for the mother to express. Squeezing increases positive pressure inside the breast, facilitating the movement of milk from an area of high pressure to an area of low pressure (the baby's mouth).

A mother will often instinctively shape her breast, provide support, and massage her breast while nursing the baby. You can point out these behaviors and praise her for instinctively knowing what to do. Affirming her intuitive behavior helps build her confidence in herself and in her body. Breast massage can be especially useful to mothers who are relactating or initiating lactation to nurse an adopted baby. The mother can massage her breasts just before a feeding, hand expression, or pumping in order to stimulate letdown. She can combine it with relaxation techniques such as deep breathing and visualization.

For a baby who seems impatient for milk to flow, the mother can massage to enhance letdown before putting her baby to breast. Performing massage before manual expression or pumping will help initiate letdown in these instances. Edema of the nipple and areola can cause the nipple to retract with a pinch test, thereby confusing mothers who had no nipple retraction prenatally. This is especially the case when mothers are induced or have long labors followed by a cesarean delivery, because of the massive fluid infusion. Massage stimulates milk flow to alleviate engorgement, a plugged duct, or mastitis—all situations in which milk stasis increases difficulty. When the baby pauses during a feeding, alternate massage will encourage sustained sucking in a sleepy baby or inefficient feeder. Alternate massage also increases the volume of fat content per feeding (Morton, 2004).

Breast Compression

Breast compression is similar to massage, but more focused on squeezing milk into the baby's mouth. Hold the breast with one hand, with the thumb on the top of the breast and the other fingers on the bottom, away from the areola. Watch for the baby's sucking. When he is no longer suckling nutritively, compress the breast by squeezing gently. This compression usually triggers another sucking burst (Newman, 2005). The mother can repeat this throughout the feeding whenever she notices the baby is not suckling effectively. Reassure her that breast compression is not something she will have to do longterm, but is helpful in the early days, especially with ineffective feeders.

Breast Massage Technique

The techniques for breast massage, or breast compression, are useful to teach mothers (Newman, 2000) and easy for mothers to learn (Figure 21.3). Beginning at her chest

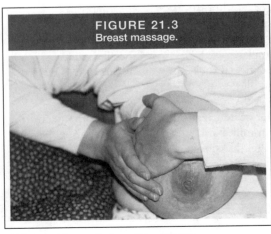

FIGURE 21.3
Breast massage.

Printed with permission of Kay Hoover.

wall, the mother uses the palm of her hand to exert gentle pressure on the breast, massaging in a circular motion from the chest wall toward the nipple. Note that she uses the palm of her hand and not her fingers. She will continue in this manner, rotating her hand around the breast. Encourage her to focus on the areas of greatest milk duct development, which are under the breast and along the side under the arm. A mother with large breasts may need to support her breast with the other hand while she massages it. Women from a culture other than your own may have variations in breast massage that accomplish the same purpose.

Reverse Pressure Softening

Practitioners have observed that many mothers who receive IV fluids in a hospital delivery have edema in their breasts and extremities. This often results in flattening of the areola, similar to engorgement. A reverse pressure softening technique helps move the fluid away from the areola so the baby can latch on. Table 21.1 shows this procedure, with instructions for the mother. The procedure has also proven helpful in relieving engorgement and triggering the mother's letdown reflex (Cotterman, 2004).

C-hold

Mothers often find it helpful in the early days of breastfeeding to support the breast for feedings. Cupping the breast with one hand forming the letter "C," referred to as the C-hold, forms the breast and nipple to help the baby latch on. Continuing this throughout the feeding will support the weight of the breast and keep the nipple from slipping out of the baby's mouth. The mother cups the breast in her hand, placing her thumb on top and her fingers below (see Color Plate 20). Make sure she places her hand well behind the areola so that her fingers do not interfere with the baby's latch. Her fingers and thumb may slightly compress the breast to help form it for her baby. The mother will compress the breast so that it matches the plane of the baby's mouth, like a "breast taco" or "breast sandwich" (Wiessinger, 1998). This is helpful for a mother to use in the beginning when her baby is just learning to latch. Some women are uncomfortable touching and handling their breasts and may need verbal encouragement and "hands-on" assistance. If the baby's chin, jaw, or lips touch the mother's hand, she will need to move her hand back toward the chest wall. When she feels her baby no longer needs assistance, she can discontinue holding her breast at feedings.

Dancer Hand Position

A slight variation of the C-hold is useful with premature infants and other babies who have weak muscle development and find it difficult to hold their jaw steady while they suck. This position, the Dancer hand position, begins in the C-hold position. The mother then brings her hand forward to support her breast with the first three fingers. She supports the baby's chin in the crook of her hand between her thumb and index finger (see Color Plate 21). The mother can bend her index finger slightly so that it gently holds the baby's cheek on one side, with the thumb holding the other cheek. This hold helps decrease the available space in the baby's mouth and increases negative pressure. The use of steady, equal pressure while holding her baby's cheeks will avoid interfering with the rooting reflex. As the baby's muscle tone begins to improve, the mother can move her thumb back on top of the breast, with her index finger supporting the baby's chin.

 ## BREASTFEEDING DEVICES

Sometimes a mother may have a special need for a breastfeeding device to assist her with feedings or the care of her breasts. After careful assessment of a situation, you can make appropriate suggestions that will be least problematic for breastfeeding. Starting with the least invasive methods for approaching a problem will lead to fewer complications and later difficulties. Mothers who use breastfeeding aids often need special counseling suggestions and close follow-up during their use. The products discussed in this chapter are available from numerous sources, which are identified in the Breastfeeding Products Guide cited in the Suggested Reading in Appendix A.

Lubricants on the Breast and Nipple

Glands within the areolar skin normally keep the nipple area soft and pliable. An artificial lubricant is necessary only if this natural lubrication has been disturbed and needs to be replaced. Prenatally, a lubricant may be necessary when a mother has excessively dry skin, eczema, or other dermatologic condition. It can also replace moisture when the improper use of drying agents or other practices have removed the natural lubrication. After breastfeeding begins, mothers may apply a lubricant if their nipples become sore or cracked. Research varies on the effect of breast lubricants (see the discussion on sore nipples below and in Chapter 16). Many mothers believe that topical treatments will reduce soreness. You can guide them in making appropriate decisions.

Lubricants to Avoid

The choice of breast lubricant must take into consideration its potential effects on the health of both the mother's breast skin and her baby. Mothers should avoid any lubricant that contains petroleum, as it will inhibit skin respiration and actually prolong nipple soreness.

TABLE 21.1

Reverse Pressure Softening Technique

K. Jean Cotterman RNC, IBCLC

You (or your helper, from in front, or behind you) choose one of the patterns pictured. To see your areola better, try using a hand mirror. Place the fingers/thumbs on the circle touching the nipple. If swelling is very firm, lie down on your back, and/or ask someone to help by pressing his or her fingers on top of your fingers. Push gently but firmly straight inward toward your ribs. Hold the pressure steady for a period of 1 to 3 full minutes.

Relax, breathe easy, sing a lullaby, listen to a favorite song or have someone else watch a clock or set a timer. It is okay to repeat the inward pressure again as often as you need. Deep "dimples" may form, lasting long enough for easy latching. Keep testing how soft your areola feels. You may also press with a soft ring made by cutting off half of an artificial nipple. Offer your baby your breast promptly while the circle is soft.

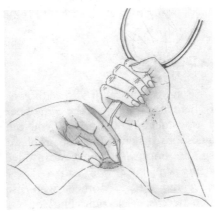

One handed "flower hold." Fingernails short, fingertips curved, placed where baby's tongue will go.

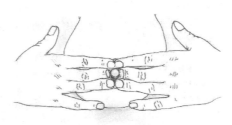

Two handed, one-step method. Fingernails short, fingertips curved, each one touching the side of nipple.

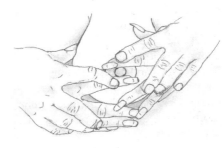

You may ask someone to help press by placing fingers or thumbs on top of yours.

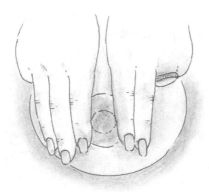

Two step method, two hands, using 2 or 3 straight fingers each side, first knuckles touching nipple. Move ¼ turn, repeat above and below nipple.

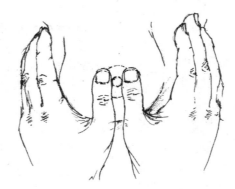

Two step method, two hands, using straight thumbs, base of thumbnail even with side of nipple. Move ¼ turn, repeat, thumbs above and below nipple.

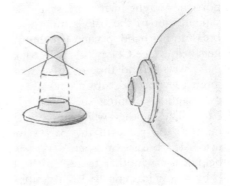

Soft ring method. Cut off bottom half of an artificial nipple to place on areola to press with fingers.

Printed by permission of Lactation Education Consultants, © 2004. May be reproduced for non-commercial purposes. Illustrations by Kyle Cotterman.

Some petroleum-based products include baby oil, petroleum jelly, vaseline based lotions, cocoa butter, A and D ointment, and dimethicone. Mothers should avoid products that contain alcohol, which are drying to the skin. They should not use vitamin E oil due to the potential for elevated levels in the baby (Marx, 1985) and sealing of an open wound with a crack.

If the baby's mother or father has a family history of allergies, the mother will want to avoid exposing him to a potential allergen such as peanut oil or massé cream. Women with a family history of wool allergy should avoid lubricants that contain wool derivatives. Some lubricants with wool derivatives contain pesticides, which may pose an additional threat to the baby (Walker, 1989). Any product the mother must wash off can further irritate sore nipples from rubbing the nipple with a washcloth. Mothers receive a variety of breast creams in the hospital that also are available in most pharmacies. Generally, although these products do no harm, they are ineffective in the prevention of sore nipples and may delay a mother from seeking early help.

Acceptable Applications

Many lactation experts suggest application of the mother's milk in the treatment of sore nipples. The prophylactic benefit of human milk to infants is well established, and it may help in the treatment of nipple soreness as well. One study found that although expressing milk did not help prevent cracked nipples, fewer mothers had nipple pain in the group that applied expressed breastmilk (Akkuzu, 2000). Hypoallergenic, medical-grade, anhydrous lanolin may help severely dry or sore nipples. This form of lanolin does not contain the concerning levels of pesticides or the alcohols that contribute to allergic response and are therefore less of a risk in allergic patients. A small amount massaged gently into the nipple and areola after a feeding is sufficient. If she prefers, the mother can express a bit of her milk and gently massage it around the nipple. When applied correctly after a feeding, the skin absorbs the lubricant before the next feeding.

Some practitioners recommend hydrogel dressings in the form of gel pads. The pads are worn between feedings to soothe sore nipples. Those designed for breast use are circular and flat, with two sides of film that the mother peels off before use. They can be stored in the refrigerator to provide the comfort of coolness on sore nipples. Some gel pads can be washed and re-used. Mothers should discontinue the use of gel pads if they experience soreness or irritation. One study found a higher infection rate with gel pads than with lanolin (Brent, 1998). Another study found the opposite, with infection in some of the lanolin users and none in the hydrogel group (Dodd, 2003). Gel pads are water based and keep the skin moist. If using gel pads, some IBCLCs recommend air drying the nipple prior to feeding.

There is no substitute for your clinical judgment and experience when you work with mothers. You should first address the root cause of soreness and determine if correcting latch and positioning will remedy the problem. If soreness persists and you perceive that the mother wants "something" to fix the problem, the use of lanolin or gel pads may help her through a period of transient soreness and extend breastfeeding duration. Instruct the mother to discontinue gel pad use and contact her physician if she sees any sign of infection.

Inverted Syringe for Flat or Inverted Nipples

Some clinicians suggest the use of an inverted syringe to help mothers evert a flat or inverted nipple. This technique can be used prenatally as well as before a feeding. In the prenatal period, the mother first will want to check with her primary caregiver to determine whether this type of nipple stimulation is safe during her pregnancy. For certain women, nipple stimulation prenatally can lead to preterm labor.

To use an inverted syringe to evert the nipple, the mother will need a syringe with a barrel that is slightly larger than her nipple. Usually a 10- to 20-ml syringe will work well. After cutting off the tapered end of the syringe, she should reverse the plunger direction to provide a smooth surface against the breast. Caution the mother not to place the cut end against her breast, as the sharp edges could damage her breast tissue. With the smooth end of the syringe placed over her nipple, the mother then pulls gently on the plunger (Figure 21.4). There are commercial eversion products, such as the Evert-It nipple enhancer. It consists of a syringe with a soft, flexible tip made of silicone. The mother may use either end to provide suction to help her nipples protrude for easier latch.

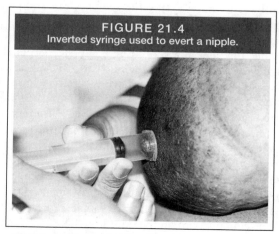

FIGURE 21.4
Inverted syringe used to evert a nipple.

Reprinted with permission of Kay Hoover.

It is important that the mother do the pulling on the syringe and not you or another caregiver, as only she can assess her comfort level. Instruct her to hold the pressure for about 30 seconds and release. The pressure should be gentle and not painful. If she experiences pain, the mother should stop the procedure. She should never pull hard enough to cause pain or color changes in the nipple. After each use of the syringe, the mother should wash it in hot, soapy water and air-dry it for the next use (Kesaree, 1993). Women can use this technique prenatally 2 or 3 times a day until the baby is born, holding the plunger out for 30 seconds 2 or 3 times in each session. After the baby is born, if he has difficulty latching on, she can use the technique before putting him to breast to help evert the nipple and improve latch. There has been debate among lactation professionals about the use of syringes for nipple eversion as a "use for which the syringe is not intended." If you practice in a hospital, ask for guidance from your administration. If you are in private practice, use your judgment to determine if this use is appropriate for a certain mother, or if a commercial device specifically for nipple eversion would be better received.

Breast Shells

Plastic breast shells have a variety of uses. Some mothers use them to relieve engorgement, wearing them for about 20 minutes before feedings. Wearing them between, or for short periods before, feedings can help shape a flat or inverted nipple to improve latch. Shells can protect a sore nipple between feedings and prevent rubbing against clothing that could irritate the skin further.

Some mothers wear breast shells in the early days postpartum to protect their clothes from milk that leaks between feedings. Make sure mothers know they cannot save milk that accumulates in a breast shell worn between feedings because of possible bacterial growth. However, a mother can collect milk in a breast shell worn on the opposite breast during a feeding. If she plans to save the **drip milk**, she must be sure the shell is clean and placed on the breast immediately before the feeding.

The mother wears the shells against her breast inside her bra. The bra should be a cup size larger than the shell to avoid pressing the shell too tightly against the breast. The shells should have several openings for air circulation in order to keep the skin from becoming softened and susceptible to chapping. Mothers can sometimes achieve a similar effect to that produced by the shell by cutting a small hole in the bra that allows the nipple to protrude.

Caution mothers not to wear breast shells while they sleep and not to use them excessively. Women have used breast shells prenatally to improve nipple protractility by gently placing pressure on the skin, stretching and pushing the nipple forward (Figure 21.5). However, research does

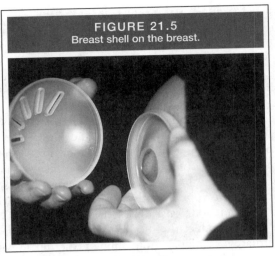

FIGURE 21.5
Breast shell on the breast.

Printed with permission of Kay Hoover.

not support the premise that wearing breast shells prenatally will produce changes in the nipples. Moreover, promoting their use prenatally may decrease breastfeeding rates because women then view breastfeeding as difficult (MAIN, 1994; Alexander, 1992). Another practice that is now questioned is the Hoffman technique for correcting nipple inversion. The mother would pull outward away from the nipple with her forefingers, in a pattern like rays of the sun, to break the adhesions. A study by the MAIN Trial Collaborative Group showed that the use of neither breast shells nor the Hoffman technique by randomly assigned women caused nipple elongation (MAIN, 1994).

Nipple Shield

A nipple shield is an artificial nipple placed over the mother's nipple during a feeding. The baby latches on to the nipple shield to nurse (Figure 21.6) and does not have direct contact with the mother's nipple. Studies with rubber and latex shields report significant decreases in the volume of milk transfer (Amatayakul, 1987; Jackson, 1987). In addition to concerns related to milk transfer and volume, nipple shields may present the dilemma of shield preference. The baby may refuse to suckle on the soft breast in preference for the rigid texture of the shield or other such rigid shape (DeNicola, 1986).

Whenever you use alternative feeding methods, the baby's preference for the method is a factor to consider. Your clinical expertise will help you gauge the best intervention for each mother and baby. Nipple shields can be a useful transitional tool for breastfeeding when used wisely (Meier, 2000; Wilson-Clay, 1996). It is important that nipple shields be used under the care of an IBCLC to assure appropriate use. Considerations when using nipple shields include selection of correct size and material (silicon, never rubber or latex), infant preference, possible breast tissue damage, adequate sucking

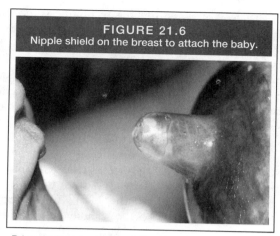

FIGURE 21.6
Nipple shield on the breast to attach the baby.

Printed with permission of Kay Hoover.

stimulation, correct shield placement during feeding, and adequate milk transfer. Never use a baby bottle nipple as a nipple shield.

Appropriate Use of a Nipple Shield

A nipple shield should not be the first intervention for latching difficulties or sucking concerns. Other techniques need to be tried first, such as a change in positioning, forming the nipple, reducing breast fullness, eversion techniques, and encouraging more sucking. As with any breastfeeding device, a nipple shield can be helpful in certain situations when appropriate instruction and follow-up care are given.

A nipple shield can help preterm infants with feedings. One study found a significant increase in milk transfer when preterm babies used a nipple shield. The mean transfer was 18.4 ml with the nipple shield, such a significant outcome that the researcher halted the control group of babies not using the nipple shield (Meier, 2000). A nipple shield appears to help preterm, SGA, and low-tone babies sustain suction within the oral cavity by holding the nipple in the mouth. It may compensate for those infants' lack of fat buccal pads and weak suckle (Wilson-Clay, 2002). It has also been used for babies with a short tongue, short frenulum or high palate. Nipple shields can help a mother who has flat or inverted nipples that have not responded to other attempts to improve latch. A shield can help the transition to direct breastfeeding when a baby has been bottle-fed and refuses the breast.

Caution mothers of the need to comply with careful follow-up when they use a nipple shield. An out-of-court settlement against a nurse and the hospital where she worked cited the potential negative outcome of reduced milk production with shield use, coupled with possible inappropriate use or inadequate instruction (Bornmann, 1986). Requiring the mother to sign a consent form for use of a nipple shield will stress the importance of follow-up. Frequent pre-feeding and post-feeding weight checks during the transition time will determine if the nipple shield allows the baby to transfer milk adequately. If a mother is considering weaning because of breastfeeding difficulties, a shield can buy the mother and baby time to work through the difficulty and preserve breastfeeding (Wilson-Clay, 2002, 1996).

Method for Using a Nipple Shield

When a mother uses a nipple shield, make sure she understands its correct use. Instruct her to fold the shield back so that it is almost inside out. Place it snugly over the nipple with the mother's nipple centered in the shield. When she smoothes the shield over the nipple, it will sometimes draw the nipple into the shield. As a rule, begin with the smallest shield possible that accommodates both the baby's mouth and the mother's nipple. This will enable the baby to compress the ducts behind the nipple. Never try to force a large, prominent nipple into a small shield.

When used appropriately, the shield will optimally be in place for only a few minutes at the beginning of the feeding. The mother should remove it after the baby begins to suckle and then quickly put him back to breast to suckle without the shield. A preterm or low-birth-weight infant may need the shield in place for the entire feeding in order to transfer milk. The mother may experience less stimulation to her breasts when the shield is in place. Reduced stimulation can lead to reduced milk production. Removing the nipple shield at some point during the feeding so the baby suckles directly on the breast and stimulates milk production will minimize this risk.

Monitoring and Follow-up

The mother needs to monitor her baby's intake and output carefully during the shield's use, with a daily record of feedings, voids, and stools. She should check her baby's weight periodically and may need to pump to maintain milk production. Encourage her to consider the shield as a temporary measure to work through a breastfeeding difficulty and to think of it as a bridge, not a crutch.

Advise the mother to wean from the shield as soon as is practical. She can put her baby to breast periodically without the shield when it "feels right" to see whether he will nurse without it. Weaning from a nipple shield is similar to learning to dance, alternating two steps forward, one step back, and one step forward, two steps back. Most infants who need time, maturity, and fattening up will transition from the nipple shield easily once they can milk the breast as effectively without it as with it. In the instances of severely inverted nipples that will not evert or uncommon infant anomalies such as a sub-mucosal cleft, the mother may need to use a shield for the entire time she breastfeeds. Give her lots of praise and affirmation for persevering in a less than optimal situation, and help her feel positive about her experience.

Nipple Shield Consent Form

Because of the potential risks associated with the use of a nipple shield, some practitioners ask the mother to sign a consent form. A consent form for use of a nipple shield, to be signed and dated by both the mother and IBCLC, may contain the wording below:

> I wish to use a nipple shield temporarily to help my baby learn to latch onto my breast and suckle effectively. I understand that improper or continuous use of a nipple shield can decrease milk production, inhibit letdown of my milk, and result in little or no weight gain for my baby. I understand that while I am using a nipple shield I should use a hospital-grade electric breast pump to stimulate and maintain milk production. I understand that while using a nipple shield my baby's weight will need to be checked once or twice a week. I understand that improper or continuous use of a nipple shield can lead to my baby becoming dependent on it in order to nurse from my breast. I understand that a nipple shield is a temporary breastfeeding aid and that I should discontinue its use as soon as possible.

Weaning the Baby from the Shield

When you and the mother decide that the time is right to work toward weaning from the shield, the mother will benefit from practical suggestions. A past recommendation of trimming the shield gradually is not advisable because the trimmed edges of silicone may lacerate the baby's mouth or the mother's nipple. Rather, the mother can watch for cues from her baby that he may nurse without the shield. Often, a sleepy baby is less likely to resist the transfer from shield to breast. Some babies will be more receptive after the initial fullness at the beginning of a feeding has decreased. Increased skin-to-skin contact with the mother will aid in the transition from shield to breast. The mother can try slipping the nipple shield out when the baby has nursed well and is in a satiated sleeping state. Often the baby will continue to nurse in his sleep. Some babies will nurse directly when cobathing with the mother.

Pacifiers

Pacifiers are often at the center of debate about their usefulness. This is especially true for babies who breastfeed. What may be an appropriate avenue for meeting the sucking needs of a bottle-fed baby is often a source of difficulty when used with a breastfeeding infant. Pacifier use correlates with a higher incidence of early weaning (Soares, 2003; Gorbe, 2002; Vogel, 2001; Aarts, 1999), particularly when sucking technique is incorrect (Righard, 1998, 1997).

There is a strong relationship between daily pacifier use and weaning by 3 months (25 percent use versus 12.9 percent non-use). While pacifier use does not necessarily cause early weaning, it may be a marker for breastfeeding difficulties or decreased maternal motivation to breastfeed (Benis, 2002). In another study, mothers who gave their babies a pacifier before 6 weeks of age nursed for an average of 6 months. Mothers who either used no pacifier or delayed its use until later than 6 weeks averaged 7 months breastfeeding duration. Those who did not use a pacifier breastfed for as long as 10 months (Ullah, 2003). Pacifier use also increases the incidence of candida and ear infections (Mattos-Graner, 2001; Warren, 2001) and can cause malocclusion (Palmer, 2004; Charchut, 2003; Zardetto, 2002; Larson, 2001). Pacifier use in the neonatal period is detrimental to exclusive and overall breastfeeding and should be avoided (Howard, 2003).

Pacifiers offer no nutritional benefit to an infant. They expend calories and, in some instances, may contribute to slowed growth. The time a baby spends sucking on a pacifier is time spent away from the breast. This interferes with the symbiotic relationship of the baby increasing the mother's milk production through suckling. Therefore, pacifiers can negatively affect a mother's milk production in relation to her baby's needs (Newman, 2000). A baby who uses a pacifier frequently may show poor weight gain from having inadequate time at the breast. Less time at the breast can also cause insufficient milk drainage, which, in turn, can result in engorgement or mastitis.

When a baby uses a pacifier, it is easy for parents to miss hunger cues. He may suck on the pacifier, and grow hungrier and hungrier, until he finally spits it out and starts crying. Crying is a late indicator of hunger (AAP, 2005). A baby who is frantic and hungry is difficult to soothe enough to latch on and nurse. Sucking on a pacifier tires some babies, especially near-term 37–38 weekers. The baby tires out, goes to sleep, and misses a feeding. If he had not had the pacifier in his mouth, the parents could have noticed him rooting, bringing his hands to his mouth, opening his mouth, and making sucking motions.

Rather than using a pacifier in response to crying, encourage parents to respond to early hunger cues. Help them learn other ways to comfort their baby (see the discussion of crying in Chapter 13). Babies whose parents "wear" them against their bodies with a baby sling cry less often and are given a pacifier less often (Hunziker, 1986). Teach parents options that are more appropriate than pacifiers for helping their crying babies. They will make better choices, decrease breastfeeding difficulties, and perhaps save on orthodontia bills in the future.

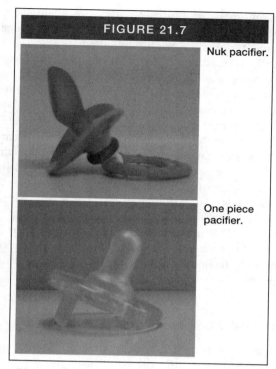

FIGURE 21.7

Nuk pacifier.

One piece pacifier.

Printed with permission of Anna Swisher.

A pacifier should not replace breastfeeding, interaction, or skin contact with the mother. It should not be offered until the baby's needs for food, comfort, and human contact are fully met. The mother needs to tune into her baby's cues. If he settles when being held, he may simply have needed comfort. If he remains unsettled and roots, urge the mother to put him to breast before offering a pacifier. If he does not want to nurse and continues to demonstrate a need to suck, a pacifier may help settle him.

Appropriate and Safe Use of a Pacifier

One appropriate and beneficial use of a pacifier is with a preterm infant. Preterm infants benefit from sucking on pacifiers during **gavage feeding** (Drosten, 1997; Wolf, 1992; Bernbaum, 1983). Accelerated maturation of the sucking reflex, decreased intestinal transit time, and increased rates of weight gain are all positive effects of pacifier use in these infants. A pacifier also helps calm infants who must undergo painful procedures and may be an especially effective way to reduce testing stress for severely ill babies. Fussy, term babies in a NICU setting may benefit from a pacifier if feedings are restricted or at times when they are NPO (Latin term, nil por os, meaning nothing by mouth) for medical reasons. Excessive crying increases blood pressure, heart rate, and calorie expenditure.

Some occupational therapists recommend pacifiers for babies with gastroesophageal reflux disease (GERD).

A pacifier allows the baby to suckle for comfort and to salivate, which coats the esophagus and reduces pain. Constant suckling at the breast can cause the baby to consume excess amounts of milk, overfilling his stomach, and aggravating the GERD (Boekel, 2000). See the discussion on GERD in Chapter 13.

Mothers need to receive instructions on safe pacifier use. Figure 21.7 shows two types of pacifiers. The first type, with an "orthodontic" shape, elicits a different sucking pattern from all other nipples (Nowak, 1994; Wolf, 1992). Additionally, the multiple parts have the potential to harbor bacteria, thrush, and mold. The second type is a solid piece of molded silicone with no separate parts. This may be a safer choice for the baby. The pacifier's material also may be an issue. Because of a growing concern about latex allergies, mothers may want to avoid latex pacifiers. A 1998 recall of one brand of pacifier occurred because it contained phthalates which can be harmful in large doses; phthalates are no longer used in pacifiers. Parents should never connect a pacifier to a cord around the baby's neck because of the potential for strangulation. If their baby has a medical or therapeutic need for a pacifier, parents can work with their occupational therapist to select one that is best for their baby's particular needs (Wolf, 1992).

▶ DIGITAL TECHNIQUES

The baby's oral cavity is extremely sensitive, with many nerve fibers and impulses. Too much inappropriate stimulation can result in an aversion to anything going into the mouth, including the breast. Inserting your finger into a baby's mouth should be done only when necessary and within your scope of practice. The use of digital techniques range from calming a baby to assessing the oral cavity to improving the baby's suck. At the most advanced level, a clinician may use digital manipulation to alter a dysfunctional suck.

Barger (1998) identifies four levels of digital intervention for infants who have difficulty suckling. When a mother needs assistance, the caregiver should start with the least intrusive method and progress to the highest degree of intervention only when other less intrusive methods have failed. Refer to Chapter 15 for further discussion on the four levels of digital intervention.

Minimal Level: Pacifying the Baby

The least invasive digital technique involves the evaluator or parent touching the baby's lips with an index finger, pad side up. The caregiver waits for the baby to latch

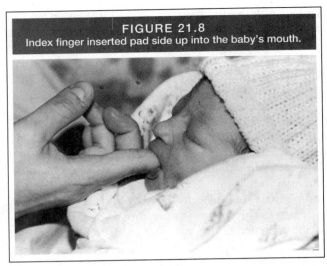

FIGURE 21.8
Index finger inserted pad side up into the baby's mouth.

Printed with permission of Kay Hoover.

onto the finger and draw it into his mouth (Figure 21.8). Parents may use this to pacify their baby or to initiate suckling at the beginning of a feeding. They can also use it in conjunction with a tube feeding system at the breast to increase the baby's calorie intake, described later in this chapter under finger feeding. Passively presenting your finger in this way is a minimal level of intervention, with the baby in total control as he sucks on your finger.

Low Level: Evaluating the Oral Cavity

Digitally evaluating the infant's oral cavity is a low-level intervention used by many clinicians when assessing an infant's suck. When he is relaxed and ready to receive your finger, insert your index finger, pad side up, very gently into his mouth. When he draws your finger into his mouth, subtly move your finger to feel the inside of the oral cavity and the palate. Assess whether the palate is normal, flat, or excessively high. As the baby suckles, notice whether his tongue covers the alveolar ridge and cups around the bottom of your finger to form a trough. Detect whether his tongue moves rhythmically from front to back. Assessing these elements will help you determine if a problem exists. This technique should only be used if you suspect a problem. It is not appropriate to do it routinely with all babies. Evaluating the oral cavity, while a bit more invasive, still places the baby in control of sucking on the finger.

Moderate Level: Suck Reorganization

It is common for a baby to exhibit an uncoordinated or disorganized suck, especially a baby who is preterm or near term. A baby's uncoordinated sucking often resolves with the passage of time as his system and reflexes become more mature. Increasing the baby's caloric intake can help resolve a disorganized suck. Use of a nursing supplementer provides fluids while the baby suckles. The flow of fluid regulates suck and therefore improves sucking for some babies. Before any digital manipulation is attempted, it should first be determined if these methods will achieve the desired result.

Digitally manipulating a baby's suck should never be done routinely and should be done only after all other solutions have been tried. Allow the baby to draw your finger, pad side up, into his mouth. Place slight downward pressure on the midline of the tongue and pull your finger out slowly to encourage the baby to suck it back in. Verbal praise will reinforce appropriate movement. This may be all the baby needs to help him organize his suck into an effective rhythm and movement. This technique places the caregiver in control rather than the baby.

High Level: Suck Training

The technique known as suck training involves tapping, stroking, and massaging the baby's tongue, gums, and palate. A baby who needs suck training should be referred to a professional who is trained and skilled in this field, such as a physical, occupational, or speech therapist with specialization in infant disorders. If there is a need for suck training, there often are other neurological problems (such as cerebral palsy), and the suck can be the first area where the problem manifests itself. Do not attempt to handle this situation alone, and do not cavalierly manipulate a baby's sucking.

Suck training is beyond the scope of practice for most nurses and IBCLCs. It involves the therapist placing an index finger in the baby's mouth, pad side up, and stimulating certain portions of the oral anatomy to train him to suck. The therapist's finger "walks" back on the tongue almost to the point of the baby gagging. This technique is highly active and controlling on the part of the therapist. If the baby appears to have neurological or other physical problems, referrals to community support and parent education groups are recommended.

▶ MILK EXPRESSION

There are times in most women's breastfeeding when they need to remove milk from their breasts. Mothers need to understand that no matter what method of milk expression they use, they cannot remove milk from their breasts as effectively as the suckling of a robust baby. The baby combines suction and rhythmic compression of the areola with his gums to obtain the milk. Just as a mother and baby need time to learn how to nurse, a mother may express several times before she becomes proficient and is able to obtain the desired amount of milk. Gentle breast massage will encourage the flow of milk and help relax and soothe the mother so she can obtain more milk.

Manual Expression

Knowing how to hand express their milk enables women to be self-reliant, no matter what circumstances arise in the course of breastfeeding. They will be able to extract milk during a brief separation and despite a broken pump, power failure, natural disaster, or low battery. Learning to be independent and to function without a need for devices can help instill further self-confidence. The mother is able to express any time and anywhere, without waiting. It is cost free and quiet, and she is in charge of the pressure applied. Milk collection by hand expression shows no difference in contamination rates as compared with milk collection using a breast pump (Pittard, 1991). Manual expression may actually be cleaner than pumping, because pumps are not always cleaned adequately.

Technique for Manual Expression

In preparing to express by hand, the mother should first wash her hands well. If she wishes, she can gently massage her breast and apply a warm, moist cloth for several minutes prior to expressing her milk. Both of these techniques will help promote milk flow. Massaging her breast throughout her expressing session will continue to promote the flow of milk.

   To begin expressing, she can lean slightly forward with her nipple aimed at the collection container, as shown in Figure 21.9. Grasping her breast as she would when using the C-hold, she places her thumb on the areola above the nipple and her index finger on the areola below the nipple. Next, she presses her thumb and index finger inward toward her chest wall a short way and then firmly presses on the ducts beneath the areola between her finger and thumb.

   The mother will continue the cycle of pressing and releasing the thumb and forefinger throughout her expressing session. Initially, it may take several attempts until milk begins to drip. Milk will spray out with greater force after the milk lets down. Rotating her thumb and forefinger around the areola will ensure that she compresses all the ducts. Caution her not to squeeze the nipple itself and not to move her fingers along her skin. Such actions have little or no benefit to expressing milk and may irritate her breast tissue.

   Many mothers find a different method of hand expression that works equally well or better. In fact, most women report that they find it difficult to master the technique as it usually is described in literature.

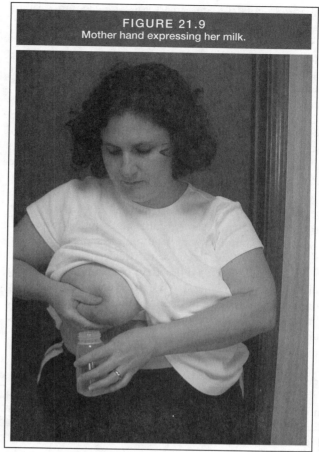

FIGURE 21.9
Mother hand expressing her milk.

Printed with permission of Anna Swisher.

Some women express by cupping the breast with the C-hold, gently massaging and applying pressure on the ducts. Encourage mothers to experiment with various hand positions until they find what works best for them. There is no one correct way for this or many other techniques. Honor individual choices by not commenting negatively or insisting on the mother's conforming to a certain technique. Practice and adaptation are keys to hand expression working for the mother. When she masters hand expression, it can be as fast and efficient as a breast pump.

Use of a Breast Pump

When a mother is using a breast pump, close contact with an IBCLC will help identify any difficulties with pumping or with maintaining milk production. Her needs are especially great when she is using a mechanical device to empty her breasts and maintain milk production without the emotional gratification of her baby nuzzling at her breast. Her reactions to using a breast pump may range from fear of possible pain to embarrassment to irritation to passive acceptance or to gratitude and relief.

If the need for a pump has resulted from a health problem, the mother may be anxious about the outcome and want to share her concerns with someone. If she will be pumping for several days, or perhaps even weeks or months, she may experience periods of discouragement and will benefit from your reassurance and support. Several electric breast pump manufacturers have instructional information available to mothers on their Web sites. A mother who is preoccupied with the situation requiring that she pump may not pay close attention to the information you provide her. Make a special effort to offer clear instructions and explanations.

Although her present circumstances may be stressful, you can help a mother view pumping as a positive tool in the resolution of her need for the device. Encourage her to regard pumping as more than a means of obtaining milk—it is her lifeline to breastfeeding her baby. By pumping regularly, she can maintain the potential to breastfeed. It is something that only she can do for her baby. In a situation in which she can do little else, pumping can help a mother to feel involved and essential.

Conditioning Letdown for Pumping

When a baby suckles at the breast, the stimulation on his mother's nipple triggers the letdown of her milk. A breast pump or manual expression does not provide the same degree of stimulation as that of the baby. Therefore, the mother may need to condition her milk externally to let down. Her emotional state may be a factor in her ability to establish letdown. She can prepare mentally for pumping and arrange to pump at times when she feels rested and unhurried. An atmosphere that is conducive to pumping will include privacy, a comfortable chair, a picture of her baby, and perhaps a tape recording of her baby's sounds to listen to while pumping. Other techniques for establishing letdown appear in Chapter 7.

When a mother finds it difficult to establish letdown while pumping, she may become tense, agitated, and upset, which inhibits her letdown even further. After first confirming that she is using a quality pump with correct pressure, and using good technique, you can encourage her to continue pumping to obtain the readily available milk. Often, the regular routine of pumping helps the mother relax and patiently work toward increasing her milk production. Ensuring that the mother's nipple has contact with the side of the flange will help provide the stimulation needed for her milk to let down.

Selecting a Breast Pump

There are many types of breast pumps available, and each has particular advantages for certain situations. In selecting a pump, the mother will want to consider her baby's age and condition and how long she will need to pump. If she will pump at work, she can consider the amount of time she has available for pumping, facilities for pumping and storage, affordability, and personal preference.

Familiarize yourself with the types of breast pumps available in your community, as well as the ease with which mothers can obtain them. Provide practical information such as descriptions and prices of various pumps, how they are used, and their advantages and disadvantages. Breast pumps manufactured by companies that sell artificial baby milk or feeding products may not be the best choice. Advise mothers to select a pump manufactured by a company whose primary mission is the support of breastfeeding. Mothers must avoid long periods of uninterrupted vacuum that could damage breast tissue. For this reason, automatic cycling pumps are a better choice. Your guidance will help mothers select the appropriate pump.

Criteria for Selecting a Breast Pump

◆ Does it cycle quickly, similar to the rhythm of the baby's suck?

◆ Is the flange shape comfortable and an appropriate size for the mother's breast?

◆ Are large (27 mm) and extra-large (30 mm) flanges available? Many mothers' nipples are too large for the standard 24 or 25 mm flanges. One manufacturer makes a 40 mm glass flange.

◆ Are inserts available for the flanges for very small areolas and nipples?

◆ Can standard-size bottles be used for collecting milk?

◆ Are the breast pump parts dishwasher safe?

◆ Is the pump easy to assemble, with few parts?

◆ Is the pump easy and comfortable to use with the type of hand or arm motion required?

◆ If the pump is electric, will the power source be adequate (i.e., type of outlet—two or three prongs—and amount of voltage)?

◆ Is the pump quiet?

◆ Is the pump easy to transport?

◆ Is the pump affordable for the length of time it is required?

◆ Are quick service and overnight replacement available?

◆ What period and what parts does the warranty cover?

◆ Are written instructions provided?

◆ Is there someone at the company who is knowledgeable in breastfeeding to answer questions and resolve problems?

◆ Is there a toll-free number to call with questions?

◆ Is there an up-to-date Web site?

Hand-Held Breast Pump

Many mothers use a hand-held breast pump as an occasional supplement to breastfeeding (see Figure 21.10). A hand-held pump consists of a collecting bottle and flange that fits over the breast. A piston, trigger, or motor provides the suction. Hand-held pumps may be either manual, battery operated, or a combination of battery and electric. A wide variety of styles and prices are available.

A manual pump that uses natural movements will be the most comfortable for the mother. Motorized hand pumps provide suction either with a control button so the mother can regulate pressure or with an auto-cycling motor that does all of the suction work. An early hand-held breast pump, still found in some stores today, was the "bicycle horn" pump. The name derives from its resemblance to the horn on a bicycle. This pump can damage a mother's nipple and harbors bacteria that could be dangerous to the baby. Mothers should not use hand pumps that use a bulb to generate suction. Those pumps belong in a museum, not in a mother's home!

Hands-free Breast Pump

One manufacturer makes a battery operated double pump that is designed for hands-free operation (Figure 21.11). There are also bras available designed to provide hands-free operation of electric breast pumps.

Electric Breast Pump

Electric breast pumps are useful in the regular absence of nursing when the mother and baby cannot be together (Figure 21.12). Electric pumps most closely mimic the baby's suckling rhythm and provide the stimulation that is necessary to maintain milk production. They offer the option of pumping both breasts at the same time, as

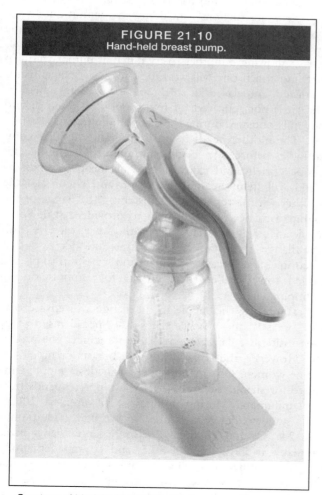

FIGURE 21.10
Hand-held breast pump.

Courtesy of Medela, Inc., McHenry, IL.

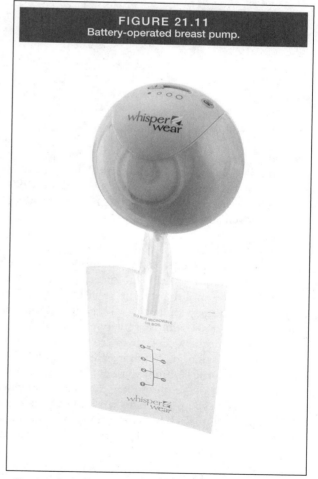

FIGURE 21.11
Battery-operated breast pump.

Courtesy of Whisper Wear, Marietta, GA.

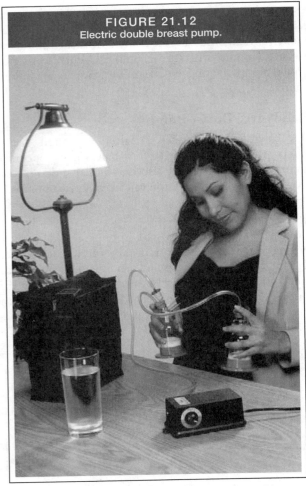

FIGURE 21.12
Electric double breast pump.

Courtesy of Bailey Medical Engineering, Los Osos, CA.

shown in Figure 21.12, thus saving time and increasing breast stimulation. In some cases, simultaneous double pumping obtains higher milk yields (Auerbach, 1990). Heavy-duty double electric breast pumps are produced for both hospital and consumer use.

Hospital-Grade Pump

Hospital-grade electric breast pumps are the best option for mothers who need the most efficient pumping. Mothers with an ill baby, a preterm baby, or multiples (who are usually preterm) will typically use this pump. Hospital-grade pumps are very expensive to purchase, so most mothers rent them from an authorized rental station. Hospital-grade pumps are approved by the U.S. Food and Drug Administration (FDA) for multiuse. This designation requires that the pump provider disinfect and clean the pump between rentals to prevent cross-contamination. Each user must purchase a personal pump kit, which should not be resold. Many women who use pumps for lengthy or regular separation, such as full-time employment, invest in a quality consumer version of the double electric pump.

Consumer Pump

Consumer pumps are FDA approved for single use. Multi-use of consumer pumps can cause cross-contamination and is therefore not appropriate. The reality is that many women trade, borrow, or buy used pumps. However, the design of the motor and diaphragm parts on the consumer pumps are not conducive to multiple use, and the pressure may be lower than needed. You can encourage mothers to research the information about used pumps. One helpful Web site, www.breastfeedingonline.com, lists the pumps rated for multiple or single use, with explanations about their ratings. If a mother insists on using a previously owned pump, you can suggest that she at least obtain a new kit and have the pressure checked.

Pumping Technique

Because the use of breast pumps accompanies an interruption in breastfeeding, the mother may need specialized counseling. For this reason, many IBCLCs have pumps and accompanying equipment readily available for demonstration and hands-on teaching. Mothers need complete instructions, including a demonstration of proper equipment use. Regardless of the type of pump the mother uses, she also needs appropriate written instructions. Allowing a mother to try different pumps will help her find which one will work best for her. She can use a sterilized, autoclaved kit solely for test pumping. Because the kit is not approved for multi-use, she should discard any milk obtained during the test pumping.

The mother needs to wash her hands and get comfortable before she begins pumping. Massaging her breasts briefly and expressing a few drops of milk by hand will help the milk let down and encourage the mother with faster results. Moistening the flange of the pump with her milk will help to provide a seal. Some clinicians suggest that the mother use olive oil on the flange to obtain a good seal and decrease skin friction. Large-breasted women find it helpful to place a rolled towel under their breasts for support during pumping.

Centering the nipple in the flange will ensure that her breast tissue touches the sides. Special inserts that rest inside the flange are available to achieve the proper fit. However, they may cause sore breasts or nipples in some women. One manufacturer provides a nipple template for sizing. Be aware that the nipple expands by a few millimeters during pumping (Wilson-Clay, 2002). The standard flange apertures for hospital-grade pumps are 24 mm and 25 mm. There are larger flange sizes available in 27, 28.5, 30, 30.5, and 40 mm depending on the manufacturer. The 40 mm flanges are glass and very expensive. Mothers who have small nipples and areolas will benefit from optional inserts.

The mother will want to use only as much suction as is needed to maintain milk flow throughout her pumping session. Advise that she begin with the suction on the lowest setting and gradually increase suction strength as necessary. Encourage mothers to tailor pumping times to their specific needs and circumstances. Mothers can expect to pump varying amounts of milk on different days and at different times of the day. Morning pumping frequently yields more milk than pumping in the afternoon or evening. If her baby breastfeeds some or most of the time, pumping can be adapted to their breastfeeding schedule. A mother may pump in place of a missed feeding, between feedings, or on one breast while feeding the baby on the other breast. Experimenting will help her find which arrangement will best suit her and her baby's needs.

A mother who is single pumping will find it helpful to alternate between breasts several times throughout her pumping session to capitalize on the multiple letdowns that occur simultaneously. She can pump 5 to 7 minutes on one breast and then switch to the other breast for another 5 to 7 minutes. She can then return to the first breast for 3 to 5 minutes of pumping and repeat that time on the second breast (massaging her breasts if necessary to promote flow). Finally, she can finish on the first breast with 2 to 3 minutes of pumping and then the second breast for the final 2 to 3 minutes. If the mother is double pumping with an electric pump or 2 battery pumps, 10 to 15 minutes total pumping time may be sufficient. You can suggest that she pump for only 10 to 15 minutes, or a minute or two after the milk stops spurting. Mothers who pump long-term have found that massaging their breasts after the milk stops flowing, and then pumping again for a few minutes, yields more milk and better drainage of the breast (Morton, 2004).

Pumping for a Hospitalized Baby

When a mother and baby are separated, she will need to pump at least eight times every 24 hours, regardless of the amount of milk she obtains. Pumping during the night will produce larger quantities of milk because prolactin levels are highest at that time. The mother also needs a four- or five-hour stretch of sleep to maintain her health and energy. She can pump during the night whenever she wakes naturally and can drink extra fluids just before bedtime to facilitate waking. As the time grows closer for her baby to come home, she can begin to pump more regularly at night.

Regular milk removal will help the mother build and maintain milk production so that she has sufficient milk when her baby is able to nurse. Initiating copious milk production helps establish long-term lactation. This is especially important in times of stress. If the mother needs to collect large amounts of milk for her baby, she can pump more frequently and try to reduce stress and get sufficient rest. A mother may find that one breast produces more milk and lets down more easily than the other. This is normal and is common in most women. Both breasts need regular milk removal in order to establish milk production and avoid complications caused by overfullness.

A mother who uses a breast pump to protect lactation can ask her healthcare practitioner to write a prescription for insurance reimbursement. More progressive insurance companies support breastfeeding, recognizing that families have fewer health claims with breastfed children (AAHP, 2001). Medicaid reimburses for electric pump rentals for preterm and ill babies. U.S. WIC clinics provide hospital-grade electric pumps for mothers of preterm and ill babies. If a mother has financial problems, encourage her to explore these avenues. The hospital NICU will have hospital-grade electric pumps there for her to use, but she will need a pump for home use as well.

Collecting and Storing Human Milk

Mothers collect milk for a variety of reasons. They may store it in the freezer for emergencies and for a regular separation, such as working or attending school. They may store it for a short-term separation such as a shopping trip, wedding, or other social outing. An infant who tires out or cannot manage every feeding at the breast may need expressed milk. Many mothers donate their milk to human milk banks to be given to other babies, children, or sick adults.

If a mother expresses her milk to relieve breast fullness or collects drip milk during a feeding, she can save it for later use. She should not save milk that accumulates in a breast shell worn between feedings. It has been against her skin for a lengthy time and could have increased bacterial growth. When the mother is taking a medication proven to be harmful to her baby, she should not give her milk to her baby. If she or her baby has a yeast infection, she should discard any collected milk since it may harbor the infection. A multiple child care setting may require varying guidelines for milk storage. The mother can review safety issues with the care provider. You can assist them by providing up-to-date guidelines and educating the child care staff.

Storage Container

Milk must be stored in a manner that preserves its quality and keeps it from spoiling. The mother must clean collection containers and any pump parts that have contact with the milk after every use. She can wash them in hot soapy water and then thoroughly rinse and air-dry them, or simply cycle them through a dishwasher.

Glass containers are the best choice for milk storage. Glass does not absorb the milk's antibodies or other proteins. It is easy to clean and offers protection against contamination of the milk during storage. A hard plastic (polypropylene) container is the next best choice for storage. A drawback to this container is that the interior surface can scratch and make cleaning difficult. Soft plastic (polyethylene) baby bottle liners are not recommended for storing milk. When milk is stored in soft plastic containers such as bottle liners, certain antibodies in the milk reduce in concentration. Additionally, such soft plastics are difficult to seal and may puncture easily.

The amount of milk stored in each container will vary as the mother determines how much her baby consumes in her absence. Initially, she should store her milk in small amounts, usually one to two ounces, to minimize waste. If the milk will be frozen, she needs to leave space for expansion during freezing.

Labeling the container with a waterproof marker will assist the mother and other caregivers. The label should include the date and time the milk was expressed, and possibly the amount of milk contained. If the milk is given to the baby by another caregiver with multiple children, the mother's and baby's full names should be written on the label. The baby's last name is important because some babies and mothers do not have the same last name. The mother may want to transport the milk in a container that is ready for feeding to reduce the possibility of the caregiver contaminating the milk while pouring.

Storage Time

Storage times vary, depending on how soon the baby will receive the expressed milk. One study suggests milk that will be used within five days can be placed in the refrigerator immediately after it is collected (Sosa, 1987). However, milk-banking experts recommend that milk be refrigerated for only three days, noting the difficulty of controlling for contamination. A three-day storage time was echoed by an expert work group (Wellstart, 1996).

Mothers do not always have immediate access to refrigeration. One study found that milk that remains at room temperature for up to eight hours has no significant increase in bacteria count (Pittard, 1985). Another recommends that milk be stored at room temperature for no more than four hours (Hamosh, 1996). This conservative approach accounts for variables inherent in milk collection such as amount of contamination and definition of "room temperature." If a mother is not sure that she will use her milk within three to five days, she should freeze it. She can place her expressed milk directly in the freezer after collecting it.

A mother's milk can be stored in the freezer for up to one year, depending on the type of freezer. In a freezer that is part of a refrigerator unit with a separate door, the milk will keep for three to six months. A deep freezer will keep the milk for six months to one year, depending on the temperature. To avoid extremes of temperature, milk should not be stored on the door of the refrigerator or freezer or near the freezer's defrosting unit. Also caution mothers not to store their milk near an automatic icemaker, which has a variance in temperature that can affect the milk. The optimal temperature in the freezer is 0 degrees F, or minus 18–20 degrees C.

A mother may complain that her milk smells bad after it has been frozen for a short while. The odor seems related to the level of lipase in the milk. The mother can prevent this by gently warming her milk before freezing, never to the point of boiling. Although warming the milk lowers some of the immunoglobulins, it prevents the mother from discarding her milk because of the smell. Her milk is always a better option for her baby than artificial milk.

Special Guidelines for the NICU Infant

Milk collection and storage guidelines vary slightly, depending on the reason the mother is collecting her milk. Guidelines often focus on mothers with healthy babies who are collecting milk for convenience or employment. Such guidelines are not appropriate in all situations. A mother who is collecting milk for her baby in the neonatal intensive care unit will need to follow more strict guidelines to ensure her baby's safety. Whenever possible, the mother should express her milk just before feeding the baby. If he will not receive the expressed milk within one hour, the milk should be refrigerated immediately. If the baby is ill or preterm and will not receive her fresh milk within 48 hours, the mother should freeze it. Mothers who collect milk for a preterm infant need to place milk from each pumping session in a separate storage container to minimize handling and contamination of the milk (HMBANA, 2004).

When a baby goes to the NICU, an IBCLC or NICU nurse should contact the mother with specific instructions on how to collect and store her milk. Mothers who are not given information about the need to begin expressing their milk within the first 24 hours after delivery may have difficulty establishing adequate production. A mother may assume that because she and her baby are separated due to prematurity or illness, breastfeeding is no longer an option for her. Encourage NICU staff to educate mothers about early pumping to help maximize their milk production potential. Guidelines vary from one hospital to another. If your hospital does not offer critical care, parents will need guidelines for milk collection and storage from the critical care NICU that will care for their baby. Make sure parents receive this information before the mother leaves the hospital.

Combining Containers of Milk

Mothers often have questions about the procedure for storing milk from more than one pumping session or from both breasts at the same pumping session. When a mother pumps both breasts at the same time for a well baby, she can combine both containers of milk for storage. She can combine milk from different pumping sessions, with the label stating the date and time of the earliest pumping. As she uses stored milk, she should select the oldest date. She can add newly pumped milk to refrigerated milk after the newly pumped milk cools. She needs to chill the newly pumped milk for at least two hours before adding it to frozen milk. Make sure the mother understands that the amount of chilled newly pumped milk cannot be greater than the amount of frozen milk. This will avoid the freshly pumped milk partially defrosting the frozen milk. The expiration date of the earliest expressed milk will determine the storage time for combined milk.

Defrosting and Warming Human Milk

Appropriate labeling makes it easy for the mother to use milk based on when she expressed it, using her oldest milk first. If she has a large stock of milk in her freezer, she can arrange the milk with the oldest containers toward the front. Frozen milk can be placed in the refrigerator to thaw and remain refrigerated for up to 24 hours before use (Pierce, 1992). To ensure the safety of the milk, the mother should not refreeze thawed milk.

Milk can be thawed or warmed either by placing it in the refrigerator overnight or by thawing it rapidly in a pan of warm water or under a stream of warm tap water. It should be used or discarded within 24 hours of thawing. A microwave oven should not be used for warming milk. Microwaving a liquid substance results in hot spots that could burn the baby's mouth (Nemethy, 1990). Additionally, microwaving substantially decreases activity of anti-infective properties in human milk (Quan, 1992).

When the mother's milk sits in the refrigerator or freezer, the fat will rise to the top of the milk. Gently swirling the milk throughout the warming process will mix the fat. After stored milk has been warmed, it needs to be used immediately and only for that feeding. Any milk that remains after the feeding may harbor bacteria from the baby's saliva and cannot be saved.

Human Milk Banks

A mother's expressed milk is more appropriate for her baby than any other alternative feeding choice. It responds to her particular baby, to his suckling, and to his environment. Occasionally, a mother may be unable to provide enough milk through either breastfeeding or expression. In such cases, the baby can receive donor milk from other women, in preference to infant formula. Human milk banks offer a safe alternative to mothers who cannot breastfeed or who cannot produce enough milk for their baby.

A milk bank is a collection point where healthy nursing mothers donate their milk (Figure 21.13). The milk bank screens all donors for infectious diseases. Donated milk is processed and pasteurized and dispensed by prescription to infants, children, and occasionally, adults with a medical need. Recipient families pay a processing fee, but the milk bank does not deny recipients who have a medical need and cannot afford to pay the fee. Most hospitals cover processing fees and shipping costs for babies receiving donor milk as inpatients.

There was a decline in the number of milk banks in the United States during the 1980s due to an increase in preterm formulas and the isolation of human immunodeficiency virus (HIV) in human milk (Balmer, 1992). Research increasingly documents improved outcomes for infants given human milk, and the risks of artificial formula now are more widely recognized by the public

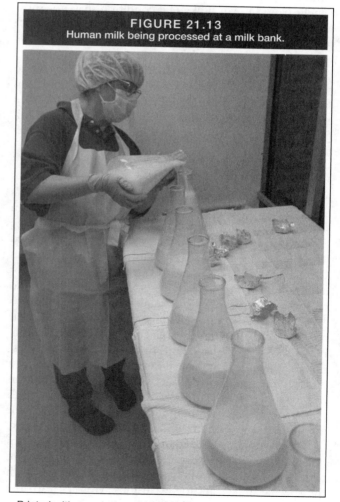

FIGURE 21.13
Human milk being processed at a milk bank.

Printed with permission of HMBANA.

and the medical community. Thus, the demand for banked human milk is skyrocketing.

There are currently eight operating milk banks in North America: Austin, Texas; Denver, Colorado; Fort Worth, Texas; Newark, Delaware; Iowa City, Iowa; Raleigh, North Carolina; San Jose, California; and Vancouver, British Columbia. Additional milk banks are slated to open in Michigan, South Carolina, Ohio, and Indiana. These milk banks have Web sites, as does the Human Milk Banking Association of North America (HMBANA) which can be found at www.hmbana.org. Donor milk can be shipped overnight anywhere in the U.S. It is important that lactation support providers know how to access this service so that parents with critically ill infants do not have to search for it (Arnold, 1998).

Babies may need donor human milk because they are temporarily unable to breastfeed, are intolerant of human milk substitutes, or suffer from digestive disorders or severe diarrhea. Some preterm or very ill infants need donor milk until their mother increases her milk production to meet their needs. Infants with auto-immune disorders or a condition such as cystic fibrosis benefit from human milk. The condition may not show up until several weeks or months after birth. The mother may be unable to relactate and therefore turns to a milk bank to help her baby survive.

Because the cost of production exceeds the cost to the recipient, nonprofit milk banks depend on donations or grants. Some milk banks receive support from an associated hospital. Mothers who are interested in additional information can contact HMBANA or an area milk bank directly.

Procedure for Donating Milk

Mothers who express and save milk for another person's baby find great emotional gratification and reward in knowing that they are helping a baby in need. Some donors are bereaved mothers whose babies have died (see the discussion on counseling grieving parents in Chapter 23). You can facilitate the use of milk banks for donors and recipients by providing information to mothers in your care who have plentiful supplies.

Learn the location of milk banks as well as their policies regarding milk collection and distribution. HMBANA provides such information for health professionals. When a mother expresses a desire to become a donor, you can provide her with general information and refer her to the nearest milk bank. Because each milk bank has slightly different procedures, it is best for the mother to communicate directly with the milk bank.

Some potential donors may be disqualified from donating milk, such as mothers who are ill or who are taking certain medications. Mothers can check with the specific milk bank for exclusions. Donors learn the clean technique for milk expression, with appropriate handwashing, washing and disinfecting of pump parts, and handling of disinfecting equipment. They learn to label their milk, proper milk storage, and proper technique for transporting their milk to the bank. Some milk banks provide containers for mothers to pump and store their milk for shipping.

Milk banks require that mothers freeze their milk and attach the label to the jar before placing it in the freezer to ensure that it will adhere. Mothers must insulate the milk well to prevent thawing, as it must stay frozen until it arrives at the milk bank. Some milk banks require that the mother collect milk in a sterile container and mark it with her name, collection date, number of ounces, and the name and dosage of any drugs she is taking. Others accept excess stockpiled milk. The individual milk bank will provide its specific collection and storage guidelines.

Screening of Donated Milk

Milk banks screen potential donors before they accept milk. After the milk arrives at the bank, the frozen milk is thawed in a refrigerator and pooled under clean conditions with **universal precautions**. The milk then undergoes heat treatment at 62.5 degrees C (**Holder pasteurization**) for 30 minutes. This kills any HIV, hepatitis, and other viruses and bacteria that may be present. Fortunately, heat-treated milk retains most of its immunologic and nutritional properties. Then the milk is rapidly cooled and refrozen. Each batch is thoroughly cultured, and any with bacterial growth is excluded from infant use. The milk bank conducts routine antigen testing similar to that of blood banks to further rule out the presence of HIV.

When a need arises for raw human milk, all parties involved consult on the decision, with potential risks carefully outlined. The milk bank screens the pool of raw milk for bacteria, which must have an acceptably low level of bacteria colonies of normal skin flora. This is true for all milk, whether or not it is to be used raw. When colonies are unacceptably high, or if any bacteria other than normal skin flora are present, the milk is excluded from both raw and pasteurized use.

Mothers should obtain donor milk through a milk bank and should be discouraged from sharing their milk on an informal basis. There are serious liability issues for healthcare providers who arrange for a mother to supply milk informally to another mother's baby. The absence of home pasteurization controls may make home pasteurization unsafe.

The Value of Human Milk: Position Paper on Donor Milk Banking is available at the HMBANA Web site. It provides an eloquent summary of the importance and value of banked human milk as the third preferred feeding alternative for infants. The preferred method is for the baby to nurse directly at the breast. The second preference is for the baby to receive his mother's expressed milk. The third preferred method is donor milk. Artificial formula is last.

▶ ALTERNATE FEEDING METHODS

When a mother needs to use an alternate feeding method, this means that her idealized view of breast-feeding has not materialized. Approach the issue of alternate feeding methods gently and with a lot of support. The mother needs an opportunity to verbalize her concerns and fears about her situation and her baby. She needs to know her options and their risks and benefits to breastfeeding. Enabling the mother to make the choice about what will fit best in her life gives her some control over an otherwise tenuous situation.

The options available for a breast alternative include a cup or spoon, a tube-feeding device used at the breast, a tube device used for finger feeding, and an artificial nipple and bottle. The mother needs to understand the appropriateness of each method to her baby's situation. She also needs to know the cost and the care and cleaning of each device. She will need thorough instructions, both verbal and written, with demonstration and close follow-up until the baby is breastfeeding without the supplemental method.

Cup Feeding

Cup feeding offers a baby-led alternative for a baby who is unable to breastfeed (Figure 21.14). The cup provides an initial sensory stimulus to the baby's lips, olfactory senses, and tongue. A younger baby will lap the milk, which promotes appropriate tongue movement used during breast-feeding. He can pace his intake, and because he is in control, respiration is easier and swallowing occurs when he is ready. A baby as young as 30 weeks' gestation is capable of maintaining his heart rate, respiration, and oxygenation while cup feeding (Lang, 1994). At 30 to 34 weeks, babies lap by protruding their tongues into the cup to obtain small boluses of milk. They often hold the milk in their mouth for some time before swallowing. As the baby matures, a sipping action begins to develop. Lang noted a positive correlation between cup feeding the preterm baby and the establishment of breastfeeding. One study found that twice as many mothers who had cup fed their babies were still breastfeeding at three months compared to those who bottle-fed (Rocha, 2002).

Cup feeding is easy for a mother and baby to learn. It may take the baby only four or five feedings to catch on to the technique. Avoiding the risk of the baby forming a preference for an artificial nipple is well worth the investment. A small cup with rounded edges works best, such as a shot glass, a medicine cup, a hollow-handed medicine spoon, or even a conventional spoon (Figure 21.15). The small plastic cups used by fast-food restaurants for catsup are a convenient choice, as are disposable small paper cups.

Mothers in India have used a small cup-like device called a paladai (Figure 21.16) for centuries. It has been trialed in the United States in cities such as Philadelphia and is gaining in popularity (Sideman, 1999). One study compared the use of a bottle, cup, and paladai in 100 newborn infants. Infants took the maximum volume in the least time and stayed calmest with the paladai. Spilling was higher with the cup, especially with preterm infants. Infants could accept feedings with the paladai or cup before the bottle, with the youngest baby at 30 weeks gestational age (Narayanan, 2002). Parents should avoid using "sippy" cups because the spout does not allow the baby to trough his tongue to mirror feeding at the breast.

FIGURE 21.14
A baby being fed by a cup.

Printed with permission of Kay Hoover.

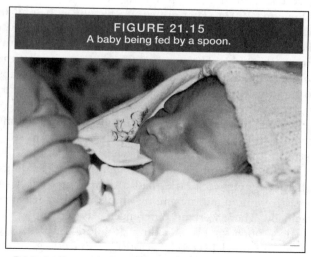

FIGURE 21.15
A baby being fed by a spoon.

Printed with permission of Kay Hoover.

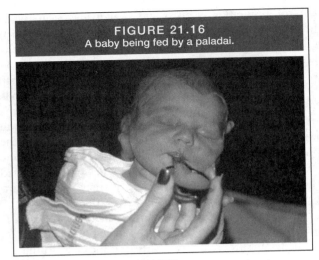

FIGURE 21.16
A baby being fed by a paladai.

Printed with permission of Kay Hoover.

Procedure for Cup Feeding

For cup feeding, the mother should fill the cup about halfway with about ½ to ⅓ of an ounce of milk. Tucking a cloth under the baby's chin will catch any spills. Holding her baby in her arms or in a semi-sitting position on her lap, the mother brings the cup to the baby's lips and rests the rim of the cup on his lower lip so that it touches the corners of his mouth. She then tips the cup until the milk touches his lips. The baby will begin to lap the milk from the cup. His tongue will form a trough to bring the milk to the back of his throat so that he can swallow it.

This method provides a low level of intervention that is much less invasive to the baby's oral cavity than finger feeding or the use of an artificial nipple. One key limitation with cup feeding, however, is that the baby does not get any practice suckling. Spillage is also greater, with one study reporting that 38.5 percent of milk taken from the cup spilled onto the baby's bib (Dowling, 2002). That aside, cup feeding is helpful in assisting the baby in learning to extend his tongue over the alveolar ridge. It also results in fewer oxygen desaturations than with other methods. It is important that the baby lap the milk. The mother needs to allow the baby to lead this activity and to rest between swallows. Pouring milk directly into his mouth increases the risk of aspiration. Slow pacing also is important for avoiding aspiration. If the baby resists the cup, it is best to stop, comfort him, and try again later when he is calmed.

A hospital study found that supplemental feedings, whether by cup or bottle, had a detrimental effect on breastfeeding duration among mothers who delivered vaginally. There were no differences between cup versus bottle groups for breastfeeding duration. Interestingly, among infants delivered by cesarean, cup feeding significantly prolonged exclusive, full, and overall breastfeed-

ing duration. Perhaps supplementation with two or more cup feedings provided calories to sustain the babies until their mothers' mature milk production, which may have been delayed due to the cesareans (Howard, 2003).

Tube Feeding

A tube-feeding device can be used during a breastfeeding to provide supplemental nutrition while the baby suckles at the breast. A commercial nursing supplementer consists of a plastic bag or bottle designed to hold fluid. The mother suspends the supplementer by a cord around her neck or clips it to her clothing at shoulder level so that it rests between her breasts. Thin, flexible tubing leads from the container to the end of the mother's nipple (Figure 21.17). Manufacturers make "starter" supplementers that attach directly to a bottle. A less expensive noncommercial supplementer can be constructed with the use of a number 5, 6, or 8 French oral gastric tube on the end of a syringe or placed in a bottle (Figure 21.18). If the syringe and feeding tube are used, exercise caution and demonstrate paced feeding to parents so the baby receives a comfortable flow.

A tube-feeding device encourages nutritive suckling. The mother can adjust it to deliver more fluid when her milk production is low and less fluid as her production

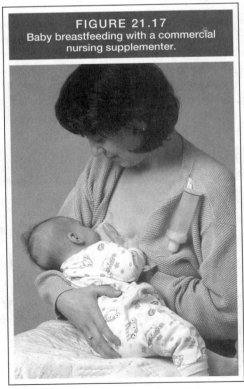

FIGURE 21.17
Baby breastfeeding with a commercial nursing supplementer.

Courtesy of Medela Inc., McHenry, IL.

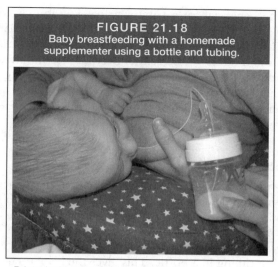

FIGURE 21.18
Baby breastfeeding with a homemade supplementer using a bottle and tubing.

Printed with permission of Anna Swisher.

increases. A mother who has been expressing milk for an ill baby may need to use a supplementer during the transition from milk expression to nursing. If the baby has been receiving the mother's milk from a bottle, the mother can replace use of the bottle with tube feeding. A mother who is relactating or inducing lactation may find this device helpful for supplementing her baby's intake while she increases production. A baby who has difficulty nursing at the breast can be encouraged by the flow of milk from the supplementer.

For a baby who will latch, a tube-feeding device is the least invasive supplemental method. It avoids the possibility of nipple preference from a bottle nipple and provides the mother with the breast stimulation she needs (Edgehouse, 1990). The baby suckles at the breast and the tip of the tube simultaneously, and the flow of supplement from the container encourages him to continue suckling. In this way, the baby receives nourishment at the same time as stimulation of his oral reflexes. Additionally, the mother receives natural stimulation of her breasts to encourage milk production.

Procedure for Tube Feeding

The substance used in tube feeding can be either expressed human milk or artificial baby milk. Some infant formulas are thick and do not flow well through the narrow tubing. If the mother uses powdered formula, she needs to shake it well to avoid clogging the tubing. Some sources suggest avoiding the use of powdered formulas in a tube-feeding device because of this potential for clogging and the infant thus receiving insufficient supplementation. Human milk fortifiers can also clog tubing. Potential for clogging may be a factor in parents' decision because of the increased cost of ready-to-feed formula.

The tube should extend a few centimeters beyond the end of the nipple. Taping it to the breast will keep it in place. The tape needs to be long enough to prevent it from coming loose in the baby's mouth. Paper tape is the least irritating to the mother's skin. Many mothers have found it more comfortable to use an adhesive bandage. The mother threads the tube through the pad part of the bandage and can leave the bandage on all day without having to remove it. She should check her baby's mouth daily to make sure that the tube is not irritating the roof of his mouth. After every use, the tubing needs to be flushed with cold water, washed with hot soapy water, and then rinsed with clear water.

The container of milk can be positioned level with, above, or below the baby's head, depending on the desired rate of flow. The level of the container initially should be adjusted so the baby has about one suck per swallow. As his suck becomes stronger and milk flow increases, the container can be lowered. Some commercial supplementers have a flow-control valve that responds to the baby's sucking, and some have various sizes of tubing to adjust flow rate. It is unnecessary to compress the tube manually in order to control milk flow. In fact, doing so may damage the device or place the baby at risk by causing him to expend energy on nonnutritive sucking.

Some babies may initially object to having the tube in their mouths and will require time to accept it. Performing alternate breast massage during the feeding will increase milk flow and encourage the baby to suckle. If the baby is not at risk, the mother can start a feeding without the supplementer and use it only when her baby needs additional nourishment. Some babies become so accustomed to nursing with the tubing that they refuse to nurse without it. Others seem to figure out that the milk is coming from the tubing, slide off the mother's breast, and suck on the tube like a straw. Taping the tubing farther back on the mother's nipple, either flush with her at-rest nipple or a few centimeters behind it, encourages the baby to grab more of the mother's breast tissue to obtain the milk. Some mothers tape the tubing below the nipple to keep the baby from sliding down the tubing.

When it is evident that the baby is receiving increasing amounts of his mother's milk, the mother can reduce the amount of supplement at each feeding. Such clues will be softer, emptier-feeling breasts after a feeding or increased amounts of milk left in the supplementer accompanied by good weight gain. Test weights will measure the intake of the mother's milk and supplement to monitor the mother's production. For example, the mother puts one ounce of expressed milk into the supplementer. She weighs the baby, nurses, and then weighs the baby again. He gained two and a half ounces and there is half an ounce left in the supplementer, indicating that he received two ounces of his mother's milk during the feeding.

Daily milk production usually seems highest in the morning, and the mother can reduce the amount of supplement accordingly. Encourage her to watch for changes in suckling rhythm and supplement flow during feedings, and to switch breasts for optimal stimulation of milk production. She can observe signs of sufficient nourishment, such as wet diapers, ample stooling, good skin turgor, weight gain, and a consistent pattern of eating and sleeping. When she and her baby's caregiver are confident that milk production is adequate, based on clinical evidence such as the baby's output and the mother's milk production, supplements can be decreased slowly and finally discontinued.

Some mothers use a nursing supplementer for the entire course of breastfeeding. These usually are either adoptive mothers or mothers with impaired milk production because of true insufficient milk supply, breast reduction, or breast augmentation. They will benefit from encouragement while they persevere in nurturing their baby at the breast (West, 2002). The adoptive breastfeeding Web site www.fourfriends.com/abrw contains many practical hints for mothers who use nursing supplementers.

Finger Feeding

Finger feeding is another means of getting nourishment to the baby (Figure 21.19). Whereas in tube feeding the tubing is placed on the end of the mother's nipple, in finger feeding the tubing is placed on the end of the caregiver or parent's finger. Finger feeding is more invasive than tube feeding. As with any alternative feeding method, if the mother uses finger feeding too long, the baby may come to prefer it to the breast. Finger feeding

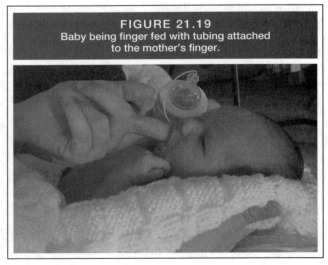

FIGURE 21.19
Baby being finger fed with tubing attached to the mother's finger.

Printed with permission of Anna Swisher.

can be beneficial for a baby who has low muscle tone, who has a disorganized suck, or who needs stimulation to elicit suckling. This is common in babies from heavily medicated births whose central nervous systems are thus depressed. Although caregivers need to use a glove when demonstrating finger feeding, most parents can finger feed without gloves. Because of the potential for allergy, latex gloves should not be used.

Procedure for Finger Feeding

As with tube feeding, you may use either a commercial nursing supplementer or number 5, 6, or 8 French oral gastric tubing on the end of a syringe that has the plunger removed. Removing the plunger allows the baby greater control over feeding. Another alternative is placing tubing in a bottle. This gives the baby total control over how much he receives and how quickly. Place the appropriate amount of expressed milk or substitute in a container attached to the tubing. Prime the tubing with the milk and crimp it to stop the flow until it is positioned. Hold the baby in an upright or semi-upright position. Place the container of milk level with, above, or below the baby's head, depending on the desired rate of flow. You can raise or lower the syringe or supplementer to achieve the appropriate flow.

Ensure that the nail of the index finger is short and smooth. If the mother has long nails, she can wear a non-latex glove to prevent scratching and protect the baby from possible bacteria under her nails. As you teach the mother, lay the tubing along the fat pad of the finger. Because the finger does not elongate as the nipple would in the baby's mouth, place the end of the tube flush with the finger or a few centimeters behind it to prevent the tubing from poking the baby. If you wish, you can tape the tubing to your finger. Gently tickle the baby's lips so he will open his mouth for your finger. Never push your finger into his mouth. Wait until the baby invites you to insert your finger, and then place the fat pad of your finger with the tube on it into the baby's mouth against the hard palate (the fingernail will be against the baby's tongue).

The baby's condition and the reason he needs finger feeding will determine the number of times this technique is used and the amount of milk he receives. If possible, hold the baby against the breast, as for breastfeeding. Be sure that he is at a 45-degree angle to avoid milk getting into his ears. The goal is to elicit one suck per swallow, as with breastfeeding. More than four sucks per swallow may be tiring to the baby.

Evaluating the baby's actions during finger feeding can be a helpful diagnostic tool. If he cannot suckle, does not respond to the finger by suckling, cannot sustain sucking bursts, or takes three or four sucks to form a bolus big enough to swallow, finger feeding is not a useful feeding method. Make sure the baby's caregiver knows that the baby is not suckling. He may need to be syringe fed, with the parent pacing the feedings, or possibly gavage fed. Increased calories through gavage or syringe feeding may help him start suckling more effectively.

Encourage the mother to check her baby's mouth several times each day to make sure the tubing is not irritating the roof of his mouth. After every use, she needs to flush out the tubing with cold water, wash with hot soapy water, and rinse with clear water. Water can be siphoned through the tube by sucking on the other end if necessary.

Syringe Feeding

Some IBCLCs use a standard or periodontal syringe either with finger feeding or at the breast (Figure 21.20). As with all alternate feeding methods, be cautious when using a syringe. Feeding a baby with a syringe places the caregiver in control, not the baby. Teach parents to deliver the milk bolus just a little bit at a time and not to squirt the milk into the baby's mouth. Squirting the milk could cause aspiration, especially when done by someone who is inexperienced with the use of a syringe.

Both the periodontal syringe and the standard syringe have sharp points, presenting the possibility of scratching or gouging the baby's tongue, gums, or palate. Teach parents to keep the syringe forward and in the middle of the baby's mouth. If using a syringe with a finger, place the syringe in the corner of the baby's mouth. Placing a small amount of milk toward the front third of the baby's tongue encourages him to extend his tongue. Some babies quickly become proficient at sucking on a syringe and learn to pace themselves. When the baby starts to suck, he can be put to the mother's breast.

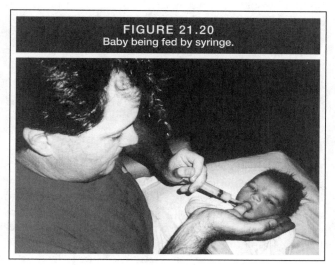

FIGURE 21.20
Baby being fed by syringe.

Printed with permission of Kay Hoover.

Spoon Feeding

Occasionally, all babies need is an infusion of calories to get them started with breastfeeding. If the baby is unable to latch on or sustain a suck, the mother can express colostrum onto a spoon. To feed the baby by spoon, she places the tip of the spoon gently at the tip of the baby's tongue and ladles the colostrum onto his tongue a few drops at a time. Most babies love the taste of colostrum and will extend their tongues to lap it. This small feeding may rouse the baby enough for the mother to put him to breast and try feeding again. You can reassure her that the range of intake for a $7\frac{1}{2}$ pound baby in the first day of life is from 10.2 ml to 108.8 ml (.3 to 3.6 oz), with an average of 13 ml/kg (.43 oz/pound) of weight, or 44.2 ml (1.47 oz) the first day (Casey, 1986).

Bottle Feeding

Baby bottles carry the powerful influence of cultural acceptance and encouragement, often to the point of excluding breastfeeding. Some mothers may lack support for the use of any alternative feeding device other than a bottle. A mother may decide she is only comfortable with the use of the bottle, or she may try another alternative feeding method for some time and decide to switch to a bottle.

Parents deserve to know the risks involved with bottle-feeding. Long-term use of artificial nipples can weaken a baby's suck and contribute to malocclusion. There is a marked difference between the breast and an artificial nipple within the baby's oral cavity during feeding. When a baby breastfeeds, he fills his entire oral cavity with breast tissue, not just with the nipple. No artificial nipple on the market can conform to the individual shape of the baby's mouth in the way a mother's breast does.

Another consideration is the difference in the baby's mouth action on the breast and with a bottle (Ramsay, 2004; Smith, 1988). On the breast, the baby is in charge. For the most part, when he suckles, the breast responds to his action with varying degrees of milk flow. When he stops suckling, the flow also stops. With bottle-feeding, the baby's action changes to one of protecting his airway. The bottle provides a continuous flow of fluid, and the baby must clamp the nipple in order to stop the flow. No bottle and nipple currently available is able to mimic baby-led feeding at the breast.

Appropriate Use of Bottles

Babies who have trouble breastfeeding frequently receive supplements in bottles. Many preterm babies receive a bottle before breastfeeding, even though studies have shown that oxygenation rates are more stable with breast-feeding (Chen, 2000; Meier, 1988). Used appropriately, a bottle can be a therapeutic tool to help a baby learn to breastfeed (Kassing, 2002; Wilson-Clay, 2002). Some IBCLCs have observed that it may not be so much the nipple that causes problems as it is the rate of flow. Even "slow-flow" nipples continue to drip when the bottle is turned upside down and will squirt when barely compressed. The mechanics of suck/swallow/breathe that feeding specialists observe in healthy babies can form a basis for appropriate bottle-feeding (Wolf, 1992).

Selecting a Bottle Nipple

Mothers who combine breastfeeding and bottle-feeding will usually want to avoid a bottle nipple that has a small base (Figure 21.21). When the baby sucks on this type of nipple, he tends to purse his lips, an action he may repeat when he is put to breast. A nipple with a large base forces the baby to open his mouth wide, as he does with breastfeeding (Figure 21.22). The wide base can help minimize latch difficulties when he switches back and forth between breast and bottle.

Some babies have difficulty pulling a nipple with a large base back far enough into the mouth to flange their lips on the wide part of the base. Instead, they slide down and purse their lips around the narrow part of the nipple. A few bottles on the market have a shorter teat, illustrated by the nipple on the left in Figure 21.22. If the mother hears smacking or clicking when the baby drinks from a bottle, she can try a different nipple, avoiding one that causes the baby to purse his lips.

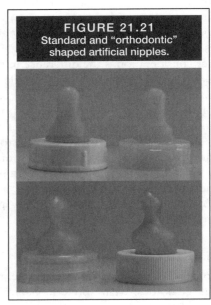

FIGURE 21.21
Standard and "orthodontic" shaped artificial nipples.

Printed with permission of Anna Swisher.

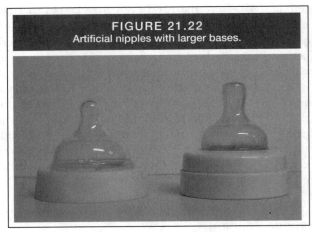

FIGURE 21.22
Artificial nipples with larger bases.

Printed with permission of Anna Swisher.

Another issue related to artificial nipples is the choice between latex and silicone. Latex nipples are cheaper and are available in more shapes than those made of silicone. They do not last as long, however. Latex nipples can become rather gummy, particularly after boiling. There is also concern that boiling latex can release nitrates, which are potentially carcinogenic. Many people are latex allergic. Using latex teats and pacifiers could precipitate this reaction in a susceptible infant. Although silicone nipples are firmer and more expensive, they withstand boiling better than the latex ones and thus last considerably longer. Silicone nipples are a potential source of silicone ingestion.

Selecting a Feeding Bottle

It probably does not much matter what type of bottle the mother uses. However, because there are no antibacterial agents in formula, it is important that the mother clean the bottle thoroughly with a bottle brush that can reach into every crevice. She probably cannot clean the elongated "0" shaped bottle designed for easy holding by the baby as well as she can clean a plain bottle. Parents should use a bottle that is easiest for the feeder to hold comfortably, especially as feedings may take a long time (Wolf, 1992). Using an angled bottle may give the baby more control, especially if he is held in an upright or semi-upright position.

Responding to the Baby's Feeding Cues

A bottle delivers milk without much effort on the baby's part. Parents will need to watch their baby for cues that he is responding favorably to the feeding and is able to nipple-feed appropriately. Table 21.2 presents the signs of stability, disorganization, and dysfunction in nipple-feeding. In addition to watching the baby's responses, parents can optimize their method of bottle-feeding in the following ways:

TABLE 21.2
Infant Cues During Nipple Feeding

Signs of Stability in Nipple Feeding	Signs of Disorganized Nipple Feeding	Signs of Dysfunctional Nipple Feeding
◆ Smooth, regular respirations ◆ Hand activity near face with good consistent postural control ◆ Organized and calm with optimal color and oxygen saturation ◆ Focused and alert ◆ Good coordination of suck, swallow, breathe ◆ Sustained awake behavior	◆ Sucking bursts vary in length consisting of usually 5–10 sucks each ◆ Flaring of nose; uncoordinated suck, swallow, breathing ◆ Worried look ◆ Extraneous movement of upper extremities ◆ Head turning ◆ Irregular jerky jaw excursions ◆ Lack of response to nipple insertion ◆ Rapid deterioration of normal sucking pattern denotes potential aversion to the nipple ◆ Difficulty latching or initiating sucking	◆ Lack of role change between non-nutritive and nutritive suck; non-nutritive is usually faster ◆ Excessively wide jaw excursions ◆ Restricted range of motion at temporal mandible joint with jaw clenching ◆ Flaccid or retracted tongue with absence of tongue groove ◆ Hyperactive gag

Adapted from Seton Healthcare Network policy on managing nipple feeding of the infant and offering developmental support, updated November 2003.

◆ Touching the corner of the baby's mouth to stimulate sucking.

◆ Allowing him to root for the nipple.

◆ Inserting the nipple into his mouth and over the tongue.

◆ Positioning the baby in a flexed position so his head is above the stomach and midline.

◆ Managing the feeding by:

  ◆ Holding the bottle at a horizontal angle to prevent a rapid rate of flow (it is okay for baby to take in some air) OR

  ◆ Pacing the feeding by removing the bottle after every two or three sucks, so the baby can order his suck/swallow/breathing, slow the feeding, and better emulate breastfeeding

◆ Avoiding a rocking motion while feeding to avoid overstimulation.

◆ Avoiding constantly moving the nipple in the baby's mouth, which may cause stress.

◆ Observing the baby for signs of stress.

Stress Cues During Bottle-Feeding

Teach parents to observe their baby during bottle-feeding and to watch for stress cues. Stress cues are avoidance behaviors that tell the parent something is bothering the baby. They include the baby frowning, wrinkling his brow, squinting, or closing his eyes as if in pain. He will appear tense and may flail or clench his fists. Milk may spill out of the baby's mouth. He may stop sucking and gag, choke, or sputter. He may become stiff and arch his back. Signs of stress during bottle-feeding include:

◆ Color change

◆ Tachypnea, or nasal flaring

◆ Shallow breathing

◆ High-pitched crowing noise

◆ Drooling

◆ Gulping

◆ Coughing

◆ Choking

◆ Changes in oxygen needs

◆ Squirming

◆ Arching

◆ Yawning

◆ Hiccuping

◆ Finger splaying

◆ Increased fussiness

◆ Saluting sign

◆ Covering face with hands

◆ Looking away from caretaker

◆ Tongue extension

◆ Falling asleep

◆ Changes in vital signs

◆ Hypertonicity or motor flaccidity

These behaviors do not mean the baby is "mad" or "stubborn." Inexperienced parents tend to ascribe cognitive behaviors to newborns that are not age appropriate. Help them see that their baby is trying to tell them that he is stressed or uncomfortable and that something about the feeding is not working. Paced feeding can calm him and help make feedings a pleasant learning experience.

Paced Feeding to Mimic Breastfeeding

Many babies feel overwhelmed by the amount of fluid and the rate of delivery with bottle-feeding. You can help parents mimic breastfeeding by teaching them **paced feeding**, a very simple technique that parents can do easily. The goal of paced feeding is for the baby to suck, swallow, and breathe as he would during breast-feeding. Babies can suck and breathe at the same time. But when they attempt to swallow and breathe at the same time, they can aspirate milk into their lungs and nasal cavity (Wolf, 1992). Paced feeding slows bottle-feeding to better mimic what the baby would do at the breast.

Parents will often observe their frantic, worried baby become calm when they use paced feeding. He may relax his hands, smooth his brow, and open his eyes. Point out this composure and alertness to parents, and teach them what to look for. Paced feeding teaches the baby that it is safe to feed and that he will be able to breathe. He will learn that feeding does not have to be an aversive experience. A baby who gulps down a full bottle quickly is doing so in an attempt to breathe. He ends up taking in air, no matter how expensive or pro-gressive the bottle.

A few minutes of slow paced feeding can raise the trust level of a baby who is unenthusiastic about feeding at the breast. It can calm him enough that the mother can then put him to the breast. A baby who cannot sus-tain a suck on the bottle, who leaks milk from his mouth, or who elicits no "pop" sound when the bottle is pulled out needs to be referred to his physician. If the baby exhibits such low tone when feeding, a physical or neurological problem may be present. Babies are born to breastfeed. When something does not work, parents need to investigate it, not ignore it, or sacrifice breast-feeding "on the altar of ignorance" (Newman, 2000). Paced feeding is a helpful diagnostic and therapeutic tool for IBCLCs. It is a gentler and healthier way to bottle-feed any baby.

Instructions for Paced Feeding

◆ Hold the baby at a 45-degree angle or greater. Pro-vide postural support to the neck, shoulders, back, and torso. Some babies calm better if they are swad-dled (Karp, 2003). This may be helpful in prevent-ing the baby from flailing his arms.

◆ Tickle the baby's upper lip, just as the mother would with her nipple. When he opens his mouth, let the baby pull the bottle's nipple into his mouth.

It is important that the baby control insertion of the bottle and that it is not forced into his mouth.

◆ Hold the bottle at an angle that is as close as possi-ble to the angle of the breast, so the baby's neck angles slightly up at its most open position, provid-ing a clear airway.

◆ When the baby begins to suck, count to three sucks and then remove the bottle. Observe what the baby does. Most babies will swallow, then breathe, and then open their mouths.

◆ Put the bottle back to the baby's mouth, count to three sucks, and then remove the bottle again. Continue in this pattern for the entire feeding.

Another method of paced feeding is to hold the bottle horizontally in the baby's mouth so that a limited amount of milk enters the nipple. The baby will take in more air, but the delivery rate will be greatly slowed, allowing the baby to breathe between swallows (Wilson-Clay, 2005). Of more concern than swallowing air should be too-rapid swallowing of fluids, which can lead to apnea, bradycardia, and fatigue aspiration. Parents may be concerned that when burped, the baby may also spit up. Encourage parents to try both pacing tech-niques and to watch their baby to see how he responds.

Bottle Feeding the "Breastfeeding Way"

The advantages of breastfeeding for the mother and baby extend far beyond nutritional and immunologic benefits. When a mother chooses to breastfeed, she is making a health choice. She is choosing a method of communicating with her infant that is unique to breast-feeding. This lifestyle and relationship is the natural and normal one for new mothers. A mother who bottle-feeds exclusively can make certain adaptations so that she and her baby will receive some of the benefits of a breastfeeding relationship.

Mothers hold their babies in several different posi-tions for breastfeeding. Babies breastfeed from both the right and left sides of the mother's body and receive a different visual perspective when they change breasts. Bottle-fed babies can receive the same advantage by being cuddled in the right arm for one feeding and in the left arm for the next feeding. Likewise, breastfeeding involves skin-to-skin contact between the mother and baby that is continuous throughout a feeding. Bottle-feeding mothers can make a point to provide frequent skin-to-skin contact with their babies.

There may be a temptation with bottle-feeding to prop the bottle rather than hold the baby. This practice is dangerous for the baby and is strongly discouraged. The baby can easily choke on or aspirate the milk. Breastfeeding mothers instinctively "groom" their babies while they nurse. That is, they stroke, pat, and otherwise touch their babies with their free hand. This is a bit more difficult to do while bottle-feeding. Bottle-feeding mothers can be encouraged to snuggle and hold the baby for at least 15 to 20 minutes after a feeding so that he can benefit from this mothering. They can also be encouraged to carry their baby in a sling or snuggli.

Breastfed babies enjoy periods of nonnutritive sucking at the breast. This usually occurs at the end of a feeding. A bottle-fed baby is unable to suck nonnutritively on a bottle because any movement of his mouth will result in milk entering his mouth. A bottle-feeding mother may want to give her baby a pacifier at this time. If she is bottle-feeding because of low milk production, encourage her to pacify the baby at her breast.

Breastfeeding does not have to be an all-or-nothing experience. With any time spent at the breast, the baby will obtain the benefits of oral musculature and dental development, skin-to-skin contact, and attachment grooming behaviors. Breastfed babies often have the opportunity to cuddle in bed with the mother during feedings, with both of them napping while the baby nurses. A bottle-fed infant does not generally have this opportunity. Taking her baby to bed with her after he is finished eating will provide this special time.

When parents choose to use artificial baby milk and bottles for feeding, it is the role of the healthcare professional to provide them with appropriate feeding guidelines to minimize the risk to their baby. This information will assist women prenatally as they make their infant feeding choice. Maternity staff who teach postpartum patients need to include complete and correct information for those who choose to bottle-feed. Often, much information regarding proper bottle-feeding and use of an artificial baby milk is glossed over or not discussed at all. This does a disservice to mothers and to their babies and does not provide true informed consent for their decisions. Parents need complete and accurate information in order to make responsible decisions.

▶ SUMMARY

There are specific uses for the various breastfeeding devices and techniques available to mothers. Practitioners should use them only when there is a clear need. If used inappropriately, some breastfeeding aids can have a negative impact on breastfeeding. Begin with the least invasive methods for dealing with a problem in order to minimize interference. Provide guidance, support, and follow-up to ensure that the mother has a clear understanding of the proper use of the device. When mothers must be away from their babies during feedings, help them select a method of milk expression that will best suit their needs. Learning hand expression may be all the mother requires. Make sure mothers know the proper collection and storage techniques for preserving the nutritional quality of their milk. Help them learn alternate feeding methods that work best for them. Above all, serve as an advocate for the mother and baby remaining together with minimal interventions. Incorporate special aids into care plans only when necessary.

▶ CHAPTER 21 — AT A GLANCE

Applying what you learned—

Counseling precautions:

◆ Begin pumping immediately when initiation of breastfeeding is delayed.

◆ Use digital techniques appropriately.

◆ Use suck training only if you have appropriate training.

Teach mothers how to:

◆ Do the pinch test to determine nipple evertion.

◆ Do breast massage to help early feedings.

◆ Use reverse pressure softening.

◆ Use the C-hold support.

◆ Use the Dancer hand position for premies and babies with weak muscle development.

◆ Apply lubricants to the breast appropriately.

◆ Use an inverted syringe or everter for flat or inverted nipples.

◆ Wear breast shells appropriately.

◆ Use drip milk safely.

◆ Use a nipple shield appropriately and wean their baby from it.

◆ Select and use a pacifier appropriately.

◆ Manually remove milk from their breasts.

◆ Select and use a breast pump.

◆ Condition letdown for pumping.

◆ Pump for a hospitalized baby.

◆ Collect and store their milk for healthy infants and NICU infants.

◆ Combine, defrost, and warm their milk.

◆ Donate milk to a milk bank.

◆ Cup feed and spoon feed as baby-led feeding alternatives.

◆ Tube feed with a supplementer.

◆ Select and use bottles and nipples appropriately.

◆ Pace bottle-feedings according to feeding cues, and watch for stress cues.

▶ REFERENCES

Aarts C et al. Breastfeeding patterns in relation to thumb sucking and pacifier use. *Pediatrics* 104(4):e50; 1999.

Akkuzu G, Taskin L. Impacts of breast-care techniques on prevention of possible postpartum nipple problems. *Prof Care Mother Child* 10(2):38–41; 2000.

Akre J. Infant feeding: The physiological basis. *WHO Bulletin* Supplement 67; 1989.

Alexander J et al. Randomised controlled trial of breast shells and Hoffman's exercises for inverted and non-protractile nipples. *Br Med J* 304:1030–1032; 1992.

Amatayakul K et al. Serum prolactin and cortisol levels after suckling for varying periods of time and the effect of a nipple shield. *Acta Obstet Gynecol Scand* 66(1):47–51; 1987.

American Academy of Pediatrics (AAP). Policy Statement on Breastfeeding and the Use of Human Milk. *Pediatrics* 115(2):496–506; 2005.

American Association of Health Plans (AAHP). Health Plans' Innovative Programs in Breastfeeding Promotion. August 2001. Available at: www.aahp.org. Accessed August 6, 2003.

Arnold L. How to order banked donor milk in the United States: What the health care provider needs to know. *J Hum Lact* 14:65–67; 1998.

Auerbach KA. Sequential and simultaneous breast pumping: A comparison. *Int J Nurs Stud* 27:257–265; 1990.

Balmer SE, Wharton BA. Human milk banking at Sorrento Maternity Hospital, Birmingham. *Arch Dis Child* 67:556–559; 1992.

Barger J. Lactation Management Course. Breastfeeding Support Consultants, Chalfont, PA; 1998.

Benis M. Are pacifiers associated with early weaning from breastfeeding? *Adv Neonatal Care* 2(5):259–266; 2002.

Bernbaum J et al. Nonnutritive sucking during gavage feeding enhances growth and maturation in premature infants. *Pediatrics* 71(1):41–45; 1983.

Boekel S. Gastroesophageal reflux: The breastfeeding family's nightmare. Presentation at ILCA Conference, Washington, DC; July 27, 2000.

Bornmann PG. *Legal Considerations and the Lactation Consultant—USA.* Lactation Consultant Series. New York: Avery Publishing Group; 1986.

Brent N et al. Sore nipples in breast-feeding women: A clinical trial of wound dressings vs. conventional care. *Arch Pediatr Adolesc Med* 152(11):1077–1082; 1998.

Casey C et al. Nutrient intake by breast-fed infants during the first five days after birth. *Am J Dis Child* 140(9):933–936; 1986.

Charchut S et al. The effects of infant feeding patterns on the occlusion of the primary dentition. *J Dent Child (Chic)* 70(3): 197–203; 2003.

Chen C et al. The effect of breast- and bottle-feeding on oxygen saturation and body temperature in preterm infants. *J Hum Lact* 16(1):21–27; 2000.

Cotterman KJ. Reverse pressure softening: A simple tool to prepare areola for easier latching during engorgement. *J Hum Lact* 20(2):227–237; 2004.

DeNicola M. One case of nipple shield addiction. *J Hum Lact* 2:28–29; 1986.

Dodd V, Chalmers C. Comparing the use of hydrogel dressings to lanolin ointment with lactating mothers. *JOGNN* 32(4): 486–494; 2003.

Dowling D et al. Cup-feeding for preterm infants: Mechanics and safety. *J Hum Lact* 18(1):13–20; quiz 46–49, 72; 2002.

Drosten F. Pacifiers in the NICU: A lactation consultant's view. *Neonatal Network* 16:47–50; 1997.

Edgehouse L, Radzyminski SG. A device for supplementing breastfeeding. *MCN* 15:34–35; 1990.

Goldblum RM et al. Human milk banking I. Effects of container upon immunologic factors in mature milk. *Nutr Res* 1: 449–459; 1981.

Gorbe E et al. The relationship between pacifier use, bottle-feeding and breast feeding. *J Matern Fetal Neonatal Med* 12(2):127–131; 2002.

Hamosh M et al. Breastfeeding and the working mother: Effect of time and temperature of short-term storage on proteolysis, lipolysis, and bacterial growth in milk. *Pediatrics* 97: 492–498; 1996.

Hopkinson J et al. Glass is container of choice. Letter to Editor. *J Hum Lact* 6:104–105; 1990.

Howard C et al. The effects of early pacifier use on breastfeeding duration. *Pediatrics* 103(3):e33; 1999.

Howard C et al. Randomized clinical trial of pacifier use and bottle-feeding or cupfeeding and their effect on breastfeeding. *Pediatrics* 111(3):511–518; 2003.

Human Milk Banking Association of North America (HMBANA). Best practice for pumping, storing and handling of mother's own milk in hospital and at home. Available at: www.hmbana.org. Accessed November 10, 2004.

Hunziker UA, Barr RG. Increased carrying reduces infant crying: A randomized controlled trial. *Pediatrics* 77:641–648; 1986.

Jackson D et al. The automatic sampling shield: A device for sampling suckled breast milk. *Early Hum Dev* 15(5): 295–306; 1987.

Karp H. *The Happiest Baby on the Block: The New Way to Calm Crying and Help Your Newborn Baby Sleep Longer.* New York: Bantam; 2003.

Kassing D. Bottle-feeding as a tool to reinforce breastfeeding. *J Hum Lact* 18(1):56–60; 2002.

Kesaree N et al. Treatment of inverted nipples using a disposable syringe. *J Hum Lact* 9:27–29; 1993.

Lang S et al. Cup feeding: An alternative method of infant feeding. *Arch Dis Child* 71:365–369; 1994.

Larson E. Sucking, chewing, and feeding habits and the development of crossbite: A longitudinal study of girls from birth to 3 years of age. *Angle Orthod* 71(2):116–119; 2001.

MAIN Trial Collaborative Group. Preparing for breast feeding: Treatment of inverted and nonprotractile nipples in pregnancy. *Midwifery* 10:200–214; 1994.

Marshall TA et al. Associations between intakes of fluoride from beverages during infancy and dental fluorosis of primary teeth. *J Am Coll Nutr* 23(2):108–116; 2004.

Marx CM et al. Vitamin E concentrations in serum of newborn infants after topical use of vitamin E in nursing mothers. *Am J Obstet Gynecol* 152:668–670; 1985.

Mattos-Graner R et al. Relation of oral yeast infection in Brazilian infants and use of a pacifier. *ASDC J Dent Child* 68(1):33–36, 10; 2001.

Meier P et al. Nipple shields for preterm infants: Effect on milk transfer and duration of breastfeeding. *J Hum Lact* 16(2):106–114; 2000.

Meier P. Bottle- and breast-feeding: Effects on transcutaneous oxygen pressure and temperature in preterm infants. *Nurs Res* 37(1):36–41; 1988.

Morton J. Breastfeeding the preterm infant, Lessons for all. Amarillo Conference, Human Lactation: Current Research and Clinical Implications, Breastmilk for Pre-term Babies; October 21, 2004.

Narayanan I, Bambroo A. Alternative methods of feeding low birthweight infants: An additional support to kangaroo mother care. 4th International Workshop on Kangaroo Mother Care. Cape Town, South Africa; November 27, 2002.

Nemethy M, Clore ER. Microwave heating of formula and breastmilk. *J Pediatr Health Care* 4:131–135; 1990.

Newman J. Handout #15. Breast Compression. January, 2005. Available at: www.breastfeedingonline.com/15.html. Accessed March 3, 2005.

Newman J, Pitman T. *The Ultimate Breastfeeding Book of Answers*. Roseville, CA: Prima; 2000.

Nowak A et al. Imaging evaluation of artificial nipples during bottle-feeding. *Arch Pediatr Adolesc Med* 148(1):40–42; 1994.

Palmer B. Sleep apnea from an anatomical, anthropologic and developmental perspective. Presentation to the Academy of Dental Sleep Medicine, Philadelphia; June 4, 2004.

Pierce K, Tully MR. Mother's own milk: Guidelines for storage and handling. *J Hum Lact* 8:159–160; 1992.

Pittard W et al. Bacteriostatic qualities of human milk. *J Pediatr* 107:240–243; 1985.

Pittard W. Bacterial contamination of human milk: Container type and method of expression. *Am J Perinatol* 8:25–27; 1991.

Quan R et al. Effects of microwave radiation on anti-infective factors in human milk. *Pediatrics* 89:667–669; 1992.

Ramsay D. Ultrasound imaging of the sucking mechanics of the term infant. Amarillo Conference, Human Lactation: Current Research and Clinical Implications, Amarillo, TX; October 22, 2004.

Righard L, Alade M. Breastfeeding and the use of pacifiers. *Birth* 24:116–120; 1997.

Righard L. Are breastfeeding problems related to incorrect breastfeeding technique and the use of pacifiers and bottles? *Birth* 25:40–44; 1998.

Rocha N, Martinez F, Jorge S. Cup or bottle for preterm infants: Effects on oxygen saturation, weight gain, and breastfeeding. *J Hum Lact* 18(2):132–138; 2002.

Sideman A. American mothers to solve breast feeding problems with some help from India. Rediff on the Net. Available at: www.rediff.com/news/1999/jun/09us2.htm. Accessed September 15, 2004.

Smith WL, Erenbert A, Nowak A. Imaging evaluation of the human nipple during breast-feeding. *Am J Dis Child* 142:76–78; 1988.

Soares M et al. Pacifier use and its relationship with early weaning in infants born at a child-friendly hospital. *J Pediatr (Rio J)* 79(4):309–316; 2003.

Sosa R, Barness L. Bacterial growth in refrigerated human milk. *Am J Dis Child* 141:111–112; 1987.

Ullah S, Griffiths P. Does the use of pacifiers shorten breastfeeding duration in infants? *Br J Community Nurs* 8(10):458–463; 2003.

Vogel A et al. The impact of pacifier use on breastfeeding: A prospective cohort study. *J Paediatr Child Health* 37(1):58–63; 2001.

Walker M. Management of selected early breastfeeding problems seen in clinical practice. *Birth* 16:148–158; 1989.

Warren J et al. Pacifier use and the occurrence of otitis media in the first year of life. *Ped Dentistry* 23(2):103–107; 2001.

Wellstart. Expert work group meeting. Washington, DC; 1996. (Personal communication from Lois Arnold.)

West D. *Defining Your Own Success: Breastfeeding after Breast Reduction Surgery*. Schaumburg, IL: La Leche League International; 2001.

Wiessinger D. A breastfeeding tool using a sandwich analogy for latch-on. *J Hum Lact* 14(1):51–56; 1998.

Wilson-Clay B, Hoover K. *The Breastfeeding Atlas*, 2nd ed. Austin, TX: Lactnews Press; 2002.

Wilson-Clay B. Clinical use of silicon nipple shields. *J Hum Lact* 12:279–285; 1996.

Wolf L, Glass R. *Feeding and Swallowing Disorders in Infancy*. San Antonio, TX: Therapy Skill Builders; 1992.

Yokoyama Y et al. Release of oxytocin and prolactin during breast massage and suckling in puerperal women. *Eur J Obstet Gynecol Reprod Biol* 53:17–20; 1994.

Zardetto C et al. Effects of different pacifiers on the primary dentition and oral myofunctional strutures of preschool children. *Pediatr Dent* 24(6):552–560; 2002.

▶ **BIBLIOGRAPHY**

Arnold L, Larson E. Immunologic benefits of breastmilk in relation to human milk banking. *Am J Infect Control* 21:235–242; 1993.

Auerbach KA. The effect of nipple shields on maternal milk volume. *JOGNN* 19:419–427; 1990.

Henderson T et al. Effect of pasteurization on long-chain polyunsaturated fatty acid levels and enzyme activities of human milk. *J Pediatr* 132:876–878; 1998.

TEMPORARY BREASTFEEDING SITUATIONS

A new mother may face an interruption or a temporary obstacle with breastfeeding and will benefit from encouragement and suggestions. Understanding the relationship of breastfeeding practices to jaundice will help parents avoid its incidence. Some babies seem to lose interest in breastfeeding or to prefer one breast to another. Parents who experience a delay in the initiation of breastfeeding or who wish to relactate will need advice and support. You can help these mothers see breastfeeding as a way of nurturing, not just feeding, their baby.

KEY TERMS

albumin	inducing lactation
alternate massage	involution
apnea	jaundice
bili-bed	kernicterus
bili-light	lactogenesis
blood incompatibility	late-onset jaundice
breast compression	near-term infant
breastfeeding-associated jaundice	normal newborn jaundice
	nursing supplementer
breastfeeding jaundice	pathologic jaundice
breastmilk jaundice	phototherapy
conjugation	physiologic jaundice
Coombs' test	prolactin receptor cells
edema	rebirthing
exchange transfusion	relactation
fiber optic blanket	remedial co-bathing
gestational age	respiratory distress
hemoglobin	syndrome
hospital-grade electric	ruptured membranes
breast pump	switch nursing
hyperbilirubinemia	transcutaneous bilimeter

▶ HYPERBILIRUBINEMIA (JAUNDICE)

Clinically, hyperbilirubinemia (jaundice) is one of the most commonly treated medical conditions in the healthy newborn (Stevenson, 2002). It is apparent in up to 50 percent of full-term infants in their first week of life (Merck, 1999; Woodall, 1992). Symptoms include a progressive yellow coloring of the skin and the whites of the eyes. In some cases, weakness and loss of appetite occur. Most jaundice is physiologic and will clear up spontaneously within a few days with no intervention and no ill effects. However, jaundice was the most common reason for rehospitalization according to two studies (Escobar, 2005; Johnson, 2002).

Types of Jaundice

At birth, the healthy newborn's bilirubin level is 1.5 mg/dl or less. Over the next 3 to 4 days, it rises to a peak of approximately 6.5 mg/dl. Bilirubin then returns to a normal level of less than 1.5 mg/dl by around the tenth day of life (deSteuben, 1992). This natural rise and fall of the newborn's bilirubin is **physiologic jaundice**. In infants with mild jaundice, the yellow coloring may be difficult to detect visually under artificial light. Physiologic jaundice needs to be distinguished from high bilirubin levels in the infant that result from mismanagement of breastfeeding, later onset of jaundice, or pathology. When the bilirubin level rises above 12 mg/dl and has no identifiable cause, it is non-physiologic jaundice. The term **pathologic jaundice** applies when a disease process causes elevated bilirubin.

Physiologic Jaundice (Normal Newborn Jaundice)

In utero, the fetus produces large amounts of red blood cells, which carry needed oxygen to him from his mother's blood via the placenta. This is his only source of oxygen until he leaves his mother's womb and draws in oxygen through his lungs. The hemoglobin portion of these red blood cells transports oxygen. Newborn infants have more hemoglobin than adults do. The healthy full-term infant is born with both fetal and adult hemoglobin. Although fetal hemoglobin is efficient in handling oxygen in utero, only adult hemoglobin is efficient after birth. Because the infant does not need fetal hemoglobin after birth, his body breaks it down, separates it, and reuses the globin portion. The heme portion undergoes many changes, the final byproduct of which is bilirubin.

Every newborn infant thus has an increased concentration of bilirubin. However, not all infants will have the high concentrations that result in the visible yellow coloring associated with jaundice. Many infants are able to dispose of bilirubin through physiologic processes. Under normal conditions, the bilirubin becomes bound chemically to proteins, such as albumin, which transport it to the liver. The liver converts the bilirubin through a process of **conjugation** into a form that can pass through the bile to the intestine. In the intestine, it undergoes further changes that enable the baby's stools and, to a much lesser extent, his urine, to excrete it.

Frequently in the newborn, red blood cells break down more quickly than the immature body can handle them, resulting in a temporary buildup of bilirubin. Physiologic jaundice occurs when, because of the infant's immature system, bilirubin production exceeds the liver's ability to process it. Bilirubin levels gradually decline as the liver matures, bacteria colonize in the intestine, and the transition from fetal to adult hemoglobin is complete.

Bruising, **blood incompatibility**, or antibodies against the baby's own red blood cells can cause a rapid rise in bilirubin level. Many diseases and drugs can lead to the production of auto-antibodies, which sometimes destroy red blood cells and cause anemia (Cohen, 2002). The direct Coombs' test is used to detect the presence of these auto-antibodies and to help diagnose the cause of anemia, jaundice, or red blood cell abnormalities.

In physiologic jaundice, there is a decreased rate of bilirubin conjugation. In conditions such as hepatitis, galactosemia, biliary atresia, or sepsis, there is an abnormality of excretion or reabsorption of bilirubin. This unconjugated bilirubin remains to circulate freely in the bloodstream. Bilirubin that is conjugated, or bound (attached to albumin), is not in itself harmful to the baby, because it remains in the bloodstream. If it is unbound, however, it can migrate to other parts of the body, such as the brain, skin, muscle tissue, and mucous membranes, where it deposits (Figure 22.1).

Unconjugated, unbound bilirubin migrates toward tissues with high fat content, including the brain and nervous system. Under certain conditions that disrupt the blood-brain barrier—such as prematurity, asphyxia, and hemolytic disease—the bilirubin can pass the blood-brain barrier and deposit in nerve cells in the brain. Bilirubin has a toxic effect on brain and nerve cells and can result in neurological damage known as **kernicterus**, or bilirubin encephalopathy. In extreme cases, it can cause death. The bilirubin level at which kernicterus occurs varies with the gestational and postnatal age of the infant, his birth weight, the presence of other disease, and the availability of albumin-binding sites. Generally, a healthy full-term

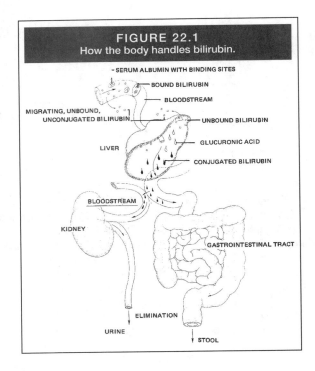

FIGURE 22.1
How the body handles bilirubin.

- SERUM ALBUMIN WITH BINDING SITES
BOUND BILIRUBIN
BLOODSTREAM
MIGRATING, UNBOUND, UNCONJUGATED BILIRUBIN
UNBOUND BILIRUBIN
LIVER
GLUCURONIC ACID
CONJUGATED BILIRUBIN
BLOODSTREAM
KIDNEY
GASTROINTESTINAL TRACT
ELIMINATION
URINE
STOOL

infant will not develop kernicterus when his bilirubin level is below 20 mg/dl (Stevenson, 2004).

All jaundice warrants investigation and follow-up. Jaundice becomes clinically significant when it develops within the first 24 hours of the baby's life, when bilirubin rates rise rapidly, when levels become exaggerated, or when it is prolonged beyond two weeks in term babies and beyond three weeks in preterm babies (Dodd, 1993). Jaundice rates are higher in babies who live at higher altitudes, perhaps because the decrease in oxygen levels at high altitudes leads to an increase in hemoglobin and number of red blood cells (Leibson, 1989).

Breastfeeding-Associated Jaundice

Breastfeeding-associated jaundice is generally a result of such iatrogenic causes as rigid hospital schedules, routine mother-infant separation, unnecessary supplementation of breastfeeding, and pacifier use. The mother and hospital staff may not understand what to expect with breastfeeding. Additionally, the use of labor medications often results in sleepy babies who then have difficulty nursing. The result of one or more of these conditions is inadequate intake of the mother's milk.

Elevated bilirubin levels in breastfeeding-associated jaundice result not from dehydration but from caloric deprivation and decreased stooling. Gartner states, "This is the infantile equivalent of adult starvation jaundice. It is breastfeeding jaundice or, to be more accurate, 'breast-nonfeeding jaundice'"(Gartner, 2001a). In extreme cases, elevated bilirubin can place the infant at risk for kernicterus. Bilirubin levels may range from 9 to

19 mg/dl, with a small number of babies experiencing higher levels (Bertini, 2001). Frequent cases of exaggerated jaundice in a hospital or community of breastfed babies may indicate a need to improve breastfeeding policies and support. "The challenge to clinicians is to differentiate normal patterns of jaundice and hyperbilirubinemia from those that indicate an abnormality or place an infant at risk"(Gartner, 2001b).

Breastfeeding-associated jaundice is preventable through appropriate breastfeeding practices. Establishing policies of obstetrical care based on the WHO/UNICEF's *Ten Steps to Successful Breastfeeding* will eliminate interference with breastfeeding that perpetuates this type of jaundice. When jaundice does occur, treatment needs to target increasing the number and quality of breastfeedings, observing the baby's attachment and positioning, and listening for swallowing. Rooming-in will facilitate an increase in the number of feedings, and frequent skin-to-skin contact at the breast will further increase feeding opportunities.

If the baby's suck is weak and ineffective, breast compression (alternate massage) will help increase the flow of milk (Newman, 2000). If this does not increase the baby's swallowing, the mother can use a tube-feeding device at the breast. If the need for tube feeding arises, she can express her milk to increase milk production and provide milk in the supplementer. She will want to allow her baby unlimited access to the breast, with no restrictions on frequency or duration.

While optimal breastfeeding does not eliminate neonatal jaundice, it leads to a "pattern of hyperbilirubinemia that is normal and, possibly, beneficial to infants" (Gartner, 2001b). There is speculation that since bilirubin is a powerful antioxidant, the occurrence of jaundice in healthy breastfed infants is normal and may provide protection against free-radical cellular damage after birth. The question to ask may be what harm formula causes artificially fed infants when they do *not* exhibit jaundice (Newman, 2000).

Late-Onset Jaundice (Breastmilk Jaundice)

Late-onset jaundice, or **breastmilk jaundice**, most likely results from a factor present in the mother's milk. Arias (1963) speculated that milk from some mothers caused jaundice in their infants by inhibiting the enzyme in the liver that conjugates bilirubin. However, later studies led researchers to believe this was not the case (Murphy, 1981). Other studies then linked breastmilk jaundice to free fatty acids in the milk (Yung, 1977) but this, too, has been disputed (Constantopoulos, 1980).

Alonso (1991) found that up to one-third of 2- to 3-week old breastfed babies had bilirubin levels over 5 mg/dl and jaundiced skin color. Another one-third had ranges of 1.5 to 5 mg/dl, without noticeable skin color changes. This shows a much higher rate of continued elevated bilirubin counts in breastfed babies than was previously believed. It may be that enhanced intestinal absorption of bilirubin contributes to jaundice.

Late-onset or breastmilk jaundice may not become apparent until between the fourth and seventh days of life, when mature milk begins to replace colostrum. Bilirubin reaches a maximum concentration by the second or third week and may persist through the sixth week of life. The baby is lively and does not appear to be sick.

Continuation of jaundice into the third and later weeks of life in a healthy breastfed newborn is actually a normal extension of physiologic jaundice. Gartner suggests that a factor in the mother's milk increases infant absorption of bilirubin from the intestines and the circulation of bilirubin (Gartner, 2001b). Breastfeeding soon after delivery and very frequently minimizes weight loss and helps the baby gain weight quickly. These optimal breastfeeding practices are associated with reducing breastfeeding jaundice and minimizing the intensity of breastmilk jaundice.

Late-onset jaundice is a self-limiting and benign condition. Most cases do not require an interruption in breastfeeding. It can be treated in the same way as physiologic jaundice, with increased feedings and exposure to sunlight. (The AAP does not recommend sun exposure. See the discussion on Vitamin D in Chapter 7.) There are no reports in the literature of kernicterus caused by late-onset jaundice. Some practitioners have the mother stop breastfeeding. Such an interruption, while it may confirm the diagnosis of late-onset jaundice, has no reported benefits to the baby.

As with any instance of jaundice, parents need the reassurance that nothing is wrong with either the mother's milk or the baby. Prepare them for a long period of resolution if the baby's skin is still yellow after the second week. There seems to be a familial tendency for this type of jaundice (Grunebaum, 1991). It is important to keep this factor in mind when counseling a mother whose previous baby experienced late-onset jaundice.

Pathologic Jaundice

Pathologic jaundice can result from conditions such as infections in the blood or liver, diseases of the liver, obstructions in the gastrointestinal system, and interference with the binding of bilirubin in the bloodstream. Many of these circumstances are also associated with jaundice in an adult. Clinical evaluations and various tests are performed to pinpoint specific diseases. Treatment of the disease, as well as treatment of the jaundice, is necessary in these situations. Because of its diverse nature, it is possible for pathologic jaundice to appear any time after birth. The baby could have any combination of jaundice types, thereby making diagnosis relatively difficult. Blood incompatibility and certain drugs can also result in pathologic jaundice.

Detection of Jaundice

Jaundice is visible when the bilirubin level reaches 5 to 7 mg/dl. Of those babies with visible jaundice, 15 percent will have a bilirubin level of 10 mg/dl or higher. Approximately 3 percent of these babies will have exaggerated or sustained bilirubin levels because of a normal development process in their ability to conjugate and excrete bilirubin (deSteuben, 1992). If the infant is ill or premature, the safe level is lower, and the jaundice requires quick treatment and close monitoring. Bilirubin levels are 3 points lower in babies who nurse more than 8 times per day compared with those who nurse less frequently (De Carvalho, 1982).

As jaundice increases, the yellowing progresses from the head down to the chest, to the knees, lower legs and arms, and finally to the hands and feet. Bilirubin levels correspond to the visual jaundicing of the baby's body. Jaundice at shoulder level correlates to a bilirubin level of 5 to 7 mg/dl. A bilirubin of 7 to 10 mg/dl will show jaundice to the level of the umbilicus. Jaundice below the umbilicus indicates a level of 10 to 12 mg/dl. Jaundice below the knees corresponds to a bilirubin level greater than 15 mg/dl (Kramer, 1969).

When clinicians suspect jaundice or detect it visually, they perform a blood test to determine the bilirubin level. Some hospitals routinely check bilirubin levels of all newborns on the third postpartum day. The decision to draw a serum bilirubin level most often depends on the assessed level of jaundice (Schumacher, 1990). The test usually consists of pricking the infant's heel to fill a very thin tube with blood for analysis. In addition, the infant is clinically evaluated to rule out disease and infection. Blood types of both the mother and baby are evaluated to rule out blood incompatibilities. Assessment of the Coombs' test performed at birth is coordinated with these other tests to check for antiglobulins in the baby's blood.

A baby with a high bilirubin count may receive multiple heel sticks throughout the course of his treatment. It has been found that breastfeeding during painful procedures is a "potent analgesic" that helps reduce crying and grimacing and lowers the babies' heart rates (Gray, 2002). Carbajal (2003) also found that breastfeeding effectively reduced pain response during minor invasive procedures. Mothers can ask hospital staff to permit them to breastfeed during heel sticks to reduce their babies' pain level.

Mothers can also request a less invasive procedure. Transcutaneous bilirubin (TcB) measurement systems are noninvasive hand-held devices similar to a small hand-held calculator or flashlight. When held over the baby's skin, usually the torso, a number appears on the screen to indicate bilirubin level. **Transcutaneous bilimeters** have been used for years as a quick, noninvasive way to screen babies. If the meter indicates a certain level, the baby will then have a heel stick for a serum test.

The newer TcB devices are reliable substitutes for serum bilirubin measurements (Maisels, 2004). The Chromatics Colormate III estimates serum bilirubin levels from skin reflectance (skin color). The BiliCheck measures transcutaneous bilirubin by analyzing the entire spectrum of visible light reflected by the skin (Bertini, 2002). If parents are concerned about repeated heel sticks, they might ask for a bili-flash, as these lights are called, first.

Treatment of Jaundice

When a bilirubin level is significant, the caregiver may rely on several types of treatment, depending on the baby's condition. For less severe jaundice, regular visual observation and periodic testing of bilirubin levels may be sufficient. Physiologic jaundice is usually very mild and causes no known lasting effects in the healthy fullterm infant. In most cases, bilirubin values rise slowly (less than a 5 mg/dl increase in 24 hours). Bilirubin reaches a noticeable level by the third day of life. It remains slightly elevated for several days and falls by the end of the first week. Active treatment is rarely required as long as levels remain within a safe range.

Increased Feeding

Increasing the frequency of feedings in the early days often helps to reduce bilirubin levels. Increased feedings provide greater stimulation of the gastrocolic reflex, which increases gut motility and stooling, thereby reducing intestinal reabsorption of bilirubin (De Carvalho, 1982; Varimo, 1985). When meconium, which is laden with bilirubin, is passed quickly, the incidence of jaundice is decreased. Because colostrum has a laxative effect on the baby, early and frequent breastfeedings will help prevent jaundice by aiding in the efficient elimination of bilirubin. Additionally, frequent feedings help the mother establish milk production, which increases fluid intake and weight gain in the early weeks.

Water supplementation shows no rate of reducing serum bilirubin levels (De Carvalho, 1981). Giving a baby water causes him to void, not stool. In the past, parents and caregivers frequently placed babies near a sunny window, as bilirubin breaks down when exposed to sunlight or its equivalent. The AAP (2004) states "Although sunlight provides sufficient irradiance in the 425- to 475-nm band to provide phototherapy, the practical difficulties involved in safely exposing a naked newborn to the sun either inside or outside (and avoiding sunburn) preclude the use of sunlight as a reliable therapeutic tool, and it therefore is not recommended."

The breastfeeding mother and baby should discontinue any drugs that contribute to the buildup of bilirubin. If the baby is not breastfeeding well, or if the mother has a delayed onset of mature milk, she can use a tube-feeding device at the breast to encourage her baby to nurse and receive the nutrition he needs. Ideally, she can supplement with her expressed milk. If she is initially unable to obtain adequate amounts from milk expression, she will need to use donor milk or artificial baby milk.

Phototherapy

When bilirubin approaches a level that requires more aggressive treatment, the baby may be placed under a special fluorescent light called a **bili-light** for phototherapy. A bili-light works in the same way as sunlight to break down bilirubin, forming products that are colorless and able to be excreted without conjugation. A full-term newborn with bilirubin levels reaching 20 mg/dl is a good candidate for phototherapy. Treatment often is begun when the level exceeds 15 mg/dl.

Oski (1992) asserted that the belief that a bilirubin level of 20 mg/dl is dangerous is based on observations made in the 1950s of newborns with Rh incompatibilities. The American Academy of Pediatrics (2004) recommends phototherapy with a bilirubin level at 15 mg/dl or above at 25 to 48 hours of life, with a bilirubin level of 18 mg/dl or above at 49 to 72 hours of life, and with a bilirubin level of 20 or above at greater than 72 hours of life. It is important to keep informed of current practice recommendations.

Types of Phototherapy

For traditional phototherapy conducted in the hospital, maximum skin exposure is desirable. Placed in an isolette to keep him warm, with his eyes covered to protect them from the light, the infant usually remains under the bili-light continuously except for brief feeding periods. Some hospitals enable parents to hold their babies while they are under the lights, in order to provide skin contact and additional opportunities for bonding.

Although phototherapy results in lowered bilirubin levels, it does have side effects for the infant. He may have an increased insensible (not perceptible) water loss that could lead to dehydration. He may have loose stools, develop riboflavin (vitamin B_2) deficiency, experience temperature instability, or develop skin breakdown or rashes. The potential exists for eye damage due to the bili lights. Apnea (failure to breathe) may develop due to displaced eye patches (deSteuben, 1992). If the infant becomes sluggish in his responses and has a noticeably weak sucking reflex, more frequent, short feedings and additional fluids are recommended.

Traditional phototherapy increases separation of mothers and infants and thus has been shown to have an impact on breastfeeding. The short period of separation associated with phototherapy can decrease the duration of breastfeeding (Elander, 1984). Less obtrusive options now include the use of the bili-bed (Figure 22.2) and the bili-blanket, a fiber optic blanket (Figure 22.3). The bili-bed provides light underneath the baby, so he is able to lie in it. No eye patches are needed and parents can hold his hand, stroke his body, and gaze into his eyes. A mother can even lean over the bili-bed to breastfeed.

Home phototherapy using a fiber optic blanket provides similar advantages to the bili-bed in the treatment of jaundice in the full-term newborn. Parents can hold their baby, and the mother can even nurse him during

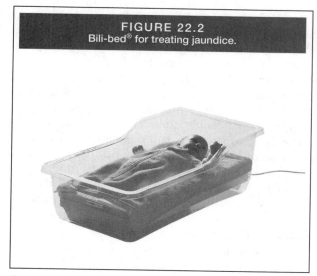

FIGURE 22.2
Bili-bed® for treating jaundice.

Courtesy of Medela, Inc., McHenry, IL.

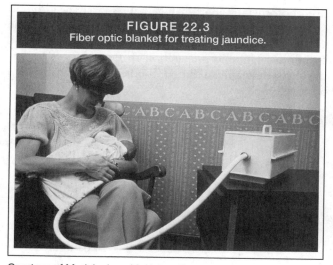

FIGURE 22.3
Fiber optic blanket for treating jaundice.

Courtesy of Medela, Inc., McHenry, IL.

treatment. A receiving blanket placed over the bili-blanket will keep him warm. Eye patches are unnecessary, and treatment can take place at home with the family's support system around them.

A comparison of home phototherapy and traditional hospital phototherapy found no difference in the decrease of bilirubin levels over time. Nor was there a difference in the number of phototherapy hours required for treatment (Woodall, 1992). Breastfeeding rates and parental satisfaction are higher for mothers who treat their baby's jaundice with home phototherapy (James, 1993). Parents with babies receiving traditional hospital phototherapy voice concern regarding the inability to hold their babies and the need for the babies to wear eye patches. Additionally, the cost of hospital phototherapy is five times higher than home treatment. Intermittent phototherapy performed one hour out of every four has been shown to be as effective as continuous phototherapy (Dodd, 1993). As in the use of a fiber optic blanket, it allows for greater mother-infant interaction and is less of an economic drain in healthcare costs.

Familiarize yourself with the availability of home phototherapy in your community. When counseling parents who face a possible extended hospital stay for their newborn due to jaundice, you can suggest they explore the option of home phototherapy with the baby's caregiver. It is helpful to point out the options of these therapies to parents, who may feel overwhelmed with the thought of their baby needing an extended hospital stay.

Exchange Transfusion

A baby whose bilirubin levels fail to drop after phototherapy may require a blood exchange transfusion. The AAP (2004) recommends this serious step for babies whose bilirubin counts reach the levels indicated in Table 22.1. Babies with dangerously high levels receive a combination of exchange transfusion and intensive phototherapy. Fortunately, babies rarely need blood exchange transfusions. They were more commonly done in the 1940s and 1950s, before the advent of RhoGam, an immunoglobulin preparation that prevents Rh negative mothers from making antibodies to their baby's Rh positive blood.

Treatment of Jaundice in the Preterm Infant

In preterm infants, jaundice that is not truly physiologic occurs more frequently and may last for up to three or four weeks. The premature infant's digestive system takes longer to mature to the point at which it can detoxify and eliminate bilirubin. Because the premature infant's brain is especially sensitive to bilirubin, photo therapy is often used to lower bilirubin levels. Bilirubin levels that are permissible in the premature infant relate inversely to the degree of prematurity.

Experience with premature infants has demonstrated that neurological impairment can occur with this type of jaundice. As the infant's liver matures and works more efficiently, physiologic jaundice decreases without treatment. Increasing the frequency of feedings will help speed the reduction in bilirubin levels. Discontinuing breastfeeding does not improve this type of jaundice and will unnecessarily disrupt the establishment of milk production.

The AAP (2004) recognizes in its jaundice management guidelines that even though newborns of 37 weeks' gestation and above are considered to be at term, they may not nurse as well as more mature infants. There is a strong correlation between lower gestational age and risk for hyperbilirubinemia. Babies born at 37 weeks' gestation are much more likely to develop a serum bilirubin level of 13 mg/dl or higher than are those born at 40 weeks' gestation. The AAP's 2004 guidelines for treating hyperbilirubinemia are available on its Web site at www.aap.org.

There is a wide variance between private practice physicians and hospital-based physicians in their protocols for treating jaundice (Gartner, 1998). Neonatologists are more likely to interrupt breastfeeding at each incremental increase of bilirubin than private practitioners. Office-based practitioners' protocols are more similar to the AAP's 2004 recommendations than the neonatologists'.

An AAP subcommittee on hyperbilirubinemia, responding to incidents of kernicterus, found several cumulative risk factors in these tragedies. Those at risk are 35 to 38 weeks' gestation, male, and Asian. They have bruising, develop jaundice within 24 hours of

TABLE 22.1			
AAP Treatment Guidelines for Jaundice			
Baby's Age	Phototherapy	Exchange Transfusion	Exchange Transfusion with Phototherapy
25–48 hours	≧15 mg/dl	≧20 mg/dl	≧25 mg/dl
49–72 hours	≧18 mg/dl	≧25 mg/dl	≧30 mg/dl
Over 72 hours	≧20 mg/dl	≧25 mg/dl	≧30 mg/dl

Source: *Pediatrics* Vol. 114 No. 1 July 2004, pp. 297–316.

birth, and remain visibly jaundiced at discharge. They have a previous sibling who had jaundice and are being exclusively breastfed (AAP, 2001).

Practitioners are urged not to treat near-term newborns as term newborns in the management of hyperbilirubinemia. Infants of 35 to 37 weeks' gestation have significantly lower birth weights, significantly higher serum total bilirubin levels on days 5 and 7, and are 2.4 times more likely to develop significant hyperbilirubinemia than are those of 38 to 42 weeks' gestation (Sarici, 2004).

Parental Concerns About Jaundice

Because newborn jaundice occurs so frequently, it is helpful for all prospective parents to learn about this condition so they are prepared if their baby develops jaundice. High bilirubin levels appear to occur more often among Asians, Native Americans, Eskimos, and babies who are born at higher altitudes.

An IBCLC involved in prenatal education is in a key position to educate parents about birthing practices that have an impact on breastfeeding (Kroeger, 2004). Let parents know that jaundice is a common newborn condition that can be resolved with great success. Reinforcing information for parents after their baby is born will help them integrate the facts and encourage them to focus on ways they can ensure continued close contact with their baby during treatment.

Optimal Birth Practices

When parents learn about the factors associated with jaundice, they can take action to minimize its occurrence. The mother can avoid the use of drugs during pregnancy. Parents can arrange for a birthing environment that promotes early, uninterrupted breastfeeding and thus minimizes the risk of high bilirubin. They can choose to deliver their baby at home or at a birthing center to reduce unnecessary interventions. If the mother chooses a hospital birth, she can arrange ahead of time to nurse her baby immediately after birth and very frequently in the early days postpartum.

A mother can refuse an elective induction performed solely for convenience and thus reduce the amount of IV fluids she receives. This helps avoid edema, which can affect a baby's ability to latch on and may delay stage II lactogenesis. Refusal of induction may also lower her risk for a cesarean section, which is implicated in delayed onset of milk production, and even more IV fluids. She can minimize the types and amounts of medications taken during labor and delivery, which pass through to her baby, and may result in depressing his central nervous system and ability to suckle effectively (Loftus, 1995).

Concerns About Their Baby

Parents can reduce emotional stress by arranging to be with their baby whenever possible. They can request treatment at the mother's bedside and intervals of interaction where eye and skin contact are possible. If the mother is discharged before her baby, parents can arrange for the mother to be "discharged to the room," meaning that she stays with her baby in his room.

Parents can explore home phototherapy rather than an extended hospital stay in order to eliminate separation from their infant. Encourage them to stay well informed of their baby's condition and treatment plans and to discuss any concerns with their baby's caregiver. You can reassure parents that the long-range outcome is excellent. Breastfeeding is the most important thing they can do for their baby during treatment. If breastfeeding is interrupted, you can assist the mother with pumping and help her return to exclusive breastfeeding after treatment has ended (see Chapter 21 for more information on pumping).

Vulnerable Child Syndrome

Vulnerable child syndrome is a psychological condition that can occur in a parent whose child was born with a medical problem or has a chronic condition. The parent subsequently sees the child as being vulnerable to illness and becomes hypervigilant. Researchers found a higher incidence of vulnerable child syndrome following treatment for newborn jaundice (Kemper, 1989). Mothers in both the **control** group and the comparison group reported similar levels of infant health problems. However, those whose babies were jaundiced were more likely to judge the health problems as serious and to take the baby to the emergency room (Kemper, 1990).

Any potential benefits of treating jaundice in an otherwise healthy infant should be weighed against the risk of his parents developing vulnerable child syndrome. Anticipatory guidance you give to parents prenatally can empower them to be proactive, prudent, and effective advocates in caring for their baby. This will reduce the new parents' feelings of powerlessness or victimization and help to reduce the incidence of perceiving their child as unusually vulnerable.

Working with the Baby's Doctor

Parents can work with their baby's doctor to develop a care plan that allows frequent feeding and access to their baby. Understanding the cause and treatment of their baby's jaundice will help them recognize that it will most likely resolve completely within a few days or weeks. They can remain in close communication with the doctor to learn which tests the baby will have, the results of the tests, and what further testing will be done. They can ask which type of screening tool the practitioner uses for detecting bilirubin levels and whether the baby can be breastfed during the procedures (Carbajal, 2003; Gray, 2002).

Parents can ask when the caregiver expects the jaundice to clear and the type of treatment the baby will receive. They can ask about options and criteria for home phototherapy and express their desire for a treatment plan that allows the baby to breastfeed during the procedure (as with a bili-blanket). If the baby will receive treatment under a bili-light, they can clarify how often he can be breastfed and how frequently the parents can have social contact with him. If breastfeeding has been interrupted, they can ask the rationale for the decision and the criteria for when breastfeeding can

resume. See Table 22.2 for further suggestions for counseling parents of a jaundiced baby.

DELAYED ONSET OF BREASTFEEDING

At times, circumstances do not permit a new mother to begin breastfeeding immediately after her baby's birth. A short-term delay from a few hours to a couple of days can result from the baby being born with a low body temperature, having aspirated meconium at birth, or having been born after a prolonged rupture of the mother's membranes. These conditions may necessitate that the baby and mother be separated until the condition is stabilized.

TABLE 22.2	
Counseling the Mother of a Jaundiced Baby	
Mother's Concern	**Suggestions for Mother**
Parents feel bewildered by procedures and other aspects of baby care	◆ Discuss questions with the baby's physician and other caregivers. ◆ Read available literature.
Separation of mother and baby	◆ Arrange for bedside treatment of baby, either from sunlight or portable bili-blanket or bili-bed. ◆ Arrange for regular intervals of interaction for eye and skin contact.
Treatment is interfering with breastfeeding	◆ Arrange for fiber optic blanket or bili-bed phototherapy. ◆ Arrange for regular contact with baby and frequent feedings. ◆ Use relaxation techniques to promote letdown. ◆ Arrange for uninterrupted feedings.
Baby has sluggish responses and a weak sucking reflex	◆ Begin more frequent feedings. ◆ Use breast compression while nursing to encourage suckling. ◆ Use a tube-feeding device. ◆ Use cup, spoon, or syringe feedings if latch is poor.
Physician is considering interruption in breastfeeding	◆ Ask for a delay in treatment while the baby is breastfed frequently to increase his intake of fluids. ◆ Ask for frequent checks of the baby's bilirubin level.
Breastfeeding must be interrupted	◆ Begin expressing milk as soon as possible to establish and maintain milk production.
Prevention of jaundice	◆ Avoid exposure to chemicals during pregnancy. ◆ Avoid jaundice-producing drugs during labor and delivery. ◆ Nurse within one hour after birth and frequently thereafter.

In the case of prolonged ruptured membranes, some hospitals isolate the mother and baby together to avoid a separation. Prematurity, **respiratory distress syndrome**, and other birth complications can require several weeks or months of hospitalization. Although breastfeeding can most likely begin at some point during the hospitalization, it may not be possible in the early days.

Many women who plan to breastfeed give up their plan when they are separated from their infant or when breastfeeding is delayed for another reason. Caregivers involved with these mothers and babies can reassure them that a temporary delay does not preclude breastfeeding. Women who understand that breastfeeding is still possible will need a great deal of encouragement, support, and information on how to establish and maintain milk production until they can breastfeed. Babies who are born with health problems need their mother's milk to aid in their recovery. The importance of this has led neonatologists around the world to encourage mothers to express milk for their babies or to nurse them.

Expressing Milk to Maintain Lactation

When a delay occurs in breastfeeding, it is important that the mother begin milk expression as soon as possible and continue to express on a regular basis in order to establish and maintain milk production. Even if the baby's prognosis and chances for survival are poor, the mother can be comforted knowing that she is providing milk for her baby. If the baby is not yet able to receive his mother's milk, the mother at least has the opportunity to be involved in a parenting role.

Advise that the mother express her milk at least eight times every 24 hours, including at least once at night when prolactin levels are highest. If she drinks fluids before bedtime, she is likely to wake during the night to urinate and can take advantage of this night waking by expressing milk. She will need to travel to and from the hospital to visit her baby if she is unable to room in or stay nearby. Expressing milk throughout the day and trying to recover physically from childbirth can add to the mother's anxiety and exhaustion. She may also have other children at home who need her. Sleep and rest will be important to her.

Establishing letdown may be difficult for a mother who is worried about her sick baby and must turn to a breast pump in place of her baby for establishing and maintaining milk production. She can tape a picture of her baby to the breast pump and play a recording of her baby's sounds while she is expressing. She may find that expressing her milk is more successful when she is at the hospital near her baby.

The type of breast pump that is used will affect the mother's milk production. High quality, hospital-grade, electric double pumps provide the best yield. Despite her best efforts, a mother's milk production may decrease with time. Some mothers find that their milk production corresponds to the baby's condition, decreasing if the baby's condition worsens. You can remind a mother that the important thing is to stimulate production of prolactin receptor cells in the breast. If she has done this, her milk supply is more likely to rebound after the baby begins nursing.

The mother may find it useful to use both an electric and a hand pump for expressing her milk. An electric pump requires less effort on the mother's part and is convenient for maintaining milk production on a long-term basis. She can arrange to rent one for use at home. A hand pump is useful when the mother's electric pump is inaccessible. Some electric pumps have battery backup or car adapters. Many women express milk manually or with a hand pump and do not use an electric pump. Knowing how to hand express will ensure that the mother is not reliant on a pump in case one is not available at a particular time. See Chapter 21 for guidelines on storing and transporting expressed milk for a hospitalized baby.

Transition to Breastfeeding

When her baby is able to begin nursing, the mother may need help in making a smooth transition from milk expression to breastfeeding. Ideally, the first breastfeeding will take place in the hospital as the baby's condition improves. However, it may not occur until after he is home. If the mother returns to the hospital for feedings, NICU staff will provide her with a place to nurse her baby.

The mother may find the first feeding to be stressful. She may feel unsure of how to breastfeed and doubt the adequacy of her milk production. Her baby may be confused about how to suckle at the breast and may have a poor sucking reflex, or he initially may appear disinterested in breastfeeding. The mother may need to increase her milk production and adjust to the difference between her baby's sucking pattern and the pump. These are all issues she can work through with varying degrees of success, depending on her baby's condition. If prematurity caused the delay in breastfeeding, the outcome for transitioning to direct breastfeeding as her baby matures can be very positive. She will benefit from your support and advice until the transition is complete.

If the mother is unable to nurse every two or three hours, she will need to continue expressing milk to maintain production. If she is nursing frequently and her baby is not transferring milk adequately, she may need to supplement with some of her stored milk or infant formula until milk transfer improves. It may take several days or even months to reach the goal of exclusive breastfeeding.

Encourage the mother to concentrate on enjoying her baby and to take things one day at a time. The following guidelines may help the mother in making the transition from expressing to breastfeeding.

Guidelines for Conditioning the Baby to Breastfeed

- Express milk onto a breast pad and place it near the baby.
- Place a picture of the mother in the baby's view.
- During gavage feeding, insert the gavage tube through a bottle nipple.
- Provide frequent skin contact.
- Conduct practice sessions at the breast.
- Shape and hold the breast for the baby with the Dancer hand position.
- Express milk into the baby's mouth.
- Use a tube-feeding device for feedings.

Mothers Who Return to Bottle Feeding

Because of the health benefits of human milk, caregivers strongly urge mothers to breastfeed their ill babies. Some of these mothers may not have planned to breastfeed and may provide their milk through expressing or nursing only as long as it is medically necessary. When the baby is out of danger, these women switch to formula. Even short-term breastfeeding can foster an intimate bond between a mother and baby. Remember that your role is to support the mother in her choices, which include guiding her through weaning when it is her wish.

▶ RELACTATION

Relactation is defined as reestablishing milk production in a mother who has greatly reduced milk production or has stopped breastfeeding. It may follow untimely weaning or separation of the mother and baby, as with a low-birth-weight infant or hospitalization of the mother or baby. One of the most common motives for relactation is a baby's allergic reaction to artificial baby milk.

A 2003 study evaluated whether mothers with babies less than 6 weeks of age can initiate or establish lactation (Banapurmath, 2003). Mothers who had either stopped breastfeeding or were not able to initiate breastfeeding received help with establishing lactation at an outpatient clinic. Within 10 days, 91.6 percent of mothers established lactation, with 83.4 percent achieving complete lactation and 8.2 achieving partial lactation. The study concluded that it is possible to help the majority of mothers with lactation difficulties when the baby is less than 6 weeks of age. Helping mothers with proper attachment at the breast is crucial for success.

Reason for Wanting to Relactate

In one study, 19 mothers were able to relactate between less than 1 day and 3 months postpartum (Marquis, 1998). Healthy babies had weaned when their mothers perceived health problems or time demands. The primary reason for relactation was the child's negative reaction to weaning (e.g., incessant crying or refusal to eat). Healthcare practitioners are urged to consider recommending relactation when mothers wean prematurely and human milk would improve the baby's nutritional and health status.

When a mother approaches you about relactating, it is important that you explore the reasons she did not initially begin or continue with breastfeeding. She may have weaned due to misinformation. Her milk production may not have been up to full potential, or the baby may have rejected the breast or suckled poorly. Her interest may result from family pressure or guilt; breastfeeding can even be used as a factor in a divorce or custody dispute. Understanding her motivation without judging it will enable you to find the best counseling approach.

Along with these considerations, it is important to look at how much time has passed since her baby was at the breast and how he has been fed since. It is important to learn about the mother's breastfeeding routine before her decision to wean. She may need to learn about breastfeeding practices and behaviors.

Realistic Expectations

A mother who is highly motivated and enthusiastic about relactation but also tempered by realistic goals is likely to be more successful with it. If her decision to relactate is at another person's urging, on the other hand, she may lack the motivation to persevere. Learn how the mother defines successful relactation and how she will react if her milk production does not meet the full needs of her baby. Consider how she will react if relactation does not work. The mother needs to assess her expectations honestly and consider possible responses to these possibilities. You can discuss these issues with her and provide a realistic and supportive picture that invites her thoughtfulness and aids in her decision.

A mother who wishes to relactate must understand what to expect and have appropriate information. She will need to determine her sources of support and how those in her immediate household feel about the process. If she has opposition to her plans to relactate, she needs to determine how she will proceed despite the lack of support. After you determine that the mother is motivated to carry through with relactation, you can address issues of milk production and how to encourage the baby to take the breast.

The Process of Relactation

Estrogen concentrations fall rapidly immediately following birth, and prolactin levels drop to normal by about 3 weeks in a woman who is not breastfeeding (Lawrence, 1999). The degree of postpartum breast involution is a factor in successful relactation. The amount of time that elapsed since weaning or the baby's birth is also a factor, with the least time being best. The window of time for prolactin receptor proliferation is narrow (Peaker, 1996; Wilde, 1996). The degree to which the breast empties in the first week determines the number of prolactin receptors laid down in the breast cells (De Carvalho, 1983). The mother may not have laid down enough receptor cells before involution set in if she did not breastfeed at birth. If she started out breastfeeding well and had lactation interrupted by poor advice or a temporary medical condition, she may have laid down a sufficient number of prolactin receptors.

Another factor in relactation success is the amount of breast stimulation, which is dependent on the baby's willingness to suckle at the breast. Frequent suckling is by far the easiest way to increase milk production. If the baby will take the breast, suckling along with the use of a tube-feeding device at the breast will provide stimulation for the mother's breasts and nourishment for the baby simultaneously. During a breastfeeding, **switch nursing** and breast massage will help increase milk flow. With switch nursing, the mother alternates between both breasts several times during a feeding.

An infant's willingness to suck corresponds to his age and to the length of time that elapses before the mother first puts him to breast (Auerbach, 1985). Frequent and continuous skin-to-skin contact in a relaxed, unpressured atmosphere may entice the baby to latch. A drowsy baby or a baby in a light sleep state may be encouraged to latch with skin-to-skin contact and some expressed milk or formula on the end of the nipple.

If the baby is unable to suckle, the mother can initiate pumping using a double electric breast pump, matching the frequency to her baby's feeding patterns. The baby may become more interested in suckling when milk is available, so breast massage can also help. Once the baby is willing to suckle, expressing milk between feedings will provide further stimulation to increase milk production.

The mother can adjust her lifestyle to give total attention to the relactation process and find practical ways to manage her life to optimize her efforts. She will need adequate daily nutrition and rest. If it is available

and affordable, a doula service can help her with household routines. Family and friends can provide invaluable support by doing simple errands, caring for other children, and preparing meals. The mother will also want to examine possible milk-reducing substances in her life, such as oral contraceptives, nicotine, or herbal teas like peppermint and sage (Humphrey, 2003). You can help her find ways to reduce or eliminate such influences. See the discussion of galactogogues in Chapter 18.

Until the mother establishes her milk production well enough to serve as her baby's sole form of nourishment, she will need to supplement with donor milk or infant formula. As the mother's milk production increases, the amount of supplement her baby receives will reduce accordingly. She must work closely with her baby's caregiver to make sure that she decreases the supplement in relation to her milk production and keeps a close check on her baby's weight as his supplement decreases.

Increasing the Mother's Success

Some mothers have success with relactation by re-creating the birth experience (Shinskie, 1998). **Rebirthing**, or **remedial co-bathing**, simulates the birth experience. The baby and mother begin with gentle, calming time together in bath water. After some time, the mother reclines and places the baby on her abdomen. She allows her baby to crawl unassisted to the breast, and root and latch on. The mother can carry out the rebirthing technique when it fits into her routine, as a means of calming both her baby and herself, and as a means of achieving a latch. See Chapters 15 and 16 for more suggestions on encouraging the baby to nurse and increasing milk production.

Because of the emotional and physical demands of relactation, the topic should be approached cautiously. Allow the mother to approach you rather than making the suggestion yourself. Encourage her to view breastfeeding as a means of nurturing her baby and not one of only feeding. Help her measure success in terms of bonding with her baby rather than the amount of milk she produces or the length of time she nurses. A support system is essential to successful relactation, so arrange for her to receive frequent contact during this period. Many mothers who are relactating benefit from the support provided by groups such as breastfeeding after breast surgery and adoptive breastfeeding groups.

▶ NURSING AN ADOPTED BABY

Nursing an adopted baby can provide emotional satisfaction for both the mother and infant as long as the mother has realistic motives and expectations. If a mother has ever had a pregnancy, she is technically considered to be relactating for the adopted baby, even if she never gave birth or breastfed a biological child. A woman who has never been pregnant and is attempting to produce milk is inducing lactation. It differs from relactation because the woman has experienced none of the mammary changes associated with pregnancy.

A mother may or may not be able to nourish her adopted baby entirely on her milk alone. If she begins breastfeeding with this goal she may feel that her attempts are unsuccessful and disappointing. If her motive is to have an emotionally gratifying experience for herself and her baby and an opportunity to develop a warm and loving bond with her baby, she will find great satisfaction in her nursing experience. Success can depend greatly on the woman's desire to nurse.

As in relactation, you would not want to suggest breastfeeding an adopted infant. A general mention in a pre-adoptive class is appropriate. Many adoptive mothers do not know it is possible to breastfeed their adopted child and welcome the opportunity eagerly. You can respond to a mother who is highly motivated and indicates an interest. When possible, point her to resources, such as the adoptive breastfeeding Web site, www. fourfriends.com/abrw, and books about nursing adopted babies well before her baby arrives.

It is time consuming to **induce lactation** in the absence of a pregnancy. Without the estrogen concentrations of pregnancy that prepare a woman's breasts for lactation, prolactin may not have a sufficiently potent stimulative effect on milk secretion (Bose, 1981). Women who have lactated previously are three times as likely to have milky secretions while attempting to induce lactation as women who have never lactated (Auerbach, 1985). If the mother's inability to conceive resulted from a hormonal imbalance, that same imbalance could affect her chances of inducing lactation (Marasco, 2000).

In a study at Massachusetts General Hospital involving five women with adopted infants, all of the women achieved some degree of lactation within eleven days of first putting the infant to breast (Kleinman, 1980). Another study reported on women who received estrogen and either metoclopramide or chlorpromazine to begin milk production, along with frequent suckling (Kramer, 1995). Women who had breastfed previously did not need estrogen. One mother in another study was able to initiate full milk production by the time her adopted baby was four months old (Cheales-Siebenaler, 1999).

The Process of Inducing Lactation

An adoptive mother may benefit from attending a support group for breastfeeding or adoptive nursing women while she waits for placement. The relactation techniques discussed earlier also apply to the process of inducing lactation for adoptive mothers. An adoptive mother can use all the same measures for nipple preparation as biologic mothers. They will want to avoid soap and other drying agents and to check for inverted nipples. Breast massage and back rubs will help increase blood circulation to and within the breast, as nerves in the breast radiate from the area between the shoulder blades. Suggest that she massage her breasts from five to eight times daily over a period of three to six months.

If she knows when the baby's birth is expected, the mother can begin pumping for up to one month before placement to stimulate milk production. A hospital-grade electric breast pump with a double setup will provide the most effective nipple stimulation. It may be some time before she sees any results from her pumping, and she can be encouraged by even the smallest amount of milk she produces.

Often, parents receive only a few days' warning, which does not allow much time for preparation. If she does have prior notice, the adoptive mother can begin pumping several times a day for ten-minute sessions. By the time placement occurs, she should be pumping every two to three hours throughout the day. Many adoption agencies cooperate with the adoptive parents' plans to breastfeed, and may arrange to have the baby fed with an alternative feeding method in order to minimize nipple preference. They may also provide for breastfeeding sessions if placement does not occur soon after birth.

The length of time it takes for the woman's milk to appear and the amount of milk produced will vary with each individual mother and baby. Regular milk removal is necessary to ensure continued milk production (Daly, 1995). Milk production will increase more rapidly after the baby begins suckling at the breast. The baby's age will also be a factor. Babies younger than three months are more likely to suckle when placed at the breast. Other factors are involved as well. In one Australian study, milk output nearly doubled when the mother massaged and expressed milk before and after feedings (NMAA, 1985). Having the baby sleep in bed with the mother so that he can suckle sleepily for comfort throughout the night will enhance milk production as well.

The milk of an adoptive mother will not, in most cases, be adequate for totally nourishing her baby. She most likely will need to supplement her baby with donor human milk or an appropriate infant formula to ensure optimal nourishment. You can encourage her to view breastfeeding primarily as a means of bonding with her baby. The mother's milk production will usually not be copious enough to sustain her baby's growth, and the quantity will increase much more slowly than that of a biologic mother. She can use a tube-feeding device at most breastfeeding sessions to provide her baby with adequate nourishment and reduce the amount of time she needs to spend supplementing. She also can save time and reduce anxiety by preparing an entire day's feeding equipment and formula at one time.

When inducing lactation, the baby's health and well-being must always take priority. Caution the mother to proceed slowly with any decrease in supplement, ensuring that the decrease corresponds with the amount of milk her baby receives directly from the breast. Make sure she understands that she must decrease the supplement rather than diluting it. As a general guide, the decrease should not exceed 25 ml per feeding and she should monitor her baby's growth and output for four to seven days before another decrease in supplement takes place. A diary of supplemental feedings and nursing sessions—with attention to frequency, duration, and the baby's disposition—will help her monitor his intake. Encourage frequent visits to the baby's caregiver for weight checks and the monitoring of other signs of growth.

The baby's suckling provides the best stimulation for establishing and maintaining milk production. His willingness to nurse will improve over time. An adopted baby's nursing schedule is similar in frequency and duration to that of a baby whose biologic mother breastfeeds him. The age at which he begins solid foods and initiates weaning is also similar to biologic babies. Because the adoptive mother will usually not produce enough milk for her baby's total nourishment, she will need extra support and encouragement. Adoptive breastfeeding support Web sites provide helpful suggestions, support, and e-mail lists (ABRW, 2004). You can help the mother educate caseworkers and other caregivers who are responsible for her baby's welfare, emphasizing the beneficial nature of the nurturing relationship between her and her baby. Suggestions for counseling a mother who is attempting to relactate or induce lactation are in Table 22.3.

▶ BABY LOSING INTEREST IN BREASTFEEDING

Some babies seem to become disinterested in nursing as early as three or four months, and most commonly around seven months of age. The baby may be happy to go to breast and mouth the nipple, but then act disinterested or cry. This may happen suddenly, or he may gradually decrease the number of feedings. Most often, such disinterest in breastfeeding lasts only a few days to a week. However, some periods of nursing abstinence may continue for three or four weeks. The mother may become uncomfortable from overfull breasts or feel emotionally drained from trying to satisfy her baby. Encourage her to relax and to be patient as she learns to manage the change in her breastfeeding pattern. She can maintain milk production by expressing her milk regularly and putting her baby to breast frequently without pressuring him to nurse.

This temporary phase is not a sign of weaning. Few infants self-wean before one year of age and toddlers are not fussy when they wean (Bengson, 2000; Bumgarner, 2000); they are simply ready to move on to their next stage of development. A baby in the throes of a nursing strike is unhappy. He is hungry but cannot settle to breastfeed. Reassure the mother that this phase will pass and that her baby will probably return to a regular nursing pattern within several days.

If a nursing strike persists for more than a few days, encourage the mother to contact her baby's caregiver. Babies sometimes refuse to nurse because they are in pain. Thrush, for example, is painful in adults (Worthington, 2002), and it is safe to assume it causes discomfort in babies as well. Babies can have ear infections or other illnesses without fever. During the time the baby is not breastfeeding, the mother will need to protect her milk supply by pumping as frequently as her baby was nursing. She also needs to feed her baby by an alternate method until he returns to breastfeeding.

Possible Causes of the Baby's Disinterest

It is sometimes difficult to pinpoint the cause of a baby discontinuing breastfeeding. You can help the mother understand her baby's changing needs as he develops. Many times, disinterest is a result of a developmental stage that will subside as the baby matures. He may simply be more efficient at nursing and can obtain more milk in a shorter period. He may be easily distracted by new objects and people, in which case the mother can either move away from the distraction or end the feeding and resume when the baby is more interested. She can shift her position so the baby faces the activity and has the best of both worlds as he nurses. She can also let him play and nurse intermittently at the breast.

Extra evening or late night feedings may make up for missed daytime feedings. The baby sometimes needs his mother's undivided attention while nursing. Late at night is quiet, and he may be too sleepy to be distracted. The mother can make a point not to talk, read, or watch television during feedings. Retiring to a quiet darkened room for these brief periods of breastfeeding can help. Some babies may show disinterest in breastfeeding if their parents manipulate their schedules in an attempt to encourage them to sleep through the night. These babies have difficulty knowing when they may breastfeed.

A baby who has an ear infection or a head cold will have difficulty nursing if he must breathe through his mouth. Nursing in an upright position or with the clutch hold takes pressure off his ears and facilitates drainage in his nose. The mother can massage her breasts and express milk before nursing to promote letdown. Performing breast compression during the feeding will prevent her

TABLE 22.3

Counseling a Mother Who Is Relactating or Inducing Lactation

Mother's Concern	Suggestions for Mother
Inadequate letdown	◆ Use relaxation techniques.
Establishing milk production	◆ Begin nursing as early as possible.
	◆ Use regular supplements and decrease the amount as milk production increases.
	◆ Use breast massage.
	◆ Breastfeed frequently.
	◆ Get sufficient rest.
	◆ Eat a nutritious diet.
	◆ Keep a diary of breastfeedings and formula feedings.
Baby is reluctant to nurse	◆ Use soothing techniques and increase skin-to-skin contact.
	◆ Apply the mother's milk or a sweet substance to the nipple (not honey).
	◆ Slowly drop the mother's milk into the side of the baby's mouth before placing the baby on the breast.
	◆ Use a nursing supplementer.
Preparation for breastfeeding	◆ Massage the mother's back and breasts.
	◆ Stimulate the nipples manually.
	◆ Stimulate milk production by using a breast pump.
	◆ Avoid soap and other drying agents on the breasts.
Low milk supply	◆ Supplement the baby with formula; do not dilute.
	◆ View breastfeeding primarily as a means of nurturing the baby's emotional health.
	◆ Have the baby checked frequently for weight gain.
	◆ Monitor the baby's weight while replacing formula with breastfeeding.
Nipple preference in the baby	◆ Use a nursing supplementer, cup, spoon, or dropper.
Mother is frustrated with partial breastfeeding	◆ Simplify bottle preparation techniques or use a nursing supplementer.
	◆ Learn to appreciate breastfeeding as a nurturing relationship with the baby.

baby having to suck as hard to obtain milk. She can also consult her baby's caregiver about medications for decreasing the production of mucus or mechanical methods for removing it before nursing.

Teething pain can make it uncomfortable for a baby to nurse and may cause him to nurse sporadically, fuss, and pull away from the breast. Comfort measures to ease the pain in his gums, such as rubbing them with a cool washcloth or allowing him to gum a cooled teether, will usually renew his interest in nursing. Pain may cause him to bite the mother when at the breast. The first time this happens, a mother may unknowingly rebuff her baby with an overwhelming reaction and he may feel rejected. He may associate nursing with his mother becoming upset because of the biting and may not want to risk trying it again. Skin-to-skin contact

between the mother and baby will help to re-establish trust. The mother can undress and take the baby to bed or into the bath with her. She can hold him close to her body with her breasts exposed so that he recalls what it feels like to be next to her skin. This may encourage him to nurse. Use of a baby sling also provides increased intimacy to build the baby's trust.

A baby may reject nursing because he is satisfying his sucking needs in some other way, such as sucking on his thumb or other object. The mother can put her baby to breast whenever he begins to do this. Sometimes receiving solid foods or supplemental bottles causes the baby to become less interested in breastfeeding. If the mother is giving her baby supplemental foods, she may want to cut back on them temporarily to rekindle his interest in the breast.

TABLE 22.4
Encouraging the Baby to Breastfeed

Issue	Advice for the Mother
Baby	◆ Check for illness or teething pain and contact his caregiver if necessary.
	◆ Discontinue any use of pacifiers.
	◆ Take a warm bath with the baby, with dim lighting, such as candles. The tranquility will relax the mother, and often, the baby as well. Co-bathing works well for newborns that cannot latch, and it often is effective for older babies who resist nursing.
Mother	◆ Cleanse the breasts with clear water before feedings to remove deodorant, lotions, or other substances.
	◆ Discontinue the use of any new brand of deodorant or lotion.
	◆ Get plenty of rest, consume adequate protein and fresh vegetables, and drink sufficient fluids to promote a feeling of well-being.
	◆ Hand express or pump between feedings to maintain milk production.
	◆ Determine if she is pregnant or taking any new medications.
Managing feedings	◆ Nurse in a quiet, dark room without distractions.
	◆ When ready to go to bed for the night, take the baby to bed with her to nurse.
	◆ Attempt to nurse when the baby is almost asleep, or put him to breast when he first falls asleep.
	◆ Express a little milk onto the nipple or the baby's lips to encourage him to feed.
	◆ Feed the baby by an alternative method for a few minutes, and then put him to breast.
	◆ Feed the baby in the presence of other breastfeeding babies.
	◆ Hold the baby in an upright position for easier breathing during feedings.
	◆ If the baby prefers one breast, transfer him to the other breast by gently sliding him over rather than turning him around.
	◆ Use breast compression while the baby is at the breast to increase milk flow.
	◆ If the baby's gums are sore, rub them with ice or a finger before the feeding.
	◆ Increase skin contact with the baby before feedings.
	◆ Use relaxation techniques and breast massage before feedings.
	◆ Increase evening and nighttime feedings.
	◆ Nurse before offering any dietary supplements.
	◆ Reduce the amount of supplements being given to the baby.
	◆ Supplement liquids with a cup or other method that avoids an artificial nipple.
	◆ Put the baby to breast when he begins sucking on his thumb or other object.

What the Mother Can Do

The mother can examine events in her life to determine if her own overexertion, tension, poor eating habits, or fatigue led to her baby decreasing his feedings. She can examine her situation and resolve to care for herself with adequate rest, nutrition, exercise, and stress reduction. During menstruation, the taste of her milk and the scent of the secretions on the mother's skin may change slightly, making feedings seem less familiar and therefore less desirable to the baby. In this situation, the baby will renew his interest in breastfeeding after menstruation has passed. The mother may have begun taking a medication that has reduced her supply, such as pseudoephedrine or birth control pills. There may be the possibility that the mother is pregnant and the taste of her milk has changed or the supply is reduced.

The mother will need to express her milk regularly to maintain milk production and prevent engorgement until her baby nurses again. She also needs to work out an alternate method of feeding her baby while she helps him through this phase. Use of a bottle and artificial nipple may cause nipple preference because of the difference between sucking at the breast and on a bottle nipple. Choosing an alternative feeding method such as cup feeding will avoid this obstacle. Your objectivity can help the mother establish priorities and work toward resuming breastfeeding with her baby. See Table 22.4 for measures to encourage the baby to breastfeed.

▶ Baby Who Prefers One Breast

It is common for a baby to display a preference for one breast over another. While it is often difficult to determine a cause, one factor may be the hand preference of the mother. If a woman is right-handed, her baby may seem to prefer her left breast. She may put him to breast on the left side more often while she uses her right hand for other tasks, unconsciously promoting a preference. By evaluating her breastfeeding patterns, she can adjust positions so that her baby will nurse equally on both breasts.

The baby may dislike the appearance or feel of one of the mother's breasts. Perhaps one breast has a mole, hair, or other difference that causes him to prefer the other one. He may dislike the smell of the skin on one side due to deodorant or perfume. You can suggest that the mother temporarily eliminate these products and wash with clear water before nursing. In rare cases, a baby may seem to dislike the taste of the milk in one breast. Feeding the milk to the baby with a cup can help rule this out. Refusal may result from a plug of thick milk that has broken loose and is traveling through the ducts and out of the nipple. As soon as the plug clears, usually after one pumping session, regular nursing usually resumes.

The mother may have engorgement on one breast and firmer tissue in the areolar area, which does not allow for a comfortable and productive suckle. Hand expressing or pumping to soften the breast tissue may encourage the baby to nurse on that breast. The baby's birth experience may have involved trauma to one side of his face, chin, neck, or shoulder, and he may be in pain when held in certain positions. Careful attention to positioning may entice the baby to nurse equally well on both sides. After the discomfort is relieved, the baby usually returns to the refused breast. A baby's preference led one woman to see her physician, who found a malignant growth in her breast tissue (Saber, 1996). You can keep this rare possibility in mind without frightening the mother with it. Simply suggest that she have her breasts examined by a physician if all other measures fail.

Encouraging the Baby to Feed at Both Breasts

The mother can try various methods to get her baby back on both breasts. She can begin feedings on the preferred breast first to promote letdown and express some milk from the other breast to start the baby on it. She could begin with the less preferred breast, after first having obtained letdown by pre-expressing her milk. She might try doing this at times when the baby is sleepy and less aware of which breast he is suckling. She can also entice the baby with expressed milk on her nipple. Using the football hold will sometimes fool him into thinking he is on the preferred breast, especially if he has an earache or other sensitive ear condition. Simply putting the baby to breast in any new position may do the trick.

The mother will need to express milk from the less preferred breast regularly to relieve discomfort and maintain milk production. Some women decide to nurse primarily or totally on one breast. One breast can produce a sufficient amount of milk for the baby. Although the breast may be slightly larger for a time, the mother can conceal this size difference with loose-fitting clothing.

▶ Summary

Temporary breastfeeding situations often present a challenge to the mother. Preserving breastfeeding may involve altering the baby's feeding routine, as with jaundice. It may mean supplementing at the breast while the mother increases her milk production. It may mean promoting milk production for relactation or adoptive nursing. It may require maintaining lactation with the use of a breast pump for a nursing strike. With your support and suggestions, mothers can navigate these challenges smoothly and achieve a satisfying outcome for the mother and baby.

▶ Chapter 22 — At a Glance

Applying what you learned—

Counseling the parents:

- ◆ Assure parents that a temporary setback does not preclude breastfeeding.
- ◆ Empower parents to be proactive, prudent, and effective advocates.
- ◆ Encourage parents to keep themselves well informed of their baby's condition and treatment plans.
- ◆ Support mothers in their choices, including weaning when it is their wish.
- ◆ Assure adoptive mothers that breastfeeding involves nurturing and not simply feeding.

Teach mothers about:

- Discontinuing drugs that contribute to the buildup of bilirubin.

- Requesting treatment at the mother's bedside, and time for eye and skin contact.

- Requesting home phototherapy with a bili-bed or bili-blanket.

- Expectations and management for relactating and nursing an adopted baby.

- Frequent and continuous skin-to-skin contact.

- Pumping frequency to match her baby's feeding patterns.

- Co-bathing to encourage self-attachment.

Teach mothers how to:

- Feed frequently (10–14 times a day) in the early days to reduce bilirubin levels.

- Use a tube-feeding device at the breast to encourage the baby to nurse.

- Establish letdown and express milk to maintain lactation.

- Transition the baby to breastfeeding and re-establish milk production.

- Proceed slowly with any decrease in supplement.

- Encourage a baby who seems disinterested in breastfeeding.

- Encourage a baby to feed at both breasts.

▶ **REFERENCES**

Adoptive Breastfeeding Resource Website (ABRW). Available at: www.fourfriends.com/abrw. Accessed June 12, 2004.

Alonso E et al. Enterohepatic circulation of nonconjugated bilirubin in rats fed with human milk. *J Pediatr* 118(3): 425–430; 1991.

American Academy of Pediatrics (AAP). Subcommittee on Hyperbilirubinemia. Clinical practice guideline. Management of hyperbilirubinemia in the newborn infant 35 or more weeks of gestation. *Pediatrics* 114(1):297–316; 2004.

American Academy of Pediatrics (AAP). Subcommitee on Neonatal Hyperbilirubinemia. Neonatal jaundice and kernicterus. *Pediatrics* 108(3):763–765; 2001.

Arias IM et al. Neonatal unconjugated hyperbilirubinemia with breastfeeding and a factor in milk that inhibits glucuronide formation in utero. *J Clin Invest* 42:913; 1963.

Auerbach KG, Avery J. Relactation: A study of 366 cases. *Pediatrics* 65:236–248; 1980.

Auerbach KG, Avery J. Induced lactation. A study of adoptive nursing by 240 women. *Am J Dis Child* 135(4):340–343; 1981.

Auerbach KG, Sutherland A. *Relactation and Induced Lactation*. Garden City Park, NY: Avery Publishing; 1985.

Banapurmath CR, Banapurmath SC, Kesaree N. Initiation of relactation. *Indian Pediatr* 30:1329–1332; 1993.

Banapurmath SC, Banapurmath CR, Kesaree N. Initiation of lactation and establishing relactation in outpatients. *Indian Pediatr* 40(4):343–347; 2003.

Bengson D. *How Weaning Happens*. Schaumburg, IL: La Leche League International; 2000.

Bertini G et al. Is breastfeeding really favoring early neonatal jaundice? *Pediatrics* 107:3:e41; 2001.

Bertini G, Rubaltelli F. Non-invasive bilirubinometry in neonatal jaundice. *Semin Neonatol* 7(2):129–133; 2002.

Bose CL et al. Relactation by mothers of sick and premature infants. *Pediatrics* 67(4):565–569; 1981.

Bumgarner N. *Mothering Your Nursing Toddler*, rev ed. Schaumburg, IL: La Leche League International; 2000.

Carbajal R et al. Analgesic effect of breast feeding in term neonates: Randomised controlled trial. *BMJ* 326:13; 2003.

Cheales-Siebenaler NJ. Induced lactation in an adoptive mother. *J Hum Lact* 15(1):41–43; 1999.

Cohen E. Coombs' test-direct. Medline Medical Encyclopedia; 2002. Available at: www.nlm.nih.gov/medlineplus/ency/article/003344.htm. Accessed June 12, 2004.

Constantopoulos A et al. Breastmilk jaundice: The role of lipoprotein lipase and the fatty acids. *Eur J Pediat* 134(1):35–38; 1980.

Daly S, Hartmann P. Infant demand and milk supply, Part 2: The short-term control of milk synthesis in lactating women. *J Hum Lact* 11:27–37; 1995.

De Carvalho M et al. Frequency of breastfeeding and serum bilirubin. *Am J Dis Child* 136:737–738; 1982.

De Carvalho M et al. Effect of frequent breast-feeding on early milk production and infant weight gain. *Pediatrics* 72(3): 307–311; 1983.

De Carvalho M. Effects of water supplementation on physiological jaundice in breastfed babies. *Arch Dis Child* 56:568–569; 1981.

deSteuben C. Breastfeeding and jaundice: A review. *J Nurse Midwife* 37:59s–65s; 1992.

Dodd KL. Neonatal jaundice: A lighter touch. *Arch Dis Child* 68:529–533; 1993.

Elander G, Lindberg T. Short mother-infant separation during first week of life influences the duration of breastfeeding. *Acta Paediatr Scand* 73:237–240; 1984.

Escobar G et al. Rehospitalisation after birth hospitalisation: Patterns among infants of all gestations. *Arch Dis Child* 90(20):125–131; 2005.

Gartner L, Herschel M. Jaundice and breastfeeding. *Pediatr Clin North Am* 48(2):389–399; 2001b.

Gartner L et al. Practice patterns in neonatal hyperbilirubinemia. *Pediatrics* 101(1 Pt 1):25–31; 1998.

Gartner L. Breastfeeding and jaundice. *J Perinatol* 21(Supp 1): S25–S29; discussion S35–S39; 2001a.

Gray L et al. Breastfeeding is analgesic in healthy newborns. *Pediatrics* 109(4):590–593; 2002.

Grunebaum E et al. Breastmilk jaundice: Natural history, familial incidence and late neurodevelopmental outcome of the infant. *Eur J Pediatr* 150:267–270; 1991.

Humphrey S. *The Nursing Mother's Herbal*. Minneapolis, MN: Fairview Press; 2003.

James JM et al. Discontinuation of breastfeeding infrequent among jaundiced neonates treated at home. *Pediatrics* 92: 153–155; 1993.

Johnson D, Jin Y, Truman C. Early discharge of Alberta mothers post-delivery and the relationship to potentially preventable newborn readmissions. *Can J Public Health* 92(4):276–280; 2002.

Kemper K et al. Jaundice, terminating breast-feeding, and the vulnerable child. *Pediatrics* 84(5):773–778; 1989.

Kemper K et al. Persistent perceptions of vulnerability following neonatal jaundice. *Am J Dis Child* 144(2):238–241; 1990.

Kleinman R et al. Protein values of milk samples from mothers without biologic pregnancies. *Pediatr* 97:612–615; 1980.

Kramer LI. Advancement of dermal icterus in the jaundiced newborn. *Am J Dis Child* 118:454–458; 1969.

Kramer P. Breast feeding of adopted infants. *Br Med J* 311: 188–189; 1995.

Kroeger M, Smith L. *Impact of Birthing Practices on Breast-feeding*. Sudbury, MA: Jones and Bartlett; 2004.

Lawrence RA. *Breastfeeding: A Guide for the Medical Profession* 5th ed. St. Louis, MO: Mosby; 1999.

Leibson C. Neonatal hyperbilirubinemia at high altitude. *Am J Dis Child* 143(8):983–987; 1989.

Loftus J et al. Placental transfer and neonatal effects of epidural sufentanil and fentanyl administered with bupivicaine during labor. *Anesthesiology* 83:300–308; 1995.

Maisels M et al. Evaluation of a new transcutaneous bilirubinometer. *Pediatrics* 113(6):1628–1635; 2004.

Marasco L et al. Polycystic ovary syndrome: A connection to insufficient milk supply? *J Hum Lact* 16(2):143–148; 2000.

Marquis G et al. Recognizing the reversible nature of child-feeding decisions: Breastfeeding, weaning, and relactation patterns in a shanty town community of Lima, Peru. *Soc Sci Med* 47(5):645–656; 1998.

Merck Manual of Diagnosis and Therapy, 17th edition. (Beers M, Berkow R eds.) Section 19, Pediatrics, Chapter 260, Disturbances in newborns and infants, metabolic problems in the newborn: Hyperbilirubinemia. Whitehouse Station, NJ: Merck Res Lab; 1999.

Murphy J et al. Pregnanediols and breast milk jaundice. *Arch Dis Child* 56(6):474–476; 1981.

Newman J, Pitman T. *The Ultimate Breastfeeding Book of Answers*. Roseville, CA: Prima; 2000.

Nursing Mothers' Association of Australia. *Adoptive Breastfeeding and Relactation* Nunawading, Victoria: Nursing Mothers' Association of Australia, 1985.

Oski FA. Hyperbilirubinemia in the term infant: An unjaundiced approach. *Contemp Pediatr* 9:148–154; April 1992.

Peaker M, Wilde CJ. Feedback control of milk secretion from milk. *J Mammary Gland Biol Neoplasia* 1(3):307–315; 1996.

Phillips V. Relactation in mothers of children over 12 months. *J Trop Pediatr* 39:45–48; 1993.

Saber A et al. The milk rejection sign: A natural tumor marker. *Am Surg* 62:998–999; 1996.

Sarici S et al. Incidence, course, and prediction of hyperbilirubinemia in near-term and term newborns. *Pediatrics* 113(4): 775–780; 2004.

Schumacher RE. Noninvasive measurements of bilirubin in the newborn. *Clin Perinatol* 17:417–435; 1990.

Shinskie D. Use of rebirthing to facilitate latch in neurologically impaired baby. *Clinical Issues* 3(1):4–5; 1998.

Stevenson D et al. The jaundiced newborn: Understanding and managing transitional hyperbilirubinemia. *Minerva Pediatr* 54(5):373–382; 2002.

Stevenson D et al. NICHD Conference on Kernicterus: Research on prevention of bilirubin-induced brain injury and kernicterus: Bench-to-bedside-diagnostic methods and prevention and treatment strategies. *J Perinatol* 24(8):521–525; 2004.

Thompson N. Relactation in a newborn intensive care setting. *J Hum Lact* 12(3):233–235; 1996.

Varimo P et al. Frequency of breastfeeding and hyperbilirubinemia. *Clin Pediatr* 25:112; 1985.

Wilde C, Hurley W. Animal models for the study of milk secretion. *J Mammary Gland Biol Neoplasia* 1(1):123–134, Review; 1996.

Wilde C et al. Breast-feeding: Matching supply with demand in human lactation. *Proc Nutr Soc* 54:401–406; 1995.

Wilson-Clay B. *External Pacing Techniques: Protecting Respiratory Stability During Feeding*. Independent Study Module. Amarillo, TX: Pharmasoft Publishing; 2005.

Woodall J et al. A new light on jaundice. *Clin Pediatr* 31(6): 353–356; 1992.

Worthington H et al. Interventions for preventing oral candidiasis for patients with cancer receiving treatment. Review. *Cochrane Database Syst Rev* (3):CD003807; 2002.

Yung FC, Cheah SS. Breastmilk jaundice: An in vitro study of the effect of free fatty acids on the bilirubin-serum albumin complex. *Res Commun Mol Pathol Pharmacol* 17(4):679–688; 1977.

▶ **BIBLIOGRAPHY**

American Academy of Pediatrics. Practice parameter: Management of hyperbilirubinemia in the healthy term newborn. *Pediatrics* 49:558–565; 1994.

Auerbach KG, Gartner L. Breastfeeding and human milk: Their association with jaundice in the neonate. *Clin Perinatol* 14(1):89–107; 1987.

Auerbach KG. Sequential and simultaneous breast pumping: A comparison. *Int J Nurs Stud* 27:257–265; 1990.

Auerbach KG. When treatment for jaundice undermines breastfeeding. *Contemp Pediatr* 105–106; 1992.

Beers M, Berkow R (eds). *The Merck Manual of Diagnosis and Therapy*, 17th ed. Hoboken, NJ: John Wiley and Sons; 1999.

De N et al. Initiating the process of relactation: An institute based study. *Indian Paediatr* 39:173–178; 2002.

De Carvalho M et al. Effect of frequent breast-feeding on early milk production and infant weight gain. *Pediatrics* 72(3): 307–311; 1983.

Drew JH, Kitchen WH. The effect of maternally administered drugs on bilirubin concentrations in the newborn infant. *J Pediatr* 89:657; 1976.

Gartner L, Lee K. Jaundice in the breastfed infant. *Clin Perinatol* 26(2):431–445, vii; 1999.

Hale T. *Medications and Mother's Milk*. Amarillo, TX: Pharmasoft; 2004.

LaTorre A. et al. Beta-glucuronidase and hyperbilirubinemia in breast-fed babies. *Biol Neonate* 75:82–84; 1999.

Madlon-Kay D. Evaluation and management of newborn jaundice by Midwest family physicians. *J Fam Pract* 47:461–464; 1998.

Maisels M et al. The effect of breast-feeding frequency on serum bilirubin levels. *Am J Obstet Gynecol* 170:880–883; 1994.

Martinez J et al. Control of severe hyperbilirubinemia in full-term newborns with the inhibitor of bilirubin production Sn-Mesoporphyrin. *Pediatrics* 103:1–5; 1999.

Mennella JA, Beauchamp GK. Maternal diet alters the sensory qualities of human milk and the nursling's behavior. *Pediatrics* 88(4):737–744; 1991.

Newman T, Maisels M. Does hyperbilirubinemia damage the brain of healthy full-term infants? *Clin Perinatol* 17:331–356; 1990.

Newman TB, Maisels MJ. Evaluation and treatment of jaundice in the term newborn: A kinder, gentler approach. *Pediatrics* 89:809–818; 1992.

Rosta J et al. Delayed meconium passage and hyperbilirubinemia. *Lancet* 2:1138; 1968.

Salariya E, Robertson C. Relationships between baby feeding types and patterns, gut transit time of meconium and the incidence of neonatal jaundice. *Midwifery* 9:235–242; 1994.

Seldman D et al. Hospital readmission due to neonatal hyperbilirubinemia. *Pediatrics* 96:727–734; 1995.

Tay C et al. Twenty-four hour patterns of prolactin secretion during lactation and the relationship to suckling and the resumption of fertility in breast-feeding women. *Hum Reprod* 11:950–955; 1996.

Whitington P, Gartner L. Disorders of bilirubin metabolism. In Nathan and Oski (eds). *Hematology of Infancy and Childhood*, 4th ed. 74–114. Philadelphia, PA: WB Saunders; 1993.

CHAPTER
23

HIGH-RISK INFANTS

When a couple plans for the birth of their baby, they anxiously anticipate bringing him home and settling in as a family. Sometimes parents must return home alone, however, leaving their baby in the special care of medical personnel. All parents will respond in their own way to such an untimely separation. Their need for support will be just as individual. Hospitalization of a **high-risk infant** creates trauma, anxiety, and uncertainty for parents. The transition from hospital to home can present another stressful and difficult time. Familiarizing parents with normal reactions and ways of coping will help them learn how to interact with their baby and plan for his homecoming. Learning what these parents are experiencing will help you fashion your counseling to meet their needs.

KEY TERMS

adipose tissue
AGA
apnea
appropriate for
   gestational age
blood sugar levels
bradycardia
cyanosis
ELBW
enteral
gastrostomy
gavage tube
glucuronic acid
grief process
high-risk infant
human milk fortifier
hyperalimentation
hypercapnia
hypoxemia

hypoxia
IUGR
kangaroo care
kangaroo transport
lactoengineering
LBW
nasogastric
near-term
NICU
orogastric
parenteral
postterm infant
preterm infant
renal solute load
SGA
small-for-date
tertiary
VLBW

▶ PROLONGED HOSPITALIZATION OF THE HIGH-RISK INFANT

Except for a brief glimpse of their baby at birth, parents of a high-risk infant may have little opportunity to interact with him in the first hours. Depending on the baby's condition, it may be several days or weeks before they can even hold him. Likewise, it may be several weeks or months before the mother is able to put her baby to breast. She will need to learn how to initiate and maintain milk production during that period, expressing her milk instead of directly breastfeeding her baby. She must also cope emotionally with the delay in her anticipated breastfeeding. More information on this topic appears in Chapter 24.

Parents' Reactions

Care of high-risk infants in a NICU is delivered in the safest and mildest way possible to achieve the best outcomes medically, nutritively, and developmentally. When parents see their high-risk infant in the nursery, he most likely will be lying in an isolette with tubes and monitors connected to his unclothed body. This can be a frightening scene, even if parents are prepared to expect it and have been given an explanation for all of the life-sustaining devices. The equipment and its correlation to their baby's chances for survival can overwhelm them.

Parents sometimes find it difficult to focus on their high-risk baby as an individual. Even with a favorable prognosis, they may wonder silently if their baby will survive. They will want to know what can be done to help him, how soon he will be out of danger and disconnected from tubes and monitors, and when he can breastfeed and go home. They will feel helpless, wanting to do something for their baby, but not knowing what or how.

You can help parents formulate questions for their baby's caregivers. Stress the importance of asking for explanations and clarification of anything they do not fully understand. They may find it difficult to absorb and process all the information they receive from you and other caregivers. You may need to continually repeat, review, and clarify important points for the mother about breastfeeding her high-risk infant.

Feelings of Detachment and Grief

Many parents of high-risk infants experience feelings of guilt, loneliness, and anxiety. They may avoid contact with parents who have healthy babies. Mothers in the hospital may detach themselves from other mothers and babies. Parents may try to avoid involvement with their own baby in an instinctive effort to protect themselves from becoming attached to a baby they may lose. This is a very common and natural reaction. Such feelings usually subside after the parents are able to accept their baby's condition.

Parents sometimes disconnect so much that they emotionally, mentally, and even physically abandon the baby. Most parents work through their loss and do not progress to this extreme. Be aware that parents will move through stages of grief, similar to those shown in Figure 23.4, as they mourn the loss of their "dream" baby, regardless of the baby's prognosis. Once the parents have grieved for and mourned the healthy baby they had expected, they can begin to accept the baby they have.

Need for Support

Parents of a high-risk infant may become overly tired and anxious, which can put a strain on their relationship. Many times crisis brings out unresolved conflicts between a couple. Thus, disagreements or arguments you observe in the parents' interactions may be unrelated to the baby's condition. The baby's condition may be a catalyst for problems rising to the surface. Encourage parents to seek out sources of support, both in the hospital and within their community. Most hospitals have chaplains trained in grief and crisis counseling. Talking with other parents who have experienced similar situations can help them realize that their reactions are typical and may give them techniques for coping.

Support groups are available in many communities for parents of high-risk infants. Attending the group's discussions can provide parents the opportunity to share their feelings and concerns and to learn to put their reactions into perspective. The hospital's social caseworkers should have a community list of resources. It may be helpful for you to compile one specifically about feeding issues. You can also refer parents to resources in their communities of faith, such as a pastor, priest, or rabbi.

Mothers of high-risk infants who have sources of support are more likely to continue breastfeeding (Meier, 2004). Familiarize yourself with available support and make appropriate referrals. Also inquire about the mother's family and friends as support systems. Because of modern mobility, many people do not live near their own parents and will need to establish a circle of support.

A high-risk infant requires a great deal of attention and care, and parents' needs often go unrecognized or unmet. You can take an interest in the mother and encourage her to talk about her labor and delivery experience. Focusing on her rather than on her baby will invite her to share her feelings about her birth, her baby, and her coping abilities. Asking about her sleep, her appetite, and any prescribed pain medication will show concern for her. She will receive information and advice from many sources and may need you to listen to her in an accepting, objective, and interested manner. Sincere and honest concern is natural. Let her know that you care and that you are there to support her.

Caring for the High-risk Infant

Tremendous medical advances have improved the morbidity and mortality rates of high-risk infants. This is due in large part to the care that is available to these infants in special care facilities. Pediatric **tertiary** care centers have the necessary equipment and specially trained staff to care for seriously ill infants. Many times babies can be cared for at the hospital where they were born. This can be a comfort to the parents when the hospital is near their home. In some instances, a high-risk pregnancy is detected early enough so the woman can deliver in a tertiary care facility that has the means to care for both her and her baby.

Parents go through a very real grief experience when it is necessary to transfer their infant to another facility. The new medical personnel who will care for their infant, although very competent, are complete strangers to them. Furthermore, they may be separated from their baby by a distance that will make visitation difficult. The very fact of transferring their baby to a special care facility underscores the seriousness of his condition.

Often, the mother of a high-risk infant has had a cesarean and will not leave the birth facility for three or four days, time in which she will be away from her new baby. NICU case managers can assist families with information on extended stay resources, such as Ronald McDonald Houses and Family Rooms. Information is available at www.rmhc.com. These corporate-sponsored facilities offer free accommodations for parents visiting sick children. Many times, as the baby improves, he can return to the hospital in the parents' community until he is ready for discharge.

The Neonatal Intensive Care Unit

The neonatal intensive care unit (NICU) is an overwhelming place for both the parents and their baby (Figure 23.1). In the baby's intrauterine environment,

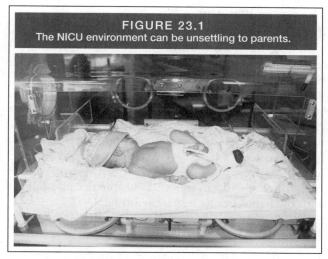

FIGURE 23.1
The NICU environment can be unsettling to parents.

Printed with permission of Kay Hoover.

his mother's voice and rhythmic body sounds comforted him. There was no sharp variation in light, and he was continuously bathed in warm amniotic fluid and rocked by his mother's movements. In contrast, the NICU can be a noisy environment with continuous white noise and harsh mechanical sounds occurring at varying times. Voices often are not distinct, and lighting has no daily rhythmicity.

There are three levels of NICUs. A Level I NICU provides routine newborn care. Level II NICUs care for newborns that may require monitoring and care beyond routine newborn care. A Level III NICU is a high-risk facility equipped to care for the smallest and sickest babies. These include preterm infants as well as full-term infants with severe or potentially life-threatening conditions. Regional Level III NICUs receive and care for babies transported from the surrounding geographic area.

Most touching that takes place with the high-risk infant in the NICU is either technical or medical in nature. He thus may learn to associate touch with unpleasant events. The baby may receive nourishment initially through **hyperalimentation**, intravenously receiving a solution of amino acids, glucose, electrolytes, and vitamins. He will then progress to gavage feedings via **nasogastric** (NG) tubing. Nasogastric tubes can damage nasal mucosa, so limiting the period of NG tube use is a NICU goal.

Imprinting affects babies' feeding abilities, and preterm or ill babies may develop oral aversions (Pinelli, 2001; Wolf, 1992). There is debate among healthcare professionals regarding how much stimulation is appropriate for the high-risk infant. (See the discussion of kangaroo care later in this chapter.) Becoming aware of current research in NICU care will help you advocate for a baby-friendly environment that encompasses the best of high-tech developmental care. You can share with the mother ways she can nurture her infant through gentle, warm, and loving touch.

Interaction Between Parents and Baby

Parents can initiate as much meaningful interaction as possible to minimize the impact of early separation from their high-risk infant. The overwhelming nature of the experience can cause parents to feel hesitant or fearful about interacting with their baby. You can help bridge this gap by inquiring about and addressing their concerns. Encourage their participation, and provide explanations in simple and concrete terms.

Privacy and Time Alone with Their Baby

Parents often are not aware of what is normal and expected for their baby in the NICU. It is helpful to point out what to expect of their baby based on his condition and gestational age. Parents feel less anxiety and more realistic expectations when they recognize their baby's behavioral capabilities (Culp, 1989). They can visit their baby in the nursery, touching and fondling him as much as allowed for his condition. Babies have better weight gains and quicker recoveries when their mothers hold and care for them during hospitalization (Hurst, 1997; Sloan, 1994). NICU infants given massage gain weight faster and are discharged sooner than infants not given massage (Vickers, 2004; Beachy, 2003; Bond, 2002).

Eye-to-eye contact between the parents and their baby is important as well. If eye patches are used, parents can ask that they be removed temporarily during their visit. They can also request time alone with their baby to interact as a family without the presence of hospital staff. Encourage them to take part in caring for their baby with feeding, bathing, and diapering. This is especially important in the days preceding the baby's discharge, so that they can gradually begin assuming their roles as caretakers.

Nyqvist (1993) studied the concerns of former NICU mothers and their advice to other mothers with babies in the NICU. Mothers expressed concern about the lack of privacy and the ability to simply sit and hold their babies and get to know them. Privacy screens and rooming in when the baby is able address these obstacles. Encourage mothers to arrange private time whenever the baby's condition permits.

Mothers in the Nyqvist study also preferred that they, not the nurses, feed their babies whenever possible. Additionally, they preferred breastfeeding to the use of gavage feeding or bottles. You can advocate for practices that protect breastfeeding, such as not using artificial nipples and not requiring successful bottle-feedings before time at the breast (Lang, 2002). These experienced mothers also advocated close physical contact and breastfeeding as soon as possible, both of which enhance the baby's well-being. Finally, they advised that mothers ask questions. You can encourage these behaviors in the mothers in your care and advocate for change in NICU policies whenever evidence-based practices would improve infant and maternal outcomes. Bottle-feeding is deeply entrenched in the NICU culture. Typically, a key developmental goal prior to discharge for NICU staff is "nippling," the ability to suck, usually on a bottle teat (Shaker, 1999; VandenBurg, 1990).

Pressure of Other Demands

When encouraging parents to interact with their baby, keep in mind possible logistical concerns, such as caring for siblings and transportation to and from the hospital. Time commitments present challenges for the mother in terms of rest, expressing her milk, and caring for other children or family members. The father, feeling overwhelmed by rising medical bills, may focus on his job because he fears losing the income and insurance on which his family depends. Many employed mothers must return to work before the baby comes home, robbing them of rest and bonding time.

Although they will want to spend as much time as possible with their baby, parents feel pressured by all these demands. They should not be made to feel guilty or negligent if they cannot visit their baby as often as you or others think is appropriate. Assume parents are doing the best they can in a difficult situation, unless you observe behaviors that indicate otherwise. For purposes of this discussion, both parents are included. The reality is that over 30 percent of births in the United States are to single mothers. In 2002, 10.57 percent of U.S. births were to teenagers aged 15 to 19 (CDC, 2003). Teens are at the highest risk for problem pregnancies and low birth weight babies, and may have little or no support. In such cases, social services become even more vital for the mother's and baby's well-being.

Taking the Baby Home

Many parents of hospitalized infants perceive their baby as needing special care. They are often anxious at the time of discharge and overwhelmed at the thought of caring for him full time. Parents often have advance notice of their baby's discharge; for others it may occur relatively quickly. Parents' emotions will be a mixture of elation, anxiety, caution, and insecurity in their roles as full-time caretakers.

Baby's Health Status

Before a high-risk baby can go home, he must be physically stable and able to maintain his body temperature. He must be able to suck on either a bottle nipple or breast and tolerate feedings by mouth. Small infants are discharged today much earlier than in the past, and babies are no longer required to reach a "magic" weight. Today, it is common for a 3½ -pound infant to go home when he meets three criteria: He must be able to maintain his temperature in an open crib, take the prescribed amount of fluid by any means, and be in stable medical condition.

Discharge Planning

The mother can prepare for her baby's homecoming by arranging for household help, freezing meals for later use, stocking up on grocery items, and any other preparations that will maximize her time with her infant. Before discharge, she will want to discuss a feeding plan with her baby's caregiver, as well as any special care procedures or restrictions. If supplements are required, she will need to know how much and how often she must feed them to her baby. Pre-scheduling a visit with the local physician who will care for her baby provides continuity of care and ensures that the physician is familiar with the baby after he leaves the hospital.

Home Priorities and Responsibilities

Today, 55 percent of U.S. mothers with small children work outside the home. Many women will have exhausted their maternity leave or personal leave options by the time their high-risk baby comes home and will have to arrange for special caregivers. This exerts an additional emotional and financial toll on the parents. Resources such as home health services, specialized day care providers, and respite caregivers may be helpful for these mothers. If the mother has lost her job, you can tactfully suggest the family check into benefits such as WIC, Medicaid, and other social services.

After the baby is home, encourage the parents to limit visitors. The baby will still be recovering physically and the mother will most likely feel drained, both physically and emotionally. Both parents need to have quiet time together with other family members, reestablishing relationships and integrating the baby into the family. Many parents experience an initial phase of excitement, followed by exhaustion, until the transition is completed and enjoyment and self-confidence return (Klaus, 2000).

Baby Care and Feeding at Home

You can assist the mother through this time of transition by increasing your contact with her before her baby's discharge from the hospital. Inquire about her most pressing concerns, and refer her to appropriate assistance as necessary. McKim (1993) found that mothers of high-risk infants are concerned about crying, breathing noises, spitting up, and infant behavior, all of which relate to feeding. It is important to address these issues with parents.

Preterm or sick infants often do not give feeding cues, and mothers may be unaware of the cues given by their babies in the early days. It is helpful to point out any subtle cues such as rooting that indicate readiness to feed. Also, teach typical infant responses that show a sign of overstimulation, such as the baby's breathing changes, frowning, arching his back, waving his arms, hiccoughing, and avoidance of eye contact (Burns, 1995; Farran, 1989). See the discussion about these cues in Chapter 13. One helpful video resource is *A Premie Needs His Mother*, by Jane Morton, MD, 2002, available at www.ibreastfeeding.com.

The crying behavior of a preterm high-risk infant will vary according to his gestational age. His cries may be more high pitched and uneven than those of a full-term baby. He will likely cry more frequently as well. A greater number of preterm babies develop colic-like symptoms than do full-term babies (Boukydis, 1989). They also have a greater incidence of reflux (Boekel, 2000). This can be very trying for parents as they adjust to and attempt to know and console their child. Anticipatory-guidance will help them learn what to expect and how to cope with crying.

Mothers who do not receive enough information regarding their babies' care and expected behavior are more anxious and less confident in caring for their babies (McKim, 1993). You can ease this anxiety and help build maternal confidence. Ongoing support through post-discharge follow-up can assist these mothers in their baby's transition to home.

▶ THE PRETERM INFANT

An infant receives a complete assessment at birth for gestational age, intrauterine growth, and such physical characteristics as skin, posture, reflexes, and fat deposits. Birth weight is also a consideration. The average gestation time for a human baby ranges from 38 to 42 weeks. A baby born before that time will typically require specialized care for a period of time. An infant born before 37 weeks' gestation is considered preterm. Most preterm infants weigh less than 5½ pounds (2500 g). The infant is deemed appropriate for gestational age (AGA) if his rate of intrauterine growth is normal. If intrauterine growth was slowed, referred to as intrauterine growth retardation (IUGR), he is considered small for gestational age (SGA). Full-term babies can also be SGA or large for gestational age (LGA). Preterm babies are classified by birth weight as:

◆ low birth weight (LBW): under 5 lb, 8 oz (2500 g) (March of Dimes, 2003);

◆ very low birth weight (VLBW): under 3 lb, 5 oz (1500 g) (March of Dimes, 2003); and

◆ extremely low birth weight (ELBW): under 2 lb, 3 oz (Siva Subramanian, 2002).

One in every 13 babies is low birth weight, and low birth weight is a factor in 65 percent of all neonatal deaths (March of Dimes, 2003). Extremely low birth weight babies, born at 27 weeks' gestational age or younger, constitute one of every ten low birth weight births. ELBW babies are highly susceptible to all the possible complications of preterm birth (Siva Subramanian, 2002). Because health problems increase with lower birth weights, it is important to learn the gestational age and birth weight of any baby you work with, even if it is months later.

Baby's Appearance and Health Status

A preterm infant's skin is loose and wrinkled, with a gelatinous appearance. Blood vessels and bony structures are visible because there is very little subcutaneous fat. Fine downy hairs may be present on the sides of his face and on his forehead, back, and extremities. Hair on his head is scanty, and he usually has no visible eyebrows. Lacking full development of the cartilage needed to support them, his ears may fold in many positions. Because skull growth is complete before other body growth, his head will appear large in proportion to the rest of his body.

The preterm infant's heart is usually well developed. However, his lungs and rib cage may not function efficiently at birth due to muscular weakness. Because his heat regulation is poorly developed, he will need his body temperature stabilized and carefully monitored. Preterm infants tend to have a higher rate of physiologic jaundice than do full-term infants. This is due to their immature liver and digestive systems as well as low levels of **glucuronic acid**. (See the jaundice discussion in Chapter 22.) Since iron stores deposit during the last six weeks of pregnancy, babies who are born before that time will probably need to receive iron supplements. All preterm infants do not automatically require iron supplements, however, and it is important to evaluate each baby for iron status.

Because of limited amounts of **adipose tissue**, SGA or preterm infants often have problems regulating their blood sugar and body temperature. They frequently exhibit early feeding problems, and may breastfeed poorly and require supplementation with their mother's expressed milk or with an artificial baby milk until their condition has stabilized and they begin to gain weight. After their condition has stabilized, these infants often desire very frequent feedings, as if they are trying to gain the weight they should have gained in utero. Mothers need to be informed that these infants "love to nurse" and will breastfeed frequently and for long periods. Such a pattern is expected and is normal for a preterm infant.

Promoting Breastfeeding of the Preterm Infant

When you work with families and staff in the NICU, it is essential that you keep current on breastfeeding recommendations for preterm infants and update staff as appropriate. Caregivers who work with NICU families must give up-to-date, correct, and referenced information, not information that is based on personal experiences. Presenting factual information to mothers does not allow for a "neutral" position regarding infant feeding. Breastfeeding is clearly the optimal way to feed a baby. Withholding the facts in order to avoid guilt fails to provide valuable information. The mother deserves to know all the facts so she can make decisions based on current, accurate information.

The personnel encountered by the mother while her baby is in the NICU can be very influential in promoting breastfeeding for her baby. Having a specific protocol that covers education, nonnutritive time at the breast, nonnutritive sucking, and the transition to breastfeeding was shown to increase the rate of breastfeeding in one NICU (Bell, 1995). The baby's caregiver is especially influential.

Meier (2004) began an evidence-based breastfeeding program to provide education and support to mothers and their VLBW infants. Two years later, breastfeeding initiation was 72.9 percent and outcomes for low-income African American women were the highest reported in the literature to that point. These outcomes approach the national health objective despite the mothers having had significant risk factors for initiating and sustaining lactation. The findings have important implications for clinicians, researchers, administrators, and policy makers.

Breastfeeding education about prematurity often focuses on the significant advantages that a mother's milk offers to her baby. It is also helpful to point out the benefits to the mother. Only her milk is the same age as her baby, and it will change to meet her baby's changing needs. At a time when she can do little else for her baby, expressing her milk is something she can do to provide a valuable contribution to her baby's health and development.

Establishing and Maintaining Lactation

A mother may feel overwhelmed by the birth of her premature baby and need help getting started with breastfeeding. Nursing staff on the postpartum unit will need to give her hands-on lessons in establishing lactation, supported by written instructions. The goal is to help her develop a plan for milk expression that will meet her and her baby's needs until the baby can be put to breast.

Expressing Her Milk

A mother who cannot breastfeed her preterm infant should begin to express milk within six hours of her baby's birth (see Chapter 21 for a discussion on pumping for a hospitalized baby). Initially, she may express only a few drops of colostrum. You can prepare her for this and reassure her that this is the normal progression for lactation. The amount will increase gradually, and the small quantities she initially has will provide essential health benefits to her baby. Her colostrum can be spoon-fed to her baby if he is able to tolerate oral feedings or can be added to his nasogastric tube. She can drip some colostrum onto a breast pad and place it in the isolette with her baby to familiarize him with his mother's scent.

It is advisable that the mother express at least 8 times every 24 hours, with one session during the late evening or early morning hours. The greatest volume of milk pumped will be in the first 10 to 12 minutes (Auerbach, 1990). Recommend that she allow at least 10 to 15 minutes of expressing time for each breast, using a hospital-grade electric breast pump (Morton, 2004; Auerbach, 1994; Stern, 1990; Stine, 1990). If she pumps both breasts at the same time, she can initially pump for 10 to 15 minutes total time.

Breast massage before and during pumping sessions can lead to faster expression of milk and may produce increased amounts, especially after the mother's milk comes in (Morton, 2004). Longer pumping sessions do not increase milk yield. To increase volume, the mother can pump more frequently throughout the 24 hours. It is very important that the mother pump as often as she can in the first few days after birth. Frequent pumping in the early weeks will determine the amount of milk she is able to produce long-term. Research suggests that mothers with smaller storage capacities may need to pump more frequently (Mitoulas, 2004). A pumping diary can help her keep track of her efforts.

Mothers delivering extremely preterm infants (babies as early as 22 weeks are now surviving) appear sometimes to have delays initiating lactation and establishing adequate milk production (Hartmann, 2004; Cregan, 2002). Betamethasone, the corticosteroid administered to hasten preterm lung development, may also have a negative impact on lactation. The effect appears to depend on how soon before birth the medication is administered (Hartmann, 2004). Since this medication is vital to the preterm infant's lung maturity, withholding it is not an option. Be aware of this connection and follow these mothers closely. More research on how to address this connection is needed.

Stimulating Letdown

Stimulating the milk ejection reflex will help the mother obtain the greatest amount of milk in the least time. Sensory stimulation through a picture of her baby or the smell of his clothing can help. The use of auditory and visual relaxation is another method (Feher, 1989). Massaging the mother's back while she is pumping can promote milk ejection as well (Lang, 2002). If these measures fail to increase the mother's yield, she can discuss with her caregiver the use of galactogogues such as fenugreek or blessed thistle or prescription medications such as metoclopramide or domperidone (Hale, 2002; Gabay, 2002; Cheales-Siebenaler, 1999; Ehrenkranz, 1986).

Fluctuations in Milk Production

The mother's milk production may fluctuate in response to her baby's condition. If her baby experiences a setback, the mother may notice a drop in milk volume. The NICU environment can be overwhelming to a mother. Although her baby may be doing well medically, there may be others nearby who have debilitating, terminal conditions. It is not uncommon for a mother of a recovering newborn to "empathize" for those mothers and babies to the point of affecting her own milk production. Encourage mothers to take frequent breaks for fluids, nutrition, pumping, and walking outside the unit if possible.

Changes in her lifestyle may also affect the mother's milk quantity. A mother who returns to work while her baby remains in the NICU may experience a decrease in supply. Over time, she may notice an unexplained decrease in milk production or increased time required for her milk to let down. Sometimes the opposite is true, and the mother produces much more milk than her baby is able to use. Any excess milk can be stored for later use or donated to a milk bank to help other preterm and ill infants. Without support, many mothers of preterm infants will encounter problems with milk production. Follow-up with these mothers is a high priority in order to support them through these fluctuations.

Human Milk for the Preterm Infant

Human milk can be vital to the progress of a high-risk infant, who is at risk for developing a variety of infections (Hylander, 1998). See the section in Chapter 9 about the reduced risk for infection for NICU infants receiving human milk. Human milk can help protect these babies through its immunologic properties. Emphasize the importance of the mother's milk for her high-risk infant, and encourage the mother to provide her milk to her baby.

Many caregivers recommend that a preterm infant receive his mother's milk whether or not the mother had planned to breastfeed. As a second option, they recommend donor milk from a human milk bank (Wight, 2001). Neurodevelopment of preterm infants fed human milk, including mature donor milk, is better than that of their artificially fed counterparts (Lucas, 1994). Human milk is associated with higher intelligence scores during childhood (Smith, 2003).

Health Benefits to the Preterm Infant

Human milk helps establish enteral (through the digestive system) tolerance and allows for an earlier discontinuation of **parenteral** (intravenous) nutrition. It has a positive effect on both direct and indirect bilirubin levels as well. Studies show long-term neurodevelopmental improvements in preterm infants who receive human milk (Gross, 1993). While breastfeeding a preterm infant poses challenges in the early days and weeks, the challenges seem less imposing when one considers the wealth of benefits provided by human milk.

In light of the health concerns that accompany prematurity, the mother's milk becomes all the more important. Human milk offers preterm infants the advantages of receiving physiologic amino acids and fat. It provides greater bioavailability of nutrients, a lower **renal solute load**, enzymes to aid digestion, and anti-infective protection. Human milk greatly diminishes the incidence of necrotizing enterocolitis. As discussed in Chapter 9, human milk has the ideal protein balance for babies weighing 1500 grams or more. Babies below that weight may need increased calories, carbohydrates, and proteins.

Human Milk Fortifiers

Concern has arisen over whether the total volume of protein and minerals such as calcium and phosphorous found in human milk is sufficient for preterm infants (Wheeler, 1990; Hall, 1989). Landers (2003), among others, has expressed concern that human milk does not provide sufficient nutrition for preterm infants, especially VLBW (under 1500 grams). At issue are the calcium and phosphorus requirements for the VLBW baby's bone growth. Without enough of these minerals, VLBW babies are at risk for **osteopenia** of prematurity, decreased bone mineral content that occurs mainly because of lack of adequate calcium and phosphorus intake. VLBW babies also require higher amounts of fat-soluble vitamins because they have not laid down adequate stores before birth.

One solution is to supplement the baby with human milk fortifiers (HMF), which contain protein, calcium, potassium phosphate, carbohydrates, vitamins, and trace minerals. Preterm infants fed human milk with HMF had improved short-term weight gain, and linear and head growth over infants not fed HMF (Kuschel, 2004). There is insufficient data to evaluate long-term neurodevelopmental and growth outcomes.

Lactoengineering

Many breastfeeding advocates propose lactoengineering for preterm infants, which is also discussed in Chapter 9. The science of lactoengineering, the engineering of human milk, holds much promise. Lactoengineering provides increased calories, carbohydrates, and proteins through the mother's hindmilk. Creamatocrits estimate the fat and energy content of milk (Meier, 2003). The hindmilk that rises to the top is skimmed off and given to the baby to increase his fat intake. Mothers can learn how to do this, thereby increasing their participation in their babies' care (Griffin, 2000). Low birth weight infants in Nigeria grew well through lactoengineering (Slusher, 2003).

Some argue that the focus with human milk fortifiers is often on weight gain rather than brain growth (Ebrahim, 1993). However, this focus ignores the fact that human milk is clearly the nutrition of choice to promote neurodevelopment. Researchers can also separate the proteins and calcium in human milk (Li, 2004; Kent, 2004). The goal is to develop human milk fortification for infants that is made from human milk, not from the milk of other species.

Lucas (1994) points out that preterm infants who receive human milk, when compared with their formula-fed counterparts, show no negative differences on Bayley psychomotor and mental developmental tests at 18 months. Further research shows that preterm infants can catch up to their expected intrauterine growth at 38 to 42 weeks postconception when they are exclusively breastfed (Ramasethu, 1993).

Preserving the Safety of the Mother's Milk

With consideration to the more fragile state of the preterm infant, a mother needs to practice good hygiene to ensure the safety of her milk. Provide the mother with written instructions for pumping hygiene and care of her milk. Encourage her to shower daily, wash her hands thoroughly with soap before every pumping session, and dry them with paper towels that she can throw away.

The mother should immediately rinse any pump parts exposed to her milk with cold water and then wash them in hot soapy water. She must boil the parts daily. Her milk should be stored in sterile hard plastic or glass containers that maintain the integrity of her milk's composition. Individual NICUs have slightly different collection and storage guidelines and usually provide the mother with the desired containers.

Unlike milk expressed for full-term infants, milk from different pumping sessions should not be combined for the preterm infant. The mother needs to store milk from each pumping session separately and label it according to the NICU's specifications. She can ask how the hospital wishes to receive her milk and whether it should be fresh or frozen.

If the baby is unable to tolerate oral feedings or if the mother is unable to deliver the milk to her baby within 24 hours after she expresses it, the hospital may request that she freeze her milk. Wrapping her milk in newspaper or a towel and transporting it in a cold insulated container will avoid thawing. Freshly expressed milk is preferred for feedings when the baby is not yet able to go to breast. The composition of fresh milk is most suitable for the baby, whereas frozen milk loses a small portion of its protective properties. However, frozen milk is still preferable to an artificial substitute in terms of the nutrition and protection afforded the preterm infant.

Feeding Expressed Human Milk

A preterm infant's initial feedings are often via gavage tubing. A gavage tube may be nasogastric, passing through the nose into the stomach, or **orogastric**, passing from the mouth to the stomach. Occasionally, the baby may have a **gastrostomy** tube placed through the skin directly into his stomach. As he is able to tolerate enteral feedings and as he grows more clinically stable, he can progress to oral feedings, including feeding at the breast. In the mother's absence, he can be fed via an alternative feeding method, such as cup, spoon, or dropper. Realistically, however, most babies in the United States will be fed by bottle due to staff time constraints and familiarity with bottle-feeding.

As discussed previously, preterm infants optimally would not receive feedings with artificial nipples and bottles. Bottle-feeding is associated with physiologic and biochemical changes in the infant such as **hypoxemia**, **hypoxia**, **hypercapnia** (high carbon dioxide levels), apnea, **bradycardia** (slow heart rate), and **cyanosis**. Effective breastfeeding is possible for babies as young as 30 weeks' gestation and as small as 1100 grams. Research shows that it is physiologically easier for a preterm infant to suckle on the human breast than on an artificial nipple (Anderson, 1993, 1989; Meier 1988). Mead (1992) showed that the preterm infant can suckle well enough at the breast to maintain good weight gain.

Every baby is different in his capabilities, and should be assessed on an individual basis. Although many preterm babies will be ineffective feeders, each should be given a chance to breastfeed directly once they are physiologically stable. In one study, 57 out of 71 preterm babies established full breastfeeding at an average of 36 weeks' gestational age, with a range of 33.4 to 40.0 weeks (Nyqvist, 1999).

Until the baby can breastfeed nutritively, he can be encouraged to suckle nonnutritively on the mother's emptied breast. This allows him to practice coordinating his pattern of suck/swallow/breathe without the theoretical risk of aspiration. He begins to associate the mother's breast with the smell of her milk and learns that her breast is a cozy, pleasant place to be. Lang encourages individual feeding plans for each baby, a formal strategy designed to progress the baby predictably from parenteral feeding through each stage until he can breastfeed directly. *Breastfeeding Special Care Babies* provides an in-depth reference for any NICU (Lang, 2002).

Preterm Infant's Ability to Breastfeed

Practices differ for determining a preterm infant's physical ability to breastfeed. Readiness to breastfeed begins when the baby becomes stable. Each preterm infant needs an individual assessment of his readiness to go to

TABLE 23.1
Preterm Infant Developmental Milestones for Feeding

26–28 weeks	◆ Receptors present for taste and smell
28 weeks	◆ Rooting, sucking, and swallow well established
	◆ Response is slow and imperfect
29–31 weeks	◆ Odors can be detected
32 weeks	◆ Gag reflex serves as a protective mechanism for feeding
32–34 weeks	◆ Can discriminate taste and show preferences
	◆ May react to smells
	◆ Suck, swallow, breathe coordination achieved
	◆ Shows signs of readiness to feed
35–37 weeks	◆ Rapid proliferation of receptor cells for taste and smell completed
38–40 weeks	◆ Can differentiate between sweet, sour, and bitter tastes
	◆ Prefers odors of the mother's milk or axillae

Source: Seton Healthcare Network policy: Managing nipple feeding of the infant and offering developmental support, rev. November 2003.

breast—irrespective of his size or ability to suck on a bottle. Premature infants are ready to breastfeed when they are able to coordinate sucking and swallowing. They will put their fists to their mouths and feed with only occasional disruptions in breathing and heart rate.

Questionable Requirements for Readiness

Some caregivers continue to withhold breastfeeding until the infant first "proves" that he is able to bottle-feed well. This practice, based on the premise that breastfeeding is more "stressful" for the preterm infant, has no basis in fact. Bottle-feeding may be less stressful for NICU staff because it is faster than breastfeeding. Preterm breastfeeding infants actually have less oxygen desaturation during a feeding than their bottle-feeding counterparts. They also have fewer episodes of apnea and bradycardia (Chen, 2000; Blaymore-Bier, 1997; Bier, 1993; Meier, 1988). See Table 23.1 for feeding developmental milestones for the preterm infant. Requiring the preterm infant to reach a certain weight before he begins to breastfeed is a questionable practice. Size does not correlate with an infant's ability to coordinate his sucking, swallowing, and breathing. Sucking motions and swallowing of amniotic fluid occur early in gestation.

Typically, babies in the NICU may breastfeed up to four times per day before discharge. They rarely progress to complete direct breastfeeding before they go home. NICU staff prefer that the baby go home as soon as possible to avoid the risk of infection inherent in a hospital setting.

Kangaroo Care

Kangaroo care, or kangaroo mother care, is a skin-to-skin care method that has moved from the fringe into the mainstream of neonatal medicine. Many studies demonstrate that infants and parents benefit from kangaroo care, a method that places the baby skin to skin with his mother in close proximity to her breasts (Browne, 2004). It allows him the opportunity to become gently familiar with his new feeding environment and explore his new feeding method.

A preterm baby can begin kangaroo care as soon as his condition permits (Anderson, 2003, 1993, 1989; Hamelin, 1993; Ludington-Hoe, 1992; Whitelaw, 1990; Weibley, 1989). Stable infants may begin kangaroo care even when they are still on a ventilator (Ludington-Hoe, 2003). Kangaroo care may actually assist in, rather than retard, recovery from respiratory distress (Swinth, 2003).

Kangaroo Method

For kangaroo care, the mother places her baby clothed only in a diaper skin to skin, upright and prone, between her breasts. He and his mother are then wrapped together to maintain his temperature adequately (Figure 23.2). The mother can wear a button-down shirt and no bra for ease of kangarooing. In order not to overstimulate her baby, she can sit quietly at first, with minimal or no talking, singing, stroking, or rocking. As her baby's condition improves, he will show an interest in maintaining eye contact. Often during this kangarooing, her baby initially will be in a quiet alert state and then settle down to sleep.

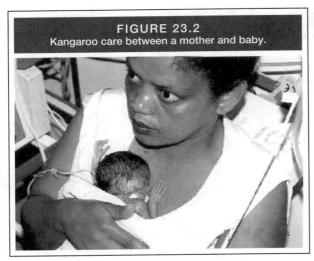

FIGURE 23.2
Kangaroo care between a mother and baby.

Printed with permission of Nils Bergman.

Benefits to Baby and Parents

Kangaroo care offers many advantages to the preterm baby and his parents. The skin-to-skin contact has a soothing effect on the baby. He cries less, his heart rate and respirations are more regular, and he has better sleep periods. He has better oxygenation and is able to maintain his temperature within acceptable levels (Ludington-Hoe, 2004). Kangaroo care is the "only effective, affordable and available method to prevent neonatal hypothermia in most developing countries" (Tunell, 2004).

Babies who receive kangaroo care tend to gain weight faster and leave the hospital earlier. The effects are long term as well, with less crying noted at six months of age and a decreased rate of serious infection in the six months following kangaroo care (Sloan, 1994). Kangaroo care effectively decreases neonatal pain from heel sticks and promotes greater parental participation in caring for and comforting the baby (Johnston, 2003). Mothers feel more attached to their babies and more confident in caring for them when they use kangaroo care (Hurst, 1997). Kangarooing provides fathers the opportunity to bond with their baby as well and should be encouraged.

Kangaroo care increases the success of breastfeeding for the preterm infant. Time spent lying quietly by the breast—becoming familiar with the scent, sight, and sensations—gradually develops into rooting, licking, and tasting. This is a very important step in the baby's progress toward exclusive breastfeeding. As he becomes stronger and more alert, kangarooing will lead to the baby latching onto the breast with active suckles. A small study showed greater improvement in milk production in mothers who practiced kangaroo care for about four hours per week than in mothers who did not practice this skin-to-skin contact (Hurst, 1997).

Kangaroo care can serve purposes other than promoting growth, facilitating feeding, and bonding. A recent study promotes the use of **kangaroo transport**, transporting neonates from their birth facility to the tertiary care center. The baby is held skin-to-skin on the parents' or doctor's chest instead of in an incubator (Sontheimer, 2004). Heart, respiratory, temperature, and oxygen saturation rates remained stable during all 31 kangaroo transports, lasting 10 to 300 minutes. Parents felt very comfortable and safe and appreciated this method of transport.

Transition to the Breast

NICU staff can support parents in their transition to breastfeeding by providing a conducive atmosphere and assisting them as needed. Parents can assist the baby's transition from gavage feedings to breastfeedings as well. The mother can continue to place drops of her milk on a breast pad and leave it in her baby's isolette to increase his familiarity with her scent. During gavage feedings, she can put her baby to breast to build his association with sucking and eating. Support and instruction from hospital staff at this critical time will ensure a smooth transition for the baby and mother as they begin breastfeeding.

Initial Feedings

Initial feedings at the breast will involve only minimal feeding, interspersed with much resting time. Assure the mother that this is normal and expected. It is a time when she and her baby are getting to know one another, and it will involve much practice at first. Ideally the location should be quiet and private, and near any needed equipment. The mother will want to avoid any unnecessary stimulation from bright lights, loud noises, or stroking, rocking, or talking to her baby. Learning his new skill of feeding at the breast will require a great deal of his attention. Too much outside stimulation can overwhelm him. If at any time during the feeding her baby seems irritated or fussy, the mother can kangaroo him near her breast and allow him the comfort of simply being there.

Encourage the mother to approach feedings in a relaxed and unhurried manner. Her baby will need frequent opportunities to rest when he begins breastfeeding. Holding her baby in the football or cross-cradle position will enable her to see and handle him with optimal control. She can begin the feeding by holding her baby at the level of the breast and supporting his entire body. Supporting her breast with the Dancer hand position will support her baby's jaw at the same time as she minimizes the weight of her breast in his mouth. This jaw and cheek support can help increase milk intake (Einarsson-Backes, 1994). The mother can massage her breast before and during the feeding to encourage her baby to nurse. Some mothers use a breast pump to initiate milk flow.

If her baby experiences gulping and choking, an adjustment in the mother's and baby's positions will improve milk flow. The mother can hold her baby with the back of his throat somewhat higher than the breast, or she may sit in a semi-reclined position. She can also express her milk before the feeding, which will allow her baby to nurse with a less intense milk flow. This enables him to "practice" sucking without being overwhelmed by milk (Naranayan, 1991).

Monitoring Intake and Weight

Your instruction and support during these early feedings are quite valuable to the mother, who may feel overwhelmed by this new experience (Gunn, 1991). Mothers frequently worry about what to expect of their preterm baby and how to know that he is getting enough milk (Hill, 1994). They will benefit from learning how to determine when the baby is in a pattern of nutritive, or high-flow, sucks and swallows. Mothers can also become familiar with the special devices used during the baby's transition to the breast. A tube-feeding device, for instance, may encourage more effective sucking at the breast.

The mother may need to follow some breastfeedings with a supplementary feeding. For increased calories, she can feed her baby the creamy portion of expressed milk that rises to the top or the hindmilk expressed after a breastfeeding (Valentine, 1994). The neonatologist may recommend test weights to determine milk intake at the breast in order to calculate supplement needs. Electronic scales provide an accurate measurement of the preterm infant's milk intake at the breast (Meier, 1994, 1990). Many mothers find test weights very reassuring and easy to perform (Hurst, 2004). You can provide mothers with encouragement about their progress with pumping and, eventually, breastfeeding.

Taking the Preterm Infant Home

When her baby is nearing hospital discharge, the mother's emotions may range from excitement and anticipation to apprehension and dread. The day she has been waiting for is finally approaching, and yet her baby still seems so fragile. Rooming in with her baby in the hospital for several days before discharge eases this transition for the mother. It allows her to function independently, with help available when she needs it. It is especially important that 24-hour rooming-in is provided for her, if possible, as nighttime care of the infant seems especially threatening to new parents.

Discharge Guidelines

Within certain parameters, preterm infants typically leave the hospital when they reach 35 weeks' gestational age.

The infant must demonstrate a sucking reflex and have few respiratory problems. There must be no signs of disease or complications, and he must exhibit a weight gain of $\frac{2}{3}$ to 1 ounce per day. Some hospitals will discharge an infant as small as $3\frac{1}{2}$ pounds (1600 grams) if he is doing well. Babies who are born with extremely low birth weight (less than 2 pounds, 3 ounces or 1000 grams) and babies who have serious medical complications such as respiratory, heart, or neurological problems will remain hospitalized for a longer time.

Special Care at Home

A preterm baby will require special care at home. Parents cannot treat him as they would a full-term baby simply because he left the hospital. He must be protected from infectious illness and other conditions that could compromise his health. His caregiver will need to supervise his progress closely, particularly when medical problems are evident. Caution parents against expecting their baby to catch up very quickly developmentally. It may take as long as two years for a preterm baby to reach the developmental state of a full-term baby of the same age. However, the overall outlook for preterm babies is excellent, and most reach their full physical and mental potential.

Test Weights

The biggest worry of mothers who take their preterm infant home is how to tell if he is getting enough milk. Kavanaugh (1997, 1995) and Meier (1994, 1990) recommend the use of electronic balance scales at home to help mothers recognize that their babies are consuming adequate milk. They believe that doing this will enable many mothers to continue breastfeeding who would have quit otherwise because their anxiety over milk transfer outweighed their desire to nurse.

Some breastfeeding supporters worry that the use of in-home test weights may imply that the mother's milk is not adequate. They see it as medicalizing breastfeeding and putting stress on the mother regarding her "performance." Parents may consider the use of in-home scales for test weights, like any breastfeeding intervention or device, as either a help or a hindrance. You can explain the rationale behind the test weights, the strengths and weaknesses associated with them, and empower the parents to choose what they wish to do.

Mothers in a recent study reported that in-home measurement of milk intake by test weighing had been or would have been helpful (Hurst, 2004). Those who used scales experienced no increased stress or lower achievement of breastfeeding goals compared to mothers who did not perform test weights. Continuing to monitor milk transfer reassures many mothers that their baby is getting enough milk.

Breastfeeding at Home

If the hospital does not provide outpatient breastfeeding follow-up, the mother should be referred to a community-based IBCLC who can help her finalize the baby's transition to direct breastfeeding. In one study, long-term breastfeeding counseling of parents of very low birth weight infants did not demonstrate a significant difference in duration of breastfeeding (Pinelli, 2001b). Both study groups were highly motivated to breastfeed and were in a relatively advantaged population with community breastfeeding resources available. There may be a new trend of longer duration of breastfeeding for preterm infants.

After she is home, the mother can continue hospital routines for the first few days to ease the transition for

TABLE 23.2	
Counseling the Mother of a Preterm Infant	
Mother's Concern	**Suggestions for Mother**
Anxiety about taking a small baby home	◆ Continue close medical supervision of the baby.
Anxiety about beginning breastfeeding	◆ Keep realistic expectations.
	◆ Allow a transition period
The baby tires easily at the breast	◆ Wake the baby frequently during breastfeeding.
	◆ Stimulate the baby to nurse.
	◆ Nurse frequently for short periods as long as the baby is suckling and swallowing.
	◆ Use a nipple shield.
Weak rooting reflex	◆ Provide skin-to-skin contact.
	◆ Turn the baby's head toward the breast.
	◆ Help the baby open his mouth.
	◆ Form the nipple and bring the baby to the breast.
Weak suck	◆ Use the Dancer hand position to increase intraoral negative pressure.
	◆ Use a nipple shield
Intermittent sucking and resting during feedings	◆ Plan to allow a lengthy time for each feeding.
Nipple preference	◆ Express milk until letdown occurs.
	◆ Avoid artificial nipples.
	◆ Use an alternate feeding method when the mother is not present for feedings.
Difficulty interesting the baby in the breast	◆ Provide frequent skin contact and nuzzling.
	◆ Familiarize the baby with the smell of the mother's milk.
Difficulty positioning the baby at the breast	◆ Use pillows to bring the baby to breast level.
	◆ Use the clutch hold for positioning and the Dancer hand position under the baby's chin.
Difficulty determining whether the baby is getting enough milk	◆ Determine with NICU staff the number of wet diapers and stools to expect each day.
	◆ Plan a schedule of follow-up visits with the baby's primary care practitioner.
	◆ Determine the minimum feeding frequency to expect and what to do if the baby does not meet that goal.
	◆ Consider renting an electronic scale for daily weights at home. Plan with baby's practitioner what weight gain to expect. Learn from nursing staff how to determine accurate weights.

both her and the baby. She needs to continue expressing her milk during this time. As her baby gradually begins to breastfeed more frequently and more efficiently, she can decrease pumping time. If her baby required supplementation or special devices when he went home, she can discontinue these gradually.

Follow-up will ease the mother's worries as she initiates these changes. She can weigh her baby periodically as the feeding routines change. Remind her that feeding cues and other infant expectations do not always apply to preterm infants. Encourage her to regard her baby's gestational age, rather than his age from birth, as an indicator of what to expect. Suggestions for counseling the mother of a preterm infant are in Table 23.2.

▶ OTHER BABIES NOT BORN AT TERM

Preterm infants are not the only ones whose gestational age requires special care at birth. Some babies—referred to as near-term—are born near the early range of 37 weeks. Others are born at the other extreme of 42 weeks—referred to as postterm or postmature. Both of these extremes call for special care of the newborn. The length of hospitalization and degree of care needed will depend on the baby's condition and the number of weeks before or after term he was born. You can familiarize parents with the typical characteristics of these babies as well as implications for breastfeeding.

The Near-Term Infant

The near-term infant is a healthy infant born at 35 to 38 weeks (Figure 23.3). He often receives the same treatment as a full-term infant, being cared for in the normal newborn nursery and going home with the mother at 48 to 72 hours postpartum. The baby is generally able to maintain body temperature, is at or above 2500 grams, and seems to breastfeed well in the hospital. A near-term baby appears healthy and competent. However, there is a 5 to 10 percent risk of readmission to the hospital due to jaundice and/or weight loss. Wight (2003) lists characteristics of near-term infants that can affect their ability to breastfeed. These include cardiorespiratory instability, poor temperature control, metabolic instability, immunologic and neurological immaturity, and immature oro-motor development.

Problems After Discharge

Problems develop for near-term infants after they leave the hospital. A near-term baby often has low muscle tone and finds it difficult to initiate and maintain the mother's milk supply due to poor lip and cheek tone. Early delivery prevents full development of buccal fat pads and masseter muscles. There may be anatomic incompatibility due to the mother's nipple being too large for the baby's small mouth, making it difficult for the baby to maintain a seal on the breast. He may be unable to attach far enough back on the breast to trigger an effective milk letdown. He tires more quickly and has difficulty drawing the nipple into his mouth, maintaining a good latch, and compressing the nipple during the suckling phase.

Near-term babies may move quickly from a hyper-alert state to deep sleep. They give very subtle feeding cues or none at all and have a difficult time tuning out excess stimulation. There is poor neurological organization, with an immature rooting reflex and difficulty coordinating the suck/swallow/breathe cycle. Early delivery results in decreased albumin sites and therefore an increased risk for jaundice. This can lead to sleepiness and additional difficulty with effective milk transfer (Wight, 2003).

Breastfeeding Precautions

Parents need clear and consistent teaching about what to expect from their near-term infant. It is important to make sure the baby nurses at least eight times in 24

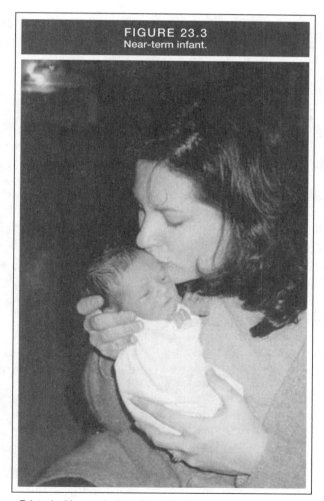

FIGURE 23.3
Near-term infant.

Printed with permission of Jan Riordan.

hours. Many of these babies do better with shorter, more frequent feedings because they tire easily at the breast. They should go no longer than three hours between feedings during the day, with one longer stretch of four hours at night if they have achieved eight feedings in 24 hours. Mothers need to watch closely for subtle feeding cues and breastfeed as often as the baby indicates a need. Realizing that feeding cues may be subtle or lacking, parents can use gentle waking techniques and plenty of skin-to-skin contact to accomplish the appropriate number of feedings in a 24-hour period.

A near-term baby should still be in utero sleeping and growing, not working for his food. Because of his compromised condition, the mother cannot expect him to initiate and maintain sufficient milk production through suckling alone. She will need to pump until the baby reaches his due date, or until he is well over birth weight and milk production is well established. The mother can aim for double pumping four times a day with a hospital-grade pump, for about ten minutes per session. The baby's weight should be checked weekly during this time.

Near-term babies may find it easier to transfer milk with the use of a nipple shield (Meier, 2000). It is important to have adequate follow-up if a nipple shield is used. Once he has grown and matured more, the near-term baby typically can breastfeed well without a shield, usually when he reaches his due date. It often helps mothers realize that most near-term babies seem to "wake up" and begin to breastfeed like term babies when they reach their due date.

The Postterm Infant

A postterm infant is one who is born after 42 weeks' gestation. The danger of postmaturity involves deterioration of the placenta, which progressively becomes less efficient after the normal gestation period of 37 to 42 weeks. Postmature infants may be appropriate for gestational age in body length but are often small-for-date because of the progressive decrease in placental function. Fetal oxygenation will be marginal or depressed before labor, and meconium may be secreted during labor. Delivery may be through induction of labor or cesarean section. The baby has difficulty tolerating the stresses of labor after he is born. He may struggle to maintain respiration, blood sugar levels, and nervous functioning. These situations generally are manageable.

The skin of some postterm infants is dry and cracked, with a texture similar to parchment paper. The skin is sagging and loose, with an absence of vernix. The baby may have profuse scalp hair, as well as long nails on his fingers and toes. Meconium secretion will produce a yellow-green staining of his skin and nails.

The baby may be sluggish during his initial attempts at breastfeeding. He may need coaxing and prodding much in the same way as a preterm baby. It is sometimes helpful to explain to the mother that even though her baby is postterm, he may behave like a preterm baby initially. The strategies used to breastfeed a near-term infant usually work well with postterm babies. As postterm babies put on weight, their feeding behaviors mature.

▶ COUNSELING A MOTHER WHOSE BABY HAS DIED

Probably the most distressing situation you will encounter professionally will be caring for a mother who has lost her baby. At such a time, it seems impossible to find the right words as you try to avoid painful remarks and show support sensitively. With appropriate counseling techniques, insight into the mother's emotions, and sincere empathy, you can approach the situation comfortably, more confident in your ability to support the mother in her grief.

What to Say to the Mother

After listening to the mother relate what happened, you can let her know how sad you feel. Avoid telling her, "I know how you must feel" or "I can imagine what you are going through." You cannot begin to know what the mother is feeling unless you experienced a similar loss. Even if you lost a child, this is *not* the time to talk about your loss. Talking about the death of your child takes the focus off this mother's grief and minimizes it.

You can reflect back to the mother how you imagine she must feel. Appropriate statements may be "You must be heartbroken" or "I can't imagine the loss you feel." You could say something like, "There is nothing more painful than what you are feeling right now." You are validating her pain without taking the focus off her and her baby.

To encourage the mother to talk, you can tell her that other mothers who have suffered similar losses have found it helpful to talk through their feelings. Unless she shares her feelings and works through them, her grief will continue without resolution. People close to the mother may feel uncomfortable listening to her relate her birth experience and the circumstances surrounding her baby's death. She may appreciate being able to turn to you, knowing that you will be concerned and interested in listening to her. Let her know that you are glad to listen, assuring her that you do not want to invade her privacy.

Having an insight into the mother's feelings will help you in your counseling. For many mothers, bonding and maternal feelings begin the day they learn they are pregnant or when they first hear their baby's heartbeat. Parents need others to acknowledge that their baby, even though born very young or stillborn, was loved before birth and was a person who meant a lot in their lives. Avoid comments such as, "At least you can have more children" or "It was for the best." The mother may rather care for an "imperfect" baby than no baby at all. The thought of replacing her deceased baby with a new one is no consolation to her right now. She is grieving for the baby she just lost. You can acknowledge her baby's importance by asking his or her name and using it during your discussion.

Grieving for Their Loss

Parental grief over the loss of a child is more intense than losing a spouse or an adult child losing a parent (Middleton, 1998). Parents will progress through several stages of grief before their loss is resolved, typically beginning with denial and ending in acceptance of the loss. The range of emotions they experience between these two extremes appears in Figure 23.4. The time it takes parents to move from denial to acceptance will vary greatly, and could take as long as three or four years (Murphy, 2003). Parents never truly "get over" the loss of a child. Their lives are irrevocably changed, and parents hold on to their relationship with their deceased child (Davies, 2004). It is never appropriate to minimize the loss of a child, even after decades have passed.

Acceptance of the loss depends on the amount of support and understanding the parents receive from friends and family. The mother may need to talk about her baby long after most people have tired of hearing it. You may be the one person she feels will be receptive, especially if you formed a bond with her. Try to key into the mother's needs and sense how often she would like to hear from you. It will be much easier for her to receive a call than to initiate a call and worry that she is bothering you. The list in Table 23.3 will help you choose your comments carefully.

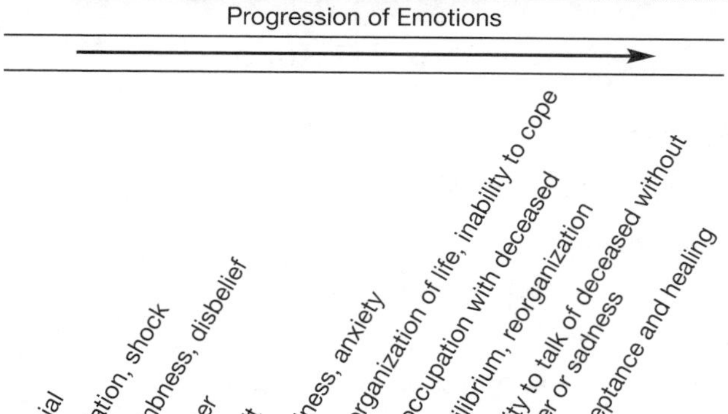

Breastfeeding Concerns

The mother may have concerns specific to breastfeeding, especially if she and her baby had begun nursing. Even if she had not begun to breastfeed, the mother's breasts may fill with milk a few days after delivery and can become engorged and painful. You can help the mother relieve the fullness without stimulating her breasts to the extent that she produces more milk. Advise her to express her milk just enough to relieve discomfort. She can use the same comfort measures for engorgement presented in Chapter 16. Continuous application of cabbage leaves to the breasts will promote the milk drying up and will offer the mother relief. Remind her to replace the cabbage leaves about every two to three hours.

A mother who had been pumping to maintain milk production for a preterm or ill baby will have more difficulty ending lactation. She may need to continue pumping and decrease slowly in a weaning pattern to avoid problems associated with abrupt weaning. A mother who had begun nursing her baby may also need to express milk to decrease milk production gradually. Mothers who had been nursing or expressing milk for their babies can be further comforted in knowing they gave their babies the best possible care, both nutritionally and emotionally. Many bereaved mothers donate their milk to a milk bank for a period of time. Donating milk to help save another baby's life can add to the mother's emotional healing. Human milk bank staff are trained to deal sensitively with these mothers. If the mother seems receptive, it is a suggestion you can offer.

Support Systems for Parents

Parents who lose a child may benefit from professional counseling, available through local clergy and social service organizations. Talking with other parents who experienced a similar loss can help them and encourage them to share feelings. As time passes, they may continue to need to talk about their loss. They will benefit from the ongoing support they receive from other parents and professionals in a support group. There are many support groups for grieving parents, often affiliated with a hospital or medical center. Compassionate Friends is one such support group (www.compassionatefriends.org).

You can help parents learn their rights and options regarding their infant. They will need time and privacy with their family to begin the grieving process. They

FIGURE 23.4
Sequence of the grief process.

Progression of Emotions

Denial
Isolation, shock
Numbness, disbelief
Anger
Guilt
Sadness, anxiety
Disorganization of life, inability to cope
Preoccupation with deceased
Equilibrium, reorganization
Ability to talk of deceased without anger or sadness
Acceptance and healing

TABLE 23.3
Counseling Grieving Parents

DO show your genuine concern and caring.

DO be available to listen and empathize.

DO say you are sorry about what happened.

DO allow the mother to express as much grief as she feels.

DO encourage parents to be patient with themselves.

DO allow the mother to talk about her baby.

DO talk about the special qualities of the baby she lost.

DO acknowledge the impact of the baby's death.

DO reassure the parents that they did everything possible for their baby.

DO refer to the baby by name.

DO show your sadness and disappointment.

DON'T let your own sense of helplessness keep you from reaching out to the mother.

DON'T avoid the mother because you are uncomfortable with her situation.

DON'T say you know how the mother feels.

DON'T suggest that the mother should be feeling better by a certain time.

DON'T tell parents what they should feel or do.

DON'T change the subject when the baby is mentioned.

DON'T try to find something positive about the baby's death.

DON'T point out that they can always have other children or suggest that they should be grateful for any other children they already have.

DON'T suggest that the baby's care by the parents or medical personnel was inadequate.

DON'T avoid using the baby's name for fear of causing pain for the mother.

DON'T be overly cheerful or casual.

Adapted with permission from a list compiled by the Compassionate Friends.

have the right to hold or see their baby after he dies. If they elect to visit with their baby prior to discharge, a staff member can wrap him in warm blankets and bring him to the mother's room. This practice is particularly helpful for parents of a stillborn infant.

Some hospitals take pictures of the deceased infant for parents to keep. This can be especially important to parents who choose not to see their infant at the time of death. Often these parents have the desire to see their baby months later, when it is too late. Pictures can help parents put their baby's death into perspective. Offering parents an opportunity to take pictures can provide them with a treasured image of their child. A staff member can cleanse, dress, and swaddle the infant for the pictures. Giving parents their infant's identification bracelet is further validation of his importance to them as a family member and another memento of their brief time with him.

Encourage parents to seek information about their options with hospital personnel and their baby's caregiver. If requested, hospital chaplains typically will baptize stillborn infants. Hospital staff will arrange for the baby's transfer to a funeral home. Caregivers, especially a midwife or labor nurse, often will attend the funeral. If you have cared for the mother and baby, your attendance would be appropriate. Attending a service acknowledges the importance of the baby. This means a lot to families, even if they are not able to express their appreciation at the time.

▶ Summary

IBCLCs are valuable resources for parents of a high-risk infant. You can help the mother provide her milk for her baby's care and make the transition to breastfeeding. You can also support the mother as she works through her feelings related to this unexpected outcome, feelings that go beyond breastfeeding. Your support will help her develop a realistic expectation in the beginning and plan for her baby's nutrition. This may occur long before her baby is able to go to the breast. You can guide the mother through the initiation of pumping and caring for her stored milk. Be available to her to support early breastfeeding and to guide her through the transition of bringing her baby home from the hospital. Compassion and experience will help you support a mother whose baby has died. Your participation in the mother's health-care team will be critical in these special circumstances.

▶ Chapter 23 — At a Glance

Applying what you learned—

Concerns of parents of a high-risk infant:

◆ Initiating and maintaining milk production.

◆ A delay in breastfeeding.

◆ Worry about the baby's survival.

◆ Feelings of guilt, loneliness, and anxiety.

◆ Strain on their relationship.

◆ Desire for privacy and time alone with their baby.

Counseling preterm parents in the hospital:

◆ Ask the baby's caregivers for explanations and clarification.

◆ Seek out sources of support and community resources.

◆ Provide gentle, warm, and loving touch.

◆ Express milk for their baby.

◆ Participate in feeding, bathing, and diapering their baby.

◆ Kangaroo their preterm infant.

◆ Encourage nonnutritive sucking on an emptied breast.

Counseling preterm parents at home:

◆ Read feeding cues and infant responses that show signs of overstimulation.

◆ Plan for unhurried, long, frequent feedings at home with long periods of rest.

◆ Stimulate letdown and manage fluctuations in milk production.

◆ Support the baby's jaw with the Dancer hand position.

◆ Monitor the baby's intake and weight at home.

◆ Base expectations on gestational age, rather than age from birth.

Counseling near-term parents:

◆ Plan for short, frequent feedings.

◆ Allow no longer than three hours between feedings during the day.

◆ Watch closely for subtle feeding cues.

◆ Use gentle waking techniques and plenty of skin-to-skin contact.

◆ Use a nipple shield as necessary.

Counseling parents who lose a baby:

◆ Help them arrange time and privacy with their baby.

◆ Express your concern and sorrow.

◆ Use reflective listening and be available.

◆ Key into the mother's needs and sense how often she would like to hear from you.

◆ Help the mother relieve fullness without stimulating more milk.

◆ Refer the mother to a milk bank if she wishes to donate milk.

◆ Refer parents to a support system and help them learn their rights and options.

▶ **REFERENCES**

Anderson G et al. Early skin-to-skin contact for mothers and their healthy newborn infants. *Cochrane Database Syst Rev* (2):CD003519; 2003.

Anderson G. Skin to skin: Kangaroo care in Western Europe. *Am J Nurs* 89:662–666; 1989.

Anderson G. Current knowledge about skin to skin (kangaroo) care for preterm infants. *Breastfeeding Review* 8:364–373; 1993.

Auerbach K, Walker M. When the mother of a premature infant breastfeeds: What every NICU nurse needs to know. *Neonatal Network* 13:23–29; 1994.

Auerbach K. Sequential and simultaneous breast pumping: A comparison. *Int J Nurs Stud* 27:257–265; 1990.

Beachy J. Premature infant massage in the NICU. *Neonatal Netw* 22(3):39–45; 2003.

Bell E et al. A structured intervention improves breastfeeding success for ill or preterm infants. *MCN* 20:309–314; 1995.

Bier J et al. Breastfeeding of very low birth weight infants. *J Pediatr* 123:773–778; 1993.

Blaymore-Bier J et al. Breastfeeding infants who were extremely low birth weight. *Pediatrics* 100(6):E3; 1997.

Boekel S. *Gastroesophageal Reflux: The Breastfeeding Family's Nightmare*. Presentation at ILCA International Conference, Washington, DC; July 27, 2000.

Bond C. Positive Touch and massage in the neonatal unit: a British approach. *Semin Neonatol* 7(6):477–86; 2002.

Boukydis Z. Crying and preterm babies. *Intensive Caring Unlimited* 7:7; 1989.

Browne J. Early relationship environments: Physiology of skin-to-skin contact for parents and their preterm infants. *Clin Perinatol* 31(2):287–298, vii. Review; 2004.

Burns K et al. Infant stimulation: Modification of an intervention based on physiologic and behavioral cues. *JOGNN* 23: 581–589; 1995.

Centers for Disease Control (CDC). Births: Final data for 2002. National Vital Statistics Report 52(10); December 17, 2003.

Cheales-Siebenaler NJ. Induced lactation in an adoptive mother. *J Hum Lact* 15(1):41–43; 1999.

Chen C et al. The effect of breast- and bottle-feeding on oxygen saturation and body temperature in preterm infants. *J Hum Lact* 16(1):21–27; 2000.

Cregan M et al. Initiation of lactation in women after preterm delivery. *Acta Obstetric Gynecol Scand* 81(9):870–77; 2002.

Culp R et al. A tool for educating parents about their premature infants. *Birth* 16:23–26; 1989.

Davies R. New understandings of parental grief: Literature review. *J Adv Nurs* 46(5):506–513; 2004.

Ebrahim G. Feeding the preterm brain. *J Trop Pediatr* 39: 1430–1431; 1993.

Ehrenkranz R, Ackerman B. Metoclopramide effect of faltering milk production by mothers of premature infants. *Pediatrics* 78:614–620; 1986.

Einarsson-Backes L. The effect of oral support on sucking efficiency in preterm infants. *Am J Occup Ther* 48:490–498; 1994.

Farran A et al. Infant stimulation in the NICU. *Intensive Caring Unlimited* 7:13; 1989.

Feher S et al. Increasing breast milk production for premature infants with a relaxation/imagery audiotape. *Pediatrics* 83: 57–60; 1989.

Gabay M. Galactogogues: Medications that induce lactation. *J Hum Lact* 18(3):274–279. Review; 2002.

Griffin T et al. Mothers' performing creamatocrit measures in the NICU: Accuracy, reactions, and cost. *JOGNN* 29(3):249–257; 2000.

Gross S, Slagle T. Feeding the low birth weight infant. *Clin Perinatol* 20:193–209; 1993.

Gunn T. Breastfeeding preterm infants. *N Z Med J* 104: 188–189; 1991.

Hale T, Berens P. *Clinical Therapy in Breastfeeding Patients.* Amarillo, TX: Pharmasoft; 2002.

Hall R et al. Hypophosphatemia in breastfed low birth weight infants following initial hospital discharge. *Am J Child Dis* 143: 1191–1195; 1989.

Hamelin K, Ramachandran C. Kangaroo care. *Can Nurse* 89: 15–17; 1993.

Hartmann P. *Initiation And Establishment of Lactation With Special Reference to Mothers Who Deliver Pre-Term.* Amarillo Conference: Human Lactation: Current Research and Clinical Implications: Breastmilk for Pre-term Babies, Amarillo, TX; October 21, 2004.

Hill P et al. Mothers of low birthweight infants: Breastfeeding patterns and problems. *J Hum Lact* 10:169–176; 1994.

Hurst N et al. Skin-to-skin holding in the neonatal intensive care unit influences maternal milk volume. *J Perinatol* 17:213–217; 1997.

Hurst N et al. Mothers performing in-home measurement of milk intake during breastfeeding of their preterm infants: Maternal reactions and feeding outcomes. *J Hum Lact* 20(2): 178–187; 2004.

Hylander MA et al. Human milk feedings and infection among very low birth weight infants. *Pediatrics* 102(3):e38; 1998.

Johnston C et al. Kangaroo care is effective in diminishing pain response in preterm neonates. *Arch Pediatr Adolesc Med* 157(11):1084–1088; 2003.

Kavanaugh K et al. Getting enough: Mothers' concerns about breastfeeding a preterm infant after discharge. *JOGNN* 24:23–32; 1995.

Kavanaugh K et al. The rewards outweigh the efforts: Breastfeeding outcomes for mothers of preterm infants. *J Hum Lact* 13:15–21; 1997.

Kent J. *Breastmilk Calcium for the Pre-term Baby.* Amarillo Conference, Human Lactation: Current Research and Clinical Implications, Breastmilk for Pre-term Babies; October 22, 2004.

Klaus MH et al. *Bonding: Building the Foundations of Secure Attachment and Independence.* New York: Perseus; 2000.

Kuschel C, Harding J. Multicomponent fortified human milk for promoting growth in preterm infants. *Cochrane Database Syst Rev* 1:CD000343; 2004.

Landers S. Maximizing the benefits of human milk feeding for the preterm infant. *Pediatric Annals* 32:5; 2003.

Lang S. *Breastfeeding Special Care Babies*, 2nd ed. London: Bailliere Tindall; 2002.

Li C. *Variations in the Composition of Breastmilk and Its Fortification for Pre-term Babies.* Amarillo Conference, Human Lactation: Current Research and Clinical Implications, Breastmilk for Pre-term Babies; October 22, 2004.

Lucas A et al. A randomized multicenter study of human milk versus formula and later development in preterm infants. *Arch Child Dis* 70:F141–F146; 1994.

Ludington-Hoe S et al. Selected physiologic measures and behavior during paternal skin contact with Colombian preterm infants. *J Dev Psych-01* 18:223–232; 1992.

Ludington-Hoe S et al. Safe criteria and procedure for kangaroo care with intubated preterm infants. *J Obstet Gynecol Neonatal Nurs* 32(5):579–588; 2003.

Ludington-Hoe SM, Anderson GC, Swinth JY, Thompson C, Hadeed AJ. Randomized controlled trial of kangaroo care: Cardiorespiratory and thermal effects on healthy preterm infants. *Neonatal Netw* 23(3):39–48; 2004.

March of Dimes. Low Birth Weight. #09-285-0; April 2003. Available at: www.marchofdimes.com. Accessed January 22, 2005.

McKim E. The information and support needs of mothers of premature infants. *J Pediatr Nurs* 8:233–244; 1993.

Mead L et al. Breastfeeding success with preterm quadruplets. *JOGNN* 21:221–227; 1992.

Meier P et al. The accuracy of test weighing for preterm infants. *J Pediatr Gastroenterol Nutr* 10:62–65; 1990.

Meier P et al. A new scale for in-home test-weighing for mothers of preterm and high risk infants. *J Hum Lact* 10(3): 163–168; 1994.

Meier P et al. Nipple shields for preterm infants: Effect on milk transfer and duration of breastfeeding. *J Hum Lact* 16(2): 106–114; 2000.

Meier P et al. Mothers' milk feedings in the neonatal intensive care unit: Accuracy of the creamatocrit technique. *J Perinatol* 22(8):646–649; 2002.

Meier P et al. The Rush Mothers' Milk Club: Breastfeeding interventions for mothers with very-low-birth-weight infants. *JOGNN* 33(2):164–174; 2004.

Meier P. Bottle and breastfeeding: Effects on transcutaneous oxygen pressure and temperature in preterm infants. *Nurs Res* 37:36–41; 1988.

Meier P. Supporting lactation in mothers with very low birth weight infants. *Pediatr Ann* 32(5):317–325; 2003.

Middleton W et al. A longitudinal study comparing bereavement phenomena in recently bereaved spouses, adult children and parents. *Aust N Z J Psychiatry* 32(2):235–241; 1998.

Mitoulas L. *Pumping Frequency and Duration and Milk Yields in Preterm Mothers.* Amarillo Conference, Human Lactation: Current Research and Clinical Implications, Breastmilk for Pre-term Babies; October 21, 2004.

Morton J. *Breastfeeding the Preterm Infant: Lessons for All.* Amarillo Conference, Human Lactation: Current Research and Clinical Implications, Breastmilk for Pre-term Babies; October 21, 2004.

Murphy S et al. Bereaved parents' outcomes 4 to 60 months after their children's deaths by accident, suicide, or homicide: A comparative study demonstrating differences. *Death Studies* 27(1):39–61; 2003.

Naranayan I et al. Sucking on the "emptied" breast: Nonnutritive sucking with a difference. *Arch Dis Child* 66:241–244; 1991.

Nyqvist K, Sjoden P. Advice concerning breastfeeding from mothers of infants admitted to a neonatal intensive care unit: The Roy adaptation model as a conceptual structure. *J Adv Nurs* 18:54–63; 1993.

Nyqvist K, Sjoden P, Ewald U. The development of preterm infants' breastfeeding behavior. *Early Hum Dev* 55(3): 247–264; 1999.

Pinelli J, Symington A. Non-nutritive sucking for promoting physiologic stability and nutrition in preterm infants. Cochrane Database Syst Rev. 2000;(2):CD001071. Review. Update in: *Cochrane Database Syst Rev* (3):CD001071; 2001a.

Pinelli J et al. Randomized trial of breastfeeding support in very low-birth-weight infants. *Arch Pediatr Adolesc Med* 155(5):548–553; 2001b.

Ramasethu J et al. Weight gain in exclusively breastfed preterm infants. *J Trop Pediatr* 39:152–159; 1993.

Shaker C. Nipple feeding preterm infants: an individualized, developmentally supportive approach. *Neonatal Netw* 18(3): 15–22; 1999.

Siva Subramanian K, Yoon H, Toral J. Extremely Low Birthweight Infant. October 31, 2002. eMedicine.com. Available at: www.emedicine.com/ped/topic2784.htm. Accessed January 22, 2005.

Sloan N et al. Kangaroo mother method: Randomised controlled trial of an alternative method of care for stabilised low-birthweight infants. *Lancet* 344:782–785; 1994.

Slusher T et al. Promoting the exclusive feeding of own mother's milk through the use of hindmilk and increased maternal milk volume for hospitalized, low birth weight infants (< 1800 grams) in Nigeria: A feasibility study. *J Hum Lact* 19(2):191–198; 2003.

Smith M. Influence of breastfeeding on cognitive outcomes at age 6–8 years: Follow-up of very low birth weight infants. *Am J Epidemiol* 158(11):1075–1082; 2003.

Sontheimer D et al. Kangaroo transport instead of incubator transport. *Pediatrics* 113(4):920–923; 2004.

Stern J, Reichlin S. Prolactin circadian rhythm persists throughout lactation in women. *Neuroendocrinology* 51:31–37; 1990.

Stine M. Breastfeeding and the premature newborn: A protocol without bottles. *J Hum Lact* 6:167–170; 1990.

Swinth J et al. Kangaroo (skin-to-skin) care with a preterm infant before, during, and after mechanical ventilation. *Neonatal Netw* 22(6):33–38; 2003.

Tunell R. Prevention of neonatal cold injury in preterm infants. *Acta Paediatr* 93(3):308–310; 2004.

Valentine C et al. Hindmilk improves weight gain in low-birth-weight infants fed human milk. *J Pediatr Gastroenterol Nutr* 18:474–477; 1994.

VandenBurg K. Nippling management of the sick neonate in the NICU: The disorganized feeder. *Neonatal Netw* 9(1): 9–16; 1990.

Vickers A et al. Massage for promoting growth and development of preterm and/or low birth-weight infants. *Cochrane Database Syst Rev* (2):CD000390; 2004.

Weibley T. Inside the incubator. *MCN* 14:96–100; 1989.

Wheeler R et al. Calcium and phosphorous supplementation following initial hospital discharge in 1800 gm birthweight breastfed infants. *Am J Perinatol* 7:389–390; 1990.

Whitelaw A. Kangaroo baby care: Just a nice experience or an important advance for preterm infants. *Pediatrics* 85:604; 1990.

Wight NE. Donor human milk for preterm infants. *J Perinatol* 21(4):249–254; 2001.

Wight NE. Breastfeeding the borderline (near-term) preterm infant. *Pediatric Ann* 32(5):329–336; 2003.

Wight NE. Breastfeeding the former NICU infant. *Breastfeeding Abstracts* 23(3):19–20; 2004.

Wolf L, Glass R. *Feeding and Swallowing Disorders in Infancy.* San Antonio, TX: Therapy Skill Builders; 1992.

▶ BIBLIOGRAPHY

Bose CL et al. Relactation by mothers of sick and premature infants. *Pediatrics* 67(4):565–569; 1981.

Bradshaw J. Breastfeeding twins, triplets and quads: Making the impossible easy. Newsletter: National Capital Lactation Center 16; Summer, 1996.

Bu'Lock F et al: Development of coordination of sucking, swallowing and breathing: Ultrasound study of term and preterm infants. *Dev Med Child Neurol* 32:669–678; 1990.

Furman L et al. Breastfeeding of very low birth weight infants. *J Hum Lact* 14:29–34; 1998.

Gross SJ et al. Nutritional composition of milk produced by mothers delivering preterm. *J Pediatr* 96(4):641–644; 1980.

Klaus M, Kennell J. *Mother-Infant Bonding*. St. Louis, MO: Mosby; 1982.

Lambert J, Watters N. Breastfeeding the infant/child with cardiac defect: An informal survey. *J Hum Lact* 14:151–155; 1998.

Lucas A, Cole TJ. Breast milk and neonatal necrotising enterocolitis. *Lancet* 386:1519–1523; 1990.

Lucas A et al: Breast milk and subsequent intelligence quotient in children born preterm. *Lancet* 339:261–264; 1992.

Mathew OP, Bhathia J. Sucking and breathing patterns during breast and bottle-feedings in term neonates. *Am J Dis Child* 143:588–592; 1989.

Measel CP, Anderson GC. Nonnutritive sucking during tube feedings: Effect on clinical course in premature infants. *JOGNN* 8(5):265–272; 1979.

Meier P, Pugh EJ. Breastfeeding behavior of small preterm infants. *MCN* 10:396–401; 1985.

Meier P. Breastfeeding in the special care nursery. Prematures and infants with medical problems. *Pediatr Clin North Am* 48(2):425–442; 2001.

Neifert M, Thrope J. Twins: Family adjustment, parenting, and infant feeding in the fourth trimester. *Clin Obstet Gynecol* 33:102–112; 1990.

Raiha N. Protein fortification on human milk for feeding preterm infants. *Acta Paediatr* 405(Suppl):93–97; 1994.

Schanler R, Abrams S. Postnatal attainment of intrauterine macromineral accretion rates in low birth weight infants fed fortified human milk. *J Pediatr* 126:441–447; 1995.

Schanler R. Suitability of human milk for the low-birthweight infant. *Clin Perinatol* 22:207–222; 1995.

Sollid D et al. Breastfeeding multiples. *J Pernat Neonat Nurs* 3:46–65; 1989.

Williams R, Medalie J. Twins: Double pleasure or double trouble? *Am Fam Phys* 49:869–873; 1994.

Woerner J. The joy of multiples. *Int J Childbirth Education* 8:35–36; 1993.

CHAPTER
24

WHEN BREASTFEEDING IS INTERRUPTED

Ideally, a breastfeeding mother and her baby are together throughout lactation with no interruption in feedings. However, in today's world, this is often not realistic, nor even desired by some mothers. Some occasions that result in separation of the mother and baby are temporary, whereas others are regular and long term. The separation may be for a few hours or a few days. The mother may be away on a daily basis because of returning to work or school, or over a long period because of illness and hospitalization. Some of these separations may not involve missed breastfeedings. Others will require milk expression and the use of an alternative feeding method during the mother's absence. Mothers who experience such separations have special needs in terms of managing feedings and maintaining milk production. They will benefit from emotional support and encouragement as well.

KEY TERMS

antibodies	reverse cycle nursing
caregiver	Ronald McDonald house
child care	short-term separation
hospitalization	working mother

MANAGING BREASTFEEDING THROUGH A SEPARATION

Separation from her baby can create stress and anxiety for a new mother, especially when the separation is a result of illness. You can help relieve some of the mother's anxieties by accepting and supporting her decisions concerning breastfeeding. If she chooses to combine breastfeeding with a daily or prolonged separation, she will need advice about expressing her milk and maintaining milk production. You can help her obtain a pump and offer her practical suggestions for its use. The mother will need to be strongly motivated to overcome any potential difficulties and pressures that may confront her. This discussion focuses on how you can help a mother whose separation from her baby affects her breastfeeding.

The Mother's Needs

When a mother is separated from her baby during usual feeding times, she may face challenges regarding attitudes of family members, child care arrangements, and family and time management. She will need to express milk regularly in order to relieve fullness and to maintain milk production. She also will need to know that her baby will accept nourishment by an alternative feeding method during her absence. This requires planning, to allow time to work through her baby's possible rejection of the chosen feeding method.

The mother may experience conflicting emotions about the separation and about continuing to breastfeed in spite of obstacles. Effective use of counseling skills will help you listen and respond to the mother's concerns about the cause of the separation, especially if her baby remains hospitalized. This can be a trying time for her family, and your support and encouragement will be helpful.

Considerations for Timing of the Separation

Mothers often have no control over the timing of a separation. A working mother may have a limited maternity leave, or hospitalization may be necessary for either mother or baby. Those who can be flexible in scheduling a separation can delay missed breastfeedings until milk production is well established. Barring any interference, most mothers will have breastfeeding well established by the time the baby is two months old. The mother can likely manage a separation at that time. The transition will be even smoother if a separation is delayed until about six months, when the baby is old enough to begin eating solid foods. At that time, there will be less need for supplemental feedings while the mother and baby are apart. There are also many factors unrelated to breastfeeding, such as the emotional needs of both the mother and baby, and separation anxiety which occurs at around nine months. The mother ideally can assess her particular situation to determine when the separation will be least disruptive.

481

Maintaining Milk Production

A mother's milk production may diminish to some extent if she experiences a substantial separation from her baby. She cannot remove milk from her breasts as effectively as a healthy, robust baby does when he nurses. You can provide her with instructions on how to hand express or use a breast pump. Many mothers who are away from their babies on a regular basis find it convenient to express milk routinely. Others prefer to express only enough to relieve discomfort during the separation and allow their milk production to diminish slightly. Their babies may receive infant formula during their absence rather than human milk. This choice will depend on each mother's preference and the circumstances of the separation. Your role is to support her decision. In either situation, you can encourage the mother in her efforts to provide milk for her baby.

Nourishing the Baby During the Absence

When a mother is away from her baby during feeding times, she must arrange for her baby's nourishment until she returns, taking into consideration the feeding method and type of food. She may choose to provide her milk or may prefer that her baby receive infant formula. Depending on the length of her absence and the baby's age, he may also receive juice, water, or solid foods. Experimenting with feeding methods for at least two weeks before the separation will help the baby learn to accept nourishment by some means other than breastfeeding.

Although a bottle may be convenient for the caregiver, it can cause a young baby to develop a nipple preference that interferes with breastfeeding. Feeding the baby with a cup will eliminate nipple preference, though it may require more time for feeding. This actually has advantages if the caregiver is willing to spend the extra time. Slowing down artificial feedings to emulate breastfeeding is a more baby-friendly option.

Choice of Bottle Nipple

If a bottle is used, those with nipples that encourage the baby to open his mouth wide can make the transition from breast to bottle easier for the very young baby. Many babies accomplish this with a nipple that has a large base. Some babies tend to clamp down on the nipple at the narrowest part and not take the bottle in deeply to the wide base. Mothers may, therefore, need to try more than one type of nipple. A bottle with a short teat is preferable to a longer one. The key factor for many babies seems to be more the rate of flow than the type of nipple (Kassing, 2002; Wilson-Clay, 2002). Be aware that even "slow flow" nipples drip milk. (See Chapter 21 for more information about selecting a nipple.)

Motivation to Continue Nursing

Motivation and determination are critical factors for a mother continuing to breastfeed despite a separation from her baby. Some mothers believe they must wean their babies when a separation occurs. You can assure mothers that breastfeeding is compatible with both short-term and long-term separations. If weaning becomes necessary, you can reassure the mother that the quality of her breastfeeding experience is important, not its duration. If the separation has prompted the mother to compromise her initial breastfeeding goals, she can still work toward a satisfying experience if she remains flexible and positive.

A mother who is not totally committed to breastfeeding may respond to a separation by weaning her baby. On the other hand, some mothers may want to continue nursing despite feeling discouraged. When mothers contact you in these situations, be sensitive to messages that signal conflicted feelings: "I guess I should wean . . ." "I will have to wean . . . ." Draw the mother out with open-ended questions. Use reflective listening skills to give feedback to help the mother clarify her situation and her options and validate her choices. By assessing her motives, you can help each mother achieve the outcome she truly wants. Mothers who deal with a separation will benefit from a great deal of support and practical suggestions, whether the decision is to continue nursing or to wean.

Coping with Difficulties

A separation between mother and baby can create physical consequences related to breastfeeding, as well as emotional tension and anxiety. The mother must remove milk from her breasts regularly in order to avoid leaking, plugged ducts, engorgement, and mastitis. Despite her diligence in expressing her milk, she may still experience problems because this does not remove milk from her breasts as efficiently as her baby does when he nurses.

The mother will be taxing her energy reserves, whether from working or from traveling back and forth to the hospital. Therefore, she will want to pay close attention to adequate rest and nutrition. If the separation is due to the mother's illness, she will have an even greater need for rest and good nutrition, to aid her recovery as well as build or maintain her milk production. The mother needs to be mindful that skimping on her nutrition can affect her sense of well-being and her ability to function efficiently. Drinking something directly before or during the times she expresses will help her remember to supply herself with adequate fluids. Sufficient rest is also important to the mother's well-being.

At times, a baby may demonstrate a strong desire to remain with his mother. Other times, he may appear to reject her and seem more attached to the person who cares for him. This can be either a source of comfort to the mother or a source of jealousy and anxiety. Many mothers experience a sense of guilt about a separation, regardless of whether it is planned or unplanned and whether it is optional or unavoidable. This feeling of guilt may relate to the mother's absence from her baby or to her original goals for breastfeeding. Such guilt can motivate a mother to reconsider her options and alter her situation. You can help a mother cope with these anxieties by supporting her when she and her baby are separated and when they reunite and resume breastfeeding.

Following the Separation

If a period of separation results in a decline in milk production, the mother can hand express or pump to rebuild it. She may be able to entice her baby to nurse by feeding her milk to him from a tube-feeding device while he is at the breast. He may need supplemental feedings for a while after he resumes breastfeeding until milk production increases to meet his requirements. Encourage the mother to arrange for help with household chores so she can renew her breastfeeding connection with her baby. (See the suggestions for getting the baby back on the breast in Chapter 21.) Table 24.1 contains suggestions for counseling a mother who is separated from her baby.

▶ SHORT-TERM SEPARATIONS

Most mothers will be away from their babies during a usual feeding time at some point. Such short-term absences sometimes help a woman adjust to her new

role as mother and caretaker of a small baby. They offer a break from the routine of baby care and can help a new mother maintain a positive outlook. A brief time away can strike a compromise between mothering and outside interests such as volunteer work, sports activities, crafts, or exercise classes. A mother may have responsibilities that necessitate a short absence, such as doctors' appointments or attending functions for other family members. She may wish to simply plan an evening out with her partner, go to the hairdresser, or shop with a friend.

A mother can try to plan events at times that will avoid missed feedings, or it may be possible for the baby to accompany her. For occasions when the baby stays home, he can receive the mother's expressed milk through an alternative feeding method. The mother can express milk in the morning and throughout the day for several days before the planned separation. She can then store her milk in the freezer. If she becomes uncomfortably full or experiences leaking during the separation, she can express milk for comfort and to avoid breast problems. She can use manual expression or carry a hand-held pump for that purpose.

Hospitalization of Mother or Baby

Whether planned or unexpected, any separation can cause emotional stress. Stress intensifies when hospitalization results from an illness or injury and the mother may need support for more than breastfeeding. Chapter 23 addresses special situations that can necessitate a baby's prolonged hospitalization following birth. The discussion in this section focuses on general aspects of hospitalization and offers guidelines to assist the mother.

TABLE 24.1	
Counseling a Mother Who Is Separated from Her Baby	
Mother's Concern	**Suggestions for Mother**
Overfullness or leaking	◆ Express milk during the absence. ◆ Wear breast pads when away. ◆ Nurse directly before and after the absence.
Low milk production	◆ Delay the separation until milk production is well-established (around 2 months). ◆ Practice milk expression so you can express regularly during missed feedings. ◆ Drink to thirst. ◆ Nurse frequently when with the baby.
Feeding the baby	◆ Have the caregiver feed the baby the mother's milk or formula. ◆ Use a cup to avoid bottles if nipple preference is a concern. ◆ Practice alternate feedings before the separation to make sure the baby will accept the method.

A mother can explore the possibility of remaining with her baby continually or being together at feeding times. If rooming-in is available, she can inquire about the cost and whether she must pay for the additional bed or meals. If the mother needs to pump to maintain milk production, she can ask about using a hospital breast pump while she is there. She will need to express milk regularly throughout the day. If the baby cannot receive the mother's milk, pumping still is important for her to maintain milk production. Table 24.2 will help a mother who must plan for a hospitalization.

When the Mother Is Ill

Whenever a mother contracts an infection—whether it be a cold, fever, or more serious illness—her body responds by producing antibodies in her milk that help to protect her breastfeeding baby (Hanson, 2003). Although some viruses will be transmitted through her milk, in most cases the presence of antibodies to counteract them offsets the potential harm to the baby. Often, a more likely mechanism of disease transmission from the mother to her baby is through touching and close mouth and nose contact, not through her milk.

When the mother becomes ill, exposure to her baby already has occurred through contact during her most contagious period. The most effective treatment for the baby is to continue to breastfeed while the mother receives any necessary medication. The mother can decrease her baby's exposure to the disease by careful hand washing before contact. In extreme cases, she can wear a mask over her nose and mouth.

Therefore, a breastfeeding mother who develops a cold or fever need not worry about infecting her baby through her milk. She will want to practice good hygiene and limit facial contact with her baby during the infectious period, if possible. She also needs to rest and follow the treatment prescribed by her caregiver in order to return to good health quickly and not compromise her milk production.

Hospitalization of the Mother

In most cases, a mother hospitalized due to illness or injury can continue to breastfeed, provided that she is not consuming medication that could be harmful to her baby. If rooming-in is permitted, she can ask to be assigned to a floor that will accommodate a young baby

TABLE 24.2	
Preparing for Hospitalization	
Points to Consider	**Suggestions for Mother**
Explore your options	◆ Learn if hospitalization is necessary. ◆ Request a second opinion. ◆ Learn if hospitalization can be delayed until the baby is older and milk production is established. ◆ Learn whether early discharge is possible if home nursing care is arranged. Contact local Visiting Nurses Association for home care.
Be assertive regarding your wishes	◆ Discuss all concerns and wishes with your physician to avoid separation or to work toward minimizing missed feedings. ◆ Examine hospital policies concerning rooming-in and the use of hospital breast pumps.
Become well informed	◆ Learn about hospital procedures and factors surrounding hospitalization. ◆ Review informed consent as discussed in Chapter 4. ◆ Contact local and Internet resource groups.
Keep clear, well-organized records	◆ Record expenses for income tax deductions for child care, travel, and breast pump rental, as these may be paid by insurance. ◆ Record all details of your care plan and provide copies for yourself, your physician, and the hospital.
Prepare for transportation to and from the hospital	◆ Arrange for someone to drive you to and from the hospital.

such as in obstetrics. Depending on the mother's condition, she may need to have another adult in the room to help her care for her baby. If rooming-in is not possible, she can arrange for someone to bring her baby to the hospital during the day and stay to care for the baby and help her during feedings if necessary. Another option is for someone to bring the baby to the hospital intermittently throughout the day to breastfeed.

A mother may be so ill that she is physically unable to breastfeed. In that case, "the nursing staff should be knowledgeable in breast care associated with establishing a milk supply, expressing milk to prevent breast engorgement, and initiating breastfeeding when the mother's condition permits" (Dauphinee, 1997). Ignoring a woman's lactation when she is in acute or emergency care can lead to more severe physical complications, such as mastitis or a breast abscess.

Family members and lactation staff need to advocate for preserving the mother's lactation until she is able to voice her wishes. In cases where the mother has severe mastitis or an abscess and decides to wean, she should recover from the mastitis before initiating weaning. It is important that she continue to remove milk from her breasts during the course of the mastitis (Berens, 2004).

Continuing to nurse through a complicated medical situation may not be the best choice for every woman. If breastfeeding would compromise her medical condition or if she finds it difficult to cope, pumping or weaning may be better alternatives. On the other hand, many mothers have continued to breastfeed throughout a hospitalization. One mother underwent a breast biopsy on an outpatient basis without ever missing a feeding. Another mother underwent a mastectomy, pumping and dumping during bouts of chemotherapy. She continued to breastfeed her two-year-old on the remaining breast when the drugs cleared from her system.

While a mother's medical condition may make nursing or caring for her baby challenging, her determination and advance planning will ease these difficulties. She will benefit from help in planning for the hospitalization, managing breastfeeding during the time she is hospitalized, and returning to a regular routine after she has returned home.

When the Baby Is Hospitalized

It is always stressful for parents of a hospitalized baby, and there are additional challenges when the baby breastfeeds. A baby may remain hospitalized for a prolonged period after birth, or he may return to the hospital due to complications, a contagious illness, or injury. Traveling back and forth to the hospital can be very tiring for a mother, especially if it occurs directly after the birth, at a time when she needs to give attention to her

own recovery. Frequently, the mother will have other children requiring her attention and care as well.

If the baby is in a high-risk center, the mother can ask about having him transferred to a facility closer to her home after his condition has stabilized, where she can visit him more easily. Many mothers will want to remain with their babies and can inquire about rooming-in policies for mothers of sick babies. Most major hospitals have corporate-sponsored housing available, such as Ronald McDonald houses or family rooms. A baby occasionally contracts a contagious illness that requires that he be isolated from other babies in a special isolation room. Most often, however, the mother would be safe rooming in with her baby and she can inquire about this option.

Breastfeeding is analgesic for painful bloodletting procedures, such as heel sticks (Carbajal, 2003; Gray, 2002). The mother can negotiate with caregivers to nurse her baby during these procedures. A baby who must undergo surgery will benefit from his mother's presence immediately before and after the procedure. Physicians generally request that a patient consume nothing within eight hours preceding surgery. However, human milk digests so quickly that a baby's stomach empties much more quickly, and he would be very hungry by the time he underwent surgery if not permitted a later feeding. An infant generally can nurse up to three hours before surgery (Litman, 1994; Tomomasa, 1987). The mother can ask her baby's caregiver how soon she can nurse before and after surgery. She can also ask to be with her baby in the recovery room.

After the Hospitalization

When the mother and baby are together at home again, they will benefit from frequent contact and support. If breastfeeding was interrupted during the hospitalization, the mother may need help increasing milk production. If the separation was for an extended period, she may need to relactate in order to continue breastfeeding. Even if the mother and baby were able to nurse during the hospitalization, they may need help re-establishing their breastfeeding routine. The anxiety and worry about the situation that precipitated the hospitalization will not necessarily subside when they settle in at home. The mother may appreciate having a compassionate and concerned listener to help her talk through her emotions.

▶ SUPPORTING THE WORKING MOTHER

The reality is that many mothers face regular separations from their baby. This most often involves a return to work or school. The majority of mothers with young children today work outside the home. In 2001, the proportion of working mothers with children under 6 years old ranged from a low of 36 percent in the Czech Republic to a high of 76 percent in Sweden. In the United States, approximately 61 percent of women with children under the age of 6 work outside the home (OECD, 2002) and 70 percent of these women work full time and have children under the age of 3. One-third of employed mothers return to work within 3 months after giving birth, and two-thirds return to work within 6 months (USBC, 2002). With almost 60 percent of children in the United States regularly in child care (Hofferth, 1998), combining working and breastfeeding will be prevalent among the mothers you see.

Obstacles to Working and Breastfeeding

Mothers who work outside the home initiate breastfeeding at the same rate as mothers who stay at home. However, the breastfeeding continuance rate declines sharply in mothers who return to work (Biagioli, 2003). You are in a position to help mothers work through the conflicting goals of motherhood and career. Greater effort with outreach will benefit younger and less educated mothers, as well as mothers who must work full time or who have shorter maternity leaves.

Unaware It Is Possible

Counseling efforts need to focus on educating women about the feasibility of combining employment with breastfeeding. A mother may assume that her circumstances can lead only in one direction. Realizing that she must return to work, she expects that she will be unable to breastfeed her baby. Number of children, plans to return to work or school by six months after birth, and maternal confidence are the three most significant factors in how long mothers plan to breastfeed (O'Campo, 1992).

A large Hong Kong study found that although the participants wanted to breastfeed, they faced many obstacles in a nonsupportive society. Mixed messages from health professionals, short maternity leaves, lack of workplace support for breastfeeding, and a lack of breastfeeding knowledge presented roadblocks for continued breastfeeding (Tarrant, 2002). To integrate the roles of breastfeeding mother and employee, women need practical advice as well as encouragement and support of healthcare providers, society, and the workplace (Meek, 2001).

Cultural Influences

The lactation consulting profession is doing an exemplary job of empowering women to initiate breastfeeding. However, many of society's attitudes, particularly those that involve a woman's return to work or school, do not support an atmosphere that is conducive to the mother continuing to breastfeed. This is evident in both attitude and action. Women often view breastfeeding as an interruption in their "real" life, with careers and lifestyles touted as a priority over the child's needs. Many times the expectation is that they will place their career or lifestyle ahead of child rearing.

The question is not whether it is possible to combine employment with long-term breastfeeding. The challenge is trying to do so in a culture that does not support breastfeeding. In Kenya, a culture supportive of breastfeeding, 94.1 percent of working mothers breastfeed and work an average of 46.2 hours per week (Lakati, 2002). Mothers in Swaziland combine hard physical labor with successful breastfeeding (Mbuli, 1993). These findings refute the belief in Western countries that a return to work is the reason breastfeeding needs to end prematurely (Lakati, 2002).

U.S. culture seems to view employment as a socially acceptable reason for mothers to wean (Van Esterik, 1981). Mothers feel there are few occupations that will allow them to combine breastfeeding with employment, despite the fact that most women believe it is desirable to work and breastfeed (Chalmers, 1990). U.S. welfare reform requires recipients to engage in work activities. Because in many states these work requirements apply to mothers whose children are only a few months old, lowered breastfeeding rates are an unfortunate consequence (Haider, 2003). Socio-cultural support and policies related to employment, health, and early childhood are important for increasing the rates of employed breastfeeding women (Galtry, 2003).

Fear of Job Loss

There is an ongoing concern about women illegally losing their jobs during maternity leave (ILO, 1999). The Maternity Protection Coalition supports women's right to breastfeed and work by advocating for improved maternity protection entitlements (WABA, 2004). The Maternity Protection Kit: A Breastfeeding Perspective provided by the Maternity Protection Coalition (MPC) is an important resource for IBCLCs and employers. The coalition is comprised of groups from the International Baby Food Action Network (IBFAN), the International Lactation Consultant Association (ILCA), the LINKAGES project, and the World Alliance for Breastfeeding Action (WABA). The Maternity Protection Kit is designed for breastfeeding advocates interested in working toward better maternity protection laws, regulations, and workplace policies. It provides information, resources, and tools for breastfeeding educators.

Unaccommodating Work Environment

Women who return to work after childbirth juggle their professional roles with their new family roles. Most put in a double day, fulfilling job requirements while striving to meet the nurturing needs of their child (Hochschild,

2003). Even well-educated healthcare professionals who understand and embrace the health importance of breast-feeding find it hard to continue breastfeeding their own children. Among physician mothers in one survey, 146 breastfed an average of 18.8 weeks, with a range of 1 to 128 weeks. The main factors contributing to weaning were a return to work (45 percent), diminishing milk produc-tion (31 percent), and lack of time to pump (18 percent). Return to part-time work was positively associated with greater duration of maternity leave and breastfeeding.

Upon returning to work, space and time for milk expression were obstacles for the majority of the physi-cian mothers. "Flexible employment arrangements may increase duration among physician mothers and provide an atmosphere of greater acceptance. Protected time and a space for milk expression could contribute to greater frequency of pumping and fewer problems associated with incomplete emptying of the breast" (Arthur, 2003).

Although employers are aware of the importance of breastfeeding for mothers and children, they generally do not place a high priority on providing breastfeeding sup-port (Brown, 2001). Less than half of employers surveyed had personal experience with breastfeeding (Libbus, 2002). While many employers are willing to help employ-ees who wish to breastfeed or express milk, they see little value to their business. An extensive social marketing campaign in Australia provided breastfeeding support materials to educate businesses. Over two-thirds of these businesses considered the marketing information and sug-gested workplace solutions sufficient to support balancing breastfeeding and working (McIntyre, 2002).

Some women discover their return to work is marked by resentment from colleagues or less favorable treatment by employers. Negative treatment may result in a lower position, job loss, verbal abuse, or social isola-tion (ILO, 1999). The ILO states: "Forfeited career opportunities represent not only long-term earnings loss for the woman and her family, but in cumulative terms, a tremendous reduction of women's potential contribu-tion to economic growth. Discrimination on the basis of maternity is costly to women, their families and society as a whole."

Combining Work and Breastfeeding

When a mother combines breastfeeding with a work sit-uation that separates her from her baby, many factors can affect her success. Statistically, women who are most likely to continue breastfeeding while working are older and more educated. They work fewer hours per week and occupy positions at a higher professional level (Hanson, 2003; Hills-Bonczyk, 1993). Timing of the mother's return to work has an impact on the length of time she breastfeeds. Employment within two or three

months postpartum appears to shorten breastfeeding duration (Galtry, 2003; Taveras, 2003; Gielen, 1991).

Family Considerations

Seeking assistance and information in the prenatal period will enable a woman to explore her options ade-quately in an unhurried manner. There are many cre-ative solutions available for incorporating motherhood and breastfeeding into her life. Help her recognize, though, that after she is home with her new baby, new goals may alter her plan. Information and classes on breastfeeding and working offer practical advice for women who plan to combine employment and breast-feeding. They can explore options that promote their productivity while keeping them with their babies and enabling them to meet their babies' needs (Greiner, 1993; Furman, 1992; Walker, 1992; Chalmers, 1990).

Exploring Options and Support at Work

Encourage the mother to explore employment options and seek input from her employer. She will want to become familiar with her employer's policies regarding maternity leave, her legal rights, and any issues involved with her return to work as they relate to her child's needs, including breastfeeding. Questions related to employment rights may include:

◆ What resources are available to her?

◆ How long can she stay on maternity leave? Are there any options for extending it?

◆ Can she alter, reduce, or eliminate hours at work?

◆ Does her employment provide flexible working options, such as job sharing, on-site child care, telecommuting from home, flex hours, or part-time hours?

◆ Does her work require separation from her baby, or is an alternative available that will keep her and her child together?

◆ Can she begin a home-based business that does not require her to leave her baby?

You can provide relevant literature to the mother to help her communicate her needs to her employer and coworkers. She can point out to them that breastfeeding gives the baby health benefits, thereby reducing the baby's number of illnesses and lost time from her work to care for him. She can discuss her plans and enlist sup-port from her employer, immediate supervisor, and coworkers. This will help her gauge the amount of sup-port she will receive when she is ready to return to work.

The mother can check the provisions of her health insurance plan for the cost of lactation assistance or a breast pump. Descriptions of model programs and breastfeeding promotion within the insurance industry are available in *Advancing Women's Health: Health Plans' Innovative Programs in Breastfeeding Promotion*. This monograph explores eight case studies of companies that promote breastfeeding coverage and provide benefits to their breastfeeding employees (AAHP, 2001).

Feeding Options

You can help the mother explore feeding options for her baby. She may be able to breastfeed on breaks throughout the day if there is child care available on-site or nearby. She can work toward reversing her child's nursing cycle by providing most or all of his feedings at times when she is with him, referred to as **reverse cycle nursing**. A mother most likely will need information about breast pumps so that she can express milk for missed feedings. Before she returns to work, she can begin collecting milk for later separations. Some women opt for artificial baby milk for feedings during the separation and breastfeed when they are with their baby. Other women choose to wean.

Child Care Options

When separation is necessary, a crucial concern for parents is the quality of substitute child care. In the United States, a variety of arrangements are used by parents. There are over 10.5 million children under the age of 5 whose mothers are employed outside the home. About 21 percent are cared for by one of the parents, about 29 percent are cared for by close relatives, 22 percent are in organized facilities, and 20 percent are in private, non-relative care (U.S. Census Bureau, 1999).

There is a wide range in the quality of care. One study examining organized facility care found that 12 percent were rated "less than minimal" in quality and 15 percent were rated "good." Only 52 percent of the sites consented to being observed. The sites that did not consent to the study seem likely to have offered lower-quality care (Helburn, 1995). One extrapolated study by the National Institute of Child Health and Human Development (NICHD) on children under age 3 estimates that 8 percent of settings are poor, 53 percent fair, 30 percent good, and 9 percent excellent (Vandell, 2000).

Addressing these issues honestly with mothers will help them make informed choices. The American Academy of Pediatrics (AAP), the American Academy of Family Physicians (AAFP) and the National Association of Child Care Resource and Referral Agencies have extensive child care checklists for parents. They can all be accessed at the National Institute of Health's website: www.nlm.nih.gov/medlineplus/childdaycare.html. When the mother interviews child care providers, she can address the needs of a breastfeeding baby, the use of her milk, and alternative feeding methods. She can also acquaint the provider with the positive aspects of breast-

feeding. Breastfed babies will be less fussy, will spit up less, and their spit-up will not stain clothing. They also will have fewer illnesses and less diaper odor.

Both the mother and her substitute child care provider will need to feel comfortable with the arrangement. You can provide information that is useful for both of them, particularly facts related to milk storage and handling. Mothers need to be aware of the increased risk of illness in the baby if they stop breastfeeding at the same time as they put him in day care.

Returning to Work

You can provide support and information to help the mother form solutions to the challenges associated with breastfeeding and employment. She is learning a new routine and integrating her maternal role with her workplace role. She is experiencing a degree of separation from her child, with its accompanying worries and doubts about how her child will fare. She will benefit from ideas to enhance her letdown and increase efficiency with her expression times.

When the time comes for the mother's return to work, several suggestions will make the transition a bit smoother for both her and her baby. Based on a traditional workweek, initially returning to work on a Thursday or Friday may allow the mother to feel less overwhelmed. If the return to work is a bit rocky, she and her baby will have the weekend to recoup and get ready for a full workweek. Packing a bag for her baby and herself the night before work will avoid a harried morning start and allow an opportunity to snuggle and feed her baby before beginning the workday. If possible, she might return to work part time, either in terms of days per week or hours per day.

Breastfeeding Routine

With employment and child care arrangements made prior to her baby's birth, the mother can focus on initiating good breastfeeding practices and using her support systems for information and encouragement. As she settles in at home, devoting her time to enjoying her new baby and forging their relationship will benefit both the mother and baby.

About two to three weeks before her return to work she can begin the hands-on planning for her baby's needs during the separation. As she familiarizes herself with breast pump use or manual expression, your assistance will help the mother learn these techniques and increase her self-confidence. She can begin expressing on the unused breast at the end of a feeding or express between feedings. In addition to practicing her technique, this enables her to begin storing milk for her baby.

Practicing for the Separation

In the weeks prior to separation the mother can begin practicing with the feeding method she has chosen. She can enlist the help of another person close to the baby to feed him her expressed milk at a comfortable temperature to encourage him to accept the new method of feeding. If she uses a bottle with an artificial nipple, she can warm the nipple. Occasionally, a baby will outright refuse any alternative method while his mother is nearby, so she may need to leave the immediate area. The baby often is more receptive when the person feeding him is someone who is very familiar. It is also best not to try a new feeding method when the baby is too hungry to deal with something new and unfamiliar.

As she becomes more proficient with expressing her milk and her baby is more accepting of his new feeding method, the mother can do several trial runs with the baby's substitute care provider. She can begin easing into a feeding routine that mimics her work schedule. As she finds herself in the midst of these intense changes, encourage her to keep open communication with those closest to her. Combining caring for a young baby with employment requires adjustments in other areas. Housework and errands may become less of a priority as the mother considers what must be done, what can wait, what can be streamlined for greater efficiency, and who is able to do it best.

Combining employment with a young baby presents challenges, regardless of how the mother feeds her baby. The special bond afforded by breastfeeding provides a unique way to reconnect before and after the day's work. The first feeding at the end of the workday provides special time for the mother and baby to be alone with one another. It helps the mother obtain the rest she needs and the baby to reconnect with his mother after having been away from her. Breastfeeding's health benefits will, in turn, reduce the working mother's stress. Breastfeeding mothers have an opportunity for rest during their nighttime hours, because breastfeeding only minimally interrupts their sleep if they keep the baby close. Mothers who encourage their babies to reverse their nursing cycle will find less of a need to express milk during working hours.

Child Care Provider

By the time the mother returns to work, she and her substitute care provider need to have decided on plans related to feeding. The mother can provide a written list of instructions related to the care of her milk and her baby's special preferences. She and her care provider can review the feeding regimen, including the feeding method. The caregiver will want to watch for signs of hunger so the baby does not become overly hungry. The mother can ask that the caregiver hold her baby in the same position as she holds him for breastfeeding. Some babies will not take a bottle in the same position as breastfeeding, however, and may do better when held on the caregiver's lap facing outward. It is important that the baby be in charge of drawing the milk or bottle nipple into his mouth rather than the caregiver controlling it. The mother can teach the caregiver paced feeding, described in Chapter 21, to avoid overfeeding and stress.

The mother and care provider need to communicate closely about the amount the baby takes at feedings, how he handles an artificial nipple, and how he is doing in general. Avoiding a feeding too close to the time the mother is to arrive will ensure that her baby is hungry and eager to nurse. This will relieve the mother's breast fullness and facilitate their coming back together at the end of the day. If the baby seems especially hungry just before the mother's return, the caregiver can provide only a partial feeding. If her baby is cared for outside the home, the mother may want a quiet place at the caregiver's site to breastfeed when she arrives. Some women prefer to drive home immediately to settle in with their baby. Together, the mother and care provider can help make the transition as smooth as possible.

Expressing Milk at Work

The mother will need to express milk regularly at work to maintain milk production and avoid engorgement, mastitis, plugged ducts, or excessive leaking. She will benefit from your support as she prepares to return to work and after she has implemented her plans. Part of this support can include information about the importance of expressing her milk. When the mother understands its importance, she is more likely to be committed to doing it. Knowing how her baby will benefit from her milk can comfort the mother when she feels discouraged. She will be reassured knowing that she is providing her baby with health and nutrition that no one can duplicate. Furthermore, she is saving money for her family by avoiding the cost of infant formula, the various feeding devices, and medical costs incurred due to more illnesses.

Pumping Routine

The expressing routine the mother developed at home may change after she returns to work. She will gradually learn to blend the expressing strategy she refined at home with her new work routine. Ideally, she can work toward matching her lactation breaks to her baby's feeding needs. At the very least, she will need to respond to any uncomfortable fullness in her breasts.

If her baby is still quite young, the mother may find it best to express milk every 3 hours. A double breast pump will decrease the mother's pumping time to about 10 minutes to stimulate milk production and remove the available milk. If she is single pumping or hand expressing, she will need about 20 minutes. As her baby grows older, the time needed for pumping will decrease.

The mother will want to express her milk in a place with privacy, a comfortable chair and room temperature, and options for passing the time while expressing her milk. Massaging her breasts and, if possible, using moist heat will help her relax. Stimulating her senses in a way that reminds her of her baby will also help. She could play an audiotape of his sounds, keep a picture of him close by, or even have an article of his clothing with her.

Storing Her Milk

The milk that the mother expresses at work can be stored in quantities her baby will take at one feeding. Initially, this amount may be uncertain. As she and her baby settle into a routine, the amount needed at a feeding will become clearer. Her freshly expressed milk can remain at room temperature safely for up to eight hours (Barger, 1987). However she cools her milk, she needs to make sure it remains cooled on her commute home. See Chapter 21 for more discussion of collecting and storing expressed milk.

Mother's Comfort and Adjustment

As the mother adjusts physically to her new routine, she may notice that her milk production fluctuates. This could be a byproduct of missed feedings as well as emotional swings associated with being separated from her baby. If she has delays in expressing her milk, her breasts can become uncomfortably full and leak. Some mothers keep a complete change of clothes at their workplace for when leaking occurs. Prints rather than solid colors will help to conceal breast fullness, leaks, or lopsidedness. The mother can keep a jacket or sweater handy and wear breast pads to absorb leaked milk. Clothing will need to allow easy breast access for pumping at work, as well as for nursing her baby just before leaving for work and on reuniting after work.

Routine After Work

Planning her time after work hours is equally as important as the mother's plans during work. Breastfeeding provides an opportunity to relax with her baby after work. Planning quiet time with her baby as a priority over other demands may help the mother deal with her after-work pressures. Some babies react to the separation by increasing the frequency and duration of feedings. This is helpful to both the mother's milk production and her need for rest. If it leads to reverse cycle nursing, the mother can be encouraged to take her baby to bed with her to meet her need for sleep.

Support for the Mother

The benefits of support for an employed breastfeeding mother extend beyond the mother and child. Employers find that employee morale and loyalty increase, with less time lost from work for a sick baby because of the protection he receives from breastfeeding (Cohen, 1995).

Fewer days off translate to lower healthcare costs for the company. When employers take an active interest in the families of their employees, they improve cohesiveness and productivity within the company.

Resources are available for women who combine motherhood and working. One book many mothers have found helpful is *Nursing Mother, Working Mother* (Pryor, 1997). Local breastfeeding support groups may offer evening or weekend meetings to accommodate working mothers. Lactation consultants and breastfeeding counselors have noticed that working mothers continue to breastfeed far longer than they originally planned, some for as long as three and four years. They will benefit from reassurance that extended breastfeeding is a biological norm, albeit not always a cultural one. You can recommend resources such as toddler nursing groups and books such as *Mothering Your Nursing Toddler* (Bumgarner, 2000).

▶ THE BABY-FRIENDLY WORKPLACE

Employers need to accommodate breastfeeding mothers so they can continue breastfeeding after they return to work (Chen, 2003). Many breastfeeding women return to work soon after the birth of their baby. Consequently, employers significantly influence a woman's ability to continue breastfeeding. There has been a trend in the workplace to create a more family-friendly environment for working parents. *Working Mother* magazine conducts an annual survey and compiles an annual list of the 100 best companies for working mothers. Figure 24.1 reflects the policies that distinguished the top 100 companies from the rest of U.S. corporations in 2003.

FIGURE 24.1
The 100 best U.S. companies compared with other companies.

National figures based on the Society for Human Resource Management's 2003 Benefits Survey:

◆ 100% offer flextime vs. 55% nationwide
◆ 99% offer an employee assistance program vs. 67% nationwide
◆ 98% offer elder-care resource and referral services vs. 20% nationwide
◆ 96% offer child-care resource and referral services vs. 18% nationwide
◆ 94% offer compressed workweeks vs. 31% nationwide
◆ 93% offer job-sharing vs. 22% nationwide
◆ 77% offer therapeutic massages vs. 11% nationwide
◆ 47% sponsor sick-child care vs. 7% nationwide
◆ 44% offer before/after school care vs. 4% nationwide
◆ 39% offer paid paternity leave vs. 12% nationwide
◆ 27% offer paid maternity leave beyond the short-term disability period vs. 14% nationwide

Source: Working Woman Media, 2003.

Employer Support for Breastfeeding

Many states promote companies that support their breast-feeding employees. An example of one such program is Texas' Mother Friendly Worksite designation. The Texas Department of Health officially designates Texas businesses as "Mother-Friendly" if they voluntarily have a written policy to support employed mothers by doing the following:

◆ Having flexible work schedules to provide time for expression of milk.

◆ Providing an accessible location that allows privacy.

◆ Providing access to a nearby clean and safe water source and a sink for washing hands and rinsing breast pump equipment.

◆ Providing access to hygienic storage for the mother's expressed milk (TDH, 2004).

Employers who support breastfeeding employees often are more positive toward breastfeeding overall (Dunn, 2004). Negative employer attitudes sometimes result from lack of experience, rather than outright opposition (Bridges, 1997). Because companies operate on a profit basis, you can educate businesses and mothers in your community about the benefits to employer support for breastfeeding employees (TDH, 2004):

◆ Cost savings of $3 for every $1 invested in breast-feeding support.

◆ Less illness among breastfed children of employees.

◆ Reduced absenteeism to care for ill children.

◆ Lower healthcare costs (an average of $400 per baby over the first year).

◆ Improved employee productivity.

◆ Higher employee morale and greater loyalty.

◆ Improved ability to attract and retain valuable employees.

◆ Family-friendly image in the community.

Simple measures can provide breastfeeding support in the workplace. The procedures are practical, safe, and easy to implement economically. A wide range of occupations has implemented them. See Table 24.3 for the components of a breastfeeding support program for the workplace.

Formula manufacturers have targeted working mothers as a hot market for their products. Ross Products has collaborated with Working Mother Media, the publisher of *Working Mother* magazine, on "Business Backs Breastfeeding." It is a marketing program represented as a "new comprehensive workplace lactation program designed to help businesses support breastfeeding mothers upon their return to work" (Abbott Labs, 2004). Business Backs Breastfeeding enables Ross entry to hundreds of businesses to create brand awareness and loyalty. This type of marketing creates "goodwill" and the perception of community service.

In reality, a program like this undermines a woman's confidence in breastfeeding and promotes the perception that infant formula is a healthy alternative to her milk. When the mother visits the Ross Web site to order breastfeeding supplies, she reaches the Infant and Toddler Nutrition page, which advertises artificial baby milks. Breastfeeding supplies appear under "specialty products." The Maternity Protection Kit described previously and other resources from breastfeeding proponents support mothers' rights to breastfeed, not to be sabotaged by a formula manufacturer.

Approaching the Employer for a Lactation Room

You can be instrumental in helping a mother achieve breastfeeding support at work by suggesting ways she can approach her employer about developing a lactation program. She can survey other employees to learn how many are pregnant, how many plan to breastfeed, and how many would use a lactation room. This will help garner support for the program as well as provide concrete data to present to the employer. She can gain support from fellow employees, another breastfeeding mother or breastfeeding advocate, the corporation's nurse, a wellness program director, or a health educator. Collaboratively, they can determine the best way to approach the employer and the necessary preparations beforehand.

Suggesting more than one option may increase the mother's chances for success with her employer. She should be prepared to discuss alternative solutions and make compromises in her original plan. It is best to present the idea of a lactation room to the employer in a written proposal that identifies the required time, space, and type of environment. The proposal should indicate potential costs and whether the company's budget can support those costs. Indicating the cost-benefit ratio will illustrate long-term savings to the company in healthcare costs. Attaching relevant research on the health savings of breastfeeding will lend further credence to the proposal. The mother can also demonstrate to the employer that the cost of a lactation program will be less than the cost of training a new employee.

Healthy People 2010 has a goal of 50 percent of mothers breastfeeding until their infants are 6 months old (Ortiz, 2004). Company-sponsored lactation programs

TABLE 24.3

Components of a Workplace Breastfeeding Support Program

Adequate	Expanded	Comprehensive
Facilities		
A clean, private, comfortable multipurpose space (that is not a bathroom) with an electrical outlet in order to pump milk or to breastfeed.	A breastfeeding mothers' break room (BMBR) for use only by breastfeeding women.	A breastfeeding mothers' break room (BMBR) (or rooms) close to women's worksites.
Employee provides her own breast pump.	Employer provides one multi-user electric breast pump, and employees provide their own collection kits.	Employer provides collection kits. Additional multi-user electric pumps are provided if needed.
Table and comfortable chair.	Improved aesthetics to promote relaxation.	Room large enough to accommodate several users comfortably.
Sink, soap, water, and paper towels. If these are very far, extra time is allowed for cleaning hands and equipment.	Items listed in "Adequate" column are available near the BMBR.	Items listed in "Adequate" column are available in the BMBR.
Employee supplies cold packs for storage of milk.	Employer makes available refrigerator space designated for food near BMBR.	Employer provides a small refrigerator in the BMBR for storage of human milk.
Written Company Policy		
Employer grants a 6-week unpaid maternity leave.	Employer grants a 12-week unpaid maternity leave (FMLA).	Employer offers a 6- to 14-week paid maternity leave (ILO).
Employer allows creative use of accrued vacation days, personal time, sick days, and holiday pay after childbirth.	In addition, employer allows part-time work, job sharing, individualized scheduling of work hours, compressed work week, or telecommuting.	In addition, mother can bring child to work, caregiver can bring child to workplace, or on-site day care is available.
Employer allows 2 breaks and a lunch period during an 8-hour work day for expressing milk or breastfeeding the child.	Employer allows expanded unpaid breaks during the work day for expressing milk or breastfeeding the child.	Nursing breaks are paid and are counted as working time.
Workplace Education		
Company breastfeeding support policy is communicated to all pregnant employees.	New employees, supervisors, and coworkers all receive training on the breastfeeding support policy.	Breastfeeding education is offered to the partners of employees who are expectant fathers.
Employer provides a list of community resources for breastfeeding support.	Employer contracts with skilled lactation care provider on an "as needed" basis.	Employer hires a skilled lactation care provider to coordinate a breastfeeding support program.

Source: USBC, 2002.

enable mothers to maintain milk production for their babies for as long as they wish. Ortiz surveyed 462 women in 5 companies and found that breastfeeding was initiated by 97.5 percent of the participants, with 57.8 percent continuing for at least 6 months. Of 435 participants, 336 were successful at maintaining lactation. They expressed milk in the workplace for a mean of 6.3 months. The average age of the baby when the mother stopped pumping was 9.1 months. Of these women, 82.2 percent were full-time employees.

Employer Breastfeeding-friendly Program

Employers can support breastfeeding mothers in many ways (Wyatt, 2002). They can provide extended paid maternity leave to allow a mother to remain at home with her baby for as long as possible. They can incorporate breastfeeding breaks into the mother's work schedule or give mothers the option of bringing their baby to work to avoid missed feedings. They can provide information about child care or, better yet, provide child care at or near the worksite. Some companies provide prenatal and postpartum programs for parents. Employers can also accommodate mothers with appropriate physical facilities and a policy of support among coworkers.

Physical Arrangements

The biggest challenge to establishing facilities for breastfeeding mothers may be finding available space that is private. The room will need a lockable door to prevent embarrassing interruptions. A screen inside the door will offer additional privacy. The room will need comfortable chairs with arm support and a table or desk on which the mother can place her breast pump, her baby's picture, a beverage, and other items she may need. Employees on maternity leave and those who are pregnant can receive information about the pumping room so they are aware their employer supports breastfeeding. This will help demonstrate the importance of the program.

Employers may find it helpful to have a sign-in book in the pumping room so they can track and report the number of employees from different departments who use the space. Employees are encouraged to provide feedback on the conditions of the station and offer suggestions for improvement. Usually, the employees express gratitude and praise.

Time to Express Milk or Breastfeed

The time allotted for mothers to express their milk needs to be valued and respected. This is not comparable to a coffee break. It is a health practice for both the mother and her baby, grounded in a significant amount of research. Most mothers express their milk about twice a day and spend under an hour when in a breastfeeding-supportive employment environment (Slusser, 2004).

Employers are encouraged to allow the mother freedom to leave her workspace when she determines the need. She requires enough time to reach the room, time for unhurried pumping, and time to return. The understanding should be that coworkers will not question her use of time and will not complain. The employer can establish this policy with the coworkers, recognizing that the mother is doing this for her baby's health. Allowing time for cigarette breaks seems to be standard in many companies. A break for breastfeeding—a healthy choice—certainly warrants the same accommodation!

Positive Environment

The support of management will be crucial to a mother's ability to balance work with breastfeeding. Some employees may make negative comments about the mother's efforts. Ironically, male coworkers often seem to support breastfeeding employees more than other women do. A positive climate established by management will encourage coworkers to support the mother in a meaningful way. Company policy needs to incorporate protection of the mother's right to pumping time and intolerance of nonsupport or sexual harassment from other employees. Even the U.S. military is studying the needs of active-duty breastfeeding mothers (Stevens, 2003).

The climate in the pumping area should be non-stressful and soothing, perhaps enhanced by quiet music and reading material. Providing a refrigerator for the mother's milk is another gesture that shows a commitment to her efforts. It would also be helpful to have a mirror so that she can check to be sure that her clothes are back in place before leaving the room. Some employers have a lactation consultant on call for any concerns or special situations that arise.

Employers are a significant contributor to mothers reaching their breastfeeding goals. Whaley (2002) found that nearly 70 percent of WIC employees who were breastfeeding reached the AAP goal of 12 months' duration or more. Whaley concluded, "It is clear that full-time employment and breastfeeding can be compatible given appropriate worksite support." You can be instrumental in helping employers in your community establish policies that support their breastfeeding employees. Stressing both the financial and health benefits will strengthen your efforts.

 ## SUMMARY

It is important to help mothers continue breastfeeding in spite of time away from their babies. A mother who is ill or whose baby is ill needs practical ways to deal with her milk production and the baby's feeding needs. Your support will be a valuable resource to a mother throughout the stress of a hospitalization. Most separations are due to social or economic needs and may allow for more planning on the mother's part. You can help the mother recognize her options and provide her milk to her baby. Continued assistance after she has implemented her plans will help her find ways to fine-tune her pumping, milk storage, use of alternative feeding methods, and other changes in her breastfeeding routine. Developing or managing a corporate lactation program, or being on call for assistance, will provide essential support and encouragement to working mothers as they blend breastfeeding with employment.

▶ CHAPTER 24—AT A GLANCE

Facts you learned—

Counseling a mother through a separation:

◆ Ensure that her baby will feed from an alternative method during her absence.

◆ Express milk regularly to relieve fullness and maintain milk production.

◆ Plan the least disruptive timing for the separation, if possible.

◆ Avoid leaking, plugged ducts, engorgement, and mastitis.

◆ Get adequate rest and nutrition.

Counseling mothers about illness and hospitalization:

◆ Pump to maintain milk production.

◆ Decrease the baby's exposure by careful handwashing before contact.

◆ Room in with another adult in the room to help her care for her baby.

◆ Have the baby brought to the hospital throughout the day to breastfeed.

◆ Nurse before and after surgery.

Counseling a mother who returns to work:

◆ Recognize conflicting goals of motherhood and career.

◆ Realize goals may change after the baby arrives.

◆ Discuss her wishes, plans, needs, and concerns with family, friends, coworkers, and employer.

◆ Contact ILCA for a Maternity Protection Kit.

◆ Explore work and child-care options that will protect breastfeeding.

◆ Breastfeed uninterruptedly and bond with baby until return to work.

◆ Practice for the separation with the child care provider and feeding method.

◆ Plan for milk expression, enhancing letdown, collection, and storage of milk.

◆ Plan for relieving breast fullness and leaking.

◆ Plan quiet time for breastfeeding after return from work.

◆ Inquire about a workplace breastfeeding support program.

▶ REFERENCES

Abbott Labs, Ross Products Division. Working Mother Media Join Forces To Promote Workplace Support for Breastfeeding. Press Release, February 20, 2004. Available at: www.abbott.com/ross/index.cfm?id=690. Accessed February 7, 2005.

American Association of Health Plans (AAHP). Health Plans' Innovative Programs in Breastfeeding Promotion. August 2001. Available at: www.aahp.org. Accessed October 6, 2004.

Arthur C et al. The employment-related breastfeeding decisions of physician mothers. *J Miss State Med Assoc* 44(12):383–387; 2003.

Barger J, Bull P. A comparison of the bacterial composition of breast milk stored at room temperature and stored in the refrigerator. *Int J Childbirth Education* 2(3):29–30; 1987.

Berens P. *Breast Complications While Breastfeeding.* La Leche League of Texas Area Conference, San Antonio, TX; June 12, 2004.

Biagioli F. Returning to work while breastfeeding. *Am Fam Physician* 68(11):2201–2208; 2003.

Bridges C et al. Employer attitudes toward breastfeeding in the workplace. *J Hum Lact* 13:215–219; 1997.

Brown C et al. Exploring large employers' and small employers' knowledge, attitudes, and practices on breastfeeding support in the workplace. *J Hum Lact* 17(1):39–46; 2001.

Bumgarner N. *Mothering Your Nursing Toddler.* Schaumburg, IL: La Leche League International; 2000.

Carbajal R et al. Analgesic effect of breastfeeding in term neonates: Randomised controlled trial. *BMJ* 326(7379):13; 2003.

Chalmers B et al. Working while breastfeeding among coloured women. *Psychol Rep* 67:1123–1128; 1990.

Chen C, Chi C. Maternal intention and actual behavior in infant feeding at one month postpartum. *Acta Paediatr Taiwan* 44(3):140–144; 2003.

Cohen R et al. Comparison of maternal absenteeism and infant illness rates among breast-feeding and formula-feeding women in two corporations. *Am J Health Promot* 10(2):148–153; 1995.

Dauphinee J et al. Support of the breast-feeding mother in critical care. Review. *AACN Clin Issues* 8(4):539–549; 1997.

Dunn B et al. Breastfeeding practices in Colorado businesses. *J Hum Lact* 20(2):170–177; 2004.

Furman L. A second look at breastfeeding and full time maternal employment. *Am J Dis Child* 146:540; 1992.

Galtry J. The impact on breastfeeding of labour market policy and practice in Ireland, Sweden, and the USA. *Soc Sci Med* 57(1):167–177; 2003.

Gielen AC et al. Maternal employment during the early post partum period: Effects on initiation and continuation of breastfeeding. *Pediatrics* 87:298–305; 1991.

Gray L et al. Breastfeeding is analgesic in healthy newborns. *Pediatrics* 109(4):590–593; 2002.

Greiner T. Breastfeeding and maternal employment: Another perspective. *J Hum Lact* 9:214–215; 1993.

Haider J. Welfare work requirements and child well-being: Evidence from the effects on breast-feeding. *Demography* 40(3):479–497; 2003.

Hanson M et al. Correlates of breast-feeding in a rural population. *Am J Health Behav* 27(4):432–444; 2003.

Helburn S et al. *Cost, Quality, and Child Outcomes in Child Care Centers.* Public Report. Denver, CO: Economics Department, University of Colorado at Denver; 1995.

Hills-Bonczyk S et al. Women's experiences with combining breastfeeding and employment. *J Nurs Midwife* 38:257–266; 1993.

Hochschild A, Machung A. *The Second Shift.* New York: Penguin Books; 2003.

Hofferth SL, Shauman KA, Henke RR, West J. *Characteristics of Children's Early Care and Education Programs: Data from the 1995 National Household Education Survey* (Report No. 98–128). Washington, DC: U.S. Department of Education, National Center for Education Statistics; 1998.

International Labour Organization (ILO). *Maternity Protection at Work.* Revision of the Maternity Protection Convention (Revised), 1952 (No. 103), and Recommendation, 1952 (No. 95). 87th International Labour Conference, 1999. Available at: www.ilo.org/public/english/standards/relm/ilc/ilc87/rep-v-1.htm. Accessed June 23, 2004.

Kassing D. Bottle-feeding as a tool to reinforce breastfeeding. *J Hum Lact* 18(1):56–60; 2002.

Lakati A et al. Breast-feeding and the working mother in Nairobi. *Public Health Nutr* (6):715–718; 2002.

Libbus M, Bullock L. Breastfeeding and employment: An assessment of employer attitudes. *J Hum Lact* 18(3):247–251; 2002.

Litman R et al. Gastric volume and pH in infants fed clear liquids and breast milk prior to surgery. *Anesth Analg* 79:482–485; 1994.

Mbuli A. Working and breastfeeding. Voices from the field: Swaziland. *Mothers Child* 12(2):1–3; 1993.

McIntyre E et al. Balancing breastfeeding and paid employment: A project targeting employers, women and workplaces. *Health Promot Int* 17(3):215–222; 2002.

Meek J. Breastfeeding in the workplace. *Pediatr Clin North Am* 48(2):461–474, xvi. Review; 2001.

O'Campo P et al. Prenatal factors associated with breastfeeding duration: Recommendations for prenatal interventions. *Birth* 19(4):195–201; 1992.

Organisation for Economic Co-operation and Development. OECD employment outlook 2002—Chapter 2. In: *Women at Work: Who Are They and How Are They Faring?* Available at: www.oecd.org/dataoecd/28/58/18960381.pdf. Accessed June 23, 2004.

Ortiz J et al. Duration of breast milk expression among working mothers enrolled in an employer-sponsored lactation program. *Pediatr Nurs* 30(2):111–119; 2004.

Pryor G. *Nursing Mother, Working Mother.* Schaumburg, IL: La Leche League International; 1997.

Ross Products Division, Abbott Labs. *Infant and Toddler Nutrition.* Available at: www.rosstore.com/pediatric.cfm. Accessed June 23, 2004.

Slusser W et al. Breast milk expression in the workplace: A look at frequency and time. *J Hum Lact* 20(2):164–169; 2004.

Stevens KV, Janke J. Breastfeeding experiences of active duty military women. *Mil Med* 168(5):380–384; 2003.

Tarrant M. Initiating and sustaining breastfeeding in Hong Kong: Contextual influences on new mothers' experiences. *Nurs Health Sci* 4(4):181–191; 2002.

Taveras E. Clinician support and psychosocial risk factors associated with breastfeeding discontinuation. *Pediatrics* 112(1 Pt 1): 108–115; 2003.

Texas Department of Health (TDH), Bureau of Nutrition Services. *Just for Grandparents.* Publication #13-06-11288; 2002.

Texas Department of Health (TDH). *Become a Mother Friendly Worksite.* Publication #13-58; March 2004.

Tomomasa T et al. Gastrointestinal motility in neonates: Response to human milk compared with cow's milk formula. *Pediatrics* 80:434–438; 1987.

United States Breastfeeding Committee (USBC). *Workplace Breastfeeding Support* [issue paper]. Raleigh, NC: Author; 2002.

U.S. Census Bureau. *Who's Minding the Kids? Child Care Arrangements: Spring 1999 Detailed Tables* (PPL-168) Historical Table: Primary Child Care Arrangements Used by Employed Mothers of Preschoolers: 1985 to 1999. Available at: www.census.gov/population/www/socdemo/child/ppl-168. html. Accessed February 9, 2005.

Vandell D, Wolfe B. *Child Care Quality: Does It Matter and Does It Need to Be Improved?* Office of the Assistant Secretary for Planning and Evaluation. Washington, DC: U.S. Department of Health and Human Services; May 2000. Available at: www.aspe.hhs.gov/hsp/ccquality00/index.htm. Accessed February 9, 2005.

Van Esterik P, Greiner T. Breastfeeding and women's work: Constraints and opportunities. *Stud Fam Plann* 12:184–197; 1981.

Walker M. Why aren't more mothers breastfeeding? *Childbirth Instr* 19–24; Winter 1992.

Whaley S et al. Predictors of breastfeeding duration for employees of the Special Supplemental Nutrition Program for Women, Infants, and Children (WIC). *J Am Diet Assoc* 102(9):1290–1293; 2002.

Wilson-Clay B, Hoover K. *The Breastfeeding Atlas.* 2nd ed. Austin, TX: Lactnews Press; 2002.

Working Mother Media, Inc. Press Release: Working mother magazine finds no drop in programs, announces 100 best companies for working mothers; September 23, 2003.

World Alliance for Breastfeeding Action (WABA). Women, work and breastfeeding: Campaigning for maternity protection at the workplace. Available at: www.waba.org.my/womenwork/campaign.html. Accessed June 23, 2004.

Wyatt S. Challenges of the working breastfeeding mother: Workplace solutions. Review. *AAOHN J* 50(2):61–66; 2002.

▶ **BIBLIOGRAPHY**

Ajusi AD et al. Bacteriology of unheated expressed breast milk stored at room temperature. *East Afr Med J* 66(6):381–387; 1989.

American Academy of Pediatrics (AAP). *New Mother's Guide to Breastfeeding*. Joan Younger Meek, ed. New York: Bantam; 2002.

American Academy of Pediatrics (AAP) Section on Breastfeeding. Breastfeeding and the use of human milk. *Pediatrics* 115(2):496–506; 2005.

Arnold L. Storage containers for human milk: An issue revisited. *J Hum Lact* 11(4):325–328; 1995.

Auerbach K. Assisting the employed breastfeeding mother. *J Nurs Midwife* 35:26–34; 1990.

Bocar D. Combining breastfeeding and employment: Increasing success. *J Perinat Neonat Nurs* 11:23–43; 1997.

Cohen R, Mrtek MB. The impact of two corporate lactation programs on the incidence and duration of breastfeeding by employed mothers. *Am J Health Promotion* 8:1–6; 1997.

Corbett-Dick P, Bezek S. Breastfeeding promotion for the employed mother. *J Pediatr Health Care* 11:12–19; 1997.

Dimico G. Teaching breastfeeding to working mothers. *Int J Childbirth Education* 20–21; 1991.

Duckett L. Maternal employment and breastfeeding: Clinical issues in perinatal and women's health nursing. *Breastfeeding NAACOG* 3(4):701–712; 1992.

Freed GL et al. National assessment of physician's breastfeeding knowledge, attitudes, training, and experience. *JAMA* 273:472–476; 1995.

Freed GL et al. Pediatrician involvement in breastfeeding promotion: A national study of residents and practitioners. *Pediatrics* 96:490–494; 1995.

Haider R, Syeeda B. Working women, maternity entitlements, and breastfeeding: A report from Bangladesh. *J Hum Lact* 11(4):273–278; 1995.

Healthy Mothers, Healthy Babies. What gives these companies a competitive edge? Worksite support for breastfeeding employees. Author: Washington, DC; July 1993.

Kavanaugh K et al. Getting enough: Mothers' concerns about breastfeeding a preterm infant after discharge. *JOGNN* 24:23–32; 1995.

Kavanaugh K et al. The rewards outweigh the efforts: Breastfeeding outcomes for mothers of preterm infants. *J Hum Lact* 13:15–21; 1997.

Lawrence RA. *Breastfeeding: A Guide for the Medical Profession.* St. Louis, MO: Mosby; 1999.

Medela Sanvita soars in Scottsdale. *Rental Roundup* 10:1–2; 1993.

Nkanginieme K. Breastfeeding: An appeal. *Afr Health* 15(3):20; 1993.

Riordan J. *Breastfeeding and Human Lactation.* 3rd ed. Sudbury, MA: Jones and Bartlett; 2005.

Rogers B, Banchy P. Establishing an employee breast pumping facility. *J Hum Lact* 10(2):119–120; 1994.

Saunders SE, Carroll J. Post partum breastfeeding support: Impact on duration. *J Am Diet Assoc* 88:213–215; 1988.

Slusser W, Powers NG. Breastfeeding update I: Immunology, nutrition and advocacy. *Pediatri Rev* 18(4):111–119; 1997.

USDA. *Breastfeeding Babies Welcome Here!* Alexandria, VA; USDA Food and Nutrition Service; Division Food and Nutrition Service, October 1993.

LONG-TERM MATERNAL AND INFANT CONDITIONS

The goal for breastfeeding advocates is to empower mothers to have positive experiences nursing their babies. Some mothers require special assistance with breastfeeding. Various health conditions—in both the mother and the infant—have the potential to affect the course of breastfeeding. When an infant is born with a health condition or neurological disorder, the effect on family members and their relationships will depend on the type and severity of the disorder. The medical expertise and emotional support available to parents will also be factors. Parents can overcome many feeding problems when they understand how to help their baby adapt to breastfeeding.

KEY TERMS

acetone
acquired immune deficiency syndrome (AIDS)
alactogenesis
anomaly
attachment parenting
autoimmune disorder
cleft lip
cleft palate
cosleeping
cystic fibrosis
cytomegalovirus
diabetes
Down syndrome
Duarte variant
endometriosis
epinephrine
Epstein-Barr
eustachian tube
exocrine system
galactosemia
goiter
grommet
hepatitis C
herpes

human immunodeficiency virus (HIV)
hydrocephalus
hypernatremic
hypertension
hyperthyroidism
hypothyroidism
infertility
insufficient milk supply (IMS)
lactogenesis
lymphocytes
multipara
multiple birth
obturator
oral aversion
otitis media
palatal repair
phenylalanine
phenylketonuria
Pierre Robin Sequence
polycystic ovarian syndrome (PCOS)
postpartum thyroiditis
primipara
propylthiouracil

Raynaud's phenomenon
rheumatoid arthritis
scleroderma
seroconversion
Sjogren's syndrome
spina bifida
submucosal cleft palate

systemic lupus erythematosus
tandem nursing
thyroid disorder
transplacental
tuberculosis
varicella zoster
vasospasm

SPECIAL MATERNAL HEALTH CONDITIONS

Some medical conditions can have an impact on a mother's breastfeeding. Any condition that requires the mother to take medication raises the question of whether she can safely breastfeed her baby. Other disorders may affect a woman's energy or otherwise impair her ability to breastfeed. Health conditions discussed in this chapter include autoimmune disorders, infertility, diabetes, thyroid disorders, cystic fibrosis, and phenylketonuria (PKU). Also addressed are several viruses that a mother may contract, including HIV/AIDS, with discussion of their safety in terms of breastfeeding.

Autoimmune Disorders

Autoimmune disease is estimated to affect up to 20 percent of the U.S. population. About 75 percent are women in their childbearing years (AARDA, 2004). Autoimmune disease is one of the 10 leading causes of all disease deaths among U.S. women aged 65 and younger (Walsh, 2000). While autoimmune diseases may not have direct impact on breastfeeding, common symptoms of many of the diseases are chronic fatigue and pain, which can affect a woman's overall health and outlook. Women are increasingly being diagnosed with one or more of these diseases, so the chances are high that some of the women in your care will have an autoimmune disease. It is even more likely that many have undiagnosed autoimmune disease, as those afflicted with a disease typically exhibit symptoms for several years before they are correctly diagnosed.

Autoimmune diseases are a result of a biological error in which the immune system misfires and attacks the cells, tissues, or organs it normally protects. Autoimmune diseases strike about three times as many women as men. Women are most vulnerable during their reproductive years, and the predominance among women may reflect the involvement of female hormones in the regulation of immune response. All autoimmune diseases show evidence of a genetic predisposition and they tend to cluster in families. Environmental triggers such as diet, sunlight, and a preceding infection may play a role in triggering the diseases in individuals with a genetic predisposition.

There are more than 80 autoimmune diseases, which clinicians now consider as a group of disorders (Hales, 2003). Some genes are specific to a certain disease, while others predispose to autoimmunity in general. Autoimmune diseases share many common symptoms, and often an individual has more than one disease. Some of the autoimmune diseases more familiar to the public are multiple sclerosis, Graves' disease, scleroderma, Raynaud's phenomenon, inflammatory bowel disease, ulcerative colitis, Crohn's disease, lupus, Sjogren's syndrome, and rheumatoid arthritis.

Fibromyalgia has recently gained recognition as a distinct clinical entity that often accompanies other autoimmune disorders. It exhibits a characteristic pattern of specific, intensely tender trigger points on the body. Chronic fatigue immune dysfunction syndrome (CFIDS) may have an autoimmune component as well, as it is often associated with circulating anti-nuclear auto-antibodies.

Counseling Implications

What does this all mean to you as a lactation consultant? First, by understanding the nature of autoimmune disease, you may recognize symptoms such as chronic fatigue and pain as potential red flags for women in your care. You can then suggest they consult their caregiver. Proper diagnosis is one of the most difficult challenges related to autoimmune disease. You can suggest that these women learn the medical history of their immediate and extended family. They can make a list of symptoms, even those that are seemingly unrelated, dating back as far as they can recall. Finding informed caregivers who have experience with autoimmune disease is one of the most important factors in obtaining a correct diagnosis. Many individuals seek second, third, and fourth opinions over several years before they finally receive an appropriate diagnosis and treatment.

Second, you can be alert to potential symptoms that could affect these women during lactation. The chronic fatigue and pain associated with many of the autoimmune diseases can affect a woman's coping abilities and mental outlook. Serotonin reuptake inhibitors (anti-depressants) relieve symptoms for some of the diseases, and you can share appropriate information about the safety of taking these and other medications while breastfeeding.

Endometriosis and Immune Disorders

Women with endometriosis have a higher incidence of autoimmune disorders than the general female population. Table 25.1 shows the relative frequency of autoimmune disorder diagnoses for women with endometriosis compared with the general population. Because 41 percent

TABLE 25.1

**Women with Endometriosis Diagnosed with Autoimmune Diseases
Compared to General U.S. Female Population**

Immune Disorder	% with Endometriosis	% of General Population
Hypothyroidism	9.6%	1.5%
Fibromyalgia	5.9%	3.4%
Chronic fatigue immune dysfunction syndrome (CFIDS)	4.6%	.03%
Rheumatoid arthritis	1.8%	1.2%
Systemic lupus erythematosus	.8%	.04%
Sjogren's syndrome	.6%	.03%
Multiple sclerosis	.5%	.07%
Allergies	61%	18%
Asthma	12%	5%
Allergies with fibromyalgia or CFIDS	88%	18%
Asthma with fibromyalgia or CFIDS	25%	5%

Source: Sinaii, 2002.

of women with endometriosis have fertility problems (Sinaii, 2002), you may see quite a few of these women who became pregnant through assisted reproduction and then have problems with lactation. A thorough medical history will help you identify markers.

Other Implications for Breastfeeding

Sjogren's syndrome is an autoimmune disease that attacks the tear, salivary, and other secretory glands and impairs their ability to produce moisture. In the majority of cases, the autoimmune response affects the tear ducts, salivary glands, and vagina (NINDS, 2003). There is no evidence that it has an effect on the mammary glands; however, because the breast is a secretory organ, the possibility of a correlation bears scrutiny. Sjogren's syndrome can be a marker for other diseases, including scleroderma. Some autoimmune diseases, such as multiple sclerosis, may improve during pregnancy. Others may worsen before or after childbirth. Lupus worsens during pregnancy and may improve afterward (Lupus Foundation, 2001). Some autoimmune diseases, such as thyroid diseases, increase the risk of infertility (Poppe, 2004, 2003a, 2003b, 2002).

As discussed in Chapter 9, human milk has protective factors that reduce the risk of autoimmune diseases. These include Crohn's disease (Thompson, 2000), ulcerative colitis (Corrao, 1998), juvenile diabetes (Young, 2002; Monetini, 2001; Kimpimaki, 2001), juvenile arthritis (Mason, 1995), multiple sclerosis (Tarrats, 2002; Pisacane, 1994), and celiac disease (Ivarsson, 2002). Multiple sclerosis is rare in countries where breastfeeding is common (Dick, 1976). Mexico has experienced a rise in the incidence of multiple sclerosis as breastfeeding has decreased (Tarrats, 2002). Because of the familial nature of the disorder, mothers would be wise to breastfeed their children to reduce the chances of their developing any of the scores of immune diseases.

Raynaud's Phenomenon

Raynaud's phenomenon is a common condition, affecting up to 22 percent of women aged 21 to 50 (Olsen, 1978). Pain in the extremities when exposed to cold is a marker for Raynaud's, which is a disorder of the small blood vessels in the skin. During a Raynaud's attack, restricted blood flow in the extremities causes numbness and pins-and-needles sensations. Sometimes a dull pain and clumsiness occur. Skin color changes of the extremities occur in a sequence of white (blanching or pallor) to blue (cyanotic) and then to red (rubor) as blood returns to the area. Raynaud's can also affect the nose and ears. A Raynaud's attack could affect a woman's dexterity and ability to relax during a feeding. Cold is more apt to cause an attack when the woman is physically or emotionally stressed. Sometimes stress alone will cause vasoconstriction without

exposure to cold. Given the stressors of birth and postpartum adjustment, it is not surprising that IBCLCs see many women with these symptoms.

Injuries such as frostbite or surgery can cause Raynaud's phenomenon. Regular use of machinery such as chain saws and vibrating drills can damage the small blood vessels. Other activities that may worsen the condition include frequent typing and piano playing (NHLBI, 2004). Certain drugs and medical conditions can cause secondary Raynaud's, including some heart, blood, and migraine headache medications. Conditions that may cause secondary Raynaud's include:

- Scleroderma—a thickening and hardening of the skin and other body tissues
- Systemic lupus erythematosus—a chronic inflammation of the skin and organ systems
- Rheumatoid arthritis—a chronic inflammation and swelling of tissue in the joints
- Blood flow reduction—problems that slow or stop blood flow in a vessel, such as inflammation and hardening of the arteries (arteriosclerosis)
- Nerve problems—problems that affect the nerves supplying the muscles
- Pulmonary hypertension—a condition in which pressure rises in the blood vessels of the lungs

Caffeine and nicotine increase the severity of Raynaud's due to increased blood vessel constriction. You can caution mothers that consuming caffeine or smoking may worsen their symptoms. Increasing intake of vitamin B_6 has helped some mothers. However, very high doses (600 mg) can lower milk production. Caution mothers that vitamin B_6 passes readily into their milk, and that too much can harm an infant's liver (Hale, 2004). Hale suggests a maximum intake of 25 mg/day of vitamin B_6. Newman (2003) recommends a dosing protocol of 150–200 mg/day once a day for 4 days, followed by 25 mg/day once a day. He advises that if vitamin B_6 fails to work within a few days it probably will not produce results. Calcium channel blockers, such as nifedipine, have been helpful for some mothers with Raynaud's (Hale, 2002b).

Raynaud's and Nipple Soreness

As described in Chapter 16, a Raynaud-like phenomenon can cause vasospasms of the nipple. Mothers describe the pain as a stinging, tingling, burning, very painful sensation that persists after a feeding. The same triphasic color change occurs on the nipple as with the extremities in true Raynaud's (Anderson, 2004; Lawlor-Smith, 1997). A poor latch and suckle is often the cause of such a vasospasm. Many mothers find that when the latch improves, the baby no longer compresses the nipple to cause vasospasm. Sometimes, however, the baby may latch without problems but the mother still experiences this kind of pain. Women who have true Raynaud's usually are aware of it prior to pregnancy, but mothers may report never having symptoms prior to the baby's birth. Some mothers with nipple vasospasms report the pain also occurs when they are exposed to cold.

For some mothers, your validation that their nipple pain has a medical cause will be a big relief. Always refer the mother to her caregiver for evaluation and treatment. If she is on any of the medications associated with secondary Raynaud's, her physician may be able to adjust or change them.

If you have helped a mother fix her baby's latch and she is still experiencing vasospasms, other comfort measures may provide relief. Applying heat immediately after breastfeeding can help to minimize the vasospasm. Some mothers prefer the dry heat of a heating pad, while others prefer moist heat. If a mother wishes to use a microwavable pad, caution her to make sure it is not too hot. She can take measures to protect her entire body from the cold, not just her hands and feet. She can wear warm socks inside the house, avoid putting her hands in cold water, and remove food from the refrigerator or freezer with gloves or potholders. She should try to avoid cuts, bruises, and other injuries to the affected areas. She may need to limit activities such as typing, sewing, or other detail work. Some people find that biofeedback helps their symptoms (NHLBI, 2004).

Diabetes

Mothers with diabetes may be highly motivated to breastfeed if they are educated about the health impact of *not* breastfeeding. Breastfeeding lowers children's risk of diabetes, depending on whether it is exclusive breastfeeding and how long breastfeeding continues (Sadauskaite-Kuehne, 2004; Kimpimaki, 2001; Monetini, 2001). The three classifications of diabetes mellitus are insulin-dependent (IDDM), noninsulin-dependent (NIDDM), and gestational diabetes (GDM). Women with diabetes generally can breastfeed safely, regardless of the type of diabetes they have. Because gestational diabetes virtually disappears following delivery, there are no special breastfeeding guidelines for these women. IBCLCs have noticed a delay in the onset of milk production with some mothers with gestational diabetes, so you will want to encourage frequent feeding of the newborn. Diet-controlled diabetic women have no breastfeeding restrictions. Most diabetic women who control their condition with oral hypoglycemic agents switch to insulin therapy during pregnancy for the safety of the fetus. Insulin-dependent women may breastfeed safely while continuing insulin therapy throughout lactation.

Understanding how diabetes affects the body will help you counsel diabetic women appropriately. Diabetes occurs because of insufficient insulin production or inefficient use of insulin by the body's cells. Unable to metabolize carbohydrates for energy, the body burns fat as its energy source. When the fat metabolizes, increased amounts of ketones are excreted into the urine. With the kidneys unable to keep up with the input of ketones, blood sugar level is affected. Uncontrolled blood sugar levels can cause coma and death.

The Diabetic Breastfeeding Mother

A diabetic mother is typically an active member of her healthcare team. She is responsible for monitoring her blood glucose levels, following a restricted diet, and administering her insulin. A woman's insulin needs will drop dramatically after the delivery of the placenta. Therefore, an insulin-dependent mother must conduct frequent blood glucose tests in the first few days postpartum to determine her requirements. Insulin levels will fluctuate erratically until lactation is established and will fluctuate again when weaning occurs. Careful monitoring is essential during these times.

There is evidence that lactogenesis is delayed by up to two to three days in insulin-dependent diabetics compared to nondiabetics. This phenomenon does not seem to interfere with the mother's overall lactation outcome. However, it is important that you be aware of the possibility of delayed lactogenesis and counsel mothers appropriately. Breastfeeding early and regularly postpartum is especially important for diabetic mothers to assist stage II lactogenesis (Arthur, 1994; Jackson, 1994; Ferris, 1993; Ostrum, 1993; Hutt, 1989).

Before the discovery of insulin in 1922, babies of nongestational diabetic mothers often died; the mothers often died as well. Risks are still higher for diabetic mothers and their babies. Babies have a higher incidence of morbidity and congenital malformations if the mother's diabetes is poorly controlled (Engelking, 1986). Fortunately, advances in diabetes management have dramatically improved health outcomes.

Diabetes treatment is highly individual. Some women may need to increase, rather than decrease, their dosage of insulin. Many diabetic women feel their healthiest and have better control over their diabetes during lactation than at any other time in their lives. In a study reported by Whichelow and Doddridge (1983), a breastfeeding mother's insulin requirement was 40 units at 3 months postpartum as compared to 45 units before pregnancy. This was true despite a daily increase of 50 grams of carbohydrates.

Because of an altered hormone balance, diabetic women may experience remission throughout lactation. Sugar is absorbed from the mother's system to produce the energy needed for milk production. Additionally, lactose is a component in the mother's milk, and the activity of breastfeeding expends more calories. This combination of factors often permits a higher caloric intake and lower insulin dosage.

During lactation, diabetic women generally require an increase in calories, carbohydrates, and protein. This varies with every woman, and precise dietary guidelines need to be part of the new regimen she plans with her caregiver. If her blood sugar climbs too high, she will release acetone and transmit it to her baby through her milk. After several days of exposure to high acetone levels, the baby can develop an enlarged liver. An increase of carbohydrates, possibly accompanied by an increased insulin dosage, will control the risk of acetone migrating into the mother's milk. If blood sugar is too low, the woman may experience diabetic shock, releasing epinephrine into her system and inhibiting letdown and milk production. Tight control of blood sugar levels will avoid these complications.

During any interruption in breastfeeding, and especially during weaning, the mother will need to adjust her caloric intake and insulin dosage to compensate for the decrease in utilization of sugar for lactation. Whenever sugar is present in her urine, she must increase her insulin dosage gradually and reduce her caloric intake to respond to her nursing schedule. If the interruption is short-lived, a simple reduction in food intake may be sufficient, with no change in insulin dosage.

Diabetic women are prone to yeast infections, which can affect both the mother's vaginal area and nipples. Moisture provides a breeding ground for fungus and can cause nipple soreness. Keeping the nipples dry between feedings will help to avoid this complication. If sore nipples fail to respond to the usual treatment, a yeast infection may be the cause (see Chapter 16 for a discussion of thrush). The delicate balance of diet, insulin, and exercise can be disturbed by an infection or by a digestive or emotional upset. During lactation, the mother will need to minimize stress and remove milk from her breasts regularly to avoid plugged ducts and mastitis. If mastitis occurs, the mother must monitor her blood sugar closely and make necessary adjustments in her treatment regimen.

With modern monitoring techniques, both in the hospital and at home, most diabetic women carry their babies to term and breastfeed with few complications. Diabetic women are often highly motivated to breastfeed and have a good working knowledge of nutrition because of their condition. By carefully monitoring her blood sugar level, working closely with her caregivers—which may include an obstetrician, a pediatrician, and an endocrinologist—and managing her breastfeeding appropriately, a diabetic woman can breastfeed without compromising her health or that of her baby. One Australian study found that diabetic mothers breastfed for a longer time than nondiabetics did, even though they did not initiate lactation as early and even though their babies received more supplements (Webster, 1995).

Some women may have insulin resistance rather than full-fledged diabetes. Symptoms of insulin resistance include high weight gain in pregnancy or preexisting obesity, gestational diabetes, high cholesterol, hypertension, acanthosis nigricans, and the development of skin tags during pregnancy. Some patients with insulin resistance receive treatment with metformin, which increases the body's sensitivity to insulin (Rao, 2001). See the following discussion on polycystic ovarian syndrome (PCOS) for more information about this medication.

Infertility and Insufficient Milk Supply (IMS)

When you take a mother's history, be sure to ask about any history of infertility or miscarriage. Miscarriages and infertility can result from thyroid disorders and are also associated with PCOS, both of which can be associated with insufficient milk supply. Many women with a history of infertility will have problems with milk production. Primary insufficient milk supply (IMS) and infertility seem to be related, although fertile mothers also can have IMS, and some mothers who conceive by reproductive technology can have ample milk supplies.

Primary IMS differs from a delay in lactogenesis. Distinguishing factors of a delay in lactogenesis include cesarean delivery, hypertension, edema, hormonal birth control, diabetes, retained placenta, obesity, or a theca lutein cyst as discussed in Chapter 7. IMS also differs from secondary lactation failure, which results from external causes such as scheduling, infrequent feedings, medications, hormonal birth control, or herbs. Secondary failure may also result from conditions in the baby, such as prematurity, ineffective latch or suck, or oral anomalies such as ankyloglossia.

When you are working with a mother with insufficient milk supply, pay careful attention to her breast development. Note the shape, symmetry, and vein prominence. Ask her about breast growth during puberty (e.g., cup size changes) and pregnancy. Ask about the level of fullness or engorgement after delivery and whether she felt her milk "coming in." Measure the space between her breasts, and palpate the breasts to determine their composition: the amount of glandular and fatty tissue and whether they are soft, flaccid, lumpy, or knotty (Marasco, 2003). Hypoplasia and spacing between the breasts (intramammary spacing) greater than 1.5 inches are markers for IMS (Huggins, 2000). (See Color Plates 4–7.)

Polycystic Ovarian Syndrome (PCOS)

Lactation consultants increasingly encounter mothers with insufficient milk supplies who have either a PCOS diagnosis or symptoms consistent with the syndrome

(Marasco, 2003, 2000). PCOS is the leading cause of infertility in women and has a constellation of possible symptoms. It is often associated with an accumulation of many incompletely developed follicles in the ovaries. The condition typically causes irregular menstrual cycles, scanty or absent menses, multiple small cysts on the ovaries (polycystic ovaries), mild to severe hirsutism (excessive hair), and infertility. Many women who have this condition may develop diabetes with insulin resistance (OMRN, 2000). Some women with PCOS conceive spontaneously, but many others require infertility assistance.

Prolactin resistance, a possible explanation for **alactogenesis** (no onset of stage II lactogenesis), may act much like insulin resistance, which suggests a possible genetic link (Zargar, 1997). Prolactin resistance may have caused alactogenesis in three births of a woman with normal breast development and an adequate pituitary prolactin reserve (Zargar, 2000). Another woman who had insufficient glandular tissue with her first child was later diagnosed with luteal phase defect and was treated with natural progesterone. She was able to exclusively breastfeed her second child, which suggests that the progesterone may have stimulated mammary gland growth (Bodley, 1999).

Medications such as metoclopramide, domperidone, and metformin have helped some women with IMS. Metformin is an insulin-sensitizing agent that has been in use for over 40 years, although it was not available in the United States until 1995. It enhances insulin sensitivity in the liver and muscle, thus improving glycemic (sugar) control. Improved metabolic control with metformin may be associated with moderate weight loss (OMRN, 2000). Very little metformin is found in the plasma of infants of mothers taking the drug (Gardiner, 2003; Hale, 2002a). Babies' birth weight, height, weight, and motor and social development at three and six months of life have been found to be normal (Glueck, 2002a).

Results of a prospective observational study of 39 women who used metformin prior to and during pregnancy suggest that metformin can help reduce the likelihood of developing gestational diabetes and prevent androgen excess in the fetus (Glueck, 2004). Early diagnosis and therapy of the underlying insulin resistance of PCOS can help reduce or reverse infertility and reduce the risk for heart disease and miscarriage with no increase in congenital defects (Glueck, 2002b).

It is difficult to predict lactation outcomes for women with PCOS. Improving insulin resistance may help to increase milk production, and treating women prenatally may improve outcomes (Gabbay, 2003). Some breastfeed easily, some experience an oversupply of milk, and some experience undersupply (Kelley, 2003). You can encourage a mother with PCOS symptoms or IMS

to have a thorough physical and hormonal work-up. There are major health risks associated with PCOS, including obesity, developing type II diabetes, a sevenfold increased risk of heart attack, and a fourfold increased risk of hypertension. Women with PCOS also have a higher risk of endometrial cancer (OMRN, 2000).

The relationship of hormonal disorders to insufficient milk production is an area of ongoing research. If you have mothers who fit these profiles and use metformin or other medications, encourage them to join the International Registry for Lactation Research at www.ibreastfeeding.com.

Mothers with PCOS are often extremely motivated to breastfeed their highly prized babies, which can help to heal a fragile body image battered from infertility and, often, repeated miscarriages. They may be discouraged when they have difficulty increasing their milk production. In working with these mothers, the same sensitivity and approaches you use with adoptive mothers and those who have had breast surgery will be helpful.

Multiparas have lower serum levels of prolactin postpartum than **primiparas**, and their babies take in significantly more milk. Multiparas are believed to have an increased number of prolactin receptors in their mammary glands to bind with circulating prolactin, which is either reflected in or results in the lower serum levels of the hormone (Zuppa, 1988). This is supported by reports of other second-time mothers who produced significantly more milk (Kelley, 2003; Ingram, 2001).

Thyroid Disorders

Thyroid disorders in women are very common and relate to a woman's reproductive cycle. Even slight hypothyroidism can increase rates of miscarriage, fetal death, and cognitive deficits in babies. Hyperthyroidism during pregnancy is a cause for concern. Redmond recommends testing thyrotropin (TSH) levels before or during pregnancy, and postpartum for mothers who complain of unusual fatigue or anxiety or who have markers for hyperthyroidism or hypothyroidism (Redmond, 2004). Because of hormonal fluctuations during pregnancy, pregnant women need close monitoring when they have thyroid therapy.

Hypothyroidism

Hypothyroidism results from a deficiency in thyroid secretion. Symptoms include sluggishness, low blood pressure, dry skin, obesity, and sensitivity to cold. Replacement therapy with natural or synthetic hormone preparations can eliminate these effects. When thyroid supplementation is properly managed, the mother can breastfeed with no risk to her baby's health. The supplementation she receives merely brings the mother's thyroid to a normal level. Therefore, the amount of thyroid secretion the baby receives through her milk is equal to that of any other breastfeeding mother.

There is one word of caution for a mother who is severely hypothyroid and receiving unusually high dosages of thyroid supplement. The additional thyroid that passes to her baby through her milk can mask latent hypothyroidism in her baby while he is being breastfed. After weaning begins and the level of thyroid intake decreases, a baby with latent hypothyroidism could suffer neurologic damage. Many hospitals routinely screen for hypothyroidism in newborns.

Although hypothyroidism is a marker for infertility, many women with thyroid disorders are able to conceive through assisted reproductive technologies (Poppe, 2003). There seems to be a link between untreated hypothyroidism and insufficient milk supply. If a mother contacts you regarding low milk production and has a history of thyroid problems, you might recommend thyroid testing. Thyroid testing may also be in order when a mother presents with low milk production that has no identifiable cause.

Goiter

Adequate iodine intake is necessary for normal thyroid function. When a woman does not have sufficient iodine, a **goiter** may result. A goiter is an enlargement of the thyroid gland, resulting in a thick-looking neck or double-chin appearance. Length of lactation does not significantly affect iodine concentrations in milk, and untreated goiters have no impact on breastmilk iodine levels (Dorea, 2002). Iodine levels in human milk respond quickly to the mother increasing her intake, either by iodine-rich foods or by supplements.

Hyperthyroidism

Hyperthyroidism is a condition in which the thyroid is overactive, producing too much thyroid hormone. Thyroid hormone controls many body processes, and excessive levels can affect heart rate and blood pressure. Hyperthyroidism is diagnosed through blood tests that reveal abnormally high thyroid hormone levels and low levels of thyroid stimulating hormone (TSH) produced by the pituitary gland. Low TSH levels in the blood are the most reliable test of most hyperthyroidism. In rare cases, the pituitary gland produces excess amounts of TSH, increasing levels of both TSH and thyroid hormones in the blood. Graves' disease is a form of hyperthyroidism in which pressure occurs on the eyes from supporting muscles, resulting in a staring, wide-eyed appearance (Martin, 1993).

Methimazole, a common medication for treatment of hyperthyroidism, is considered compatible for use in breastfeeding mothers (Azizi, 2002, 2000, 1996; Rylance, 1987; Lamberg, 1984). Propylthiouracil (PTU) is also used in lactating women (Momotani, 2000, 1989) and may be preferable because only small amounts are secreted into the mother's milk (Hale, 2004). Breastfeeding awareness needs to improve in all sectors of the health profession. As late as 2000, 44 percent of the endocrinologists studied failed to recommend breastfeeding during PTU therapy (Lee, 2000). Educate your client regarding treatment options and available literature. Encourage her to share information with her caregivers to help protect her breastfeeding plans.

As part of the diagnostic process, a radioactive picture of the thyroid can help identify if the thyroid gland is overactive. In one case, a mother pumped and dumped until the radioactive iodine 131 and technetium fell below measurable levels. She then resumed breastfeeding (Saenz, 2000).

Postpartum Thyroiditis

Postpartum thyroiditis (PPT) causes a mother's thyroid function to fluctuate, resulting in either transient hyperthyroidism or hypothyroidism. This transient dysfunction usually resolves within a year after birth. The prevalence of PPT ranges from 1.1 to 16.7 percent of all mothers, with a mean prevalence of 7.5 percent. PPT may be an immunologic flare following the immune suppression of pregnancy (Stagnaro-Green, 2004). Insulin-dependent diabetics have a threefold increase in the prevalence of PPT. Approximately 25 percent of women with a history of PPT will develop permanent hypothyroidism within 10 years. If you see a mother with markers for either hyperthyroidism or hypothyroidism, encourage her to contact her doctor for further evaluation and care.

Cystic Fibrosis

Cystic fibrosis (CF) is an inherited disease that affects the exocrine system. In most people, mucus, sweat, saliva, and digestive juices are thin and watery. The defective gene in CF makes these secretions thick and sticky. They clog ducts and tubes throughout the body, including the pancreas and lungs. There are about 30,000 American adults and children with CF (Mayo, 2004). Many young adults with CF are now marrying and having children. Women with mild cystic fibrosis can maintain a normal pregnancy with appropriate weight gain and can deliver infants of normal weight. During lactation, they can maintain their weight and support growth in healthy infants (Michel, 1994). Breastfeeding duration for mothers with CF tends to be less than three months (Luder, 1990). Breastfeeding experiences among mothers in several CF centers were not always positive, suggesting a need for criteria to predict and ensure a successful outcome.

One study found a higher rate of miscarriage, preterm births, and perinatal deaths among mothers with CF. People with CF may have **hypernatremia** (too much salt in the blood). However, their milk was not hypernatremic, and researchers concluded that breastfeeding is possible (Kent, 1993). The disease may compromise the mother nutritionally, and the caloric requirements of breastfeeding may further compromise her nutritional status. Breastfeeding women with cystic fibrosis must give careful attention to their nutritional requirements. Adults with cystic fibrosis are at increased risk for diabetes mellitus (Mackie, 2003).

Some researchers question the amount of bacterial exposure to the breastfeeding infant because people with cystic fibrosis are usually chronic carriers of *Staphylococcus aureus*, a potential pathogen (Welch, 1981). However, the infection passes to the baby not through the mother's milk but by close contact with the mother. Consequently, exposure also occurs in formula-fed babies of mothers with cystic fibrosis. The infection risk is not limited to the breastfed baby. Furthermore, lymphocytes in the mother's milk become sensitized to pathogens and provide protection to her baby. The milk of mothers with cystic fibrosis has tested normal except for a decrease in macronutrients during lung infections. This warrants routine monitoring during lung flare-ups (Shiffman, 1989).

Maternal Phenylketonuria

Phenylketonuria, commonly known as PKU, is a rare inherited disease that can cause brain damage if not detected and treated immediately after birth. The success of newborn screening for PKU has led to many babies with PKU growing to maturity normally and having children of their own. This has led to a new dilemma: maternal PKU, a situation with potential dangers for a developing fetus. A woman who had PKU as an infant will need to return to a special PKU diet during her pregnancy. The phenylalanine overload in her body resulting from a regular diet would affect her fetus' growing brain. The brain damage occurs before the baby is born, regardless of whether the baby has inherited PKU (ACOG, 2000; Hanley, 1999).

A woman may not even be aware that she had PKU as an infant. The phenylalanine overload during infancy may not have been high enough to cause the disease, although it still could be high enough to cause brain damage in her developing fetus. She also simply may not remember that she had PKU because she would probably have been on a regular diet from the age of five years. When a woman becomes pregnant or, better yet, when she plans to begin a family, she should ask her parents about her medical history as an infant. She can also request that her caregiver perform a simple test for PKU.

A woman with PKU will optimally discuss breastfeeding with her physician prior to conceiving or at least during her pregnancy. In one case, twin sisters with PKU initiated special diets before conception and during pregnancy. Both sisters breastfed for several months. Although the phenylalanine in both mothers' milk was higher than in that of mothers without PKU, their breastfed babies maintained normal phenylalanine levels (Fox-Bacon, 1997).

Tuberculosis

Tuberculosis (TB) is a bacterial disease caused by *Mycobacterium tuberculosis*. The bacteria usually attacks the lungs, although it can attack other body parts as well. Breast tuberculosis is a rare form of tuberculosis seen mostly in developing countries. It comprises between .025 and .1 percent of all surgically treated breast diseases (Kalac, 2002). TB was once the leading cause of death in the United States, and more than 16,000 cases were reported in 2000 (CDC, 2004). TB kills about 2 million people annually, mostly in nonindustrialized countries. The occurence of TB has increased in Africa over the past decade, primarily because of HIV infection. TB has also increased in southeast Asia and the former Soviet Union due to the decline of the healthcare system and socioeconomic changes (Frieden, 2003; WHO, 2002).

A mother with active tuberculosis may breastfeed with certain precautions. When maternal disease is discovered before birth, treatment must begin immediately during pregnancy and infant prophylaxis must begin at birth. When active maternal disease is discovered after the baby is born, all contact between the mother and baby will need to be suspended until appropriate therapy is initiated (AAP, 2000) and continued for at least two weeks. This contact includes breastfeeding. During the interruption in breastfeeding, the mother can express and discard her milk every two to four hours to establish milk production (Lawrence, 1999; Freed 1996).

Hepatitis C

The risk of mothers transmitting hepatitis C to their infants through breastfeeding appears to be quite low (Hale, 2004). No difference is apparent in transmission at one year between breastfed and formula-fed infants (Hale, 2002b). Some sources state that if mothers of newborns know they have hepatitis C, they should not breastfeed. That recommendation stems from the fact that the risks are unknown, not from evidence of transmission of the infection (Freed, 1996). The AAP states, "There is no evidence that hepatitis C is transmitted by breastfeeding. Mothers with chronic hepatitis C are often advised that they can nurse their infants, but they should discuss this with their caregiver" (AAP, 2000). There is also evidence to suggest that human milk, even if it contains the virus, does not cause infection in newborns (Lin, 1995).

Herpes

Herpes can pose a major health hazard to an infant, including blindness and death. There are several diseases in the herpes family, and the degree of danger varies among them. Herpes infections all share a common structure, have similar biologic behavior, are transmitted by a virus, and are highly contagious. Several herpes infections manifest themselves as skin lesions that begin as small red pimples. They develop into fluid-filled blisters, and then dry up and heal. Varicella zoster and the herpes simplex viruses fall into this group. During the active phase, the blisters cause a burning, tingling, and itching sensation, often accompanied by fever and enlarged lymph nodes.

Exposure to active herpes lesions can be fatal to a neonate, so all active lesions must be covered to prevent exposure. The AAP does not include herpes in their list of conditions that contraindicate breastfeeding. Avoiding possible transmission by covering lesions on the breast is a wise precaution. Breastfeeding is acceptable if there are no herpetic lesions in the area or if active lesions on the breast are covered (AAP, 2003b; Lawrence, 1999, 1997). If a lesion is present on the nipple, however, the mother cannot breastfeed or feed her milk to her infant from that breast until the lesion heals. She will need to express milk to maintain production in that breast. The milk should be discarded.

Epstein-Barr

The Epstein-Barr virus (infectious mononucleosis) affects mostly young adults up to age 35 and rarely affects people beyond that age. Huang found no detectable risk factors for breastfeeding associated with primary Epstein-Barr virus (Huang, 1993). Epstein-Barr virus may trigger rheumatoid arthritis, but no conclusions have been reached (Silman, 2002).

Varicella Zoster

The two zoster viruses are shingles and chicken pox. Chicken pox is usually contracted by children, whereas shingles is generally an adult affliction. Both zoster infections are contracted through direct contact or through droplets from the nose or mouth. If the mother is infected at the time of delivery, she must be isolated from her infant until the lesions heal completely. With either of the zoster viruses, unless there are lesions on her breast, she can feed her milk to her baby (Lawrence, 1999, 1997; Frederick, 1986).

A baby whose mother develops chicken pox up to 7 days before delivery or up to 28 days after delivery must receive zoster immunoglobulin (ZIG), the chicken pox vaccine. Mothers may breastfeed when their baby has a chicken pox infection or exposure. After delivery, a mother who contracts chicken pox or shingles does not need to be isolated from her baby. If children at home have chicken pox and the mother does not test positive for antibodies, the newborn needs to receive the vaccine. The baby does not need to be isolated from siblings with chicken pox, regardless of whether he received ZIG (Heuchan, 2001).

Herpes Simplex

Both of the herpes simplex viruses are contracted through direct exposure to the lesions. The infection tends to reside in the skin or tissues of the nervous system, remaining there without symptoms until it becomes active. Common activating agents are fever, physical or emotional stress, exposure to sunlight, and certain foods or drugs. The infection can be present in the infant without any maternal history of herpes, usually presenting with upper and lower respiratory symptoms, a hoarse cry, and fever.

Herpes simplex I (cold sore or fever blister) usually appears on the mouth and nose areas. Herpes simplex II (genitalis) is usually transmitted through sexual contact. It produces painful blisters on the skin and the moist lining of the sex organs. In addition to the other herpes simplex symptoms, herpes genitalis causes painful intercourse, urinary problems, and swelling in the groin area. Neonates who contract the disease usually do so through direct contact with the infected tissue. Mortality rates are extremely high for infants exposed to herpes genitalis during vaginal birth. If a woman has had active lesions within three weeks of delivery, she will need a cesarean delivery to ensure her baby's safety.

Cytomegalovirus

The sixth member of the herpes family is cytomegalovirus (CMV). Although nearly all adults are infected with CMV by the age of 50, the infection rarely causes symptoms. Symptoms include fatigue, fever, swollen lymph glands, pneumonia, and liver or spleen defects. When contracted in early infancy, the usual source is the infant's mother. The breast is the most frequent site of CMV reactivation in postpartum women. Excretion of CMV in the mother's milk seems to peak after 2 to 12 weeks (Ahlfors, 1985). The virus is not usually active during the first 8 days following birth, and few positive samples occur after 2 months.

Term infants can be breastfed even when the mother is shedding the virus in her milk (Lawrence, 1999). Breastfed babies may receive passive immunity to CMV through their mothers' milk. The cumulative rate of transmission was 37 percent in one study of mothers breastfeeding preterm babies. The babies had an average incubation time of 42 days. About 50 percent of the infected infants had no symptoms, and 4 had sepsis-like symptoms (Hamprecht, 2001).

Infants acquire immunity to CMV through **transplacental** antibodies and can contract CMV in utero (Nelson, 1997). The greatest danger of CMV to breastfeeding infants is the possibility of **seroconversion** if the infant of a **seronegative** mother receives donor milk from a **seropositive** mother (Dworsky, 1982). Because the infant will not have received transplacental antibodies, the infection could be life threatening. This is especially dangerous for premature infants or infants who are immunologically impaired. Pasteurization at 62 degrees C for 8 minutes can destroy CMV in human milk. Although pasteurization destroys some of the milk's immunologic properties as well, it provides donor recipients protection from CMV and is the standard for milk bank processing. See Chapter 21 for more on human milk banking.

Human Immunodeficiency Virus

Human immunodeficiency virus (HIV) is a retrovirus that destroys the human immune system. It can lead to acquired immune deficiency syndrome (AIDS), in which the body cannot fight off viral, mycobacterial, and fungal pathogens. Today HIV/AIDS is a major global health emergency that affects all regions of the world. It causes millions of deaths and causes suffering to millions more. An estimated 3 million people died from AIDS-related complications in 2003, and an estimated 5 million people acquired HIV. This brings to an estimated 40 million the number of people living with the virus globally (UNAIDS, 2004). However, estimates may be overstated, with many nations now cutting HIV estimates by half or more (Donnelly, 2004). Research and policy development about HIV infection in women and their children tends to be focused in developing countries, especially in sub-Saharan Africa. Within those countries, those most vulnerable to exploitation are low-income, uneducated women (Liles, 2004).

When left untreated, HIV usually quickly leads to infection, disease, and death. AIDS has orphaned an estimated 14 million African children. Only about 400,000 of the almost 6 million people requiring treatment in developing countries actually received it in 2003. In late 2003, WHO and UNAIDS declared the inequity in access to HIV/AIDS antiretroviral (ARV) treatment a global public health emergency and launched the initiative dubbed "3 by 5," which aims to treat 3 million people living with HIV in developing countries by the end of 2005 (WHO, 2004). The "3 by 5" initiative increased ARV treatment to 720,000 people in 2004 (WHO, 2005).

Safety of Breastmilk

HIV is transmitted through sexual contact, contaminated body fluids, and intravenous drug use. It is transmitted from mother to infant during pregnancy, delivery, and (it is believed) breastfeeding. The AIDS pandemic has enabled formula manufacturers to reach new markets where government enforcement of the International Code of Marketing of Breastmilk Substitutes has previously hampered their marketing efforts. Thought-provoking research has caused some researchers to rethink the role of infant feeding in the containment of HIV.

Extended breastfeeding may account for approximately 40 percent of infant HIV infections worldwide. However, most breastfed infants remain uninfected, despite prolonged and repeated exposure. There is evidence that human milk may provide some protection to the infant (Kourtis, 2003). Lactobacillus, commonly found in the mouth and in breastmilk, can bind to sugars on the surface of HIV and prevent it from infecting cells. This finding could play a role in preventing **vertical transmission** of HIV from the mother to her child (Tao, 2004).

Dangers of Promoting Formula Feeding

Two current approaches to reducing or preventing the risk of postnatal transmission are to either avoid all breastfeeding and give artificial milks, or to breastfeed exclusively with no mixed feedings and with early and rapid weaning at around four to six months of age. Coutsoudis (2002) suggests that while use of formula may prevent HIV transmission "it incurs the risk of increased mortality, whereas breastfeeding has multiple benefits but entails risk of HIV transmission."

HIV Studies

One clinical trial found that although breastfed children had a twofold increase in HIV transmission over formula-fed children, both groups experienced similar rates of mortality during the first two years of life (Mbori-Ngacha, 2001). Breastfed infants had better nutritional status than the artificially fed ones, especially during the first six months of life (although the overall prevalence of malnutrition was not different in the two study groups). Another study found that HIV-infected infants who were never breastfed had a poorer outcome than those who were breastfed. The researchers concluded that the extra illness experienced by never-breastfed infants and by HIV-infected nonbreastfed babies should be considered "in all decisions by mothers, health workers and policy makers so as not to offset any gains achieved by decreasing HIV transmission through avoiding breastfeeding" (Coutsoudis, 2003).

Inactivating HIV in the mother's milk would allow infants to receive human milk while reducing the risk of transmission of HIV (Rollins, 2004). A simple method of home pasteurization, maintaining milk between 56 degrees and 62.5 degrees C for 12 to 15 minutes, has proved reliable under a wide range of conditions. There was no evidence of viral replication in any of the study specimens that underwent this Pretoria Pasteurization process (Jeffery, 2001). Pasteurization also kills other bacteria (Jeffery, 2003) and retains properties that may be helpful to infants of HIV-1–positive mothers. In developed countries that do not recommend breastfeeding, babies can receive banked milk that has been pasteurized to destroy HIV (Black, 1996). Previous studies have found pasteurization effective as well (Orloff, 1993).

In one study, researchers predicted child lives likely to be saved by age 10 by using combined prenatal testing and antiretroviral (ARV) treatment. They then compared this to increases in deaths due to more uninfected mothers choosing to use artificial feeding. In poor countries the use of ARV alone would result in an estimated gain in child survival of around 0.36 percent. However, adding artificial feeding would reduce the gain, to 0.03 percent. In middle-income countries, the gain from antivirals was estimated at 0.26 percent, but a spillover of artificial feeding by uninfected women would more likely result in a net *increase* in child deaths of up to 1.08 percent (Walley, 2001). Researchers in the Coutsoudis study call for the use of affordable ARV to reduce transmission; high-quality, widely available HIV counseling; support for the mothers' choice of feeding; and exclusive breastfeeding for those who choose to breastfeed (Coutsoudis, 2002).

Another simulation model compared the risk of HIV from breastfeeding with the risk of death from artificial feeding. Breastfeeding during the first 6 months by HIV-positive mothers increases HIV-free survival by 32 per 1000 live births compared to artifical feeding. The authors concluded that replacement feeding by HIV-infected mothers should wait until the baby is about 6 months old (Ross, 2004). The cumulative probability of late postnatal transmission at 18 months is 9.3 percent, with a significantly higher risk to male babies (BHITSG, 2004). Girls may have an increased risk (1.5 times) of intrauterine transmission compared with boys (Thorne, 2004).

WHO Guidelines

The World Health Organization guidelines state, "when replacement feeding is acceptable, feasible, affordable, sustainable and safe, avoidance of all breastfeeding by HIV infected mothers is recommended. Otherwise, exclusive breastfeeding is recommended during the first months of life." WHO recommends weaning as soon as feasible after the first month, emphasizing that the primary need is to prevent HIV infection in the parents (WHO, 2003; Newell 2001). Researchers concur, urging that "the key to prevention of paediatric HIV infections is adequate prevention of infection in women of reproductive age" (Thorne, 2003).

AAP Guidelines

The official position of the AAP is that "complete avoidance of breastfeeding by HIV-1-infected women remains the only means by which prevention of breastfeeding transmission of HIV-1 can be absolutely ensured. In settings such as the U.S., with virtually universal access to clean water and with widespread cultural acceptance of formula feeding as an alternative to breastfeeding, avoidance of breastfeeding by HIV-1-infected women is possible. In other parts of the world where breastfeeding is the norm, affordable, feasible, and culturally acceptable interventions to decrease the risk of breastfeeding transmission of HIV-1 are urgently needed" (AAP, 2003a).

AnotherLook

AnotherLook, a nonprofit organization started by La Leche League International founder Marian Tompson, is dedicated to gathering information, raising critical questions, and stimulating research about breastfeeding in the context of HIV and AIDS. Their 2003 "Call to Action" (Figure 25.1) aims to ensure the best maternal and infant health outcomes. AnotherLook asserts that current research, policy, and practice that focus on reducing transmission neglects the impact of not breastfeeding on morbidity, mortality, and health.

You can present current information, recommendations, and guidelines to HIV-positive women and encourage them to discuss options with their physician. Because of the impact of AIDS on breastfeeding and the financial stake that pharmaceutical and formula manufacturers have in decreasing breastfeeding, it is important that you stay current with HIV/AIDS research. Search past the popular press articles to the original research studies behind them. Filter them through the lens of your critical thinking and research skills, as presented in Chapter 27.

▶ SPECIAL INFANT HEALTH CONDITIONS

You may encounter an infant whose physical condition becomes an issue with breastfeeding. The nutritional benefits derived from human milk are especially important to a compromised baby. It may help a mother accept a challenging situation when she knows she is

---

FIGURE 25.1
Infant feeding and HIV/AIDS: A call to action.

We acknowledge the possibility that HIV may be transmitted through breastfeeding and that there is an urgent need for feeding guidelines. However, there is currently no published scientific evidence showing that infants born to mothers who are HIV-positive would be healthier and/or less likely to die if they were not breastfed. In light of the above, we call for immediate action to provide:

◆ Clear, peer-reviewed research, with careful ongoing follow-up, which will provide sound scientific evidence of optimal infant feeding practices that lead to the lowest morbidity and mortality.

◆ Concise, consistent definitions of feeding methods, testing methods, HIV infection and AIDS.

◆ Development of research-based infant feeding policies which are feasible to implement in light of prevailing social, cultural and economic environments; which address breastfeeding (particularly exclusive breastfeeding) as a critical component of optimal infant health; and which fully consider the impact of spillover mortality/morbidity associated with infant formulas.

◆ Epidemic management from a public health perspective, with the focus on primary prevention, careful, unbiased surveillance, and the achievement of overall population health with the lowest rates of morbidity and mortality.

◆ Evidence-based practices which protect the rights of both mothers and infants including education, true informed consent, support of a mother's choice, and avoidance of coercion.

◆ Funding to support the above actions and those programs which improve maternal/child health in general such as prenatal and postnatal care, nutrition, basic sanitation, clean water, and education, as well as exclusive breastfeeding until clear scientific evidence supporting the abandonment of breastfeeding is available.

◆ Continued commitment by local and global researchers, policy makers, health workers, and funding bodies to basic scientific, medical, public health, and fiduciary principles in responding to this critical issue.

In summary, we call for answers to critical questions not currently being addressed that will foster the development of policies and practices leading to the best possible outcomes for mothers and babies in relation to breastfeeding and HIV/AIDS.

Source: AnotherLook, 2003.

---

doing everything possible to comfort and nurture her baby and when she recognizes that her baby depends on her. The bonding associated with breastfeeding can lessen emotional stress and help the family through this difficult time. Infant conditions presented here include phenylketonuria (PKU), cleft lip, cleft palate, and neurological impairment.

Parents typically respond with shock and some degree of guilt at having a baby born with a defect. They often progress through a cycle of grief, including denial, anger, rejection, and mourning for the "perfect" child. There is no set pattern or time progression for these emotions. You can be most helpful by listening and taking cues from the parents. Allow the mother to work freely through her feelings until she reaches a point of acceptance.

Phenylketonuria

Phenylketonuria (PKU) is a genetic disease that affects 1 in every 10,000 to 14,000 live births (Purnell, 2001). An infant with PKU appears healthy at birth. Diagnosis is made through a simple blood test and is required by law, with exceptions made for religious beliefs. Diagnosis and treatment initiated promptly during the first weeks of life can avoid permanent damage. PKU results from the infant lacking an enzyme needed to change phenylalanine, an amino acid in food protein, into a form the body can use. If PKU remains untreated, the body becomes overloaded with phenylalanine. Skin rashes, convulsions, mental impairment, and other problems can result.

The infant must immediately begin a diet that restricts the level of phenylalanine intake while providing an amount sufficient to allow him to grow appropriately. Phenylalanine intake requires strict monitoring. Continuing this diet regimen throughout the person's lifetime will preserve normal cognitive function.

The level of phenylalanine in human milk is low (approximately 40 mg/dl) when compared to cow's milk and other artificial baby milk, which range from 73 to 159 mg/dl. The infant's diet is adjusted for phenylalanine based on weekly blood tests. After control has been established, 20 ounces of human milk daily, along with a supplement of phenylalanine-free formula, will meet his requirements of phenylalanine. Direct breastfeeding and supplementation with a phenylalanine-free formula gives good metabolic control and improves the growth and development of PKU children with early diagnosis (Cornejo, 2003).

Breastfeeding will maintain the mother-infant bond and ensure adequate milk production. It also will help reduce the emotional stress for parents after they learn that their baby has a chronic illness. There is evidence that PKU babies initially fed human milk subsequently have higher IQs than those who receive no breastmilk (Riva, 1996). Developmental outcomes are better for breastfed infants than for those exclusively fed low-phenylalanine formulas (Lawrence, 1997; Riva, 1996).

Breastfed infants with PKU exhibited higher blood levels of arachidonic acid than bottle-fed infants. Researchers found a weak positive association between plasma long-chain polyunsaturated fatty acids at diagnosis, which is higher in breastfed infants, and neurodevelopmental indices through the first year of life (Agostoni, 2003).

Physicians may interrupt breastfeeding while they stabilize phenylalanine levels and determine the infant's diet prescription. The mother can express her milk during this time to maintain production. After control is established (with the level of phenylalanine below 10 mg/dl) and the amount of phenylalanine-free formula needed has been determined, the mother's milk can be added to the diet. Some physicians may recommend an alternative that allows the mother to continue breastfeeding without interruption while control is being established, using one of two procedures. One method is to allow the infant to continue nursing and to offer a phenylalanine-free formula at each feeding, while maintaining a consistent daily intake of a prescribed volume of human milk and phenylalanine-free formula. The other method is to substitute a phenylalanine-free formula for one or two breastfeedings per day, with the mother expressing her milk at the missed feedings. A drawback to both methods is the infant's prolonged exposure to potentially toxic levels of phenylalanine. However, frequent analysis of the infant's serum can monitor this closely (Duncan, 1997).

Low-phenylalanine or phenylalanine-free formula was designed to be supplemented with cow's milk or a cow's milk–based formula. Consequently, vitamin and mineral supplements may be required to augment the nutrients present in the mother's milk. If not, the addition of phenylalanine-free formula to the infant's diet could result in a decrease of nutrient absorption. Additional fluid requirements may be minimal because of the lower solute load of human milk.

Between three and twelve months of age, the baby will receive a phenylalanine load to reconfirm the diagnosis. He will receive a natural protein load calculated to provide a specific amount of phenylalanine for three days. This is usually in the form of cow's milk or an evaporated milk formula. If the mother does not wish to interrupt breastfeeding during this time, she will need to have the phenylalanine content of her milk measured to minimize error.

Managing Breastfeeding

When unique circumstances place restrictions on a mother's nursing pattern, she will need a great deal of support, as well as advice on how to manage feedings and monitor her baby's intake. She may have difficulty maintaining milk production, and the additional worry about her baby may affect her letdown reflex. She may be prone to plugged ducts or mastitis because of restricted feedings, so she will want to express milk whenever necessary. Periodic test weighing will be necessary to track the amount of breastmilk the baby has consumed. Amounts of phenylalanine-free formula can be measured before the feeding. Daily weight checks of the baby with an electronic scale will measure his average intake of the mother's milk.

The standard approach for supplementing babies with PKU is to give the baby phenylalanine-free formula within 15 minutes of any supplemental food containing protein, such as human milk. This approach is used to ensure efficient use of amino acids. Feeding the prescribed amount of phenylalanine-free formula through a tube-feeding device at the breast will save the mother time. Although powdered formula can clog the tubing, mixing the formula with warm water and reblending it just before pouring it into the container can avoid this. The use of a tube-feeding device at the breast can be an effective way of preserving the quality of the breastfeeding bond.

If the phenylalanine formula is given separately from the breast, absorption of nutrients in the mother's milk may be less efficient. The baby may fill up on the mother's milk and not take the second feeding well. If he falls asleep at the breast at the end of a feeding, he will need to be disturbed to receive the supplement.

A new approach to supplementing babies with PKU is advocated (Van Rijn, 2003). It was found that alternating breast and phenylalanine-free formula feedings enables babies to drink to satiety and receive hindmilk. There was no statistically significant difference in metabolic control and growth within the first six months in the study. This study suggests that such an approach is more convenient for parents and safe for otherwise healthy babies with PKU. Managing PKU with a combination of breastfeeding and low-phenylalanine formula provides easier maintenance of satisfactory phenylalanine blood levels. This diet helps avoid long-term neurological deficits and the adverse effects of uncontrolled maternal PKU in babies born of mothers with the disease (Purnell, 2001).

If levels of phenylalanine are high during the initial prescription phase, the baby could be breastfed once or twice a day after pumping. Although he will not get much milk, he will stimulate milk production and receive the emotional benefits of being at the breast. After pumping, the mother can feed the phenylalanine-free formula to her baby and then put him to breast. This will avoid the baby becoming frustrated from hunger. The mother can also use a tube-feeding device while the baby nurses on a breast she just pumped. If the volume of the mother's milk increases too rapidly, she can reduce feedings on a just-pumped breast or use only one breast at a feeding. If the mother's milk volume is low, she can nurse more frequently to increase milk production.

Dietary Changes

As an infant with PKU grows, his dietary requirements will change. The mother can ask for an evaluation of the energy content of her milk to determine if a dietary adjustment is required. Guidelines for introducing solid foods are mostly the same as for any other breastfeeding infant. High-phenylalanine foods such as eggs, meat, cheese, and milk should be avoided.

Weaning a baby with PKU from the breast requires more structure than weaning other breastfeeding babies. The mother must monitor phenylalanine intake closely by replacing each dropped feeding with the appropriate amount of phenylalanine-free or low-phenylalanine formula or solid foods in order to maintain a balance. Weaning may need to occur earlier than usual if physicians have difficulty controlling the baby's phenylalanine levels. When considering weaning, the mother will want to designate a target date and estimate what her baby's weight will be in order to determine his requirements for phenylalanine, protein, and energy at that time. She can then consult with a nutritionist specializing in PKU to calculate the amounts of phenylalanine-free or low-phenylalanine formula and other supplements needed.

Mothers can breastfeed their PKU infant safely with appropriate monitoring and special care. It requires motivation, access to daily or weekly blood checks for the baby, a support system, and a cooperative medical team. Many medical professionals have learned more about breastfeeding PKU babies and work with mothers toward a positive outcome. The AAFP (2001) supports breastfeeding of PKU infants.

Galactosemia

Galactosemia is an inherited disease in which the liver enzyme that changes galactose to glucose is absent. Galactose is a simple sugar found in lactose, referred to as milk sugar. An infant with galactosemia is unable to metabolize lactose. Without treatment, the infant would progress from lethargy to cerebral impairment and, ultimately, to mental retardation. The AAFP (2001) breastfeeding position states that "infants with galactosemia are unable to breastfeed and must be on a lactose-free diet." Galactosemia requires immediate and total weaning from all milk—including human milk—as well as other foods that contain galactose. The infant is placed on a special formula that is free of galactose. Infants with galactosemia are unable to breastfeed altogether, except for infants with a form of galactosemia known as the Duarte variant (Ono, 1999). With Duarte's, it is possible

to breastfeed, although the baby's galactose levels must be carefully monitored, with some non-dairy formula probably provided (Ganesan, 1997).

Cleft Lip and Cleft Palate Defects

A cleft lip or cleft palate can affect the infant's ability to generate suction and thus his ability to obtain adequate nourishment. A cleft is an opening in the upper lip or palate, or both, caused when these oral structures fail to fuse during the first trimester of pregnancy. A cleft in the palate results in an opening to the nasal cavity in the roof of the mouth. Clefts can occur on one side of the mouth (unilateral) or both sides (bilateral). They can be a cleft of the lip only, a cleft of the palate only, or most commonly, a cleft of both the lip and palate (Figure 25.2 and Figure 25.3). Clefts can occur as part of other congenital anomalies, syndromes, and medical complications. One study found that over 40 percent of infants with clefts had other malformations (Shah, 1980). These require specialized medical care and often preclude breastfeeding.

Approximately 1 in 700 children are born with a cleft, ranking it as the fourth most common birth defect. A child born with a cleft usually faces continuous treatment until adulthood, involving plastic surgery, orthodontics, management of ear fluid, and sometimes speech therapy. Each child's condition is unique, and treatment plans will vary. Cleft palate treatment centers specialize

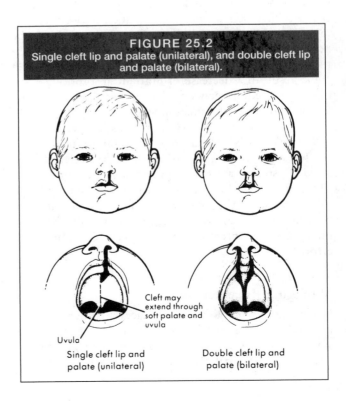

FIGURE 25.2
Single cleft lip and palate (unilateral), and double cleft lip and palate (bilateral).

Cleft may extend through soft palate and uvula

Uvula

Single cleft lip and palate (unilateral)

Double cleft lip and palate (bilateral)

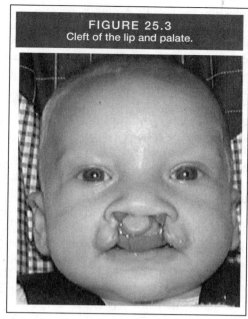

FIGURE 25.3
Cleft of the lip and palate.

Printed with permission of Dr. Scott Franklin.

in treating clefts and offer a comprehensive team approach to each child's needs. The child's prognosis and outcome, as well as his potential, are generally excellent.

Parents' Reactions to a Cleft

The type of cleft a baby has can have some impact on parents' reactions. Facial visibility of an unrepaired cleft lip, with or without a cleft palate, leads to an immediate emotional response. A cleft palate is visible only when the infant cries. Generally, surgery to repair a cleft lip is performed much sooner (at about three months of age) than that of a cleft palate (at about one year).

You can provide encouragement by commenting on how well a mother is doing in her maternal role and on her baby's positive attributes. Avoid comments that minimize the parents' concerns or deny the mother's reactions. It is unrealistic to tell parents that surgery performs such miracles that afterward no one will ever know their child had a cleft. Despite tremendous surgical advances and remarkable results, traces of the cleft will exist.

It is helpful to give parents information in gradual doses during the newborn period. They may benefit from the repetition of facts as they progress through the range of emotional reactions and become more receptive to explanations and suggestions. Support is crucial and extremely valuable. In one study, parents described first seeing their child, their adaptation to a child with cleft, support from professionals, and other people's reactions. They generally regarded the craniofacial team with satisfaction, but they often received poor feeding advice from other caregivers, who had low levels of knowledge and difficulty handling the situation. These findings can promote staff understanding of parental experiences and ways to improve assistance (Johansson, 2004).

Breastfeeding Adjustments with a Cleft

The optimal food for babies with clefts, like all babies, is human milk. The baby will have fewer ear infections, and milk that leaks into the nasal cavity will be less irritating than artificial formula. Breastfeeding, whether nutritive or not, will aid in proper oral-facial development. Comfort and non-nutritive sucking will enhance bonding between the mother and baby (Mick, 2002).

Methods of feeding infants with clefts are often difficult and time consuming, especially in the early weeks. Parents may be apprehensive about feeding their baby and will appreciate support in overcoming their fears and dealing with obstacles. Mothers may be discouraged from initiating breastfeeding despite the fact that breastfeeding can be a positive technique for these children. Children with a cleft palate are apt to have fluid in the middle ear and thus are prone to ear infections. Therefore, the immunologic properties of human milk can be particularly valuable (Paradise, 1994). Additionally, breastfeeding offers these children improved speech development and aids in their visual development as discussed in Chapter 9.

The birth order of the infant can have some effect on breastfeeding outcome. Multiparas, who typically establish milk production better initially than primiparas, may have an easier time lactating. The support and assistance a mother will need depends on the type of cleft her infant has.

Breastfeeding with a Cleft Lip

An isolated cleft lip presents no physiologic impediment to breastfeeding. The baby can usually nurse at the breast as well as his non-cleft peers can. He may actually be able to mold his open cleft around a breast more easily than around a small rubber nipple. In many cases, the breast tissue will fill the cleft to seal it off. The mother can place her thumb over a cleft lip while her baby nurses to improve the seal if necessary (Figure 25.4). The mother will benefit greatly from support and encouragement, despite the relative ease with which she can accomplish breastfeeding.

Breastfeeding with a Cleft Palate

A cleft palate poses challenges with breastfeeding. When an infant breastfeeds, he uses his tongue to draw the nipple into his mouth. The tongue and palate create a vacuum that holds the breast in his mouth, and his

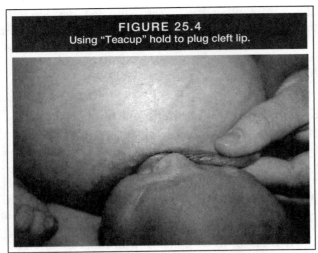

FIGURE 25.4
Using "Teacup" hold to plug cleft lip.

Printed with permission of Kay Hoover and Barbara
Wilson-Clay.

gums compress the breast to promote milk flow. With a cleft palate, because of the opening between the baby's mouth and nose, the baby is unable to hold the breast in his mouth and create a vacuum. To compensate for this inability, the mother can cup her breast as she brings her baby toward her to latch on. She will need to continue holding her breast in the baby's mouth throughout the feeding.

Milk transfer may be easiest at the beginning of a feeding when the breast is firmer. The mother may not feel that the sucking sensation is particularly strong, especially if she has had the experience of breastfeeding other children. Extracting the hindmilk is sometimes difficult. Massaging her breasts before and during the feeding will increase milk flow and make it easier for her baby to transfer milk.

Encourage the mother to put her baby to breast on cue and with great frequency in the newborn period—at least every two hours during the day if he doesn't cue. With a unilateral cleft, the breast needs to enter the baby's mouth on the side of the cleft in such a way that the cheek on the side of the defect touches the breast. When the cleft is bilateral, the breast should enter the baby's mouth at midline. Holding the baby upright, with his nose and throat higher than the breast, can minimize milk leaking into his nasal cavity. He can straddle the mother's body while she holds him upright or in a football position.

Some babies with a cleft palate will choke often during feeding. Choking and milk leaking through the nose occur frequently with babies with cleft palates, regardless of feeding method. Although feeding can be time-consuming and frustrating in general, it often becomes easier after the first month. Breast pumping will maintain

milk production, make milk readily available at the beginning of a feeding, and remove milk that remains in the breast after a feeding. Short, frequent feedings will prevent the infant from tiring. If he is reluctant to nurse, skin-to-skin contact with the mother and initiating a feeding before he is completely awake will help.

Because having a cleft of the palate prevents the baby from creating a vacuum in the oral cavity, he cannot create the suction required in breastfeeding (Wilson-Clay, 2002). Specialty feeders such as the Pigeon Cleft Palate Nurser, the Hazelbaker Feeder, and the Medela Haberman Feeder are available. Familiarize yourself with such alternative feeders so you can counsel parents about their use. Parents may find that spoon-feeding results in too much spillage or that tube-feeding takes too long and tires the infant. You can help them find a feeding method that will work best for them and their baby. The parents' cleft palate team will instruct them to be very attentive to their baby's weight pattern and to monitor weight gain with weekly weight checks. The mother will feed her expressed milk to her baby to supplement his feedings at the breast.

Breastfeeding with a Cleft Lip and Palate

If the baby has both a cleft lip and palate, the techniques discussed relative to a cleft palate will apply. Long-term use of a breast pump for expressing hindmilk is likely to be even more necessary. The more extensive the cleft, the more difficult the feeding will be. Many mothers pump exclusively and provide their milk through an alternative feeding method until the cleft palate is repaired. Putting her infant to breast as often as possible will enhance bonding and nipple stimulation for milk production. Being at the breast also provides a nice time for "comfort" nursing.

Otitis media is common among children with cleft palates despite cleft repair and early treatment with feeding plates, called **grommets** or **obturators**, probably because of **eustachian tube** dysfunction. Aniansson (2002) found a significant correlation during the first 18 months of life between longer duration of feeding with breastmilk and a lower incidence of otitis media. Children with a cleft palate and those with a cleft lip and palate were breastfed for an average of 2.8 months, compared with 3.6 months for those with a cleft lip only and 7.5 months for the controls (babies without clefts). The researchers found that terminating breastmilk might contribute to increased incidence of otitis media. A Brazilian study found a low prevalence of breastfeeding in cleft babies, mainly due to sucking inability. Complete cleft lip and palate was the primary cause that affected sucking. The authors observed that dietary habits in babies with cleft lip and palate are more risky, with some of these babies receiving fruit juices and sugar (da Silva, 2003).

Breastfeeding with a Submucosal Cleft Palate

Submucosal clefts of the soft palate can escape the newborn screening process. A layer of skin covers a cleft in the soft palate, which sometimes appears as a bluish midline discoloration. The salivary glands may be involved and can cause drooling. A bifid (forked) uvula, a short soft palate with muscle separation (furrow) in the midline, and a bony notch in the posterior of the hard palate are markers for a submucosal cleft (McWilliams, 1991).

Sometimes an occult (hidden) submucosal cleft is not discovered until the child begins speaking and hypernasal speech is noted, or because of feeding difficulties or recurrent otitis media (Stal, 1998). At times the cleft is never diagnosed. A submucosal cleft makes it difficult for the newborn to sustain a suck. If you work with an infant with breastfeeding difficulties and you observe the above symptoms, refer the mother to her baby's physician. Encourage an evaluation by a specialist such as an ear, nose, and throat (ENT) specialist. A submucosal cleft can be a symptom of other more serious problems, such as velocardiofacial syndrome or chromosomal defects. Surgical repair, when performed, consists of a single procedure (Lilja, 2000).

Surgical Repair

Infants with a cleft lip, with or without a cleft of the palate, will usually have lip repair surgery between two and three months of age. Some physicians permit infants to resume breastfeeding immediately following surgery. If the mother is not able to breastfeed during this time, she can be encouraged to express her milk and feed it to her baby through an alternative method. She can freeze milk in preparation for the surgery. When an infant with a cleft lip and palate has lip repair, his nursing ability will probably not be altered significantly. Any breastfeeding difficulties lie more with the palate than with the lip. However, lip repair may provide an important psychological lift to the mother.

Some cleft palate teams fit obturators over part of the cleft palate to assist in feeding (Figure 25.5). The baby still cannot create negative intra-oral pressure, so assisted feeding is required (Choi, 1991). The use of nasal stents helps minimize deformities and stretches the skin for repair. Obturators are used to position the palate for repair and to prevent dental arch collapse. Although experts dispute its effectiveness for this purpose, an obturator sometimes produces psychological benefits for parents. In Japan, a modified plate helped

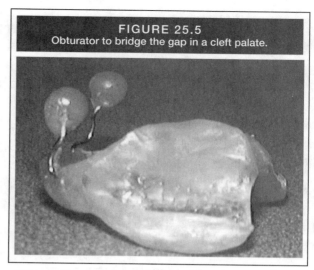

FIGURE 25.5
Obturator to bridge the gap in a cleft palate.

Printed with permission of Dr. Scott Franklin.

partially breastfed babies gain weight at a similar rate to that of formula-fed babies. One baby breastfed for 14 months (Kogo, 1997).

Some surgical teams perform lip repair during the first few weeks postpartum. Early **palatal** repair is also more frequent. Palatal growth determines when the surgery may be performed (Franklin, 2002). Earlier surgery can produce a smoother transition to full breastfeeding. While many mothers find it difficult to transition to breastfeeding, it is important to offer the parents hope (Mick, 2002). Clinicians and parents should consider each baby's feeding strengths and limitations and never automatically dismiss the possibility of breastfeeding (Wolf, 1992).

You can work with the mother following lip or palate repair surgery to help her and her baby learn to breastfeed nutritively. If the baby is unable to achieve nutritive breastfeeding, any breastfeeding has value for both comfort and bonding. You can encourage the mother to continue to provide her milk to minimize her child's risk for ear and respiratory infections. Practical feeding suggestions from other mothers can offer insights into managing breastfeeding in this situation (Stockdale, 2000; Crossman, 1998), so support groups can be helpful.

Pierre Robin Sequence (Syndrome)

Pierre Robin Sequence is an **anomaly** characterized by a receding lower jaw and displacement at the back of the tongue, as well as a cleft palate and an absence of the gag reflex (Figure 25.6). Pierre Robin Sequence, not to be confused with a simple cleft palate, is not very common. An infant with Pierre Robin can suffer severe respiratory

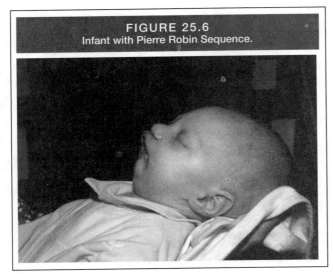

FIGURE 25.6
Infant with Pierre Robin Sequence.

Printed with permission of Linda Kutner.

distress and have difficulty maintaining an airway, particularly during the newborn period. He can also have difficulty thriving (Wolf, 1992). Some of these babies require endotracheal intubation and gavage feeding. Pierre Robin is associated with genetic syndromes, most commonly Stickler's syndrome, a connective tissue disorder that can cause blindness (Mayo, 2003; Ziakas, 1998). The possible severity of airway obstruction and concerns over survival usually make direct breastfeeding unlikely.

Pierre Robin Sequence occurs in varying degrees. An infant with a very slight case may be able to breastfeed. An infant who cannot breastfeed initially can receive his mother's expressed milk. After the infant with Pierre Robin Sequence gets through the crucial early stages of his life and has developed sufficiently so that he can maintain an airway without difficulty, the outcome is positive for him. At this time, the mother may be able to put him to breast, depending on the recommendations of his caregiver. Sometimes Pierre Robin is caused by deformity because of the baby's position in utero. When this is the cause, jaw growth usually catches up to normal by four to six years of age.

Support for the Parents

In a retrospective survey, 95 percent of parents wanted to see the normal aspects of their baby's exam results, and 87 percent wanted reassurance that the cleft defect was not their fault. Using proper terms to describe abnormal findings was important, as well as assurance that their child was not in pain. Many healthcare providers do not discuss these issues with parents (Young, 2001). Parents need direct information about expected difficulties in feeding and care. They need to know signs and symptoms of illness, possible complications, and information on deferring

future treatment. Parents report being overwhelmed with too much information during a time of initial emotional stress. Learning how to deal with the feelings of friends and family is also a concern (Mick, 2002).

Many new parents, especially those of first-born children with clefts, tend to attribute all behavior and problems of the infant to the cleft rather than realizing that much is part of the usual newborn pattern. You can help parents put the cleft into proper perspective and to view their child as normal in other respects. Encourage the mother to become an advocate for her child and to become comfortable with questioning and understanding all aspects of her child's treatment. It is very important that you avoid evaluating or judging their breastfeeding experience. The cleft palate feeding regimen can be trying, frustrating, and extremely time consuming. Help the mother recognize success in every effort.

Some mothers are unable emotionally or physically to continue breastfeeding for as long as they might have wished. If it becomes necessary for the mother to wean, her disappointment over losing the nursing relationship may require special counseling. You can assist the mother by providing support and information about weaning. Remind her that her baby benefited from the breastfeeding relationship and the human milk he received. Additionally, support groups for parents of children with cleft palates exist in many parts of the country. They can give parents a unique, useful opportunity to relate to others who have dealt positively with the experience. One recommended Internet resource is the Web site for Wide Smiles Cleft Lip and Palate Resource at www.widesmiles.org. See Table 25.2 for counseling tips for parents about cleft lip and cleft palate and Appendix A for resources for parents.

Spina Bifida

Spina bifida, a nerve defect present at birth, results in a gap in the bone that surrounds the baby's spinal cord. It is relatively common, occurring in about 20 of every 1000 births. Surgical repair is unnecessary if the gap is very small. If it is large enough to allow parts of the spinal cord to protrude, surgery may be required. Most of these infants will have weakness or paralysis of the lower extremities. Surgery to repair the defect usually occurs as soon as possible—within 24 to 48 hours after birth. The infant will be in the NICU following surgery, and the mother will need help expressing and transporting her milk.

The baby can go to the breast as soon as it is allowable. After the mother positions herself comfortably, a helper can carefully lift the baby and bring him to her, supporting him with pillows. The mother's position will need to avoid pressure on the baby's spinal column.

TABLE 25.2
Counseling Mothers About Cleft Lip and Cleft Palate

Mother's Concern	Suggestions for Mother
Nursing with a cleft lip	◆ Lip will usually mold around the breast. ◆ If necessary, cover the cleft with a finger to ensure good suction.
Ensuring adequate nourishment	◆ Massage the breasts before nursing to promote milk flow. ◆ Hold the breast in the baby's mouth. ◆ With a unilateral cleft, the breast enters on the side of the defect. The baby's cheek on the side of the defect should touch the breast. ◆ With a bilateral cleft, the breast enters at midline. The baby's body straddles the mother. ◆ Use a feeding plate (obturator) to partially cover the cleft.
Maintaining milk production	◆ Closely monitor weight gain, wet diapers, and frequency of feedings. ◆ Express milk after feedings and during surgical repair; feed the milk to the baby with the appropriate feeding device. ◆ Pump or hand express after feedings to adequately remove milk from the breast and stimulate milk production. ◆ Wear breast shells between feedings to stimulate milk production.
Managing breastfeeding	◆ Feed the baby in an upright position to avoid choking or milk leaking from the baby's nose. ◆ Push the baby's chin to his chest to stop choking and then resume the feeding. ◆ Use short frequent feedings. ◆ Nurse while the baby is still sleepy. ◆ Use a tube-feeding device at the breast to encourage the baby to nurse.

Feeding times will be brief until the baby has recovered, with longer feedings beginning after the baby grows stronger. The recovery process may take several weeks. You can support the mother as she pumps to provide milk for her baby, and you can be available to assist her after the baby arrives home.

Neurological Impairment

A healthy, full-term infant has a mature suck and swallow reflex, which is essential for transferring milk from the breast. A neurologically impaired infant rarely has a fully developed or strong suck and swallow reflex. Consequently, breastfeeding is more challenging, and feedings will take more time. The degree of difficulty will depend on the severity of the impairment and the mother's ability to cope with the emotional stress and practical aspects of breastfeeding. Babies who are born with a neurological impairment have a higher percentage of premature births and therefore may require longer

hospitalization than most babies. The mother may need to deal with separation from her baby, as well as possible nipple preference because of bottle-feeding. Generally, these mothers will need assistance and support to compensate for their babies' low muscle tone and will need patience while the baby learns and relearns how to suckle.

Infant with Down Syndrome

Down syndrome is a congenital anomaly that afflicts one out of every 1000 infants. Its cause is the presence of an extra chromosome, resulting in an infant who has oval eyes that slant slightly upward, a protruding tongue that seems too large for his small mouth, small ears, a wide flattened nose, muscular weakness, hypotonicity (low muscle tone), and a short stature (Figure 25.7). His growth and development, although slower than that of an uncompromised child, usually will allow him to do most physical activities other children can do. Physically, he may have incomplete heart and gastrointestinal

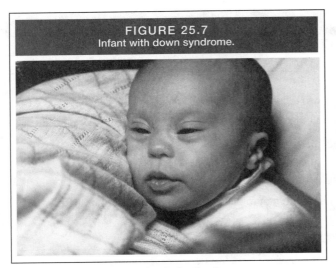

FIGURE 25.7
Infant with down syndrome.

Printed with permission of Sarah Coulter Danner.

development, respiratory infection, digestive upset, and obesity. An infant with Down syndrome benefits from the immunologic factors in human milk and its easy digestibility. He may have a lower tendency toward obesity if he receives human milk in his infancy (Martin, 2004; Grummer-Strawn, 2004; Toschke, 2002).

Pisacane (2003) found a 30 percent breastfeeding rate among infants with Down syndrome admitted to the neonatal unit. Reasons given by mothers for not breastfeeding include infant illness, frustration or depression, perceived milk insufficiency, and difficulty with suckling. A Dutch study found no significant difference in breastfeeding rates for children with and without Down syndrome, and the adequacy of energy and nutrient intakes were similar (Hopman, 1998). Down syndrome significantly delays the age at which the baby begins receiving solid food, which can be deleterious to oral-motor development.

Most babies with Down syndrome are able to breastfeed. In a study of 59 breastfed infants with Down syndrome, 31 had no difficulty establishing sucking, 4 were slow for less than 1 week, 8 took 1 week to establish sucking, and 16 took longer than 1 week. Severe cardiac anomaly was associated with poor sucking ability. The authors concluded that Down syndrome does not cause initial feeding problems in all infants and stated that their mothers need a lot of support (Aumonier, 1983).

The mother can minimize the effort her baby needs to make by paying careful attention to positioning and supporting his body and by watching for signs of fatigue. Cardiac complications may be present, most likely in a mild form that will allow breastfeeding to take place with little difficulty. At the other extreme, however, a cardiac condition may be so severe that the activity required for breastfeeding is too stressful and may be contraindicated.

The infant's hypotonia will cause his head, arms, and legs to be loose and floppy. He may also have difficulty rooting and sucking because of weak reflexes. He may be sluggish in his nursing and become easily fatigued at the breast, making it difficult for him to remove milk sufficiently. Although he will require extra assistance and patience in the early days, his muscle tone will improve as he learns to nurse and as he exercises and stretches his muscles. Encourage the mother to view early breastfeedings as practice sessions. She and her baby can get to know one another, and the mother can learn how to hold and rouse her baby. If she needs to stimulate her baby to an alert state for nursing, the rousing techniques presented in Chapter 14 will be helpful.

Any of the conventional breastfeeding positions work well for an infant with Down syndrome. With his head and body well supported, he can reserve energy for nursing. His head should be slightly flexed but not drooped too far forward. Positioning him so that his throat is slightly above the level of the nipple will prevent choking and gagging, especially if the mother leans back slightly to allow her nipple to tilt upward. The side-lying position seems to work well for many of these babies, with the baby supported by several pillows and the baby's head propped higher than the rest of his body. The football hold gives the mother more ability to form and control her breast.

Pressing down on her baby's chin will help him open his mouth. When he latches on, the mother can check that his bottom lip turns outward and not inward over the alveolar ridge. His flaccid, flat tongue initially may be unable to cup around the nipple and form a trough to carry the milk to the back of his throat. The mother can press down on the center of his tongue with her finger several times before each feeding to help him learn to shape his tongue appropriately. With the Dancer hand position, she can cup her baby's chin and hold his cheeks lightly with her thumb and index finger. Her other three fingers can support her breast during the feeding.

To help her baby obtain milk more easily, the mother can massage and express milk to initiate letdown before putting him to breast. Her goal is to nurse for at least ten to twelve minutes on each breast every two to three hours if her baby does not give cues. If her baby has difficulty suckling, she will need to express milk after the feeding and feed it to her baby. Because her baby may be passive, the mother will need to initiate feedings frequently. She can learn to observe her baby for subtle signs of wakefulness, such as lip and eye movements, that will signal her to pick him up and put him to breast.

Typically, an infant with Down syndrome will gain weight and grow in length more slowly than the average infant, regardless of feeding method. There are special growth charts for children with Down Syndrome to reflect this. Slow weight gain by itself is not an indication that breastfeeding is providing insufficient nourishment. If the mother expresses milk after every feeding to ensure adequate stimulation for good milk production, and if she feeds her baby the expressed hindmilk, she will probably be able to meet her baby's nutritional needs through her milk.

Parents of babies with Down syndrome may experience shock and grief at the birth of their "less than perfect baby." Breastfeeding will help them form an attachment to their baby as they work through their emotions. These mothers benefit from a great deal of support and encouragement. Praise them for their efforts and remind them of all the beneficial aspects of breastfeeding for an infant with Down syndrome. Referral to a Down syndrome support group will help them deal with their grief in the company of other parents who are in the same situation.

Hydrocephalus

Hydrocephalus is an excessive accumulation of cerebrospinal fluid in the intracranial cavity. It results from interference in the flow or absorption of fluid through the brain and the spinal canal. The infant's head enlarges as fluid increases. In most cases, he will have a high-pitched cry, muscle weakness, and severe neurological defects. Breastfeeding is possible with adjustments in positioning. The infant's head needs to be slightly higher than the breast and he needs frequent feedings to avoid reflux.

Neurological Impairment

Infants with neurological damage or impairment can have varying degrees of mental deficiency and learning ability. A severely brain-damaged infant will be unable to maintain concentration because of an extremely poor attention span. He will soon forget reflexes that were instinctive at birth, and the mother will have to teach them to him. He also will require constant and continual reinforcement of learned abilities. Thus, infants with neurological damage may require ongoing techniques and assistance to accomplish effective attachment and suckling (McBride, 1987). This will call for patience and perseverance on the part of the parents.

The severity of brain damage will determine the degree to which an infant is able to breastfeed. In many cases, the infant's brain mechanism does not pick up the impetus to perform specific functions. Although reflexes may be present, he may not have the ability to coordinate them with the stimulus. Although the reflexes for rooting and sucking are satisfactory in an uncompromised infant, they may be insufficient to enable an infant with brain damage to breastfeed. In the early months, he may respond to these reflexes. However, as the months pass, the reflexes regress from instinct to a learned ability. The mother must be prepared to coax her baby to nurse because he may continually forget how to nurse. Additionally, the baby may have difficulty swallowing, resulting in gagging and choking. Nursing the baby in an upright position and stroking downward under the chin to aid his swallowing may help (Wolf, 1992).

Because a brain-damaged infant may not maintain his level of concentration, he can lose interest in nursing before he transfers milk adequately. The mother can try nursing for brief five-minute periods and nurse more frequently. Because her infant may become very frustrated waiting for milk to release, the mother can express her milk to initiate letdown before putting him to breast. A tube-feeding device may also be useful for nourishing the baby while he suckles at the breast. These babies need to be followed closely to assure adequate intake. Supplementation with the mother's expressed milk may be necessary.

Sensory Processing Disorder

Sensory integration is the process of our brain taking input from our five senses and forming a functional composite that enables us to comprehend the world around us. When sensory integration does not develop normally, problems in learning, development, or behavior may result (Sensory Integration International, 2004). A hypo-responsive baby, one with low registration of sensory input, may fail to suckle when put to the breast. A hyper-responsive baby, one with high registration of input, also called sensory defensive (Kranowitz, 1998), may be hypertonic, easily overstimulated, and aversive to the breast.

If you observe a baby with feeding difficulties who exhibits any or some of these behaviors, referral back to the baby's physician and a list of occupational or physical therapists who specialize in sensory integration is appropriate. Special feeding strategies may help both hypo- and hyper-responsive babies transition to breastfeeding more effectively. A hypo-responsive infant may respond to finger feeding; gentle massage to the face, mouth, and palate; and being held upright. Strategies for the hyper-responsive baby include deeper pressure touch, swaddling, swinging the baby gently from head-to-toe in a blanket before feeding, or self-attachment (Watson-Genna, 2002).

Sensory processing disorder is complex, and the baby will need the care of an occupational or physical therapist. If you are able to attend the baby's evaluation or therapy, you will learn a lot from the therapist's expertise. You can offer valuable insights from a feeding perspective and help the mother advocate for continued breastfeeding. Many occupational and physical therapists have little experience working with breastfeeding infants.

TABLE 25.3	
Counseling the Mother of a Neurologically Impaired Infant	
Mother's Concern	**Suggestions for Mother**
Baby has difficulty grasping the breast	◆ Position the baby close to the breast and adequately support his body. ◆ Position the baby's lower lip outward from his gum. ◆ Press the baby's tongue down to create a groove for the nipple. ◆ Use the Dancer hand position to support the breast and the baby's chin.
Baby has difficulty sucking	◆ Feed milk by a cup, dropper, or spoon.
Baby gags or chokes during feedings	◆ Position the baby's head so his throat is slightly above the nipple. ◆ Stroke downward under the chin to aid swallowing.
Baby loses interest after several minutes of nursing	◆ Pre-express milk to initiate letdown. ◆ Express milk onto the nipple or into the corner of the baby's mouth. ◆ Nurse more frequently for 5-minute periods at a time. ◆ Use a tube-feeding device to maintain milk flow and encourage sucking.

This interdisciplinary approach will benefit everyone on the team, especially the mother and baby (Weiss-Salinas, 2001).

Support for the Parents

Parents of neurologically impaired infants will need an extensive network of support, and you will be an important part. Reinforce the mother's commitment to breastfeed, and praise her for her diligence in coping with difficulties. She may need help dealing with the loss of her normal healthy baby and accepting a new, imperfect baby. Encourage parents to draw on each other for strength and support, and put them in touch with special support groups for parents of challenged children. See Table 25.3 for counseling suggestions.

One study of babies with the rare disorder of Rubenstein-Taybi syndrome found that 59 percent of mothers breastfed for an average of 7.1 months. Overall, 48 percent felt their child had a good to fair suck and 50 percent rated their breastfeeding experience as fair to very pleased. Problems included poor weight gain (46 percent), poor latch (35 percent), failure to thrive (34 percent), and infant fatigue (33 percent). The authors noted the importance of "instruction, proper positioning, close nutritional follow-up and strong encouragement by the healthcare team" (Moe, 1998).

It is common for a mother to experience negative feelings sometimes about her compromised baby. This mother's depression can be much more severe than postpartum depression, and she will need a great deal of support. (See Chapter 19 for more information on postpartum depression.) You may be the only person with whom she can express her true feelings. She needs to know you are there for her and that you genuinely care. It may be difficult for you to deal with a situation like this, and you will need to draw upon support from those close to you. You cannot "fix" the baby. Your role is to provide lactation support.

▶ SUMMARY

Mothers in challenging circumstances are often able to reach their breastfeeding goals despite obstacles. Your assistance will be valuable to them as they learn to manage breastfeeding and meet the needs of their babies. Despite health conditions, mothers can establish sound breastfeeding practices that do not compromise the health of either the mother or her baby. Breastfeeding helps normalize the relationship between a mother and her compromised baby and optimizes the baby's health through human milk.

▶ CHAPTER 25—AT A GLANCE

Facts you learned—

Counseling mothers with special health needs:

◆ Autoimmune diseases such as chronic fatigue, Sjogren's, and Raynaud's may affect breastfeeding.

◆ There is a correlation between endometriosis, infertility, and autoimmune disorders.

- Breastfeeding may reduce the risks of children developing an autoimmune disease.

- Insulin levels in diabetic women may fluctuate erratically until lactation is established and may fluctuate again when weaning is initiated.

- Diabetic women are prone to yeast infections.

- Some mothers with primary IMS take metoclopramide or domperidone.

- Decreasing insulin resistance may help increase milk production for women with PCOS.

- Properly managed thyroid supplementation is not a risk to an infant's health.

- Thyroid that passes to the baby through his mother's milk can mask latent hypothyroidism.

- Mothers with cystic fibrosis can breastfeed, with attention to special nutritional needs.

- Mothers with tuberculosis can breastfeed with certain precautions and treatment.

- Mothers are at low risk of transmitting hepatitis C to their infants through breastfeeding.

- Active herpes lesions must be covered to prevent infant exposure.

- A mother with chicken pox at delivery must be isolated from her newborn until the lesions heal; her milk can be given to her infant unless there are lesions anywhere on her breast.

- Breastfed babies may receive passive immunity to CMV through breastmilk and transplacental antibodies.

- Recommendations for HIV-positive women in developed countries are that they should not breastfeed if they can safely formula-feed or obtain donor milk.

Counseling the mother of a compromised infant:

- Breastfeeding with a cleft lip may be easier than bottle-feeding.

- Breastfeeding with a cleft palate presents more breastfeeding challenges.

- Massaging her breasts before and during the feeding will increase milk flow and make it easier for the baby to transfer milk.

- Phenylalanine intake for an infant with PKU must be strictly monitored throughout breastfeeding and through structured weaning.

- Mothers can feed their PKU baby phenylalanine-free formula through a tube-feeding device at the breast.

- A baby with complete galactosemia cannot consume human milk.

- A baby with Duarte's form of galactosemia may be able to breastfeed with careful monitoring and some nondairy formula.

- In a neurologically impaired infant, rooting and sucking regress from instinct to a learned ability, requiring continual teaching and coaxing.

Breastfeeding a compromised infant:

- Put the baby to breast with great frequency in the absence of cues—at least every two hours—in the newborn period.

- Hold the baby upright with his nose and throat higher than the breast.

- Provide skin-to-skin contact.

- Begin a feeding before the baby is completely awake.

- Nurse for brief periods, more frequently, to avoid tiring the baby.

- Recognize signs of fatigue, cardiac complications, hypotonia, and difficulty rooting and sucking.

- View early breastfeeding as practice sessions.

- Press down on the center of the tongue, and use the Dancer hand position to assist the baby as needed.

Applying what you learned—

Counseling mothers of babies with special health needs:

- Help parents deal with emotions and stages of grief for the "perfect" child.

- Avoid comments that minimize parents' concerns or deny a mother's reactions.

- Give parents information in gradual doses during the newborn period.

- Help parents view their child as normal in other respects.

- Avoid judging their breastfeeding decisions.

- Help the mother with pumping and provide follow-up care after discharge home.

- Recognize symptoms of hypo-responsive and hyper-responsive babies; teach parents coping mechanisms, and refer to specialists.

▶ **REFERENCES**

Agostoni C et al. Plasma long-chain polyunsaturated fatty acids and neurodevelopment through the first 12 months of life in phenylketonuria. *Dev Med Child Neurol* 45(4):257–261; 2003.

Ahlfors K, Ivarsson S. Cytomegalovirus in breast milk of Swedish milk donors. *Scand J Infect Dis* 17:11–13; 1985.

Alioum A et al. Estimating the efficacy of interventions to prevent mother-to-child transmission of human immunodeficiency virus in breastfeeding populations: Comparing statistical methods. *Am J Epidemiol* 158(6):596–605; 2003.

Alioum A et al. Estimating the efficacy of interventions to prevent mother-to-child transmission of HIV in breast-feeding populations: Development of a consensus methodology. *Stat Med* 20(23):3539–3556; 2001.

American Academy of Family Physicians (AAFP). *AAFP Policy Statement on Breastfeeding.* Breastfeeding Position Paper; 2001.

American Academy of Pediatrics (AAP). Special challenges to breastfeeding: Maternal illness. Medical Library; 2000. Available at: www.medem.com/medlb/article_detaillb_for_printer.cfm?article_ID=ZZZHCCBXQ7C&sub_cat=1. Accessed June 23, 2004.

American Academy of Pediatrics (AAP). Committee on Pediatric AIDS. Human milk, breastfeeding, and transmission of human immunodeficiency virus type 1 in the United States. *Pediatrics* 112:1196–1205; 2003a.

American Academy of Pediatrics (AAP). *Red Book: Report of the Committee on Infectious Diseases*, 26th ed. Elk Grove, IL: AAP; 2003b.

American Autoimmune Related Diseases Association, Inc. (AARDA). Autoimmune disease in women: The facts, 2004–2005. Available at: www.aarda.org/women.php. Accessed February 6, 2005.

American College of Obstetricians and Gynecologists (ACOG). Committee on Genetics. *Maternal phenylketonuria.* Committee Opinion, Number 230; January 2000.

Anderson J et al. Raynaud's phenomenon of the nipple: A treatable cause of painful breastfeeding. *Pediatrics* 113(4): e360–e364; 2004.

Aniansson G et al. Otitis media and feeding with breast milk of children with cleft palate. *Scand J Plast Reconstr Surg Hand Surg* 36(1):9–15; 2002.

AnotherLook. Infant feeding and HIV/AIDS: A call to action; 2003. Available at: www.anotherlook.org. Accessed March 7, 2005.

Arthur P et al. Metabolites of lactose synthesis in milk from diabetic and nondiabetic women during lactogenesis II. *J Pediatr Gastroenterol Nutr* 19:100–108; 1994.

Aumonier M, Cunningham C. Breast feeding in infants with Down's syndrome. *Child Care Health Dev* 9(5):247–255; 1983.

Azizi F, Hedayati M. Thyroid function in breast-fed infants whose mothers take high doses of methimazole. *J Endocrinol Invest* 25(6):493–496; 2002.

Azizi F et al. Thyroid function and intellectual development of infants nursed by mothers taking methimazole. *J Clin Endocrinol Metab* 85(9):3233–3238; 2000.

Azizi F. Effect of methimazole treatment of maternal thyrotoxicosis on thyroid function in breast-feeding infants. *J Pediatr* 128(6):855–858; 1996.

Black R. Transmission of HIV-1 in the breast-feeding process. Review. *J Am Diet Assoc* 96(3):267–274; 1996.

Bodley V, Powers D. Patient with insufficient glandular tissue experiences milk supply increase attributed to progesterone treatment for luteal phase defect. *J Hum Lact* 15(4):339–343; 1999.

Breastfeeding and HIV International Transmission Study Group (BHITSG). Late postnatal transmission of HIV-1 in breast-fed children: An individual patient data meta-analysis. *Infect Dis* 189:2154–2166; 2004.

Budin P. Le Nourisson, Paris: Octave Doin; 1900 (Malony WJ, transl): The nursling: The feeding and hygiene of premature and full-term infants; Lecture 3. London: Caxton Publishing Co; 1907. Available at: www.neonatology.org/classics/nursling/nursling.html. Accessed December 5, 2004.

Centers for Disease Control (CDC). Births: Final data for 2002. *National Vital Statistics Report* 52(10); December 17, 2003.

Centers for Disease Control and Prevention (CDC), National Center for HIV, STD, and TB Prevention, Division of Tuberculosis Elimination. Questions and answers about TB. Available at: www.cdc.gov/nchstp/tb/faqs/qa_introduction.htm#Intro. Accessed June 5, 2004.

Choi B et al. Sucking efficiency of early orthopaedic plate and teats in infants with cleft lip and palate. *Int J Oral Maxillofac Surg* 20(3):167–169; 1991.

Cornejo V et al. Phenylketonuria diagnosed during the neonatal period and breast feeding. *Rev Med Chil* 131(11): 1280–1287; 2003.

Corrao G et al. Risk of inflammatory bowel disease attributable to smoking, oral contraception and breastfeeding in Italy: A nationwide case-control study. *Int J Epidemiol* 27(3):307–404; 1998.

Coutsoudis A et al. Free formula milk for infants of HIV-infected women: Blessing or curse? *Health Policy Plan* 17(2): 154–160; 2002.

Coutsoudis A et al. Morbidity in children born to women infected with human immunodeficiency virus in South Africa: Does mode of feeding matter? *Acta Paediatr* 92(8):890–895; 2003.

Crossman K. Breastfeeding a baby with a cleft palate: A case report. *J Hum Lact* 14(1):47–50; 1998.

da Silva Dalben G et al. Breast-feeding and sugar intake in babies with cleft lip and palate. *Cleft Palate Craniofac J* 40(1):84–87; 2003.

Dick G. The etiology of multiple sclerosis. *Proc R Soc Med* 69:611; 1976.

Donnelly J. Estimates on HIV called too high. *Boston Globe*: A1; June 20, 2004.

Dorea J. Iodine nutrition and breast feeding. *J Trace Elem Med Biol* 16(4):207–220; 2002.

Duncan LD, Elder S. Breastfeeding the infant with PKU. *J Hum Lact* 13(3):231–235; 1997.

Dworsky M et al. Persistence of cytomegalovirus in human milk after storage. *J Pediatr* 101:440–443; 1982.

Engelking C, Page-Lieberman J. *Maternal Diabetes and Diabetes in Young Children: Their Relationship to Breastfeeding*. La Leche Leche League, International Lactation Consultant Series Unit 5. Wayne, NJ: Avery Publishing Group; 1986.

Ferris A et al. Perinatal lactation protocol and outcome in mothers with and without insulin-dependent diabetes mellitus. *Am J Clin Nutr* 58:43–48; 1993.

Fox-Bacon C et al. Maternal PKU and breastfeeding: Case report of identical twin mothers. *Clin Pediatr* 36:539–542; 1997.

Franklin S. *Cleft Palate: A Team Approach*. 5th Annual Texas Breastfeeding Summit. San Antonio, TX; October 1, 2002.

Frederick I et al. Excretion of varicella herpes zoster virus in breast milk. *Am J Obstet Gynecol* 154:1116–1117; 1986.

Freed G, Clark S. Breastfeeding and maternal illness. *Contemporary Pediatrics* 13(4):49–61, 1996.

Frieden T et al. Tuberculosis. *Lancet* 362(9387):887–899; 2003.

Gabbay M, Kelly H. *Use of Metformin to Increase Breastmilk Production in Women with Insulin Resistance: A Case Series*. Abstract submitted to the Academy of Breastfeeding Medicine, Eighth International Meeting Physicians & Breastfeeding: Controversy, Challenge & Change. Chicago, IL; October 16–20, 2003.

Ganesan R. Borderline galactosemia. *New Beginnings* 14(4): 123–124; 1997.

Gardiner S et al. Transfer of metformin into human milk. *Clin Pharmacol Ther* 73(1):71–77; 2003.

Glueck C et al. Pregnancy outcomes among women with polycystic ovary syndrome treated with metformin. *Hum Reprod* 17(11):2858–2864; 2002a.

Glueck C et al. Treatment of polycystic ovary syndrome with insulin lowering agents. *Expert Opinion on Pharmacotherapeutics* 3:1177–1189; 2002b.

Glueck C et al. Metformin during pregnancy reduces insulin, insulin resistance, insulin secretion, weight, testosterone and development of gestational diabetes: Prospective longitudinal assessment of women with polycystic ovary syndrome from preconception throughout pregnancy. *Hum Reprod* 19(3): 510–521; 2004.

Grummer-Strawn L et al. Does breastfeeding protect against pediatric overweight? Analysis of longitudinal data from the centers for disease control and prevention pediatric nutrition surveillance system. *Pediatrics* 113(2):e81–e86; 2004.

Hale T et al. Transfer of metformin into human milk. *Diabetologia* 45(11):1509–1514; 2002a.

Hale T, Berens P. *Clinical Therapy in Breastfeeding Patients*. Amarillo, TX: Pharmasoft; 2002b.

Hale T. *Medications and Mother's Milk*. Amarillo, TX: Pharmasoft; 2004.

Hales, D. When the body attacks itself. *Parade Magazine*; October 12, 2003.

Hamprecht K et al. Epidemiology of transmission of cytomegalovirus from mother to preterm infant by breastfeeding. *Lancet* 357(9255):513–518; 2001.

Hanley WB et al. Undiagnosed maternal phenylketonuria: The need for prenatal selective screening or case finding. *Am J Obstet Gynecol* 180(4):986–994; 1999.

Heuchan A, Isaacs D. The management of varicella-zoster virus exposure and infection in pregnancy and the newborn period. Australasian Subgroup in Paediatric Infectious Diseases of the Australasian Society for Infectious Diseases. *Med J Aust* 174(6):288–292; 2001.

Hopman E et al. Eating habits of young children with Down syndrome in The Netherlands: Adequate nutrient intakes but delayed introduction of solid food. *J Am Diet Assoc* 98(7):790–794; 1998.

Huang L et al. Primary infections of Epstein-Barr virus, cytomegalovirus, and human herpesvirus-6. *Arch Dis Child* 68(3):408–411; 1993.

Huggins K et al. Markers of lactation insufficiency: A study of 34 mothers. *Current Issues in Clinical Lactation*. Sudbury, MA: Jones and Bartlett, 25–35; 2000.

Hutt P. The effects of diabetes on lactation. *Breastfeed Rev* 14: 21–25; 1989.

Ingram J, Woolridge M, Greenwood R. Breastfeeding: It is worth trying with the second baby. *Lancet* 358(9286): 986–987; 2001.

International Lactation Consultant Association (ILCA). *Core Curriculum for Lactation Consultant Practice* (M Walker, ed.). Sudbury, MA: Jones and Bartlett; 2002.

Ivarsson A et al. Breast-feeding protects against celiac disease. *Am J Clin Nutr* 75(5):914–921; 2002.

Jackson M et al. Total lipid and fatty acid composition of milk from women with and without insulin-dependent diabetes. *Am J Clin Nutr* 60:353–361; 1994.

Jakobsen M et al. Termination of breastfeeding after 12 months of age due to a new pregnancy and other causes is associated with increased mortality in Guinea-Bissau. *Int J Epidemiol* 32(1):92–96; 2003.

Jeffery B et al. Determination of the effectiveness of inactivation of human immunodeficiency virus by Pretoria pasteurization. *J Trop Pediatr* 47(6):345–349; 2001.

Jeffery B et al. The effect of Pretoria Pasteurization on bacterial contamination of hand-expressed human breastmilk. *J Trop Pediatr* 49(4):240–244; 2003.

Johansson B, Ringsberg K. Parents' experiences of having a child with cleft lip and palate. *J Adv Nurs* 47(2):165–173; 2004.

Kalac N et al. Breast tuberculosis. *Breast* 11(4):346–349; 2002.

Kelley C. *PCOS and Breastfeeding: Breastfeeding Update*. San Diego County Breastfeeding Coalition 3(3):1,3; September 2003. Available at: www.breastfeeding.org/newsletter/v3i3/page1.html. Accessed June 8, 2004.

Kent F, Farquharson D. Cystic fibrosis in pregnancy. *CMAJ* 149(6):809–813; 1993.

Kimpimaki T et al. Short-term exclusive breastfeeding predisposes young children with increased genetic risk of Type 1 diabetes to progressive beta-cell autoimmunity. *Diabetologia* 44(1): 63–69; 2001.

Kogo M et al. Breast feeding for cleft lip and palate patients, using the Hotz-type plate. *Cleft Palate-Craniofac J* 34: 351–353; 1997.

Kourtis A et al. Breast milk and HIV-1: Vector of transmission or vehicle of protection? *Lancet Infect Dis* 3(12):786–793; 2003.

Kranowitz C. *The Out-of-Sync Child: Recognizing and Coping with Sensory Integration Dysfunction*. New York: Perigee; 1998.

Kriess J. Breastfeeding and vertical transmission of HIV-1. *Acta Paediatr* 421(Suppl):113–117; 1997.

La Leche League International. *Breastfeeding and HIV*. Franklin Park, IL; July 4, 2001.

Lamberg et al. Antithyroid treatment of maternal hyperthyroidism during lactation. *Clin Endocrinol* (Oxf) 21(1):81–87; 1984.

Lawlor-Smith L, Lawlor-Smith C. Vasopasm of the nipple: A manifestation of Raynaud's phenomenon. *BMJ* 314:644–645; 1997.

Lawrence R. A review of the medical contraindications to breastfeeding. *Technical Information Bulletin*. Washington, DC: National Center for Education in Maternal Child Health, USDHHS; October 1997.

Lawrence R. *Breastfeeding: A Guide for the Medical Profession*, 5th ed. Philadelphia, PA: Mosby; 1999.

Lee A et al. Choice of breastfeeding and physicians' advice: A cohort study of women receiving propylthiouracil. *Pediatrics* 106(1 Pt 1):27–30; 2000.

Liles C, Tompson M. *Breastfeeding and HIV/AIDS*. La Leche League of Texas Conference. San Antonio, TX; June 13, 2004.

Lilja J et al. Isolated cleft palate and submucous cleft palate. *Oral Max Surg Clinic N A* 12(3):455–468; 2000.

Lin H et al. Absence of infection in breast-fed infants born to hepatitis C virus-infected mothers. *J Pediatr* 126:589–591; 1995.

Luder E et al. Current recommendations for breast-feeding in cystic fibrosis centers. *Am J Dis Child* 144(10):1153–1156; 1990.

Lupus Foundation of America. *Pregnancy and Lupus*, 2001. Available at: www.lupus.org/education/pregnant.html. Accessed February 5, 2005.

Mackie A et al. Cystic fibrosis-related diabetes. *Diabet Med* 20(6):425–436; 2003.

Marasco L et al. Polycystic ovary syndrome: A connection to insufficient milk supply? *J Hum Lact* 16(2):143–148; 2000.

Marasco L. *Insufficient Milk Supply Explored: Causes, Recent Research, and Theories*. La Leche League International 2003 Lactation Specialist Workshop Series XVIII. Austin, TX; March 29, 2003.

Martin I. *The Thyroid Book*. New York: St. Martin's Press; 1993.

Martin L et al. *Presence of Adiponectin and Leptin in Human Milk*. 2004 Pediatric Academic Societies' Annual Meeting. San Francisco, CA; May 2, 2004.

Mason T et al. Breast feeding and the development of juvenile rheumatoid arthritis. *J Rheumatol* 22(6):1166–1170; 1995.

Mayo Clinic, Mayo Foundation for Medical Education and Research. Stickler's syndrome. November 5, 2003. Available at: www.mayoclinic.com/invoke.cfm?objectid=0B7B773A-A6F5-4DCE-A70C8AD6696E6E56. Accessed June 12, 2004.

Mayo Clinic, Mayo Foundation for Medical Education and Research. Cystic fibrosis. April 8, 2004. Available at: www.mayoclinic.com/invoke.cfm?id=DS00287. Accessed June 12, 2004.

Mbori-Ngacha D, Nduati R, John G, et al. Morbidity and mortality in breastfed and formula-fed infants of HIV-1-infected women: A randomized clinical trial. *JAMA* 286: 2413–2420; 2001.

McBride M, Danner S. Sucking disorders in neurologically impaired infants: Assessment and facilitation of breastfeeding. *Clin Perinatol* 14:1:109–130; 1987.

McWilliams B. Submucous clefts of the palate: How likely are they to be symptomatic? *Cleft Palate Craniofac J* 28(3): 247–249; discussion 250–251; 1991.

Michel S, Mueller D. Impact of lactation on women with cystic fibrosis and their infants: A review of five cases. *J Am Diet Assoc* 94:159–165; 1994.

Mick V. *Cleft Palate: A Team Approach*. 5th Annual Texas Breastfeeding Summit. San Antonio, TX; October 1, 2002.

Moe J et al. Breastfeeding practices of infants with Rubinstein-Taybi syndrome. *J Hum Lact* 14(4):311–315; 1998.

Momotani N et al. Recovery from foetal hypothyroidism: Evidence for the safety of breast-feeding while taking propylthiouracil. *Clin Endocrinol (Oxf)* 31(5):591–595; 1989.

Momotani N et al. Thyroid function in wholly breast-feeding infants whose mothers take high doses of propylthiouracil. *Clin Endocrinol (Oxf)* 53(2):177–181; 2000.

Monetini L. Bovine beta-casein antibodies in breast- and bottle-fed infants: Their relevance in Type 1 diabetes. *Diabetes Metab Res Rev* 17(1):51–54; 2001.

Morris S. Developmental implications for the management of feeding problems in neurologically impaired infants. *Sem in Speech Lang* 6:293–315; 1985.

National Heart Lung and Blood Institute (NHLBI). Facts about Raynaud's Phenomenon. Bethesda, MD. Available at: www.nhlbi.nih.gov/health/public/blood/other/raynaud.htm #what. Accessed June 12, 2004.

National Institute of Neurological Disorders and Stroke (NINDS). *NINDS* Sjogren's Syndrome information page, December 3, 2003. Available at: www.ninds.nih.gov/disorders/sjogrens/sjogrens.htm. Accessed February 5, 2005.

Nelson C, Demmler G. Cytomegalovirus infection in the pregnant mother, fetus, and newborn infant. *Review Clin Perinatol* 24(1):151–160; 1997.

Newell M. Prevention of mother-to-child transmission of HIV: Challenges for the current decade. *Bulletin of World Health Organization* 79:1138–1144; 2001.

Newman J. Handout #3b. *Treatments for sore nipples and sore breasts.* January 2003. Available at: www.breastfeedingonline. com. Accessed March 12, 2004.

Obesity Meds and Research News. Hot topic of the month: Metformin and weight loss 4(2); 2000. Available at: www. obesity-news.com/absmet.htm. Accessed June 28, 2004.

Olsen N, Nielson S. Prevalence of primary Raynaud's phenomenon in young females. *Scand J Clin Lab Invest* 37:761–776; 1978.

Ono H et al. Transient galactosemia detected by neonatal mass screening. *Pediatr Int* 41(3):281–284; 1999.

Orloff S et al. Inactivation of human immunodeficiency virus type I in human milk: Effects of intrinsic factors in human milk and of pasteurization. *J Hum Lact* 9(1):13–17; 1993.

Ostrum K, Ferris A. Prolactin concentrations in serum and milk of mothers with and without insulin-dependent diabetes. *Am J Clin Nutr* 58:49–53; 1993.

Paradise J et al. Evidence in infants with cleft palate that breastmilk protects against otitis media. *Pediatrics* 94(6):853–860; 1994.

Pisacane A et al. Breastfeeding and multiple sclerosis. *Br J Med* 308:1411–1412; 1994.

Pisacane A et al. Down syndrome and breastfeeding. *Acta Paediatr* 92(12):1479–1481; 2003.

Poppe K et al. Thyroid dysfunction and autoimmunity in infertile women. *Thyroid* 12(11):997–1001; 2002.

Poppe K et al. Assisted reproduction and thyroid autoimmunity: An unfortunate combination? *J Clin Endocrinol Metab* 88:4149–4152; 2003a.

Poppe K, Glinoer D. Thyroid autoimmunity and hypothyroidism before and during pregnancy. *Hum Reprod Update* 9(2):149–161; 2003b.

Poppe K, Velkeniers B. Female infertility and the thyroid. *Best Pract Res Clin Endocrinol Metab* 18(2):153–165; 2004.

Purnell H. Phenylketonuria and maternal phenylketonuria. *Breastfeed Rev* 9(2):19–21; 2001.

Rao G. Insulin resistance syndrome. *Am Fam Physician* 63: 1159–1163, 1165–1166; 2001.

Redmond G. Thyroid dysfunction and women's reproductive health. *Thyroid* 14 Suppl 1:S5–S15; 2004.

Riva E et al. Early breastfeeding is linked to higher intelligence quotient scores in dietary treated phenylketonuric children. *Acta Paediatr* 85:56–58; 1996.

Rollins N et al. Preventing postnatal transmission of HIV-1 through breast-feeding: Modifying infant feeding practices. *J Acquir Immune Defic Syndr* 1:35(2):188–195; 2004.

Ross J, Labbok M. Modeling the effects of different infant feeding strategies on infant survival and mother-to-child transmission of HIV. *Am J Public Health* 94(7):1174–1180; 2004.

Rylance G et al. Carimazole and breastfeeding. *Lancet* 1(8538):928; 1987.

Sadauskaite-Kuehne V et al. Longer breastfeeding is an independent protective factor against development of type 1 diabetes mellitus in childhood. *Diabetes Metab Res Rev* 20(2): 150–157; 2004.

Saenz R. Iodine-131 elimination from breast milk: A case report. *J Hum Lact* 16(1):44–46; 2000.

Sensory Integration International. Resource information for sensory integration dysfunction. Available at: //mmm1106. verio-web.com/sensor/index.htm. Accessed June 15, 2004.

Sensory Processing Disorder Network. Resource information for sensory processing disorders; May 28, 2004. Available at: www.spdnetwork.org. Accessed June 15, 2004.

Shah C, Wong D. Management of children with cleft lip and palate. *CMA J* 122:19–24; 1980.

Shiffman M et al. Breastmilk composition in women with cystic fibrosis: Report of two cases and a review of the literature. *Am J Clin Nutr* 49:612–617; 1989.

Siega-Riz A, Adair L. Biological determinants of pregnancy weight gain in a Filipino population. *Am J Clin Nutr* 57(3): 365–372; 1993.

Silman A, Pearson J. Epidemiology and genetics of rheumatoid arthritis. Review. *Arthritis Res* 4 Suppl 3:S265–S272; 2002.

Sinaii N, Cleary SD, Ballweg ML et al. High rates of autoimmune and endocrine disorders, fibromyalgia, chronic fatigue syndrome and atopic diseases among women with endometriosis: A survey analysis. *Hum Reprod* 17:2715–2724; October 2002.

Stagnaro-Green A. Postpartum thyroiditis. *Best Pract Res Clin Endocrinol Metab* 18(2):303–316; 2004.

Stockdale H. Long-term expressing of breastmilk. *Breastfeed Rev* 8(3):19–22; 2000.

Tao L et al. *Lactobacillus Traps HIV by Mannose-Specific Binding L.* American Society for Microbiology, 104th General Meeting. New Orleans, LA; May 25, 2004.

Tarrats R et al. Varicella, ephemeral breastfeeding and eczema as risk factors for multiple sclerosis in Mexicans. *Acta Neurol Scand* 105(2):88–89; 2002.

Thompson N et al. Early determinants of inflammatory bowel disease: Use of two national longitudinal birth cohorts. *Europ Jnl Gastroenter Hepatology* 12(1):25–30; 2000.

Thorne C, Newell M. Mother-to-child transmission of HIV infection and its prevention. *Curr HIV Res* 1(4):447–462; 2003.

Thorne C, Newell M. Are girls more at risk of intrauterine-acquired HIV infection than boys? *AIDS* 18(2):344–347; 2004.

Toschke A et al. Overweight and obesity in 6- to 14-year-old Czech children in 1991: Protective effect of breast-feeding. *J Pediatr* 141(6):764–769; 2002.

UNAIDS. *AIDS epidemic update, December, 2004.* Global summary of the HIV/AIDS epidemic. Available at: www.unaids.org. Accessed February 5, 2005.

Van Rijn M et al. A different approach to breast-feeding of the infant with phenylketonuria. *Eur J Pediatr* 162(5):323–326; 2003.

Walley J et al. Simplified antiviral prophylaxis with or without artificial feeding to reduce mother-to-child transmission of HIV in low and middle income countries: Modelling positive and negative impact on child survival. *Med Sci Monit* 7(5):1043–1051; 2001.

Walsh S, Rau L. Autoimmune diseases: A leading cause of death among young and middle-aged women in the United States. *Am J Public Health* 90(9):1463–1466; 2000.

Watson-Genna C. Tactile defensiveness and other sensory modulation difficulties. *Leaven* 37(3):51–53; 2001.

Watson-Genna C. Sensory integration and breastfeeding. *Medela Messenger* 12(1):11–16; 2002.

Webster J et al. Breastfeeding outcomes for women with insulin dependent diabetes. *J Hum Lact* 11:195–200; 1995.

Weiss-Salinas D, Williams N. Sensory defensiveness: A theory of its effect on breastfeeding. *J Hum Lact* 17(2):145–151; 2001.

Welch M et al. Breast-feeding by a mother with cystic fibrosis. *Pediatrics* 67:664–666; 1981.

Whichelow M, Doddridge M. Lactation in diabetic women. *Br Med J* 287:649–650; 1983.

Wide Smiles Cleft Lip and Palate Resource. Available at: www.widesmiles.org. Accessed June 12, 2004.

Wilson-Clay B, Hoover K. *The Breastfeeding Atlas,* 2nd ed. Austin, TX: Lactnews Press; 2002.

Wolf L, Glass R. *Feeding and Swallowing Disorders in Infancy.* San Antonio, TX: Therapy Skill Builders; 1992.

World Health Organization (WHO). Tuberculosis Fact Sheet #104. August; 2002.

World Health Organization (WHO). HIV and infant feeding: Framework for priority action. WHO; 2003.

World Health Organization (WHO). WHO's HIV/AIDS strategy under the spotlight. *Bulletin of the World Health Organization* 82(6): 399–478; 2004.

World Health Organization (WHO). "3 by 5" Progress Report, December 2004. *WHO and AIDS; 2005.* Available at: www.unaids.org. Accessed February 5, 2005.

Young J et al. What information do parents of newborns with cleft lip, palate, or both want to know? *Cleft Palate Craniofac J* 38(1):55–58; 2001.

Young T et al. Type 2 diabetes mellitus in children—prenatal and early infancy risk factors among native Canadians. *Arch Ped Adol Med* 146(7):651–655; 2002.

Zargar A et al. Familial puerperal alactogenesis: Possibility of a genetically transmitted isolated prolactin deficiency. *Br J Obstet Gynaecol* 104(5):629–631; 1997.

Zargar A et al. Puerperal alactogenesis with normal prolactin dynamics: Is prolactin resistance the cause? *Fertility and Sterility* 74(3): 598–600; 2000.

Ziakas N et al. Stickler's syndrome associated with congenital glaucoma. *Ophthalmic Genet* 19(1):55–58; 1998.

Zuppa A et al. Relationship between maternal parity, basal prolactin levels and neonatal breast milk intake. *Biology of the Neonate* 53(3):144–147; 1988.

▶ BIBLIOGRAPHY

Abbott Laboratories. Global care initiatives & product access program. Available at: www.abbott.com/citizenship/access/global_access.cfm. Accessed February 5, 2005.

Bobat R et al. Breastfeeding by HIV-1 infected women and outcome in their infants: A cohort study from Durban, South Africa. *AIDS* 11:1627–1633; 1997.

Braun, Palmer (eds). *Early Detection and Treatment of the Infant and Young Child with Neuromuscular Disorders.* New York: Therapeutic Media; 1992.

Curtin G. The infant with cleft lip or palate: More than a surgical problem. *J Perinat Neonatal Nurs* 3:80–89; 1990.

Cutting W. Breastfeeding and HIV infection. *Br Med J* 305: 788; 1992.

Danner S. Breastfeeding the neurologically impaired infant. *NAACOG Clin Issu Perinat Womens Health Nurs* 3(4): 640–646; 1992.

Danner S, Cerutti E. *Nursing Your Neurologically Impaired Baby.* Rochester, NY: Childbirth Graphics; 1984.

Danner S, Wilson-Clay B. *Breastfeeding the Infant with a Cleft Lip/Palate.* Lactation Consultant Series, La Leche League International, Unit 10. New York: Avery; 1986.

Datta P et al. Mother-to-child transmission of human immunodeficiency virus Type I: Report from the Nairobi study. *J Infect Dis* 170:1134–1140; 1994.

Dunn D, Newell M. Quantifying the risk of HIV-I transmission via breastmilk. *AIDS* 7:134–135; 1993.

Dunne W, Jevon M. Examination of human breast milk for evidence of human Herpes virus 6 by polymerase chain reaction. *J Infect Dis* 168:250; 1993.

Edwards M, Watson ACH (eds). *Advances in the Management of the Cleft Palate.* Edinburgh: Churchill Livingstone; 1980.

Ehrenkranz R, Ackerman B. Metoclopramide effect on faltering milk production by mothers of premature infants. *Pediatr ICS* 78:614–620; 1986.

Ekvall S. *Pediatric Nutrition in Chronic Diseases and Developmental Disorders: Prevention, Assessment, and Treatment.* London: Oxford University Press; 1992.

Fernhoff P, Lammer E. Craniofacial features of isotretinoin embryopathy. *J Pediatr* 105(4):595–597; October 1984.

Forbes A et al. Composition of milk produced by a mother with galactosemia. *J Pediatr* 113:90–91; 1988.

Grady E. Breastfeeding the baby with a cleft of the soft palate. *Clin Pediatr* 16(11):978–981; 1977.

Greve L et al. Breastfeeding in the management of the newborn with phenylketonuria: A practical approach to dietary therapy. *J Am Diet Assoc* 94:305–309; 1994.

Hira S et al. Apparent vertical transmission of human immunodeficiency virus type I by breastfeeding in Zambia. *J Pediatr* 117:421–424; 1990.

Hutt P. The effects of diabetes on lactation. *Breastfeed Rev* 14:21–25; 1989.

Jacobson S et al. Incidence and correlates of breast-feeding in socioeconomically disadvantaged women. *Pediatrics* 88(4): 728–736; 1991.

Jain L et al. Energetics and mechanics of nutritive sucking in the preterm and term neonate. *J Pediatr* 111(6):894–898; 1988.

Kampinga G et al. Primary infections with HIV-1 of women and their offspring in Rwanda: Findings of heterogeneity at seroconversion, coinfection and recombinants of HIV-1 subtypes A and C. *Virology* 227:63–76; 1997.

Kent G, Crowe D. Infant feeding and HIV: The importance of language in shaping policy. Evanston, IL: AnotherLook; October 14, 2002.

Lewis MB, Pashayan HM. Management of infants with Robin anomaly. *Clin Pediatr* 19(8): 519–528; 1980.

Mosca F et al. Transmission of cytomegalovirus. *Lancet* 357(9270):1800; 2001.

National Institutes of Health. National Institute for Child Health and Human Development Conference Statement: Phenylketonuria Screening and Management. *Pediatrics* 108: 972–982; 2001.

Newberg D et al. A human milk factor inhibits binding of immunodeficiency virus to the CD4 receptor. *Pediatr Res* 31:22–28; 1992.

Nommsen-Rivers L, Heinig M. HIV transmission via breastfeeding: Reflections on the issues. *J Hum Lact* 13:179–181; 1997.

Numazaki K et al. Transmission of cytomegalovirus. *Lancet* 357(9270):1799–1800; 2001.

Orloff S et al. Inactivation of human immunodeficiency virus type I in human milk: Effects of intrinsic factors in human milk and of pastuerization. *J Hum Lact* 9:13–17; 1993.

Oxtoby M. Human immunodeficiency virus and other viruses in human milk: Placing the issues in broader perspective. *Pediatr Infec Dis J* 7:825–835; 1988.

Palasanthiran P et al. Breastfeeding during primary maternal human immunodeficiency virus infection and risk of transmission from mother to infant. *J Infect Dis* 167:441–444; 1993.

Posnick J. *Craniofacial and Maxillofacial Surgery in Children and Young Adults.* Philadelphia, PA: WB Saunders Co.; 2000.

Townsend D. Nursing after cleft lip surgery. *New Beginnings* 6:147–148; 1989.

United Republic of Tanzania (URP). National Policy on HIV/AIDS; September 2001. Available at: www.tanzania.go.tz/hiv_aidsf.html. Accessed June 18, 2004.

Watson A et al. *Management of Cleft Lip and Palate.* Edinburgh: Whurr; 2001.

Weatherly-White RCA et al. Early repair and breast-feeding for infants with cleft lip. *Plast Reconstr Surg*: 879–885; 1987.

ROLE OF THE IBCLC

PROFESSIONAL CONSIDERATIONS

Contributing Authors: Jan Barger, Linda Kutner, and Carole Peterson

A lactation consultant is an integral member of the breastfeeding mother's healthcare team, a position accompanied by tremendous responsibilities. Your professional growth will take you through a progression of stages as you acquire the role of lactation consultant. The process is similar to the acquisition of the parental role described in Chapter 19. As you navigate through this journey, you will learn to appreciate the importance of formal lactation education and extensive clinical experience. This chapter explores **networking** with colleagues and participating in your professional association, as those resources will form an essential part of your support system. Safeguards for providing appropriate care to mothers and babies are discussed in terms of professional certification and standards of practice. You will learn to recognize your limitations and when you need assistance. This awareness will help you maintain a positive perspective that will enable you to give the best of yourself to mothers and infants.

KEY TERMS

care plan	internship
certification	job description
client relationship	legal considerations
clinical experience	liability
code of ethics	networking
curriculum vitae	pitfalls
documentation	professional burnout
follow-up	record retention
HIPAA	referral system
informed consent	role acquisition
IBCLC	standards of practice
IBLCE	universal precautions
ILCA	

▶ ACQUIRING THE ROLE OF LACTATION CONSULTANT

Moving into a new role is a dynamic process, whether it involves a new career or parenthood. *Acquiring the Parental Role* describes four stages of role acquisition—the Anticipatory Stage, the Formal Stage, the Informal Stage, and the Personal Stage (Bocar, 1987). This process from novice to expert was adapted to the context of entering the lactation profession (Barger, 1998). Examining the role of a lactation professional within this framework will help you understand the elements involved in assuming the role of International Board Certified Lactation Consultant (IBCLC).

Anticipatory Stage

In the Anticipatory Stage, the aspiring IBCLC collects information about the profession from many sources. Contact with an IBCLC during your breastfeeding experience may have sparked in you an interest in the profession. You may be a health professional seeking to expand your role with women and children, or perhaps your interest arose from having breastfed your own children. Your perception of being an IBCLC may be somewhat idealized at this early stage. You may envision balancing work at home with family responsibilities. Perhaps you anticipate making a substantial salary doing something you love. You may seek the "perfect" job in a clinic or hospital setting.

Whatever the source of your interest, you will gather information from other IBCLCs, your professional association, the certification board, providers of lactation education, and professional journals. You will soon recognize how much there is to learn and the need for formal training. This will direct you to enroll in a lactation management course and then become a lactation consultant intern. Interns are those who have completed the didactic segment of their lactation management education and are involved in acquiring the clinical experience necessary toward becoming certified. Internship begins the Formal Stage of the IBCLC's role acquisition.

Formal Stage

The Formal Stage begins when the lactation consultant intern begins to care for mothers and babies. Formalized expectations define the intern's role in objective, written terms. Expectations are based on three seminal documents in the lactation profession, available on the Internet. The International Lactation Consultant Association (ILCA) maintains standards of clinical practice (ILCA, 1999). The International Board of Lactation Consultant Examiners (IBLCE) monitors a code of ethics that governs the IBCLC's actions (IBLCE, 2004). IBLCE also has identified a list of clinical competencies to guide interns as they acquire the necessary skills (IBLCE, 2003). Most institutions in which an IBCLC works will have a written job description to define the role within that particular institution.

Using these documents to guide you through the Formal Stage, you begin to break down preconceived ideas and teachings. It will become clear that there is conflicting advice among the "experts" on many aspects of breastfeeding care. Wanting to do everything the "right" and "best" way, you will begin to choose from more than one method to determine your own practices. You may practice rigidly and formally according to your perceived "rules" as you try to do everything right. It can be difficult during this time for you to make decisions based on the needs of an individual mother and baby. You may still view your execution of a care plan as black and white. For example, you may have learned that bottles contribute to a baby developing a preference for an artificial nipple, or that a "good" IBCLC never uses a nipple shield. Therefore, you may be reluctant to use either of them, not recognizing when they might be appropriate.

Although you are eager to work independently, you will prefer the security of a mentor to guide you during this stage. Reactions and comments from the mentor will have a great impact on you, and you will appreciate your mentor's moral support and affirmation as you progress toward independence. This is an excellent time to join local breastfeeding coalitions and your professional association. You will be learning how to apply your knowledge in order to individualize your practices for each mother and baby. You will soon believe you are adequately performing the essential plans of care and will begin to feel comfortable caring for new mothers. You will gain confidence in sharing your knowledge and skills with colleagues. You no longer think that you must know everything and will gain confidence to move on to the next stage of role acquisition, the Informal Stage.

Informal Stage

As you enter the Informal Stage, you will begin to modify the rigid rules and directions you had sought out and used during the Formal Stage. You are comfortable considering all the different approaches to care and weighing various options. Networking with other IBCLCs will help you mature in your role, as you continue to learn

that there may be many ways to approach various aspects of breastfeeding care. Attending professional conferences will increase your knowledge and vary your exposure to many different styles and ways of practicing as a professional lactation consultant. Your interactions with mothers and other IBCLCs will become more spontaneous, and you will have less fear of imperfection. If you are not already certified, you will now sit for the certification exam provided by the International Board of Lactation Consultant Examiners. After passing the exam, you will be a qualified IBCLC. You then enter the Personal Stage.

Personal Stage

Having reached the Personal Stage, you evolve further in your role to a style that is consistent with your personality. You are better able to understand the motives and whims of new mothers. You recognize that mothers are responsible for their choices, and you learn not to feel guilty for undesirable outcomes. Consequently, you are more accepting of a mother who chooses a path that you regard as less than optimal.

Although you seek other opinions, you are quick to discard them if they are incompatible with your approach. You look critically at research and adapt it to your practice. You are comfortable in your role as an IBCLC and enjoy opportunities to teach others through inservice and conference presentations. You may become involved with assisting your professional organization in leadership capacities. This is also the stage in which you take the lead in helping to create coalitions and in advocating for breastfeeding. You will promote the IBCLC credential and may become active at leadership levels in your professional association.

Facilitating Role Acquisition

Aspiring IBCLCs will progress through these stages at their own pace. The speed with which you progress will be determined by your comfort level at each stage. Other IBCLCs can be valuable as mentors during your Formal Stage. It is through such exposure to a variety of lactation practitioners that you will emerge with your own unique approach. You might model yourself after an experienced IBCLC whom you have observed. The flexibility you learn to adopt in your approach will carry through to enable you to remain flexible in developing your plans of care for mothers and babies. In the Personal Stage, you may serve as a model to other aspiring IBCLCs.

Recognizing this dynamic process of role acquisition illustrates that there are few hard-and-fast rules about working with mothers and babies. You will learn to adapt theory and book knowledge to each new situation.

Clinicians who have not changed their practices substantially during the past five years have failed to remain current with new information that has surfaced during that time. As researchers and practitioners continue to discover and understand more about breastfeeding and human lactation, practices will continue to change.

▶ PREPARING FOR THE PROFESSION

Preparing for any new profession can seem daunting. Most likely, you have already come a long way in the process. In its short existence, the lactation profession has laid much groundwork for establishing standards. Entry-level education and assessment, standards of practice, and clinical competencies are in place and provide a well-grounded starting point for lactation professionals. The profession will continue to evolve and be further refined.

New practices and recommendations appear continually, sometimes making it difficult to remain current. You need to be aware of controversies regarding new practices and to consider them with respect to basic information and solid research. You will then be able to decide carefully whether newer ideas are better than older ones. Anyone who wishes to work in a helping role with breastfeeding mothers has a professional responsibility to give optimal, evidence-based care. Remaining current is essential to your growth and development as a clinician.

The knowledge and skill base in the lactation field is broad and extensive. In the early years of the profession, many lactation consultants gained their knowledge through self-directed education. As the profession continues to evolve past its infancy, its members recognize the value of formal education in lactation management. The International Lactation Consultant Association (ILCA) provides a list of educational programs offered throughout the world, including distance instruction available over the Internet. Even the experienced health professional will benefit from specialized instruction in lactation management.

General Education

The lactation profession and the public are best served when an individual entering the profession has additional education related to healthcare. IBLCE requires that exam candidates must have completed courses in anatomy and physiology, sociology, psychology or counseling, child development, and nutrition. Courses in adult learning and counseling techniques are especially important, as you will use these skills frequently when interviewing mothers and educating families and professionals.

A curriculum of basic college courses in a 2-year program may include the courses identified in Table 26.1.

TABLE 26.1

Basic College Courses in a Two-Year Program*

Discipline	Semester credit hours
Communications	9 credit hours (English composition and speech)
Math and Science	20 credit hours
Humanities	6 credit hours (languages, fine arts, literature, and philosophy)
Social Sciences	6 credit hours (psychology, sociology, and anthropology)
Contemporary Studies and Life Skills	3 credit hours (art, music, and computer science)
Electives	18 credit hours

In addition to basic education are courses that complement the lactation field and that are especially helpful to IBCLCs. Those who do not have a health-related degree will benefit from these courses to fill the gap in their education. Table 26.2 identifies courses that would be helpful as well.

Lactation Management Program

A lactation management program needs to include information and discussions specific to the practice of lactation consulting. Ideally, instruction would include documentation; developing private, hospital, clinic, or public health–based practices; and review of the standards of practice as defined by the profession. The program should emphasize preparing the practitioner for practice as an IBCLC, with a focus on practical aspects of lactation management. It should also provide information and guidance for obtaining clinical experience (Kutner, 2002).

A comprehensive lactation management course will address the subjects defined in the grid for the IBLCE exam. They include:

- Maternal and infant anatomy, physiology, and endocrinology
- Maternal and infant nutrition, biochemistry, immunology, and infectious diseases
- Maternal and infant pathology, pharmacology, and toxicology
- Psychology, sociology, and anthropology
- Growth parameters and developmental milestones from preconception to beyond 12 months
- Reading and interpretation of research
- Ethical and legal issues related to the practice of lactation consulting

TABLE 26.2	
Courses Helpful to IBCLCs*	
Introduction to Anatomy and Physiology	4 credit hours
English Composition I	3 credit hours
English Composition II	3 credit hours
Fundamentals of Speech	3 credit hours
Microbiology	4 credit hours
Introduction to Psychology	3 credit hours
Child Psychology	3 credit hours
Introduction to Sociology	3 credit hours
Family in Society	3 credit hours
Computer Basics	3 credit hours
Medical Terminology	2 credit hours
Medical Law and Ethics	3 credit hours
Basic Nutrition	3 credit hours
Introduction to Human Disease	3 credit hours
Psychology of Human Development	3 credit hours
Child Development	3 credit hours
Marriage and the Family	3 credit hours
Counseling	3 credit hours
Pharmacology	4 credit hours
Chemistry	4 credit hours
Biology	4 credit hours

*These lists of courses (Tables 26.1 and 26.2) will assist the aspiring lactation consultant in identifying areas that will strengthen her knowledge and skills in the field. The lists are reprinted with permission from the text, *Clinical Experience in Lactation: A Blueprint for Internship*, by Kutner and Barger, 2002.

◆ Technology related to breastfeeding
◆ Public health issues surrounding lactation

Clinical Experience

Armed with the knowledge and skills learned in your formal didactic education, along with your own personal enrichment, you will be prepared to acquire hands-on clinical experience. Requirements for candidates of the IBLCE certification exam include extensive clinical hours. You may be able to arrange with a hospital-based lactation consultant to mentor and supervise you in providing services for mothers while you gain experience. Some hospitals have lactation clinics located within their facilities that offer extended postpartum experiences. You might also volunteer or work in a physician's office, WIC agency, or other clinic.

IBLCE's *Clinical Competencies for IBCLC Practice* identifies specific experiences needed to prepare for the certification exam and to work as an International Board Certified Lactation Consultant. The text *Clinical Experience in Lactation: A Blueprint for Internship* gives clear guidelines for finding broad-based clinical experiences (Kutner, 2002). It includes worksheets and study questions that cover the essential elements in each clinical experience. Both of these publications ensure balance in preparing for the profession. A well-rounded IBCLC needs clinical experience in the various settings that care for breastfeeding mothers and babies, as well as clinical experience with various infant ages. This can be acquired in community support groups, health clinics, home visits, and maternity/infant care areas in the hospital such as the NICU, labor and delivery, and mother-baby units.

Certification

Many professionals who work in the maternal and infant health fields incorporate their knowledge of breastfeeding into an existing practice. A pediatric nurse practitioner, physician, midwife, or hospital staff nurse may wish to become more skilled in helping breastfeeding mothers and babies. Some may decide to specialize in the care of breastfeeding mothers and infants through certification as an IBCLC. A comprehensive course in lactation management is essential to anyone who plans to specialize in lactation. However, completion of a course does not provide the safeguards and standards that the official IBLCE certification does. Although some courses may bestow the title "certified" to their graduates, this title is not recognized by the lactation profession. Any recognized certification must be subject to criterion-referenced testing and requirements for periodic recertification through testing or continuing education.

Presently, the only certification that meets the standards of the profession is that received by successfully completing the exam provided by the IBLCE. Candidates for the exam must meet minimal requirements regarding education in lactation management and clinical experience. Successful completion of the exam allows the candidate to use the title "International Board Certified Lactation Consultant" (IBCLC). Recertification is required every five years, with retesting every ten years. See Appendix A for IBLCE's contact information to get current requirements.

▶ ## STANDARDS OF PRACTICE FOR THE LACTATION PROFESSION

Practicing as a lactation professional means providing quality care to the public and accepting responsibility for that care. Quality and service constitute the core of a profession's responsibility to the public. Supporting that belief, ILCA developed the *Standards of Practice for Lactation Consultants* (ILCA, 1999). ILCA believes that "all individuals representing themselves as lactation consultants, whether or not they are IBCLC, should adhere to these standards of practice in any and all inter-actions with the clients' families." Standards of practice identify "stated measures or levels of quality" that serve as models for the conduct and evaluation of practice (AWHONN, 1991). Those who describe themselves as lactation consultants should provide the level and qual-ity of care described in the ILCA Standards of Practice.

As an IBCLC you work in concert with primary prac-titioners who care for the infant and mother. You provide a level of care that facilitates continued health and well-ness, particularly as it relates to breastfeeding and early parenting. You focus on helping breastfeeding women and their families achieve their breastfeeding goals. The next section includes summaries of the standards of practice (Kutner, 2001). See Appendix D for the full document.

Standards for Plan of Care

No matter what your practice setting, you will assess, plan, implement, and evaluate a variety of situations, both simple and complex. You are expected to individualize your approach and to prioritize practices to meet the physical and emotional needs of the mother and infant.

Assessment and History

You must assess the mother and child individually, eval-uate the physical appearance and findings of the mother and child, and document the findings appropriately. This includes taking a formal history on both a general level and one specifically related to lactation. You then need to consider carefully the information you have gathered and develop a plan of care based on the mother's needs and goals. Part of this plan of care must include appropriate documented follow-up.

Plan of Care

In implementing a plan of care, you must provide appropriate guidance to the mother, which includes dis-cussing the risks and benefits of any suggested interven-tions. Mothers should receive demonstrations of all suggested techniques, along with written instructions for reinforcement. Any plan of care must include provi-sions for safety, hygiene, infection control, and universal precautions. Chapter 12 further explores the plan of care for breastfeeding.

Documentation

After you and the mother have worked out an agreeable plan, you must inform the primary caregiver of the mother or child, or both, of the interaction and plan. This should be in writing, with a verbal report as well, depend-ing on the immediate needs of the mother or child. You also have a responsibility to make referrals to other care providers and support groups whenever appropriate. All steps involved in implementing the mother's plan of care must be included in your documentation.

Follow-up and Evaluation

An important final step is to evaluate the outcome of any plan of care you and the mother have implemented. This evaluation will identify any intervention that is not work-ing so you can modify the plan. Knowing whether the intervention is working will help in similar situations in the future. Document the evaluation of the care plan in the mother's record for consistency and future reference.

Standards for Education and Counseling

You will educate mothers and families in a variety of set-tings as you guide them to make informed decisions regarding infant feeding. Providing anticipatory guidance promotes optimal breastfeeding and minimizes breast-feeding difficulties. When difficulties arise, you will pro-vide support and education that encourage the mother and her family to continue breastfeeding through to res-olution. Your role as an educator will extend to col-leagues, as well. You have the responsibility to educate other caregivers—professional and paraprofessional—in order to optimize breastfeeding care for mothers and their babies. To do this effectively, it is important that you understand different types of learning styles and use a variety of methods in teaching adults.

Standards for Professional Responsibilities

In addition to adhering to your profession's standards, you must function within the broader standards of the healthcare industry. You have a responsibility to practice in an ethical manner, realizing that you are an advocate for the mother and child at all times. You must remain current with any changes in your profession's standards as well as with clinical research. You must be clinically competent and accountable for your professional actions, which include:

- Respecting the privacy of the mother-child rela-tionship.
- Maintaining awareness of changing practices and of professional or ethical issues.
- Recognizing limitations in your knowledge or skills.
- Obtaining clients' written consent before providing care.

◆ Communicating relevant information to the primary caregiver (or caregivers).

◆ Collaborating with and referring to other healthcare professionals as appropriate.

◆ Participating in appropriate professional organizations.

◆ Lending support to colleagues.

Standards for Legal Considerations

You must practice within the laws of the geopolitical region in which you live and must respect the mother's and baby's rights to privacy and issues that are confidential in nature. It is imperative that you obtain liability insurance before practicing as a lactation consultant. If you work for a hospital or government agency and are not performing duties beyond that scope of practice, your employer's liability insurance should provide sufficient coverage. Privately employed IBCLCs need to secure some form of liability insurance. See Appendix A for source information.

HIPAA Regulations

In 1996, the United States passed the Health Insurance Portability and Accountability Act (HIPAA). HIPAA provides federal protections for the privacy of patients' protected health information. The act prohibits use or disclosure of protected health information unless authorized by the patient. HIPAA also ensures privacy and confidentiality of research participants unless they authorize use or disclosure of the information. It prohibits reuse or disclosure of the information unless required by law.

The act allows certain incidental uses and disclosures that occur as a by-product. You can guard against violating a client's privacy through incidental disclosure by speaking quietly and avoiding use of client names when in public areas. If you email or fax client reports, a confidentiality notice such as the one in Figure 26.1 will ensure that your transmittal complies with HIPAA regulations. You can further protect privacy by isolating or locking file cabinets that contain client records, using a password on your computer, and destroying research identifiers at the earliest opportunity. Suspected child neglect or abuse does not fall within HIPAA privacy restrictions. You still have authorization and a legal duty to report such instances to appropriate public health authorities.

If practicing privately, you should have a HIPAA Notice of Privacy Practices posted in your office or on your Web site. Provide a copy to your clients when you make home visits. Clients should sign a form acknowledging receipt of the HIPAA information. ILCA's *Core Curriculum for Lactation Consultant Practice* (2002)

FIGURE 26.1
Confidentiality notice.

The attached pages are my report of a recent lactation consultation. **If you received this transmission in error,** please respect the privacy of the people involved. Contact (your name, phone or fax number, or email address) to tell me I have sent it to the wrong recipient. **Destroy the report** you received by mistake.

This report contains information which falls under the privacy sections of the Health Insurance Portability and Accountability Act of 1996. When you read it, you will see personal information and details about a mother and her baby. I have obtained consent from the mother involved to transmit this report to her healthcare providers, as required by the International Board of Lactation Consultant Examiners Code of Ethics and the International Lactation Consultant Association Standards of Practice.

Printed with permission of Elizabeth C. Brooks, JD, IBCLC.

contains detailed information for meeting HIPAA requirements, along with sample forms. There are also software education and forms available. See Appendix A for these.

Client Relationships

When you accept a client, you create certain expectations and duties that are contractual in nature. Those duties exist regardless of whether clients pay for your services. You will have a duty to render the appropriate level of care unless the client authorizes your withdrawal. You have a duty to refer the client to another caregiver, and not to abandon the client if you are unable to render appropriate care.

Establishing a Relationship

A relationship is established whenever you and the mother have contact, whether in person or over the telephone. In some cases, you create a client relationship simply by the act of making an appointment. When a mother arrives by previous appointment, you are obligated to give her care or to make alternate arrangements by referring her to another competent practitioner. If you discover a problem that is beyond your competency during an examination, you must advise the mother of your concerns. Make sure she understands she will need follow-up care, and refer her to a competent practitioner when the problem is beyond your level of competency.

Telephone Contacts

Telephone conversations can create a client relationship if you indicate acceptance or give comments in the nature of treatment. The content of the conversation will determine whether it constitutes a relationship. You can avoid creating this relationship through several measures. First, when receiving a call, identify yourself and obtain the name of the person who is calling. You may listen to the caller's complaints. If the mother makes an appointment, clarify that the appointment is to evaluate whether you can accept her as a new client. If the mother makes no appointment, you can inform her of her options, such as going to the emergency room or contacting an appropriate caregiver or another lactation consultant without creating a relationship. Bear in mind that as soon as you give comments in the nature of advice you have created a relationship with the client.

Where No Relationship Exists

There are interactions that do not create a client relationship. If a physician requests that you see a patient or review a patient's record, this does not constitute a relationship. However, if the physician relies on you for lactation advice and you are aware of this, a relationship between you and his or her patient is implied, and you will want to see the patient as soon as possible. If you work at a hospital, generally no relationship exists between you and mothers who were once in that hospital. However, this rule will not apply if the mother contacts you through a hospital telephone contact.

Duration of a Relationship

Whenever you have an established relationship with a client, you are legally required to continue care until the need for your services no longer exists, until the mother withdraws from your care, or until you withdraw in a manner that does not constitute "abandonment" of the mother. If you choose to withdraw from the relationship, you must give the mother appropriate notice of your intentions, either by talking with her or by sending a certified letter with a return receipt requested. In the letter, you should state the mother's status, any need for follow-up care, and your intention to withdraw by a definite stated date that will allow the mother time to seek alternative care. You must indicate that until the stated date you will be available for emergencies. In addition, you must state that the mother's physician can obtain a copy of all records with written permission of the mother. Be aware that a client's failure to pay will not justify your withdrawal without giving her sufficient opportunity to obtain alternative care. After notifying the mother of your intent, you must refer her to a competent replacement or to a specialist if her problem is outside the lactation consultant's competence.

You can avoid the potential of abandonment by performing services when needed. When a physician asks you to evaluate a patient, you can tell the patient verbally, "I have been contacted by Dr. _____ to evaluate you and your baby." Also, write this in the patient's chart. When you terminate the relationship, tell the patient, and write in the chart, "I am signing off this case and will no longer follow this patient. However,

I will remain available if I am notified that additional consultations or assistance are required."

Substituting your services with those of another lactation consultant does not constitute abandonment. To avoid problems, you can notify the replacement IBCLC of case details, both verbally and in writing. If possible, notify the client about the replacement as well. If a client fails to keep a follow-up appointment or to follow your advice, there are safeguards to ensure that the client understands the nature of the condition and the risks of failing to seek medical attention. Provide her with an opportunity to visit you for counseling or care. While you will share all of this verbally with the client, you also need to follow it up in writing with a certified letter.

Informed Consent

It is important that you obtain informed consent before providing care to mothers. Although informed consent may not be a legal requirement in some places of residence, you are wise to discuss specific topics with mothers so they are fully informed. You will want to discuss the nature of the mother's problem, the proposed treatment, and reasonable alternative treatments. Inform the mother of the chance of success with the proposed treatment, as well as any inherent risks. Make sure she understands the consequences of failing to undergo treatment. You can explore alternative treatments and risks with colleagues to learn what they explain to their clients. Consult current medical literature as well to document frequency and severity of risks so you can include this in your consent form.

Standard consent forms ordinarily do not provide sufficient information about disclosures made to the patient or client to establish that consent was adequately informed. Lactation consultants in a busy practice can ensure adequate legal protection by preparing an information sheet for the courses of treatment. Both you and the mother should sign the form, attesting to the fact that the mother acknowledges receipt of the information. Retain one copy for your files and give another copy to the mother. Generally, competent adults are capable of giving valid consent for infants. Therefore, the mother's signed consent covers both her care and that of her infant. In addition to consent forms for treatment, you may want to include permission for photographs to use for educational purposes. You can also attach photographs to the mother's chart to document the status of her breasts and nipples before and after treatment.

Record Retention

Your geopolitical region will define how long you must retain records. Client records provide a history of the mother's and infant's health that will be helpful to other care providers. Records will help comply with statutes and other regulations, obtain third-party payment by substantiating fees, and defend against professional negligence suits. In addition, patient records (with identifiers removed) are a great source of research projects and are useful when preparing teaching presentations.

If you work in a physician's office, the state's medical practice act or licensing statutes may dictate the type of information to be included in a patient's record. In the United States, these typically include a written record of patient history, examination results, and test results. To remain accredited, a hospital's records must contain identification data, patient medical history, reports of relevant physical examinations, diagnostic and therapeutic orders, evidence of appropriate informed consent, clinical observations, reports of procedures and tests, and conclusions at the termination of hospitalization or evaluation of treatment. You will want to keep a record of every telephone call, long-distance telephone bills, if this applies, written correspondence, and appointment calendars. These will demonstrate that you followed up on a mother's care or responded to a complaint in a timely fashion. They will also demonstrate dates of appointments or the mother's failure to keep an appointment.

Avoiding Liability

You can avoid placing yourself at risk for liability in several ways. ILCA's *Core Curriculum for Lactation Consultant Practice* contains important reading on the topic of liability (ILCA, 2002). Become familiar with your local laws regulating the practice of medicine. Familiarize yourself with protocols in your practice setting. Obtain professional liability insurance, and keep it in force continuously. Building a positive relationship with patients and being knowledgeable are safeguards against lawsuits. Be sure not to guarantee results or create unrealistic expectations, and empower parents to make informed decisions rather than relying on you to direct their actions.

Recognize when a case may be beyond your level of competence or when you may not have time to handle it. Document everything you do, as well as what you chose not to do and why. Avoid making any negative notations in the mother's record that could be seen later. Remember that the mother can request to see her records at any time. Organize your workspace and keep necessary paperwork accessible to make it convenient for documenting what you do. Keep a copy of everything you document. If you are in private practice, consider incorporating your practice to limit your personal liability. Consulting a business attorney before you open your practice is a worthwhile investment.

Standards for Ethics

As a member of the healthcare team, it is important that you work with both the mother's and baby's caregiver and that you send appropriate reports. Be careful not to undermine the caregiver's position, and try to work within the parameters of the caregiver's advice as much as possible. If you disagree, discuss the discrepancy with the caregiver. If a mother asks you for a referral to another physician, lactation consultant, or other caregiver, make it a practice to suggest at least three names.

If you work in private practice, inform the client of your fees before you initiate an assessment. You may wish to post fees in your office. When asked over the telephone what the fees will be, you can respond, "As a lactation consultant in private practice, my fees are similar to those of a physician visit. An office or home visit is $_____ and generally lasts about _____ hours. You may pay by cash or check at the end of the consultation." If you make breastfeeding equipment available as a service to mothers, you are expected to charge the standard fees for each item. Inform mothers of all fees at the beginning of the consultation so that there are no surprises later. Also, make sure that rental equipment such as breast pumps are scrupulously cleaned and in good working condition. Pumps in rental stations should be returned to the manufacturer for servicing within two years. Check with the manufacturers of the pumps you are interested in carrying to find out their current requirements for a rental station. If you rent digital scales, you should invest in a calibration weight and check them before and after each rental for accuracy.

Examples of Ethical Situations

A variety of situations can occur that require a lactation consultant to consider possible ethical consequences of an action or practice. A few are presented here as examples (Barger, 1998). Questions appear at the end of each scenario to identify relevant issues and serve as a catalyst for you to consider how you would respond in similar circumstances.

Situation One

A pediatrician refers Tracy and her son Michael to you. Michael is six weeks old and is about five ounces over birth weight. As you are taking a history and doing a breastfeeding assessment, Tracy tells you that she is feeding Michael on a three-hour schedule during the day. He sleeps about eight hours at night and breastfeeds about six times in a 24-hour period. You suggest that she feed Michael more often and wake him at night to increase his weight and Tracy's milk production. You talk with her about watching for hunger cues and trying to get more feedings in each day.

Tracy tells you it is important that Michael stay on their schedule. She explains that she took a parenting class at her church that discourages the use of cue-related feedings. The program taught her that babies should sleep through the night at 6 to 8 weeks of age, and she is pleased that Michael is doing so. In addition, she learned that to increase the numbers of feedings would cause Michael's metabolism to "go into chaos." You probe a bit further and learn that for the first 4 or 5 weeks, Michael would cry for up to 40 minutes at a time. Tracy learned from the program that babies will not eat well if mothers feed them more frequently than every 3 hours. Therefore, she left Michael in his crib to "cry it out." She tells you, "It is important for the baby to learn that the parents are in control."

You share your concerns about Michael's weight and suggest that Tracy use a supplemental feeding device. You recommend that she express her milk between feedings to increase milk production. Tracy rejects both suggestions. She does agree to supplement Michael after each feeding until his weight improves.

Issues to Consider:

◆ How much do you "push" to salvage breastfeeding for this mother and baby?

◆ What will you say to her about her parenting methods?

◆ What follow-up will you provide?

◆ What information will you provide to her physician?

Situation Two

You have started lecturing about breastfeeding in several areas of your state. A hospital in a city about four hours from you has invited you to present a one-day conference. During the process of planning your presentation, you learn that a major manufacturer of infant formula is one of the conference sponsors. Although there is nothing that specifically forbids you from taking money from the formula industry, you feel uncomfortable speaking at the conference. As you discuss it with one of your colleagues, she says to you, "You ought to go ahead with it. It would be better that you give the presentation rather than a formula representative. At least that way you will know the attendees receive appropriate information."

Issues to Consider:

◆ If you speak at the conference, what underlying message does it send?

◆ Do the ends justify the means? You know you would give good information, but at what cost to your ethics?

◆ How can you participate in the conference without taking formula money and without forgoing compensation?

Situation Three

You are a newly certified IBCLC working in your community hospital. On several occasions, mothers have told you that their pediatrician gave them information about breastfeeding that is terribly outdated. You have witnessed this same prominent physician speak sarcastically with staff who do not agree with him. Most pediatricians in your community are supportive of breastfeeding and have been receptive to learning more about appropriate breastfeeding care. You are working with a mother who has this pediatrician for her baby. How can you help her within the context of her relationship with her pediatrician?

Issues to Consider:

◆ If you speak with the pediatrician, what approach will you take?

◆ How will you correct the misinformation mothers receive?

◆ If the pediatrician continues to give misinformation, what actions can you take without jeopardizing your new job?

▶ DEVELOPING RESOURCES

You are not alone in your efforts to promote, protect, and support breastfeeding. The field of lactation consulting has grown tremendously since the creation of ILCA and IBLCE in 1985. By 2004, there were over 15,000 lactation consultants certified as IBCLCs worldwide. Opportunities abound for networking with others for advice on a particular issue. It is important to make sure you know experienced IBCLCs with whom you can network. With the growth of the lactation consulting profession, there are increasing numbers of knowledgeable and skilled IBCLCs who may serve as a mentor for you until you feel competent and confident in your abilities. Even after becoming a qualified IBCLC, you will continue to benefit from mentoring and networking with other experienced clinicians.

Continuing Education

Becoming a member of ILCA will bring you in contact with over 4000 lactation professionals worldwide. You will have access to a Members Only side of the ILCA Web site that provides a wealth of resources. With your membership, you will receive the *Journal of Human Lactation* and the association's online newsletter. These periodicals share new research and practical tips, case studies, and innovative approaches. Appendix A lists other professional newsletters and journals.

Professional conferences provide networking opportunities for lactation professionals and other breastfeeding advocates. The ILCA Web site contains discussion boards that enable members to network on a variety of topics. Lactnet, a listserve on the Internet designed for lactation professionals, provides breastfeeding information and the opportunity to ask questions of a large number of people at one time. Many Lactnet members share unusual cases and their resolution. See Appendix A for instructions on how to subscribe to Lactnet. Once subscribed, you will immediately begin receiving up-to-date posts from colleagues around the globe.

Professional Referral Sources

You frequently will need to seek assistance during your career in the lactation profession. There may be an unusual breastfeeding situation, a medical question, or some other circumstance that you do not believe you can address adequately with your existing information. In order to offer women the services and support that will aid them in breastfeeding, you will need to develop resources to help you deliver complete and correct information. Develop contacts with people in areas that will enhance your consulting. Establish an advisory relationship so that you may call on them when questions arise. Hospitals, physicians, dietitians, pharmacies, medical libraries, service organizations, and colleges can be valuable resources for you.

It is important to keep these resources in mind and to cultivate contacts with others in related fields so that mothers in your care will have access to the information and services they need. Keep a list of referral resources such as physical therapists, occupational therapists, speech and language therapists, physicians and dentists who will clip a frenulum, craniosacral therapists, acupuncturists, chiropractors, herbalists, and other specialists. In addition to establishing personal resources, you need to develop a reference library with current breastfeeding texts and periodicals. You can also keep a lending library or an updated list of books and other materials that may be of interest to parents.

▶ PROMOTING YOUR SERVICES

Conducting a needs assessment will help you determine the market for IBCLCs in your community. Learn how many already work in local hospitals, physician's offices, and clinics. Determine how many are in private practice within comfortable driving distance for parents in your community. After you have settled on the best potential settings for employment, decide which services you can offer that will fill the needs of your target market. Establish baseline data on breastfeeding statistics in order to demonstrate a need for your services. Record how many mothers initiate breastfeeding and how long they continue. Identify current policies, practices, and attitudes.

Determine the breastfeeding resources that are currently available for parents and caregivers and fill the gap.

Referral System

Maintaining a referral system is integral to the quality of your assistance to breastfeeding women. Women who receive breastfeeding education and support prenatally are more likely to achieve their goals. Therefore, if you work in a hospital setting, you want to ensure that mothers who give birth in your hospital will receive this exposure before they deliver. IBCLCs in private practice will depend on referrals for their entire practice. Mothers need to know how to access your services, and all areas of your community need to be aware of your services as well. This includes hospitals, birthing centers, physicians, midwives, childbirth educators, breastfeeding support groups, community groups, pharmacies, providers of breastfeeding accessories, and others who encounter expectant or new mothers. Chapter 2 presents referral suggestions specific to individual practice settings.

Community Awareness

Regardless of your work setting, you want your community to be aware of your services. If you are in private practice, you can develop an attractive logo that identifies you easily to prospective clients and referral sources. Use the logo on printed brochures, business cards, letterhead, postcards, and other materials that promote your services. A consistent, professional look to all printed material will speak well for you. A professional appearance and demeanor will also have a great impact on the impressions you make.

You can obtain free exposure in the community in a variety of ways. Consider providing outreach programs to educate the public about breastfeeding. You can offer to present breastfeeding information to high school classes as part of their health curriculum. Newspapers will often print an article about members of the community who have recently achieved special honors. Participating in health fairs, trade shows, and charities will further advertise your services. World Breastfeeding Week offers an ideal time for you to sponsor a breastfeeding program in your community. A local radio or television station may be willing to conduct an interview.

Offering to speak in the community will help you develop a reputation as an authority on breastfeeding. You can produce promotional items such as pens, note pads, magnets, and buttons that advertise your services. Providing inservice education to childbirth educators and other health professionals in your area will open doors for later referrals and relationships. Offer professional discounts or in-kind services to groups such as your local breastfeeding coalition, ILCA affiliate, or support group.

Something as simple as bringing refreshments or breast-feeding literature when you visit other healthcare professionals may make a personal impression that will bring you to their mind later.

Résumé or Curriculum Vitae

A well-written résumé or curriculum vitae (referred to as a CV) will help you make a professional impression to a potential employer. Employment agencies and computer software programs can help you develop this document. You can begin by taking a personal inventory of your background, work experience, and strengths. There are distinct differences between a résumé and curriculum vitae. Your choice will depend on what you have learned about the facility and which format you feel will pique their interest. The purpose of both documents is to highlight your talents. Include a cover letter that states the kind of position you are seeking and why you are applying to the particular facility. Follow up with a telephone call a short time later to request an interview.

Résumé

A résumé is a brief, one-page, promotional piece that identifies a specific job or interest. Personal data to include are name, address, telephone number, fax number, and e-mail address. Begin with a brief statement of your objective or career goal and any skills and abilities that may be useful in the position you are seeking. This may include such things as years of IBCLC experience, knowledge of foreign languages, public speaking abilities, artistic talents, and computer capabilities. Follow this with a history of your education, employment, formal education, and other professional training. List dates of graduation, degrees or certificates received, major and minor subjects, and any scholarships or honors. You can organize your work history either by job or by function.

Work History by Job

List each job separately, even if you held more than one position at the same facility. List dates of employment, name and address of the employer, nature of the business, the position that you held, specific job duties, any special assignments or use of special equipment, your scope of responsibility (e.g., how many people you supervised, the degree of supervision you received), and noteworthy accomplishments (backed up by concrete facts and figures).

Work History by Function

List functions, fields of specialization, and types of work you performed related to your present employment objectives. Describe briefly the work you have done in each of these fields, without breaking it down by jobs.

You could also list volunteer activities related to your present objectives, such as breastfeeding counseling.

References

In this day of résumé inflation and fraud, it is imperative that you represent your experience and skills honestly. References should be former employers or mentors who have worked with you in clinical or internship settings, and have seen your skills and mother-baby interaction firsthand. Four or five references are usually appropriate. Many people, in order to keep the résumé short, state "References provided upon request" and take the reference sheet with them to give the prospective employer at the face-to-face interview.

Curriculum Vitae

A CV is an extensive, scholarly piece that reflects all of your professional activity. It will begin with your name, address, telephone number, fax number, and e-mail address. List your educational background, professional practice, academic appointments, memberships to professional associations, and any publications or articles you have written. Indicate outside professional interests and related community and consultant activities. Include all professional presentations and licensure. If your CV has several pages, you can prepare a one-page abbreviated version with a note at the bottom that the complete CV is available on request. Conference planners often request a CV from potential speakers.

Job Description or Proposal

In addition to a complete CV, you can approach a facility with a formal job proposal. A prospective employer may be receptive if you request a position on a trial basis for a period of six months. During that time, you can train staff, establish breastfeeding protocols, and collect data to justify the continuation of your position. Below is a list of possible elements to include in a job description or a proposal for a position as an IBCLC. Items are categorized in terms of the type of activity and expertise required. Not all will apply to a particular position. Determine what the specific needs are of the facility so that you can personalize your proposal based on their needs. Try to identify the appropriate person to receive the proposal, which is often the person in charge of maternity services.

Cover Letter or Introductory Remarks

Begin with rationale for establishing an IBCLC position. Give a brief description of your role in the mother's and infant's healthcare team, and describe how you see yourself functioning in the facility. Focus on the benefits to the hospital of having an IBCLC on staff. You might also indicate the cost-benefit issues to the hospital for your services.

Objectives

Demonstrate that the establishment of an IBCLC position will enhance the facility's reputation in the community as a provider of healthcare to mothers and babies. Point out that the increased number of mothers who will choose to deliver there because of the facility's reputation will fund your position. Cite that with an IBCLC on staff the facility will:

◆ Provide a positive breastfeeding experience for both the mother and baby.

◆ Promote bonding between the mother and her baby.

◆ Promote healthier babies and mothers.

◆ Provide consistent breastfeeding teaching and support.

◆ Increase the incidence of mothers choosing to breastfeed.

◆ Increase the incidence of mothers continuing to breastfeed at six months.

◆ Decrease the incidence of unresolved breastfeeding problems.

Teaching Services

Indicate the educational programs you can provide to both parents and staff:

◆ Teach prenatal infant feeding classes.

◆ Teach in-hospital breastfeeding classes.

◆ Teach postpartum classes.

◆ Provide inservice education for staff.

◆ Assist with orientation of staff.

◆ Maintain a resource center for patient and staff materials.

◆ Conduct bedside teaching of staff through a mentorship or preceptor program.

Services to Mothers and Infants

Identify the services you can offer to mothers:

◆ Individual consultation during the hospital stay, which may include:

  ◆ Conduct daily rounds with breastfeeding mothers.

  ◆ Give anticipatory guidance to mothers.

  ◆ Perform a breastfeeding assessment.

  ◆ Revisit mothers who are experiencing problems.

◆ Develop a plan of care with the mother.

◆ Provide problem-solving advice and support.

◆ Document teaching and progress on patient charts.

◆ Coordinate or provide home follow-up through telephone calls, postcards, or visits.

◆ Provide a 24-hour hotline where mothers can call and have their questions answered immediately, or a 24-hour warm line where mothers leave a message on an answering machine or voice mail and the call is returned later.

◆ Refer mothers to a support group and other community resources.

◆ Coordinate counseling and support of mothers who wish to provide their milk for a high-risk infant.

◆ Coordinate dispensing of breastfeeding devices.

◆ Provide an outpatient lactation clinic for weighing infants and discussing problems.

Working with Staff

Indicate the manner in which you will work with staff:

◆ Initiate case conferences and confer with staff on patient needs.

◆ Serve as a resource for staff, physicians, and support group counselors.

◆ Consult with the mother's and baby's primary care providers.

◆ Discuss appropriate referrals with primary care providers.

◆ Provide on-call service for consultations with staff.

◆ Participate as a team member with staff and physicians to provide comprehensive care.

◆ Coordinate or participate in a breastfeeding committee.

Writing, Reviewing, and Revising Printed Materials

A lactation consultant needs the writing and editing skills necessary for developing and revising printed materials and protocols. Indicate the materials you can provide:

◆ Standards of care that support breastfeeding.

◆ Breastfeeding policies.

◆ Breastfeeding care plans.

◆ A charting system for documentation, teaching, and progress notes.

◆ Patient literature.

- Monthly breastfeeding newsletter for staff.
- Statistics to assess the effectiveness of your services.

Professional Requirements

Learn the preferences in the facility regarding credentials as well as experience that would be required for an IBCLC to practice there. Some facilities may require a degree in another area of healthcare. Be sure to include any education and experience that will complement the position you are seeking. This serves the purpose of a conventional résumé by identifying skills and abilities that will make you attractive for the position you are seeking. Stress the importance of hiring a board-certified lactation consultant as opposed to someone without the IBCLC credential. Your list may include:

- IBCLC-certified through the International Board of Lactation Consultant Examiners.
- Member of the International Lactation Consultant Association.
- Graduate from a lactation management course (name the course).
- Graduate from a school of nursing or other facility (name the school).
- Current licensure in the state in a related field.
- College degree(s).
- Skills, knowledge, and attitude to promote breast-feeding.
- Communication skills for interactions with patients, families, and colleagues.
- Knowledge of cultural, psychological, psychosocial, nutritional, and pharmacological aspects of breast-feeding.
- Understanding of current breastfeeding practices and research findings.
- Participation in continuing education through seminars, workshops, networking, and relevant professional journals.
- Support for the facility's philosophy and policies.

Fee for Services

The reality in any business is that the bottom line is profit. This is no different in healthcare. You have identified in previous sections of the job proposal how your services will enhance the facility's delivery of care. You now need to demonstrate how the facility can cover the cost of your services. Better yet, you can show how your services will actually generate new revenue for the facility. One way to do this is to indicate areas in which the facility can charge a fee for your services. Some insurance companies will reimburse for lactation services. Check the status of the insurance carriers for women in your community and in the facility. Fee-for-service offerings may include:

- In-hospital assistance.
- Prenatal classes.
- Home or outpatient follow-up (including telephone counseling with an unlimited 24-hour hotline, an office visit, or a home visit).
- Outpatient consultation services.

Equipment and Other Resources

The facility will want to know the additional expenses your position will require. Therefore, in your proposal, indicate the initial investment that will be required in terms of equipment and other resources. The list may include:

- Office space.
- Desk and chair.
- File cabinets.
- Computer and printer.
- Telephone and fax machine.
- Answering machine or voice mail.
- Internet access.
- Beeper.
- Comfortable cushioned armchair or sofa.
- Electric breast pumps and other breastfeeding devices.
- Infant scale.
- Secretarial support.
- Funds for reference books and continuing education.
- Dictation services.

▶ STAFF EDUCATION

An important goal for lactation professionals is to achieve a continuum of supportive breastfeeding care for mothers and babies. If you are the breastfeeding expert in your facility and everyone saves all the breastfeeding problems for you to handle, then you are not doing your job! You need to train others to help you and to carry through with consistent care. By empowering others, you will be helping yourself. It will give you the ability to remain creative and energized, as well as minimize the number of problems mothers experience.

Teaching Breastfeeding Care

In order for breastfeeding mothers to receive the best possible healthcare and advice, their providers must be knowledgeable in lactation and have the necessary skills to facilitate learning. A knowledge deficit regarding breastfeeding exists in all areas of healthcare (Hellings, 2004; Taveras, 2004; Beal, 2003; Power, 2003). Professional education often includes little or no meaningful breastfeeding education. When health practitioners must refer routine situations to an IBCLC for help, the mothers, infants, and staff can lose valuable time. The longer a mother has a problem, the longer it takes to resolve it.

You can provide other members of the healthcare team with necessary knowledge through group inservice programs and individual clinical mentoring. If a staff member expresses concern regarding a specific mother and baby, you can accompany that staff member to the mother's room and involve the staff member in the consultation (Figure 26.2). Scheduled inservices need to meet the needs of both new and experienced staff. You might consider holding occasional seminars with more involved information and short breastfeeding updates at unit meetings or on bulletin boards. You can also participate in the orientation of new staff members (Stokamer, 1993).

Creating Enthusiasm Among Staff

Staff education can take many forms. You could launch a breastfeeding initiative with a motivational program for the staff. A workshop or conference will energize people and generate enthusiasm for learning more about

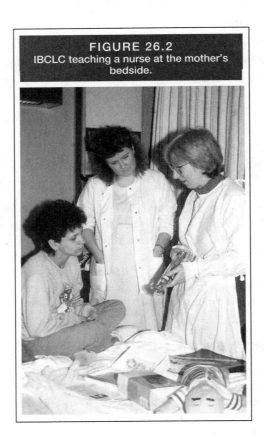

FIGURE 26.2
IBCLC teaching a nurse at the mother's bedside.

breastfeeding. A breastfeeding bulletin board with monthly updates can include highlights of particular staff members who have done something noteworthy related to breastfeeding. Post breastfeeding messages where people are likely to read them, such as in the locker room or on the back of the stall door in the restroom. When staff attends a breastfeeding program, you can show your appreciation with a small token such as a badge that reads, "Ask me about breastfeeding." In addition to serving as a token of thanks, it identifies the staff member to mothers and other staff as someone who can help them with their breastfeeding questions.

You can begin a class with a needs assessment or a quiz to whet their appetites. Let them know that the purpose is to receive their input in order to design a program that will meet their needs. It is important that time be planned for questions and comments. Disgruntled members may need to voice negative feelings or raise contentious issues. Many times these people can become your most supportive allies when they know you have heard them and respect their feelings and concerns.

A receptive learning climate enhances your effectiveness in teaching other staff members about breastfeeding care. Chapter 4 discussed the use of humor as a communication tool. In many ways, humor is simply allowing your humanness to come through. Be willing to make mistakes in front of colleagues. You are a role model to them. Let them see that in the real world we all make mistakes, and show them how we recover from our mistakes. Weave humor into your teaching. Humor is graphic and creates mental images that help the learner remember better and longer. Modeling the use of humor is a first step to teaching staff how to use humor themselves as a communication tool with mothers. Providing opportunities to role-play situations in the classroom helps relieve anxiety and makes the anticipated situation less awkward in reality.

▶ MATURING THROUGH EXPERIENCE

At times, lactation consulting may present discouraging experiences. There will be times when something unfavorable happens that you cannot correct. At these times it is helpful to talk with a colleague to express your frustrations or doubts. The following sections describe some circumstances that may occur during your career.

Lack of Compliance

You will invariably encounter mothers who do not follow through on your advice. Some of these outcomes may result in what you consider inappropriate or ill-advised action by the mother. A mother may wean unexpectedly or earlier than you would advise. Another may supplement with formula or introduce solid foods at an early age. It is discouraging when a mother fails to follow your advice. It is equally frustrating to see breastfeeding deteriorate because a mother has chosen not to follow suggestions and advice that were in her baby's best interest. Keep in mind that what a mother does with your advice is her responsibility, as are the consequences of her actions. As long as you have given the appropriate support and information, you have fulfilled your obligation to the mother. You must then step back and respect her choice.

Medical Complications

It is discouraging for both you and the mother when a mother is unable to breastfeed for medical reasons. When a highly motivated and determined mother is unable to breastfeed, you may view it as failure on your part. Other times, more tragic events may leave you feeling helpless, such as a baby dying or a mother having had radical breast surgery that prevented breastfeeding. These tragedies can affect you deeply because you have learned to cultivate warmth and caring, and you may find it difficult to remove yourself emotionally from the situation. You may need to work through the grief process just as the mother does.

External Interference

Some discouraging situations may involve people other than the mother in your care. Perhaps her partner is unsupportive and resents your involvement. A member of the medical community may be unsupportive of your efforts or may consistently give incorrect breastfeeding information. These situations can make it difficult to provide necessary help and advice to a mother. Yet at the same time, they offer challenges. You can educate the partner or caregiver and try to determine the cause of the misinformation or lack of support. You can be open and frank with the mother about her partner's feelings and arrange follow-up contacts at times when he is not at home. You can give literature to the mother to share with her caregiver and encourage her to also share the positive aspects of her breastfeeding with her caregiver. You can suggest she seek another caregiver's opinion.

Professional Burnout

Working in a caring profession such as the medical field carries a risk of stress and burnout. Burnout may occur any time that you become overly involved in your work. Although almost everyone feels burned out to some degree at times, idealists who have high standards and believe that they must do all the work themselves tend to burn out more quickly in their efforts to achieve perfection. When this happens, there is a lack of enthusiasm to perform tasks. Accompanying this may be a low tolerance level and a loss of creativity and openness to change.

Recognize the Signs of Emotional Burnout

When burnout occurs, caregivers may distance themselves from the patient. By releasing your feelings and tension, you can return to the mother and give compassionate care. Case conferences, similar to those used by social workers, will help IBCLCs learn and grow. Sharing concerns with colleagues will help you recognize if you are too emotionally or unprofessionally involved with a client. Signs of emotional burnout include:

- Tunnel vision
- Loss of coping skills
- Lack of focus and concentration
- Inability to manage time
- Irrational behavior; a feeling of being on an "emotional roller coaster"
- Irritation
- Avoiding obligations and other avoidance behaviors
- Feeling that life is out of control
- Unexplained physical pain
- Physiological reactions such as fatigue, insomnia, depression, or anxiety attack

Understand the Cause of Burnout

In order to progress past emotional burnout, you first need to recognize that the problem is with your job and not with you. Emotional burnout can occur when you fail to achieve a balance. It is a response to unrelieved stress. Lactation professionals and others who care for breastfeeding mothers are often available to clients 24 hours a day. The nurturing nature of the lactation profession impels many caregivers to provide constant access to mothers whenever a concern or problem arises. One practitioner described her burnout as "compassion fatigue syndrome." When we give continually to our clients and fail to achieve a balance between professional responsibilities and personal needs, we are in danger of professional burnout.

Accept your limitations, and acknowledge that this particular situation is too much for you to handle at the time. It is often difficult for us to admit to our limitations. You need to establish personal boundaries. Trying to be everything for everyone is unrealistic and impractical. This makes it especially important that you empower others to give breastfeeding mothers the help they need. Trained people can certainly help with the first levels of care, and this will help minimize the types of problems that cause stress.

Learn how to take a short time-out. Visualization and slow, deep breathing will help you relax and reclaim your strength and perspective. Physical exercise or a massage can also help rejuvenate you. Your ability to maintain perspective and find humor in situations will be especially important during times of stress.

Make Time for Yourself and Your Family

Women, and especially mothers, feel torn by all the demands on their time. They can spend so much effort trying to please everyone else that there is little or no time or energy left for their own needs. You need to learn how to balance all that you do. Determine what is important, and then prioritize your list. When you attempt to do too many things, you cannot give your best to what is most important. Learn to delegate responsibilities so that you can put your valuable time and energy into the most important functions. Train others on the staff to take calls and answer basic breastfeeding questions. This gives ownership to others and enables everyone to focus on priorities. When you multiply yourself by delegating and training staff, you will recognize that you do not have to shoulder the responsibility alone.

If you are in private practice, develop a referral list of two or three other private practice IBCLCs whose abilities you respect. When you feel overwhelmed, ask one of them to take your referrals. You can record a message on your answering machine letting callers know you are not available and refer them to your colleague.

Recapturing some personal time to enjoy your family and friends will help you overcome burnout. Take the time to cultivate and nurture relationships with the important people in your life. You also need time for the most important person in your life—you! Plan special time to relax, pamper yourself, and enjoy activities that your busy schedule has not allowed. You might spend the entire time reading a favorite book, knitting, or watching a movie. The goal is to relax and rejuvenate yourself. Do something unrelated to healthcare, like rollerblading or taking an art class. This small break can clear your thinking when you return to work. You will then be able to give your best to others.

You cannot give the best of yourself when you feel stressed and stretched to the limit. Learn to say no when others ask more of you than you can give. Use an answering machine to screen telephone calls and take messages at times when you feel unprepared to answer the telephone. Limit the commitments you place on your time. Moreover, keep your sense of humor! People with a sense of humor are healthier, happier people.

Renew Enthusiasm

Try to be aware of situations that make you feel uncomfortable and why. Learn how to work out these kinds of problems by discussing them with a colleague. Networking at conferences and affiliated meetings is a perfect opportunity for getting rejuvenated in the lactation field. Spending time with others in similar situations and learning new techniques can help breathe new life into a job that is wearing you down. You can expand your learning further by reading journals and technical books. You can increase networking by serving on committees and becoming active in your professional association.

If lack of cooperation and support from others creates stress, you may need to use a new approach or find other avenues for garnering their support. If you enjoy community outreach, you could speak to clinics, high school health classes, and local organizations. If you enjoy writing, you could write a newsletter or weekly column on breastfeeding for your local newspaper. If you enjoy teaching, you can teach lay counselors in the community or mentor new lactation consultant interns. You can work at the local, state, national, or global level in breastfeeding promotion efforts. When you redefine your goals and relate them to your actions in this manner, you will be on your way toward developing a satisfying new role for yourself.

Avoiding Pitfalls in Counseling

Every mother is unique, with her own personality and personal limitations. Approaching each mother with a focus on her individual needs will ensure that you help her reach her goals. Being aware of your own potential pitfalls will help you deliver effective care.

Not Accepting Your Limitations

Acknowledge to a mother when you do not have all the answers and need to get help from outside sources. Realize that your influence on a mother's behavior is limited. Encourage her to determine her own solutions. Recognize when a mother needs referral to another caregiver, and do not attempt to handle a situation that is beyond your expertise.

Getting Overly Involved

If a mother seems to rely on you too much, encourage her to take charge of her own decisions. Build her confidence, and offer her information with minimal guidance. When problems are serious and outside the realm of breastfeeding, encourage her to contact her physician, mental health professional, religious advisor, or other sources of advice and support. You are not the mother's professional guidance counselor. Help her understand that your services are restricted to breastfeeding and related topics.

If you are a licensed counselor or psychologist, have been counseling a mother in breastfeeding, and the nature of the contact changes, you need to renegotiate your relationship formally. It is not a good practice to counsel family members or close friends. Because of the emotional ties, you may have very strong emotions about the choices the parents make. If breastfeeding goes well, the mother may become overly dependent on you and fail to mature in her mothering experience as quickly as she otherwise might. If breastfeeding does not go well regardless of the reason, she may blame you, thus harming your relationship. It is usually wise to refer family members or friends to another IBCLC and maintain your present role as a loving family member or friend. "A prophet is without honor in her own country" is often true in any profession when it comes to family or friends.

Discussing Your Breastfeeding

If a mother asks how long you breastfed, it is important to maintain a professional relationship with her. It is doubtful that she really wants to know about your breastfeeding experience. More likely, she has a question about her own breastfeeding. Capitalizing on your counseling skills will help you determine the real purpose of the question. You might say, for example, "You're wondering how long to breastfeed your baby." Discussing aspects of your life diminishes the mother's experience. Keep the discussion focused on her. At times, it may be appropriate to give a short answer and immediately return the focus to her, without elaborating on your personal experience.

Making Value Judgments

At times, it may be challenging to remain objective and avoid conveying value judgments to mothers. Remember that your role with mothers is to empower them as informed consumers. You are responsible for giving correct and appropriate information and advice. What the mother does with that advice is her choice and her responsibility. Encourage mothers to make decisions that fit into their lifestyle, and then support their choices. Always leave mothers with a graceful exit if they are not comfortable with your suggestions. Clearly state, "Only *you* know what you and your family can deal with at this time"—and mean it!

Interrupting

Becoming an effective listener and using counseling skills will draw out the mother and engage her in conversation. Resist the urge to interject comments before the mother finishes her train of thought. Do not change the subject until you are sure the mother has explored it sufficiently. This pitfall is common in many social and professional interactions. Avoiding it will often require practice and careful attention to your communication skills. The BestStart 3-Step Counseling Strategy provides an easy tool to remember: (1) ask open-ended questions, (2) reflect feelings, and (3) educate.

Overwhelming the Mother

Avoid falling into the trap of overwhelming mothers with too much advice and information. Remember to restrict the amount of information you give to a mother at any one time. As a rule, offer only three suggestions at a time. As in the art world, less is more! You can always follow up a contact with a telephone call or e-mail. Clearly explain to the mother that there are more options and if this suggestion does not work, she can call you for more help.

Being Too Solution-Oriented

Being in a helping role within the health profession, there is always the risk of focusing too much on solutions at the expense of other issues in the mother's life. This is especially true in a hospital, where staff time is limited. You can avoid this by listening carefully for feelings and concerns the mother expresses. Gather impressions from what she is *not* saying and read her body language. Allow the mother time to define her situation and work out solutions. Enter into problem solving only after you have gathered sufficient information and impressions. The entire consultation should follow the mother's and baby's pace, not yours.

Failing to Provide Follow-up

Routine follow-up with clients will indicate whether your advice has been helpful. Always follow through to learn if the situation has improved and to give the mother support. Encourage her to contact you if she needs further help. If there are times when you will not be available, make sure to arrange for someone to receive your calls. This is especially important if you will be away for an extended period of time. Refer the mother to community resources when it is apparent that you cannot resolve her problem while she is in your care. Make it a practice to consider a consultation unfinished until appropriate follow-up is arranged.

▶ SUMMARY

The IBCLC, an integral member of the mother's healthcare team, must continually grow and thrive in the profession. Appropriate education and clinical experience will prepare you to enter the profession. Understanding the stages of role acquisition will help you anticipate each new challenge. Availing yourself of the networking and support from colleagues and your professional association will enhance your effectiveness with mothers and babies. Becoming certified and adhering to the profession's standards of practice and ethics will ensure that you provide appropriate care. Finally, you will give your best effort to mothers when you recognize your limitations and seek assistance when appropriate.

▶ ## CHAPTER 26—AT A GLANCE

Applying what you learned—

Your growth as a lactation professional:

◆ Recognize your growth through the stages of role acquisition.

◆ Complete a lactation management course.

◆ Acquire clinical experience with a mentor, using the IBLCE clinical competencies.

◆ Become IBCLC certified.

◆ Obtain liability insurance.

◆ Follow the code of ethics and standards of practice for the profession.

◆ Network with other lactation professionals to mature in your own role.

◆ Attend conferences and read professional journals to learn new clinical practice and research.

◆ Join the International Lactation Consultant Association and use its resources.

Your role with mothers:

◆ Recognize what constitutes a client relationship and provide appropriate care.

◆ Obtain informed consent and retain records appropriately.

◆ Build positive relationships with the mothers in your care.

◆ Never guarantee results or create unrealistic expectations for mothers.

◆ Empower parents to make their own decisions, and accept their choices.

◆ Work within the parameters of the caregiver's advice as much as possible.

Establishing yourself in the profession:

◆ Develop resources and contacts in areas that will enhance your consulting.

◆ Determine the market for IBCLCs in your community.

◆ Provide prenatal breastfeeding education and support.

◆ Market your services through brochures, business cards, postcards, health fairs, and other community events.

◆ Offer to speak in the community to build recognition as an authority.

◆ Develop a résumé or curriculum vitae and a job proposal based on the needs of the facility where you wish to work.

◆ Teach breastfeeding care to all members of the healthcare team in order to provide consistency.

◆ Launch a breastfeeding initiative with a motivational program for the staff.

◆ Use creativity and humor to create a receptive learning climate.

◆ Learn how to deal with misinformation and lack of support.

◆ Achieve a balance between professional responsibilities and personal needs.

◆ Recognize signs of emotional burnout and learn how to minimize it.

◆ Find new challenges and goals to renew your enthusiasm.

◆ Accept your limitations and avoid becoming overly involved, discussing your own breastfeeding, making value judgments, interrupting, or overwhelming mothers.

◆ Use counseling skills to avoid being too solution-oriented.

◆ Provide follow-up to mothers.

▶ ## REFERENCES

Association of Women's Health, Obstetric and Neonatal Nursing (AWHONN). *Standards for the Nursing Care of Women and Newborns.* Washington, DC: AWHONN; 1991.

Barger J. *Acquiring the LC Role.* Lactation Management Course, BSC Center for Lactation Education. Chalfont, PA; 1998.

Beal A et al. Breastfeeding advice given to African American and white women by physicians and WIC counselors. *Public Health Rep* 118(4):368–376; 2003.

Bocar DL, Moore K. *Acquiring the Parental Role.* Lactation Consultant Series #16. New York: Avery Publishing Group; 1987.

Hellings P, Howe C. Breastfeeding knowledge and practice of pediatric nurse practitioners. *J Pediatr Health Care* 18(1): 8–14; 2004.

International Board of Lactation Consultant Examiners. *Clinical Competencies for IBCLC Practice.* Falls Church, VA: IBLCE; 2003.

International Board of Lactation Consultant Examiners. *The Code of Ethics: International Board Certified Lactation Consultants.* Falls Church, VA: IBLCE; 2004.

International Lactation Consultant Association (ILCA). *Standards of Practice for Lactation Consultants.* 2nd ed. Raleigh, NC: ILCA; 1999.

International Lactation Consultant Association (Walker M, ed.). *Core Curriculum for Lactation Consultant Practice.* Sudbury, MA: Jones and Bartlett; 2002.

Kutner L, Barger J. *Clinical Experience in Lactation: A Blueprint for Internship.* 2nd ed. Wheaton, IL: Lactation Education Consultants; 2002.

Kutner L. *Lactation Management Course.* Chalfont, PA: BSC Center for Lactation Education; 2001.

Power M et al. The effort to increase breast-feeding. Do obstetricians, in the forefront, need help? *J Reprod Med* 48(2):72–78; 2003.

Stokamer C. In-service breastfeeding program development: Needs assessment and planning. *J Hum Lact* 9:253–256; 1993.

Taveras E et al. Mothers' and clinicians' perspectives on breast-feeding counseling during routine preventive visits. *Pediatrics* 113(5):e405–411; 2004.

▶ **BIBLIOGRAPHY**

Bagwell J et al. Knowledge and attitudes toward breast-feeding: Differences among dietitians, nurses, and physicians working with WIC clients. *J Am Diet Assoc* 93:801–804; 1993.

Bocar DL. The lactation consultant: Part of the health care team, Clinical issues in perinatal and women's health nursing: Breastfeeding. *NAACOG* 3(4):731–737; 1992.

Freudenberger HJ. *Burnout: The High Cost of High Achievement.* New York: Bantam Books; 1980.

Hancock L et al. Breaking point. *Newsweek* 56–62; March 6, 1995.

Maslach C. *Burnout: The Cost of Caring.* Cambridge, MA: Malor Books; 2003.

Nelson DS. Humor in the pediatric emergency department: A 2–year retrospective. *Pediatrics* 89:6, 1089–1090; 1992.

Schaef AW. *The Addictive Organization: Why We Overwork, Cover Up, Pick Up the Pieces, Please the Boss, and Perpetuate Sick Organizations.* San Francisco, CA: Harper; 1990.

Schaef AW. *Meditations for Women Who Do Too Much.* San Francisco, CA: Harper; 1996.

Skovholt T. *The Resilient Practitioner: Burnout Prevention and Self-Care Strategies for Counselors, Therapists, Teachers, and Health Professionals.* Cranbury, NJ: Pearson Education—Allyn & Bacon; 2000.

CRITICAL READING AND REVIEW OF RESEARCH

Contributing Author: Sandra Breck

There are three kinds of truths: lies, damn lies, and statistics.
—*Attributed to Benjamin Disraeli by Mark Twain*

By studying this and other texts, you learn a lot of state-of-the-art information and many techniques to use in your practice as a lactation consultant. One more skill you need so that your practice remains current is the skill of critically reading scientific literature. This chapter provides background information on the processes of science used in scientific journal articles. A "how-to" section on the structure and critical reading of scientific articles is aimed at readers who have little previous experience. Two mock articles with commentary provide an opportunity to practice the techniques presented. Then you will be ready to tackle a real article and savor the satisfaction of knowing you are offering families the most carefully considered, evidence-based practice they can receive from a thoughtful lactation professional.

KEY TERMS

abstract
anchors
assumptions
average
bell curve
bias
blinded
case studies
case-control study
chi-square
Cohen's kappa
cohort
confidence intervals
confounding variables
control group
convenience
correlation
Cronbach's alpha
cross-sectional study
dependent variable
descriptive study
distribution and range

evidence-based practice
experiment
generalize
homogeneity
human subjects review
hypothesis
independent variable
instruments
internal validity
Likert scale
mean
meta-analysis
nonprobability
normal distribution
odds ratio
operationalize
outcome
output variables
oximeter
peer review
population
probability

prospective study
P-value
qualitative study
random assignment
randomized clinical trials
regression
relationship
reliability
research reports
retrospective study
review articles
sample

slope
speculation
spurious
statistically significant
subjects
theory
tools
true assumptions
T-test
validity
variables
variation

TYPES OF ARTICLES IN SCIENTIFIC JOURNALS

Scientific journals contain many types of articles. Commonly, the first prose to appear is an editorial, and some journals will print more than one. Editorials are very interesting and important to read. The editor is a prominent person in the field whose knowledge is broad and whose perspective on how the field is changing is often insightful. It is important to recognize that editorials are not studies and do not report on a particular study. Therefore, they cannot be subjected to the kind of critical analysis which this chapter addresses.

Case Studies

Case studies are a type of article published by many biomedical journals. They report on one or more **cases** of a problem, diagnosis, or treatment. A case study often appears because there is interest in a particular topic; however, because the diagnosis is unusual or treatment would be risky, it is unlikely that any **experiments** will take place. An example of this in lactation literature is a case study of mothers who need to use a medication not often prescribed during breastfeeding. Typically, the physician who treated the mother will describe her medical history and circumstances that led to the decision to try the medication. This will be followed by a description of the **outcome** for the mother and baby. Such a case study has a **sample** of one mother and one baby. The absence of comparison subjects or comparison treatment prevents critical analysis. It is still important information to retain because it may be the only information available on the use of a particular drug in breastfeeding. The information may help guide an especially difficult decision in clinical practice. However, because of its limited nature, a case study cannot form the basis for generalizing to most breastfeeding mothers and babies.

Meta-Analysis

Meta-analysis is a technique that combines the data and results of several studies in order to improve the strength of the conclusions. Although meta-analyses are important studies, the analysis approach discussed in this chapter does not apply to them. If you read a meta-analysis, you may want some help from a researcher or statistician before you implement the recommendations made in the study. Scientific journals still publish a lot of debate questioning the validity of the criteria for a good meta-analysis. Since this type of study relies heavily on statistical **assumptions**, clinicians often need help in judging their quality. Often such articles contain the words "meta-analysis" in their titles or abstracts, so you should be able to identify them fairly easily.

Review Articles

Review articles are written by one or more experts in the field who summarize and often critique the best and worst studies published on a topic. They differ from a meta-analysis in that they do not combine the data and results as a meta-analysis does. The opinions of the experts clearly play a role in the selection and the critical analysis of the articles to review. Little or no original data appears in a **review** article. Therefore, this chapter does not cover critical reading of this type of article.

If you wish to learn about an area of clinical research that is new to you, reading a review article can be very productive. You will discover some of the most recent information, some of the important scientists in the field, and some of the current controversies. Most of these articles will contain the word "review" in the title or abstract. If you want to find a review article, you can use the word "review" in your database search or in your request to the librarian.

Clinical Practice

Clinical practice articles often appear in journals for applied sciences such as nursing, dietetics, physical therapy, and medicine. Authors with experience in a particular

diagnosis, problem, deficit, or preventive technique write these articles to share their accumulated wisdom with other clinicians. The *Journal of Human Lactation*, for example, usually has several of these articles in each issue, offering valuable insights from one lactation consultant to another.

Because such articles do not study a problem scientifically, there are usually no presentations of data in graphs, tables, or figures. There also are no hypotheses or research questions. There may be some summary information about how, for example, mothers who followed Protocol X coped with Problem Y. However, there is no comparison group or an attempt to show that Protocol X is better than some other protocol. Although these articles are helpful, there is no substantive test of the authors' ideas. Therefore, they do not constitute the same quality of evidence for changing care practices as research does.

Research

Research articles put a long-held belief or new idea to a scientific test. Researchers subject themselves and their work to the processes of scientific investigation and to the scrutiny of their peers. They take the risk that their colleagues may find their work wanting. Therefore, as lactation consultants, we must approach the work of our colleagues respectfully. Each article deserves careful attention, both for the growth of our human understanding about lactation and for the benefit of the families in our care. Research articles follow the basic structure described in the following sections.

▶ STRUCTURE OF A SCIENTIFIC ARTICLE

Most scientific articles follow a format that provides a maximum amount of information in a limited amount of journal space. You will learn to appreciate well-written journal articles that condense information effectively. You will come away knowing exactly what the researchers did and why. They will have explained what they wish they had done differently and what they can justifiably conclude from their work. With practice, you will derive a clear sense of whether or not you agree with their conclusions, and you will be able to give clear reasons for your decisions. The growth of the science of lactation depends on this clear communication and on feedback to researchers.

Identifying Information

At the very top of many scientific journals, especially the European ones, is information identifying the journal using its standard abbreviated name. For example, *Acta*

Paediatr is the abbreviation for the journal *Acta Paediatrica*, a Scandinavian journal. Although the format for the name, volume number, pages, and year of publication varies from one journal to another, the format used by *Acta Paediatrica* illustrates the commonalities. All of this information is very handy to have at the top of the first page of the article. Those journals that do not put it at the top usually put it at the end of the abstract or somewhere else on the first page.

Example: *Acta Paediatr* 91(3):267–274; 2002.

◆ Acta Paediatr is the journal's abbreviation.

◆ 91 is the volume of the journal. Most journals publish one volume every year; however, some publish two volumes per year.

◆ 267–274 are the pages where the article is located. Most journals paginate continuously for one year. Volume 91 begins with page 1. If the first issue for that year ends at page 112, then the second issue begins at page 113, and so on. This continuous pagination is the reason many journals do not include the issue number in the identifying information; it is not necessary. However, some do include it, usually right after the volume. In the example, (3) is the volume number. Many journals publish an issue monthly. Some, like the *Journal of Human Lactation*, publish quarterly. Others, like *Lancet*, publish weekly. When you look up an article or request one from a library, it is important to copy the numbers from the reference list carefully.

◆ 2002 is the year of publication. In some journals, the year appears directly after the name of the journal.

Title of the Article

A well-chosen title will tell you a lot about an article. In some journals, the title explains the main finding and may be two sentences long. This helps busy readers choose which articles are highest priorities for their reading.

Authors

As you read research regularly, you will begin to recognize the research interests of particular lactation scientists who publish several articles on aspects of a limited scope of problems. Many times, you can acquire a good reference list on a single topic just by knowing a few researchers' names and noting the references in their articles. If you do not have a library where you can perform a computer search and do not have Internet access, you can build your own library of articles by authors' names. This will help when you are preparing a presentation or documenting the need for a practice change.

Abstract

Most journals ask authors to write a brief summary of (1) the reason they performed the study, (2) a description of the main subjects and methods, (3) the findings, and (4) the conclusion. This is the abstract. The abstract is often the best guide for deciding whether the article is worth reading. Although it will not answer all of your questions about the study, it will indicate what the authors thought was most important about their study. Abstracts vary in length and format and from one journal to another. Each journal sets its own requirements.

Introduction

The authors usually will spend a few paragraphs explaining why they chose to study the problem cited in the article. Many studies receive funding from a particular source. The authors will need to justify their acceptance of funding from the source, and that kind of justification is often contained in the introduction. You may also find clues to why the authors made certain decisions, such as why they only studied infants under six weeks old or collected data only during a particular season.

Review of the Literature

The purpose of this section of the article is to explain the issues surrounding the problem studied and review past research. Many funding sources will not support a study on a question that has received a great deal of past research. Therefore, the researcher must either identify an aspect of the problem that was not covered or demonstrate that past research has not clarified an important point. The literature review narrows down the subject of interest. It cites previous studies and their findings and shows how the current study is different or better. Authors sometimes will also explain weaknesses of past studies that their current study will correct.

In some journals (the *New England Journal of Medicine*, for example), the review of the literature is combined with the introduction. There may not even be a heading to identify this first part of the article. Nearly all articles contain a discussion of the research problem and of past studies before they begin to explain the current research. Literature reviews could be very long, and journals usually want them to be limited to the most relevant studies. If you read such a review and do not find a study cited there that you know is available, space considerations could be the reason.

Methods

The goal of the methods section is to tell the reader how the scientists **operationalized** the hypotheses and questions they studied. This section often begins with a description of subject recruitment. A member of the research team may have recruited subjects with certain criteria in mind (such as a previous preterm birth or giving birth to twins). Alternatively, subjects may have volunteered to be part of the study after hearing about it through a childbirth class or a newspaper advertisement. Sometimes the study relied on charts or other records and the subjects were unaware of the study. Usually, journals require that the authors state that the study obtained approval from a **human subjects review group** and that the subjects gave informed consent.

Instruments

The methods section describes the tools (**instruments**) used to measure the outcome under study. The instrument may be a written questionnaire or survey, an electronic balance scale, a chemical test, biopsy, or ultrasound. The authors often explain the methods in much detail, including the way in which different measurement instruments led to the results. For example, a milk sample collected early in a feeding will probably not have the same proportion of hindmilk as a sample from a breast that was drained more fully. One study takes early samples of milk and finds low vitamin A levels. The other study takes a sample after a complete feeding and finds higher vitamin A content. The difference might be due to the greater fat content in the complete feeding sample because vitamin A is fat-soluble.

Definition of Terms

The methods section defines the terms used in the study. When the authors include "breastfeeding dyads," they need to define what they mean by breastfeeding. Was it exclusive breastfeeding or partial breastfeeding? Did they ask mothers about the amount of supplemental formula the baby consumed, or did they actually measure it?

Statistical Methods

Statistical methods usually appear in the methods section. The authors will tell what methods they used and why they chose those particular ones. They may explain that they applied more than one statistical test to the data to strengthen the conclusions. This can be the least familiar part of the article to read. However, if you keep track of statistical terminology, you can develop a list of tests that you can look up in a text. Appendix A lists some texts that explain statistics without the use of calculus.

Results

The most important study results often appear in graphs, tables, or charts. The title of the table or graph will explain its topic. A key below the table explains the statistical significance of the results. Another helpful use of tables is to summarize information about the subjects. Tables often compare the experimental group to the control group on relevant characteristics.

Most authors will phrase their results very carefully. Because their article has been through **peer review**, they usually cannot claim findings that are not fairly well supported by the work they present. However, reading only the results or the abstract of a study can limit the reader's understanding of both the general problem and this particular study's approach to it. Many clinicians are tempted to read just the results because it seems like so much work to wade through the methods. Making the effort to understand the methods, though, may prevent clinicians from inappropriately adopting a recommended change in practice that does not really fit their clinical practice. The results of a study, in other words, need to be considered in the context of the rest of the article so that the findings can be judged based on the specifics of that study.

Discussion

The discussion is the easiest part of the article to read. The authors explain their reason for conducting the study, review more of the relevant literature, sum up their most important results, and suggest applications and further research. They also explain any weaknesses or problems with the project. Some of these explanations are in response to the comments of peer reviewers. These can be very helpful to a reader who is too unfamiliar with a particular area of research to think of alternative methods or interpretations. Although the earlier parts of the article are standard and prescribed by the journal itself, the discussion shows more of the authors' thinking and creativity. By the time a study is complete and ready for publication, the researchers have raised many questions in their minds, which they often explore in the discussion.

References, Literature, and Bibliography

In this final section, you will find the articles that the authors cite in their review of the literature. It will include any article cited in their methods section if they used a method described in a separate article. Many journals also permit the listing of additional articles related to the main topic.

CRITICAL READING OF A SCIENTIFIC ARTICLE

This discussion of critical reading will suggest an order in which to read the parts of an article. For beginners, it might be helpful to use this standard approach with the first several articles you read. Using this method will help you compare in a defined way the strengths and weaknesses of a study. This will improve your ability to determine why studies differ in their findings and clarify why you find a particular study unsatisfying. As you acquire more experience, you will create your own approach.

The process of critical reading does not lend itself to a "recipe" format. If it did, you and another reader would come to the same conclusions every time. By reading critically, your opinion will differ from other readers. If you reread an article at a later time, you may assess its strengths and weaknesses differently from the first time you read it. This is where the fun lies in critical reading, in the challenge of the puzzles the science investigates.

Some readers will be frustrated that they cannot clearly label a given study as "good" or "bad" and they will either reject it entirely or apply every finding. Most studies are a mixture of well-done science and things that merit improvement. Honest investigators admit this in the discussion section. These imperfections reveal the nature of science. Science is a process, not a body of facts written in a textbook. The evidence for or against "truth" accumulates over time, as the result of many imperfect studies. Clinicians who want to find the best science to use in their practice will find that they must keep reading because there is no final story. The process of following the development of our human understanding of a particular problem is fascinating and exciting once you are familiar with the **tools** scientists use to share their work with one another.

After the following discussion of critical reading, you will read two mock articles. Using the format described, you will stop to answer each question for yourself as you progress through each article. You will get more out of this process if you actually try to be critical at each stage rather than just reading the answers the text provides (of which you should also be critical!). Finally, you will review some general themes of critical reading. They are not the final words on the subject, as your own experiences are valuable, too. Expect to grow as a reader and as a clinician from your continuing efforts to consider the science of lactation carefully. The following sections describe the steps to critical reading.

Step 1: Look at the Title

A well-written title will indicate the subject of the article. From reading the title, determine what you expect the article to present. Sometimes, a title may lead your thinking along one track and the article turns out actually to be about a different facet than you were expecting. When you are aware of what you had expected, you can adjust more readily to what the authors really meant.

What Do You Know About the Topic?

Consider what you already know about the subject. Try to be specific in terms of what you know from other studies, textbooks, lectures, and experience. Do you know, for example, that sore nipples usually decrease by day five to ten postpartum? Do you know that in the Hispanic community, support for breastfeeding from the mother's mother may be more important than support from the baby's father? Have sources taught you that processing at high temperatures decreases immunoglobulins?

Taking time to review what you know will help you recognize discrepancies between your knowledge and what the authors claim later in the article. There may be legitimate reasons for those discrepancies. The scientists may have learned something new, for instance. Your reading will be more critical if you identify your own knowledge before you begin. Usually, this does not take very long. You may have chosen to read the article because of its importance for a problem that already interests you and that you have encountered several times in practice. What you already know about it will be easy to recall. With new subject matter, your knowledge will be limited, so that review does not take very long either!

How Would You Have Studied the Topic?

Consider how you would have studied the topic. If you are new to reading research, you may not have many ideas. Nevertheless, try this step anyway. If the topic were breastfeeding twins, where would you have gone to find subjects? Would you want any specific age of twins? Would gender of the babies be relevant? If a mother had other children, would that affect the findings? If the twins were born before 35 weeks, could that complicate the causes of problems you are studying? Do you need to find twins who were exclusively breastfed?

For the question you are asking, is it possible to do an experiment, or can you simply observe mothers and babies who have made their own choices? Will it be easy to come up with 20 or more twin sets that meet the criteria, or is the problem so unusual that the number of subjects will be small? Does the problem occur in one ethnic or cultural group more than in other groups? If so, do you want to do a comparative study or focus more on just one group? The more questions you ask yourself about how you would have done the study, the more readily you will grasp the significance of the choices the researchers made.

What Will You Expect to Find?

What should result from your brief review is a short list of aspects you expect to find in the study. For example, you may expect the study to include both first-time breastfeeders and experienced ones. On the other hand, you may expect it to include only preterm infants weighing over 2500 grams. If the result turns out to be different from your expectations, you will be very interested in the reasons. This may lead you to uncover a deficiency in the study.

Step 2: Read the Authors' Names

Noting author names is helpful, especially if you have read a previous work by the author or authors and found the work to contain a problem. You will want to determine whether the authors corrected the problem in this study. If the authors studied a related problem previously in a way that you thought was valuable, it will alert you to any changes in their methods or focus. If you have never read work by these authors, noting their names will give you a reference point for future reading.

Step 3: Read the Abstract

Reading the abstract will be the first point at which you confirm whether your assumptions about the study are correct. The abstract should briefly tell you the main characteristics of the subjects and methods. If a study's colicky babies are older than six months of age and you wanted information for six-week-old infants, you may stop reading and look for a different article. If the abstract proclaims an article to be about treating engorgement but does not mention the use of cabbage leaves, you will want to read the introduction and literature review to determine the reason for the omission.

The article may report a finding that contradicts what you know about the subject. Do not let this cause you to stop reading. Reading the abstract will alert you to the importance of specific aspects of the study that may justify the unexpected findings. The abstract may give you your first hint of the results the investigators believe warrant their recommendations. Knowing the direction in which they want to apply their findings prepares you to read for specific inclusions or exclusions in their work. For example, they may state in the abstract that they believe all new mothers should receive a video or DVD on positioning to take home with them. You may want to determine whether they included any low-income women in their study. They may suggest that all new mothers need a visit from a lactation consultant before discharge. You may question whether they measured the lactation knowledge of the nursing staff or whether they included any mothers who had nursed previous babies.

Reading the abstract will heighten your awareness of what the scientists believe is most important about their study. The abstract does not include much rationale for decisions made by the investigators. You must read the entire study for that. However, questioning while you read the abstract will help you get more out of the article itself.

Step 4: Study the Tables and Graphs

Make a quick overview of the tables and graphs to determine how many there are, their titles, and whether they are understandable. The most helpful tables have a title that tells the main idea, a source of the data (e.g., from a survey or from patient charts), and clear labels on each column and row, including the units of measurement (i.e., ml, kg, sec, and so on). Some will provide percentages of the total that each subgroup represents as well as statistical test results.

For each table or graph, ask yourself why the authors chose to put this particular information in a summary form. Often, it is to save space, as there is not enough space in many journals for the authors to present their "raw" data (the actual numbers they collected or measured). They therefore summarize quantitative information in tables, graphs, and charts. Tables are often the simplest way to capture a large amount of quantitative information in concise form. A table or graph may highlight an unusual aspect of their sample, method, or results. If a treatment produced a dramatic improvement in the patients' problems, for example, a graph may show that most clearly.

Take special note of graphs or tables that display results you consider minor while ignoring results that seem to be more important. You may become aware of a **bias** in such a presentation. Also, ask yourself if the table agrees with the text. This seems very basic. However, sometimes the text will portray one picture and the table another. If you cannot explain this in a plausible way, it may be a flaw in the article or an editorial error. Evaluate tables first by their clarity of presentation. Then, as you read the article, make sure the table agrees with the text.

Pay particular attention to whether the number of subjects reported in the tables is the same as described in the text. The number of subjects who gave consent to participate initially is often greater than the number who participated in any particular aspect of the study. For example, the authors may have explained their study to several childbirth preparation classes and obtained consent from 50 couples to observe the first breastfeed. What could happen to reduce that number? The researchers might have been out of town when two of the couples delivered. Perhaps two mothers were so tired after delivery that they refused to allow the researcher to observe them. Maybe three mothers decided not to breastfeed. This reduces the sample size to 43 couples. Therefore, if you read that 50 couples granted consent, and then see that the total number of observations was 43, you might need to reread the part of the article that describes what happened to the other seven couples. As long as the tables and text agree and there is an explanation of any apparent discrepancies, you will be able to use the information in the tables to decide if your clients or patients are similar to the ones studied. You will also be able to decide whether the tables and figures support the findings and reasoning claimed by the researchers.

Graphs should have clear titles and labels, designed to portray the data accurately. You will need to look carefully at the scale of the graph. In the graph in Figure 27.1, the scale goes from 0 to 20, so the height of the curved lines looks lower and less impressive than the height of the curves in the graph in Figure 27.2, in which the scale goes from 0 to 7. Either scale could be appropriate depending on the definition of the pain scale. However, the graphs create different reactions in the viewer. Because the **slope** or angle of the lines in Figure 27.2 is steeper than that of Figure 27.1, it appears that the change in pain was different from that shown in Figure 27.2. Actually, both are the same. Therefore, although graphs can be very helpful, they can also be misleading and require careful scrutiny.

Second, suppose this study was one in which each woman was her own control, randomly assigned to treat one nipple and not the other. Suppose further that the authors claim that the treated nipple was in pain for less total time than the untreated nipple. Although you might agree with that conclusion, you might wonder if it was a fair test. Perhaps some of the babies sucked more vigorously on the untreated nipple, causing it to be more painful than the treated nipple on Day One. This example is probably not what the authors would publish because it represents only one subject. You can

see that the details of a graph can both clarify and confuse your understanding!

There are many additional kinds of tables, graphs, and charts. Their purposes range from summarizing basic information to clarifying complex patterns found in the data. When you read the results to decide whether the evidence supports the findings, you will want to look closely at these graphics. Critical analysis includes judging their clarity and consistency with the rest of the article.

Step 5: Read the Results

Read the results to get firmly in your mind what the authors claim to find. You need to understand their claims in order to read about their methods effectively. Pay particular attention to the subjects in the study and the relationships between variables. The first time you read the results section, determine whether the results are what the authors expected based on their theories and hypotheses. Before you read the article any further, get the results clear in your mind, whether those results were predicted or not.

Subjects

This section of the article will tell you what their final sample was. Identify the subjects who actually ended up in the study. Perhaps the researchers intended an equal portion of first-time breastfeeding mothers and experienced breastfeeding mothers. You then need to decide

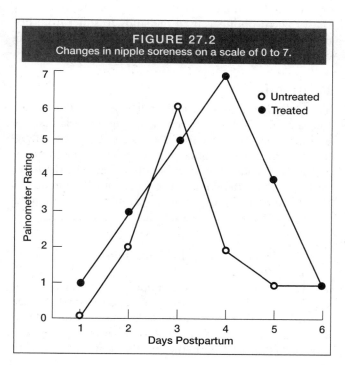

FIGURE 27.2
Changes in nipple soreness on a scale of 0 to 7.

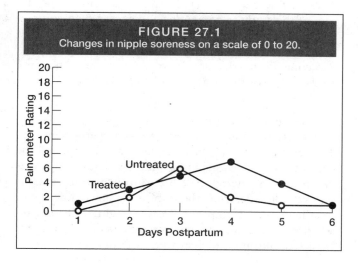

FIGURE 27.1
Changes in nipple soreness on a scale of 0 to 20.

whether the sample was appropriate for the question they asked and whether the results are justified based on the kind of subjects they acquired. Most researchers try very hard to anticipate a certain number of study dropouts. However, they are sometimes unlucky (or plan poorly), and more subjects drop out from one group than from the other. Consider whether their results could have been different if their original plan had worked. Dropouts can affect the results. Some leave the study because their problem resolves quickly and they no longer need the treatment. Some leave because there are side effects of the treatment they cannot tolerate. Others drop out because the research process is a burden. Some families move before the study is completed.

Consider the implications of each reason for dropping out of the study. If the dropouts had remained in the study, might the findings have been different? Suppose a study of women who returned to employment at six weeks postpartum was trying to determine what factors made it likely that they would continue breastfeeding to twelve weeks. One factor to study might be employer support. The researchers might enroll women in the hospital who were planning to return to work at six weeks and continue nursing until at least twelve weeks. If a few women drop out because they expect lack of support from their employer, the remaining subjects would disproportionately include more mothers who expect support from their employers. It would then be likely that both those who continued and those who stopped expected support. This might lead the researchers to conclude that there was no difference between the two groups in terms of support. In reality, a higher proportion of those who expected no support simply left the study. The dropouts caused the study to suffer from **homogeneity** with respect to employer support, preventing detection of a difference in the "employer" factor.

Relationships

The investigators will usually tell you that their study found a relationship between two or more variables. For example, they may have found a relationship between giving discharge packs containing formula to new mothers and early discontinuation of breastfeeding. The discharge packs are the **independent variable**, and the duration of breastfeeding is the **dependent variable**. Think about all the logical steps needed to substantiate that finding.

The Data Needs to Be Consistent with the Claims

In the discharge pack example, one result could be that more of the mothers who received discharge packs needed to stop breastfeeding earlier than did the mothers who did not receive packs. The number of mothers who stopped compared with those who continued must be significantly different in a statistical sense—statistically significant. It also needs to be convincingly different to you. Similarly, "early" weaning must be meaningfully different from "late" weaning.

There Must Be No Other Equal or Better Explanation

In the discharge pack example, determine whether the data can rule out other possible competing explanations. Did more mothers in the discharge pack group have sore nipples? Was there a higher proportion of preterm infants? Were there more mothers who only intended to breastfeed for six weeks or less? Ruling out these possible explanations makes it more likely that the discharge pack itself is the cause of the early weaning.

There Must Be a Plausible Mechanism That Links the Two Variables

In the discharge pack example, the mechanism for this causation might be that a discharge pack is a subtle signal to the mother that her healthcare professionals do not really believe she can make sufficient milk for her baby. Because she then doubts the adequacy of her milk supply, she weans early.

Step 6: Read the Methods (or Subjects and Methods)

The topics covered in this section are the most important to your critical reading because they determine whether the authors can justify their conclusions. The design of the study, the definitions of terms, the tools for measurement, and the statistical tests all contribute to your evaluation and are covered in the next section.

Design of the Study

There are several shorthand ways of describing the design of the study to a scientific audience. When you recognize these basic study designs, you will be able to understand aspects of subject selection, data gathering, and comparisons that are drawn. You also will know the kinds of conclusions warranted by the study's design.

Retrospective Study

A **retrospective study** uses two comparison groups. The cases have the problem under examination, and the controls do not. Designing a study by designating cases first results in a design based on **output variables**. Output variables describe the subjects after follow-up or treatment. For example, the cases might be babies readmitted to the hospital with weight loss in excess of that expected during the first week of life. The controls would be babies without such weight loss, possibly found by a search of the charts in a pediatric practice. The purpose of such a comparison might be to determine whether there were any differences in the number of feedings or stools in the first four days of life or differences in the highest bilirubin level achieved that could be associated with the need for readmission. Such a retrospective study is a case-control study.

When the methods section declares that the design is retrospective, you would expect to read a description of the groups chosen for comparison. You then would want to decide whether the groups were appropriate. Retrospective studies greatly depend on records kept before researchers conducted the study. If a retrospective study concluded that babies who had stooled only once during their first 24 hours were at higher risk of readmission, you would want to know whether the record keeping of stools passed was accurate. In a retrospective study, the use of existing records may be all that is possible. The evidence gained from such a study may not be as strong as when the record keeping is more deliberate and planned.

Prospective Study

In a prospective study, subjects are sampled based on input variables that are believed to influence the outcomes. A prospective study might be one in which the authors held staff education classes and designed new record-keeping tools before data collection began. From the starting date forward in time, the staff would be asked to keep careful count of the number—and perhaps color and size—of the stools on a certain **cohort** of babies designated as infants born from January 1 to June 30, 2005. If the number of stools related to the risk of readmission for weight loss, there would be greater confidence in this prospective study than in the retrospective one. The researchers ensured the accuracy of data collection before the study. Another term for prospective studies is **cohort studies**.

Cross-Sectional Study

A **cross-sectional study** relies on record keeping or memory, much as a retrospective study does. However, researchers do not begin by identifying an affected group. Rather, they gather data from everyone at the same time. In a study about stooling and readmission rates in a cross-sectional design, for example, researchers might collect data at the time of all infants' two-month visits. After gathering data, researchers identify the affected group (readmitted infants, in this example). Researchers compare the information about their stools, feedings, and bilirubin levels, with the same information for the unaffected group. Cross-sectional studies are adequate for suggesting causative factors and relevant variables. The possibility that the data collection was too dependent on

recall or missed too many possible subjects on the collection day or days limits confidence in their findings.

Descriptive Study

A **descriptive study** will list many relevant variables of a defined sample rather than compare two groups. A family practice office might want to know the characteristics of its childbearing families before designing a preconception class. The study might describe how many families in the previous year had borne a first child, how many had a second child, how many breastfed and for how long, and so on. Even though researchers gathered the information from one particular sample, they might publish their findings so that other family practices with similar types of families might benefit from the information. Descriptive studies require a thorough and careful description of the sample. Readers can then understand the degrees of similarity and difference between their own groups of families and the one studied.

Qualitative Study

Another type of descriptive study is the qualitative study. In this type of study, researchers will observe subjects and events in a natural setting rather than establishing a control. These researchers are often looking for the meaning of an event or practice to the person experiencing it. Variables in a qualitative study usually are not measured in numbers, and differences between variables are not expressed numerically. Qualitative variables are often words that the researcher believes will change together, that is, category labels. For example, as "ethnic heritage" changes, so does the "critical support person."

Qualitative research emphasizes getting a sense of the whole or comprehending the emergent properties of an experience instead of breaking down a phenomenon or experience into parts. Qualitative studies in breastfeeding, for instance, have described the feelings of women who breastfed a child for several years, as well as the empowerment of low-income women through breastfeeding. When you are evaluating such studies, you can use the more general ideas in this chapter. Because qualitative work by itself does not claim that practice should change in a particular way, qualitative research critique is discussed separately later in this chapter.

Experiments and Trials

In research about breastfeeding, it is less common to find studies designed as experiments. Problems that involve humans are difficult to conduct as experiments. However, researchers might study comparisons of equipment or differences between animals experimentally. The best information about a problem that involves humans comes from studies called **randomized clinical trials**. They are similar to experiments. These trials attempt to avoid bias in the comparisons they draw. If the trial is

blind as well, then knowledge of which treatment the patient received remains secret until analysis of the data begins. In that way, the patient's or lactation consultant's assessment of the effectiveness of treatment is not influenced by knowing to which treatment group the patient belonged. Treatment groups are as similar as possible at the beginning of the study, with great effort to identify any differences that exist. Furthermore, the groups are treated the same in all ways except for the treatment itself.

Suppose there were a new drug to eliminate mastitis caused by *staphylococcus aureus*. To conduct a blinded study, researchers would disguise the new and old drugs, perhaps by using identical capsules, and administer them in the same manner. In that way, no one could tell which was which. Only a system of codes would be able to detect the difference for later analysis. Both groups are otherwise healthy first-time breastfeeders of babies two to six months old. Therefore, the groups are as similar as possible. The mastitis is diagnosed and its severity graded by strict criteria and by the same two clinicians for all the subjects. Recommendations for other aspects of treatment (pain relief, treatment of baby, and so on) are the same for all subjects. In a tightly controlled study like this, differences in cure rates between the two drugs are more likely to be attributable to the drugs than in a case-control or other less controlled study.

There are several reasons why more studies are not blinded, randomized trials. First, ethical concerns preclude **random assignment** of people to potentially poorer treatments. Second, it is difficult to control many of the variables about people that result in comparison groups of humans who are different in many ways. Third, very large numbers of subjects are required when a trial attempts to study prevention of problems. Fourth, precision in measuring "soft" outcomes—such as quality of mother-child attachment—is lower. Funding and recognition for researchers tend to be greater when their study outcomes are "harder" and more quantifiable. Your critical analysis of clinical trials involves judgments about the researchers having adequately identified and controlled important variables.

Definitions

You will need to identify the important terms used in the article. These will be the key concepts of the study. They may include *breastfeeding, supplementation, multipara, infant, pain, treatment, exercise*, and so on. In this section of the article, the authors should define these terms clearly enough that you know who or what was included and excluded.

If the authors studied only multiparas, were they women with previous breastfeeding experience, or did the authors assume they had previously breastfed without specifically asking them? If they identified experienced breastfeeders, does it matter to the study's conclusions whether the previous experience was positive or negative? Is the age of the multiparas important? Is their experience coping with other stressful situations or child rearing problems significant?

Not all multiparous women are the same. You will need to keep in mind what the results were and consider how the definition of *multipara* in the study might affect the results. All of the possible differences in multiparas are variables. Critically reading the definitions includes being able to state how a different or clearer definition could change the results or the interpretation of the results.

Tools (Instruments)

Scales for weighing babies, survey questions, diet diaries, and pain ratings are examples of tools. Some tools may be intimidating if you are not familiar with them. You may not be able to analyze the tool completely if it is new to you. Still, you want to read the study because you may encounter similar tools in later reading. In addition, you will need to have some basic idea of how a defined term was measured in order to decide its applicability to your situation.

In the better studies, the tool will have undergone testing. Good tools should measure the dependent variable consistently. The **reliability** of the measurement from one time to the next may be part of the reason the investigators chose to use this tool. Authors may assume some familiarity with the type of tool without explaining the general type in much detail. For example, they would expect healthcare professionals to know what a **Likert scale** is and how a pulse **oximeter** is used. Although they do not describe their Likert scale in detail, they should tell how it is different from others (whether it is a 5-point or a 7-point scale, for example). They should also tell whether the placement of the pulse oximeter was on a finger or toe. Any details about the tool itself or its use should be described clearly, so that you do not have serious questions about whether the quirks of their method are more responsible for their results than the explanation for the results that they expound.

It is not necessary that the authors publish the entire tool in the article. Its length, developmental status, or potential profitability may prevent its publication. Examples or short versions of a survey's questions may help you decide whether the tone or complexity of the questions could have influenced the way subjects answered them. If you have serious concerns about the quality of the questions, you can often write to the authors through the journal and request more information. Even if you agree with a study's conclusions, you may not want to use the study in a formal presentation until you have learned more about the tool so that you can adequately answer your audience's questions.

Operationalizing

When you put together the definitions and the tools, you should understand how the researchers operationalized their concepts. Suppose they are studying the change in pain after the application of a treatment. They should tell you how they define pain. It often will be the subject's verbal or written report of her pain. Alternatively, the definition might involve videotaping subjects before and after the treatment and watching for changes in facial expression.

A different tool will measure each definition of pain. The tool for verbal reports might be a 10-point scale in which the **anchors** (words used at specific points on the scale to describe what that number means) are "1 = no pain" and "10 = the worst pain you can imagine." You can then understand that the researchers operationalized the concept "pain" by asking the subject herself to place a mark on the scale that best represented her pain before the treatment and again at a specified time afterward.

The critical reading of this operationalization involves both its clarity and your judgment about its validity. The validity of a pain measure is often supported by expert review or by comparing the current pain tool with an older one and finding that the two agree. Although pain is very difficult to measure due to its subjectivity, what is important is the person's determination of the amount of pain and whether that determination changes.

A scale that reflects the changes is the operationalization of the pain. The construction of measurement scales is the subject of many research articles. You may want to investigate previously tested tools if you decide to design a scale yourself. Below are several common methodological concerns in lactation research.

Methodological Concerns in Lactation Research

♦ Test weighing is not uniform. At present, this is usually resolved by careful instruction of the people who weigh the babies and by the use of electronic balance scales.

♦ It is difficult to equate the volume of expressed milk to the volume produced. Such volumes can be quite different unless good quality pumps are used, pumping duration is adequate, milk lets down, and the study accounts for time of day.

♦ Observing and measuring the breastfeeding process disturbs the natural process.

♦ It is difficult to obtain a representative milk sample. Milk composition varies by length of time postpartum, time of day, proportion of breast drained, and gestation of the infant.

♦ Changing method of feeding is a one-direction change. With rare exceptions, mothers do not usually switch from formula to breastfeeding. If a mother changes feeding methods, it is a change from human to artificial. Therefore, when studies encompass babies who have been fed for any length of time, some in the group will usually have breastfed at some point and then bottle-fed. None will have fed in the reverse order. This can make it difficult to interpret growth differences. To improve growth, mothers may try to switch to formula, but they cannot switch to breastfeeding. Most researchers believe that there are ways to overcome this built-in direction, but that may complicate interpretation.

♦ Studies of environmental contaminants often use human milk because it is easier to obtain than blood or other body tissue and because milk fats promote the accumulation of some chemicals in milk. However, the media may misunderstand the use of milk, implying that finding a pollutant in milk automatically means that feeding human milk is harmful.

♦ Studies of effects of breastfeeding on women's bone mineralization have sometimes been misunderstood because the time it takes to recover bone mass that was mobilized during lactation has been longer than the length of the study.

When you have read and thought about the methods, think back to the results. Do the study design, definitions, tools, and operationalizations allow for the conclusions the scientists made? How could they have done the study differently to make you believe that the conclusions were more justified? What additional information about the methods would help you evaluate the findings even more thoroughly?

Statistics

A brief description of the main statistical approach used to evaluate the data is usually found within the methods section of the article. For lactation consultants, this section may be the most difficult to decipher because the language is so specialized. As you have learned, a lot of meaningful critical analysis can occur, even without judging the statistical techniques used. To some extent, you must rely on the peer review process to catch any major problems in the statistics. The more you read breastfeeding research, the more you will become familiar with some of the common approaches used in certain research designs. The examples presented in the following sections will help you understand some of these more common statistical ideas and tests.

Statistical Theory

Statistical theory is based on probability, a mathematical discipline that focuses on trying to precisely answer finely tuned questions about uncertain events.

Statistical theory uses probability to answer real questions based on real data. For example, if one is wondering whether the new Euro coin is biased (i.e., will tend to land heads more often than tails or vice versa) you might flip the coin, say, 100 times and record how often heads results from those 100 flips. Statistics would then allow you to take the observed number of heads (the data) and see if there is convincing evidence of a bias. For example, if you observe only 37 heads in the 100 flips, a pattern that would happen less than 1 percent of the time if you were flipping a fair coin, you would conclude that the coin has some bias. Sample size (the number of data points) is important. If there is an interesting trend (for example, if low-birth-weight babies tend to have lower IQ scores later in life), the larger the sample, the more likely we would see this pattern in the data in a way that convinces us of the reality of what was observed.

Study Frequency

When you study the frequency of breastfeeding by mothers and their babies at 10 days of age in your city, you are studying a sample of the whole **population** of 10-day-old breastfed babies and their mothers (in the world, and maybe throughout human history). If your goal in studying the frequency in this sample was to publish in a textbook that the "normal" or "usual" or "**average**" frequency for all human babies at 10 days was X, then you would be trying to make a statement about the population by studying a sample of it. If your sample is large (500 subjects or more) there will be far less chance of an error in your estimate of X than if your sample is only 20 subjects.

Good studies will aim for the largest sample size they can reasonably get. The statistical analysis will tell what the **power** of that sample size was. Power relies on more than sample size. However, sample size is what researchers have the most control over, so they try to maximize it. For most purposes, researchers want a power of 0.80 (80 percent) or higher. If the power of a test is low, then the reason for failing to find a significant difference between two groups could be that the sample selected was too small for that difference to show up, not that there is no real difference. A power of 80 percent means that the data have an 80 percent probability of correctly rejecting the null hypothesis.

Statistical Tests

Statistical tests are valid only when applied correctly. In order to be valid, each test assumes certain things about the data. If those assumptions are not **true**, the test should not be used. Sometimes in the methods section there will be a brief statement about why a certain test was used and whether or not a particular assumption was met. There are few hard-and-fast rules in statistical analysis.

Statisticians disagree, just as lactation consultants do, about which should be the first solution to try.

Discussions about assumptions often speak to potential readers who are researchers and statisticians who might disagree with the choice of statistical test. One such discussion sometimes centers on whether or not the assumption of a **normal distribution** of the data is true. A normal distribution describes much of the infinite data we could collect about the natural world. A normal distribution, plotted on a graph, looks like a **bell curve**. Look, for example, at the graph entitled "How much milk the one-month-old infant takes at a single episode at breast" (Figure 27.3).

The left end of the graph shows a few babies who take very tiny amounts, perhaps when nursing is very frequent and short. The right end shows a few babies who take a very large amount. Assuming that most babies take in about 120 ml, the center of the graph (the large hill or bell) represents what the bulk of babies do. Between the center and each extreme is a gradual slope.

Now, instead, suppose the data on milk intake actually comes from a distribution that looks like the graph in Figure 27.4. Here, the bulk (greatest number of values) of the data is at one extreme, not in the middle. The left side rises quickly with a long slope off to the right. Perhaps this is a group of preterm infants at one month of age whose intake tends to be less than that of full-term infants. A statistical test that was attempting to predict what happens in the bulk of this distribution by expecting it to be a normal distribution would be way off. The middle in this distribution is far to the left of where it would be with normal distribution of the data. The data in Figure 27.4 would require a statistical test designed for this particular distribution. It is very important that researchers and statisticians carefully choose which tests

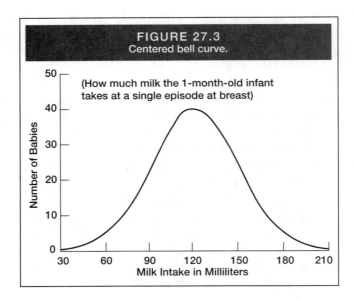

FIGURE 27.3
Centered bell curve.

(How much milk the 1-month-old infant takes at a single episode at breast)

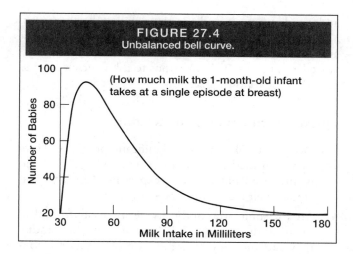

FIGURE 27.4
Unbalanced bell curve.

to use, and that they look at all the underlying assumptions, including distribution of the data.

Statistical Significance

Statistical significance, or lack of significance, is determined by applying a statistical test to a fact about the data (a result) and calculating the probability of obtaining that result (or more extreme result). The probability is reported as a **p-value**. Most researchers want p-values that are 0.05 or lower. The p-value measures the risk of rejecting a true null hypothesis. Researchers want the chance of falsely stating that there is a real difference between two groups to be 5 percent or less.

Confidence intervals (CIs) provide information about the statistical significance of a result. CIs are the range within which a population's true value is expected to be found. Usually, a 95 percent CI is reported. This describes the other possible results that are close to the one that actually came from the data and that are likely to contain the true population value. So, if the mean (average) of the weight gain from the study's sample was 200 g and the 95 percent CI was 185 to 215 g, then it is likely that the population's true weight gain is somewhere between 185 and 215 g.

Large confidence intervals (from 50 to 350 g, for this example) do not tell you very much. Nearly every weight gain will fall somewhere in that interval, so you cannot tell the difference between a usual one and a more extreme one. Large confidence intervals often arise when the sample size is small. Furthermore, if you are trying to compare, for example, the weight gains in two different groups and you expect them to be different, you will not want their CIs to overlap. So, if the mean for group A (breastfed) is 200 g (95 percent CI 185 to 215 g) and the mean for group B (formula-fed) is 220 g (95 percent CI 205 to 235 g), the intervals share the values 205 to 215 g. These shared values mean that the real average weight gain could be the

same for both groups. These confidence intervals would not allow you to claim you had found a statistically significant difference between the two groups. (See "odds ratio" below for another example of the use of a confidence interval.)

Common Statistical Tests and Terms

This section on common statistical tests and terms can help you understand some of the tests you are most likely to encounter. For greater depth, you can consult a statistics text such as one listed in Appendix B.

Chi-Square. There are several slightly different versions of the **chi-square** test. Its use is usually to determine whether the proportions in two groups are significantly different. You may want to determine, for example, if the proportion of experienced breastfeeders who have mastitis is the same as the proportion of first-time breastfeeders who have mastitis. Large chi-square values usually lead to low, statistically significant p-values.

Cohen's Kappa. Cohen's kappa is calculated when two observers rate the same event on a scale and the researcher wants to show that the two raters are in close agreement. Values at 0.7 or higher are considered good.

Cronbach's Alpha. A Cronbach's alpha test is often reported when the researcher is trying to give evidence of the reliability of an instrument. Values can range from 0.0 to 1.0. The closer they are to 1.0, the better the reliability.

Odds Ratio. Odds ratio is not a statistical test; rather, it is a way to summarize the relative proportion of illness in two different groups. For example, you may want to compare the proportion of breastfed babies who get otitis media with the proportion of artificially fed babies who do, under certain similar conditions. If you found that 2 out of 10 breastfed babies developed otitis media and 4 out of 10 formula-fed babies did, the ratio of those odds is 0.2/0.4 = 0.5. The odds of the breastfed baby getting an ear infection were one-half the odds of the baby who failed to receive human milk's protection.

The only way an odds ratio could equal 1 is if the odds for both groups are the same. CIs for odds ratios might be written like this: "0.5 (95% CI, 0.35–0.60)." This means that the best estimate of the odds ratio could be anywhere from 0.35 to 0.60. Significant CI for the odds ratio should not contain "1" (0.90–1.05, for example) because that would mean the odds ratio could be 1. This is another way of saying that the odds for the breastfed baby were the same as the odds for the artificially fed baby. In studies comparing breastfed infants, bottle-fed infants, and differing risks, we would expect to find that the breastfed babies had less risk.

Regression. Regression is a technique used to try to understand the relationship between variables. Simple regression relates one **predictor variable** (or independent variable) to one outcome variable (or dependent variable). Multiple regression relates several variables to one outcome variable. **Logistic regression** relates one or more variables to a **dichotomous outcome** (two-possibility) variable. This addresses a question such as, "Do maternal satisfaction, infant weight gain, and family support with the first breastfed child relate to the decision to breastfeed or not breastfeed [dichotomous outcome] the next child?" Regression methods usually try to estimate how much change there is in the outcome variable for a one-unit change in the predictor variable. For example, "How much change occurs in infant crying time for each additional half-hour of being carried in a baby sling?"

T-test. Use of a **t-test** is to decide between two contradictory hypotheses about the mean of a sample. For example, you may want to know if the average weight gain of breastfed infants in Hospital A is the same as the average weight gain for all breastfed babies in the United States (where the national average is often considered a "norm" or "true" population value). A slightly different t-test could be used to compare the average gain of babies in Hospital A with that of babies in Hospital B.

Step 7: Read the Introduction and Literature Review

You now will read the introduction and literature review to understand some of the decisions the researchers made in light of the results they found and the methods they used. You can ask yourself whether the authors' justification for doing the study seems adequate to you. Most articles start out by stating that some expert bodies recognize the superiority of breastfeeding. They may then say that although breastfeeding by all mothers would be preferable, there is such-and-such a problem that prevents near-universal breastfeeding. They might claim that their study is going to address that problem, shed light on it, and help move humankind toward more breastfeeding.

Often, the authors explain and reference the theory underlying their approach to the problem and the hypothesis they want to test. Somewhere in this line of reasoning is the explicit or implicit statement of why the authors chose this particular problem to study.

The literature review is used to show how their study is different from what has been done before and how their study is an improvement. If they have done a good job of this reasoning, they will convince you that (1) the problem is significant, (2) no one has adequately

addressed it before, and (3) their approach is superior. You can use your experience and your reading of other articles and books to decide whether they have convinced you of this. The questions to ask yourself are discussed in the following section.

Questions to Guide Your Reading

◆ Do you think this is a significant problem? Have they explained why? If you were a professional who is interested but not very experienced in lactation, would their explanation be convincing?

◆ Are the summaries of the articles they cite to explain their study accurate? If you know the studies they cite, did they do a good job of stating the conclusions?

◆ If you know any of the studies, do you think they are appropriate ones to use? For example, if the new study you are reading is about colic-like symptoms in fully breastfed babies, but the cited studies included partially breastfed babies, what parts can legitimately be compared and what parts have to be different? Suppose the new study wants to use removal of dairy products from the mother's diet as a treatment. That could be a clear change in an exclusively breastfed baby's diet. But in a baby who is also receiving some cow's milk formula, a comparable change in diet would need to include removal of the formula. On the other hand, the older study may have found that firstborn infants suffered more colic-like symptoms and the new study might want to examine birth order. That aspect of both studies would be more similar than exposure to cow's milk because birth order does not directly relate to cow's milk or maternal diet. If you do not know any of the studies cited, you will not be as able to judge their appropriateness. You will grow in your ability to do this as you read more.

◆ Did they omit any studies that you would have included? Do you know about previous research (even if you do not know the exact title or authors' names) that also addresses this problem but that the authors left out? If it is an area of research with several previous studies, lack of space may be the cause. However, it may happen by design if the authors do not want to mention contrary studies, especially if those studies rejected what the authors wish to convey. Leaving out relevant studies may also result from an inadequate literature search. However, usually peer reviewers demand that prospective authors read and include the most important articles. Leaving out relevant studies may not be too damaging to readers who know the background information well. It can portray a misleading picture of the state of knowledge to those unfamiliar with the background information.

♦ Are the methods that were used in previous studies explained fully enough that you can judge whether the authors' use or rejection of them in the new study is appropriate? For example, in a study of infection rates in children who attend day care versus those who do not attend day care, the literature review may describe the use of "written parental diaries" as the method. The authors may tell you that they propose to use the same method as previous studies, having parents record weekly whether the child had fever, sore throat, medical visits, and so on. Suppose they find that children in day care have no different infection rates than stay-at-home children, although previous studies have found a difference. The authors may have failed to mention that in the older study parents recorded symptoms on a daily basis and received biweekly calls and cards to remind them to do so. That may explain why the older study found differences in rates while the new study does not. You are looking for ways in which the current study is different from and similar to the older studies cited in the literature review. The authors should be clear about those aspects that are relevant to the current study.

Step 8: Read the Discussion

There usually is a link between the literature review and the discussion. The authors may explain the link in the beginning of the discussion section. You should ask yourself whether the intentions the researchers declared based on their review of the current state of knowledge carried through to the methods and results. Ask if they did something different from the earlier cited studies and, if so, whether it was an improvement.

In the discussion, the researchers may summarize their results in a less formal way. They may offer an interpretation of the results that puts their findings into the context of other studies conducted on the same problem. You should consider whether their findings are as important as the authors claim and whether the state of knowledge about the problem is now more complete or clearer.

Speculation

The authors may stretch the interpretation of their findings into a more speculative understanding of some aspect of the problem. An example of this would be a study that found that peanut butter and jelly sandwiches **correlated** with higher milk production. Suppose the authors had found evidence in the literature review that a chemical in peanuts could cause an appetite increase in

lab animals. They put these two ideas together to suggest that the reason peanut butter and jelly sandwiches are associated with higher milk production is that the sandwiches stimulated appetite in breastfeeding mothers who eat them. Their study did not really look at either the chemistry of peanuts or the overall calorie intake of mothers. Nevertheless, they speculate that such a causal mechanism exists.

It is your job, as a critical reader, to judge how plausible, realistic, and rational that link is. You do not know if the link is correct, but you need to think about whether it could be real and whether further suggestions by the authors along this line of reasoning are worth considering.

Suggestions for Further Research

Often, the next step the researchers take is to suggest further research. Some suggestions will be to test the speculations that they have made. Other suggestions will be to fill in the gaps in the understanding of the problem that remain in spite of the knowledge gained from their study.

Flaws or Weaknesses

The authors may acknowledge in the discussion some of the flaws or weaknesses you detected in reading the article. You can decide whether your assessment of the flaws (and their impact on the confidence you have in the results) is the same as that of the authors. If you think that the problems are more serious than the authors acknowledge, you will want to read their justification as generously as you can. On the other hand, if the authors fail to note a flaw you have uncovered, you should try to understand why. This may be just another opportunity to reinforce your critique, but it could be that the goal or methods as explained further in the discussion are different from your original understanding of them.

Step 9: Read the Results Again

When you first read the results section, you were trying to understand what the authors claimed to have found. This time, you will read to decide whether you think those claims were justified. You probably have formed some judgments about this already, having read the methods and discussion. The following suggestions will lead you to look even more closely at the logic of the relationships between variables that the authors claim to have found. Recall the three steps discussed previously:

1. The data need to be consistent with the claims.
2. There must be no other equal or better explanation.
3. There must be a plausible mechanism linking the two variables.

Data Consistent with Claims

Are the data consistent with the claims? Consider again the example of the study testing the effect of discharge packs on the duration of breastfeeding. If the study had 100 subjects (50 in the pack group and 50 in the nonpack group), and if 15 in the pack group weaned "early" but only 5 did in the nonpack group, is that a convincing difference to you? This difference would be statistically significant at $p < 0.05$. That is, there is only a 1 in 20 chance that a difference of 15 versus 5 (or a more extreme difference) would have occurred by chance. Therefore, statistically speaking, it is probable that the difference between the numbers of early weaners in the two groups is a real difference and not a chance occurrence. However, you could ask whether that difference is clinically important. Do 10 more "late" weaners out of 50 achieve enough additional health and relationship benefits to warrant discontinuing discharge packs?

This question is not just about statistics, but also about values. Many healthcare providers would probably consider this valid and important evidence against discharge packs. Skeptics, however, might say, "Well, if discharge packs are so bad, then how did 35 out of 50 mothers go on to wean late in spite of them?" Considering answers to such questions will help you think about the study and formulate responses you could use if you presented this study to skeptics.

Another Possible Explanation for Relationship

Is there another possible explanation for the claimed relationship between variables? To continue looking at the logical steps, think about another way of presenting the numbers. Instead of defining "early" and "late" and comparing the proportions in each group, suppose the average number of weeks of breastfeeding was computed in the pack group versus the nonpack group.

You need to take a close look at whatever numbers the authors present. Usually, you will find that they have chosen appropriate ways to measure and summarize their data. Nevertheless, you may find that you have questions about their numbers that make you reluctant to agree with their conclusions.

Averages and Distribution Range

If the study found that those who received packs breastfed for 18 weeks and those who did not breastfed for 20 weeks, would you think this was an important difference? This could be a statistically significant difference between the groups, depending on the group sizes and the degree of **variation** in the averages. Whenever an average (mean) is reported, you may want to know the distribution and range of each group's length of breastfeeding. An average can be misleading if one subject (or a small

---

FIGURE 27.5
Ten subjects who breastfed an average of 18 weeks.

Group 1	Group 2	Group 3
25 weeks	50 weeks	29 weeks
20 weeks	19 weeks	27 weeks
18 weeks	18 weeks	26 weeks
18 weeks	17 weeks	25 weeks
18 weeks	16 weeks	24 weeks
18 weeks	16 weeks	23 weeks
18 weeks	15 weeks	22 weeks
18 weeks	14 weeks	2 weeks
16 weeks	13 weeks	1 week
11 weeks	2 weeks	1 week
180 weeks	180 weeks	180 weeks

---

number) has an extremely short or extremely long duration. Figure 27.5 demonstrates the number of different ways a group could breastfeed for an average of 18 weeks.

Group 1 had many people who actually breastfed for 18 weeks and 4 people who breastfeed for a shorter or longer amount of time. In this kind of distribution, the average gives a good representation of the typical behavior in the group. The range is $25 - 11 = 14$ weeks. Group 2 had only 1 person who breastfed the "average" length of time and 2 people whose duration was very different from the average (**outliers**), 2 and 50. The range in this data is 48 ($50 - 2 = 48$). The range in Group 1 was smaller.

You might legitimately question whether the extremes in Group 2 had much in common with the "average." Specifically, you might wonder whether the 2-week person had a difficult problem, such as a baby with ankyloglossia and a severe cardiac defect, so that she would have breastfed only 2 weeks regardless of whether she received a discharge pack. After asking yourself that question, you should look in the results section to determine whether the authors describe the mothers' reasons for weaning. If that information is absent or not collected, the authors cannot claim that discharge packs alone made a difference in the groups.

Looking closely at the numbers to determine if they are consistent with the claims may suggest a possible alternative explanation for the study's findings. At least a few mothers may have had an extremely difficult problem that would have led to short breastfeeding, regardless of whether or not they received a pack. Excluding these mothers' durations from the calculation of duration might change the study's results. Of course, you cannot know that the results would change. Nevertheless, if the authors' data make you suspicious, you might ultimately be less willing to accept and apply their findings.

Another example of looking closely at the "average" is the other extreme in Group 2. Suppose the mother who breastfed for 50 weeks was in the discharge pack group. You might ask, "If discharge packs are so bad, how did this woman manage to continue to breastfeed for so long?" Several possible explanations exist, and you might wonder whether the authors asked what the mothers did with the packs. Did they use them? If yes, how old was the baby? Did they discard the pack? If you read some of the real studies of discharge packs, you will find that the authors rarely ask this question. Instead, there is an assumption that mere receipt of a pack probably encourages formula use. Although this may be true, the results would be stronger with data collected on actual use of the packs as well as formula use in the nonpack group.

Hidden Differences Between Groups

In Group 3, no one breastfed to 18 weeks and there is quite a clear separation into two subgroups, one who nursed for 2 weeks or less and the other who nursed for at least 22 weeks. Such a split might make you think about the possibility of a major difference within the group. Perhaps, for example, the two subgroups received substantially different amounts of support. The subgroup who breastfed longer may have had three or more support people, whereas the subgroup who breastfed less may have had two or fewer support people. So, although this entire group breastfed for an average of 18 weeks, that average does not well represent the real story about the group. By trying to explain the duration of breastfeeding using an average, the authors may have missed an alternative explanation for their findings related to differences in support.

Many studies try to avoid potential alternative explanations for their findings by avoiding major hidden differences between groups (like the difference in support cited earlier) through random assignment of subjects to groups. The idea is that if mothers are assigned by chance to receive a discharge pack, differences other than receipt of a pack between groups will be approximately the same in both groups. Differences that could confuse the explanation of findings are called **confounding variables**. In randomized assignment to groups, there will be approximately the same number of multiparas, people with good support, people with inverted nipples, and so on in both groups. Therefore, all the reasons they could have stopped breastfeeding early would be the same in both groups except for receipt of a discharge pack. Random assignment, then, allows researchers to conclude that the reason the women stopped breastfeeding must be the single relevant difference between the groups—receipt of a discharge pack.

The best studies go even further and check whether random assignment worked. In such studies, the authors will report whether the groups were different at baseline in some important ways. As their colleague, you need to consider whether they checked on the right things. For example, if you think lack of support is important in early weaning, did the scientists check their groups to be sure that, say, the average number of support people reported by mothers in the pack and nonpack groups was not statistically different? This checking for the differences and similarities achieved by random assignment is reported in the methods or results section. It is not possible to check for all differences. However, it is important to check for a few major ones, and it is up to you to decide whether the researchers omitted anything critical. If they did, you will be less likely to use the findings of the study.

Most articles related to the practice of helping women with breastfeeding do not have randomized groups. Rather they use a **convenience** (**nonprobability**) sample. Therefore, for a study about discharge packs, the sample might be the first 100 breastfeeding mothers after the starting date (in which mothers 1 to 50 do not get packs and 51 to 100 receive packs). Checking the basic similarity of groups is even more important in convenience samples than in randomized ones.

Plausible Mechanism for Relationship

Is there a plausible mechanism for the claimed relationship between variables? This may be the most difficult of the logical steps for which to find clear evidence in the article. Sometimes authors will have addressed the reason lanolin seems to help heal sore nipples, for example, in the literature review or in the discussion section. They usually do not address this in the results section unless they have studied the possible mechanism along with the relationship between variables.

For example, along with testing whether lanolin led to faster healing, they may have taken microscopic photos of cell changes in nipple skin to see if the differences in cell changes might explain healing differences. In many studies, researchers hypothesize the mechanism itself and do not study it directly. This is especially true when the variables are not physiologic but rather psychological or sociological.

Demonstrating a plausible mechanism for how peer support enables longer durations of breastfeeding than professional support does is not straightforward. Yet many mechanisms for important relationships between variables related to breastfeeding are in the "not straightforward" category. Instead of dismissing research because of an inability to demonstrate mechanisms convincingly, most scientists and clinicians instead require plausibility and thoughtful consideration of mechanisms. In your critical reading, you will want to consider whether a mechanism is discussed and whether you judge that mechanism to be reasonable. If there is very little consideration of how and why the variables are related as the study found them to be, you may be less likely to accept the study's findings.

Spurious Relationships

Sometimes there is little discussion of mechanism because the mechanism is obvious. The greatest danger in the lack of a plausible mechanism is the acceptance of a relationship that is actually **spurious**. Spurious relationships between variables are those that look statistically significant but have resulted from a correlation with no underlying meaning.

Suppose that lactation consultant Lila Cecilia found that, of her last 500 clients, the ones whose babies' home nurseries were painted lavender had a statistically significantly longer duration of breastfeeding than those whose nurseries were any other color. Suppose, further, that Lila had determined that no alternative explanations adequately fit her data. She really did not know why the color of the nursery mattered but she claimed that breastfed babies should have their nurseries painted lavender.

Many readers might guess Lila had failed to study hard enough to find the explanation. Most readers would not rush out and tell their clients to repaint their nurseries! They would not be convinced because there is no plausible relationship between nursery color and breastfeeding duration. The numeric relationship Lila found was probably spurious.

Any time a study finds a relationship for which the authors present no plausible mechanism, it could be spurious. This most often happens when researchers just happen to notice some correlation in their data that was not the main relationship they were studying. In doing a variety of manipulations of the data, sometimes a relationship will surface that is statistically significant. Although the authors may mention this "finding" in their article, it is not good science to claim it as a major result. Instead, they can consider the mechanisms and recommend further research.

▶ PRACTICING CRITICAL READING SKILLS

Now you are ready to practice using the ideas and the steps for critical reading presented earlier. Using Steps 1 through 9 read the following two mock articles in the suggested order. You will want to consider the questions presented in each section. You may find it helpful to make notes to yourself as you go through the process so that you can compare your ideas with those presented in the commentary that follows each mock article.

Before you read the commentary, return to the beginning of the Critical Reading section and apply the process to the article. Consider each part separately and in the order suggested, and make notes to yourself about the strengths and flaws you find. Then compare your ideas to those that follow. You probably will have some ideas not mentioned here. As long as you can justify them logically or by reference to other studies, your commentary is valuable.

Sore Nipple Treatments: Gooeypaste Works Best

I.M. Wright

Journal of Supposed Things, Vol. 21, pp. 5–10, 2005.

Abstract

Sore nipples are one of the obstacles many women need to overcome in order to continue breastfeeding. Thirty women began using Gooeypaste, warm water compresses, or lanolin when their nipples became sore. After 3 days, Gooeypaste provided more pain relief than the other treatments as measured on the Pain Relief Self-Rating. Gooeypaste should become the standard treatment for breastfeeding-related nipple soreness.

Introduction

Breastfeeding is acknowledged by health care professionals worldwide as the best way to feed infants.[2-4] However, women who intend to breastfeed for many weeks or months are sometimes stopped by the development of nipple soreness, which makes breastfeeding intolerable.[4-5] No single measure or combination of measures has been found to reliably reduce pain and increase healing. Although prevention is surely the best policy, the need for treatment is evident. This study was designed to investigate the effectiveness of a new product against two standard treatments.

Review of the Literature

Pain with breastfeeding has been shown to be an important reason for early weaning in several studies[1,4,5] and may include pain due to engorgement or candidiasis as well as sore nipples. Positioning is important to the prevention of soreness. Sometimes, comfortable positioning is not achieved with the first few feedings and, by then, enough nipple damage is done that pain results. In addition, nipple pain may occur later in breastfeeding when the baby tries to interact with the world at the same time as he feeds, or when solid foods begin. Cando and associates[6] found that warm water compresses applied for 15 minutes after every feeding relieved pain better than two other measures. In a study by Workhard and colleagues,[7] lanolin felt soothing to mothers with nipple soreness.

Relief from pain has been measured in many different ways. In keeping with the Ouchless[8] theory of pain perception, tools that measure the patient's perception of pain were reviewed for possible use. The Painometer, a self-rated 5-question scale, was believed to be the most convenient for a busy, new mother to use. The scale has been used before in postoperative patients and was found to correlate with the use of medication. In addition to the questions about degree of pain, there are three questions about coping with the pain.

In Helpful Hospital's Mother-Baby Unit, obstetricians prescribed lanolin for routine use by breastfeeding mothers. Some nurses encouraged mothers to use warm water, but mothers' actual use of these products and the relief provided by them had never been evaluated. When the new product, Gooeypaste, developed by Phunny Pharmaceuticals, became available, the staff decided it was time to conduct a study.

Subjects and Methods

Table 27.1 describes the subjects of the study. Subjects were recruited from the Mother-Baby Unit on the day of their post-partum stay when they first began to develop sore nipples. Except for mothers who had undergone cesarean births, most were discharged by 24 to 48 hours. When a nurse identified a mother with soreness who agreed to participate in the study, an envelope was pulled from the enrollment drawer. The envelopes were in random order (10 envelopes each for warm water, lanolin, and Gooeypaste), and each contained instructions for the mother and nurse on which treatment was to be used. Each also contained three copies of the Painometer that the mother was to complete at 24, 48, and 72 hours after she first started using her assigned treatment.

While the subjects were hospitalized, nurses reminded them to complete the scale. The nurses collected them and stored them anonymously with codes that identified the treatment used and whether this was the 24-, 48-, or 72-hour scale. For subjects who went home before all scales were completed (this included almost all subjects), nurses called mothers to remind them to complete the scales and return them in the envelopes provided. If the mother seemed especially unlikely to return her scales, nurses asked mothers the scale's questions over the telephone and recorded them. Results were analyzed by odds ratios for the odds of experiencing less pain by Day 3. In addition, the mother's responses on the questions about coping were analyzed by comparing means.

Results

Thirty new mothers agreed to participate in the study. Of these, 28 went home before they completed all the scales. All mothers were called at the appropriate follow-up times for reminders. As a result, all 30 had completed scales for all three measurement times.

For 15 of the mothers, pain worsened from 24 to 48 hours after the first treatment. Three of those were using Gooeypaste, 5 warm water, and 7 lanolin. Pain remained the same for 2 mothers from each group. It improved for 5 of the mothers using Gooeypaste, 3 using warm water, and 1 using lanolin. By 72 hours, 8 of the mothers using Gooeypaste noted improvement, whereas 6 using warm water, and 4 using lanolin reported improvement in pain.

The odds ratio for decreased pain at 72 hours comparing Gooeypaste to lanolin was 1.3. The odds ratio comparing Gooeypaste to warm water was 2.0. Both were statistically significant at $p = 0.05$.

The average score for optimism was higher in the Gooeypaste group than in the other treatment groups (see Table 27.2). Although that trend was nonsignificant, optimism remains an important part of pain relief.

Discussion

Although this is a small study, Gooeypaste appears to be an important measure to consider for the treatment of sore nipples. Further studies with larger groups of patients are needed to confirm these findings. Because the Gooeypaste mothers were also more optimistic, they will probably go on to breastfeed in greater numbers to meet their personal goals. The nursing staff at Helpful Hospital is currently working with the obstetric staff to include Gooeypaste as an alternative treatment for sore nipples in breastfeeding mothers.

References

1. Healthy World Alliance. Breastfeeding best for babies. *HWA* 56:123–125; 2003.
2. Bet U, Wynn R. Nutrition experts endorse breastfeeding. *Nutrition Group Reports* 25:2–5; 2004.
3. Up G. Support for breastfeeding grows. *Child Health Studies* 50: 3–9; 2000.
4. Rocks M. A study of engorgement. *Human Nurturing* 23:21–28; 1999.
5. Complete D. Weaning from breast. *Feeding Babies Journal* 11:335–339; 2002.
6. Cando Y. Providing relief for breast-feeding problems. *HA* 58:130–140; 2003.
7. Workhard S. The many uses of lanolin. *Journal of the Natural Products Industry* 12:22–26; 2000.
8. Ouchless T. A theory of pain: The patient knows. *Human Nurturing* 1:70–80; 1998.

Note: The author wishes to express gratitude to Phunny Pharmaceuticals for the provision of Gooeypaste, lanolin, and copies of the Painometer.

TABLE 27.1

The Subjects of the Study

	Gooeypaste	Warm Water	Lanolin
Maternal age (mean)	22.3 yrs	25.3 yrs	24.2 yrs
Breastfed previous baby	8	5	4*
Female infants	5	7	3
Infant birthweight (mean)	3500 g	3405 g	3200 g
Number of infants who had alternative feedings prior to starting the study	1	2	3

*No statistically significant differences between groups, p = 0.15.

TABLE 27.2

Pain Score

	Mean Pain Score at Each Time*		
	24 hours	48 hours	72 hours
Gooeypaste	7	8	5
Warm water	6	8	6
Lanolin	7	9	7

*Mean for the 10 mothers using that method.

Discussion of First Practice Article

Sore Nipple Treatments: Gooeypaste Works Best

Title

Your considerations of this article can begin by asking yourself what you think the article is about just from reading the title. Because this article focuses on treatment, information about the cause of the soreness will certainly be important. Will the authors have looked at causes? Will the results vary depending on the cause? Sore nipples due to continued pacifier use and resultant tongue movements would be expected to take longer to resolve than the initial tenderness of getting started breastfeeding. Therefore, if the authors did not ensure that the causes were the same in the comparison groups, the results might differ for that reason alone, no matter what the treatment was.

Also, consider what you already know. Because early soreness is often due to poor positioning, will the authors measure attempts at correct positioning? Other studies demonstrate that much nipple soreness will diminish with time. However, no treatments to date have reduced that time dramatically. A control group that does not use any treatment might be important to determine the baseline pain experience, in order to judge whether any of the treatments is better than just the passage of time.

Does the title suggest surprises? What is Gooeypaste? It must be a new product and so may be available only to researchers. In addition to measuring pain, will the study attempt to document wound healing as some research has done?

If you had designed a study on nipple soreness, would you have limited the ages of the babies? Would you have limited the previous experience of the mothers? Both of these factors might influence the expected duration and ability to cope with the pain. If the groups have underlying differences in such variables, the expectation that their pain experience would be the same is not justifiable.

Authors' Names

This author is not one you have read before (since he or she is fictitious!). You would ordinarily want to keep this name in mind for future reading.

Abstract

Which of the aspects of the study that you thought about from looking at the title does the abstract clarify? For one, the abstract does not clarify much about the mothers' experience or the babies' ages. Because the abstract recommends Gooeypaste, you would expect to find a strong relationship (documented later in the results) between its use and pain relief.

Tables and Graphs

Table 27.1 tells more about the subjects. You may have many questions after you look at this table. The average maternal age is not the same in the groups, and the authors report no tests to check whether the differences are statistically significant. The authors, and you, may decide that there is no clinically significant difference; that is, that age differences like these are not likely to contribute in important ways to how the mothers respond to treatment.

You are probably more concerned about the differences between the treatment groups in the numbers who have breastfed previously. The Gooeypaste group has twice as many mothers who previously breastfed as does the lanolin group. Although the statistical test showed the groups to be not statistically significantly different, that may be because each treatment group has only ten subjects, a small sample. Before you apply the results of this study to your practice, you might want to see a study in which the experienced breastfeeders are represented equally (or closer to equally) in each treatment group.

A further consideration, not clear from this table and seldom considered in the literature, is whether those previous breastfeeding experiences were favorable. Many women, when asked if they breastfed a previous child, will say "Yes" even if they only breastfed for one week and that week was full of problems. The level of confidence and the interpretation of pain for such women are likely to be different from that of an experienced breastfeeder who met her goals and overcame problems.

The number of female infants looks different in each group as well. However, unless you know of research that links gender of the infant to pain perception or treatment effectiveness, it probably does not matter. Do you think that infant birth weight could be an important difference between treatment groups? None of these groups has an average that makes us think about preterm babies. However, if you reread the abstract, there is no statement that all babies were full term. Therefore, it is possible that any of the groups could have a preterm baby in it.

We might be especially concerned that the lanolin group had more preterm babies than the other two groups. Preterm babies may take longer to learn effective suckling and, thereby, affect their mother's pain perception. We do not know for sure (1) that there are preterm babies in the lanolin group or (2) that preterm babies necessarily correlate with differences in healing sore nipples. Nevertheless, we do know that many preterm babies are more difficult to nurse in the first few days. Therefore, we wonder whether there might be a hidden difference between the treatment groups, such as prematurity, for example. The difference could alter the explanation for the reported faster pain relief in the Gooeypaste group. Such an unanswered question may be serious enough that we may not want to apply this study's findings without more information.

The authors also report the number of infants who received alternative feedings before starting the study. The table does not clarify whether the feedings were by bottle or cup, so we hope that information will be in the text. Statistical tests are absent, so you must consider the possibility that the differences are important clinically. How might bottle-feeding or cup feeding affect the mothers' pain perception? Notice that the table does not tell how many times each of the babies who received an alternative feeding were fed that way. It only tells how many babies (out of ten in each group) were fed by some other method.

Now take your critical reading of this table another step further. By now, you may have collected doubts about the underlying similarity of the lanolin group and the Gooeypaste group. That is, you may be concerned that (1) the number of mothers who previously breastfed differs; (2) there may be more small, possibly preterm, babies in the lanolin group; and (3) there are more babies who had alternative feedings in that group as well. Before reading the text of the article, you have begun to suspect that the groups may have started differently, both before they developed sore nipples and before they used treatments. These differences are potentially associated with sore nipples (unlike gender of the infants, which, while different between groups, is probably not related to pain). It is possible that these differences could be an alternative explanation for the different pain perceptions between the groups rather than the different treatments. Keep these doubts in mind as you read the next table and the remainder of the text.

Table 27.2 reports average pain scores for each group. Does this seem to you to be the most meaningful way to analyze the data? Could the authors instead have shown a table of improvement versus no improvement? Do we know enough about the Painometer to know what a "7" means? There was no discussion of how many points were on the scale, or what the descriptive anchors were at each end. We would also expect a table like this to report whether the pain score averages are different for each treatment group.

Looking at the numbers—without a statistical analysis—would you anticipate a clinically important difference to be demonstrated for Gooeypaste? That is, is there a big difference between Gooeypaste and the other treatments? With experience, you will come to answer that question for yourself, even without statistics, and then can compare your impression to what the statistical

tests demonstrate. In fact, there does not seem to be a very remarkable difference between the groups at any of the times. If the mothers are rating their pain on a 1–10 scale and they are reporting, on average, pain of 5, 6, or 7 at 72 hours after their pain started, they are probably still having an important amount of pain that might affect their overall breastfeeding experience.

A more difficult judgment to make is whether averaging the pain levels makes any sense. Often, when using scales like this that require people to mark specific defined anchor points, it is difficult to know what an intermediate point represents. It will be important to look at the instructions the author gave to the subjects about completing the scale. It could be that they were encouraged to mark a place anywhere along the line. In that event, the author would also need to explain how a quantity was assigned to a mark that fell between two points, such as between 3 and 4. Instead of averaging, some studies might try to sum the amount of time each woman spent at each pain level and compare the sums between groups.

One other aspect of the study is evident from this table. In thinking about designing a sore nipple study after reading the title, the need for a no-treatment group was identified. Yet, no such group appears to have been used for comparison. You might also wonder why the pain scores do not appear in a table because that was the focus of the study. You can reasonably expect that the author will explain this omission in the text.

Results

What do the authors claim? First, they claim that the Gooeypaste group was 2.7 times as likely to experience decreased pain at 72 hours as the lanolin group and 6 times as likely as the water group. This finding was statistically significant. Second, they claim that the optimism level of the Gooeypaste group was higher than that of the other groups, but statistical significance was not attained.

Independent variables in this study include Gooeypaste, lanolin, and water. Dependent variables include nipple soreness and optimism. Potential confounding variables are the cause of pain, experience of the mothers, quality of positioning, and age of the babies. Applying the three logical steps to this article:

1. The statistical significance of the odds ratios means the data on pain is consistent with the first claim. The claim about optimism is less clear.
2. From the results section, are you reassured that the authors have ruled out other possible explanations? Probably not, because the author did not show in the results that the three groups were similar in their potential confounding variables. As you read the rest of the article, you will be interested to determine

whether the subjects had enough in common that the only important difference between them was the treatment they were using.

3. Does the author suggest a plausible mechanism for how the treatment affects pain? Not to this point in the article, though that is often reserved for either the review of the literature or the discussion. The kinds of mechanisms you might be expecting to read later in the article are topical anesthesia, faster wound healing, anti-inflammatory effects, or others.

Subjects

We do not know whether the mothers were first-timers or experienced breastfeeders because the author did not report this. The proportion of these mothers in each treatment group could be significant if more experienced mothers persisted simply because they had been through similar pain before or had a higher level of confidence, or both. We do not know age and education level of the mothers or their intended breastfeeding duration, factors related to general commitment to breastfeeding.

Cesarean birth may differ from vaginal birth in several ways: (1) general rate of recovery from birth, (2) difficulty of birth, (3) more professional breastfeeding help for mothers who have undergone cesarean birth due to longer stays, and (4) possibly later milk induction.

We do not know how many times each mother breastfed before pain developed. Nor do we know how often she breastfed afterward. These factors might affect pain intensity and duration and, therefore, the likelihood of relief. The effectiveness of feeding by the baby might also tell something about the quality of latch. There is no mention of routine help with and observations of positioning.

Nurse or physician preferences for the older treatments do not seem to have prevailed, and neither were they accounted for in the design. If nurses who favored warm water encouraged its use before group assignment, for example, the mothers might have continued with that as well as with their other assigned treatment.

The Painometer was not administered at a baseline time. This means that it is possible that the Gooeypaste mothers actually started the study with a lower pain level than the other groups, so their level of pain might indeed be lower at 72 hours for that reason alone. Because we know little about the scale, we do not know if it tries to measure absolute levels of pain ("the worst pain I've ever felt . . . the least pain I've ever felt") or if it just measures changes in pain perception over time.

Methods

The design of this study followed the outline of a clinical trial with randomly assigned treatments. However, it is not a good example of a clinical trial because of its failure to control for several variables. Thus, the design of a study alone is not sufficient to guarantee the quality of the resulting evidence.

Telephoning mothers was a good way to increase compliance with the scale. However, investigators should separately have analyzed the scales for which the nurses asked the questions from the mailed ones to be certain there was no tendency to answer differently when speaking directly to a nurse. Compliance with the treatment plan was not reported as validated in any way. Often, if patients do not affirm that they have indeed followed the treatment plan a certain amount of the time, it is not considered an adequate test of the treatment and the data is discarded. Assuming that they followed the plan could lead to invalid conclusions.

What do you think of the operationalization of the variables? The independent variables were not thoroughly described. As has been addressed, the ingredients in Gooeypaste were not discussed to help us understand its pharmacologic action. It would also have been helpful to have an explanation of the way mothers were instructed to use the warm water and vitamin E. Did they use these after every feeding or four times a day? Before the lanolin was applied, were they instructed to air dry their nipples? Was the Gooeypaste to be removed before the next feeding or allowed to soak in? (If its ingredients had been explained, we might have this answered.)

In some studies, the difference between the effectiveness of treatments turns out to be related to the ease of using the treatment rather than any specific action of the treatment itself. As already discussed, the lack of detail about the Painometer makes it difficult to judge what the measurements mean in Table 27.2. However, operationalization of "pain" and "optimism" via such a scale is an accepted way to measure these dependent variables.

The confounding variables are not defined sufficiently or even acknowledged. Even though random assignment was used, it is a small sample. The researcher should have checked on whether some basic variables occurred in similar proportions in all the groups. In addition to the experience of the mothers and the quality of positioning already discussed, several more potential influences on treatment effect could confuse the interpretation of the data. Were any of the mothers experiencing problems establishing milk production, either because of the pain or for some other reason? If so, they might be inclined to feed more often, possibly necessitating more uses of a treatment. Conversely, they might have been so discouraged that they used the treatment less often.

Some readers of this study might ask why there is such a seemingly common problem with early sore nipples in this hospital. (It would have helped if the author had defined the percentage of all mothers that the 30 subjects represent). Could it be that the nurses have very different skills in helping breastfeeding mothers and that poor positioning is not detected early? Or, contrary to the author's intent, could it be that many of the mothers had only the initial nipple tenderness that improves without actual treatment beyond attention to positioning? Perhaps a hospital postpartum unit would be a good place to test Gooeypaste.

When analyzing a study, it is important to step back from its original premises and ask these basic questions. However, it is often difficult to answer them. Instead, we usually have to accept some of the assumptions and choices the author made and then build a critique based on that. Even when the initial conditions of the study are not ideal, the results can still have value.

Literature Review

Nipple pain is a widely acknowledged problem for breastfeeding mothers. There is no great need to establish this from the literature, although there are articles the author could have cited. Types or causes of pain may not all respond to the same treatment. It is therefore important that the literature review be related to the type of pain in the proposed subjects. In this study, it is not likely that *Candidiasis* is a common cause of pain so early postpartum, so it is unclear why the authors mentioned it. Superficial treatment is not likely to relieve engorgement, so its inclusion seems inappropriate.

The article by Cando was the only reference for warm water treatment. It is likely that the author intended to follow the protocol for its use described therein. However, there are no details about frequency of use, fabric used for application, temperature of the compresses, or air-drying afterward. These omissions make it more difficult to judge whether it was a more complex or time-consuming regimen to follow than that for Gooeypaste or lanolin.

Similarly, there is no description of the protocol for lanolin use. Although the author reports that mothers found lanolin to be soothing, there is no finding presented about its effect on healing or continuation of breastfeeding. Apparently the main reason that lanolin was compared was that some of the obstetricians favored it.

For both of these studies, it would be helpful to know whether the subjects studied were similar to those in the current study. Further, did pain relief correlate with longer duration of breastfeeding or more satisfaction with breastfeeding? Many studies do not report longer outcomes such as duration or satisfaction. However, as lactation science matures, it will be important to include these as dependent variables because they are the more important goals.

Readers may not be familiar with the Ouchless theory of pain cited by the authors. They need more description before they can judge its applicability to postpartum nipple soreness. Even if we agree that patient perception of pain is very important, there are other aspects of the pain that are also important—its severity, its duration, its association with an obvious wound, and its meaning to the mother. If the theory suggests that some other aspects of the mother's perception are important to the ultimate resolution of the pain, the authors should have measured those aspects as potential confounding variables.

Discussion

Readers cannot judge how adequately the author used the literature reviewed (see Methods, earlier), so the link to the discussion is missing. In addition, the author does not introduce any further literature in this section and has not delved into the problem of sore nipples to try to understand the causes. Instead, the scope of the study has been limited to treatment. This is not necessarily bad. It does mean that the implications for practice are more difficult to derive because we cannot generalize to any causes of sore nipples except those that occurred in the study. Because we do not learn what those are, the best we can do is to apply the findings to patients whose soreness develops during their hospital stay. Had the author sought to define the causes of the subjects' pain, she might have used the discussion to speculate about why Gooeypaste was especially helpful to these mothers.

In light of the finding that optimism scores were not statistically significantly different between the treatment groups, is the following statement justified: "Since the Gooeypaste mothers were also more optimistic . . . "? No, it is not. The lack of significance means that Gooeypaste could appear higher on the optimism scale simply by chance. Watch carefully for such claims. If you had not read the results, the discussion might mislead you. The suggestion that optimism may lead to longer nursing is reasonable. However, it would have provided even better evidence for Gooeypaste's effectiveness if the researcher had also studied the proportion of mothers in each group who breastfed until at least three months, for example, or who met their goals. The author does admit the need to replicate these findings in a larger sample, and that is an important admission.

Results Revisited

The data do seem consistent with the claim that soreness decreases faster for those women who use Gooeypaste. Nevertheless, the control of confounding variables (alternative explanations) was unknown. Remember that when they started treatment there was no assurance that the groups were similar and no information about variables such as breastfeeding experience, adequacy of positioning, or many others. The author depended heavily on the random assignment of this small sample but did not check on its effectiveness. Therefore, something else may explain why Gooeypaste seemed to work so well. There is also no plausible mechanism discussed.

The data on optimism are not consistent with the claim that Gooeypaste mothers are more optimistic because of the lack of statistical significance. What are the implications for your practice? You would not begin using Gooeypaste immediately in your postpartum clients. You might design a better randomized trial in your work setting and write up a research report. You might investigate Gooeypaste further by contacting the manufacturer for ingredients, mechanism of action, and any studies they conducted. When you find this number of flaws in a study and when they are so basic, you should not adopt the practice change recommended by the author without considerable further investigation.

References

Because these references are fictitious, it is difficult to determine whether important ones were included or not. Some of these references are older, but that is not necessarily negative. The most important deficiency is the lack of a reference for the Painometer. See also the "Note" following the reference list. It tells you that a manufacturer of Gooeypaste partially funded the study. Although that is not necessarily an indication of bias,

you should think about that possibility. Notes about sources of funding are not always present in articles, but it is important to pay attention when they are.

Comments

You may have uncovered other questionable aspects of this sore nipple study that make you uncomfortable in applying its findings. Critical reading can lead to many questions. This study would probably never have made it to publication in its present form because of the deficiencies identified. It illustrates questions that took the process of critical reading in whatever direction occurred to you. You undoubtedly found still more criticism within the commentary.

Peer review of this article would, no doubt, have required that the author provide a citation for the Painometer, additional data about the pain scores and other ways of comparing them, a change in the wording about the claim that Gooeypaste was related to higher optimism, and more information about the potential confounding variables. That is the purpose of peer review—to present to readers a good-quality article without fundamental flaws so that what remains is valuable information (though not perfect), and so that the judgments required of readers are about more subtle or more arguable dimensions of the study.

Nursing Strikes—Identifying Patterns

by Emma Halter and Makit Gogh

Journal of Intermittent Phenomena 13: 44–47; 1992.

Abstract

A questionnaire was distributed to over 700 breastfeeding mothers in two suburban pediatric practices. Of this group, 200 reported having had experience with their babies refusing to nurse. There was a great deal of variation in reasons for refusing—in measures tried, in other life events, and in mothers' feelings. Stress and biting may be two types of events that precipitate refusals. Teaching mothers about possible nursing refusals in prenatal classes may help them realize that they can overcome such discouraging events.

Introduction

Breastfeeding mothers often report[1,2] that their babies display a sudden lack of interest in breastfeeding that persists long enough to cause concern about hunger and dehydration. The mothers also experience engorgement. These "nursing strikes" can be the reason for the introduction of formula; and weaning may follow soon after. For mothers who intended to continue breastfeeding longer, such unplanned weaning is emotionally difficult. Pediatric experts agree that continuing breastfeeding for 6 months to 1 year is best for infant health.[3] Some scientists have found that mothers believe that nursing strikes are related to the return of their menses[2] or to starting oral contraceptives.[4] There has been little attempt to study this phenomenon. As a first step, we collected data on breastfeeding couplets in two private pediatric practices and looked for patterns. The study was approved by the Review Board of Busy Hospital and subjects gave written, informed consent.

Subjects and Methods

Participants were mothers of currently breastfeeding infants who were recruited by lactation consultants, nurses, and nurse practitioners in two large, suburban group pediatric practices. From March 1, 2004 to May 31, 2004, all nursing mothers whose babies had appointments for any reason were invited to complete a questionnaire while they waited to see their providers. Those who needed help with childcare in order to complete the survey received that help.

The questionnaire (Appendix A—Figure 27.6) was developed by the authors after reviewing the books for mothers and professionals that suggest causes and remedies. It was designed to be concise so that mothers could finish it while they waited for their appointments (about 10 minutes to complete). Descriptive statistics were calculated for most responses. Correlations were determined for demographic characteristics and responses.

Results

During the 3-month period, the combined practices had 1032 breastfeeding couplet visits. Because some couplets had multiple appointments, 955 different couplets

FIGURE 27.6
Appendix A: Questionnaire for Nursing Strikes.

Your help with this questionnaire is greatly appreciated. We are trying to understand why some babies occasionally stop breast-feeding for a few feeds. Please answer as fully as you can, and feel free to add any comments you would like.

1. Are you currently breastfeeding? ____ Yes ____ No
2. How old is your breastfed baby? ____ How old are you? ____
3. Is this your first breastfed baby? ____ Yes ____ No
   A. If yes, do you have other children? ____ Yes ____ No
      If yes, how many? ____
   B. If no, how many other children have you breastfed? ____
4. With your currently breastfeeding baby, if you have had any of the following problems at *any* time, please check:
   ____ Difficulty latching on
   ____ Sore nipples
   ____ Teething
   ____ Engorgement
   ____ Breast infection
   ____ Plugged milk ducts
   ____ Baby refused to breastfeed
   ____ Baby had a cold or stuffy nose that interfered with feeding
   ____ Biting
5. Since your baby was born, have you resumed your menstrual periods? ____ Yes ____ No
   A. If yes, how old was your baby when the first period started? ____
6. Please check any of the following birth control methods you have used since this baby was born and the age of the baby when you started using it:

Method	Age of baby when started use
____ Condoms (male or female)	____
____ Natural family planning	____
____ Lactational amenorrhea	____
____ Depo-Provera shots	____
____ Birth control pills	____
____ Intrauterine device (IUD)	____
____ Tubal ligation	____

7. Has your baby ever stopped breastfeeding for at least 24 hours? ____ Yes ____ No
   If no, you have finished this questionnaire. Thank you very much.
   If yes, how old was your baby at the time? ____
   If yes, please check all of the following which you feel apply to your situation, or write a brief description of why you think the baby stopped nursing:

Breastfeeding stopped for at least 24 hours because:
   ____ Mother needed a medicine and was advised to temporarily stop nursing.
   ____ Mother and baby were separated by a trip, a storm, or other unexpected event.
   ____ Baby had surgery.
   ____ Baby was too ill to breastfeed.
   ____ Baby was jaundiced.
   ____ Mother had sore nipples that needed rest.
   ____ Baby was teething.
   ____ Mother returned to work.
   ____ Baby had bitten mother and stopped nursing soon after.
   ____ Baby refused to nurse but would take other food.
   ____ Unknown. The reason for stopping was never clear.
   ____ Other: Please describe why you think your baby stopped nursing:

8. If your baby had stopped nursing for at least 24 hours, please check all of the following that describe your feelings during the time your baby did not breastfeed:
   ____ Concerned breastfeeding was finished for good.
   ____ Worried about hunger or dehydration.
   ____ Concerned about breasts becoming engorged.
   ____ Relieved to have a short break.
   ____ Confused about what was happening.
   ____ Confused about the cause of the refusal to nurse.
   ____ Thought baby might be sick.
   ____ Other. Please describe:

9. If your baby had stopped nursing for at least 24 hours, please check all of the following actions you tried to help resume feeding:
   ____ Just kept trying to nurse in the usual ways.
   ____ Just gave my baby time to feel better.
   ____ Called the lactation consultant, physician's office, or breastfeeding counselor (e.g., La Leche League).
   ____ Talked to a family member or friend.
   ____ Nursed my baby when he/she was very sleepy.
   ____ Increased the amount of skin-to-skin contact we had.
   ____ Took a bath with my baby.
   ____ Used a sling or pack.
   ____ Tried to reduce the stress in my life.
   ____ Other. Please describe:

Thank you so much for your help. If you would like to learn the results of this study, please let us know at your next appointment.

---

were offered a questionnaire. Of those, 780 agreed to complete the survey. For various reasons, only 600 questionnaires were actually complete enough to use. Of these, 400 had never had the problem of the baby refusing to nurse for 24 hours. Of the 200 refusers, 30 had stopped nursing at a few days old because of jaundice in the infant. Another 70 mothers identified medication, surgery, illness, separation, and maternal sore nipples (see Table 27.3). Teething was the cause 30 mothers indicated.

These causes, although stressful and needing remedies, were not the most perplexing. The nursing strikes of interest were those that 70 mothers marked as unknown reason, other reason, or preference for another food. Of course, because these mothers were nursing at the time of the appointment, they had overcome the strike. Many of the events that occurred near a nursing strike also occurred in couplets that never experienced a strike. The two strongest correlations were an increase in

TABLE 27.3	
Reasons for Stopping Nursing as Determined by Mothers	
Newborn jaundice	30
Medication	10
Surgery	12
Illness of baby	20
Maternal sore nipples	15
Separation of mother and baby	13
Teething	30
	130

TABLE 27.4		
Correlations between Unexplained Nursing Strikes and Recent Events in the Lives of the Breastfeeding Dyads		
Event	Number of Dyads	r (Correlation)
Resuming menses within 1 week of strike (<3 mo old)	5	0.21
Resuming menses	3	0.15
Starting birth control within same month	2	0.09
Increase in family stress	15	0.55
Biting	16	0.59

TABLE 27.5	
Remedies Used by Mothers to Overcome Nursing Strikes	
Remedy	% of Mothers Who Used It
Time and patience	83
Calling lactation professional	80
Nursing during sleep	50
Skin-to-skin soothing	55
Bathing together	30
Sling or pack	34
Trying to reduce stress	42

family stress and biting (see Table 27.4). However, together these included only 15 percent of couplets who experienced nursing strikes.

Discussion

Mothers need lactation professionals who are aware of the potential for nursing strikes and who can encourage them to not give up. That is probably the most important message of this study. Short periods of refusal to nurse are common. Determining a cause is very difficult. Based on this survey, we suggest educating mothers in prenatal classes about possible refusals. Cautioning them against responding strongly to biting and emphasizing the importance of stress management may be the most specific strategies that emerge from this data (see Table 27.5). There is no evidence herein that resuming menses or starting the birth control pill, as suggested by others, is causal.

References

1. Complete D. Weaning from breast. *Feeding Babies Journal* 14:120–125; 2000.
2. Empp A. Common concerns of breast-feeding mothers in a food assistance program. *Nutrition Group Reports* 55:37–41; 1996.
3. Healthy World Alliance. Breastfeeding best for babies. *HA* 56:123–125; 2000.
4. Wilgot E. Postpartum menstrual cycles. *Annals of Families* 33:293–255; 1991.

Discussion of Second Practice Article

Nursing Strikes—Identifying Patterns

Title

How will the authors define "nursing strike"? Although experienced breastfeeding mothers may speak of this phenomenon as though everyone agrees on it, a clear definition is necessary in order to determine clearly associated variables. What do you think should be included and excluded? You might expect to see refusal to nurse by the baby for a certain length of time (more than one feeding) and for no obvious reason. Would it be reasonable to allow certain probable causes and disallow others?

When attempting to explore a previously understudied phenomenon like this, there are many possible choices for the definition, none of which is right or wrong. Rather, clarity is the most important criterion for judging the choices—so that investigators, subjects, and readers all agree on which breast refusals constitute nursing strikes.

What "patterns" do you consider, based on the title? Do the authors intend to see whether babies at a particular age are more likely to go on strike? Will they study whether increased bottle use or separation (common when babies start day care) often precede strikes? For mothers who have breastfed other children, is it likely that prior instances of strikes in the older child correlate with more strikes in the current nursing baby? Many patterns are possible, and you can compare the patterns you would like to see investigated to what the researchers chose.

What study design does the title suggest? Is this a trial to determine whether certain events cause or specific treatments cure nursing strikes? Do you know of other studies of this phenomenon that have gained enough basic information to conduct such a trial? For this exercise, the topic of nursing strikes was chosen because there is not much literature on it. Therefore, a descriptive study of some sort is more likely at this point in the development of knowledge.

If the authors intended to conduct a qualitative study, what kind of data might they collect? They might ask mothers to tape-record the feelings they remember having and the effect on their confidence when the baby went on strike. Alternatively, they might try to include mothers from many different cultures and compare the ways the mothers describe the experience of nursing strikes. If they do a quantitative study, they might try to find patterns by using correlation between variables as an outcome measure.

Authors' Names

Again, because this is a mock article, you will not be able to find these authors' names in any database. However, for an actual article, if you wanted to know whether the authors had published on this topic previously, you could search *Index Medicus* or an online database such as *PubMed* (www.pubmed.org) by author name. That would be a worthwhile effort if you need the most complete information available.

Abstract

The fact that 200 mothers claim experience with breast refusal might be surprising. This should start you thinking about the definition again. The definition may indicate that many more mothers have had strikes than your experience suggests. Alternatively, it could be that this problem is much more widespread than anyone realizes simply because no one has sought to study its prevalence before.

The source of subjects was two pediatric suburban practices. Will the authors provide more demographic data on maternal income, education, race, ethnic heritage, and type of insurance? If the sample population is primarily white, married, and middle class, will the results apply to mothers in other groups? The authors used a questionnaire, which requires literacy. Did they determine whether any subjects had trouble reading English? Did they provide the questions in another language? Did the nature of the tool exclude mothers with visual disabilities or language barriers? Why did they single out biting and stress as events to mention in the abstract? Were these especially strong findings, or the only findings that mothers can modify? What is their reasoning for suggesting that prenatal education might help?

Table 27.3

Reasons for stopping nursing as determined by mothers: Note first that only 130 of the 900 mentioned in the abstract appear in this table. You will want to read why in the text. Are there reasons for nursing strikes that you had thought of that are not in this list? The investigators should explain their reasons for these choices. Note that no descriptive statistics, such as percentages, or any tests of significance appear in this table.

Table 27.4

Correlations: Why the focus on "unexplained" strikes, and how was that defined? Why do the events listed in this table differ from the "reasons" given in Table 27.3? Although the correlation statistic r is presented, no statistical significance is reported. None of the correlations is high ($r = 0.7$ or above) in many definitions. Do moderate correlations like 0.55 and 0.59 represent the most powerful of the possible variables associated with strikes? Has something been left out of the study inadvertently? The text of the article should address all of these questions. The explanations may be too complex to include as footnotes to the table.

Table 27.5

Remedies: Did all of the mothers who completed this survey successfully overcome nursing strikes? If so, they do not represent all of the mothers who have experienced strikes, because weaning occurs after strikes in some unknown proportion of cases. How would limiting the data collection to mothers who have successfully overcome strikes limit the applicability of the findings? Are there other remedies the authors should have included?

Results

First, note that the mothers targeted by the researchers were breastfeeding at the time of the appointment. Apparently, mothers who had stopped breastfeeding after a strike were not included. Regarding the claims, the strongest correlations between variables included in the questionnaire were the correlation between strike and biting and between strike and stress. The descriptive data appear to support the claim, but there is no report of statistical tests. In terms of ruling out alternative explanations:

1. Do the investigators offer any analysis of whether mothers who did not agree to participate were similar to or different from the mothers who participated? (This problem is similar to the "dropout" problem discussed in the Critical Reading section under "Results.") Some of these mothers may be unable to read English. Without knowing more about the nonparticipants, it is difficult to know how to apply (**generalize**) the results.
2. Is the list of preceding events such as medication, surgery, and jaundice in Table 27.3 sufficiently explanatory to exclude them from the study of nursing strikes? They are potential confounding variables if the essence of a nursing strike is that there is no "obvious" explanation. This is where definitions and the purpose of the investigation need to be very clear in order to interpret the data properly.
3. Are there plausible mechanisms suggested or investigated for the relationships the authors found? Typically, the results section does not discuss the mechanism unless it was the focus of the study. In a descriptive study, it is important to think about how the relationships might work in order for the results to be taken seriously. Even if no strong evidence is available for a mechanism, if it does not violate known principles of physiology or human behavior, it is plausible. Both biting and stress could plausibly relate to a nursing strike in a baby. As you read more of the article, you will be able to determine whether you believe the authors' explanations.

Methods

What is the design of this study? It is descriptive and cross-sectional. It takes a snapshot of the couplets in one area on a limited-time basis and contacts them only once, so it looks at a cross-section of the population. It is also correlational; the researchers used a structured instrument to measure variables and then sought statistically significant relationships.

Was the definition of nursing strike clear and appropriate? From the questionnaire itself, rather than from the article, you can determine that the definition was "stopped nursing for at least 24 hours." Knowledgeable professionals could disagree with this definition. Some might prefer a different time period or different wording. What is crucial is that the authors and mothers mean the same thing when they use this definition.

If there were a big discrepancy in understanding, the **internal validity** of the study would be in jeopardy. Because this is such a new area of research, the investigators could have done some work before this big study to be more certain about the meaning of this definition. They could have conducted a pilot study and talked in more depth with women about their experiences with nursing strikes. They might have suggested different definitions until the mothers and researchers agreed that they were identifying the same phenomenon. They also could have asked lactation and child development experts for their opinions on the definition.

If you were to use this study to try to convince childbirth educators or pediatricians to address nursing strikes, it is very important that you discuss nursing strike as defined in this article and that you not extend the findings to some other looser or stricter definition. The choices listed in the questionnaire are not defined for mothers, but most are probably reasonably clear. If you can think of multiple, significantly different interpretations for any of the phrases, you may have identified a less valuable part of the data.

Questionnaire

Look at the questionnaire itself. There are entire courses on how to design questionnaires in order to obtain unbiased information. You could ask many questions about the quality of this one. Even if reasonable people would disagree, it is important to think about some aspects of it. Here are just a few ideas about specific questions:

1. Item 1 does not ask whether the mother is breastfeeding exclusively or partially. With a baby younger than six months of age, the nursing strike could have been the cause of a switch to partial breastfeeding. The investigators will not be able to determine such a switch from this question.
2. Questions such as Item 3 about previous breastfeeding experience often fail to ask whether the experience overall was positive or negative.

3. In Item 4, it is not clear what information or relationship the investigators were seeking. It might have been useful to ask the age at which the mother experienced the problem in order to determine whether it was close in time to the strike. It should probably have an "other" category in case the mother wants to list problems she has had. Among ones that might bear some relationship to nursing strikes would be those in which the baby has had some frustration in getting enough milk. These may include delayed lactogenesis, delayed or overactive milk ejection, nipples that needed reshaping, or bottle-feeding that led to poor breast suckling.
4. In Item 6, some of the contraceptive methods listed may not be familiar to all mothers, but those who had used them would probably recognize them.
5. Item 7 does not allow for multiple instances of nursing strikes. As a result, some mothers may list multiple causes, intending them to refer to separate events. Often, researchers ask mothers to reflect the most recent occurrence in their answer.
6. In Item 8, the age of the baby greatly influences the mother's concern about a nursing strike. With babies who are taking solid foods and other liquids, a 24-hour nursing strike may not be alarming. Therefore, it might be important to discuss the correlations separately for different age groups.

Subjects could be characterized by age, the number of children they have, the number of children they breastfed, return of menses, use of contraception, and problems experienced. Other variables that might influence their nursing strike experience and interpretation, such as ethnic group or planned duration of breastfeeding, are not included. This often will happen in descriptive studies. You will have to decide whether the information is useful to you even with some deficiencies.

Introduction and Literature Review

Because there is little research on this topic, the review is somewhat limited. Some authors will seek what they believe is related research from other topics that cover the hypotheses they wish to highlight. For example, if they related nursing strikes to stress in the mother, they might study other research on mother-infant stress responses. These authors chose to look for patterns in a large number of couplets without a specific hypothesis. If you knew of articles they failed to include, you might judge their effort to be incomplete.

Discussion

If this is a representative cross-section of breastfeeding mothers, the authors' statement that nursing strikes are common is probably true. However, we are not sure just what group this sample represents, and we know that it does not represent mothers who weaned after a nursing strike. Therefore, it can only be a piece of the puzzle. On the other hand, if nursing strikes are very common and most nursing mothers handle them smoothly, then it would be very important to understand how they coped in order to help those who wean as a result.

The suggestion to educate mothers about nursing strikes is difficult to argue with, although doing it in the usual childbirth class may not be the best time. Similarly, although education about biting and stress are appropriate, we cannot expect them to resolve the problems of nursing strikes based on this study alone. Furthermore, although the authors claim to have found no evidence that resuming menses or starting birth control pills caused strikes, this does not constitute the best evidence. We would believe that a prospective study that queried mothers about strikes beginning shortly after birth and carefully recorded other possibly relevant variables on a regular basis would more likely detect a relationship.

Results Revisited

Depending on how convinced you are that this sample resembles your patients, you may want to initiate research yourself. At the very least, you could include questions about nursing strikes in more of your routine follow-up calls. This study, like many descriptive studies, raises more questions than it answers. To review, the moderate correlation of stress and biting with strikes (although the statistical significance is unknown) is consistent with the claim that these are two of the more common preceding events. The biggest failure of this study is its inability to rule out alternative explanations because of study design, poorly characterized sample, and inadequate definitions. Although the authors discuss implications for practice, there could be a lot of disagreement on clinical implications because of the degree of uncertainty about so many possible confounders.

References

This appears to be a relevant list. Even though the mothers in reference 2 may be a different sample than the ones in this study, the authors use that reference only to suggest what others have noted, which is appropriate.

▶ SUMMARY

The process of critique presented in this chapter is structured around the parts of a scientific article because that is how most clinicians will use it. However, the more general themes of the process of critical reading, as outlined in the following list, are not determined solely through the article's sections. As a clinician who wants to decide whether to apply the results of a study to your work, you want to determine the following:

1. What did they choose to include and exclude in their literature review, in their subjects, in the survey questions, and in the comparisons they made in data analysis? Did they adequately explain and justify their choices? Did their choices make the sample patients or study situation so different from your practice that you cannot justifiably use the results?

2. What else could they have done? Why did they not do that? Could they have included more mothers? Could they have studied them for a longer period? Could there have been a more diverse ethnic base? Could they have included a control group?

3. For every limitation of the study identified by answering questions 1 and 2, what might have been the impact on the study's findings? For example, if you think that the authors should have included more low-income women, how might that have affected the finding that intending to breastfeed more than twelve weeks is the best predictor of continuing to breastfeed at least six weeks? You may be reasoning that the low-income women in your practice must return to work by six weeks. Therefore, very few even plan to breastfeed past six weeks and some other predictor variable would tell you more about what enables them to continue to six weeks. When critically reading your scientific colleagues' work, it is not enough to say what they should have done differently. You need to justify your critique by stating how that might have changed the study's results.

Critically reading a scientific article is a skill that grows with experience and strengthens your practice as a lactation consultant. Learning how to read and analyze scientific articles opens many doors for your continued learning. Self-direction and self-education are hallmarks of the professional lactation consultant. You are well along on the road of lifelong education.

▶ CHAPTER 27—AT A GLANCE

Facts you learned—

- ◆ Editorials, while insightful, are not studies or critically reviewed.

- ◆ Case studies report on instances of a problem, diagnosis, or treatment; they cannot be used to generalize.

- ◆ Meta-analysis combines data from several studies to test conclusions.

- ◆ Reviews are written by experts who analyze the best and worst studies, with little or no original data.

◆ Clinical practice articles are reports of applications in real life.

◆ Research reports put a long-held belief or new idea to a scientific test.

◆ Titles explain main findings and may be two sentences long.

◆ Authors tend to publish profusely in a specific, narrow discipline.

◆ Abstracts are brief summaries that explain a study.

◆ Introductions contain the purpose, parameters, and restraints of the study.

◆ Literature reviews explain previous research.

◆ Methods describe how researchers operationalized the hypothesis, how subjects were recruited, tools used to measure outcomes, surveys, scales, tests, definition of terms, and statistical methods.

◆ Results are often displayed in graphs, tables, and charts; they are peer reviewed for accuracy.

◆ Discussion reviews study reasons and other relevant literature, summarize results, and suggest applications and further research.

◆ References and the bibliography list all citations referred to in the article.

◆ Study design may be retrospective, case-control, prospective, cross-sectional, survey, descriptive, qualitative, experiment, or trial.

◆ Tools (instruments) measure dependent variable consistently.

◆ Statistical theory is based on probability.

◆ Study frequency is based on samples of populations.

◆ Statistical tests include distributions, centered and unbalanced bell curves, confidence intervals, chi-square, Cohen's kappa, Cronbach's alpha, regression, and T-tests.

◆ Odds ratio is a summary of relative proportion in two different groups.

Applying what you learned—

◆ Look at the title of the article and consider what you know about the topic, how you would have studied it, and what you expect to find.

◆ Read the authors' names and the abstract.

◆ Identify terms and key concepts.

◆ Study the tables and graphs and read the results.

◆ Read the methods to determine whether the authors can justify their conclusions.

◆ Read the introduction and literature review and consider significance, accuracy, appropriateness of studies, omissions, and thoroughness of explanations.

◆ Read the discussion and watch for speculation, suggestions for further research, and flaws or weaknesses.

◆ Read the results again to check that data is consistent with claims and that there is no other equal or better explanation.

◆ Watch for spurious relationships.

◆ Determine what the researchers chose to include and exclude and why.

▶ BIBLIOGRAPHY

Bekelman J et al. Scope and impact of financial conflicts of interest in biomedical research: A systematic review. *JAMA* 289:454–465; 2003.

Bhandari M et al. Association between industry funding and statistically significant pro-industry findings in medical and surgical randomized trials. *CMAJ* 170(4):477–480; 2004.

Candy D. Funding of research by infant formula companies. *Br Med J* 318:260; 1999.

Carr JJ. *A Crash Course in Statistics*. Solana Beach, CA: High Text Publishers; 1994.

Goldbeck-Wood S. Evidence on peer review: Scientific quality control or smokescreen? *Br Med J* 318:44–45; 1999.

Hicks C. Bridging the gap between research and practice: An assessment of the value of a study day in developing critical research reading skills in midwives. *Midwifery* 10:18–25; 1994.

Jenken J et al. Changing nursing practice through research utilization: Consistent support for breastfeeding mothers. *Appl Nurs Res* 12:22–29; 1999.

Labbok M. Toward consistency in breastfeeding definitions. *Stud Fam Plan* 21(4):226–230; 1990.

Martens P. A mini-lesson in statistics: What causes treatment groups to be deemed "not statistically different?" *J Hum Lact* 11(2):117–121; 1995.

Massey V. *Nursing Research: A Study and Learning Tool*. Springhouse, PA: Springhouse Publishers; 1991.

Porter A. Positive messages on breast feeding would result in need for infant formula decreasing (Letter). *Br Med J* 318:260–261; 1999.

Rothenberg R I. *Probability and Statistics*. New York: Harcourt Brace Jovanovich; 1991.

Sackett D et al. *Evidence-Based Medicine*. New York: Churchill Livingstone; 1997.

Shaughnessy A et al. Clinical jazz: Harmonizing clinical experience and evidence-based medicine. *J Fam Pract* 47:425–428; 1999.

Smith G, Egger M. Meta-analyses of observational data should be done with due care (Letter). *Br Med J* 318:56; 1999.

vanRooyen S et al. Effect of open peer review on quality of reviews and on reviewers' recommendations: A randomised trial. *Br Med J* 318:23–27; 1999.

Waterston T et al. Researchers must recognise damage done by overt association with formula manufacturers. *Br Med J* 318:260; 1999.

▶ WEB SITES

www.ahcpr.gov—Evidence-Based Practice Centers, Agency for Health Care Policy and Research.

www.lalecheleague.org—La Leche League International Center for Breastfeeding Information.

www.nlm.nih.gov—MEDLINE and PubMed.

www.angelfire.com/in/pedscapes/index.html—Links to clinical journal home pages.

www.nofreelunch.org—Web site for healthcare professional education on pharmaceutical industry influence peddling.

BREASTFEEDING PROMOTION AND CHANGE

Excellence can be attained if you
Care more than others think is wise,
Risk more than others think is safe,
Dream more than others think is practical,
And expect more than others think is possible. —*Anonymous*

Promoting breastfeeding presents unique challenges in societies where artificial feeding is the norm. Undertaking the challenge of breastfeeding promotion requires strong, confident leadership. In order to enlist the support of colleagues and administrators, you will need to understand other points of view and work toward everyone's mutual benefit. This approach will enable you to build a strong team that can arrive at creative solutions. Being an effective change agent requires skills in assertiveness and persuasion and an appreciation for the importance of giving recognition and praise. Understanding why others resist change will help resolve conflicts and identify common goals, so that you can move on to define problems, goals, and strategies.

Capitalizing on various personality styles will contribute to productive group dynamics. Major international initiatives will support your promotion efforts as you seek to remove obstacles toward achieving baby-friendly practices. Chapter 1 of this text began with a historical perspective on infant feeding and highlights of the major initiatives to support, protect, and promote breastfeeding. This final chapter focuses on ways you can provide leadership in breastfeeding promotion and facilitate change that will continue to empower women to breastfeed.

KEY TERMS

Ad Council
assertiveness
Baby-Friendly Hospital
  Initiative
Breastfeeding Awareness
  Campaign
breastfeeding committee
breastfeeding promotion
change agent
conflict resolution
difficult people

formula manufacturer
  advertising
Global Strategy for Infant
  and Young Child
  Feeding
International Baby Food
  Action Network
  (IBFAN)
Infant Feeding Action
  Coalition Canada
  (INFACT)

International Code of
  Marketing of Breast-
  milk Substitutes
Joint Commission on
  Accreditation of
  Healthcare
  Organizations
  (JCAHO)
Media Watch
National Alliance for
  Breastfeeding Advocacy
  (NABA)
paradigm

personality types
persuasion
resistance to change
Seven Habits of Highly
  Effective People
team building
Ten Steps to Successful
  Breastfeeding
World Alliance for
  Breastfeeding Action
  (WABA)
World Health Assembly
  (WHA)

▶ TRAITS OF A STRONG LEADER

It is not surprising to learn that people prefer to work with people they like! Human nature draws us to people who are cheerful, generous, and considerate of others. People who possess these qualities find it easier to generate cooperation from those around them. Others may need to make a concerted effort to present themselves in a manner that will achieve the same results.

Part of being an effective leader is instilling confidence in others. People respond well to a leader who is self-confident, assertive, and forthright. The key to being influential is to focus on solutions, priorities, and action. An effective problem solver will look for problem areas and then focus on solutions. After establishing goals, be aware of the priorities that will help you achieve them, and be willing to take risks to put your ideas into action. Be approachable, listen well, and guard against snap judgments. All of these attributes will help you build a strong team and garner support for your breastfeeding and other healthcare initiatives.

The approach that Stephen Covey (1990) presents in his book *The 7 Habits of Highly Effective People* provides a helpful structure for examining ways to promote breastfeeding. Covey states that an effective person is proactive, establishes goals, sets priorities, and is genuinely open to others' ideas. The effective person works toward mutual benefits for both sides of an issue, promotes unity, and actively seeks self-renewal, both physically and mentally. These practices will contribute to your success in facilitating real change. Each of the seven habits are explored below within the context of breastfeeding promotion.

Choose to Be Effective

Steven Covey writes, "Our behavior is a function of our decisions, not our conditions." It is human nature to react immediately to events. However, there is always a gap between a stimulus and our response to that stimulus. The key to our effectiveness is how we use that gap. A spontaneous response is usually impulsive and based on feelings that are aroused by particular conditions. Such an impetuous reaction lacks forethought and may not lead to responsible action.

A proactive person recognizes that we have the ability to choose our responses. As Eleanor Roosevelt said, "No one can make you feel inferior without your permission." It is not what happens to us but our response to what happens to us that determines the outcome. We can take the initiative to create circumstances and make things happen by first reflecting on our options and thinking through possible actions. Our responses may not always produce the desired results. When we make mistakes, it is important to acknowledge them, learn, and go on. Making mistakes is part of being a leader and a problem solver. Making mistakes simply means we are trying! Baseball players know they have scores of strikeouts for every home run they hit. Leadership is a learning process, strengthened as much by every failure as by every success.

In bolstering your effectiveness as a leader, consider how you respond to questionable practices or unsupportive coworkers. A reactive response might be to defend what you are trying to accomplish by arguing your position and backing up your argument with research articles and other documentation. In a proactive response, you might first try to learn the reasons for resistance to or disinterest in your proposal. Understanding what has led to a situation is an important first step to finding appropriate solutions.

Start with a Blueprint

An effective planner thinks first and then acts. Imagine if an architect were to begin building a new structure without first having created a blueprint. Where would a traveler be without first mapping out a route? Knowing what you want the end result to be will dictate how you plan to arrive there. First, visualize the process of getting to where you want to be. Map it out on paper with specific goals. Then determine how you will accomplish those goals to arrive at your destination. Leadership and vision must always precede any action. You may be the person to provide that leadership and vision to others in your mission to promote breastfeeding.

Creating a mission statement will help guide your actions. WHO and UNICEF have provided a blueprint for breastfeeding promotion with the *Ten Steps to Successful Breastfeeding* and the *Global Strategy for Infant and Young Child Feeding*. These seminal documents will help focus your efforts and will guide the development of appropriate breastfeeding policies and protocols. They will help you identify practices that can stay in place and areas that need improvement. Your end goal is healthy mothers and babies. Keeping this result in mind will help you determine how to get there.

Focus on What Is Important

People often become so overinvolved in what they perceive to be urgent that the important issues get little or no attention. Do not let the tyranny of the urgent get in the way of the important. To spend time doing what is important usually requires that you learn to say "no" to others and "yes" to yourself. An effective person practices self-management, makes decisions, and then acts on them. Learn to distinguish between what is urgent and what is important, recognizing that they are often not the same. Prioritize important changes, develop a time line, and stay committed to your goals. Focusing on what is important will help you prevent your efforts from being diverted to distractions, crises, or obstacles.

There are a variety of ways to organize and execute goals and tasks around priorities, ranging from notes and checklists to calendars (both print and electronic), appointment books, and daily planners. Delegate tasks to a particular time and person. Becoming comfortable with delegating tasks to others requires that you trust others to come through for you. Such trust brings out the best in people. You may need to settle for things being done differently than you would have done them. The only way to build a strong team is to bring out the best in the other team members.

Teach other members of your staff how to assist breastfeeding mothers and babies so that you can delegate this responsibility to others. You cannot expect cooperation and compliance until you ensure that others are equipped to carry through appropriately. Time is at a premium in healthcare, especially in hospitals and health clinics, where staffing is low. With effective time management, supportive breastfeeding practices need not tax an already busy day for maternity staff or caregivers with other responsibilities. Identify the essential elements breastfeeding mothers need to learn, and focus on those areas.

Work Toward Mutual Benefit

Initiating change and planning promotion efforts requires strong teamwork. It is important that you help create mutual benefits for both sides of an issue. Success cannot be achieved at the expense of others. All parties need to feel good about the outcome. If two opposing sides are unable to compromise, be creative and try to find an acceptable third alternative. Help each side understand that, "The end result may not be your way or my way, but a better way." As a team, you can work together to determine acceptable results and identify new options to achieve those results.

All members of the team need to be on an even playing field. Establishing the expectation that everyone leaves their credentials and personalities at the door will help to achieve this. Identify the key issues and concerns and keep everyone focused on topics rather than on personalities or job titles. In planning and decision making, you want to include those who are receptive to the change as well as those who you anticipate will resist. List the needs and concerns of people on both sides of an issue, and work toward everyone's mutual benefit. If there appear to be losers on a particular issue, look for ways that both parties can benefit so that there are only winners.

Understand Other Points of View

Attempting to see an issue from another person's point of view will enhance communication. People do not generally listen with the intent to understand. Consequently, the way a problem is viewed often *is* the problem. Effective listening involves patience, openness, and a desire to understand. When you are genuinely open to other people's ideas, they are more likely to be open to yours. Listen until you can explain their point of view as well as they can. Remain open to allowing others' arguments and points of view to influence your thinking. The better you understand, the more you can appreciate others' views. Reflective listening will help you listen with intent and openness, paving the way to mutually developed, creative solutions.

In order to successfully motivate other people to change, it is important that you understand their reasons for resistance. The changes you propose may conflict with the way things "have always been done." Attempt to understand specific concerns and worries and to see the issue the way others see it. One effective method for doing this is to role-play the discussion of an issue with another colleague, placing yourself in the role of the resistor. Such an exercise will help you more clearly see the concerns and determine counterarguments. Listen attentively and with an open mind to others' arguments and concerns. Although it can be easy to assign negative motives to those with whom you disagree, it may be helpful to remember that most healthcare professionals enter the healthcare field because they care deeply about helping others. Everyone's end goal in breastfeeding is healthy mothers and babies. There may simply be differences of opinion on what that constitutes and how to get there. Remain open to flexibility and compromise.

Build a Strong Team

Covey tells us that the whole is greater than the sum of its parts. Work toward achieving unity and building a strong team. An effective team builds on each person's strengths and compensates for weaknesses. Help team members learn to sidestep negative energy and to resist taking criticism personally. Communicating back and forth until you reach a solution that is mutually comfortable fosters trust and cooperation. When others begin to feel ownership of a problem, they become more engaged and ultimately become part of the solution. Remaining open to new alternatives and compromises will help you facilitate team members taking ownership of the proposed changes.

An effective team-building climate is one in which it is safe and comfortable for everyone to air disagreements and concerns. Differences in point of view can provide valuable resources, insights, and perceptions. A variety of opinions and approaches will add to your knowledge and understanding. Two people can disagree, and both can be right—they just interpret differently. Validating everyone's perspective will help the team achieve its goals.

Take Care of Yourself

Covey says that in order to be an effective person you need to be healthy, both physically and mentally. This means paying attention to exercise, nutrition, and stress. Using your value system to guide what you say and do will help to keep you focused in a positive direction. Getting and staying in touch with your inner self will help you draw on your innate enthusiasm and energy. Continue to learn and share information with the staff, helping them stay focused on the vision and bringing out the best in each of them. Cultivate relationships, especially with people you perceive as adversaries, while keeping the team on track and working cooperatively.

 ## INCREASING SELF-CONFIDENCE

Self-confidence is an essential factor in actively facilitating change. How you perceive yourself and your abilities has a tremendous influence on how you project yourself to others. Additionally, "your attitude will determine your altitude." In other words, how successful you view yourself to be often determines your level of success. If you focus on your faults rather than your strengths, you may prevent yourself from soaring to great heights. The principles outlined in this section will help you maintain perspective and increase your ability to take action in a self-assured manner (Browder, 1994).

Much of your attitude involves the vocabulary you use in self-talk. Replace negative phrases such as, "I hope I don't . . . ," with positive self-talk such as, "I will. . . ." Tell yourself how confident you are. Rather than saying, "I wish I were . . ." or "I should be . . . ," tell yourself, "I am. . . ." Table 28.1 contains powerful statements to replace those that convey less positive messages. Positive and negative thinking are both learned habits. Simply stated, if you continually expect to fail, you probably will fail! You can recondition your mind to think positively by replacing negative thoughts with positive ones. Approach every situation with the belief that you will succeed. Focus on the best way to do the job right, and visualize yourself doing it!

Do not allow fear of failure to undermine your self-confidence. If you want good things to happen, you have to make them happen. Sometimes that means taking a risk. If you make mistakes along the way, congratulations! That means you took a risk. Learn to view your mistakes as lessons, not failures, and to regard a mistake as just another way of doing things. To borrow a phrase from a colleague, making mistakes is proof that someone out there is trying! When you make a mistake—and you will—acknowledge it and regard it as a learning experience. Trust in your ability to learn, and help others trust in their ability to learn as well. This is especially important when your efforts to change practices will require others to learn new skills. Coping with failure builds strength

and wisdom. Help others learn from their mistakes and recognize that every defeat is another step toward success.

The concept of "emotional intelligence" describes factors that come into play when people with high IQs fail while people with average IQs succeed. Emotional intelligence includes such attributes as self-awareness, impulse control, persistence, zeal, self-motivation, empathy, and social deftness (Goleman, 2002, 1997). These qualities can help you succeed in your goals, earning breastfeeding support and optimized health outcomes for mothers and babies.

▶ INCREASING ASSERTIVENESS

Caregivers who serve breastfeeding women are predominantly female. Women often are concerned that others may perceive their assertiveness negatively and interpret it as aggressive behavior. Considering assertive behavior a strong asset will help you become comfortable with your assertiveness when presenting your ideas to others. An important first step is to analyze assertive behavior in others. Identify what it is about others that you admire. Observe what they say and how they say it, and decide which approaches and traits you would like to emulate.

Next, analyze your behavior and the ways you respond in situations that call for assertiveness. Are you able to get others to comply with your wishes? Do others listen when you have something important to say? Analyze times when you were assertive and times when you were not. Think back on times when you came across as aggressive. What language did you use in each situation? What nonverbal messages did you convey? Go a step further and record your behavior, writing down how you behaved in various situations. What worked? What could you have done differently in order to be more effective?

The next step is to rehearse assertive behavior. Practice assertiveness in your interactions with family, friends, coworkers, neighbors, and store clerks. Visualize yourself being assertive, and role-play situations with others. When you feel confident that you can approach an issue with assertiveness, just do it! Undertake an easy challenge first, one you feel certain will succeed. If it does not go as well as you had planned, reflect on what you can do differently. Examine why it did not go the way you wanted. Keep a positive attitude, and adjust your approach the next time. The important thing is that you not allow one setback to discourage you from trying again.

▶ BECOMING A CHANGE AGENT

Healthcare professionals are in an ideal position to plan and implement changes that will benefit mothers and babies. Recognizing the need for change is the first step

---

TABLE 28.1

Powerful Language

Don't Say	Do Say
I have to . . .	I'll be glad to . . .
I'm no good at . . .	I'm getting better . . .
I failed . . .	Here's what I learned . . .
I'm going under . . .	I'm bouncing back . . .
This drives me crazy . . .	I can find a better way . . .
I can't do anything about it . . .	It's my responsibility to change . . .
We should have it ready by . . .	We will have it ready by . . .
Generally speaking, I tend to think . . .	I believe . . .
Do you have any questions?	What questions do you have?
It's not my fault. I couldn't help it.	I'm sorry. It was my responsibility.

in the process of planned change (Ellis, 1992). A need for change is exemplified in the way in which U.S. culture perceives infant feeding. Examining breastfeeding in a cultural context involves both the mother's culture within her family and support system and the cultural expectations and beliefs within her birth environment. Because most U.S. infants are born in hospitals, this requires attention to the culture and traditions within the hospital as it relates to infant feeding (Mulford, 1995).

Cultural beliefs evolve from the way in which members of that culture perceive their world. Figure 28.1 illustrates how two people can look at something and perceive it very differently. One person readily sees an aristocratic young woman with a stylish hat. Another sees a haggard old woman wearing a scarf. Neither perception is right or wrong; each person simply sees the illustration differently. One image stands out more clearly than the other and is recognized more easily. However, another more subtle image also is present and can be perceived with greater effort.

Understanding this duality in perception sheds light on the challenge inherent in breastfeeding promotion. There are two very different perceptions of infant feeding in the world. In much of the Western world, baby bottles

FIGURE 28.1
Both a young aristocratic lady and an old woman can be seen in this illustration.

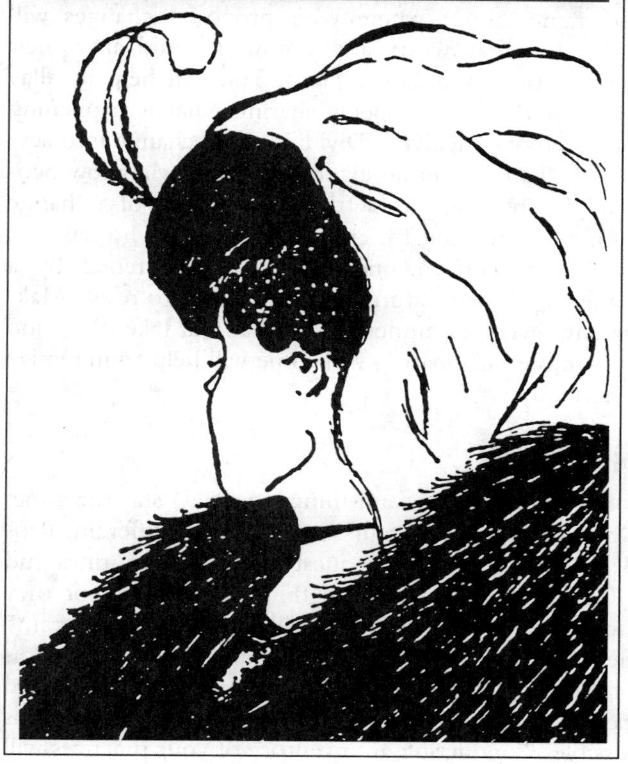

are the readily perceived method of infant feeding. Bottle-feeding is the norm and expectation of the general population. In order to increase breastfeeding rates and acceptance, society therefore needs to change how it therefore perceives infant feeding. In your efforts to promote breastfeeding, you need to recognize this perception of bottle-feeding for infants. You cannot persuade others to change their perceptions and beliefs. Change must happen from the inside out and at a pace that is comfortable for those who are undergoing the change. Understanding why others may be resistant will help you in your efforts to facilitate meaningful change.

Anticipating Resistance to Change

Not everyone will share your enthusiasm for making dramatic changes in breastfeeding policies and practices. You will undoubtedly meet with some degree of resistance in your efforts to institute changes. As common as change is, people do not always receive it well. A change in routine can be very unsettling, creating tension and stress. Unless a change is handled effectively, the changed practice can be undermined or sabotaged. It could result in employee turnover, political battles, and a drain on money and time. There are substantial financial issues at stake in U.S. hospitals, most of which receive "free" formula from manufacturers in return for serving as the manufacturers' unpaid marketing arm to consumers (Walker, 2001; Merewood, 2000). Recognizing that resistance is a natural part of the change process will help you capitalize on it and use it as a tool.

The Seven Stages of Resistance to Change

There is a descending scale of resistance to change. The most resistant person argues, "There is no problem." People who are most likely to embrace the change will acknowledge the problem and enthusiastically help to bring about the desired outcome. The stages of resistance below are adapted from educational materials developed by SARAR International and published by World Neighbors in Action (Anand, 2005). Some possible arguments against breastfeeding promotion appear with each stage. With some minor adaptations from the original version, the seven stages are:

1. There is no problem. I know human milk is good for babies, but artificial baby milk is perfectly safe. Formula has fed babies for decades. Furthermore, women have a right to choose how they want to feed their babies and they shouldn't be made to feel guilty if they choose to bottlefeed.

2. I recognize there is a problem, but it's not my responsibility. I accept that breastfeeding is superior to artificial feeding. But I can't get involved. I don't have the time. Someone else will do it.

3. I accept that there is a problem, but I doubt anyone's ability to change it. We have a problem with infant feeding, but the formula companies are too strong and influential and our society does not see a problem. Society will never embrace a breastfeeding culture.

4. I accept that there is a problem, but I'm afraid to get involved. We have a problem, but I'm afraid to try to do anything about it. If I make too many waves, I might lose my job. I'm afraid of what others will think of me. I'm afraid of the time commitment.

5. We believe we can do something about it and I will begin to look for solutions. We have a problem with infant feeding. I want to empower women and help improve infant health. I will get involved, but I'm still unsure it will make a difference.

6. We know we can do it and obstacles will not stop us. I know I can make a difference. Working together we can change things. Let's get started!

7. We did it! Now we want to share our results with others. We finally have policies and procedures that promote breastfeeding, and our staff is following the guidelines. We have returned control to mothers and babies and are empowering women to reach their breastfeeding goals.

Within any group of people, it is likely that several of these stages of resistance are represented among the various group members. It is important to recognize that progress for each individual in the group will take place one step at a time. Each member needs time and patience to progress at his or her own rate. A group goal will be to foster a climate in which each person advances to Stage 5, where the focus is on group effort rather than a single person taking responsibility. When individuals reach this stage, they are on their way to achieving the desired goal of empowerment.

Every member of the group needs to respect the process of change their colleagues undertake. Each person enters the process at varying stages in their acceptance of the anticipated change. No one can be expected to progress from Stage 1 to Stage 5 all at once. Everyone must be allowed to progress in their own way. Some individuals may slide backward during the period of change, depending on specific issues or information that surface. Some people will never change their opinions or beliefs. The group needs to be patient and flexible.

Resistance to the Ten Steps to Successful Breastfeeding

As discussed earlier, the *Ten Steps to Successful Breastfeeding* can serve as your guide to instituting changes in breastfeeding policies and practices. By anticipating the reasons people may resist these guidelines, you can select an approach that will help resolve issues before they

become obstacles. Table 28.2 identifies the types of responses that may occur relative to each of the steps for breastfeeding promotion. (BSC, 1996).

Reasons for Resistance to Change

The previous section described the stages of resistance people experience when confronted with the prospect of change. It will also be helpful to understand the possible *source* for resisting the idea of change. An awareness of individual motives will help you determine your most effective approach.

Loss of Control

How people greet a change will depend on the degree to which they feel they are in control of it. Some people who resist a change in routine may worry about losing their feeling of control or power. Just as loss of control can lead to resistance, ownership typically leads to commitment. It is important at every step in the process to recognize that change is exciting when it is done *by* us, and it is threatening when it is done *to* us. Increasing each person's involvement and participation and empowering them with legitimate choices will promote ownership of the change.

Uncertainty

Avoid springing decisions on others without groundwork or preparation. Some people may have a sense of uncertainty about where your proposed changes will lead. They may worry about how it could alter their daily routines and career plans. You can help to allay doubts and fears by openly sharing what is happening with everyone involved. Dividing a big change into several small steps over an extended period will allow people the opportunity to settle into one part of a change before experiencing the next step. People who have no time to prepare mentally can feel threatened by a change, and their natural reaction will be to resist. Making sure everyone understands what will take place and when more information will come will help to minimize uncertainty.

Difference

Some people simply want things to always stay the same. Whenever a change occurs, things will be different. People will be obligated to question familiar routines and habits. They must begin to think about behavior they had taken for granted and will need to "reprogram" their daily routines. You can help others find their comfort level by minimizing the number of changes and leaving as many habits and routines unchanged as possible. Conducting an inventory of your practices will

TABLE 28.2

Responses to Arguments Against the Ten Steps to Successful Breastfeeding

Step 1	Have a written breastfeeding policy that is routinely communicated to all health care staff.
Stage of Resistance	**Argument**
There is no problem	We've had a policy for years. It's working well enough. We've been functioning well enough without one.
It's not my responsibility	I have too much to do already. I wouldn't know where to even begin writing a policy.
No one can do it	Even if we had a policy, no one would follow it. Mothers aren't motivated enough to breastfeed, so why bother.
I can't get involved	There are too many on the staff opposed to it. I wouldn't be able to get support from the supervisor or manager.
Let's begin	I can explore policies in other hospitals. I can contact ILCA to locate resources.
We can do it	Let's bring people together from all departments to work on it. Let's survey our patients to learn how satisfied they are.
We did it!	**We accomplished our goal!**

Step 2	Train all health care staff in skills necessary to implement this policy.
Stage of Resistance	**Argument**
There is no problem	We have IBCLCs, so we don't need to train the rest of the staff. Our nurses know what they need to know about breastfeeding.
It's not my responsibility	I don't have time to train everyone. I wouldn't know where to even begin with training.
No one can do it	The staff would never agree to 18 hours of training. We don't have enough money or time to train the entire staff.
I can't get involved	Staff would resent my suggesting that they need the training. I wouldn't be able to get support from the supervisor/manager.
Let's begin	I can explore how other hospitals do their training. I will take an extensive course in lactation.
We can do it	Let's survey staff to find out what they know about breastfeeding. Let's form a committee with people from several departments.
We did it!	**We accomplished our goal!**

(continued)

Table 28.2 (continued)	
Responses to Arguments Against the Ten Steps to Successful Breastfeeding	

Step 3	*Inform all pregnant women about the benefits and management of breastfeeding.*
Stage of Resistance	**Argument**
There is no problem	We give help and advice to mothers when they are in the hospital. Teaching breastfeeding will create guilt in those who don't.
It's not my responsibility	Mothers learn what they need to know in their childbirth classes. It's the mother's responsibility to read and seek information.
No one can do it	We realize we need to, but we don't have the resources. If women want to bottle-feed, it's our responsibility to help them.
I can't get involved	I don't have time to do prenatal teaching with everything else. I wouldn't be able to get support from the supervisor/manager.
Let's begin	I can explore breastfeeding initiation rates in other hospitals. I can make a questionnaire to screen mothers with difficulties.
We can do it	Let's survey our patients to find out how satisfied they are. Let's explore what we can improve in the labor and delivery department.
We did it!	**We accomplished our goal!**

Step 4	*Help mothers initiate breastfeeding within a half-hour of birth.*
Stage of Resistance	**Argument**
There is no problem	We start breastfeeding as soon as the mother gets to her room. Most babies are too sleepy to breastfeed right away.
It's not my responsibility	If she breastfeeds after delivery, relatives will have to wait to see the baby. Babies get too cold in the delivery room.
No one can do it	The labor and delivery staff would never support such a policy. There are too many procedures that need to be done at that time.
I can't get involved	The staff is getting tired of all my suggestions about breastfeeding. I'm not very good at persuading people.
Let's begin	I can find someone in labor and delivery who will be receptive to change. I can teach the staff about the importance of early initiation of breastfeeding.
We can do it	Let's try it on a short-term trial basis and then evaluate it. We can find ways to keep babies warm.
We did it!	**We accomplished our goal!**

TABLE 28.2 (CONTINUED)

Responses to Arguments Against the Ten Steps to Successful Breastfeeding

Step 5	*Show mothers how to breastfeed and how to maintain lactation, even if they should be separated from their infants.*
Stage of Resistance	**Argument**
There is no problem	Breastfeeding is a natural instinct; we don't need to teach it. There are plenty of support groups who will help them.
It's not my responsibility	If the baby is in the NICU, those nurses are responsible for it. I can't possibly see every breastfeeding mother.
No one can do it	We don't have enough staff to spend the time required for this. A lot of our staff don't believe in pushing breastfeeding.
I can't get involved	I wouldn't get support from my supervisor for the time it will take. Staff won't spend so much time with breastfeeding mothers.
Let's begin	I can encourage staff to accompany me on rounds. I can propose telephone follow-up for breastfeeding mothers.
We can do it	Let's survey our patients about what would have helped them. Let's explore a program to mentor staff in breastfeeding.
We did it!	**We accomplished our goal!**

Step 6	*Give newborn infants no food or drink other than breastmilk, unless medically indicated.*
Stage of Resistance	**Argument**
There is no problem	We never do anything unless it is medically indicated. I am legally responsible to see that the baby is not dehydrated.
It's not my responsibility	I can't influence physician policies. Purchase of formula is an administrative decision, not mine.
No one can do it	Administration will never agree to begin purchasing formula. Formula companies will withdraw other funding if we make this change.
I can't get involved	I would not be able to get support from the supervisor/manager. What about jaundice? This could be dangerous.
Let's begin	I can explore how other hospitals have begun purchasing formula. I can teach staff the importance of exclusive breastfeeding.
We can do it	Let's review reasons we have been giving formula and water. Let's invite some mothers in to discuss how they managed.
We did it!	**We accomplished our goal!**

(continued)

TABLE 28.2 (CONTINUED)

Responses to Arguments Against the Ten Steps to Successful Breastfeeding

Step 7	*Practice rooming-in—allow mothers and infants to remain together—24 hours a day.*
Stage of Resistance	**Argument**
There is no problem	We have better security if babies are kept in the nursery. Babies could choke if they stay in the mother's room.
It's not my responsibility	Mothers are tired after laboring and delivering. That is an administrative decision.
No one can do it	If babies stay with their mothers, nursery staff will lose their jobs. Mothers do not want to keep their babies in the room.
I can't get involved	I will never get support from administration. The pediatricians will not examine babies in the mothers' rooms.
Let's begin	I can explore rooming-in policies at other hospitals. I can teach staff the importance of keeping babies with mothers.
We can do it	Let's invite pediatricians to meet with the breastfeeding committee. Let's record how much time babies spend away from their mothers.
We did it!	**We accomplished our goal!**

Step 8	*Encourage breastfeeding on demand.*
Stage of Resistance	**Argument**
There is no problem	It is more efficient having scheduled feeding times. Babies need to get on a schedule as early as possible.
It's not my responsibility	I can do it with the mothers I see, but I can't see all of them. The babies must be fed at least two times on every shift.
No one can do it	Staff routines would be disrupted too much. It would be too hard to monitor babies for hypoglycemia without a schedule.
I can't get involved	Staff routines would be disrupted too much. This would be much too confusing.
Let's begin	I can teach staff the importance of the mother and baby setting the pace. I can help staff learn to recognize and teach feeding cues.
We can do it	Let's keep statistics to see if schedules make a difference. Let's try it for 6 months to see how it works.
We did it!	**We accomplished our goal!**

Table 28.2 (continued)	
Responses to Arguments Against the Ten Steps to Successful Breastfeeding	
Step 9	*Give no artificial teats or pacifiers (also called dummies or soothers) to breastfeeding infants.*
Stage of Resistance	**Argument**
There is no problem	We have to test to see if the baby can suck and swallow. Babies have strong sucking needs and need pacifiers to keep calm.
It's not my responsibility	If parents want them, it is not my position to discourage it. Everyone uses pacifiers, so what's the big deal?
No one can do it	I'm the only one in the hospital who considers this to be a problem. Pacifiers are a part of our culture, just like baby bottles.
I can't get involved	The staff will think it takes too long to feed with a cup or spoon. There is nothing to document the use of cups for feeding babies.
Let's begin	I can teach staff about sucking preference and confusion. I can teach the staff how to cup feed a baby.
We can do it	Let's review why we give formula and water. Let's teach mothers to put the baby to breast rather than give a pacifier.
We did it!	**We accomplished our goal!**
Step 10	*Foster the establishment of breastfeeding support groups and refer mothers to them on discharge from the hospital or clinic.*
Stage of Resistance	**Argument**
There is no problem	We have the information at the desk if the patient requests it. Women in those groups make mothers feel guilty if they wean early.
It's not my responsibility	It is the mother's responsibility to seek help. The physician will refer her if there is a problem.
No one can do it	We don't have enough resources to start a support group here. The counselors do not always give sound advice and information.
I can't get involved	If I do this, I'll have to do it on my own time. I don't have time to keep updating the referral list.
Let's begin	I can visit community support groups and foster a strong link. I can offer to train mother-to-mother support counselors.
We can do it	Let's give a name and telephone number to breastfeeding mothers. Let's explore an outpatient clinic and/or support group.
We did it!	**We accomplished our goal!**

ILCA, International Lactation Consultants Association; LC, lactation consultant; NICU, neonatal intensive care unit.
Printed by permission of Breastfeeding Support Consultants from their publication "Creating Change in the Face of Resistance," 1996.

help you identify what you are doing right and what needs to be adjusted.

Loss of Face

Some people may believe that a proposed change implies that the old ways were wrong. They may fear looking foolish because of past actions and may feel embarrassed and self-conscious. Some people can have deeply personal reasons for resisting breastfeeding promotion. Help them put past actions into perspective. We all do what we perceive to be appropriate at the time. Explain that now times are different, and we understand the needs of mothers and babies better. As new research and new knowledge about breastfeeding become available, practices evolve and change. Practices five or ten years ago may have been appropriate at the time. There are now new skills and knowledge to improve the way we help mothers and babies. Praise others for their accomplishments under the old conditions, and thank them for their willingness to change to meet present needs. Help them understand that you, too, have changed your practices, and help them view the change positively.

Competence

Understandably, the prospect of change may cause concerns about future competence. People may worry about their ability to be effective after the change. They may wonder, "Can I do it?" or "How will I do it?" New ways often demand an entirely new set of competencies. Some people will feel forced to start over again with a new way of doing things. Equipping everyone with the necessary knowledge and skills for doing their jobs under the new rules will be critical to the success of your new practices. You can ensure that others will feel competent by providing sufficient training and giving positive reinforcement. Provide ample opportunity for them to practice new skills without judgment. A formal mentorship program or other method of supervised training will allow people to observe and practice in a nonthreatening setting.

Disruption

It is important to acknowledge that a proposed change can be disruptive to some of the people involved. It may interrupt plans or projects that others believe are as worthy as the one you propose. Meeting a deadline or attending a meeting may intrude on people's personal time. It could interfere with days they are not scheduled to work and with planned family activities. Staff members may be concerned that instituting the change will require more energy, time, and mental preoccupation. It will require that they go "above and beyond" their usual efforts. Be sure to give support and recognition for this extra effort. Introduce changes with flexibility, and be sensitive to the effect the process will have on those who must implement the change and operate in a new way.

Past Grievances

The goal of leaving personalities and positions at the door is for everyone to enter the process on even footing and with an open mind. In reality, this rarely happens. Unresolved grievances from the past will surface as you approach others with your proposed changes. Perhaps one person sought your support for a previous activity and was not satisfied with your response. Undercurrents of professional jealousy or other resentments may obstruct your efforts at achieving unity within the group. Perhaps your predecessor alienated staff with an offensive approach. It is important to address past issues that could color attitudes and responses to your proposed change. When the air has cleared, everyone will be better able to focus on the present issues.

Real Threat

When your change is in place, it most likely will alter people's routines. A new set of expectations will challenge people to modify their practices. The traditional way of doing things will be replaced with new routines. The process that took place may transform relationships with colleagues. Despite your efforts at collaboration and unity, instituting the change may have created winners and losers, resulting in people losing status or power.

For example, if a proposed change would institute 24-hour rooming-in as a standard in your facility, babies would no longer remain in a central nursery. A particular nurse may have worked in the central nursery for the past 20 years. Her greatest enjoyment is taking care of "her" babies. If babies spend the majority of their time in the mothers' rooms, this nurse's daily routine will change dramatically. She may consider the change too difficult and resign.

It is important that you avoid any pretense or false promises. Be sensitive to the loss of routines, comforts, traditions, and relationships. Everyone needs a chance to let go of the past and will need a supportive climate in which to do so. Accept that a perceived threat sometimes may be real. A person may find the change too difficult or too disruptive.

Conflict Resolution

Introducing change results in a certain degree of conflict. On the surface, it may seem helpful to try to avoid conflict or pretend that it does not exist. However, this attitude can actually lead to further conflict (Dana, 2000; Mayer, 2000). Embracing conflict as a natural part of the change process will enable you to manage it more rationally and productively. You need to bring conflicts out in the open in order to overcome them. This will allow you to develop honest, frank, and positive relationships with others. Conflict can actually be very constructive; it makes people revved up and more receptive to finding creative solutions. Conflict helps us realize and validate our values. It is through conflict that people learn to understand others and recognize the value of working together.

Inevitably, further conflicts will surface as the process of change continues. It is better to address these issues as they arise, no matter how minor they may seem. You want to foster an environment in which honesty prevails and where neither side keeps an "account" of grievances against the other. Recognize that people work to satisfy their own personal needs, often a need for money, power, or identity. People generally want others to accept them as they are and to like and appreciate them. In order to resolve conflict, you must meet the other person's needs as well as your own.

Be Sensitive to Others

Sensitivity to another person's circumstances is important in all communication. When conflict arises, it is critical. Avoid confronting conflict in a public setting or in the presence of others who are uninvolved. Keep in mind that you are attempting to change behaviors, not people. In order to establish and maintain solid relationships, you need to remain focused on the solution rather than on individual problems. Find ways you can all join together to work through any conflicts that stand in the way of reaching your goals. Recognize that conflict involves both issues and feelings. You must get emotions out of the way before you can solve problems. When emotions surface, reflecting them back through active listening will help to recognize and validate them. It is only then that you can move on to address problems and work toward solutions

Identify Common Goals

In addressing a conflict, it may help first to determine basic goals that you share with the other person. Establishing common ground can help set the stage for debating respective strategies for achieving your goals. One common objective is empowering mothers and babies to achieve their goals. With that as a starting point, you can begin to discuss strategies to accomplish it. You know what you have in common. Now you need to figure out how you can meet on common ground with other related issues. Find ways you can both benefit by the outcome. Operating in this manner sets a tone of cooperation and problem solving and puts both of you on the same side, instead of remaining adversaries.

Coping with Difficult People

Invariably, you will have at least one person on your team who others regard as difficult. You have tried everything in your arsenal to work with this person

cooperatively. You have validated feelings, acknowledged concerns, and yet you continually meet with resistance. A change in approach may achieve more positive results. Recognize that you cannot change the other person. Moreover, you cannot directly change the way that person responds to you. What you can change is the way you relate to that person. Finding a more effective way to communicate and present yourself can indirectly influence how the other person will respond.

Approaching a Difficult Person

- Be positive. Give recognition and praise for accomplishments, and avoid placing blame.

- Prepare for interactions by writing down exactly what you plan to say. In addition to helping you prepare, this will help release any negativism that has built up before an actual confrontation.

- Use appropriate body language. Face the person squarely, sit or stand erect, and lean forward to demonstrate a desire to interact and communicate in a meaningful way.

- Give your undivided attention and respond both verbally (I see . . . , I'm with you) and nonverbally (nodding, smiling, maintaining eye contact).

- When you are speaking, avoid distractions. Do not focus on what you anticipate the other person will say. Focus on your goal, and keep an even pace.

- Recycle the other person's message to make sure you understood it correctly. After you have sent the message, pause for a response before continuing to speak.

The Aggressor

Some difficult people are aggressive to the point of being hostile. They have a strong sense of what others should do and how they should do it. They can be abrasive, abrupt, intimidating, and relentless. Their goal is to prove that you are wrong and they are right. You need to stay as dispassionate as possible with such a person. An angry person cannot stay overtly angry for long if you remain calm. Listen attentively, look them directly in the eye, and be ready to interrupt them. On the other hand, if they interrupt you, hold your ground and say, "You interrupted me, let me finish." It is important not to allow an aggressor to take control with negative energy.

The Saboteur

You may find yourself dealing with someone who sabotages your efforts from behind the scenes. This person does not engage in direct confrontation, yet can be as divisive as one who confronts you openly. Never ignore a sniper! You need to expose their undermining efforts either privately or in a group setting. Otherwise, they will continue to breed discontent among everyone at every turn.

In a hospital setting, sabotage may come in the form of opposition or threats from formula manufacturers (Merewood, 2000). One formula company ceased printing a hospital's mother/baby care booklet because breastfeeding rates were getting too high to justify their "free" printing. One manufacturer labels its water bottles with the words "do not use for breastmilk storage." They are able to promote brand awareness, while at the same time creating negative imagery about breastfeeding.

The Wet Blanket

A wet blanket can infect others by dampening enthusiasm and undermining positive thinking. This person argues, "It won't work" or "It's no use" and refuses to buy into what the group is trying to accomplish. One way to challenge such a person is to ask them for ideas on positive, realistic ways to solve problems. Take their complaints seriously, and ask, "What's the worst possible scenario?" Put the matter back in their hands and engage them in considering solutions. Capitalize on the strength they bring to the group for identifying things that can go wrong with implementation of any policy or procedure. Engaging their talents in this way gives them value and enables them to contribute to the process.

The Expert

Be aware of people who consider themselves the experts. Although their demeanor may seem pompous and arrogant, they are usually very productive and talented. Show that you respect their opinion and ask them to explain their point further. Be prepared and accurate in your interactions with these people. Avoid trying to assert yourself as the expert, as well. Allowing them to be the expert may be more productive if it helps you accomplish your goal. If their opinion is at odds with your recommendations, make sure what you recommend is evidence based and has peer-reviewed research to support it. You can ask politely for the same evidence for their recommendations as well.

Divisiveness in a Meeting

Meeting dynamics can help neutralize the efforts of a difficult person. When you are confronted by a difficult person in a meeting, try to get involvement from others in the group. Obtain their input and support before the meeting. During the meeting, you might ask for their reactions, for example, "How would you . . . What do you think of . . . How many would agree?" Even where you sit in a meeting can help to reduce divisiveness. If you expect conflict with a particular person, arrange to sit directly next to them. Avoid placing yourself directly across from the person, as this heightens the potential for conflict. It is more difficult to spar with someone who is sitting immediately next to you.

Food is a great neutralizer in meetings. Sales organizations have used "free" food to capture attendance for years (Stolberg, 2000). The social dynamics of passing through a line, handing a plate of cookies to someone, or commenting on food increases goodwill. So do the mechanics of eating. It is socially acceptable to finish chewing and swallowing and then take a drink of water before answering. That pause gives you time to think and reduces impatience.

Using Humor as a Tool for Change

Humor is an invaluable tool for facilitating change and diffusing resistance. Humor makes it possible for us to survive in "the system." It leads toward a greater awareness of the strengths and weaknesses in the present system, new ways to respond and express creativity, and the survival and productivity of valuable human resources (Jackson, 1985). The comic relief of humor injected into a situation often presents a new perspective and leads to compromise. A leader who maintains a good sense of humor will inspire tremendous loyalty and enthusiasm (Yerkes, 2001). Humor leads to the creation of a positive climate and fosters an energized work environment. Learn how to maintain humor in your quest for change and to infuse humor in others.

▶ BEGINNING THE PROCESS OF CHANGE

The first step to creating change is to believe that you can do it! In the words of Margaret Mead, "Don't ever say one person can't change the world. It is the only thing that ever has." As described earlier, change takes place on a continuum, and everyone involved in the change enters the process at varying stages. Each person progresses at their own pace and within their own level of comfort. Many times, the greatest resister becomes one of the staunchest advocates when given the opportunity to progress through the necessary stages that will lead to understanding and embracing the change.

The Art of Persuasion

Benjamin Franklin said, "The aim of persuasion is not to confront other people, but to appreciate their points of view and try to move them generally in your direction." Franklin used the acronym TALKING to describe his success at persuasion, with each letter standing for one of seven keys for successful persuasion (Humes, 1992).

◆ Timing—It's not good enough to have the right message. You must also choose the right moment.

- Appreciation—Anyone who wants someone else to accommodate his request should learn to appreciate the other one's problems and concerns.
- Listening—Learn to listen well enough to find out what you need and how best to sell it to the other person. Feed back their own words, using their words to sell the point.
- Knowledge—Learn where the other person is coming from and how to get them where you want to go.
- Integrity—Never misrepresent your fundamental beliefs or motives.
- Need—The three most persuasive words in the English language are "I need you." When you must ask people for something, the best way to convince them is to show them that they are uniquely qualified to give it to you.
- Giving—Learn the value of giving. If you insist on everything, you may wind up with nothing.

Doing Your Homework

Your effectiveness in initiating change will depend on your preparation before you approach others with your ideas. For example, say that you want to work toward your facility becoming baby friendly. You start by considering the many policies and procedures that need to be changed. Before you approach anyone with your ideas, you need to collect as much supporting data as possible for each change you have in mind. Appropriate and adequate preparation before approaching others will be central to your success.

Gather Data

First, you will need to gather supporting research, and lots of it! Accumulate any information you will need to support your proposed change, including documentation and hospital statistics. What are your current policies and practices? What are the consequences of the way you are operating presently? What are breastfeeding initiation rates? How many women are still breastfeeding at two weeks? At three months? At six months? How do your rates compare with other hospitals in your community? Survey mothers about the breastfeeding support they received in your hospital. What was good or bad? What could have been improved?

Record all the data you collect and incorporate it into your goals for change. For example, if 68 percent of mothers in your hospital initiate breastfeeding, you might state that, "The goal is that by October of next year, the breastfeeding initiation rate will be 70 percent. The following year, the rate will be 72 percent, with increases each year to meet the U.S. Healthy People goal of 75 percent by 2010." You can do the same for

breastfeeding duration and any other statistics related to breastfeeding care.

Evaluate Your Facility

Next, you need to assess which of your present policies and protocols are research based and in line with current recommendations. Where you determine a need for change, prepare detailed rationale for the change. Write down anticipated arguments, along with your possible responses to each one. Identify alternative approaches and methods in case you experience obstacles. This careful evaluation is an essential step in the process of change. It will prepare you for responding to those who present obstacles and arguments. The best defense is a strong offense, shored by evidence-based research. After the change has been proposed and discussed, write down any unanticipated arguments that surfaced and note changes needed in your approach. Then go back to the drawing board and try again!

A Model for Planned Change

An important part of your process will be developing a systematic plan for structuring the change. Most models begin by defining a problem and goal, determining the change agent, and then designing a well-defined plan of action. In your plan for your facility to become baby friendly, you can refer to other hospitals that have achieved official Baby-friendly Hospital designation. You can use resources such as WIC, Loving Support, Best Start, and Wellstart as models for your ideas and adapt them to fit your hospital's needs.

Define the Problem

For every change you wish to institute, define the problem that makes that change necessary. Rather than stating a problem globally in terms of lack of support for breastfeeding, define each specific problem area where changes need to occur. For example, you may cite low initiation rates, high rates of engorgement, or large numbers of babies who have difficulty latching on. Next, determine the change agents, the people who will be the most effective leaders in proposing and instituting the change. Then identify all the people and positions the change will affect. Be sure to involve representatives from all of the affected areas in the process so that everyone has ownership in the change.

Define Goals and Strategies

Determine whether you hope to change behavior, attitudes, values, procedures, policies, or perhaps the entire structure. You will then be able to identify specific objectives and develop a time line for planning and implementing the change. Some objectives will be short term, some will be intermediate, and some will be long term. The goal of increasing the incidence of breastfeeding, for instance, may have a short-term objective of increasing the rate to 58 percent, an intermediate objective of 68 percent, and a long-term objective of 75 percent to meet the U.S. Healthy People 2010 goals. Reflect all of these objectives in the time line.

With objectives established, you are ready to develop an action plan and strategies. Try to think through all the issues involved in each individual objective. Be sure to address the education that will be required for empowering the staff to implement the change. In addition, determine how the change will be communicated. Decide which procedures and policies need to be altered. Consider how the changes will affect people's levels of authority or power.

Implement the Change

After you have defined the problems, goals, and strategies, you will be ready to implement the change. As you do so, be sure to monitor everyone's responses to learn if any unanticipated problems arise. If problems occur, resolve them immediately so you can maintain a high level of commitment to the change among the staff. Evaluate both the positive and negative outcomes. Too often, this step of evaluation receives little attention. Failing to evaluate the outcomes associated with the change could jeopardize long-term success. When the change has become ingrained procedurally, you can take the final step of linking it to the overall organizational structure and standardizing it.

Planning a Breastfeeding Committee

Your chances of success will be greater when change occurs through some form of concerted group effort. A breastfeeding committee or task force can serve this purpose. If you do not already have a breastfeeding committee in your facility, you may want to consider establishing one. You can approach the person in charge of maternity services to discuss how breastfeeding is going in that facility. In a hospital, this may be the nurse manager or nursing director. In a low-key manner, you can ask, "Have you noticed that our breastfeeding initiation rate is 20 percent lower than in the hospital across town?" You might then invite that person to have lunch with you to discuss some of these issues. This marks the beginning of your committee and the beginning of your initiative for change!

Members of the Team

Put a great deal of thought into the makeup of the members on a committee. You will want the committee to be large enough that if a couple of members are absent, the meeting can still go on as planned. Each person's level of support for breastfeeding is important. You will want to include people whom you have identified as allies, those you expect will resist, and those who seem to be neutral. It is important to have this diversity in the group and to get buy-in from potential resistors. This will help avoid sabotage or a perception that the cards are stacked in favor of one group over another. Many times, the greatest resistors become some of the most avid supporters after they understand the issues involved.

A quality improvement representative will be a valuable member of your breastfeeding committee. All U.S. hospitals accredited by the **Joint Commission on Accreditation of Healthcare Organizations** (JCAHO) are required to have a process in place for quality improvement. This motivates hospitals to identify problem areas and make improvements. Quality improvement efforts aim to increase customer satisfaction. In healthcare, the customer is the patient. In obstetrics, the baby is the customer (Cadwell, 1997), as is the mother. Consequently, quality improvements in obstetrics will focus on what is best for the baby and mother.

Attempt to have the group represent all the areas the change will affect. In a hospital, areas affected may include obstetrics, labor and delivery, postpartum, neonatal intensive care, and pediatrics. Consider other areas and people who have contact with breastfeeding mothers and babies as well. These may include technicians, housekeeping personnel, and management, as well as community professionals in home care, pharmacy, and speech pathology. Bringing together representatives of all these groups to form an interdisciplinary team will enable all those affected by the change to participate equally in the process. Changes in breastfeeding practices and policies are ideally suited to a quality improvement approach.

Types of Personalities

The personalities of the specific people you have in mind for your committee will be important to group dynamics. Every personality type contributes positive traits to a group. The variety of personal attributes and diversity with which people approach issues demonstrates the value of including the entire range of personalities in a group process. Capitalizing on the best of each style will contribute to the group's dynamics and productivity.

Kahler (1992) identified six basic personality types among Americans (see Table 28.3). The six types are reactors, workaholics, rebels, persisters, dreamers, and promoters. Reactors form the largest group, about 30 percent of the population. They are emotional and react quickly to the feelings of others. Reactors will respond to assurances that you are happy to have them on your team. Workaholics comprise 25 percent of the

	TABLE 28.3	
	Six Personality Types of Americans	
Personality Type	**Percent of Population**	**Characteristics**
Reactors	30%	◆ Emotional ◆ React quickly to feelings of others ◆ Will respond to assurances that you are happy to have them on your team
Workaholics	25%	◆ Logical and organized ◆ Will want you to get to the point and just tell them the facts
Rebels	20%	◆ Creative, spontaneous, and playful ◆ Enjoy stimulating contact with other people ◆ Dislike rigid schedules
Persisters	10%	◆ Conscientious, observant, and dedicated ◆ Strong beliefs make it difficult to accept criticism from others ◆ Let them know how much you value their character and accomplishments
Dreamers	10%	◆ Imaginative ◆ Like solitude and quiet surroundings ◆ May need to take the initiative with them and give them personal space
Promoters	5%	◆ Persuasive and charming ◆ Action oriented ◆ Like to bend rules

Source: Kahler T. Six Basic Personality Types. BottomLine; September 15, 1992.

population. They are logical and organized and want you to get to the point and just tell them the facts. Rebels, another 20 percent of the population, are creative, spontaneous, and playful. They enjoy stimulating contact with other people and dislike rigid schedules. Persisters are conscientious, observant, and dedicated. Representing 10 percent of the population, their strong beliefs make it difficult for them to accept criticism from others. It will help to let them know how much you value their character and accomplishments. Dreamers, another 10 percent of the population, are imaginative and like solitude and quiet surroundings. You may need to take the initiative with them and give them personal space. Promoters form the final 5 percent of the population. They are persuasive, charming, action oriented, and like to bend rules. It is easy to see that each of these personalities will contribute positively to group dynamics.

Another method of comparing personality types divides them into five categories: synthesist, idealist, pragmatist, analyst, and realist. Synthesists are often labeled as troublemakers. They seek conflict and provide debate and creativity. Idealists have extremely high standards and, because of this, they can suffer deep disappointments.

They are good at articulating goals and providing a broad view of issues. Pragmatists look for immediate results and find it difficult to focus on long-range plans. They are resourceful, adaptable, and willing to experiment. They are sensitive to what appeals to others and are willing to settle for small gains. Analysts look for one best way to do something. They rationalize and are stubborn and strong-minded. They are methodical, accurate, thorough, and persistent. Realists provide drive and momentum, and are interested in concrete results. They are confident, practical, and good at delegating. Realists focus on both facts and opinions. Others can count on them to get the job done and to rarely be wrong. They are forthright, dogmatic and sometimes seem domineering. It is easy to see the strengths each of these personalities offer to the group.

Dynamics of a Team Meeting

After committee members are in place, the group can begin to meet regularly. Not all members of the team will share a common purpose, but this should not prevent them from cooperating to reach group goals. The ultimate group goal is to find creative solutions that are mutually beneficial. A smoothly functioning team requires empathy and a willingness to encourage the best from others. Members of the group can be asked to identify specific problems and then determine how and where to start making changes.

As a group leader, withholding your own agenda until the group has processed the issues will help you learn their needs. In the process, your agenda may take a different shape if you are open to hear what others say. Avoid the trap of beginning with a rigid preplanned agenda. Know when to keep quiet, sit back, and let the discussion flow. After you have stated your position or proposal, stop and let others respond. In order for group members to take ownership of a change, they each need to be a part of designing it. It is important that you learn as much as possible about the needs of each member before proposing solutions.

Take It Slow and Easy

It is important that you not try to change everything all at once. Many routines and practices can probably remain in place. First, then, you must identify what is right with the present system and congratulate yourselves for that! Underscore with members of the group all of the positive policies and practices that already provide good care to mothers and babies. Help them to recognize the strengths of the organization.

During your evaluation, you will have targeted areas where improvements are needed. Make sure everyone has realistic expectations for how the changes will occur. Major change does not take place overnight. It may take as long as ten years for your facility to reach its full potential in protecting, supporting, and promoting breastfeeding. Give careful attention to prioritizing the changes and deciding which ones to tackle first.

Consider the anticipated level of difficulty in convincing others to support each change. Starting with a change that people are likely to find most acceptable will give you a greater chance of success. For example, it may be much easier in a hospital setting to begin regular breastfeeding rounds than to eliminate mothers being given discharge packs of infant formula. Consider which proposed changes are least disruptive to routines or least controversial. Those changes are likely to meet with greater acceptance. Move slowly to issues perceived as more complicated or potentially problematic. At the same time, recognize that the change that seems easiest to you may not be the one that will garner the least resistance from others.

Establishing a record of accomplishment with several of the easier changes will prepare you for going on to the more challenging ones. Leave the toughest hurdles until you have several of the less controversial and less difficult changes in place. The success of instituting the earlier changes will instill a greater level of self-confidence for moving on to the others. Additionally, after some of the changes are in practice, people may be better able to see the larger picture and be more willing to support the tougher changes.

Give Recognition and Praise

Everyone likes to be recognized for doing something correctly. That is especially true when they believe they have gone out of their way to provide good care. People respond well to positive feedback and expressions of gratitude. Sharing the praise with others gives well-earned recognition as well. Make sure others know the progress they made. For example, "Did you hear how much Mrs. Robinson appreciated Sheryl's help in getting her baby to latch?"

Creative incentives or rewards can encourage everyone's participation and compliance. You might award a button or pen for completing a breastfeeding module or attending an inservice program, a pizza party when a breastfeeding course is completed, or a designated breastfeeding counselor of the month. You can post a breastfeeding bulletin board with items such as lactation updates, new policies, and reports from breastfeeding committee meetings. Summarize professional articles of interest and post them. Cut out articles from newspapers, magazines, and professional journals. Publish a newsletter to send to physician offices. Such efforts can create cooperation and goodwill among those who care for breastfeeding women and their babies.

Ultimately, people have very basic needs they want to meet through their work. While priorities may vary, most people share many of the same desires. They want work that is interesting and challenging. They want appreciation expressed for their efforts. They want to be involved in and important to the overall scheme. They want job security and commensurate pay. They want opportunities for career growth and advancement. Helping them meet these needs will reap the support and cooperation necessary for meeting your own needs.

▶ MAJOR PROMOTION INITIATIVES

There is a great deal of support for breastfeeding promotion among the international healthcare community, governments, and organizations committed to protecting the health of infants and young children. To understand the challenges inherent in breastfeeding promotion, the obstacles need to be clear. Examining the motives and actions of the infant formula industry provides a clear picture of the obstacles in breastfeeding promotion. Breastfeeding promotion initiatives recommend restrictions on inappropriate marketing of infant formula, citing the health risks inherent in the aggressive promotion.

The Infant Formula Industry

The infant formula industry is eager to promote breast-feeding. Breastfeeding mothers are typically very health conscious. When they wean their babies from the breast, they are more likely to wean to an infant formula rather than immediately to cow's milk. Their babies will probably receive formula until an older age than babies who received formula from birth. They are more likely to use "toddler formulas" or "add-on formulas." Formula-feeding mothers are more likely to wean their babies to cow's milk at an earlier age. As with any industry, individual formula manufacturers are in fierce competition with each other for customers. The one that looks best will win more breastfeeding mothers. They acknowledge that breastfeeding is best, and they promote their product under the guise of promoting breastfeeding. They tell the public what they know they want to hear and couch it in language that will appeal to them. That is simply good advertising.

Infant Formula Advertising Practices

Infant formula manufacturers worldwide advertise their infant foods in medical journals and to the lay public. Hospitals receive infant formula for their nurseries at no charge, a practice that originated in the 1930s and has been criticized by health experts ever since. Mothers also receive free samples when they leave the hospital (Donnelly, 2000). Hospitals receive no other product routinely without being charged (Merewood, 2000). They should be required to pay for infant formula just as they do all other supplies. Any gifts given to hospitals should be legitimate, in the form of documentable research or teaching grants. Gifts should not go through the hospital's purchasing agent (Barness, 1987).

Manufacturers do not stop at giving free formula to hospitals. Families receive discount coupons and even cases of free formula at their homes (Howard, 1994). Aggressive marketing campaigns target physicians and hospital maternity units. Hospitals and healthcare practitioners receive free equipment, architectural planning, calendars, office supplies, and other giveaways. Funding is provided for airline tickets to conferences, medical fellowships, scholarships, educational grants, and other rewards that are common to the industry, such as tickets to sporting events, dinners, and fishing trips. Company representatives present themselves as experts in infant nutrition. They educate parents through videos and literature and physicians through continuing education programs (Moynihan, 2003; Young, 1990).

Many healthcare providers are naïve about the practices of the infant formula industry. One study sought to determine how problematic experienced physicians and residents viewed common pharmaceutical marketing activities. Although activities permitted under their guidelines troubled some respondents, the views reported by others violated the guidelines (Brett, 2003). The entire May 2003 issue of the *British Medical Journal*, "No More Free Lunches," focuses on the issue of pharmaceutical industry marketing. Available online at www.bmj.bmjjournals.com/content/vol326/issue7400, it discusses marketing tactics and how those tactics influence the behavior of healthcare providers.

Another eye-opening and educational resource, www.nofreelunch.org, urges healthcare practitioners to provide high-quality care based on unbiased evidence rather than on biased pharmaceutical promotions. The pharmaceutical industry's actions mirror the actions of the infant formula industry. This is to be expected since most formula manufacturers are owned by pharmaceutical companies. They promote their products in an effort to influence prescribing. They exert significant influence on provider behavior through samples, gifts, and food. They provide promotional materials and presentations that are often biased and non-informative (No Free Lunch, 2004).

Pharmaceutical company marketing efforts have traditionally focused on influencing prescribing decisions. Now, attention increasingly targets potential patients. Drug companies are sponsoring patient groups, fuelling debate about standards of disclosure. A "third-party" marketing strategy uses an apparently independent spokesperson to create higher credibility with a company's target audience (Burton, 2003). The failure of doctors, patients, and journalists to demand disclosure of potential conflicts of interest often reinforces the lack of disclosure by third-party messengers. Tactics aimed at shaping important decisions on healthcare continue to flourish.

Breastfeeding advocates see this ploy frequently, as formula companies offer "medical education" seminars and lectures for continuing nursing and medical education credits. One recent "medical lecture" featured a physician extolling the virtues of the addition of the long-chain polyunsaturated fatty acids DHA and AA to the manufacturer's infant formulas. Yet, what the audience may not have learned was that Mead Johnson was forced by the Canadian Health Department to remove its claims about DHA and AA improving IQ and vision from its Canadian advertising. They probably did not learn that these acids are made from algae and soil fungus (Sterken, 2004; Agennix, 2002). Such marketing seminars occur every day under the guise of continuing education.

One study investigated the issue of pharmaceutical companies invoking peer-reviewed studies to support their claims and add credence to their advertising. Of 125 citations claimed, the majority were from randomised clinical trials. In 45 claims, the reference did not support the promotional statement, most frequently because the slogan recommended the drug in a patient group other than the one assessed in the study. The reviewers concluded that "doctors should be cautious in assessment of advertisements that claim a drug has greater efficacy, safety, or convenience even though these claims are accompanied by bibliographical references to randomised clinical trials published in reputable medical journals and seem to be evidence-based" (Villanueva, 2003).

Ties between associations such as the American Academy of Pediatrics (AAP) and the American Medical Association (AMA) run deep (Petersen, 2002; Stolberg, 2000). In 1996, Nestlé sued the AAP, Ross Laboratories, and Mead Johnson's parent company, Bristol-Myers Squib, claiming a conspiracy to restrict trade. The suit stated that the AAP accepted millions from these manufacturers, including funds to help pay for the AAP's headquarters. In 2001, Ross was one of the top three corporate sponsors of the AAP's $65 million operating budget, contributing $500,000 or more (Petersen, 2002).

In 2002, drug companies and physicians fought a government plan to restrict gifts and other rewards that pharmaceutical manufacturers give physicians and insurers to encourage the prescribing of particular drugs. The Department of Health and Human Services observed that many gifts and gratuities have the appearance of illegal kickbacks. Drug makers admitted they "routinely made payments to insurance plans to increase the use of their products, to expand their market share, to be added to lists of recommended drugs or to reward doctors and pharmacists for switching patients from one brand of drug to another" (Pear, 2002).

A prime example of name identification, referred to as "branding" in marketing, is the Ross logo and teddy bear trademark prominently displayed on the AAP's new breastfeeding book, *New Mother's Guide to Breastfeeding*. Members are increasingly concerned about the influence that corporations have on the academy (Petersen, 2002). AAP members have urged the academy to develop a policy to ensure that commercial logos never again appear on its books and other educational materials. Some believe that pharmaceutical companies—which includes formula companies—spend more on marketing, advertising, and administrative budgets than on research and development efforts (Families USA, 2002).

Healthcare professionals need to recognize that accepting a "gift" implies an obligation on the receiver's part to look favorably at the giver. It causes the receiver to feel obligated to treat that person well and, ultimately, to promote his product. Editors of the *British Medical Journal* called for an end to the acceptance of "free" lunches. The University of California is considering ending free lunches sponsored by drug companies and is asking American medical students to take a revised Hippocratic Oath that forbids accepting money, gifts, or hospitality (Abbassi, 2003). The International Lactation Consultant Association (ILCA) urges lactation consultants to refuse funding from formula companies and

others who violate the International Code (ILCA, 2002). There is no such thing as a free lunch, and someone eventually pays. For parents, it is higher costs on the retail market and increased medical bills. For infants, it is a higher incidence of illness, chronic disease, and death. For the public, it is higher taxes and overall healthcare costs.

Global Response to Formula Advertising

The World Health Assembly created the International Code of Marketing of Breastmilk Substitutes in 1981, which all Member States of the World Health Organization affirmed. In 2004, more than 20 years later, the Code still awaits enactment into legislation or enforceable regulations at the national level in many countries. The United States delayed signing on to the Code for many years and was the last nation to sign it. Table 28.4 reflects the main points of the Code, which calls for regulating the marketing and distribution of products represented to be suitable as a partial or total replacement for human milk. Any product that is promoted for use during the exclusive breastfeeding period below the age of about six months will have the effect of replacing human milk in the child's intake.

You can protect breastfeeding by urging colleagues and facilities to adhere to the International Code of Marketing of Breastmilk Substitutes and its subsequent resolutions. Help colleagues develop an awareness of instances in which a facility violates the Code. Remove posters, videos, and leaflets that advertise products marketed or otherwise represented to be suitable as substitutes for human milk. Make sure instruction on the use of infant formula targets only mothers who have chosen not to breastfeed. Remove videos on artificial feeding from the hospital's television channel, for instance, and loan them individually to mothers who need the instruction. You can obtain information and educational materials about the Code on the ILCA Web site.

When you encounter violations of the Code, take action to make others aware. Ask administrators to reject anything that does not comply with the Code. Discuss the violations with colleagues, and take steps to change practices that do not comply. Refuse any gifts or samples of formula and prevent others from giving them to mothers, if you have the power to do so. Be aware that sponsorship of a conference by formula companies often may not be clear and you will need to ask before agreeing to participate in the program. Formula companies own subsidiaries that sell other products. If asked to speak or participate in a conference, find out if the sponsor or organizer has an affiliation with the pharmaceutical or infant formula industry. The Code is in place to promote, protect, and support breastfeeding. You are in a good position to help protect the interests of breastfeeding mothers and babies.

TABLE 28.4
The International Code of Marketing of Breastmilk Substitutes

Code Provision	Implications to Consider
Under the scope of the Code, items marketed or otherwise represented to be suitable as human milk substitutes can include foods and beverages such as: ◆ Infant formula ◆ Other milk products ◆ Cereals ◆ Vegetable, fruit, and other puréed preparations ◆ Juices and baby teas ◆ Follow-on milks ◆ Bottled water	Whether or not a product is considered to be within this definition will depend on how it is promoted for infants. Any products that are marketed or represented as suitable substitutes to human milk will fall into this category. Since babies should receive *only* human milk for the first six months, any other food or drink promoted for use during this time will be a human milk substitute.
Regarding advertising and information, the Code recommends that: ◆ Advertising of human milk substitutes, bottles, and teats to the public not be permitted ◆ Educational materials explain the benefits of breastfeeding, the health hazards associated with bottle feeding, the costs of using infant formula, and the difficulty of reversing the decision not to breastfeed ◆ Product labels clearly state the superiority of breastfeeding, the need for the advice of a healthcare worker, and a warning about health hazards; and they show no pictures of babies, or other pictures or text idealizing the use of infant formula	Health workers such as lactation consultants and breastfeeding counselors need to press their legislators for measures that will implement the Code in full. This would protect mothers from advertising in parent magazines and on television. It would also prevent direct company contact with mothers through hot lines, Internet sites, mailings, home-delivered supplies of formula, and baby clubs.
Regarding samples and supplies, the Code recommends that: ◆ No free samples be given to pregnant women, mothers, or their families ◆ No free or low-cost supplies of human milk substitutes be given to maternity wards, hospitals, or any other part of the healthcare system	Under the Code, free or low-cost supplies can be distributed only outside of the healthcare system and must be continued for as long as the infant needs them. In the United States, this is usually for one year. Elsewhere, it is for at least six months. The healthcare system encompasses healthcare workers, including lactation consultants *and* breastfeeding counselors.
Regarding healthcare facilities and healthcare workers, the Code recommends that: ◆ There be no product displays, posters, or distribution of promotional materials ◆ No gifts or samples be given to healthcare workers ◆ Product information for health professionals be limited to what is factual and scientific	This provision also covers bottles that are provided and shown in advertisements by breast pump companies that are clearly feeding bottles, even when no teats are shown. Pens and pads of paper with the name of a formula company are examples of gifts.

Baby-friendly Hospital Initiative

Achieving a baby-friendly environment may seem to be a daunting task. Yet the benefits are immense. If you give more than is asked of you, you will reap great rewards.

What an exhilarating feeling to be part of such a positive health-affirming effort! To get where you want to go, you must have a definite vision of your overall goal. UNICEF and WHO have provided the vision with their *Ten Steps to Successful Breastfeeding* and Baby-friendly

Hospital Initiative. The aim of the initiative is to make healthcare providers the "prime movers in recreating a world environment that supports, protects, and promotes the practice of breastfeeding—a world environment that is friendly to babies and their mothers" (Kyenkya-Isabirye, 1992). The success of the initiative will depend on countless small changes enacted one person at a time, hospital by hospital, and country by country.

A Baby-friendly Health Profession

Changes are occurring in healthcare around the globe. In the United States, for example, the length of stay following birth has altered dramatically in the past decade in response to new trends in health insurance. These changes affect everyone working in the healthcare field. Promotion of breastfeeding must fit into the context of the healthcare system. Many mothers receive marginal or no in-hospital breastfeeding care. Conflicting advice, misconceptions, and inconsistencies between theory and practice affect the course of breastfeeding for mothers. Maternity nurses may acknowledge, for example, that suckling promotes milk production, yet they may advise formula supplements if a mother appears not to have enough milk. Mothers need consistent technical assistance from caregivers who will empower them to reach their goals and follow the health guidelines of exclusive breastfeeding for at least six months.

Baby-friendly healthcare requires the commitment of all health professionals. Despite a universal recognition of the health benefits of breastfeeding, many physicians fail to support breastfeeding mothers (Taveras, 2004; Donnelly, 1994). One study showed that 48 percent of practicing pediatricians did not recommend breastfeeding to their patients. They also reported few interventions to assist breastfeeding women. These same physicians overwhelmingly reported favorable attitudes toward breastfeeding promotion (Michelman, 1990).

The absence of formal training in breastfeeding accounts for much of this lack of tangible caregiver support. Pediatricians, obstetricians, and family practice physicians need formal instruction in breastfeeding during their residency programs, with a focus on three main areas. First, the program must provide information regarding medical rationale, techniques, and problem solving. Second, it needs to address expectations, beliefs, and an acceptance of data that demonstrate the health benefits of breastfeeding. Finally, the program needs to build the physicians' confidence that they can provide effective counseling and support to breastfeeding women (AAFP, 2001; Saenz, 2000; Freed, 1993). Breastfeeding information in pediatric textbooks needs updating and expansion as well (Philipp, 2004).

Breastfeeding support requires a genuine commitment on the part of the caregiver. Physicians need to recognize that when they distribute infant formula or vouchers to parents, they place themselves in the position of advertising and promoting a product. In addition, this promotion contributes to the failure of women in their practice to breastfeed their infants (Donnelly, 2000; Howard, 1993). Physicians who support breastfeeding can be encouraged to educate their peers. UNICEF developed a pledge for physicians to sign, attesting to their commitment to protect, promote, and support breastfeeding, as presented in Figure 28.2 (Grant, 1994). Signing such a pledge demonstrates physicians' desire to support breastfeeding women in their practices.

The development of baby-friendly breastfeeding policies can further formalize this support. See the examples of baby-friendly policies for hospitals (Figure 28.3), pediatric practice (Figure 28.4), obstetric practice (Figure 28.5), home health practice (Figure 28.6), and a pediatric unit (Figure 28.7). Mothers whose care is coordinated by a healthcare team from these types of baby-friendly practices will receive optimal support and care in their breastfeeding efforts.

Official "Baby-friendly" Designation

Health facilities worldwide are being designated as "Baby-friendly," with the initiative being adopted more slowly in some countries than in others. By 2002, there

---

FIGURE 28.2
Physician's pledge to protect, promote, and support breastfeeding.

Recognizing that breastfeeding plays a uniquely important role in the healthy development of infants and young children;

that no substitute can provide the complex balance of nutrients, antibodies and growth factors that make human milk the perfect food for infants;

that women have the right to make infant feeding decisions based on complete and accurate information;

that my role as a physician is one of influence, authority and trust;

that current marketing practices—including the free and low-cost distribution of human milk substitute supplies to hospitals and other parts of the healthcare system—compete against and discourage breastfeeding;

that my Government, at the 1994 World Health Assembly, affirmed that the marketing and promotion of human milk substitutes should not be conducted anywhere in the healthcare system; and

that the promotion of health and the prevention of disease are my duties and the mandates of responsible healthcare providers everywhere;

I hereby pledge to do my part to protect, promote and support breastfeeding and to work to end the free and low-cost distribution of human milk substitutes to our healthcare systems.

Signature _____

FIGURE 28.3
Baby-friendly hospital breastfeeding policy.

1. All pregnant women and new mothers will be informed of the nutritional and health benefits and basic management of breastfeeding.
2. Staff will presume the mother is breastfeeding unless the mother informs the staff otherwise.
3. Mothers will be helped to initiate breastfeeding within an hour of birth unless maternal or neonatal complications intervene.
4. All nursing mothers will be given instructions on hand expression of milk. If they should be separated from their infants, nursing mothers will be given specific instructions on breastfeeding and how to maintain lactation (pumping). Mothers who have not begun breastfeeding within 8 to 12 hours of birth will begin milk expression.
5. Breastfeeding newborns will be given no food or drink other than human milk unless medically indicated and a specific order is written by the physician. A list of medical indications for using human milk substitutes is provided.
6. Breastfeeding babies will be given pacifiers only at the direction of the mother. The risks and benefits of using artificial nipples (pacifiers, bottles) will be explained to the mother.
7. Infants who need supplementation will be tube fed at the breast or cup fed unless medically contraindicated.
8. Rooming-in will be encouraged; babies are to be kept with their mothers 24 hours a day. Mothers will be taught how to cosleep with their infants safely.
9. Mothers will be taught to watch for infant feeding cues, and will breastfeed their babies on demand rather than on a predetermined schedule. Mothers will be encouraged to breastfeed their babies a minimum of 8 times in 24 hours.
10. Mothers will be given information about breastfeeding support groups and lactation consultants prior to discharge from the hospital.
11. Each healthcare professional who cares for mothers and infants at this facility is expected to maintain the skills and knowledge necessary for implementation of this policy.

Printed with permission of Marsha Walker.

FIGURE 28.4
Ten steps to a baby-friendly pediatric practice.

1. Develop or implement a current breastfeeding protocol for use in your practice that is communicated to all staff. Provide copies to those who cover for you.
2. Arrange for all staff to attend inservices that teach the skills necessary to implement the protocol.
3. Inform all pregnant women about the benefits and management of breastfeeding. Give written, noncommercial prenatal information on breastfeeding, refer parents to breastfeeding classes, and encourage fathers to attend.
4. Help mothers initiate and maintain breastfeeding during hospital rounds. Perform newborn exam in the mother's room, showing her how well-designed her baby is for breastfeeding.
5. If mother and baby are separated due to illness, prematurity, and so on, confirm that an electric breast pump is available for expressing milk, and that milk is expressed at least 8 times in 24 hours. A prescription may be written for human milk, if necessary, to cover the cost of renting an electric breast pump.
6. Avoid the use of sterile water, glucose water, or formula for breastfeeding newborn infants, unless medically indicated. Adequate amounts of milk are present at delivery in the form of colostrum.
7. Encourage mothers to room-in 24 hours a day in the hospital. This protects the baby from disease in the nursery, provides opportunities for unrestricted contact and feeding, and encourages mothers to become aware of their baby's needs and rhythms.
8. Advise mothers to feed their infants on cue, 8 to 12 times each 24 hours. Teach behavioral feeding cues to avoid underfeeding or overhunger, with resulting infant behavioral disorganization.
9. Avoid the use of artificial nipples and pacifiers in newborn breastfeeding infants. This approach decreases the incidence of nipple preference and its sequelae.
10. Have available on staff a nurse practitioner or lactation consultant whose responsibility can include prenatal teaching, hospital rounds, call-in times, and visits for breastfeeding questions or problems. Or refer such situations to a lactation consultant in the community. Refer mothers to breastfeeding support groups for mother-to-mother support.

Printed with permission of Marsha Walker.

were 15,000 facilities globally that were officially designated as Baby-friendly. Less than 2 percent of those facilities were in developed countries such as the United States, Canada, and Australia. By 2004, there were 42 Baby-friendly facilities in the United States.

A Baby-friendly designation means that a facility meets high global standards and has at least 75 percent of mothers exclusively breastfeeding at discharge. The global process for receiving Baby-friendly recognition involves an internal assessment, an external assessment by outside evaluators, and a presentation of the findings by UNICEF. The process may vary from one country to another, as government officials make adaptations that will complement their country's standards.

A Baby-friendly World

The baby-friendly initiative goes far beyond the health community. Many regard breastfeeding as an important woman's, human rights, and feminist issue. On the surface, feminism and breastfeeding may appear to be incompatible because breastfeeding is associated with traditional roles for women. However, breastfeeding is a holistic act that is intimately connected to all domains of life—sexuality, eating, emotion, appearance, sleeping, and parental relationships (Van Esterick, 1994). Breastfeeding confirms a woman's power to provide nutrition and nurture for her baby and challenges views of the

---

FIGURE 28.5
Ten steps to a baby-friendly obstetric practice.

1. Create and implement a breastfeeding promotion and support policy for use in your practice that is communicated to all staff. Provide copies to those who cover for you.
2. Arrange for all staff to attend inservices that teach the skills necessary to implement the protocol.
3. Inform all pregnant women about the benefits and management of breastfeeding. Give written, noncommercial information on breastfeeding. Recommend that parents attend prenatal breastfeeding classes that include fathers. Refer parents to childbirth education classes.
4. Help mothers initiate breastfeeding within ½ hour of birth. Place and leave the infant on the mother's chest to promote the prefeeding sequences of behavior that leads to proper latch, suck, and organization of breastfeedings.
5. If mother and baby are separated due to illness, prematurity, and so on, confirm that an electric breast pump is available for expressing milk; that milk is expressed at least 8 times in 24 hours; that no nipple soreness, engorgement, or breast problems arise from the use of the pump.
6. Avoid the use of sterile water, glucose water, or formula for breastfeeding newborn infants, unless medically indicated. Adequate amounts of milk are present at delivery in the form of colostrum.
7. Encourage mothers to room-in 24 hours a day in the hospital. This protects the baby from disease in the nursery, provides opportunities for unrestricted contact and feeding, and encourages mothers to become aware of their baby's needs and rhythms.
8. Advise mothers to feed their infants on cue, 8 to 12 times each 24 hours. Teach behavioral feeding cues to avoid underfeeding or overhunger, with resulting infant behavioral disorganization.
9. Avoid the use of artificial nipples and pacifiers in newborn breastfeeding infants. This approach decreases the incidence of nipple preference and its sequelae.
10. Have available on staff a nurse practitioner or lactation consultant whose responsibility can include prenatal teaching, hospital rounds, call-in times, and visits for breastfeeding questions or problems. Or refer such situations to a lactation consultant in the community. Refer mothers to breastfeeding support groups for mother-to-mother support.

Printed with permission of Marsha Walker.

FIGURE 28.6
Ten steps to a baby-friendly home health practice.

1. Create a written breastfeeding policy that is research based, and provide copies of the policy to all home health staff. Include the WHO/UNICEF Code for Marketing Breastmilk Substitutes in the policy.
2. Train all healthcare staff in the Maternal-Child Services using the WHO/UNICEF 18 Hour Course. Update staff as new or revised research-based information becomes available. New staff will be given the 18-hour course beginning during orientation and completed within 1 year.
3. Inform all pregnant women about the benefits and management of breastfeeding; weave breastfeeding information into every visit. Provide written information that complies with the WHO Code. Refer all pregnant women to the prenatal breastfeeding classes within the community.
4. Inform all pregnant women of the importance of initiating breastfeeding within the first hour of life.
5. If postpartum mothers are separated from their babies, be sure they have proper equipment for milk expression and provide instruction as needed. Teach hand expression to all breastfeeding mothers. Assess breastfeeding during each home visit.
6. Give the child (ages newborn to about 6 months) no food or drink other than human milk unless *medically* indicated. Instruct mothers (prenatal and postpartum) about the risks of artificial baby milks. A list of acceptable medical reasons for human milk substitutes is included in the breastfeeding policy.
7. Encourage a "rooming-in" home environment. Explain the importance of close mother-infant contact 24 hours a day by the use of a sling, bathing together, sleeping together and so on.
8. Teach mothers the importance of their babies' cues. Explain the importance of baby-led feedings, rather than placing limitations and times on feeds. Advise mothers that 8 to 12 or more feeds in 24 hours is normal and expected.
9. Give no artificial teats or pacifiers to breastfeeding infants. Discourage their use, and instead direct the mother to breastfeed for suckling satisfaction. Explain the negative consequences of such devices.
10. Foster the establishment of breastfeeding support groups within the community, and refer mothers to them at any time.

Printed with permission of Debbie Shinskie.

---

breast as primarily a sexual object (Stuart-Macadam, 1995). Women's groups are encouraged to commit resources and time to breastfeeding promotion. Artists can portray the beauty and power of breastfeeding through paintings, photographs, poems, and plays. The media can present breastfeeding as a natural part of our culture.

Promotion of breastfeeding at the government level increases the incidence and duration of breastfeeding (Merewood, 2004; Mitra, 2003). Successful government campaigns share several characteristics. They have a long-term plan for sustaining the program, and sound administrative and financial management. Staff and funds are devoted exclusively to the promotion program to identify key obstacles and strategies for overcoming them. A mass media program conveys appropriate messages and materials to the target audience.

Richard Reid (1993), then the Director of Public Affairs for UNICEF, cautioned that "every culture that abandons breastfeeding is inviting upon itself sicklier children, weaker mothers, poorer families, strained national economies, and more polluted environments." He urged a global return to breastfeeding as an urgent moral, health, social, and economic imperative. Long-term strategies for achieving a baby-friendly world appear in the following list. These efforts to return breastfeeding to its rightful

---

FIGURE 28.7
Optimal breastfeeding in the pediatric unit.

1. Have a written breastfeeding policy, and train healthcare staff caring for breastfeeding infants in skills necessary to implement thepolicy.
2. When the sick infant is admitted, ascertain the mother's wishes about infant feeding, and assist mothers to establish and managelactation as necessary.
3. Provide parents with written and verbal information about the benefits of breastfeeding and human milk.
4. Facilitate unrestricted breastfeeding and frequent human milk expression by mothers who wish to provide milk for their children, regardless of age.
5. Give breastfed children other food or drink only when age appropriate or medically indicated.
6. When medically indicated, use only those alternative feeding methods most conducive to successful breastfeeding, and restrict the use of any oral device associated with breastfeeding problems.
7. Provide facilities that allow parents and infants to remain together 24 hours a day, that encourage skin-to-skin contact as appropriate, and that avoid modeling the use of artificial feeding.
8. Administer medications and schedule all procedures so as to cause the least possible disturbance of the breastfeeding relationship.
9. Maintain a human milk bank that meets appropriate standards.
10. Provide information about community breastfeeding support groups to parents at the time of the infant's discharge from the hospital or clinic.
11. Maintain appropriate monitoring and data collection procedures to permit quality assurance and ongoing research.

Printed with permission of Maureen Minchin from *Breastfeeding Matters*; 1999.

---

place as the cultural norm will empower women to nurture their babies in the manner that nature intended.

Long-term Strategies for Achieving a Baby-friendly World

◆ Ensure that all maternity centers practice all of the Ten Steps to Successful Breastfeeding.

◆ Take action to implement fully all articles of the International Code of Marketing of Breastmilk Substitutes and its subsequent World Health Assembly resolutions.

◆ Enact and enforce legislation to protect the breastfeeding rights of working women.

◆ Educate communities to value women's contributions to the health of their children and thus the health of the community and the world.

◆ Encourage institutions to ease the tasks of motherhood with convenient antenatal care, respect from caregivers, good obstetric services, and patient-focused delivery procedures.

◆ Provide women with counseling and clinical services for breastfeeding and birth spacing.

◆ Enlist community, health, religious, and political leaders to promote the primary healthcare principles of preventive health education and empowerment of mothers.

Global Strategy for Infant and Young Child Feeding

In 2002, the World Health Assembly and UNICEF endorsed the Global Strategy for Infant and Young Child Feeding. The strategy builds on the Baby-Friendly Hospital Initiative, the International Code of Marketing of Breastmilk Substitutes, and the Innocenti Declaration on the Protection, Promotion and Support of Breastfeeding. It places those initiatives in the overall context of national policies, programs on nutrition and child health, and a number of other declarations and conventions. The Global Strategy addresses appropriate, evidence-based feeding practices for infants and young children that are essential for attaining and maintaining proper nutrition and health. Major components of the Global Strategy include:

◆ Development of comprehensive national policies on infant and young child feeding.

◆ Use of an evidence-based, integrated, comprehensive approach.

◆ Consideration of the physical, social, economic, and cultural environment.

◆ Healthcare support of exclusive breastfeeding for six months.

◆ Supportive work environments to increase exclusive breastfeeding rates.

◆ Support of breastfeeding with complementary foods up to two years and beyond.

◆ Provision of adequate, timely, safe complementary foods.

◆ Guidance to families in exceptionally difficult circumstances.

◆ Legislation and regulations to ensure adherence to the International Code of Marketing of Breastmilk Substitutes and subsequent World Health Assembly resolutions.

Lactation professionals can be instrumental in advancing the goals of the Global Strategy by developing breastfeeding protocols, challenging traditional procedures, and removing barriers that erode the mother's confidence in her ability to breastfeed. You have enormous potential to facilitate consistent care by instituting care plans for managing breastfeeding problems and conducting staff inservice education. UNICEF and the World Health Organization have provided healthcare professionals and administrators with very clear guidelines for the establishment of policies and procedures that will promote, protect, and support breastfeeding. ILCA and other breastfeeding advocacy organizations support the global initiatives. Hospitals, clinics, and physician offices throughout the world are incorporating the global guidelines into their policies and practices. With collaborative efforts of everyone in the healthcare system, the 21st century can turn the tide of infant health and ensure optimal growth of young children.

Turning the Tide in Breastfeeding Promotion

Breastfeeding promotion is a form of social marketing. Use of effective marketing strategies will increase awareness of breastfeeding's importance. Marketing involves promotions used by businesses to convert people's needs and wants into profitable company opportunities (Kotler, 2002). Social marketing became popular when marketers applied the same principles used to sell products to "sell" ideas, attitudes, and behaviors. Social marketing seeks to influence social behavior and benefit the target audience and society as a whole (Weinreich, 1999). Hospitals, physician practices, and employers are in the business of satisfying customer needs. In this regard, breastfeeding promotion is no different from the marketing of any other health practice that improves the consumer's well-being. An institution can add value to its services by adopting a consumer-focused marketing strategy. Parents and infants are the consumers whose needs must be met. Baby-friendly practices provide a framework within which they can achieve their goals.

Studies have demonstrated the global success of the baby-friendly approach in increasing breastfeeding rates. Several countries report increased breastfeeding rates when any of the baby-friendly steps were used. They include Australia (Oddy, 2003), Brazil (de Oliveira, 2003; Bicalho-Mancini, 2004), Germany (Dulon, 2003), Italy (Banderali, 2003; Cattaneo, 2001), Saudi Arabia (Fida, 2003), Switzerland (Merten, 2004), Taiwan (Gau, 2004), and the United States (Merewood, 2003; Philipp, 2003, 2001).

National Breastfeeding Awareness Campaign

It is fitting to end the text with an exciting advertising campaign launched in June 2004, in the United States. The Office of Women's Health in the United States Department of Health and Human Services designed a National Breastfeeding Awareness Campaign, the first of its kind since 1911. The goal of the campaign is to encourage exclusive breastfeeding for six months and increase breastfeeding rates to 75 percent (Merewood, 2004).

The Ad Council, a private, nonprofit organization, accepted the task of communicating the campaign messages to the public. Previous Ad Council campaigns include "Rosie the Riveter," "Smokey Bear," "Crash Test Dummies," and "This is your brain on drugs." All of the ads for this campaign drive home the message, "Babies were born to be breastfed." Public service announcements target the general market as well as the African American community, as rates of breastfeeding are lowest among this population. Print ads for placement in periodicals and newspapers are available from the National Women's Health Information Center Web site at www.4woman.gov, or the Ad Council's Web site at www.adcouncil.org/campaigns/breastfeeding. The public is directed to www.4woman.gov or to call (800) 994-WOMAN to talk with trained information specialists who can help with breastfeeding issues.

Concerns raised by infant formula industry executives about the campaign's content and approach delayed the campaign launch by several months. They took exception to describing the risks of *not* breastfeeding rather than the benefits of breastfeeding. Protests from the medical community, breastfeeding advocates, and AAP members—particularly the AAP Section on Breastfeeding Executive Committee—put the campaign back on track with some modifications in content. However, the main thrust and approach of the campaign remained intact. Launch of the campaign represents a major step forward for breastfeeding advocacy in the United States. The campaign serves as a model to the international community for promotion in other countries. The May 2004 issue of the *Journal of Human Lactation* contains contact information for 18 U.S. communities that facilitates contact with local media and dissemination of campaign materials.

The formula industry will continue to use its money and political power to fight against the basic truth that human milk is for human babies and cows' milk is for baby calves. Lactation professionals, physicians, nurses, and all other members of the healthcare profession and breastfeeding support community can use the Breastfeeding Awareness Campaign as a springboard for action to return breastfeeding to the cultural norm and to ensure every child's right to be breastfed. You can do this by contacting the public service director at your local media outlets and encouraging them to air or print the public service announcements frequently. You can use the controversy surrounding the formula industry's fight against the campaign to raise public awareness of the risks of *not* giving human babies human milk.

Much as the fight against the tobacco industry took more than 40 years, this fight will not be finished quickly. Report violations of the Code and deceptive advertising and trade practices to the U.S. Food and Drug Administration or the equivalent governmental agency in your country. Groups such as the National Alliance for Breastfeeding Advocacy, Media Watch, INFACT, IBFAN, and WABA can help hold companies accountable. Your involvement with local ILCA affiliates and local breastfeeding support groups will energize and motivate you to continue to help mothers and babies realize their birthright to breastfeed and be breastfed, and to work toward producing healthier families and a healthier world.

▶ SUMMARY

We wish you great success in your helping role with mothers and in your promotion of breastfeeding. We encourage you to be an active agent for change, working toward making your community baby friendly in all areas—hospitals, clinics, health workers, and the general public. Baby-friendly healthcare extends beyond the baby to create an environment that is mother friendly and family friendly. Breastfeeding is an endangered practice that needs an entire culture to support and nurture it back to its full, potent strength. You are not alone in your work toward promoting optimal nutrition for infants and young children. Major international initiatives are in place to guide and support your efforts.

▶ CHAPTER 28 — AT A GLANCE

Applying what you learned—

◆ Increase your effectiveness as a leader by choosing to be effective, making a blueprint, staying focused, working toward mutual benefit, and building a strong team.

◆ Use positive self-talk, and view mistakes as lessons.

◆ Increase your assertiveness by practicing assertive behavior.

◆ Plan and implement change, and anticipate resistance.

◆ Recognize reasons for resistance, and resolve conflicts.

◆ Gather data, and evaluate your facility.

◆ Define problems, goals, and strategies.

◆ Form a breastfeeding committee with members from areas affected by the change and different personality types.

◆ Take change slow and easy, and give recognition and praise.

◆ Be aware of marketing practices of the infant formula industry, and refuse funding from them.

◆ Learn the provisions of the International Code of Marketing of Breastmilk Substitutes, follow them, and report violations.

◆ Promote the Baby-friendly Hospital Initiative.

◆ Learn components of the Global Strategy for Infant and Young Child Feeding.

◆ Be familiar with the U.S. National Breastfeeding Awareness Campaign, and ask local media outlets to air or print the public service announcements frequently.

◆ Work as an active agent for change to promote optimal nutrition for infants and young children.

▶ REFERENCES

Abbassi K, Smith R. No more free lunches. Editorial. *BMJ* 326:1155–1156; 2003.

Agennix, Inc. Available at: www. rhlf.com. Accessed January 5, 2005.

American Academy of Family Physicians (AAFP). *AAFP Policy Statement on Breastfeeding.* Breastfeeding Position Paper; 2001.

Anand RK. *Transforming Health Colleagues into Breastfeeding Advocates.* WABA Activity Sheet No. 3. Available at: www.waba.org.my/activitysheet/acsh3.htm. Accessed February 7, 2005.

Banderali G et al. Monitoring breastfeeding rates in Italy. *Acta Paediatr Suppl* 91(441):6–8; 2003.

Barness LA. Nothing is free. *Contemp Pediatr*, May 1987.

Bicalho-Mancini P, Velasquez-Melendez G. Exclusive breastfeeding at the point of discharge of high-risk newborns at a Neonatal Intensive Care Unit and the factors associated with this practice. *J Pediatr (Rio J)* 80(3):241–248; 2004.

Breastfeeding Support Consultants (BSC). *Creating Change in the Face of Resistance.* Chalfont, PA; 1996.

Brett A et al. Are gifts from pharmaceutical companies ethically problematic? A survey of physicians. *Arch Intern Med* 163(18):2213–2218; 2003.

Browder S. Super-confidence and how to get it. *New Woman Magazine*; July 1994.

Burton B, Rowell A. Education and debate: Unhealthy spin. *BMJ* 326:1205–1207; 2003.

Cadwell K. Using the quality improvement process to affect breastfeeding protocols in United States hospitals. *J Hum Lact* 13:5–9; 1997.

Cattaneo A, Buzzetti R. Effect on rates of breast feeding of training for the baby friendly hospital initiative. *BMJ* 323(7325): 1358–1362; 2001.

Covey S. *The 7 Habits of Highly Effective People.* New York: Simon and Schuster; 1990.

Dana D. *Conflict Resolution.* New York: McGraw-Hill; 2000.

de Oliveira M et al. A method for the evaluation of primary health care units' practice in the promotion, protection, and support of breastfeeding: Results from the state of Rio de Janeiro, Brazil. *J Hum Lact* 19(4):365–373; 2003.

Donnelly A et al. Commercial hospital discharge packs for breastfeeding women. *Cochrane Database Syst Rev* (2): CD002075; 2000.

Donnelly BW. Are we really doing all we can to promote breastfeeding? *Contemp Pediat*; July 1994.

Dulon M et al. Breastfeeding promotion in non-UNICEF-certified hospitals and long-term breastfeeding success in Germany. *Acta Paediatr* 92(6):653–658; 2003.

Ellis DJ. Supporting breastfeeding: How to implement agency change. Clinical Issues in Perinatal and Women's Health Nursing. *NAACOG* 3(4):560–564; 1992.

Families USA. *Profiting from Pain: Where Prescription Drug Dollars Go.* #02-105. Washington, DC: Families USA; July 2002.

Fida N, Al-Aama J. Pattern of infant feeding at a university hospital in Western Saudi Arabia. *Saudi Med J* 24(7):725–729; 2003.

Freed GL. Breast-feeding: Time to teach what we preach. *JAMA* 269(2):243–245; 1993.

Gau M. Evaluation of a lactation intervention program to encourage breastfeeding: A longitudinal study. *Int J Nurs Stud* 41(4):425–435; 2004.

Goleman D et al. *Primal Leadership: Realizing the Power of Emotional Intelligence.* Boston, MA: Harvard Business School Press; 2002.

Goleman D. *Emotional Intelligence.* New York: Bantam; 1997.

Grant JP. Physician's pledge to protect, promote and support breastfeeding. New York: UNICEF; 1994.

Howard C et al. Antenatal formula advertising: Another potential threat to breast-feeding. *Pediatrics* 94:102–104; 1994.

Howard F et al. The physician as advertiser: The unintentional discouragement of breastfeeding. *Obstet Gynecol* 81:1048–1051; 1993.

Humes JC. Life lessons from Ben Franklin. *Bottom Line/Personal*; June 15, 1992.

International Board of Lactation Consultant Examiners. *The Code of Ethics: International Board-Certified Lactation Consultants.* Falls Church, VA; 2004.

International Lactation Consultant Association (Walker M ed.). *Core Curriculum for Lactation Consultant Practice.* Boston, MA: Jones and Bartlett; 2002.

Jackson M. The comedy of management. In Simms L, et al. *The Professional Practice of Nursing Administration.* New York: Wiley, pp. 339–351; 1985.

Kahler T. Six basic personality types. *Bottom Line/Personal*; September 15, 1992.

Kotler P. *Marketing Management.* 11th ed. Englewood Cliffs, NJ: Prentice Hall; 2002.

Kyenkya-Isabirye M. UNICEF launches the Baby-Friendly Hospital Initiative. *MCN* 17(4):177–179; 1992.

Mayer B. *The Dynamics of Conflict Resolution: A Practitioner's Guide.* San Francisco, CA: Jossey-Bass; 2000.

Merewood A, Heinig J. Efforts to promote breastfeeding in the United States: Development of a national breastfeeding awareness campaign. *J Hum Lact* 20(2):140–145; 2004.

Merewood A, Philipp B. Becoming baby-friendly: Overcoming the issue of accepting free formula. *J Hum Lact* 16(4):279–282; 2000.

Merewood A et al. The baby-friendly hospital initiative increases breastfeeding rates in a US neonatal intensive care unit. *J Hum Lact* 19(2):166–171; 2003.

Merten S, Ackermann-Liebrich U. Exclusive breastfeeding rates and associated factors in Swiss baby-friendly hospitals. *J Hum Lact* 20(1):9–17; 2004.

Michelman DF et al. Pediatricians and breastfeeding promotion: Attitudes, beliefs and practices. *American Journal of Health Promotion* 4:181–186; 1990.

Mitra A et al. Evaluation of a comprehensive loving support program among state Women, Infants, and Children (WIC) program breast-feeding coordinators. *South Med J* 96(2):168–171; 2003.

Moynihan R. Who pays for the pizza? Redefining the relationships between doctors and drug companies. 1: Entanglement. *BMJ* 326(7400):1189–1192; 2003.

Mulford C. Swimming upstream: Breastfeeding care in a non-breastfeeding culture. *JOGNN* 24(5):464–474; 1995.

No Free Lunch. Available at: www.nofreelunch.org. Accessed June 23, 2004.

Oddy W, Glenn K. Implementing the Baby Friendly Hospital Initiative: The role of finger feeding. *Breastfeed Rev* 11(1): 5–10; 2003.

Pear R. Drug makers battle plan to curb rewards for doctors. *NY Times* Late Edition—Final, Section A, Page 1, Column 6; December 26, 2002.

Petersen M. Pediatric book on breast-feeding stirs controversy. *NY Times* Late Edition—Final, Section C, Page 1, Column 3; September 18, 2002.

Philipp B et al. Baby-friendly hospital initiative improves breastfeeding initiation rates in a US hospital setting. *Pediatrics* 108(3):677–681; 2001.

Philipp B et al. Sustained breastfeeding rates at a US baby-friendly hospital. *Pediatrics* 112(3 Pt 1):e234–e236; 2003.

Philipp B et al. Breastfeeding information in pediatric textbooks needs improvement. *J Hum Lact* 20(2):206–210; 2004.

Reid R. The baby-friendly hospital initiative: A global movement for humankind. *International Child Health* 4(1):41–47; January 1993.

Saenz R. A lactation management rotation for family medicine residents. *J Hum Lact* 16(4):342–345; 2000.

Sterken E. Director, INFACT, Canada. Personal e-mail correspondence; April 27, 2004.

Stolberg S, Gerth J. High-tech stealth being used to sway doctor prescriptions. *NY Times*; November 16, 2000.

Stuart-Macadam P, Dettwyler K (eds). *Breastfeeding: Biocultural Perspectives*. New York: Aldine de Gruyter; 1995.

Taveras E et al. Opinions and practices of clinicians associated with continuation of exclusive breastfeeding. *Pediatrics* 113(4):e283–e290; 2004.

Van Esterick P. Breastfeeding and feminism. *Int J Gynecol Obstet* (Supp 1):S41–S54; 1994.

Villanueva P et al. Accuracy of pharmaceutical advertisements in medical journals. *Lancet* 361(9351):27–32; 2003.

Walker M. *Selling Out Mothers and Babies: Marketing of Breast Milk Substitutes in the USA*. Weston, MA: NABA REAL; 2001.

Weinreich N. *Hands-on Social Marketing: A Step-by-Step Guide*. Thousand Oaks, CA: Sage Publications; 1999.

Yerkes L. *Fun Works: Creating Places Where People Love to Work*. San Francisco, CA: Berrett-Koehler; 2001.

Young D. Breastfeeding: Can it compete in the marketplace? *Birth* 17:119–120; 1990.

▶ BIBLIOGRAPHY

Apple R. The medicalization of infant feeding in the United States and New Zealand: Two countries, one experience. *J Hum Lact* 10:31–37; 1994.

Armstrong HC. Breastfeeding promotion: Training of mid-level and outreach health workers. *Int J Gynecol and Obstet* 31(Suppl 1):91–103; 1991.

Auerbach K. Breastfeeding promotion: Why it doesn't work. *J Hum Lact* 6:45–46; 1990.

Auerbach KG. The many ways of marketing artificial baby milk. *J Hum Lact* 8:61–62; 1992.

Bell ML. *A Portrait of Progress: A Business History of Pet Milk Company from 1885 to 1960*. St. Louis, MO: Pet Milk Company, pp. 102–104; 1962.

Chezem J et al. Lactation duration: Influences of human milk replacements and formula samples on women planning post-partum employment. *JOGNN* 27:646–651; 1998.

Gunnlaugsson G, Einarsdottir J. Colostrum and ideas about bad milk: A case study from Guinea-Bissau. *Soc Sci Med* 36:283–288; 1993.

Hardin B. Project Bestfeeding receives the first ICEA Special Projects Grant. *Int J Childbirth Education* 8:15; 1993.

Heinig J. Breastfeeding and the bottom line: Why are the cost savings of breastfeeding such a hard sell? *J Hum Lact* 14:87–88; 1998.

Howard C et al. Infant formula distribution and advertising in pregnancy: A hospital survey. *Birth* 21(1):14–19; 1994.

International Board of Lactation Consultant Examiners. *Clinical Competencies for IBCLC Practice*. Falls Church, VA; 2003.

International Lactation Consultant Association (ILCA). *Standards of Practice for Lactation Consultants*. 2nd ed. Raleigh, NC; 1999.

Kutner L, Barger J. *Clinical Experience in Lactation: A Blueprint for Internship*. 2nd ed. Wheaton, IL: Lactation Education Consultants; 2002.

Merewood A, Phillip B. Peer counselors for breastfeeding mothers in the hospital setting: Trials, training, tributes, and tribulations. *J Hum Lact* 19(1):72–76; 2003.

Merewood A, Philipp B. Promoting breastfeeding in an inner-city hospital: How to address the concerns of the maternity staff regarding illicit drug use. *J Hum Lact* 19(4):418–420; 2003.

Minchin M et al. Expanding the WHO/UNICEF Baby Friendly Hospital Initiative (BFHI): 11 steps to optimal breastfeeding in the pediatric unit. *Breastfeeding Rev* 4:87–91; 1996.

Minchin M. *Breastfeeding Matters: What We Need to Know about Infant Feeding*. Victoria, Australia: Alma Publications; 1998.

Mitra A et al. The loving support breastfeeding campaign: Awareness and practices of health care providers in Mississippi. *J Obstet Gynecol Neonatal Nurs* 32(6):753–760; 2003.

National Association of Pediatric Nurse Practitioners. *NAPNAP Position Statement on Breastfeeding*; 2001. Available at: www.napnap.org/practice/positions/breastfeeding.html. Accessed June 18, 2004.

Newton E. Breastfeeding/lactation and the medical school curriculum. *J Hum Lact* 8:122–124; 1992.

Palmer G. The politics of infant feeding. *Mothering* 73–85; 1991.

Palmer G. *The Politics of Breastfeeding*. London: Pandora Press; 1993.

Radford A et al. Breast feeding: The baby friendly initiative. *Br Med J* 317:1385; 1998.

Sonstegard L. A better way to market maternal-child care. *MCN* 13:395–402; 1988.

UNICEF. *Take the Baby-Friendly Initiative!* New York.

UNICEF/WHO. Breastfeeding management and promotion in a baby-friendly hospital: An 18-hour course for maternity staff; 1993.

U.S. Dept of Health and Human Services. Office of the Inspector General, OIG Compliance Program Guidelines for Pharmaceutical Manufacturers. Fed Reg 68(86); May 5, 2003.

Valaitis R, Shea E. An evaluation of breastfeeding promotion literature: Does it really promote breastfeeding? *Can J Public Health* 84:24–27; 1993.

Williams E, Pan E. Breastfeeding initiation among a low income multiethnic population in Northern California: An exploratory study. *J Hum Lact* 10:245–251; 1994.

Young D. The baby friendly hospital initiative in the U.S.: Why so slow? *Birth* 20(4):179–181; 1993.

GLOSSARY

▶ A

abscess   Localized collection of pus that forms from an infection that has no opening for drainage.

acculturation   Integration into a new culture.

acinus   Any small saclike structure, as one found in a gland. Also called alveolus.

acrocyanosis   Bluish tinge of the hands and feet.

acrodermatitis enteropathica   A rare long-term disease of infants. Symptoms are blisters on the skin and mucous membranes, hair loss, diarrhea, and failure-to-thrive.

active immunity   See immunity, active.

active listening   A counseling skill that involves paraphrasing a message and reflecting it back to the sender.

adhesion   Tissue layers that adhere, or stick, to one another.

adipose tissue   Tissue made of fat cells arranged in lobes.

afterpains   Menstrual-like pains that occur in the first few days after birth as the uterus contracts to return to normal size.

alactogenesis   Absence of the onset of stage II lactogenesis.

allergen   A foreign substance that can cause an allergic response in the body.

alpha-lactalbumin   Protein in the whey portion of human milk that assists with synthesis of lactose. Bactericide against *Streptococcus pneumoniae*.

alternate massage   Technique in which the mother compresses the breast when the baby pauses during a feeding. Used to encourage suckling and increase milk production. Also called breast compression.

alveolar ridge   The bony ridge of the jaw that contains the tooth sockets.

alveoli   Tiny glands in the breast that produce milk.

amenorrhea   The absence of the monthly flow of blood and discharge of mucous tissues from the uterus through the vagina (menstruation).

amino acids   The basic building blocks that make up proteins in the body. They are the end products of protein digestion.

amylase   An enzyme that aids the breakdown of starch in digestion.

analgesia   Absence of the normal sensation of pain.

anchor   A word or phrase used at the numerical endpoints of a written scale to describe the extremes of feeling or thought measured by the scale.

anemia   A decrease in red cells in the blood, in hemoglobin, or in total volume, reducing the blood's ability to carry oxygen. Anemia occurs in about half of all pregnancies.

anesthesia   Partial or complete loss of sensation with or without memory loss as a result of disease, injury, or administration of an anesthetic agent, usually by injection or inhalation.

ankyloglossia   Tight lingual frenulum; defect of the mouth in which the membrane under the tongue is too short, limiting movement of the tongue.

anomaly   Change from what is regarded as normal; inherited problem with growth of a structure.

anovulatory   Failure of the ovaries to produce, mature, or release eggs.

anoxia   Lack of oxygen.

antibody   A protein substance that is developed in response to and interacts specifically with an antigen to form the basis of immunity.

anticipatory guidance   A form of counseling that provides encouragement, help, and guidance in order to prevent or minimize problems.

anticipatory stage   The first of four stages in role acquisition. The time in which one collects information and begins learning about the new role.

antigen   A substance foreign to the body, often a protein.

antimicrobial   Preventing or destroying the development of microorganisms.

apnea   Failure to breathe.

approach behavior   Signals the baby sends to indicate a willingness to interact, such as tongue extension, bringing the hand to the mouth, or rooting.

areola   The dark, circular area surrounding the nipple.

artificial baby milk   See human milk substitute.

artificial feeding   Feeding an infant anything other than human milk.

assessment   An evaluation of a patient that includes physical examination and medical history.

assimilate   (1) The process of incorporating nutrition into living tissue. (2) Becoming incorporated into a culture other than one's own.

assumption   In statistics, a condition that must be true of the data in order for the statistical test to be used accurately.

asymmetry   Disparity in size or shape.

atopic dermatitis   Allergic tendency (possibly inherited) to rash or inflammation of the skin.

atresia   Absence of a normal body opening.

atrophy   Loss of size of a part of the body because of disease or other influences; a natural occurrence in the final stage of lactation (involution).

attachment parenting A form of parenting that creates strong, healthy emotional bonds between children and their parents by nurturing a child's need for trust, empathy, and affection, providing a lifelong foundation for healthy, enduring relationships.

attending A counseling skill that involves listening and observing in a noninterfering manner.

attentive listening A counseling skill in which the listener actively focuses on the words that are heard.

augmentation, breast Surgical procedure performed to increase the size of the breast. It can interfere with milk production.

autocrine control Local control within a gland. In the case of the breast, the control agent is a secretory product from one type of cell that influences the activity of the same type of cell. This suggests that milk that is left in the breast acts to inhibit the production of more milk.

autonomic nerves Nerves that have the ability to function independently without outside influence.

average The sum of the values (in the group being averaged) divided by the number of members of the group.

avoidance behavior Signals the baby sends to indicate an unwillingness to interact, such as frowning, wrinkling his brow, squinting, closing his eyes, or clenching his fists.

axilla Pyramid-shaped space forming the underside of the shoulder between the upper part of the arm and the side of the chest. Also called the armpit.

B

baby blues The mild depression some women feel for several weeks following birth, frequently appearing around the third day postpartum. The mother may have bouts of tearfulness and sadness mingled with happiness and excitement. It is more common in women having their first baby.

baby friendly Maternity care that protects, promotes, and supports breastfeeding.

Baby-friendly Hospital Initiative Health initiative of the World Health Organization and UNICEF launched in 1991 to protect, promote, and support breastfeeding.

baby-led weaning Weaning initiated by the baby, according to the baby's own timetable.

baby training Popular term for feeding and putting infants to sleep at specific times, including feeding on a clock schedule; emphasizes making infants go to sleep on their own without sleep 'props' such as breastfeeding, rocking, bottles or pacifiers.

bactericidal Having the ability to destroy bacteria.

bacteriostatic Capable of restraining the development of bacteria.

basal Referring to the fundamental or basic, as in the lowest body temperature or lowest prolactin level.

baseline The starting value or values before a treatment or test is applied.

Bauer's response Reflex in which pressure on the soles of the feet will elicit spontaneous crawling efforts and extension of the baby's head.

bell curve The shape of the normal distribution on a graph, resembling the shape of a bell.

bias In sampling, bias refers to the tendency of a sample to misrepresent the whole population because some of the sample did not answer the questions. In statistics, unbiased estimators of the true value are usually desired because biased ones tend to consistently overestimate or underestimate the true value.

bifidus factor A carbohydrate present in human milk that has anti-infective properties.

bifurcated Splitting into two branches or parts.

bili-light Fluorescent light used to treat jaundice.

bilirubin A byproduct of the breakdown of the hemoglobin portion of red blood cells.

bioavailability The amount of a nutrient, drug, or other substance that is active in the tissues.

blind A characteristic of a study in which the treatment is kept secret from the person receiving it and, often, from those giving the treatment as well.

blood incompatibility jaundice A condition resulting from blood incompatibility between a mother and her baby that appears within the first 24 hours of life.

body language Nonverbal messages sent by body position and gesture.

body mass index (BMI) A measure of the body that takes into account a person's weight and height to gauge total body fat in adults.

bolus A round mass of food or liquid ready to be swallowed; a dose of a substance given intravenously.

bonding Interaction between parents and infant to form a unique lasting relationship.

bradycardia An abnormal condition in which the heart contracts steadily but at a rate below normal.

breast compression See alternate massage.

breast infection See mastitis.

breast massage Manual massage of the breast used to facilitate letdown and expression of milk.

breast shell A plastic cup worn over the nipple during pregnancy and between feedings to increase nipple protractility and protect sore nipples.

breastfeeding-associated jaundice Neonatal jaundice caused by mismanagement of breastfeeding. Also called lack-of-breastfeeding jaundice.

breastfeeding counselor A lay counselor who assists breastfeeding mothers at a peer level.

breastfeeding diary Daily log of the baby's feedings, wet diapers, and stools.

breastmilk jaundice See late-onset jaundice.

breastmilk substitute See human milk substitute.

buccal pad A fat pad over the main muscle of the cheek. It is very evident in infants and is also called a sucking pad. It is not fully developed in preterm infants.

building hope A counseling skill used to encourage the mother by offering hope for improvement.

burnout A condition of becoming bored, discouraged, or frustrated.

C

Candida albicans A tiny, common yeastlike fungus normally found in the mouth, digestive tract, vagina, and on the skin of healthy persons.

candidiasis A yeastlike fungal infection, commonly afflicting the vagina that produces a thick vaginal discharge; can be transmitted to the baby at birth and result in candidiasis in his mouth and digestive tract, which appears as white patches or ulcers. May also occur on the mother's nipples.

capillaries Tiny blood vessels in the system that link the arteries and the veins.

caput succedaneum A collection of fluid between the scalp and skull of a newborn. It is usually formed during labor as a result of the pressure of the cervix on the infant's head. The swelling begins to recede soon after birth.

case A person who has the problem under study.

case-control study Research in which cases (people who have the disease or problem of interest) are identified first, and then controls (people who are similar to cases but do not have the problem) are identified.

case study An article in a journal describing one (or a few) instances of a diagnosis, problem, or situation that arose in practice.

casein Component of the proteins in milk.

categorical data Data that can be classified but not quantified, such as survey responses "very satisfied," "satisfied," "unsatisfied," "very unsatisfied."

catheter A tubular medical device for insertion into canals, vessels, passageways, or body cavities usually to permit injection or withdrawal of fluids or to keep a passage open. Usually used during labor to drain the bladder when the mother has received anesthesia.

Centers for Disease Control (CDC) An agency of the U.S. Public Health Service established in 1973 to protect the public health of the nation by providing leadership and direction in the prevention and control of diseases and other preventable health conditions and to respond to public health emergencies.

cephalhematoma Swelling caused by the pooling of blood under the scalp. It may begin to form in the scalp of a baby during labor and may slowly become larger in the first few days after birth. It may be a result of trauma, often from forceps or vacuum extraction.

certification Process that attests to having met certain standards of the profession.

chi-square A statistical term that can describe a distribution of data; can be the name for a test of categorical data.

C-hold Technique in which the mother cups her free hand to form the letter "C," with her thumb on top and her fingers curved below the breast, well behind the areola; used to help support the breast with positioning and attachment.

cholecystokinin (CCK) A gastrointestinal hormone that enhances digestion, sedation, and a feeling of satiation and well-being. It is released in both the infant and mother during suckling.

clarifying A counseling skill used to make a point clear.

clavicle The collarbone. It is a long, curved horizontal bone just above the first rib, forming the front portion of the shoulder.

cleft lip A birth defect consisting of one or more clefts (splits) of the upper lip. This results from the failure of the upper jaw and nasal areas to fuse in the embryo.

cleft palate A birth defect in which there is a hole in the middle of the roof of the mouth (palate). The cleft may be complete, going through both the hard and soft palates into the nasal area, or it may go only partly through. It is often linked to a cleft in the upper lip.

clinical practice The day-to-day work of healthcare professionals rather than the kind of care that might be given in an experimental setting.

clustered feedings Period of almost constant wakefulness and suckling at some time of the day, generally the early evening. Also referred to as bunched feedings.

clutch hold A breastfeeding position in which the mother places the baby along her side with his feet toward her back; also known as the football hold.

cognitive learning The process of learning which includes perception and judgment.

Cohen's kappa A statistical test, designed by J. Cohen (1960) to measure concordance for dichotomous data. Experts differ, but kappa values of .7 or higher are considered evidence of excellent agreement.

cohort A group studied together because of some characteristic or experience they have in common.

cohort study A type of research that examines the effect or effects of belonging to a particular group on some result or outcome of interest.

colic Extreme fussiness in the baby that is characterized by a piercing cry, severe abdominal discomfort, and inability to be comforted.

colostrum Breastmilk secreted during pregnancy, after childbirth, and before the onset of secretion of mature milk.

community outreach Reaching the community through programs and services.

complementary feeding New foods added to the growing breastfed infant's diet to meet the energy and nutrient needs that are not met by human milk alone. Introduction of solid foods. In some cases, this term is interpreted as "topping off" the breastfed infant with liquids other than human milk but that is technically referred to as supplementing.

complete protein See protein, complete.

complex carbohydrates Carbohydrates that contain important vitamins and minerals. Complex carbohydrates take longer to digest than simple carbohydrates and do not stimulate a craving for more food. Foods in this category include vegetables, fruits, whole-grain cereals, rice, breads, and crackers.

compliance In healthcare, the act of a patient following the plan of care or treatment prescribed.

confidence interval (CI) A statistical term that states the range within which a population's true value is expected to be found.

confounding variable A characteristic or attribute of the people in the study or their experiences that could confuse the interpretation of the study's results.

congenital Present at birth, such as a congenital defect.

conjugation The process by which the liver converts bilirubin into a form that can be broken down and pass into the intestine.

consent Permission to perform a procedure.

contraception A technique or device for preventing pregnancy.

contraindicate To give indication against the advisability of, as in "In very few instances is breastfeeding contraindicated."

control (1) The group in the study to whom the treatment was not given (in an experiment) or who do not have the problem of interest (in a case-control study). (2) The amount or type of regulation of study conditions the researchers can exercise.

convenience Refers to a type of sample selected by the researcher that is not random or carefully defined but rather readily accessible.

Coombs' test Test that measures the presence of antibodies to red blood cells in the blood.

Cooper's ligaments Ligaments that run vertically through the breast and attach the deep layer of subcutaneous tissue to the dermis of the skin.

cord blood Blood that remains in the umbilical cord at birth.

correlated Shown, by a specific statistical test, to be associated.

cosleeping Practice in which the infant sleeps with the parents.

cradle hold The traditional sitting position whereby the mother sits with her baby's body across her abdomen. She places his head in the crook of her arm and supports his body with her hand.

craniosacral therapist Specialist who very subtly and gently manipulates the skull, spine, and sacrum to help with minor aches and pains through to severe and persistent health problems.

creamatocrit   Percentage of cream, used to estimate the fat and energy content of human milk.

Cronbach's alpha   A special test applied to determine whether the items on a scale or tool are internally consistent, or that they measure the same concept in a similar way.

cross-cradle hold   The same holding technique as the dominant hand hold but used for the less dominant hand as well. See dominant hand hold.

cross-sectional study   Research that examines a question at one point in time (such as surveys of a neighborhood all collected within the same week).

culture   The environment that surrounds us and influences our beliefs and attitudes.

cup feeding   Alternate feeding method in which the baby is fed with a cup.

cyanosis   Bluish coloring of the skin or mucous membranes due to low oxygen levels.

cytokines   A unique family of growth factors secreted primarily from leukocytes. Cytokines stimulate humoral and cellular immune responses, as well as the activation of phagocytic cells.

 D

Dancer hand position   Position that begins in the C-hold position. The mother then brings her hand forward so that her breast is supported with only three fingers. She bends the index finger slightly so that it gently holds the baby's cheek on one side, with the thumb holding the other cheek. This helps the baby's tongue form correctly for suckling and provides stability to help the baby stay latched. Originated by Sarah Danner and Ed Cerutti.

dehydration   Large loss of water from the body tissues.

demographics   Variables that describe basic characteristics of the subjects such as age, gender, place of residence, income, education, and ethnicity.

dependent variable   The aspect or characteristic of the subjects, or of their experience, that the researcher is trying to understand or explain. In a study of the effect of calories on weight gain, weight gain is the dependent variable.

dermis   The layer of skin just below the outer layer (epidermis). It contains blood and lymph vessels, nerves and nerve endings, glands, and hair follicles.

descriptive study   Usually, a study that begins to explore a phenomenon by describing it in detail rather than trying to control any aspects of it.

detoxify   Speed up the removal of harmful substances from the body.

diabetes   A variable disorder of carbohydrate metabolism resulting from inadequate secretion or utilization of insulin.

dichotomous outcome   A result or answer that has only two possibilities such as "Yes, No" or "True, False."

discharge planner   Hospital staff person evaluates a patient to determine readiness for discharge and gives the patient instructions until the first follow-up visit.

disorganized suck   Temporary sucking difficulty due to illness, prematurity, drugs given to the infant or mother, a delay in the first breastfeeding at birth, a neuromotor dysfunction, variations in oral anatomy or nipple preference due to the introduction of an artificial nipple.

distribution   A description of the way the values of a variable (independent or dependent) range; how many values are small, medium, and large. Often, this is shown graphically.

dominant hand hold   Position in which the mother holds her baby with her dominant hand to nurse. She holds the baby's head in her hand and supports his body with her forearm. She can nurse on the nearest breast and then move her arm with the baby across her body to the opposite breast.

donor milk   Human milk that is expressed and donated to a human milk bank to be given to another baby.

dopamine   A hormone made in the adrenal gland that acts as a prolactin inhibitor.

doula   An experienced woman who helps other women immediately before, during, and/or after delivery.

Down syndrome   A form of congenital mental retardation caused by an extra chromosome; also called trisomy 21.

drip milk   Milk that leaks from a breast without direct stimulation.

duct system (ductwork)   A system of ducts and ductules through which milk flows from the point of production out to the nipple pores.

ductule   Small duct in the mammary gland that drains milk from the alveoli into larger ducts that terminate in the nipple.

dyad   Two individuals who form one unit, each dependent on the other, such as a mother and baby.

dysfunction   Inability to function normally.

dysfunctional suck   Sucking anomaly that requires a referral to a physical, occupational or speech therapist with specialization in infant disorders.

 E

eclampsia   Coma and convulsive seizures occurring in a woman between her 20th week of pregnancy and the end of the first week postpartum.

eczema   Swelling of the outer layer of skin that may be itchy, red, have small blisters, and weep.

edema   A local or generalized condition in which body tissues contain excessive amounts of fluid.

Edinburgh postnatal depression scale   Scale for rating the degree of postnatal depression.

ELBW   Extremely low birth weight infant, born weighing under 2 lb, 3 oz (1000 gm).

emergency weaning   Weaning abruptly, with no preparation or forethought.

empathetic listening   A counseling technique in which the counselor listens with the intent to understand emotionally and intellectually.

empowerment   The act of promoting or influencing self-actualization.

endocrine   Pertaining to a gland that secretes directly into the bloodstream.

engorgement   Swelling or congestion of body tissues; overfullness of the breast.

enteral   Within or by way of the intestines.

environmental contaminant   Impurity in human milk that results from contamination of the environment by such chemicals as DDT, PBB, and PCB that then enters the food chain and is consumed by the mother.

enzyme   A protein that speeds up or causes chemical reactions in living matter.

epidermis   The outer layers of the skin. It is made up of an outer, dead portion and a deeper, living portion. Epidermal cells gradually move outward to the skin surface, changing as they go, until they become flakes.

epidural anesthesia   Anesthesia produced by injection of an anesthetic into the epidural space of the spinal cord.

epiglottis   The cartilage-like structure that overhangs the trachea like a lid. It prevents food from entering the trachea by closing during swallowing.

episiotomy A surgical incision made to enlarge the vaginal opening during childbirth.

epithelium The covering of the organs of the body.

erythema toxicum Pink to red macular (raised) area in newborns with a center that is yellow or white. It has no apparent significance and requires no treatment.

estrogen The hormone that stimulates growth of the reproductive organs, including alveoli and ducts in the breasts.

ethics The discipline dealing with what is good and bad and with moral duty and obligation; a set of moral principles or values.

eustachian tube Tube lined with mucous membrane that joins the nose-throat cavity (nasopharynx) and the inner ear (tympanic cavity).

evaluating A counseling technique used to examine the quality of a counseling contact.

evert Protrude outward.

exclusive breastfeeding Breastfeeding in which the baby receives no drinks or foods other than human milk, not even water; is given no pacifiers or artificial nipples; has no limits placed on frequency or length of a breastfeeding; and receives at least 8 to 12 breastfeedings in 24 hours, including night feedings.

excoriated Surface of the skin that is scraped or chafed.

exocrine Pertaining to a gland whose secretion reaches an epithelial surface either directly or through a duct.

exogenous Derived from outside the body.

experiment A type of research in which the scientist selects a sample and applies some treatment or performs some action on part of the sample in order to measure the differences between treated and untreated parts.

extrauterine Occurring or located outside the uterus.

F

facilitating A counseling technique used to direct a conversation in such a way that encourages the other speaker to provide information and define the situation.

failure-to-thrive (FTT) Condition in which an infant's weight is seriously compromised. Signs are failure to regain birth weight by three weeks of age, weight loss of greater than ten percent of birth weight by two weeks of age, deceleration of growth from a previously established pattern of weight gain, and evidence of malnutrition on examination, such as minimal subcutaneous fat or wasted buttocks.

fat-soluble vitamins Vitamins A, D, E, and K.

fat stores Layers of fat laid down during pregnancy that provide a reserve to help nourish the breastfeeding baby.

feedback inhibitor of lactation (FIL) A human whey protein that enables the mammary gland to regulate its milk production; it acts to inhibit milk synthesis when milk is left in the breast.

feeding cues A progression of signs that indicate a desire to feed. The baby will begin to wriggle his body, and his closed eyes will exhibit rapid eye movement (REM). He will then make mouthing movements. He will pass one or both of his hands over his head and will bring his hand to his mouth.

fibrocystic breast A common type of benign breast condition that causes lumpiness in the breast.

finger feeding An alternate feeding method in which the baby sucks on the mother's or examiner's finger. A 5, 6, or 8 French oral gastric tube that leads to the liquid is placed along the fat pad of the finger, extending a few centimeters beyond the tip of the finger. The fat pad of the finger with the tube on it is placed into the baby's mouth far enough to elicit suckling. See also tube feeding.

fistula An abnormal passage from an internal organ to the body surface or between two internal organs.

flange To extend outward, to flare, as in the baby's lips being flanged when attached at the breast; a portion of a breast pump that is placed against the breast to form suction.

flatulence Excessive gas in the stomach and abdomen causing pain in the abdomen or intestines.

flexion A state of being bent or curved.

flora Normal bacteria and other microbes.

focusing A counseling skill that is used to concentrate on a point that should be explored.

follow up Provide further contact or resources.

fontanel A space between the bones of an infant's skull covered by tough membranes.

football hold See clutch hold.

forceps Instruments used to help a difficult childbirth, to quickly deliver a baby with breathing problems, or to shorten normal labor. The blades of the forceps are put into the vagina one at a time and applied to opposite sides of the baby's head, with the baby's head held firmly between the blades.

foremilk The lower-fat milk that is present at the beginning of a breastfeeding.

formal stage The second of four stages in role acquisition. A time in which the role is viewed more personally.

frenulum A fold of skin or mucous membrane that is attached to a part of the body and checks or controls its motion, as in the fold under the tongue.

frenum A fold of skin that anchors the upper lip to the top gum.

G

galactocele A cyst that is caused by the closing or blockage of a milk duct. It contains a thick, creamy milklike substance that may be discharged from the nipple when the cyst is compressed.

galactogogue Food or drink that is believed to increase milk production. Also spelled galactagogue.

galactopoiesis Stage III lactogenesis, which marks the establishment and maintenance of mature milk.

galactorrhea Secretion and release of milk unrelated to childbirth or breastfeeding; excessive or inappropriate milk production; also called spontaneous lactation.

galactose A simple sugar produced by the breakdown of lactose (milk sugar).

galactosemia An inherited disease of inability to process galactose, caused by lack of an enzyme.

gastroenteritis Inflammation of the stomach and intestines.

gastroesophageal reflux (GER) A backflow of acidic contents of the stomach into the esophagus that produces burning pain. It is often the result of failure of the lower esophageal sphincter to close.

gastrostomy Gavage feeding in which a tube is placed through the skin directly into the stomach.

gavage feeding A method for feeding an infant in which a tube is passed through the nose, mouth, or skin into the stomach.

generalize To extend the results of a study not just to the people studied but also to a larger group who are more or less similar to them.

gestation The time period from conception to birth.

gestational age   The age of a fetus or a newborn, usually stated in weeks dating from the first day of the mother's last menstrual period.

gestational ovarian theca lutein cyst   A cyst that develops in the ovary during gestation. During a woman's menstrual cycle, a mound of yellow tissue (corpus luteum) forms in the wall of the ovary where an egg has just been released. Its purpose is to release hormones to help prepare the body for pregnancy. If the egg is not impregnated, it shrinks and is shed during menstruation.

glucuronic acid   An agent that conjugates bilirubin in the liver.

goiter   Enlargement of the thyroid gland, resulting in a thick-looking neck or double-chin appearance.

grommet   See obturator.

grooming   Gently stroking an infant's body during a feeding. This increases a mother's prolactin level.

growth spurt   A period of sudden growth when the baby nurses more frequently than usual.

guiding method   A counseling method that provides emotional support and encourages the sharing of feelings and concerns.

 H

half-life   The time needed for a drug's level in the bloodstream to go down to one-half of its beginning level.

hand expression   Removal of milk from the breast by manual manipulation.

health consumerism   An informed person who is a responsible decision maker concerning healthcare.

hematocrit   A measure of the number of red cells found in the blood, stated as a percentage of the total blood volume.

hemoglobin   The portion of the red blood cell that transports oxygen to all parts of the body.

high-risk infant   An infant born at risk due to a particular medical condition or social situation.

hindmilk   The high-fat milk resulting from the letdown reflex, which forces milk from the alveoli and washes the fat from the walls of the ducts.

Hirschsprung's disease   A condition in which a part of the infant's intestines lacks proper nerve innervation and the stool is not passed easily beyond that point. These infants frequently have large, bloated abdomens from the collection of stool and gas.

HIV   See human immunodeficiency virus.

HMBANA   Human Milk Banking Association of North America, a multidisciplinary group of health care providers that sets the standards and guidelines for donor milk banking in Canada, Mexico and the United States.

Hoffman technique   A technique used to train the nipple to become graspable by manually stretching the tissue surrounding the nipple.

Holder pasteurization   Heat treating at either 56°C or 62.5°C.

home visit   A form of consultation in which the counselor or practitioner visits the mother in her home.

homogeneity   Sameness. In studies that hope that two groups are different in important ways, finding sameness between them invalidates the results.

human immunodeficiency virus (HIV)   Virus that slowly weakens the body's immune system, thus allowing viruses, bacteria, parasites, and fungi that usually don't cause problems to cause illness and death.

human milk   Milk secreted in the human breast.

human milk bank   A service established for the purpose of collecting, screening, processing, and distributing donated human milk to meet the specific medical needs of individuals for whom it is prescribed.

human milk fortifier (HMF)   Nutrients added to expressed human milk to enhance the growth and nutrient balances of VLBW infants and ELBW infants.

human milk substitute   Any food being marketed or otherwise represented as a partial or total replacement for human milk. Also called artificial baby milk.

human subjects review group   Groups of people in research institutions and healthcare agencies who study a research proposal to be sure it does not violate people's rights or jeopardize their safety.

humoral   Immunity against invaders, as with bacteria and foreign tissue. Humoral immunity is the result of the development and continuing presence of circulating antibodies that are produced by the body's defense system.

hydration   The water balance within the body.

hyperalimentation   The administration of nutrients by intravenous feeding, especially to patients who cannot ingest food through the alimentary tract, such as preterm infants.

hyperbilirubinemia   A yellow coloring of the tissues, membranes, and secretions due to the presence of bile pigments in the blood; a symptom in the body. Also referred to as jaundice.

hypercapnia   High carbon dioxide levels.

hyperemesis   Excess vomiting that can result in weight loss and fluid and electrolyte imbalance.

hypernatremia   Overconcentration of sodium in the blood, caused by an excess loss of water and electrolytes resulting from diarrhea, excessive sweating, or inadequate water intake.

hyperprolactinemia   Elevated prolactin levels.

hypertension   A common disorder often without external symptoms, marked by high blood pressure persistently exceeding 140/90.

hypertonia   Abnormally high tension or tone, especially of the muscles.

hypocalcemia   Too little calcium in the blood.

hypopituitarism   See Sheehan's syndrome.

hypoplasia   Incomplete or under developed organ or tissue, usually the result of a decrease in the number of cells.

hypothalamus   The portion of the brain forming the floor and part of the side wall of the third ventricle. It triggers the release of hormones.

hypothesis   An expected relationship between two variables expressed before a study and around which the study is designed.

hypothyroidism   A condition caused by a deficiency of thyroid secretions causing low metabolism.

hypotonia   Abnormally low tension or tone, especially of the muscles.

hypoxemia   An abnormal lack of oxygen in the blood in the arteries.

hypoxia   Too little oxygen in the cells, characterized by rapid heartbeat, high blood pressure, contraction of blood vessels, dizziness, and mental confusion.

 I

iatrogenic   Induced inadvertently by a physician or surgeon or by medical treatment or diagnostic procedures.

IBCLC International Board Certification Lactation Consultant.

IBFAT Infant Breastfeeding Assessment Tool, which assesses the infant's behavior during a breastfeeding.

ICD-9 International Classification of Diseases.

identifying strengths A counseling skill that helps the mother focus on positive qualities.

ignoring The lowest level of listening.

immunity The quality of being protected from disease organisms and other foreign bodies.

immunity, active Long-term immunity that protects the body from new infection; gained from the production of antibodies.

immunity, passive Immunity from antibodies carried through the placenta to the fetus or through breastmilk.

immunization Any injection of weakened bacteria given to protect against or to reduce the effects of related infectious diseases; vaccination.

immunoglobulin Group of five distinct antibodies in the serum and external secretions of the body that provide immunity. Immunoglobulins include: IgA, IgD, IgE, IgG, and IgM.

immunologic Providing immunity to disease by stimulating antigens.

incomplete protein See protein, incomplete.

independent variable The aspect of the subjects or their experience that the researcher suspects may explain or predict the result or outcome. In a study of the effect of calories on weight gain, calories are the independent variable.

induce lactation Initiate breastfeeding in a woman who has not given birth, as with an adoptive mother. Milk production is prompted by frequent nursing and other measures rather than by the delivery of the placenta.

inert A chemically inactive substance.

influencing A counseling technique used to produce positive action in the mother through the use of special skills.

informal stage The third of four stages in role acquisition. A time of modifying, blending, and individualizing one's role.

informed consent Consent to medical care based on sufficient education and information.

informing A counseling technique used to educate the mother by offering her explanations to increase her understanding of situations and suggestions.

innervation The distribution or supply of nerve fibers or nerve impulses to a part of the body.

Innocenti Declaration Declaration to promote, protect and support breastfeeding, produced and adopted by WHO/UNICEF policymakers at the Spedale degli Innocenti, Florence, Italy in 1990.

insensible Small amount; not perceptible.

instruments Also called tools. Can be a variety of things used to measure such as questionnaires, photographs, tape measures, stopwatches, and so on.

intercostal Situated or extending between the ribs.

internal validity The assurance that extraneous variables are not responsible for the observed results.

International Board of Lactation Consultant Examiners (IBLCE) A nonprofit corporation established in 1985 to develop and administer certification for lactation consultants.

International Code of Marketing of Breastmilk Substitutes A set of resolutions developed in 1979 by WHO and UNICEF that regulate the marketing and distribution of any fluid intended to replace human milk, devices used to feed such fluids, and the role of healthcare workers who advise on infant feeding.

International Lactation Consultant Association (ILCA) A global association founded in 1985 for health professionals who specialize in promoting, protecting, and supporting breastfeeding. The professional association for lactation consultants.

internship In the field of lactation, a program for acquiring clinical practice hours toward becoming a certified lactation consultant (IBCLC).

interpreting A counseling skill making use of an analysis of what the mother is saying.

intraductal papilloma Benign tumor within a duct. It is often associated with a spontaneous bloody discharge from one breast.

intramuscular (IM) Referring to the inside of a muscle, as of an injection into a muscle to administer medicine.

intrauterine Within the uterus.

intrauterine growth rate Normal rate of fetal weight gain; used to describe growth rate for premature infants.

intrauterine growth retardation (IUGR) Abnormal process in which the development and maturation of the fetus is delayed by

genetic factors, maternal disease, or fetal malnutrition caused by placental insufficiency.

intravenous (IV) Referring to the inside of a vein, as of a tube inserted into a vein to provide nutrients or medication directly into the bloodstream.

intubation Passing a tube into a body opening, as putting a breathing tube through the mouth or nose or into the trachea to provide an airway for anesthetic gas or oxygen.

inverted syringe Device for everting the mother's nipple. The tapered end of a syringe is cut off and the plunger direction is reversed to provide a smooth surface next to the breast. The mother places the smooth end of the syringe over her nipple and pulls gently on the plunger.

involution A normal process marked by decreasing size of an organ, as in involution of the uterus after birth.

isolette Specialized, clear-covered infant crib that allows the infant to maintain appropriate body temperature and receive appropriate treatment; allows for continuous observation of the infant by healthcare providers; stablelet.

 J

jaundice See hyperbilirubinemia.

Joint Commission on Accreditation of Healthcare Organizations (JCAHO) An independent, not-for-profit organization that evaluates and accredits more than 18,000 healthcare organizations in the United States, including hospitals, health-care networks, managed care organizations, and healthcare organizations that provide home care, long-term care, behavioral healthcare, laboratory, and ambulatory care services in order to improve the quality of healthcare for the public by providing accreditation and related services that support performance improvement in health-care organizations.

 K

kangaroo care Technique in which the baby is held skin to skin upright and prone between his mother's breasts, wearing only a diaper. He and his mother are then wrapped together to maintain his temperature appropriately.

kangaroo transport Transporting neonates from their birth facility to the tertiary care center with the baby held skin to skin on the parent's or doctor's chest instead of in an incubator.

kappa See Cohen's kappa.

kcal The amount of heat needed to raise the temperature of 1 kg of water 17°C.

Kegel exercises Exercises to tighten muscles surrounding the vagina, urethra, and rectum.

keratin The tough surface layer of dead skin developed in response to pressure.

kernicterus Brain damage caused by excessive bilirubin.

 L

lactase An enzyme that increases the rate of the conversion of milk sugar (lactose) to glucose and galactose, carbohydrates needed by the body for energy.

lactation Breastfeeding; secretion of human milk.

lactation consultant A health professional who is board certified (IBCLC) in lactation.

lactational amenorrhea method (LAM) Method of contraception that must meet three conditions: the mother's menses has not yet returned, the baby is breastfed around the clock without other foods in the diet, and the baby is younger than six months.

lactiferous Mammary, as in lactiferous duct.

lactiferous duct Tube that collects milk from the ductules and carries it to the nipple.

Lactobacillus bifidus Organism in the intestinal tract of breastfed infants that discourages the colonization of bacteria.

lactocyte Epithelial cells.

lactoengineering Process of fortifying human milk to meet the needs of very and extremely low birth weight infants, through separating the fat and giving the fatty portion to the infant.

lactoferrin An iron-binding protein that increases absorption of iron.

lactogenesis The phase during which milk production and secretion are established. Lactogenesis occurs in three stages. Stage I is the initiation of milk synthesis, and Stage II marks copious milk production. Stage III, also called galactopoiesis, refers to the establishment of a mature milk supply.

lactose Milk sugar, the type of sugar present in human milk.

lactose intolerance A disorder resulting in the inability to digest milk sugar (lactose) because of an enzyme (lactase) deficiency.

larynx Part of the air passage connecting the throat with the windpipe (trachea) leading toward the lungs. The infant's larynx rises and is closed off by the epiglottis during swallowing.

LATCH method Acronym for system to assess the infant's ability to latch onto the breast and evaluate audible swallowing as a determinant of milk intake; Latch, Audible swallow, Type of nipple, Comfort, and Hold.

late-onset jaundice A rare type of neonatal jaundice caused by an unknown factor in the mother's milk; this condition appears between the fourth and seventh day of life. Also called breastmilk jaundice.

lay counselor Counselor who helps others on a peer level.

LBW Low birth weight. Baby born weighing less than 5 lb, 8 oz (2500 g).

leading method A counseling method that entails directing a conversation to help identify options and resources, as well as to aid in developing a plan of action.

leaking The involuntary release of human milk that usually occurs in the un-nursed breast while the baby is feeding from the other breast, the seepage of milk from a very full breast, or the expulsion of milk from the breast due to the milk letting down.

leaky gut syndrome A condition in which the intestinal lining becomes inflamed and then thin and porous. Proteins that are incompletely digested may cross from the intestines into the bloodstream.

learning climate The prevailing influence or set of conditions characterizing the setting in which learning takes place.

lesion An abnormal change in structure of an organ or part due to injury or disease.

letdown Milk ejection from the breast triggered by nipple stimulation or as a conditioned reflex.

leukocytes Cells present in human milk that fight infection.

LGA Large for gestational age, determined by size and weight at birth in the top ten percent of the growth rate appropriate for gestational age.

Likert scale A type of commonly used attitude measure that asks respondents to "strongly agree" or "strongly disagree."

lingual Pertaining to the tongue, as in lingual frenulum.

lipase A digestive system enzyme that increases the breakdown of fats (lipids).

lobule A small lobe, a cluster of 10 to 100 alveoli.

lochia Discharge that is composed of blood, mucus, and tissue caused by the gradual renewal of reproductive structures following childbirth. Its color transforms from red to pink and then to white in about two to four weeks.

logistic regression A statistical technique for studying relationships between variables that can be used when the dependent (outcome) variable is dichotomous (only two possibilities).

lymph A thin, clear, slightly yellow fluid present in the lymphatic system. It is about 95 percent water with a few red blood cells and variable numbers of white blood cells.

lymph nodes Small, rounded masses that function as filters in the lymph vessels to trap bacteria and cast-off cell parts. Each is a potential dam to arrest the spread of infection. They may swell and be painful when functioning in this way.

lymphatic system Complex network of capillaries, thin vessels, valves, ducts, nodes, and organs. The lymphatic system absorbs the excess blood fluids from the tissue spaces and eventually returns them to the heart.

lymphocyte A lymph cell or white blood cell.

lysozyme An enzyme with antiseptic actions that destroys some foreign organisms.

 M

macrophage Any large cell that can surround and digest foreign substances in the body.

macrosomia Large size at birth, associated with increased risk of diabetes and cardiovascular disease in later life and an increased risk of some cancers.

macular Of, relating to, or characterized by a spot or spots; raised.

malnutrition Inadequate nutrition due to improper diet, regardless of the number of calories consumed.

mammary organ Exocrine gland that functions and develops independently to extract materials from the blood and convert them into milk.

mammary ridge The line extending from the armpit to the inner thigh of the fetus, sometimes the site of an extra nipple. Also called milk line.

mammogenesis Stage during which the breast develops to a functioning state.

mammoplasty Breast reduction; see reduction, breast.

manual expression   See hand expression.

masseter muscle   The muscle that closes the mouth and is the principal muscle in chewing.

mastitis   An inflammation of the breast, usually resulting from a plugged duct left untreated or from a cracked nipple. Also referred to as a breast infection.

mature milk   Composition of human milk after seven to ten days postpartum.

MBA   Mother Baby Assessment, which evaluates the progress of a mother and baby as they learn to breastfeed by observing signaling, positioning, fixing, milk transfer, and ending.

mean   The average of an array of numbers.

meconium   The first stool of a newborn, greenish black to dark brown with a tarry consistency.

meta-analysis   A method of putting together the results of many studies and reanalyzing them as if they had all been parts of one big study.

metabolic   Referring to metabolism, the sum of all chemical processes that take place in the body as they relate to the movement of nutrients in the blood after digestion.

mg/dl   Milligrams per deciliter.

milk bank   See human milk bank.

milk bleb   A blocked nipple pore; milk blister.

milk blister   A blocked nipple pore; milk bleb.

milk ejection reflex   A normal reflex in a nursing mother, caused by stimulation of the nipple and resulting in the release of milk from the breast.

milk/plasma ratio   The quantity of a given drug or its metabolite in human milk in relation to its quantity in the maternal plasma or blood.

milk supply   The quantity of milk that a woman is currently producing, usually compared with the baby's requirements for milk.

milk synthesis   The process of making a compound (human milk) by joining together several elements.

minimal breastfeeding   Breastfeeding between one and three times a day, with complementary or supplementary feedings providing the remaining nourishment. Typical scenario for gradual weaning.

mixed message   A communication or impression that is indistinct or confused.

molding   Asymmetric appearance of the baby's head after birth due to the overlapping of skull bones.

Montgomery glands   Small raised areas around the nipple that enlarge during pregnancy and lactation and secrete a fluid that lubricates the nipple.

morbidity   An illness or an abnormal condition or quality. The number of ill persons or diseases in a population.

Moro reflex   A normal reflex in a young infant caused by a sudden loud noise. It results in drawing up of the legs, an embracing position of the arms, and usually a short cry.

mortality   The number of deaths in a population.

mother-led weaning   Weaning initiated by the mother without cues from the baby.

motility   Power of motion, spontaneous motion.

mucin   A glycoprotein found in mucus; it is present in human milk, saliva, bile, salivary glands, skin, connective tissues, tendon, and cartilage.

multipara   Woman who has given live birth to more than one child.

myelin   A fatty substance found in the coverings of various nerve fibers. The fat gives the normally gray fibers a white, creamy color.

myoepithelial cells   Smooth muscle layers that enclose the alveoli and ducts of the breast.

 N

nasogastric   Gavage feeding with a tube passing through the nose into the stomach.

nasopharynx   Part of the throat behind the nose and reaching from the back of the nasal opening to the soft palate.

necrotizing enterocolitis (NEC) Inflammation of the intestines and especially of the human ileum that results in tissue death.

need feeding   Feeding the baby whenever he indicates a need, in response to feeding cues. Sometimes referred to as demand or cue feeding.

neonate   The newborn infant up to six weeks of age.

networking   Communicating among people with common interests or needs.

neuromotor dysfunction   Impaired or abnormal functioning of the brain and motor function.

neurotransmitter   Chemical released from a nerve terminal that changes or results in the sending of nerve signals across spaces separating nerve fibers.

NICU   Neonatal intensive care unit.

nipple   The protruding part of the breast that extends and becomes firmer on stimulation.

nipple, common   A nipple that protrudes slightly when at rest and becomes erect when stimulated.

nipple, cracked   A nipple that has a crack or fissure lengthwise or crosswise along it.

nipple, flat   A nipple with a very short shank that does not become erect in response to stimulation.

nipple, inverted   A nipple that remains retracted, both when at rest and on stimulation.

nipple, inverted appearing   A nipple that appears inverted but becomes erect when stimulated.

nipple pores   Openings on the end of the nipple through which milk flows.

nipple preference   A preference by the baby for an artificial nipple over the breast, resulting from sucking alternately on the breast and an artificial nipple, which require two completely different mechanisms.

nipple, retracted   A nipple that appears graspable but retracts on stimulation.

nipple shield   An artificial nipple used over the mother's own nipple during nursing.

nonnutritive sucking   Alternate bursts of sucking and resting.

nonprobability   Refers to a type of sampling other than random. Convenience sampling is nonprobability.

normal distribution   The dispersal of data that comes from measuring many natural phenomena. It is a common assumption in statistical tests.

normal fullness   Increased amounts of blood and lymph necessary for milk production that cause the breasts to become fuller, heavier, and slightly tender; not to be confused with engorgement.

nosocomial   Hospital-acquired, as in a nosocomial infection.

nucleotides   Compounds derived from nucleic acid and secreted by mammary epithelial cells. They play key roles in function and growth of the gastrointestinal and immune systems.

nursing strike   Nursing abstinence; a baby's refusal to breastfeed.

nutritive sucking   An organized continuous sequence of long drawing sucks that produces a regular flow of milk.

 O

obturator   A feeding plate placed over a cleft palate to aid in feeding the baby. Grommet.

odds ratio   A descriptive measure of the association between two variables. Because it is composed of the odds of one group in the numerator and the odds of another group in the denominator, if the odds are greater in the numerator, the odds ratio will be greater than one.

oligosaccharide   A carbohydrate present in human milk that discourages the growth of pathogens in the intestinal tract.

open-ended question   A form of question used in counseling which cannot be answered by "yes" or "no"; questions beginning with who, what, when, where, why, how, how much, and how often.

operationalize   The process of defining the concepts to be studied in terms of measurable variables and relationships, including choosing instruments or tools.

orbicularis oris muscle   Circular muscle surrounding the mouth that closes the lips.

orogastric   Gavage feeding with a tube passing through the mouth to the stomach.

osteopenia   Condition where the bone lacks sufficient minerals, usually because the number of bone cells dying exceeds the number of new ones being made by the body.

osteoporosis   A loss of normal bone density, marked by thinning of bone tissue and the growth of small holes in the bone.

otitis media   Swelling or infection of the middle ear, a common disease of childhood that is less frequent in breastfed babies.

outcome   In the context of research, outcome is usually the same as the dependent variable. More broadly, outcomes are the results of any treatment or action, whether or not that treatment is part of a research study.

outliers   Unusually small or large values for one of the variables being measured. Outliers can distort an average. Researchers often try to offer explanations for why a few values are so different from most others.

output variable   Like an outcome variable, this data element is a result or effect. In some studies, the sample is selected based on an "effect" of interest such as jaundice. Babies would be studied only if they are jaundiced, or jaundice

would be the output variable that divides babies into two comparison groups.

outreach counseling   To reach out to mothers, contacting them on a regular basis to offer support and anticipatory guidance to circumvent problems.

oximeter   A small clip-on instrument that noninvasively estimates the oxygen saturation of a person's blood.

oxytocin   The hormone that stimulates the smooth muscles to contract, specifically those surrounding the alveoli in the breast (causing the release of milk) and those in the uterus (causing uterine contractions); a synthetic form is Pitocin.

 P

paced feeding   Bottle-feeding method that allows the baby to suck, swallow, and breathe as he would during breastfeeding.

paladai   Cup-feeding device used to feed babies in India that is gaining recognition in the Western world.

palatal   Referring to the palate.

palate, hard   The hard portion of the roof of the mouth.

palate, soft   The soft portion of the roof of the mouth.

palliative care   Care that will lessen or relieve pain or other uncomfortable symptoms but not provide a cure.

Palmar grasp   A reflex that curls the fingers when the palm of the hand is tickled.

paradigm shift   A change from one way of thinking to another.

parenchyma   Functional parts of an organ. In the breast, it includes alveoli and lactiferous ducts.

parenteral   Nongastrointestinal, intravenous.

passive immunity   See immunity, passive.

passive listening   A type of listening such as attending.

pathogen   Any microorganism able to cause a disease.

pathologic   That which is caused by disease.

pathologic jaundice   Jaundice that results from such conditions as infections in the blood or liver, diseases of the liver, obstructions in the gastrointestinal system, and interference with the binding of the bilirubin in the bloodstream.

peer review   A process conducted by scientific journals in which an article submitted for publication must be read and approved by several scientists with relevant knowledge. They are peers of the authors, and they can suggest improvements or reject the article.

peptide   A molecule chain of two or more amino acids.

perception   A mental image or awareness; a judgment on or inference from what one has observed.

perineum   An area of tissue that marks externally the approximate boundary of the pelvic outlet and gives passage to the urogenital ducts and rectum; also the area between the anus and the posterior part of the external genitalia, especially in the female.

periosteum   A fiber-like covering of the bones. It has the nerves and blood vessels that supply the bones.

peripheral   Referring to the outside surface or surrounding area of an organ or other structure.

peristalsis   The wavelike, rhythmic contraction of smooth muscle.

personal stage   The final of four stages in role acquisition. The time in which one's style evolves to be consistent with one's personality.

phagocyte   A cell that can engulf particles such as bacteria, other microorganisms, aged red blood cells, and foreign matter.

pharynx   The throat; passage for the breathing and digestive tracts.

phenylalanine   An amino acid present in food protein that can accumulate to dangerous levels in a baby with phenylketonuria.

phenylketonuria (PKU)   A hereditary disease that, if not treated early, can cause brain damage or severe mental retardation in the baby.

phototherapy   Use of a bili-light to treat infantile jaundice.

phthalates   Estrogen-mimicking compounds found in various plastics that infants can be exposed to by artificial feeding.

physiologic jaundice   A common type of neonatal jaundice resulting from the normal breakdown of red blood cells and the delay in removing their byproducts from the bloodstream; it appears by the third day of life.

phytoestrogen   Estrogen present in a plant, as in the phytoestrogen in cabbage (used to treat engorgement).

Pierre Robin sequence   A condition of the newborn that consists of an unusually small jaw combined with a cleft palate, downward displacement of the tongue, and absence of a gag reflex.

PIF   See prolactin inhibitory factor.

pilot study   A small, trial run of a study conducted before the main study in order to test processes or instruments planned for use in the main study so that problems can be worked out.

Pincer grasp   Use of the thumb and forefinger to pick up objects, usually occurring at about eight to nine months of age.

pinch test   A test for inverted nipples, performed by gently compressing the nipple between the thumb and forefinger and observing the amount of protrusion that results.

Pitocin   A synthetic form of oxytocin.

pituitary   A small, rounded body at the base of the brain that secretes hormones. The anterior pituitary secretes prolactin; the posterior pituitary secretes oxytocin.

placenta   The spongy structure that grows on the wall of the uterus during pregnancy and by which the baby is nourished.

plugged duct   Blockage in a milk duct caused by accumulated milk or cast-off cells.

pneumothorax   Collection of air or gas in the chest causing the lung to collapse.

polycystic ovarian syndrome   A variable disorder marked by amenorrhea, excessive hair, obesity, infertility, and ovarian enlargement; usually initiated by an elevated level of luteinizing hormone, androgen, or estrogen which results in an abnormal cycle of gonadotropin release by the pituitary gland. Also called polycystic ovarian disease, polycystic ovarian syndrome, polycystic ovary disease, and Stein-Leventhal syndrome.

pooled milk   Donor human milk that is pooled and heat treated to ensure the absence of HIV, hepatitis, and other viruses and bacteria.

population   The whole group of people who have some characteristic(s) under study of which the sample actually studied is just a part.

postmature   Born after 42 weeks' gestation.

postpartum   The six-week period following childbirth.

postpartum depression   A mild to moderate depression that lasts from one to six weeks postpartum. It is characterized by mood changes, sleep disturbances, and fatigue. The mother feels unable to cope with life and may have unexplained physical symptoms such as abdominal pains or headache. She may feel no attachment to the baby and worries that something is not "right." The mother may entertain occasional thoughts of suicide.

postpartum psychosis   Postpartum depression that can lead to a loss of control, rational thought, and social functioning. The mother may experience overwhelming confusion and hallucinations. She may attempt to harm herself or her child.

posture feeding   Feeding position in which the baby is positioned above the breast and has better control over milk flow. The mother lies flat on her back with her baby lying tummy to tummy on top of her. Also called prone position feeding.

power   A mathematical term that represents the degree of likelihood that a given sample size and test will find a difference between comparison groups when there really is a difference.

ppm   Parts per million.

praising   Counseling skills used to give emotional support and encouragement to mothers.

predictor variable   Independent variable; the characteristic that is believed to influence the result.

premature infant   See preterm infant.

prepared childbirth   Conscious cooperative birth in which the woman is aware of and able to cooperate with her body.

pretending   A type of listening in which the listener gives a noncommittal response, trying to be polite and really not giving any attention to the speaker.

preterm infant   Infant born before 37 weeks' gestation; premature.

prevalence   Frequency of disease in the population.

primipara   A woman who has completed one pregnancy.

probability   A probability sample is one selected by random sampling.

problem solving   A counseling technique that follows a step-by-step process to arrive at a solution to a problem.

progesterone   The hormone responsible for the development of the placenta and mammary glands.

projectile vomiting   See vomiting, projectile.

prolactin   The hormone that stimulates breast development and formation of milk during pregnancy and lactation.

prolactin inhibitory factor (PIF)   A factor produced in and released from the hypothalamus that prohibits the release of prolactin.

prolactinoma   A pituitary tumor that secretes prolactin.

prone   Referring to the position of the body when lying face downward.

prospective study   A study in which events to be studied have not yet happened, so data can be collected as the events happen rather than from old records or memory.

prostaglandin   One of several strong hormone-like fatty acids that act in small amounts on certain organs.

protein, complete   A protein that contains all the essential amino acids.

protein, incomplete   A protein that does not contain all the essential amino acids and must be combined with a complementary protein to become complete.

protractility   The ability of the nipple to be drawn out.

pustule   A small blister that usually is filled with pus.

p-value   The observed significance level of a statistical test; it measures how strong the evidence is against the hypothesis that there is no relationship.

pyloric stenosis   A condition in which the outflow valve of the stomach will not open satisfactorily to permit the contents of the stomach to pass through. It is most common in firstborn white male infants and is characterized by projectile vomiting.

 Q

qualitative study   A study in which the measurement of variables is less important than a description of phenomena or experiences. Statistical analysis is not usually used and changes in practice are not often recommended, except at a conceptual level. Often, such studies lead to further studies.

 R

random assignment   The process of fairly designating participants in a study to be in a treatment or control group. The fairness is achieved by a process that cannot be influenced by the scientists or participants, such as a coin flip or use of a special random number chart.

randomized clinical trial An experiment or experiment-like type of research in which the scientist controls many aspects of the study. Subjects are randomly assigned to their groups. Potential confounders are measured and analysis is planned before data collection.

range The number that results from subtracting the lowest from the highest value in the data.

Raynaud's phenomenon Sporadic attacks of interruptions in blood flow to the extremities (fingers, toes, ears, and nose), resulting in tingling, numbness, burning, and pain. Nipple vasospasms can mimic Raynaud's.

RDI Reference Daily Intake.

reassuring A counseling skill used to restore confidence through pointing out the normalcy of a situation.

rebirthing Simulating the birth experience. The baby is placed on the mother's abdomen in a bath of warm water and allowed to find the breast on his own; remedial co-bathing.

recall Bring to mind or think of again.

reduction, breast Surgical procedure to decrease the size of the breast. It can interfere with milk production. Mammoplasty.

reflective listening See active listening.

relactation Resumption of lactation beyond the immediate postpartum period.

reliability The property possessed by good-quality measurement tools that ensures that they measure a concept or characteristic the same way each time.

remedial co-bathing See rebirthing.

renal solute load Amount of solutes (i.e., glucose, amino acids, potassium, sodium, and chloride) handled by the kidneys.

replicate To repeat a study that has already been done. Often the study is conducted on a different sample of people or in a different setting.

resection Removal of part of an organ or structure by surgery.

respiratory distress syndrome A condition present, usually at birth, that is characterized by delayed onset of respiration and low Apgar score; caused by the lungs not being fully developed.

respiratory syncytial virus (RSV) Multi-strain virus that causes severe respiratory disease including bronchitis and pneumonia in infants and children.

retention A preservation of the after-effects of experience and learning that makes recall or recognition possible.

retrospective study A study in which the result of interest is identified in a group of subjects and then the past experiences of those subjects are examined to see what might have led to the result.

reverse cycle nursing A nursing pattern in which a mother who has regular separations from her baby provides most or all of her baby's feedings at the breast at times when she and the baby are together.

reverse pressure softening Breast massage method to help soften the areola to help the baby latch on effectively.

review In research, a type of study published in a journal that usually does not present any new results but rather summarizes several previous studies.

rickets Condition caused by lack of vitamin D, calcium, and phosphorus; marked by abnormal bone growth.

rooming-in Mother and baby sharing the same hospital room, beginning as soon as possible after birth.

rooting reflex The natural instinct of the newborn to turn his head toward the stimulation when touched on the cheek.

rotavirus Class of viruses that cause diarrheal illness and lead to hospitalization.

 S

sample The group of people or subjects who are selected to participate in a study. The sample is only part of the whole population of subjects who could be studied.

sebaceous Fatty, oily, or greasy, usually referring to the oil-secreting glands of the skin or to their secretions.

secretory Having the function of secretion.

secretory IgA One of the most common antibodies, found in all secretions of the body. IgA combines with protein in the mucosa and defends body surfaces against invading microorganisms.

selective listening Form of listening in which the listener hears only certain parts of what is said.

self-image One's conception of oneself or of one's role.

sensory input A message, perception, or awareness the mind receives while processing information.

sepsis Infection.

seroconversion The process by which serum shows the presence of a factor that previously had been absent, or vice versa.

seronegative Serum that does not demonstrate the presence of a factor for which tests were conducted; tested negative.

seropositive Serum that demonstrates the presence of a factor for which tests were conducted; tested positive.

serum The clear yellowish fluid that remains from blood plasma after clotting factors have been removed by clot formation.

SGA Small for gestational age, determined by size and weight at birth in the bottom ten percent of the growth rate appropriate for gestational age. Infant whose growth was retarded and who was delivered before 37 weeks (premature) or after 42 weeks (postmature).

Sheehan's syndrome A condition occurring after giving birth in which the pituitary gland is damaged. It is caused by a lessening of blood circulation after hemorrhaging of the womb. Also called hypopituitarism.

sibling A brother or sister.

simple carbohydrate The simplest sugars that can cause a sudden rise in blood sugar level after ingestion, followed by a rapid drop and a craving for more food. When consumed in the absence of nutritional foods, simple carbohydrate foods may cause fatigue, dizziness, nervousness, or headache.

sling An apparatus worn by an adult to carry and comfort a baby.

slope The slope of a line on a graph as defined by its angle relative to the horizontal axis or by making a ratio of the units of rise over the units of run.

smooth muscle The type of muscle that provides the erectile tissue in the nipple and areola.

social toxicant Mood-changing toxicant such as tobacco, coffee, tea, alcohol, marijuana, and other social drugs.

soporific Sleep-inducing agent, e.g., warm milk.

sphincter A circular band of muscle fibers that narrows a passage or closes a natural opening in the body.

spina bifida A neural tube defect present at birth that results in a gap in the bone that surrounds the spinal cord.

spitting up Baby expelling a small amount of milk from the mouth during or after feedings; common in most babies.

spontaneous lactation See galactorrhea.

spurious The relationship between two variables when statistical significance is found, but the significance is actually caused by a third variable that is hidden or unclear.

standards of practice   Stated measures or levels of quality that serve as models for the conduct and evaluation of practice.

stasis   A slowing or stoppage of the normal flow of a bodily fluid or semifluid.

statistical theory   The mathematical ideas about probability and infinite cases that underlie the applied tests commonly used by researchers.

statistically significant   Description of an outcome that did not happen by chance; there is some underlying relationship that caused the event.

subcutaneous   Under the skin.

sublingual   Under the tongue.

suck   To draw into the mouth by forming a partial vacuum with the lips and tongue.

suck reorganization   Technique in which the examiner places the index finger in the baby's mouth pad side up and places slight pressure on the midline of the tongue, pulling the finger out slowly to encourage the baby to suck it back in.

suck training   Technique in which the therapist places the index finger in the baby's mouth and stimulates certain portions of the baby's oral anatomy to train him to suck.

sucking pad   See buccal pad.

suckle   To suck and at the same time to rhythmically compress the gums together around the areola to strip milk from the breast.

summarizing   A counseling skill that entails making a summary of the important points in a conversation.

supernumerary nipple   Extra nipple, other than the one normally found on each breast, which may be present along the milk lines.

supine   Lying flat on the back.

supplementary feeding   Foods other than human milk fed to the infant in place of or following a breastfeeding. Some refer to this as "topping off" the breastfed infant with liquids other than human milk.

supply and demand   The process by which the baby increases the mother's milk production to meet his needs.

suppressor peptides   Inhibiting peptides in human milk that bring about the cessation of milk secretion during milk stasis and engorgement.

swaddle   Wrapping the baby, confining his arms and legs to inhibit the startle reflex and provide a feeling of warmth and security.

switch nursing   Frequently altering between breasts during a feeding.

syringe feeding   An alternate feeding method in which a syringe is placed into the corner or middle of the baby's mouth. Depressing the syringe releases milk into the baby's mouth.

systemic   Of or relating to the whole body rather than to a single area or part of the body.

 T

tail of Spence   Breast tissue that extends into the axilla.

tandem nursing   A mother nursing more than one child of different ages.

teachable moment   A time of optimal attention and capacity for learning.

tertiary   Third in order of use; belonging to the third level of sophistication of development, as in a specialized, highly technical tertiary-level healthcare facility.

thrush   See candidiasis.

tonic neck reflex   A normal infant reflex present until three or four months of age; also referred to as the "fencer position." When the baby lies on his back, he extends the arm and leg on the side of his body opposite to the direction his head is turned. This prevents him from rolling over until adequate neurologic and motor development occurs.

tool   In research, used interchangeably with instrument.

trachea   A nearly cylindrical tube in the neck by which air passes to and from the lungs; windpipe.

transcutaneous bilimeter   Device that indicates bilirubin levels in the blood by measuring intensity of skin coloration.

transient nipple soreness   Nipple soreness in the first week postpartum that is temporary.

transitional milk   Milk that is present at Stage II lactogenesis, around the second or third day postpartum. Blood flow within the breast increases, and copious milk secretion begins. The milk that is between colostrum and mature milk.

transplacental   Across or through the placenta.

transplantation   Removal and reattachment.

trimester   A period of three months, particularly used when referring to pregnancy.

trough (for mother's milk)   Channel through which the mother's milk travels formed in the center of the infant's tongue during suckling.

trough level   The lowest blood or milk level achieved by a drug during its dosing period.

true   In statistics, "true" value is used to refer to a population value. For example, if we knew the weight of every human baby born in the last 100 years, we could say, "The true value of the mean of the population is 3020.57 grams." Since we do not know the true value of the mean, we try to estimate it using research and statistics.

t-test   A statistical test used on data that can be averaged, like height. It determines whether two means are significantly different from one another.

tubal ligation   One of several sterilization processes in which the fallopian tubes are blocked to prevent conception from occurring.

tube feeding   An alternate feeding method in which tubing that leads to liquid is placed against the mother's breast with a few centimeters extending beyond the end of the nipple. The baby suckles at the breast and the tip of the tube simultaneously. The flow of supplement from the container encourages him to continue suckling. See also finger feeding.

turgor   Normal strength and tension of the skin caused by outward pressure of the cells and the fluid that surrounds them.

 U

unconjugated   In jaundice, bilirubin that is not bound to albumin and circulates freely in the bloodstream; it can migrate toward tissues with high fat content, including the brain and nervous system.

United Nations Children's Emergency Fund (UNICEF)   An agency of the United Nations, established in 1946 and charged with protecting the lives and health of children.

universal precautions   Guidelines observed in healthcare that help control the transmission of infection.

urethra   The canal for discharge of urine, located in women between the vagina and the clitoris.

U.S. Department of Agriculture (USDA) The government agency that oversees the Special Supplemental Food Program for Women, Infants, and Children, referred to as WIC.

uvula   Small cone-shaped process suspended in the mouth from the middle of the back edge of the soft palate.

 V

vaccine   Weakened or dead microorganisms given to a person to produce antibodies against the virus.

vacuum extraction   Vaginal delivery of the infant assisted by the use of a machine that applies suction to the infant's head.

validity   A property of research methods that conveys how well they capture or measure the phenomenon or concept under study.

variable   A characteristic or effect of either the hypothesized "causes" or "outcomes" under study. If feeding is a partial cause of jaundice, the number and amount of feedings are variables, and the possible bilirubin levels are also variables.

variation   In statistics, it is expected that most phenomena will not be exactly the same when measured over time or when measured in different individuals. The variation in the number of times each day that a breastfed baby wants to nurse and the variation in the number of feedings between different babies on the same day are both examples.

vasospasm   Sharp and often persistent contraction of a blood vessel reducing blood flow. Observed in breastfeeding mothers as nipple vasospasm. See Raynaud's phenomenon.

ventral   On the abdomen; draped on the hand.

vernix   The creamy protective coating on the newborn.

vertical transmission   The transfer of a disease, condition, or trait from a mother to her child, either in the genes or at the time of birth, as in the spread of an infection through human milk or through the placenta.

virus   A tiny organism that can grow only in the cells of another organism.

VLBW   Very low birth weight. Infant born weighing less than 3 lb, 5 oz (1500 g).

voice tone   Pitch level, rate of speech, and volume when speaking.

vomiting   Expelling the contents of the stomach with force.

vomiting, projectile   Violent expulsion of the contents of the stomach with force enough to send it over a foot.

 W

warm line   A telephone line that is answered by a machine or voice mail, asking the mother to leave a message for a return call.

water-soluble vitamins   Vitamin C and the B vitamins.

weaning   Discontinuation of breastfeeding by substituting other nourishment.

wet nursing   Breastfeeding an infant other than one's own.

whey   Clear fluid when milk stands, when curds are removed.

WIC   Special Supplemental Food Program for Women, Infants, and Children that helps pregnant women in the United States choose nutritious foods to have healthier babies and provides services to breastfeeding mothers, infants, and children up to five years of age.

witch's milk   Milk sometimes secreted by the newborn infant's breasts that disappears shortly after birth.

World Health Organization (WHO)   An agency of the United Nations charged with planning and coordinating global healthcare and assisting member nations to combat disease and train healthcare workers.

 Y

yeast infection   See candidiasis.

PROFESSIONAL RESOURCES

► INTERNATIONAL LACTATION CONSULTANT ASSOCIATION

The International Lactation Consultant Association (ILCA) is the professional association representing the IBCLC (International Board Certified Lactation Consultant) worldwide. ILCA's mission is to advance the profession through leadership, advocacy, professional development, and research. ILCA sponsors international and regional conferences to provide education and networking for members and others interested in the lactation field. ILCA also publishes the *Journal of Human Lactation*, policy and practice statements, and independent study modules. A wide variety of resource materials and professional networking is available through the association Web site.

International Lactation Consultant
Association (ILCA)
1500 Sunday Drive, Suite 201
Raleigh, NC 27607
Phone: 919-787-5181
Fax: 919-787-4916
E-mail: ilca@ilca.org
www.ilca.org

► INTERNATIONAL BOARD OF LACTATION CONSULTANT EXAMINERS

The International Board of Lactation Consultant Examiners (IBLCE) develops and administers the international certification examination for lactation consultants. The IBLCE examination is the premier, internationally recognized measure of competence in lactation consulting. Founded in 1985, the IBLCE has certified more than 15,000 IBCLCs in multiple languages and at numerous sites around the world. IBLCE is accredited by the U.S. National Commission for Health Certifying Agencies.

International Board of Lactation Consultant
Examiners (IBLCE)
The Americas and Israel
7309 Arlington Boulevard, Suite 300
Falls Church, VA 22042-3215, USA
Phone: 703-560-7330

Fax: 703-560-7332
E-mail: iblce@iblce.org
www.iblce.org

IBLCE Australia
Asia Pacific, Southern Africa,
Ireland, Great Britain
P.O. Box 13
South Hobart TAS 7004, Australia
Phone: +61 3 6223 8445
Fax: +61 3 6223 8665
E-mail: admin@iblce.edu.au
www.iblce.edu.au

IBLCE Europe
Europe, Middle East, North Africa
Steinfeldgasse 11
A-2511 Pfaffstaetten, Austria
Phone: +43 2252 206595
Fax: +43 2252 206487
E-mail: office@iblce-europe.org
www.iblce-europe.org

► MEDICAL AND LACTATION-RELATED ORGANIZATIONS

Academy of Breastfeeding Medicine
191 Clarksville Road
Princeton Junction, NJ 08550, USA
Toll-Free Phone: 877-836-9947 ext. 25
Fax: 609-799-7032
Local/International: 609-799-6327
E-mail: ABM@bfmed.org
www.bfmed.org

American Academy of Family
Physicians (AAFP)
P.O. Box 11210
Shawnee Mission, KS 66207-1210, USA
Phone: 800-274-2237
        913-906-6000
E-mail: fp@aafp.org
www.aafp.org

American Academy of Pediatrics (AAP)
141 Northwest Point Boulevard
Elk Grove Village, IL 60007-1098, USA
Phone: 800-433-9016
        847-228-5005
Fax: 847-228-5097
E-mail: kidsdocs@aap.org
www.aap.org

American College of Nurse-Midwives
(ACNM)
8403 Colesville Road, Suite 1550
Silver Spring, MD 20910-6374, USA
Phone: 240-485-1800
Fax: 240-485-1818
www.acnm.org

American College of Obstetricians and
Gynecologists (ACOG)
409 12th Street, P.O. Box 96920
Washington, DC 20090-6920, USA
Phone: 202-638-5577
Fax: 202-484-5107
E-mail: resources@acog.org
www.acog.org

American Dietetic Association (ADA)
120 South Riverside Plaza, Suite 2000
Chicago, IL 60606-6995, USA
Phone: 800-877-1600, 312-899-0040
Fax: 312-899-1979
E-mail: cdr@eatright.org
www.eatright.org

American Heart Association
7272 Greenville Avenue
Dallas, TX 75231-4596, USA
Phone: 214-373-6300, 800-242-8721
TTY: 800-654-5984
Fax: 214-706-2221
www.americanheart.org

American Medical Association (AMA)
515 North State Street
Chicago, IL 60610, USA
Phone: 312-464-5000
Fax: 312-464-4184
www.ama-assn.org

American Public Health
Association (APHA)
Clearinghouse on Infant Feeding and
Maternal Nutrition
800 I Street, NW
Washington, DC 20001, USA
Phone: 202-777-2742
Fax: 202-777-2534
E-mail: comments@apha.org
www.apha.org

AnotherLook
P.O. Box 383
Evanston, IL 60204, USA
Phone: 847-869-1278

E-mail: MT@anotherlook.org
www.anotherlook.org

Association of Women's Health, Obstetric
and Neonatal Nurses (AWHONN)
2000 L Street, NW, Suite 740
Washington, DC 20036, USA
Phone: 202-261-2414
Fax: 202-728-0575
E-mail: customerservice@awhonn.org
www.awhonn.org

Australian Breastfeeding Association
P.O. Box 4000
Glen Iris, Victoria 3146, Australia
Phone: +61 3 98850855
Fax: +61 3 98850866
E-mail: info@breastfeeding.asn.au
www.breastfeeding.asn.au

Baby Friendly USA
327 Quaker Meeting House Road
East Sandwich, MA 02537, USA
Phone: 508-888-8092
Fax: 508-888-8050
E-mail: info@babyfriendlyusa.org
www.babyfriendlyusa.org

Best Start Social Marketing
4809 E. Busch Blvd., Suite 104
Tampa, FL 33617, USA
Phone: 800-277-4975
E-mail: beststart@beststartinc.org
www.beststartinc.org

Centers for Disease Control
Breastfeeding Web page
www.cdc.gov/breastfeeding

Coalition for Improving Maternity Services
P.O. Box 2346
Ponte Vedra Beach, FL 32004, USA
Phone: 888-282-CIMS, 904-285-1613
Fax: 904-285-2120
E-mail: info@motherfriendly.org
www.motherfriendly.org

Department of Health and Human Services
Office on Women's Health
200 Independence Avenue, SW
Room 730B
Washington, DC 20201, USA
Phone: 202-690-7650
Fax: 202-205-2631
www.4woman.gov/owh

Doulas of North America
P.O. Box 626
Jasper, IN 47547, USA
Phone: 888-788-DONA
Fax: 812-634-1491
E-mail: Doula@DONA.org
www.DONA.org

Healthy Mothers, Healthy Babies
121 North Washington Street, Suite 300
Alexandria, VA 22314, USA
Phone: 703-836-6110
Fax: 703-836-3470
www.hmhb.org

Healthy People 2010
www.healthypeople.gov

Human Milk Banking Association of North
America, Inc. (HMBANA)
1500 Sunday Drive, Suite 102
Raleigh, NC 27607, USA
Phone: 919-861-4530 ext. 226
E-mail: aprather@olsonmgmt.com
www.hmbana.com

Infant Feeding Action Coalition
INFACT Canada
6 Trinity Square
Toronto, Ontario M5G 1B1, Canada
Phone: 416-595-9819
E-mail: infact@ftn.net
www.infactcanada.ca

Institute for Reproductive Health
Georgetown University Medical Center
4301 Connecticut Avenue, NW,
Suite 310
Washington, DC 20008, USA
Phone: 202-687-1392
Fax: 202-537-7450
E-mail: irhinfo@georgetown.edu
www.irh.org

International Baby Food Action
Network (IBFAN)
212 Third Avenue North, Suite 300
Minneapolis, MN 55401, USA
E-mail: babymilkacti@gn.apc.org
www.ibfan.org

International Childbirth Education
Association (ICEA)
P.O. Box 20048
Minneapolis, MN 55420, USA
Phone: 612-854-8660
Fax: 612-854-8772
E-mail: info@icea.org
www.icea.org

International Labour Office
4, route des Morillons
CH-1211 Geneva 22, Switzerland
Phone: +41-22-799-6111
Fax: +41-22-798-8685
E-mail: ilo@ilo.org
www.ilo.org

International Society for Research in
Human Milk and Lactation
Meriter Hospital Perinatal Center
202 S. Park Street
Madison, WI 53715, USA
Phone: 608-262-6561
Fax: 608-267-6377
E-mail: frgreer@facstaff.wisc.edu
www.isrhml.org

Joint Commission on
Accreditation of Healthcare
Organizations (JCAHO)
601 13th Street, NW, Suite 1150N
Washington, DC 20005, USA
Phone: 202-783-6655
Fax: 202-783-6888
E-mail: customerservice@jcaho.org
www.jcaho.org

La Leche League International, Inc.
P.O. Box 4079
1400 N. Meacham Road

Schaumburg, IL 60173-4048, USA
Phone: 800-525-3243
        847-519-7730
Fax: 847-519-0035
E-mail: lllhq@llli.org
www.lalecheleague.org

Linkages Academy for Educational
Development
United States Agency for International
Development (USAID)
1825 Connecticut Avenue, NW
Washington, DC 20009, USA
Phone: 202-884-8000
Fax: 202-884-8977
E-mail: linkages@aed.org
www.linkagesproject.org

March of Dimes
1275 Mamaroneck Avenue
White Plains, NY 10605, USA
Phone: 914-428-7100
Fax: 914-428-8203
www.modimes.org

National Alliance for Breastfeeding
Advocacy (NABA)
254 Conant Road
Weston, MA 02493-1756, USA
Phone: 781-893-3553
Fax: 781-893-8608
E-mail: Marsha@naba-
breastfeeding.org
www.naba-breastfeeding.org

National Association of
Neonatal Nurses
4700 W. Lake Avenue
Glenview, IL 60025-1485, USA
Phone: 847-375-3660, 800-451-3795
Fax: 888-477-6266
International Fax: 732-380-3640
E-mail: info@nann.org
www.nann.org

National Association of WIC
Directors (NAWD)
2001 S. Street, NW, Suite 580
Washington, DC 20009, USA
Phone: 202-232-5492
Fax: 202-387-5281
E-mail: nawdnutri@aol.com
www.wicdirectors.org

National Perinatal Association
3500 E. Fletcher Avenue, Suite 209
Tampa, FL 33613, USA
Phone: 813-971-1008
Fax: 813-971-9306
E-mail: npa@nationalperinatal.org
www.nationalperinatal.org

Sudden Infant Death Syndrome (SIDS)
Mother-Baby Behavioral Sleep Laboratory
University of Notre Dame
Department of Anthropology
Notre Dame, IN 46556, USA
E-mail: James.J.Mckenna.25@nd.edu
www.nd.edu/~jmckenn1/lab

Support for the Breastfeeding Employee
National Maternal and Child Health
Clearinghouse

Health Resources and Services
Administration
Parklawn Building
5600 Fishers Lane
Rockville, MD 20857, USA
Phone: 888-275-4772
www.hrsa.gov

UNICEF
3 United Nations Plaza
New York, NY 10017, USA
Phone: 212-888-7465
Fax: 212-303-7911
E-mail: information@unicef.org
www.unicef.org/programme/breastfeeding

UNICEF Canada
Canada Square
2200 Yonge Street, Suite 1100
Toronto, Ontario M4S 2C6, Canada
Phone: 416-482-4444
Fax: 416-482-8035
E-mail: secretary@unicef.ca
www.unicef.ca

United States Breastfeeding
Committee (USBC)
1500 Sunday Drive, Suite 102
Raleigh, NC 27607, USA
Phone: 919-861-5589
Fax: 919-787-4916
E-mail: info@usbreastfeeding.org
www.usbreastfeeding.org

U.S. Committee for UNICEF
333 East 38th Street, 6th Floor
New York, NY 10017, USA
Phone: 212-686-5522
Fax: 212-779-1679
E-mail: information@unicefusa.org
www.unicefusa.org

Wellstart, International
P.O. Box 80877
San Diego, CA 92138-0877, USA
Phone: 619-295-5192
Fax: 619-574-8159
E-mail: info@wellstart.org
www.wellstart.org

WIC Supplemental Food Programs Division
Food and Nutrition Service
United States Department of Agriculture
3101 Park Center Drive
Alexandria, VA 22302, USA
Phone: 703-305-2746
Fax: 703-305-2196
www.fns.usda.gov/wic

World Alliance for Breastfeeding
Action (WABA)
P.O. Box 1200, 10850
Penang, Malaysia
Phone: 604-6584-816
Fax: 604-6572-655
E-mail: secr@waba.org.my
www.waba.org.my

World Health Organization (WHO)
Avenue Appia 20
1211 Geneva 27, Switzerland
Phone: 22-791-2111
Fax: 22-791-3111
E-mail: info@who.int
www.who.int

▶ PROFESSIONAL NETWORKING

Breastfeeding and Medications Forum:
www.neonatal.ttuhsc.edu/lact/

www.ezzo.info
A comprehensive Web site detailing medical, behavioral, theological, and other concerns about Growing Families International (GFI). Many published articles and links. Many of the professional concerns about GFI apply to the other baby training books/programs. This Web site is a good reference for analyzing any baby-training approach.

HIPAA and the IBCLC with Privacy Documents for the IBCLC (CD-ROM in PC format only)
Elizabeth C. Brooks, JD, IBCLC
7906 Pine Road
Wyndmoor, PA 19038, USA
Phone: 215-836-9088
E-mail: ecbrks@yahoo.com

ILCA Discussion Board: www.ilca.org

Lactnet E-mail:
Listserv@library.ummed.edu

Professional Liability Insurance:
Maginnis and Associates
P.O. Box 543
Reynoldsburg, OH 43068, USA
Phone: 800-345-6917

Marsh Affinity Group Services
A service of Seabury & Smith
1440 Renaissance Drive
Park Ride, IL 60068-1400, USA
Phone: 800-503-9230

Superbill for reimbursement
UCLA Lactation Alumni Association
2021 Grismer #17
Burbank, CA 91504, USA
Phone: 818-841-4182
Fax: 818-848-2882
E-mail: cfolling@fmsn.com

▶ DOMESTIC AND SEXUAL ABUSE

Parents Anonymous, Inc.
675 W. Foothill Blvd., Suite 220
Claremont, CA 91711-3416, USA
Phone: 909-621-6184
Fax: 909-625-6304
E-mail: palmelendez@juno.com
www.parentsanonymous.org

Adult Survivors of Child Abuse
P.O. Box 14477
San Francisco, CA 94114-0038, USA
Phone: 415-928-4576
E-mail: tmc_asca@dnai.com
www.ascasupport.org

National Domestic Violence Hotline
Phone: 800-799-SAFE (7233)
TTY for the deaf: 1-800-787-3224
E-mail: ndvh@ndvh.org
www.ndvh.org

Texas Council on Family Violence
P.O. Box 161810
Austin, Texas 78716, USA
Phone: 512-794-1133

More than 1200 indexed links to domestic violence resources on the Internet:
www.growing.com/nonviolent/research/dvlinks.htm

▶ CLEFT LIP AND CLEFT PALATE

American Academy of
Otolaryngology-
Head and Neck Surgery (AAO-HNS)
One Prince Street
Alexandria, VA 22314, USA
Phone: 703-836-4444
TTY: 703-519-1585
Fax: 703-683-5100
E-mail: webmaster@entnet.org
www.entnet.org

American Cleft Palate-Craniofacial
Association (ACPA)
104 S. Estes Drive, Suite 204
Chapel Hill, NC 27514, USA
Phone: 919-933-9044
        800-24-CLEFT
Fax: 919-933-9604
E-mail: cleftline@aol.com
www.cleftline.org

American Society of Human Genetics
9650 Rockville Pike
Bethesda, MD 20814-3889, USA
Phone: 301-571-1825
Fax: 301-530-7079
www.faseb.org/genetics

American Speech-Language-Hearing
Association (ASHA)
10801 Rockville Pike
Rockville, MD 20852, USA
Phone: 301-897-5700, 800-638-8255
TTY: 301-897-0157
Fax: 301-571-0457
E-mail: actioncenter@asha.org
www.asha.org

Children's Craniofacial Association (CCA)
P.O. Box 280297
Dallas, TX 75228, USA
Phone: 972-994-9902, 800-535-3643
Fax: 972-240-7607
www.ccakids.com

FACES—National Craniofacial Association
P.O. Box 11082
Chattanooga, TN 37401, USA
Phone: 423-266-1632, 800-3FACES3
Fax: 423-267-3124
E-mail: faces@mindspring.com
www.faces-cranio.org

National Foundation for Facial
Reconstruction
317 East 34th St. #901
New York, NY 10016, USA
Phone: 212-263-6656
Fax: 212-263-7534
E-mail: nffr@earthlink.net
www.nffr.org

National Institute of Child Health and
Human Development
Building 31, Room 2A32
31 Center Drive MSC 2425
Bethesda, MD 20892-2425, USA
Phone: 301-496-5133
        800-370-2943
Fax: 301-496-7102
E-mail: NICHDClearinghouse@ mail.nih.gov
www.nichd.nih.gov

National Institute of Dental
and Craniofacial Research
Building 45, Room 4AS-19
45 Center Drive MSC 6401
Bethesda, MD 20892-6401, USA
Phone: 301-496-4261
Fax: 301-496-9988
E-mail: nidrinfo@od31.nidr. nih.gov
www.nidcr.nih.gov

National Organization for Rare
Disorders (NORD)
P.O. Box 8923
New Fairfield, CT 06812, USA
Phone: 203-746-6518
        800-999-NORD
TTY: 203-746-6927
Fax: 203-746-6481
E-mail: orphan@rarediseases.org
www.rarediseases.org

Velo-Cardio-Facial Syndrome
Educational Foundation, Inc.
P.O. Box 874
Milltown, NJ 08850, USA
Phone: 866-VCFSEFS, 800-823-7335
Fax: 732-238-8803
E-mail: info@vcfsef.org
www.vcfsef.org

WIDESMILES
P.O. Box 5153
Stockton, CA 95205-0153, USA
www.widesmiles.org

▶ **RELEVANT PUBLICATIONS**

Apple RD. *Mothers and Medicine: A Social History of Infant Feeding 1890–1950.* Madison, WI: University of Wisconsin Press; 1987.

Auerbach KG and Riordan J. *Clinical Lactation: A Visual Guide.* Sudbury, MA: Jones and Bartlett Publishers; 2000.

Auerbach KG and Riordan J. *Current Issues in Clinical Lactation.* Sudbury, MA: Jones and Bartlett Publishers; 2000.

Baumslag N and Michels D. *Milk, Money and Madness: The Culture and Politics of Breastfeeding.* Westport, CT: Bergin & Garvey; 1995.

Cadwell K. *Reclaiming Breastfeeding for the United States: Protection, Promotion, and Support.* Sudbury, MA: Jones and Bartlett Publishers; 2002.

Chamberlain D. *Babies Remember Birth.* New York: Ballantine Books; 1988.

Fildes V. *Breasts, Bottles and Babies: A History of Infant Feeding.* Edinburgh: Edinburgh University Press; 1986.

Fildes V. *Wet Nursing.* Oxford, UK: Basil Blackwell Ltd; 1988.

Gladwell, M. *The Tipping Point: How Little Things Can Make a Big Difference.* Boston, MA: Little, Brown and Company; 2000.

Greenlagh T. *How to Read a Paper: The Basics of Evidence-Based Medicine.* London: British Medical Journal Publishing; 1997.

Hale T. *Medications in Mothers' Milk,* 11th ed. Amarillo, TX: Pharmasoft Publishing; 2004.

Hale T and Berens P. *Clinical Therapy in Breastfeeding Patients.* Amarillo, TX: Pharmasoft Medical Publishing; 2002.

Hale T and Ilett K. *Drug Therapy and Breastfeeding.* Amarillo, TX: Pharmasoft Medical Publishing; 2002.

Heller S. *The Vital Touch.* New York: Henry Holt and Company; 1997.

HMBANA. *Best Practice for Pumping, Storing and Handling of Mother's Own Milk in Hospital and at Home.* Raleigh, NC: HMBANA; 2004.

HMBANA. *Guidelines for the Establishment and Operation of a Donor Human Milk Bank.* Raleigh, NC: HMBANA; 2004.

IBLCE. *Clinical Competencies for IBCLC Practice.* Falls Church, VA: International Board of Lactation Consultant Examiners; 2003.

ILCA. *Core Curriculum for Lactation Consultant Practice.* (M. Walker, ed.). Raleigh, NC: International Lactation Consultant Association; 2002.

ILCA. *Evidence-Based Guidelines for Breastfeeding Management During the First Fourteen Days.* Raleigh, NC: International Lactation Consultant Association; 1999.

ILCA. *Standards of Practice for IBCLC Lactation Consultants.* Raleigh, NC: International Lactation Consultant Association; 1999.

ILCA. *Summary of the Hazards of Infant Formula.* Raleigh, NC: International Lactation Consultant Association; 1992.

ILCA. *Summary of the Hazards of Infant Formula: Part 2.* Raleigh, NC: International Lactation Consultant Association; 1998.

ILCA. *Summary of the Hazards of Infant Formula: Part 3.* Raleigh, NC: International Lactation Consultant Association; 2004.

Klaus M et al. *Mothering the Mother.* Reading, MA: Addison-Wesley Publishing Company; 1993.

Klaus M, Kennell J and Klaus P. *Bonding: Building the Foundations of Secure Attachment and Independence.* Reading, MA: Addison-Wesley Publishing Company; 1995.

Klaus M and Klaus P. *The Amazing Newborn.* Reading, MA: Addison-Wesley Publishing Company; 1985.

Knowles MS. *Self-Directed Learning: A Guide for Learners and Teachers.* New York: Association Press; 1975.

Knowles MS. *The Modern Practice of Adult Education: From Pedagogy to Andragogy.* New York: Association Press; 1980.

Kroeger M and Smith L. *Impact of Birthing Practices on Breastfeeding.* Sudbury, MA: Jones and Bartlett Publishers; 2004.

Kutner L and Barger J. *Clinical Experience in Lactation: A Blueprint for Internship.* Wheaton, IL: Lactation Education Consultants; 2002.

Lang S. *Breastfeeding Special Care Babies.* London: Bailliere Tindall; 2002.

Lawrence R. *Breastfeeding: A Guide for the Medical Profession,* 5th ed. St. Louis, MO: Mosby; 1999.

Mager F. *Preparing Educational Objectives.* Belmont, CA: Lake Publishing Company; 1984.

McKenzie JF, McKenzie JC and Smelter J. *Planning, Implementing and Evaluating Health Promotion Programmes.* New York: Macmillan; 1993.

Merewood A and Philipp B. *Breastfeeding: Conditions and Diseases.* Amarillo, TX: Pharmasoft Medical Publishing; 2001.

Minchin M. *Breastfeeding Matters.* Victoria, Australia: Alma Publications; 1998.

Mohrbacher N and Stock J. *The Breastfeeding Answer Book.* Schaumburg, IL: La Leche League International; 2003.

Montagu A. *Touching: The Human Significance of the Skin.* New York: Harper Row; 1986.

Palmer G. *The Politics of Breastfeeding.* London: Pandora Press; 1993.

Riordan J. *Breastfeeding and Human Lactation.* Sudbury, MA: Jones and Bartlett Publishers; 2004.

Royal College of Midwives. *Successful Breastfeeding.* London: Churchill Livingstone; 2002.

Simkin P. *The Birth Partner.* Boston, MA: Harvard Common Press; 2001.

Small M. *Our Babies, Ourselves: How Biology and Culture Shape the Way We Parent.* New York: Anchor Books; 1998.

Smith L. *Comprehensive Lactation Consultant Exam Review.* Sudbury, MA: Jones and Bartlett Publishers; 2001.

Smith L. *The Lactation Consultant in Private Practice: The ABCs of Getting Started.* Sudbury, MA: Jones and Bartlett Publishers; 2003.

Stuart-Macadam P and Dettwyler K. *Breastfeeding: Biocultural Perspectives.* New York: Aldine De Gruyter; 1995.

Thevenin T. *The Family Bed: An Age Old Concept in Childrearing.* Garden City Park, NY: Avery Publishing Group; 1977.

UNICEF and WHO. *Breastfeeding Management and Promotion in a Baby-Friendly Hospital: An 18-Hour Course for Maternity Staff.* New York: UNICEF; 1993.

Van Esterik P. *Beyond the Breast-Bottle Controversy.* Piscatawny, NJ: Rutgers University Press; 1989. (Published in the United Kingdom under the title *Mother Power and Infant Feeding.*)

Van Esterik P. *Women, Work, and Breastfeeding.* Ithaca, NY: Cornell Division of Nutritional Sciences; 1992.

Walker M. *Selling Out Mothers and Babies: Marketing of Breast Milk Substitutes in the USA.* Weston, MA: National Alliance for Breastfeeding Advocacy; 2001.

Wilson-Clay B and Hoover K. *The Breastfeeding Atlas*, 2nd ed. Austin, TX: LactNews Press; 2002.

Worthington-Roberts B and Rodwell-Williams S. *Nutrition in Pregnancy and Lactation*, 6th ed. New York: McGraw-Hill Science/Engineering/Math; 1996.

▶ WORLD HEALTH ORGANIZATION PUBLICATIONS

These documents are available from WHO in Geneva or from the U.S. distributor in New York (listed under Sources for Products later in the appendix). Several are available from the WHO Web site: www.who.int.

Breastfeeding: The Technical Basis for Recommendations and Action. Geneva, Switzerland: WHO; 1993.

Breastfeeding and Child Spacing: What Health Workers Need to Know. Geneva, Switzerland: WHO; 1988.

Evidence for the Ten Steps to Successful Breastfeeding. Family and Reproductive Health, Division of Child Health and Development. Geneva, Switzerland: WHO; 1998.

Innocenti Declaration on the Protection, Promotion and Support of Breastfeeding. Geneva, Switzerland: WHO; 1990.

Infant Feeding: The Physiological Basis. Geneva, Switzerland: WHO; 1990.

International Code of Marketing of Breastmilk Substitutes. Geneva, Switzerland: WHO; 1981.

Nutrient Adequacy of Exclusive Breastfeeding for the Term Infant During the First Six Months of Life. Geneva, Switzerland: WHO; 2002.

Protecting, Promoting and Supporting Breastfeeding: The Special Role of Maternity Services. A Joint WHO/UNICEF Statement. Geneva, Switzerland: WHO; 1989.

The Global Strategy for Infant and Young Child Feeding. Geneva, Switzerland: WHO; 2002.

▶ JOURNALS AND NEWSLETTERS

Acta Paediatrica, Editorial Office, Building Z6:04, Karolinska Hospital, SE-171 76, Stockholm, Sweden. www.tandf.co.uk

American Journal of Obstetrics and Gynecology, C.V. Mosby Co., 11830 Westline Industrial Dr., St. Louis, MO 63141, USA. www.mosby.com/ajog

Birth: Issues in Perinatal Care and Education, Blackwell Publishing Ltd. www.ovid.com/site

Breastfeeding Abstracts, La Leche League International, P.O. Box 4079, Schaumburg, IL 60173-4048, USA. www.lalecheleague.org

Breastfeeding Review, Australian Breastfeeding Association. www.breastfeeding.asn.au

British Medical Journal, BMJ Publishing Group, PO Box 299, London WC1H 9TD, United Kingdom. www.bmj.com

Journal of Human Lactation, International Lactation Consultant Association. Sage Publications, 2455 Teller Road, Thousand Oaks, CA 91320, USA. 800-818-7243. www.sagepub.com

Journal of Obstetric, Gynecologic, and Neonatal Nursing, Suite 200, 600 Maryland Ave., SW, Washington, DC 20024, USA. www.jognn.awhonn.org

Journal of the American Dietetic Association, 430 N. Michigan Ave., Chicago, IL 60611, USA. www.eatright.org

Journal of the American Medical Association, 535 N. Dearborn St., Chicago, IL 60610, USA. www.jama.ama-assn.org

New England Journal of Medicine, 10 Shattuck St., Boston, MA 02115, USA. www.nejm.org

Obstetrical and Gynecological Survey, Williams and Wilkins, 428 East Preston St., Baltimore, MD 21202, USA. www.obgynsurvey.com

Pediatrics, P.O. Box 1034, Evanston, IL 60204, USA. www.pediatrics.com

Science, American Association for the Advancement of Science, 1515 Massachusetts Ave., NW, Washington, DC 20005, USA. www.scienceonline.org

The Harvard Medical School Health Letter, Department of Continuing Education of Harvard Medical School, 79 Garden St., Cambridge, MA 02138, USA. www.health.harvard.edu

The Journal of Pediatrics, C.V. Mosby, II 830 Westline Industrial Dr., St. Louis, MO 63141, USA. www.us.elsevierhealth.com

The Lancet, North American Editor: Little, Brown and Co., 34 Beacon St., Boston, MA 02106, USA. www.thelancet.com

▶ VIDEOS

Fathers Supporting Breastfeeding. U.S. Department of Agriculture, Food and Nutrition Service, WIC Program. 17 minutes; 2002. www.fns.usda.gov.wic

Delivery and Self Attachment, Dr. Lennart Righard. 6 minutes; 1992. www.geddesproductions.com

Breastfeeding: Coping with the First Week. Royal College of Midwives. 30 minutes; 1996. www.growingwithbaby.org

Breastfeeding: A Guide to Successful Positioning. Royal College of Midwives. 12 minutes; 1997. www.childbirthgraphics.com

Follow Me Mum. Rebecca Glover. 20 minutes; 2002. www.ibreastfeeding.com

From Bottles to Breasts to Baby Friendly: The Challenge of Change. Anne Merewood and Barbara L. Philipp. 15 minutes; 2001. www.ibreastfeeding.com

Mother and Baby Getting It Right. Australian Breastfeeding Association. 1996. www.ibreastfeeding.com

A Premie Needs His Mother: First Steps to Breastfeeding Your Premature Baby. Jane Morton, MD. 51 minutes; 2002. DVD and video. www.ibreastfeeding.com

Kangaroo Mother Care. Nils Bergman, MD. 26 minutes; 2001. www.geddesproduction.com

VIDEO CLIPS ONLINE

There are many fine childbirth and breast-feeding videos available. We suggest you check with your health department or ministry for regional or local titles. These Internet video clips from bona fide breast-feeding Web sites are a starting point for your library.

www.breastfeeding.com/helpme. Several clips on benefits, working, premies, pumping hunger cues, latching, and cup feeding.

www.pumpstation.com/frmvideos-1.cfm. Clips on feeding cues, latch, and finishing the feeding.

www.healthyarkansas.com/breastfeeding/training.html. Anita Baker, "Giving you the best that I've got, baby."

www.ci.bridgeport.ct.us/departments/health/breastfeedin.aspx. Several clips on benefits, working, preemies, pumping, hunger cues, latching, and cup feeding.

▶ **POWERPOINT PRESENTATIONS AND CD-ROMS**

Breastfeeding and Human Lactation, 3rd ed. Jan Riordan. Sudbury, MA: Jones and Bartlett Publishers; 2004. (CD-ROM of breastfeeding images is included with text.)

Breastfeeding Answer Book, 3rd rev ed. No. 1277-30; 2003. www.lalecheleague.org. (Available in a CD-ROM version.)

Breastfeeding Support and Promotion: A Speakers Kit. Produced by the AAP Section on Breastfeeding, 2003. Set of 77 PowerPoint slides for a basic talk about breast-feeding. www.aap.org

HIPAA and the IBCLC. CD with privacy documents for LCs by © Elizabeth C. Brooks, JD, IBCLC, July 2004. CD-ROM (PC format only). Elizabeth C. Brooks, JD, IBCLC, 7906 Pine Road, Wyndmoor, PA 19038, USA; 215-836-9088; 215-836-0591 Email: ecbrks@yahoo.com

The Breastfeeding Atlas: Images from the Second Edition. Kay Hoover and Barbara Wilson Clay. LactNews Press; 2003. CD ROM. www.ibreastfeeding.com

The ILCA Web site has PowerPoint presentations on ethics, the International Code of Marketing of Breast Milk Substitutes, evidence-based practice, and more. www.ilca.org

▶ **SOURCES FOR PRODUCTS**

Resources are available from many of the organizations listed above. In addition, the following businesses and organizations offer a variety of resources. There may be other product sources available. A search on the Internet will help you find everything that is available.

Books, Videos, and Other Products

Birth and Life Bookstore
a division of Cascade Health Care Products
Cascade Health Care
1826 NW 18th Avenue
Portland, OR 97209, USA
Phone: 503-595-1720
Fax: 503-595-1726
E-mail: info@1cascade.com
www.1cascade.com

Buttons Plus
2279 Nord Avenue, Chico, CA 95926
(530) 345-6049
buttons@now2000.com
www.northvalley.net/buttonsplus

Childbirth Graphics
Division of WRS Group, Inc.
P.O. Box 21207
Waco, TX 76702-1207, USA
Phone: 800-299-3366, ext. 287
Fax: 888-977-7653
E-mail: sales@wrsgroup.com
www.wrsgroup.com

Injoy Birth Videos, Inc.
1435 Yarmouth Ave
Suite 102
Boulder, CO 80304, USA
Phone: 303-447-2082
E-mail: custserv@injoyvideos.com
www.injoyvideos.com

Noodle Soup
Childbirth and parenting education—low literacy
4614 Prospect Ave #328
Cleveland, OH 44103, USA
Phone: 800-795-9295
www.noodlesoup.com

Pharmasoft Publishing
1712 N. Forest St.
Amarillo, TX 79106, USA
Phone: 806-376-9900
Phone: 800-378-1317
Fax: 806-376-9901
E-Mail: books@ibreastfeeding.com
www.ibreastfeeding.com

WHO Publications
49 Sheridan Ave
Albany, NY 12210, USA
Phone: 518-436-9686
Fax: 518-436-7433
E-mail: qcorp@compuserve.com
www.who.int

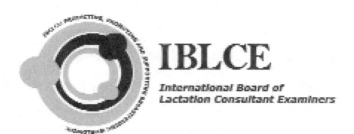

IBLCE
International Board of
Lactation Consultant Examiners

CLINICAL COMPETENCIES FOR IBCLC PRACTICE

Much of the clinical practice of the International Board Certified Lactation Consultant (IBCLC) consists of systematic problem solving in collaboration with breastfeeding mothers and other members of the health care team. This checklist includes most of the clinical/practical skills that an entry level IBCLC needs in order to be satisfactorily proficient to provide safe and effective care for breastfeeding mothers and babies. The list is designed to encompass common breastfeeding situations and the challenges that are encountered most frequently by lactation consultants. Clinical instructors will be able to use this checklist as an appropriate guide in providing individualized education. A list of possible sites for obtaining clinical/practical experience appears at the end of the list of competencies.

Students are encouraged to become familiar with other documents that address the role of the IBCLC. The knowledge, skills, and attitude inherent in the role of an IBCLC are summarized in a list of 16 "Competency Statements" contained in the *International Board of Lactation Consultant Examiners Candidate Information Guide*. A more detailed description of the role is provided in the *Standards of Practice for IBCLC Lactation Consultants* published by the International Lactation Consultant Association (ILCA). Optimal breastfeeding care is clearly presented in 24 management strategies with rationales and references in *Evidence-Based Guidelines for Breastfeeding Management During the First Fourteen Days*, also published by ILCA.

▶ COMMUNICATION AND COUNSELING SKILLS

In all interactions with mothers, families, health care professionals and peers, the student will demonstrate effective communication skills to maintain collaborative and supportive relationships.

The student will:
☐ Identify factors that might affect communication (i.e., age, cultural/language differences, deafness, blindness, mental ability, etc.)
☐ Demonstrate appropriate body language (i.e., position in relation to the other person, comfortable eye contact, appropriate tone of voice for the setting, etc.)
☐ Demonstrate knowledge of and sensitivity to cultural differences
☐ Elicit information using effective counseling techniques (i.e., asking open-ended questions, summarizing the discussion, and providing emotional support)
☐ Make appropriate referrals to other health care professionals and community resources

The student will provide individualized breastfeeding care with an emphasis on the mother's ability to make informed decisions.

The student will:
☐ Assess mother's psychological state and provide information appropriate to her situation
☐ Include those family members or friends the mother identifies as significant to her
☐ Obtain the mother's permission for providing care to her or her baby
☐ Ascertain mother's knowledge about and goals for breastfeeding
☐ Use adult education principles to provide instruction to the mother that will meet her needs
☐ Select appropriate written information and other teaching aides

▶ HISTORY TAKING AND ASSESSMENT SKILLS

The student will be able to:
☐ Obtain a pertinent history
☐ Perform a breast evaluation related to lactation
☐ Develop a breastfeeding risk assessment
☐ Assess and evaluate the infant relative to his ability to breastfeed
☐ Assess effective milk transfer

▶ DOCUMENTATION AND COMMUNICATION SKILLS WITH HEALTH PROFESSIONALS

The student will:
☐ Communicate effectively with other members of the health care team, using written documents appropriate to the geopolitical region, facility and culture in which the student is being trained, such as: consent forms, care plans, charting forms/clinical notes, pathways/care maps, and feeding assessment forms
☐ Use appropriate resources for research to provide information to the health care team on conditions, modalities, and medications that affect breastfeeding and lactation
☐ Write referrals and follow-up documentation/letters to referring and/or primary health care providers that illustrate the student's ability to identify:
   ☐ The mother's concerns or problems, planned interventions, evaluation of outcomes and follow-up
   ☐ Situations in which immediate verbal communication with the health care provider is necessary, such as serious illness in the infant, child, or mother
☐ Report instances of child abuse or neglect to specific agencies as mandated or appropriate

Source: International Lactation Consultant Association (ILCA) and International Board of Lactation Consultant Examiners (IBLCE)

SKILLS FOR FIRST TWO HOURS AFTER BIRTH

The student will:
- ☐ Identify events that occurred during the labor and birth process that may negatively impact breastfeeding
- ☐ Identify and discourage practices that may interfere with breastfeeding
- ☐ Promote continuous skin-to-skin contact of the term newborn and mother through the first feeding
- ☐ Assist the mother and family to identify newborn feeding cues
- ☐ Help the mother and infant to find a comfortable position for latching-on/attachment during the initial feeding after birth
- ☐ Identify correct latch-on (attachment)
- ☐ Reinforce to mother and family the importance of:
    - ☐ Keeping the mother and baby together
    - ☐ Feeding the baby on cue—but at least 8 times in each 24 hour period

POSTPARTUM SKILLS

Prior to discharge from care, the student will observe a feeding and effectively instruct the mother about:
- ☐ Assessment of adequate milk intake by the baby
- ☐ Normal infant sucking patterns
- ☐ How milk is produced and supply maintained, including discussion of growth/appetite spurts
- ☐ Normal newborn behavior, including why, when and how to wake a sleepy newborn
- ☐ Avoidance of early use of a pacifier and bottle nipple
- ☐ Importance of exclusive breast milk feeds and possible consequences of mixed feedings with cow milk or soy
- ☐ Prevention and treatment of sore nipples
- ☐ Prevention and treatment of engorgement
- ☐ SIDS prevention behaviors
- ☐ Family planning methods and their relationship to breastfeeding
- ☐ Education regarding drugs (such as nicotine, alcohol, caffeine and illicit drugs) and folk remedies (such as herbal teas)
- ☐ Plans for follow-up care for breastfeeding questions, infant's medical and mother's postpartum examinations
- ☐ Community resources for assistance with breastfeeding

PROBLEM-SOLVING SKILLS

The student will be able to:
- ☐ Identify problems
- ☐ Assess contributing factors and etiology
- ☐ Develop an appropriate breastfeeding plan of care in concert with the mother
- ☐ Assist the mother to implement the plan
- ☐ Evaluate effectiveness of the plan

SKILLS FOR MATERNAL BREASTFEEDING CHALLENGES

The student will be able to assist mothers with the following challenges:
- ☐ Cesarean birth
- ☐ Flat/inverted nipples
- ☐ Yeast infections of breast, nipple, areola, and milk ducts
- ☐ Continuation of breastfeeding when mother is separated from her baby
    - ☐ Milk expression techniques
    - ☐ Maintaining milk production
    - ☐ Collection, storage and transportation of milk
- ☐ Cultural beliefs that are not evidence-based and may interfere with breastfeeding, (i.e., discarding colostrum, rigidly scheduled feedings, necessity of formula after every breastfeeding, etc.)

- ☐ Medical conditions that impact breastfeeding
- ☐ Adolescent mother
    - ☐ Strategies for returning to school
    - ☐ Maintaining milk production
- ☐ Nipple pain and damage
- ☐ Engorgement
- ☐ Plugged duct or blocked nipple pore
- ☐ Mastitis
- ☐ Breast surgery/trauma
- ☐ Overproduction of milk
- ☐ Postpartum psychological issues including transient sadness ("baby blues") and postpartum depression
    - ☐ Appropriate referrals
    - ☐ Medications compatible with breastfeeding
- ☐ Insufficient milk supply, differentiating between perceived and real
- ☐ Weaning issues
    - ☐ Safe formula preparation and feeding techniques
    - ☐ Care of breasts

SKILLS FOR INFANT BREASTFEEDING CHALLENGES

The student will be able to assist mothers who have infants with the following challenges:
- ☐ Traumatic birth
- ☐ 35–38 weeks' gestation
- ☐ Small for gestational age (SGA) or large for gestational age (LGA)
- ☐ Multiples/plural births
- ☐ Preterm birth, including the benefits of kangaroo care
- ☐ High risk for hypoglycemia
- ☐ Sleepy infant
- ☐ Excessive weight loss, slow/poor weight gain
- ☐ Hyperbilirubinemia (jaundice)
- ☐ Ankyloglossia (short frenulum)
- ☐ Yeast infection
- ☐ Colic/fussiness
- ☐ Gastric reflux
- ☐ Lactose overload
- ☐ Food intolerances
- ☐ Neurodevelopmental problems
- ☐ Teething and biting
- ☐ Nursing strike/early baby led weaning
- ☐ Toddler nursing
- ☐ Nursing through pregnancy
- ☐ Tandem nursing

MANAGEMENT SKILLS

The student will demonstrate the ability to:
- ☐ Perform a comprehensive breastfeeding assessment
- ☐ Assess milk transfer with:
    - ☐ AC/PC weights, using an electronic digital scale
    - ☐ Use of balance scale for daily weights
- ☐ Calculate an infant's caloric and volume requirements
- ☐ Increase milk production

SKILLS FOR USE OF TECHNOLOGY AND DEVICES

The student will have up-to-date knowledge about breastfeeding-related equipment and demonstrate appropriate use and understanding of potential disadvantages or risks of the following:
- ☐ A device to evert nipples
- ☐ Nipple creams/ointments

- ☐ Breast shells
- ☐ Breast pumps
- ☐ Alternative feeding techniques
  - ☐ Tube feeding at the breast
  - ☐ Cup feeding
  - ☐ Spoon feeding
  - ☐ Eyedropper feeding
  - ☐ Finger feeding
  - ☐ Bottles and artificial nipples
- ☐ Nipple shields
- ☐ Pacifiers
- ☐ Infant scales
- ☐ Use of herbal supplements for mother and/or infant

▶ SKILLS FOR BREASTFEEDING CHALLENGES WHICH ARE ENCOUNTERED INFREQUENTLY

The following issues are encountered relatively infrequently, and may not be seen during the student's training. The entry-level lactation consultant would not be expected to be proficient in these situations. The student will need to use basic skills to assist the mother and infant while seeking guidance from a more experienced IBCLC.

Infant:

- ☐ Infant with tonic bite/ineffective/dysfunctional suck
- ☐ Cranial-facial abnormalities, such as micronathia (receding lower jaw) and cleft lip and/or palate
- ☐ Down syndrome
- ☐ Cardiac problems
- ☐ Chronic medical conditions, such as cystic fibrosis, PKU, etc.

Mother:

- ☐ Induced lactation and relactation
- ☐ Coping with the death of an infant
- ☐ Chronic medical conditions, such as MS, lupus, seizures, etc.
- ☐ Disabilities which may limit mother's ability to handle the baby easily, such as rheumatoid arthritis, carpal tunnel syndrome, cerebral palsy, etc.
- ☐ HIV/AIDS: understanding of current recommendations based on the mother's access to safe replacement feeding

▶ SKILLS FOR MEETING PROFESSIONAL RESPONSIBILITIES

The student will demonstrate the following professional responsibilities:

- ☐ Conduct herself or himself in a professional manner, by complying with *the IBLCE Code of Ethics for International Board Certified Lactation Consultants* and the *ILCA Standards of Practice*; and by adhering to the *International Code of Marketing of Breastmilk Substitutes* and its subsequent World Health Assembly resolutions.

- ☐ Practice within the laws of the setting in which s/he works, showing respect for confidentiality and privacy.
- ☐ Utilize current research findings to provide a strong evidence base for clinical practice, and obtain continuing education to enhance skills and obtain/maintain IBCLC certification.
- ☐ Advocate for breastfeeding families, mothers, infants and children in the workplace, community and within the health care system.
- ☐ Use breastfeeding equipment appropriately and provide information about risks as well as benefits of products, maintaining an awareness of conflict of interest if profiting from the rental or sale of breastfeeding equipment.

▶ SITES FOR ACQUISITION OF SKILLS

The student may acquire clinical/practical skills in the following settings:

- ☐ Private practice IBCLC office
- ☐ Private practice OB, pediatric, family practice or midwifery office
- ☐ Public health department; Women, Infants and Children (WIC) Program (in the US)
- ☐ Hospital
  - ☐ Lactation services
  - ☐ Birthing center
  - ☐ Postpartum unit
  - ☐ Mother-Baby unit
  - ☐ Level II and Level III nurseries: Special Care Nursery, Neonatal Intensive Care Nursery
  - ☐ Pediatric unit
- ☐ Home health services
- ☐ Out-patient follow-up breastfeeding clinics
- ☐ Breastfeeding hotlines and warmlines
- ☐ Prenatal and postpartum breastfeeding classes
- ☐ Home births (if legally permitted)
- ☐ Volunteer community support group meetings

International Lactation Consultant Association (ILCA)
1500 Sunday Drive, Suite 102
Raleigh, NC 27607, USA
Phone: (919) 787-5181
Fax: (919) 787-4916
E-mail: info@ilca.org
Web: www.ilca.org

International Board of Lactation Consultant Examiners (IBLCE)
7309 Arlington Blvd, Suite 300
Falls Church, VA 22042, USA
Phone: (703) 560-7330
Fax: (703) 560-7332
Email: info@iblce.org
Web: www.iblce.org

APPENDIX

C

THE CODE OF ETHICS
International Board Certified Lactation Consultants

▶ PREAMBLE

It is in the best interests of the profession of lactation consultants and the public it serves that there be a Code of Ethics to provide guidance to lactation consultants in their professional practice and conduct. These ethical principles guide the profession and outline commitments and obligations of the lactation consultant to self, client, colleague, society, and the profession.

The purpose of the International Board of Lactation Consultant Examiners (IBLCE) is to assist in the protection of the health, safety, and welfare of the public by establishing and enforcing qualifications of certification and for issuing voluntary credentials to individuals who have attained those qualifications. The IBLCE has adopted this Code to apply to all individuals who hold the credential of International Board Certified Lactation Consultant (IBCLC).

▶ PRINCIPLES OF ETHICAL PRACTICE

The International Board Certified Lactation Consultant shall act in a manner that safeguards the interests of individual clients, justifies public trust in her/his competence, and enhances the reputation of the profession.

The International Board Certified Lactation Consultant is personally accountable for her/his practice and, in the exercise of professional accountability, must:

1. Provide professional services with objectivity and with respect for the unique needs and values of individuals.
2. Avoid discrimination against other individuals on the basis of race, creed, religion, gender, sexual orientation, age, and national origin.
3. Fulfill professional commitments in good faith.
4. Conduct herself/himself with honesty, integrity, and fairness.
5. Remain free of conflict of interest while fulfilling the objectives and maintaining the integrity of the lactation consultant profession.
6. Maintain confidentiality.
7. Base her/his practice on scientific principles, current research, and information.
8. Take responsibility and accept accountability for personal competence in practice.
9. Recognize and exercise professional judgment within the limits of her/his qualifications. This principle includes seeking counsel and making referrals to appropriate providers.
10. Inform the public and colleagues of her/his services by using factual information. An International Board Certified Lactation Consultant will not advertise in a false or misleading manner.
11. Provide sufficient information to enable clients to make informed decisions.
12. Provide information about appropriate products in a manner that is neither false nor misleading.
13. Permit use of her/his name for the purpose of certifying that lactation consultant services have been rendered only if she/he provided those services.
14. Present professional qualifications and credentials accurately, using IBCLC only when certification is current and authorized by the IBLCE, and complying with all requirements when seeking initial or continued certification from the IBLCE. The lactation consultant is subject to disciplinary action for aiding another person in violating any IBLCE requirements or aiding another person in representing himself/herself as an IBCLC when she/he is not.
15. Report to an appropriate person or authority when it appears that the health or safety of colleagues is at risk, as such circumstances may compromise standards of practice and care.
16. Refuse any gift, favor, or hospitality from patients or clients currently in her/his care which might be interpreted as seeking to exert influence to obtain preferential consideration.
17. Disclose any financial or other conflicts of interest in relevant organizations providing goods or services. Ensure that professional judgment is not influenced by any commercial considerations.
18. Present substantiated information and interpret controversial information without personal bias, recognizing that legitimate differences of opinion exist.
19. Withdraw voluntarily from professional practice if the lactation consultant has engaged in any substance abuse that could affect her/his practice; has been adjudged by a court to be mentally incompetent; or has an emotional or mental disability that affects her/his practice in a manner that could harm the client.
20. Obtain maternal consent to photograph, audiotape, or videotape a mother and/or her infant(s) for educational or professional purposes.
21. Submit to disciplinary action under the following circumstance: If convicted of a crime under the laws of the practitioner's country which is a felony or a misdemeanor, an essential element of which is dishonesty, and which is related to the practice of lactation consulting; if disciplined by a state, province, or other local government and at least one of the grounds for the discipline is the same or substantially equivalent to these principles; if committed an act of misfeasance or malfeasance which is directly related to the practice of the profession as determined by a court of competent jurisdiction, a licensing board, or an agency of a governmental body; or if violated a Principle set forth in the Code of Ethics for International Board Certified Lactation Consultants which was in force at the time of the violation.
22. Accept the obligation to protect society and the profession by upholding the Code of Ethics for International Board Certified Lactation Consultants and by reporting alleged violations of the Code through the defined review process of the IBLCE.
23. Require and obtain consent to share clinical concerns and information with the physician or other primary health care provider before initiating a consultation.
24. Adhere to those provisions of the International Code of Marketing of Breast-milk Substitutes which pertain to health workers.

▶ TO LODGE A COMPLAINT

IBCLCs shall act in a manner that justifies public trust in their competence, enhances the reputation of the profession, and safeguards the interests of individual clients.

To protect the credential and to assure responsible practice by its certificants, the IBLCE depends on IBCLCs, members of the coordinating and supervising health professions, employers and the public to report incidents which may require action by the IBLCE Discipline Committee.

Only signed, written complaints will be considered. Anonymous complaints will be discarded. The IBLCE will become involved only in matters that can be factually determined, and will provide the accused party with every opportunity to respond in a professional and legally defensible manner.

Complaints which appear to fit the scope of the Discipline Committee's responsibilities should be sent to: IBLCE Chair of the Discipline Committee, 7309 Arlington Blvd., Suite 300, Falls Church, VA 22042-3215 USA.

D

STANDARDS OF PRACTICE FOR IBCLC LACTATION CONSULTANTS INTERNATIONAL LACTATION CONSULTANT ASSOCIATION

Preface

This is the second edition of *Standards of Practice for IBCLC Lactation Consultants* published by the International Lactation Consultant Association (ILCA). ILCA recognizes the certification conferred by the International Board of Lactation Consultant Examiners (IBLCE) as the professional credential for lactation consultants. All individuals representing themselves as IBCLC lactation consultants should adhere to these *Standards of Practice* and the *Code of Ethics for International Board Certified Lactation Consultants* in any and all interactions with clients, clients' families and other health care professionals.

Introduction

Quality practice and service constitute the core of a profession's responsibility to the public. Standards of practice have been defined as stated measures or levels of quality that serve as models for the conduct and evaluation of practice. Standards promote consistency by encouraging a common systematic approach. They also are sufficiently specific in content to meet the demands of daily practice. These standards are presented as a recommended framework for the development of policies and protocols, educational programs, and quality improvement efforts. They are intended for use in diverse settings, institutions, and cultural contexts.

Standard 1. Clinical Practice

The clinical practice of the IBCLC lactation consultant focuses on providing lactation care and clinical management. This is best accomplished within the framework of systematic problem solving in collaboration with other members of the health care team and the client. IBCLC lactation consultants are responsible for decisions and actions undertaken as a part of their professional role, including the:

- assessment, planning, intervention, and evaluation of care in a variety of situations

- prevention of problems

- complete, accurate, and timely documentation of care

- communication and collaboration with other health care professionals

1.1   Assessment

1.1.1   obtain and document an appropriate history of the breastfeeding mother and child.

1.1.2   systematically collect objective and subjective information

1.1.3   discuss with the mother and document as appropriate all assessment information

1.2   Plan

1.2.1   analyze assessment information to identify concerns and/or problems

1.2.2   develop a plan of care based on identified concerns or problems

1.2.3   arrange for follow-up evaluation

1.3   Implementation

1.3.1   implement the plan of care in a manner appropriate to the situation and acceptable to the mother

1.3.2   exercise principles of safety and universal precautions

1.3.3   demonstrate procedures, techniques, equipment, and devices

1.3.4   provide appropriate instruction

1.3.5   provide a written report to the primary health care provider as appropriate, including:

assessment information

suggested interventions

instructions provided

1.3.6   facilitate referral to other health professionals, community services, and support groups as needed

1.4   Evaluation

1.4.1   evaluate outcomes of planned interventions

1.4.2   modify the plan based on the evaluation of outcomes

1.4.3   document and communicate to the primary health care provider(s) as appropriate:

-   evaluation of outcomes

-   modifications in the plan

-   follow-up

Standard 2.
Breastfeeding Education and Counseling

Breastfeeding education and counseling are integral parts of the care provided by the lactation consultant.

2.1   provide education to parents and families to encourage informed decision making about infant and child feeding

2.2   provide anticipatory teaching to:

-   promote ideal breastfeeding practices

-   minimize the potential for breastfeeding problems or complications

2.4   provide emotional support for continued breastfeeding in difficult or complicated circumstances

2.5   share current evidence-based information and clinical skills with other health care providers

Standard 3.
Professional Responsibilities

The IBCLC lactation consultant has a responsibility to maintain professional conduct and to practice in an ethical manner, accountable for professional actions and legal responsibilities.

3.1   adhere to these *Standards of Practice* and the IBLCE *Code of Ethics*

3.2   practice within the scope of the *International Code of Marketing of Breast-milk Substitutes* and subsequent relevant resolutions, maintaining an awareness of conflict of interest when/if profiting from the rental or sale of breastfeeding equipment

3.3   act as an advocate for breastfeeding women, infants, and children

3.4   assist the mother in maintaining an intact breastfeeding relationship with her child

3.5   use breastfeeding equipment and devices appropriately by:

· refraining from unnecessary or excessive use

· discussing the risks and benefits of recommended use

· evaluating safety and effectiveness

· assuring cleanliness and good operating condition

3.6   maintain and expand knowledge and skills for lactation consultant practice by participating in continuing education

3.7   undertake periodic and systematic appraisal for evaluation of one's clinical practice

3.8   support and promote well-designed research in human lactation and breastfeeding, and base clinical practice, whenever possible, on such research.

Standard 4. Legal Considerations

IBCLC lactation consultants are obligated to practice within the laws of the geopolitical region and setting in which they work. They must practice with consideration for clients' rights of privacy and with respect for matters of a confidential nature.

4.1   work within the policies and procedures of the institution where employed, or if self-employed, have identifiable policies and procedures to follow

4.2   clearly state applicable fees prior to providing care

4.3   obtain informed consent from all clients prior to:

· assessing or intervening

· reporting relevant information to the primary health care provider or other health care professional(s)

· taking photographs for any purpose

· seeking publication of information associated with the consultation

4.4   protect client confidentiality at all times

4.5   maintain records according to legal practices within the work setting

Glossary

Client - the party for whom professional services are rendered; the breastfeeding woman employing the services of the lactation consultant.

Lactation Consultant - a health care professional who is an IBCLC.

Primary health care provider - a health professional such as a physician, nurse practitioner, or midwife, who manages, directs, and coordinates the health care of a client.

Universal precautions - a method of infection control involving the use of personal protective equipment, e.g., gloves, gown, goggles, for the handling of blood and selected body fluids.

Sample Care Plans

BREASTFEEDING TEACHING AND PROBLEM SOLVING CHECKLIST

Practitioner: Check off the measures for the mother to try. Follow up with the mother to evaluate whether further help is needed.

☐ Breastfeed 8 to 12 times in a 24-hour day, alternating the breast you feed from first.

☐ Finger feed, bottle-feed, cup feed, or spoon feed as instructed 8 to 12 times in 24 hours.

☐ Supplement your baby at breast with:
_____

☐ At _____ pounds your baby needs about _____ ounces of breastmilk and/or formula every 24 hours.

☐ Keep a record of

   ☐ Number of feedings
   ☐ Number of times you pump
   ☐ Amount of breastmilk expressed
   ☐ Number of your baby's diapers
   ☐ Amount of formula/breastmilk taken

☐ Wake your baby, if he or she does not wake enough to get at least 8 feedings in 24 hours.

☐ Breastfeed until your baby lets go of the first breast on his/her own, burp your baby, change the diaper, if needed, and then

   ☐ Offer 2nd breast until your baby lets go.
   ☐ Offer 1st breast again until your baby lets go.

☐ Express breastmilk after breastfeeding your baby _____ times a day.

☐ Express your breastmilk _____ times or more every 24 hours.

☐ Larger pump flanges may be more comfortable for you.

☐ Hold your baby skin to skin as much as possible.

☐ Offer your finger for pacification, as instructed.

☐ Train your baby to suck, as instructed.

☐ Position yourself comfortably with pillows to support your arms throughout the feeding. Use a footstool to bring your knees higher than your hips.

☐ Position your baby at the breast, as instructed with nose opposite nipple. Be sure your baby's head is free so your baby can lift his/her nose away from the breast.

☐ Position your baby in this position:
_____

☐ Make sure your baby opens his/her mouth wide and gets a big mouthful of breast.

☐ Make sure the baby's lips are flanged.

☐ Discontinue use of a pacifier until your baby is breastfeeding better.

☐ Massage your breasts during feedings/while pumping.

☐ Massage your breasts toward the end of a feeding before the baby lets go.

☐ Hand express into the baby's mouth toward the end of the feeding while the baby is breastfeeding.

☐ Take a nap every day.

☐ Drink to thirst.

☐ Eat nutritious meals and snacks so that you will feel well. (You will have good milk for your baby even if you do not have an ideal diet.)

For Engorgement:

☐ Express your milk to soften the breast just before feedings.

☐ Apply cool compresses if your breasts are uncomfortable between feedings. (A bag of frozen peas or corn, or ice wrapped in a towel, as instructed.)

☐ Lie flat on your back to elevate your breasts above the level of your heart.

For Sore Nipples:

☐ During the feeding, if the nipple starts to hurt, remove the baby, and then start again.

☐ After feedings, rinse the nipples with warm water, pat dry, and then air dry.

☐ Apply lanolin that states it is safe for the baby to ingest.

☐ Talk to your primary care practitioners about taking a pain medication.

☐ Talk to your primary care practitioners about topical medications.

☐ Wash gently with soap and water once daily, if there is a crack in the skin of the nipple.

☐ Wear breast shells for comfort when dressed. (Do not wear breast shells while sleeping.)

☐ Call your primary care practitioner for:
_____.

☐ Call me every day to keep me posted on your progress and to readjust our plan of action.

☐ Call me any time you have any questions or problems.
_____

☐ _____

☐ _____

_____
Mother's signature

_____
Date

_____
Practitioner signature

_____
Date

CARE PLAN FOR TREATING SORE NIPPLES

> **Practitioner:** Check off the measures for the mother to try. Follow up with the mother to evaluate whether further suggestions are needed.

Sore nipples are not a normal part of breastfeeding. If your nipples are tender beyond a few seconds when your baby latches on, or so painful that you cannot breastfeed, the suggestions below may help.

COMFORT MEASURES:

☐ Identify and correct the cause of your sore nipples.
☐ Treat any engorgement you may have.
☐ Call your primary care practitioner to ask for a topical medicine for your nipples, possibly an over-the-counter antibiotic ointment such as:

_____

BEFORE AND AFTER FEEDINGS:

☐ Rinse your nipples with clear water before nursing.
☐ Wear a breast shell with large multiple holes to allow air to circulate between feedings and promote healing.
☐ Start feedings on the least sore side first.
☐ Massage your breasts before nursing.
☐ Let your nipples dry well after each feeding and/or pumping.
☐ Apply a small amount of pure anhydrous lanolin to your nipples after each feeding, with lanolin that states it is safe for the baby to ingest.
☐ Wear hydrogel pads between feedings (do not use lanolin if you use gel pads).

AT FEEDINGS:

☐ Position yourself sitting upright with a pillow behind you and your knees higher than your hips.
☐ Position your baby at the breast so that he or she is able to get a large amount of the breast into his or her mouth, and not latch on just to the nipple.
☐ Reposition your baby's lips on the breast if they are not flanged out.

FEEDING PLAN:

☐ Nurse your baby at the breast every ____ hours.
☐ Pump with an electric breast pump every ____ hours for _____ minutes for the other feedings.
☐ Apply olive oil to the nipple and areola before pumping to prevent discomfort and pulling on sore areas.
☐ Begin with the suction setting on low and increase suction as your pain tolerance allows. It is not necessary to turn it to maximum pressure.
☐ Feed your baby by the _____ method.
☐ As your nipples begin to heal, you can increase the number of feedings at the breast and pump for the other feedings. Continue to increase time at the breast until you are breastfeeding exclusively again. If your nipples start to become sore again, cut back on time at the breast for another day or so. Don't push too quickly to return to full breastfeeding . . . take your time!!

SPECIAL INSTRUCTIONS:

_____   _____
Mother's signature   Date

_____   _____
Practitioner signature   Date

Adapted with permission of Jan Barger and Linda Kutner.

CARE PLAN FOR TREATING PLUGGED DUCTS

Practitioner: Check off the measures for the mother to try. Follow up with the mother to evaluate whether further suggestions are needed.

A plugged duct can occur when something causes milk to remain in the breast. When pressure is applied to the breast, it restricts the flow of milk. A change in the breastfeeding or pumping routine can also cause a plug. A small white "milk blister" may be found on the end of a nipple pore, indicating a plug in that milk duct. By using the following suggestions you should be able to relieve the swelling by 24 hours, and within 48 hours the area should no longer be tender. Consult your primary care practitioner if symptoms persist beyond 2 days.

COMFORT MEASURES:

☐ Consult with your primary care practitioner for permission to take acetaminophen for pain and a non-steroidal antiinflammatory drug (NSAID) such as ibuprofen.

- ◆ Acetaminophen: 650–1000 mg at 12–6–12–6 o'clock
- ◆ NSAID: 400 mg at 9–3–9–3 o'clock (remember to take with food)

☐ Check the end of your nipple for a small white "milk blister," which can indicate a plug in the duct beneath. If you find such a blister you can apply moist heat to the nipple area and then gently rub the area to remove the thin layer of skin covering it. Afterwards gently massage from the base of your breast out to the nipple to help force out the trapped milk and plug. Many women find it easiest to do this while taking a hot shower.

☐ If the milk bleb or blister does not resolve, call your health care practitioner. It may need to be opened with a sterile needle.

BETWEEN FEEDINGS:

☐ Gently massage the area over the plug to help release it.
☐ If the breast is still full after nursing, use a hospital-grade electric breast pump to remove milk.
☐ Apply olive oil to the nipple and areola before pumping to prevent discomfort when it pulls on the skin of the breast.
☐ Pump for 5 to 10 minutes while applying continuous pressure slightly above the plugged area.
☐ Gently massage the area over the plug while you are pumping.

FEEDING PLAN:

☐ Apply moist heat for 10 to 15 minutes just before nursing to help with the release of the milk. A disposable diaper run under hot water makes a quick and easy moist compress.
☐ Start each feeding on the breast with the plug.
☐ Try positioning the baby so that his chin is pointed toward the plug.
☐ Gently apply continuous pressure slightly above the plugged area pushing in the direction of the nipple while the infant is nursing.
☐ If the plug persists, try nursing with the baby lying on his back while you lean over him with your breasts hanging down. In this position, gravity can be used to help get the plug out.

SPECIAL INSTRUCTIONS:

_____   _____
Mother's signature   Date

_____   _____
Practitioner signature   Date

Adapted with permission of Jan Barger and Linda Kutner.

CARE PLAN FOR TREATING ENGORGEMENT

> **Practitioner:** Check off the measures for the mother to try. Follow up with the mother to evaluate whether further suggestions are needed.

As your milk "comes in," your breasts should feel heavier and full. This normal fullness should not prevent your baby from being able to latch on easily. Your breasts should also be pain free. Breasts that become engorged are very hard, and the nipples can be flattened out because of the swelling inside of the breasts. The breasts may be tender or quite painful. The skin may appear shiny. Engorgement, if left untreated, can cause loss of some or all the milk supply. It is important to treat engorgement quickly. Heat increases swelling. The goal is to decrease swelling and enable the baby to latch on effectively. Icy cold compresses and cabbage reduce swelling.

COMFORT MEASURES:

☐ Apply icy-cold compresses to your breasts and under your arms. (Compresses can be made from pouring water onto disposable diapers and placing them in the freezer for 15 to 20 minutes. Or use a bag of frozen vegetables.)

☐ Apply compresses for _____ minutes every _____ hours.

FEEDING PLAN:

☐ Hand express some milk from the breast to soften the areola before putting your baby to breast.

☐ Use Reverse Pressure Softening as shown by practitioner.

☐ Try to breastfeed every 2 hours around the clock.

☐ Try to breastfeed at least 15 minutes on the first breast before offering the other breast.

☐ Feed your baby with just a diaper on in order to keep him or her awake and stimulated.

BETWEEN FEEDINGS:

☐ Lie flat on your back between feedings to elevate your breasts.

☐ Pump your breasts after nursing to remove the milk that comes out quickly and easily or for _____ minutes.

☐ Pump between feedings for comfort if necessary, but only as long as the milk comes out quickly and easily.

☐ Apply olive oil to your nipple and areola before pumping to help prevent pulling and soreness.

☐ Take a warm shower and hand express milk in the shower. Have the water flow against your back rather than onto your breasts.

CABBAGE:

If the areola is swollen and hard and the nipple is flattened and/or the baby cannot latch on, apply green cabbage leaves to your breasts:

◆ Discard the outer leaves from the cabbage.

◆ Remove the inner leaves. Rinse and dry them. They can be kept in the refrigerator.

◆ Crush the leaves slightly with your hands.

◆ Cover the breasts entirely with the leaves (and under your arms if needed). Put your bra on over the leaves to hold them in place.

◆ Change the leaves every two hours or more frequently if they become wilted.

◆ Check your breasts often. As soon as you feel the milk begin to drip, or if your breasts begin to feel "different," remove the leaves and try to pump.

◆ Pump enough to soften the breast and areola. Put baby to breast.

◆ Reapply cabbage as needed. You can use the icy compresses over the cabbage.

◆ Use only the green leaves. The white inner leaves do not work.

◆ As soon as your breasts are soft enough to nurse comfortably, stop using cabbage leaves.

☐ Call _____ if you are not getting any relief or if you have any questions.

SPECIAL INSTRUCTIONS:

_____   _____
Mother's signature   Date

_____   _____
Practitioner signature   Date

Adapted with permission of Jan Barger and Linda Kutner.

Care Plan for the Baby Who Won't Latch on

> **Practitioner:** Check off the measures for the mother to try. Follow up with the mother to evaluate whether further suggestions are needed.

Occasionally there are times when a baby has difficulty latching on to the breast. Having a step-by-step plan to guide you will help you through those feeds. The goal is to help your baby learn to breastfeed while at the same time stimulating your milk production and ensuring that your baby has adequate nourishment. Keep breastfeeding a pleasant experience for both you and your baby. Resist the temptation to resort to using a bottle for feeds. A baby who is having difficulty latching on to the breast will develop nipple preference very quickly. This may make transitioning to the breast more challenging.

Before Feedings:

☐ Spend time snuggled with your baby skin to skin, with no attempt to latch on.

☐ Undress your baby to his or her diaper and yourself down to the waist to maximize skin-to-skin contact. This will help keep your baby awake and more alert during feeds.

☐ Make sure you are comfortable, with supporting pillows under both arms.

During Feedings:

☐ Work with your baby for short periods of time.

☐ Watch your baby closely for feeding cues. Babies demonstrate an interest in feeding by putting their hands to their mouth and sucking on them. When you see these cues, put your baby to your breast. Wait for a wide open mouth and make sure your baby's tongue is down. You can gently tickle your baby's upper lip with your nipple to encourage a wide open mouth. Express a bit of milk onto the nipple to entice your baby. Quickly pull your baby to the breast, leading with the chin to get a big mouthful of breast tissue.

☐ Your baby's tongue must be down and covering the lower gum line, with the mouth open wide, to facilitate the latch. If he or she is crying, the tongue will be up and back, and if pulled onto the breast, he or she may have difficulty breathing.

☐ Use your dominant hand to pull your baby to the breast quickly:

Right handed:

◆ Football (clutch) hold on the right side
◆ Cross cradle (dominant hand) hold on left side

Left handed:

◆ Football (clutch) hold on the left side
◆ Cross-cradle (dominant hand) hold on right side

☐ If your baby cries, arches away, or pulls back, stop immediately. You can allow your baby to suck on your finger with your nail against his or her tongue. When sucking becomes rhythmical and your baby is calm, try again. Try only a few times at each feeding.

☐ Continue as long as your baby is calm and willing to go to breast. Do not push past the tolerance level or try to get your baby to attach to the breast while crying.

☐ Try feeding with both breasts and in different nursing positions—you never know which one will work.

☐ Use positive verbal reinforcement when your baby latches on or tries to do so.

☐ Attempt to put your baby to breast at every feeding at least _____ times in each 24-hour period.

☐ Attempt to feed your baby before he or she is fully awake or crying to feed. A successful latch during the night is common.

Between Feedings:

☐ If your baby does not latch on at a feeding, pump your breasts for _____ minutes and feed your expressed breastmilk with _____.

☐ When your baby shows an interest in the breast, try again. As long as you continue to pump your breasts for _____ minutes _____ times a day, you will be able to maintain your milk production.

☐ Keep a diary of feedings, wet and soiled diapers, and any supplements your baby receives.

Special Instructions:

_____   _____
Mother's signature   Date

_____   _____
Practitioner signature   Date

Adapted with permission of Jan Barger and Linda Kutner.

CARE PLAN FOR TUBE FEEDING AT THE BREAST

Practitioner: Check off the measures for the mother to try. Follow up with the mother to evaluate whether further suggestions are needed.

Tube feeding at the breast is one way you can provide additional nourishment for your baby when milk production is low or when your baby is not taking in enough milk. This feeding method has benefits for both you and your baby. The baby continues to suckle at the breast, which provides the stimulation needed to increase milk production. Feeding your baby at the breast avoids the nipple confusion or preference that is caused by using an artificial bottle nipple.

Tube feed your baby at the breast:
- ☐ At every feeding
- ☐ Every _____ hours
- ☐ At least _____ times in every 24-hour period

☐ Try to have your baby take at least _____ ounces of supplement. As your milk production increases or the ability of your baby to take the milk from your breast increases, the amount of supplement the baby takes will decrease.

☐ Position the container of breastmilk at a height that will permit your baby to swallow after every one to two sucks. If the container is too low he or she will need to suck many times before he or she has enough milk to swallow. This may tire him or her too much to finish the feeding.

☐ After each use flush out the tubing first with cold water and then with hot soapy water. Rinse it with clear hot water.

☐ Check the roof of your baby's mouth every day to make sure that the tubing is not causing any irritation.

SPECIAL INSTRUCTIONS:

Mother's signature

Date

Practitioner signature

Date

Adapted with permission of Jan Barger and Linda Kutner.

CARE PLAN FOR TREATING THRUSH

Practitioner: Check off the measures for the mother to try. Follow up with the mother to evaluate whether further suggestions are needed.

Thrush is a yeast infection that can be transferred between an infant's mouth and the mother's nipples. A yeast infection of the nipples can cause severe pain on the nipple or breast. Nipple pain may range from slightly reddened to cracked and bleeding. Yeast infections are easily spread among family members and are difficult to cure. For best results, and to prevent recurrence, it is important to treat both the mother and baby at the same time. Thrush in the baby's mouth looks like milk curds on the insides of the cheeks, gums, and palate. It cannot be rubbed off without causing bleeding.

THRUSH MAY BE PRESENT:

- ☐ In your infant's mouth
- ☐ In your vaginal area
- ☐ On your nipples
- ☐ On your partner's genitals
- ☐ On your infant's diaper area

CONTACT HEALTH CARE PRACTITIONERS

Obtain assessment and treatment for:
- ☐ You
- ☐ Your baby
- ☐ Your partner

COMFORT MEASURES:

- ☐ Dry your nipples after nursing and expose them to air/light for a while after feeding.
- ☐ Wear a breast shell with large multiple holes between feedings to allow air to circulate and promote healing.
- ☐ If comfortable, go without a bra to reduce moist environment.

PRECAUTIONS:

- ☐ Wash your hands with hot soapy water:
  - ☐ **Before** you nurse.
  - ☐ **Before** and **after** you use the toilet (before . . . so you don't spread the yeast to your vagina).
  - ☐ **After** changing your baby's diaper.
  - ☐ **After** nursing or touching your breasts.
- ☐ Boil all pacifiers, bottle nipples, and pump flanges every day for five minutes.
- ☐ Avoid using breast pads unless necessary. If they are used, change them as soon as they become damp and use only disposable ones. Absorbent paper towels also work well.
- ☐ Wash all bras, underpants, towels, and washcloths in very hot water with bleach. Dry them in the sun or in a dryer on a hot setting.

- ☐ Wash all teething toys daily in the dishwasher or in very hot soapy water. Boil if possible.
- ☐ Dispose of all pacifiers and bottle nipples used during yeast infection.

MEDICATIONS:

- ☐ If you are to use a medicated cream after nursing, apply a **small amount** to the nipples and areolas and rub in well.
- ☐ Medicated creams generally need to be applied after every feeding or at least every three hours to stop the growth of yeast cells.
- ☐ If the medication has not been absorbed when it is time to nurse or pump, rinse off with warm water. (A squirt bottle works very well; **do not rub**.)
- ☐ If your practitioner prescribed a systemic medication, take the complete course as directed, even if symptoms improve.
- ☐ Before giving an oral thrush medication to your baby, rinse his or her mouth with clear water or wipe out his or her mouth with a moist cloth to remove any residue of breastmilk.
- ☐ Medications given to the infant for oral thrush must make contact with the thrush to be effective. Use your finger or a cotton swab to *paint* the inside of your baby's mouth, gums, lips, and tongue with the medication.
- ☐ If your baby sucks his thumb, consider applying medication to his or her thumb also.
- ☐ If the infant has a yeast diaper rash, wash his or her bottom with warm soapy water, dry well, and apply the medicated cream with every diaper change. Change the diaper **frequently**. Consider letting baby nap without diaper on.
- ☐ Adding acidophilus to your diet if you have been on antibiotics helps replenish the beneficial flora in your intestinal tract and reduce yeast overgrowth.

SPECIAL INSTRUCTIONS:

Mother's signature   Date

Practitioner signature   Date

Adapted with permission of Jan Barger and Linda Kutner.

CARE PLAN FOR CUP FEEDING YOUR BABY

> **Practitioner:** Check off the measures for the mother to try. Follow up with the mother to evaluate whether further suggestions are needed.

Cup feeding avoids the use of tubing and artificial nipples. It may take four or five feedings by cup for your baby to learn this new way to obtain milk. Cup feeding used exclusively for an extended period of time can lead to the baby stopping sucking.

- ☐ Use a small cup with rounded edges such as a medicine cup, a hollow-handled medicine spoon, or a small plastic cup (like those used for catsup or mustard).
- ☐ Tuck a cloth under your baby's chin to catch drips.
- ☐ Hold your baby either cradled in your arms or sitting semi-upright on your lap.
- ☐ Pour a small amount of supplement into the cup—about $\frac{1}{2}$ ounce.
- ☐ Bring the cup to your baby's lips. Tip it slightly until a few drops of supplement enters his or her mouth.
- ☐ After the supplement enters his or her mouth, lean your baby back slightly to allow the fluid to flow to the back of the throat where it can be swallowed. Your baby may begin to "lap" the supplement from the cup, forming a trough with the tongue as in breastfeeding, and then swallowing.
- ☐ Go at your baby's pace, allowing time to rest between swallows.
- ☐ Watch to be sure your baby is ready to swallow and willing to continue the feeding. Your baby needs to be in control of the feeding. If there is resistance, stop, comfort your baby, and try again later.
- ☐ Burp your baby frequently to release any air that enters the stomach.
- ☐ "Sippy cups" should be avoided. The small spout does not allow the baby to trough his or her tongue.

SPECIAL INSTRUCTIONS:

_____   _____
Mother's signature   Date

_____   _____
Practitioner signature   Date

Adapted with permission of Jan Barger and Linda Kutner.

CARE PLAN FOR A BABY WHO CANNOT NURSE

> **Practitioner:** Check off the measures for the mother to try. Follow up with the mother to evaluate whether further suggestions are needed.

Giving your baby your breastmilk directly from your breast is the best way you can feed your baby. When that is not possible, you can pump milk from your breasts to give to your baby. Your baby may receive your milk from a cup, bottle, or special feeding tube.

Why not feed my baby artificial formula?

Artificial infant formulas are not the same as your milk. They all state that they are closest to breastmilk in one particular nutrient or mineral, but none of them contain the hundreds of other components in breastmilk. Infant formula will provide a baby with necessary calories, but it does not provide any protection against illness or infections. Babies who are fed artificial infant formulas are sick more often than babies who receive only their mother's milk.

PUMPING TO PROVIDE MILK:

☐ Make sure that your pumpings are spaced out equally throughout each 24-hour period. This is much more effective than grouping them during part of the day.

☐ The more frequently you remove milk from your breasts, the more milk you will produce. Pumping more frequently will produce more milk than pumping for long periods of time at less frequent intervals.

☐ Using a timer or clock when you are pumping will help you to pump long enough. When milk stops flowing, turn off the pump and massage your breasts. Then turn the pump back on and continue pumping.

☐ Pump 8 to 10 times in each 24-hour period.

☐ Pump for 12 to 15 minutes using a double pumping set-up.

☐ Pump at least once during the night.

DECREASING PUMPING TIME:

☐ When your milk production is greater than your baby's intake by at least 4 ounces for several days, you can decrease your pumping time to 10 to 12 minutes each time you pump.

☐ If your milk production continues to be greater than your baby's intake, you can decrease the number of times that you pump in each 24-hour period.

☐ Only decrease one pumping every 4 to 5 days. Cutting back on too many pumpings at one time may cause your milk production to fall below what your infant needs, and then you will need to work on building it back up.

LONGTERM PUMPING:

☐ As your breasts become more efficient in making milk, you will find that you may not need to pump as often. Some mothers have found that after several months they can decrease their pumpings to 4 to 6 times in 24 hours. Every mother is different.

☐ Some mothers find that they can decrease their pumping time to 8 to 10 minutes at each session and still maintain their supply. Others will need to pump the full 15 minutes each time, but can decrease the total number of pumpings. Just as each baby is an individual and nurses differently from another baby, so must each mother pump to meet her individual milk-making needs.

PUMPING TIME DURING GROWTH SPURTS:

☐ When babies are nursing at the breast, they go through days when they want to nurse more often. As babies grow, they need more milk. During a growth spurt, the baby will nurse very frequently for 1 to 2 days. This increases the mother's milk supply to meet the baby's new needs. When you suddenly find your baby drinking more milk than you are producing, you will need to increase your production by pumping more frequently.

☐ Try pumping your breasts every hour or two for 15 to 20 minutes. Attempt to get in 10 pumpings in a 24-hour period for 1 to 2 days.

☐ After your milk supply increases to match your baby's needs, go back to your old pumping routine. If it seems to decrease somewhat, try pumping a little more frequently than you normally would until the amount stabilizes at the amount your baby is happy with.

_____   _____
Mother's signature   Date

_____   _____
Practitioner signature   Date

Adapted with permission of Jan Barger and Linda Kutner.

Care Plan for Storing and Feeding Breastmilk

There may be times when you wish to feed your baby your milk without nursing. You can take expressed milk with you by pumping right before you leave. The milk will be good for several hours in moderate temperature. Or you can freeze your milk and then thaw and warm it just before you feed it to your baby. These guidelines are for healthy, full-term infants.

Saving Your Milk:

- ☐ Newly pumped milk is safe at moderate room temperature for several hours.
- ☐ Newly pumped milk is safe in the refrigerator for up to 5 to 8 days.
- ☐ Milk that has been in the refrigerator for 2 days or less can be frozen.
- ☐ Milk that has been in the refrigerator longer than 2 days, but less than 8 days, can be fed to your baby but cannot be frozen for later use.
- ☐ Milk is safe in the refrigerator's freezer for 3 to 6 months or in a separate deep freeze for at least 12 months.
- ☐ Always store your milk in the back behind other food. Do not store near icemaker.
- ☐ Do not store frozen milk in the door or near the refrigeration unit, to avoid extremes of temperature.

Summary—Breastmilk can sit at a moderate room temperature for 4 to 8 hours and then be put into the refrigerator for 2 days. If it has not been used in 2 days, put it into the freezer for 3 to 12 months, depending on the type of freezer. Newly pumped breastmilk is good for 5 days, but it should only be frozen if it is less than 2 days old.

Combining Milk from Different Pumpings:

- ☐ When you pump both breasts at the same time, you can combine the two bottles of milk into one when you have finished pumping.
- ☐ You may add new milk to milk that you pumped previously. First, chill both containers of milk in the refrigerator for at least 2 hours. Then you can pour them together.
- ☐ If you wish to add milk to some that is already frozen, chill the new milk for at least 2 hours in the refrigerator. Then pour it on top of the frozen milk. Make sure the amount of new milk you are adding does not exceed the amount already frozen.

Summary—You can combine breastmilk that is pumped at the same time, add cold breastmilk to cold breastmilk, or add cold breastmilk to frozen breastmilk.

Storing Your Milk:

- ☐ Store your milk in either a glass or hard plastic container. You may use glass and plastic baby bottles, or most kinds of food jars, such as peanut butter.
- ☐ Wash the containers in hot soapy water and rinse well in hot water, or wash and dry them in a dishwasher.
- ☐ Plastic baby bottle bags are not recommended for storage. Some of the cells in breastmilk that protect your baby from infection stick to the insides of the bags. Also, some mothers report that they were unable to feed the breastmilk stored in these bags to their babies because it smelled and tasted bad.

Defrosting and Heating Your Milk:

- ☐ If you plan to use frozen breastmilk, remove it from the freezer the night before and put it in the refrigerator to thaw. Warm it before you feed it to your baby.
- ☐ When your breastmilk sits in a container, the fat in it will rise to the top. Gently swirl the container to mix the fat with the rest of the milk. If the milk was chilled, do this after it is warmed. Do not shake the milk, as it will break the walls of the live cells that are in the milk.
- ☐ To warm cold or frozen breastmilk, place it in a pan of warm water or hold it under warm tap water. The warm water should feel comfortable to your hand. Gently swirl the container several times as it warms.
- ☐ After breastmilk has been thawed in the refrigerator, use it within 24 hours or throw it away. Do not freeze it a second time.
- ☐ Have caregiver feed your baby in small incremental amounts to avoid waste.
- ☐ Once you begin feeding a bottle of breastmilk to your baby, it should be finished with that feeding or discarded.

_____   _____
Mother's signature   Date

_____   _____
Practitioner signature   Date

Adapted with permission of Jan Barger and Linda Kutner.

Sample Documentation Forms

Prenatal Breastfeeding Assessment

Name _____ Today's date _____ Due date _____ Current week of pregenancy _____

Breastfeeding History
Were you breastfed?   ☐ Yes ☐ No
Have you breastfed any of your children?   ☐ First child   ☐ Yes ☐ No
How many?_____ For how long?_____
How did breastfeeding go for you?

What problems, if any, did you have?

With this baby will you be working away from home?   ☐ No ☐ Yes
What are your plans?

Breasts
During your life, have your breasts experienced any trauma, burns, or radiation?   ☐ No ☐ Yes
Did you have a chest tube as a premature baby?   ☐ No ☐ Yes
Have you had any breast surgery?   Date?_____   ☐ No ☐ Yes
____implants ____biopsy ____reduction ____cysts ____abscess
Other:_____

Any changes in nipple sensation from the surgery?   ☐ No ☐ Yes
Type of incision: axillary   periareolar   subglandular   transumbilical
Have you noticed your breasts have gotten larger since you became pregnant?   ☐ Yes ☐ No
Have you noticed your breasts have gotten tender since you became pregnant?   ☐ Yes ☐ No

Breast Anomalies: ____extra nipples ____extra breast tissue ____asymmetry ____conical ____hypoplasia
Other:

R   L

Draw in surgical scars or other anomalies.

Space between breasts _____

Nipples
At rest	With compression	**Nipple or Areola Anomalies**	
☐ everted	☐ everted	☐ skin tag	OK
☐ flat	☐ flat	☐ Need to remove?	☐ hair on areola
☐ dimpled	☐ dimpled	☐ nipple ring	☐ double nipples
☐ inverted	☐ inverted	☐ Explain need to remove.	☐ unusual nipple
	☐ retracting	☐ other:	

Right nipple diameter _____mm   Right nipple length _____mm
Left nipple diameter _____mm   Left nipple length _____mm

Breast tissue: ☐ inelastic (firm)   ☐ elastic (soft)
Nipple tissue: ☐ inelastic (firm, meaty)   ☐ elastic (soft)

Printed with permission of Kay Hoover, M Ed, IBCLC, Philadelphia Department of Public Health, Division of Maternal, Child and Family Health, 1101 Market Street, 9th Floor, Philadelphia, PA 19107.

Nipple Pain Questionnaire

1. When did you start to have sore nipples?
   - ☐ The first time the baby breastfed.
   - ☐ During the first day at the hospital.
   - ☐ When my milk supply increased (usually day 3 or 4).
   - ☐ Other _____.

2. Is the pain on one or both nipples?
   - ☐ One nipple   ☐ Both nipples

3. Does one nipple hurt more than the other, or are both about the same?
   - ☐ One nipple hurts more than the other.
     Which side?   ☐ Right   ☐ Left
   - ☐ Both about the same.
   - ☐ Fluctuates day to day.

4. When does the nipple pain occur?
   - ☐ As the baby latches on.
   - ☐ During the entire feeding.
   - ☐ Starts out OK, then hurts more as feeding goes on.
   - ☐ Hurts on and off throughout the feeding.
   - ☐ Hurts after the feeding.
   - ☐ Hurts at times unrelated to a feeding.
   - ☐ Hurts all the time.

5. Describe the pain
   - ☐ tugging   ☐ itching
   - ☐ tingling   ☐ pinching
   - ☐ irritating   ☐ sharp
   - ☐ rubbing   ☐ biting
   - ☐ scraping   ☐ stinging
   - ☐ aching   ☐ shooting
   - ☐ throbbing   ☐ burning

6. Describe nipple shape when baby comes off the breast.
   - ☐ normal   ☐ peaked
   - ☐ elongated   ☐ smashed
   - ☐ creased   ☐ pointed
   - ☐ ridged   ☐ stepped on
   - ☐ pinched   ☐ flattened
   - ☐ like a new lipstick   ☐ squished

7. Does your nipple turn white at the end of the feeding?
   - ☐ Yes   ☐ No

8. Do your nipples turn white at any other time?
   - ☐ Yes   ☐ No

9. Is your nipple a different color from usual?
   - ☐ no change   ☐ red
   - ☐ lighter than normal   ☐ purple
   - ☐ pink   ☐ blanched white
   - ☐ deep pink   ☐ has a white stripe

10. Is there any nipple damage?
    - ☐ Yes   ☐ No

    If yes, what kind of damage?
    - ☐ abrasion   ☐ scab
    - ☐ crack   ☐ piece missing
    - ☐ blister   ☐ bleeding

11. Does it hurt to wear clothing?
    - ☐ Yes   ☐ No   ☐ Sometimes

12. Does it hurt when you use a breast pump?
    - ☐ Yes   ☐ No   ☐ Do not know

    What brand and type of pump are you using?

    _____

    - ☐ I am not using a breast pump.

13. On a scale from zero to ten, if zero is no pain and ten is the most pain **you have ever experienced**, please circle on the line where you would rate your nipple pain.

    0 1 2 3 4 5 6 7 8 9 10

14. Where is the nipple pain occurring?

    - ☐ On the face of the nipple
    - ☐ On the side of the nipple
    - ☐ At the base of the nipple

    - ☐ All over the nipple

    - ☐ On the areola

Draw where you feel the pain.

15. Breastfeeding Sensation Scale
    ☐ No sensation
    ☐ Strong pulling and tugging that feels good
    ☐ Strong pulling and tugging that causes no discomfort
    ☐ Strong pulling and tugging that causes some discomfort
    ☐ Pinching that is somewhat uncomfortable
    ☐ Really hurts or feels like biting
    ☐ Unbearable, excruciating pain—had to take baby off

16. What have you been doing to deal with the nipple pain?
    ☐ Applying a topical preparation. If so, what?

    _____
    ☐ Wearing breast shells.
    ☐ Wearing breast pads.
    ☐ Taking pain medication. If so, what?

    _____
    ☐ Stopped breastfeeding. How long ago?

    _____
    ☐ Pumping and feeding my baby my breast milk.
    For how long? _____
    ☐ Nothing; waiting for it to get better.
    ☐ Suffering through the pain.
    ☐ Other _____

17. Do you have a rash anywhere on your body?
    ☐ Yes   ☐ No If, yes, where?
    _____

18. Do your nipples itch?   ☐ Yes   ☐ No

19. What do you think is causing your sore nipples?

20. How is your baby doing?

21. Are you now or have you recently taken any medications?
    ☐ Yes   ☐ No
    If so, what?

22. Is your baby now or has your baby recently taken any medications?
    ☐ Yes   ☐ No
    If so, what?

23. Does your baby have oral thrush?
    ☐ Yes   ☐ No

24. Does your baby have a diaper rash?
    ☐ Yes   ☐ No

25. Are you experiencing breast pain?
    ☐ Yes   ☐ No
    If no, you are finished with the questionnaire.

26. If yes, how would you describe your breast pain?
    ☐ aching all over
    ☐ tingling sensation
    ☐ shooting pain
    ☐ burning pain
    ☐ the pain radiates down my arm
    ☐ the pain radiates around the side to my back

27. When does the breast pain occur?
    ☐ after feedings
    ☐ during feedings
    ☐ all the time
    ☐ at times not related to feedings

28. On a scale from zero to ten, if zero is no pain and ten is the most pain **you have ever experienced**, please circle on the line where you would rate your breast pain.

    0 1 2 3 4 5 6 7 8 9 10

29. Draw where on the breast you are experiencing the pain.

Right breast   Left breast

Mother's Breastfeeding Checklist

Please check off each item as you accomplish it.
Make sure you ask someone to help you with any item you are not sure about.

☐ I know holding my baby skin to skin is good for both of us.

☐ I know how the baby tells me it is time for a feeding.

☐ I know how to latch my baby onto both breasts.

☐ I know I should take turns with the breast I feed from first.

☐ I know when my baby is finished breastfeeding and that my baby needs to finish on the first breast before I feed the baby on the other breast.

☐ I can hear my baby swallowing milk during the breastfeeding sessions.

☐ I know breastfeeding should not hurt after 30 seconds.

☐ I know when and where to call if I have any breastfeeding questions.

☐ I know how to squeeze milk out of my breasts.

☐ I know my baby should eat only my milk for the first six months.

☐ I know how to tell that my baby is getting enough milk.

☐ I know how to fill out the feeding record for the first week.

    ☐ I know a wet diaper is as heavy as three tablespoons of water.

    ☐ I know my baby should gain about five to eight ounces each week (for the first two months).

☐ I have an appointment to see the pediatrician or family doctor in two or three days after we leave the hospital.

☐ I know my baby should be back to birth weight by ten days.

My baby's birth weight   _____

My baby's discharge weight   _____

My baby's weight two to three days after discharge   _____

My baby's weight at ten days   _____

BABY FEEDING REQUIREMENTS

Pounds	Ounces	Required Milk	Pounds	Ounces	Required Milk	Pounds	Ounces	Required Milk
5	0	13.3	7	8	20.0	10	0	26.7
5	1	13.5	7	9	20.2	10	1	26.8
5	2	13.7	7	10	20.3	10	2	27.0
5	3	13.8	7	11	20.5	10	3	27.2
5	4	14.0	7	12	20.7	10	4	27.3
5	5	14.2	7	13	20.8	10	5	27.5
5	6	14.3	7	14	21.0	10	6	27.7
5	7	14.5	7	15	21.2	10	7	27.8
5	8	14.7				10	8	28.0
5	9	14.8	8	0	21.3	10	9	28.2
5	10	15.0	8	1	21.5	10	10	28.3
5	11	15.2	8	2	21.7	10	11	28.5
5	12	15.3	8	3	21.8	10	12	28.7
5	13	15.5	8	4	22.0	10	13	28.8
5	14	15.7	8	5	22.2	10	14	29.0
5	15	15.8	8	6	22.3	10	15	29.2
			8	7	22.5			
6	0	16.0	8	8	22.7	11	0	29.3
6	1	16.2	8	9	22.8	11	1	29.5
6	2	16.3	8	10	23.0	11	2	29.7
6	3	16.5	8	11	23.2	11	3	29.8
6	4	16.7	8	12	23.3	11	4	30.0
6	5	16.8	8	13	23.5	11	5	30.2
6	6	17.0	8	14	23.7	11	6	30.3
6	7	17.2	8	15	23.8	11	7	30.5
6	8	17.3				11	8	30.7
6	9	17.5	9	0	24.0	11	9	30.8
6	10	17.7	9	1	24.2	11	10	31.0
6	11	17.8	9	2	24.3	11	11	31.2
6	12	18.0	9	3	24.5	11	12	31.3
6	13	18.2	9	4	24.7	11	13	31.5
6	14	18.3	9	5	24.8	11	14	31.7
6	15	18.5	9	6	25.0	11	15	31.8
			9	7	25.2			
7	0	18.7	9	8	25.3	12	0	32.0
7	1	18.8	9	9	25.5			
7	2	19.0	9	10	25.7			
7	3	19.2	9	11	25.8			
7	4	19.3	9	12	26.0			
7	5	19.5	9	13	26.2			
7	6	19.7	9	14	26.3			
7	7	19.8	9	15	26.5			

First Week Diaper Diary

1. Circle the hour closest to when your baby starts each breastfeeding.
2. Circle a **W** when your baby makes a wet diaper.
3. Circle a **P** when your baby makes a poopy diaper.
   Some babies make more diapers each day than shown. This is great!

Sample Record for Day 4

Feedings: ⑫ 1 2 ③ 4 5 ⑥ 7 ⑧ 9 ⑩ 11 Noon ① 2 ③ 4 ⑤ 6 7 ⑧ 9 10 11

Wet Diapers: Ⓦ Ⓦ Ⓦ Ⓦ Ⓦ Ⓦ

Green or Yellow Poops: Ⓟ   Ⓟ   Ⓟ   P

In this sample, the baby had nine feedings, six wet diapers, and three poopy diapers. By Day Four, most babies breastfeed 8 to 12 times each day.

Birth Date: _____/_____/_____ Time: _____ AM PM
Birth Weight: _____ Discharge Weight: _____
Baby's weight at one week: _____
For breastfeeding help call:

Call your doctor, nurse, midwife, or breastfeeding helper if:
  1. **Your baby is not making enough wet or poopy diapers**
  2. **There is dark colored pee after Day 3**
  3. **There is dark colored poop after Day 5**

Day 1

Feedings: 12 1 2 3 4 5 6 7 8 9 10 11 Noon 1 2 3 4 5 6 7 8 9 10 11

Wet Diapers: W

Black Tarry Poops: P

Day 2

Feedings: 12 1 2 3 4 5 6 7 8 9 10 11 Noon 1 2 3 4 5 6 7 8 9 10 11

Wet Diapers: W   W

Black Tarry Poops: P   P

Day 3

Feedings: 12 1 2 3 4 5 6 7 8 9 10 11 Noon 1 2 3 4 5 6 7 8 9 10 11

Wet Diapers: W   W   W

Green Poops: P   P   P

Day 4

Feedings: 12 1 2 3 4 5 6 7 8 9 10 11 Noon 1 2 3 4 5 6 7 8 9 10 11

Wet Diapers: W   W   W   W

Green or Yellow Poops: P   P   P   P

Day 5

Feedings: 12 1 2 3 4 5 6 7 8 9 10 11 Noon 1 2 3 4 5 6 7 8 9 10 11

Wet Diapers: W   W   W   W   W

Yellow Poops: P   P   P   P

Day 6

Feedings: 12 1 2 3 4 5 6 7 8 9 10 11 Noon 1 2 3 4 5 6 7 8 9 10 11

Wet Diapers: W   W   W   W   W   W

Yellow Poops: P   P   P   P

Day 7

Feedings: 12 1 2 3 4 5 6 7 8 9 10 11 Noon 1 2 3 4 5 6 7 8 9 10 11

Wet Diapers: W   W   W   W   W   W

Yellow Poops: P   P   P   P

Orders: Barbara Wilson-Clay, 12710 Burson Drive, Manchaca, TX 78652
Phone: 512-292-7227   Fax: 512-292-7228   E-Mail: bwc@lactnews.com
50 sheets/pad. $15 per pad. Bulk rate in quantities of 20. $13 per pad plus shipping.
© 2002 K Hoover/B Wilson-Clay.
See Color Plate 18 for accompanying photographs.

Birth to 36 months: Boys
Length-for-age and Weight-for-age percentiles

NAME _____

RECORD # _____

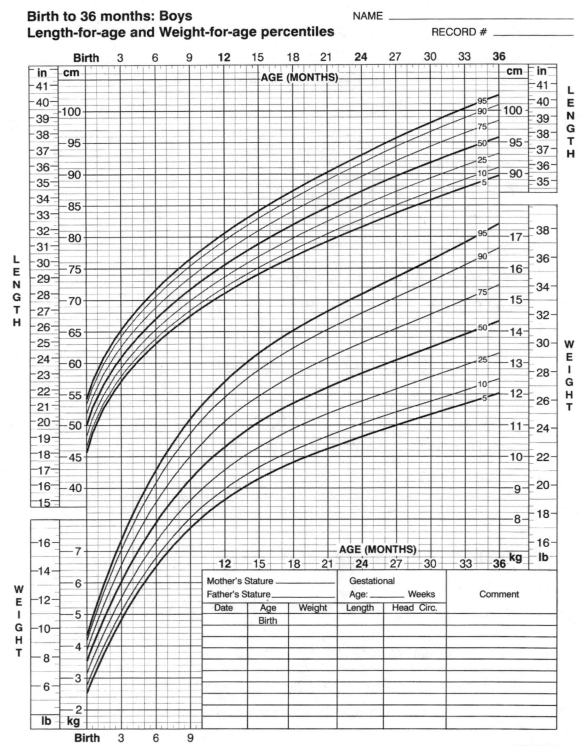

Published May 30, 2000 (modified 4/20/01).
SOURCE: Developed by the National Center for Health Statistics in collaboration with
the National Center for Chronic Disease Prevention and Health Promotion (2000).
http://www.cdc.gov/growthcharts

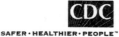

SAFER · HEALTHIER · PEOPLE™

Birth to 36 months: Girls
Length-for-age and Weight-for-age percentiles

NAME _____

RECORD # _____

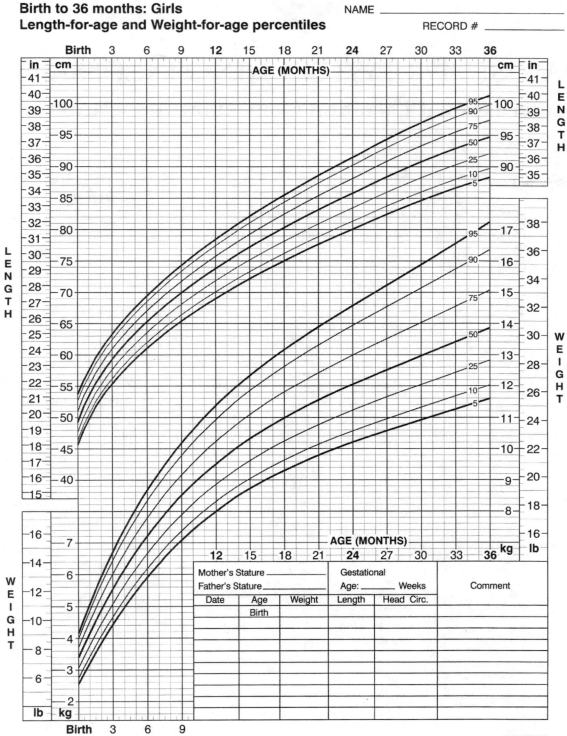

Published May 30, 2000 (modified 4/20/01).
SOURCE: Developed by the National Center for Health Statistics in collaboration with
the National Center for Chronic Disease Prevention and Health Promotion (2000).
http://www.cdc.gov/growthcharts

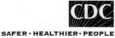

SAFER · HEALTHIER · PEOPLE™

APPENDIX
J

SPANISH BREASTFEEDING GLOSSARY
International Lactation Consultant Association

▶ GENERAL SPANISH TERMS

alcohol	alcohol
allergy	alergia
at least	por lo menos
aunt, uncle	tía, tío
cigarette	cigarillo
cousin	primo, prima
do not use	no usar
doctor	doctor
each day	cada día
enough	suficiente
family	familia
father	padre
good afternoon	buenas tardes
good evening	buenas noches
good morning	buenos días
grandmother	abuela
grandfather	abuelo
healthy	saludable
help you	ayudarla
hospital	hospital
how long	cuánto tiempo
how many times	cuántas veces
how many	cuántos
how much	cuánto
how often	cada cuando
husband	esposo
it's important	es importante
it's necessary	es necesario
medication	medicina
mother	mama, madre
mother-in-law	suegra
nurse (person)	enfermera
nutritionist	nutricionista
parents	padres
please	por favor
problem	problema
sister, brother	hermana, hermano
sister-in-law	cuñada
thank you	gracias
the more	cuanto más
upset	alterado
usually	usualmente
you're welcome	de nada

▶ TERMS RELATED TO THE BABY

baby	bebé
baby (your)	su bebé
baby blues	tristeza posparto
bonding	el apego, la bondad
bottle	biberón
bottle-fed	alimentado con biberón
burp your baby	eructe su bebé
cleft lip	labio leporino
cleft palate	paladar hendido
crying	llanto
cuddle	acurrucar abrazar
diaper rash	irritación de la piel causada por el pañal
dirty diaper	pañal(es) sucio(s) (con evacuación)
failure to thrive	retraso en el crecimiento
feeding	toma, alimentación, mamada
food allergy	alergia a las comidas
formula	fórmula
frenulum	frenillo
gain weight	aumento de peso; (ganar) peso
infant	infante
jaundice	ictericia
newborn	recién nacido
pacifier	chupete, chupón
premature	prematuro
return to work	regresar al trabajo
sleep	dormir
sling	cargador tipo hamaca
spit up	regugita
stool	evacuación
toddler	bebé mayorcito
twins	gémelos
weigh your baby	pesar el bebé
weight gain	aumento de peso
wet diapers	pañales mojados

▶ TERMS RELATED TO BREASTFEEDING

areola	areola
breast	el pecho; el seno
breastfeeding	amamantar, dar el pecho
breastmilk	leche materna
colostrum (first milk)	calostro (la primera leche)
cue feeding	seguir la señal del bebé
dropper	gotero
flat nipples	pezones planos
good latch-on	bien prendido; buen agarre
hold (to)	tomar en brazos
hormones	hormonas
inverted nipples	pezones invertidos
lactation consultant	consultora en lactancia
latch on (to)	agarrar
leaking	se sale la leche
letdown	reflejo de eyección de la leche
lump in breast	masa en el pecho
meconium	meconio, popó negro y espeso
milk expression	extracción de la leche
night feedings	tomas nocturnas
nipple	pezón
nurse (to)	amamantar; mamar
nursing	mamada
plugged duct	conducto obstruido
pump breasts	succionar los pechos
relactation	relactancia
rooting	señales de búsqueda
sore nipples	pezones adoloridos
spoon, teaspoon	cuchara; cucharadita
sucking bursts	ráfagas de succión
suckle (to)	dar el pecho; amamantar mamar
suckling	niño lactante, que toma pecho
swallow (to)	tragar
swallow(s)	trago(s)
thrush	cándida; infección de hongo
wean	destetar
weaned	destetado
weaning	destete

▶ **HELPFUL PHRASES:**

4 or more	cuatro o mas
5 to 6	cinco a seis
8 to 12 times	ocho a doce veces
attachment to the breast	prenderse al pecho
breast engorgement	congestión mamaria pechos hinchados
breast infection	infección mamaria; infección del pecho
breast massage	masaje del pecho
breast pads	protectores absorbentes para el pecho; pañalitos para el pecho
breast pump	sacaleches
breast shells	conchas plásticas; duras para pezones
close contact	contacto cercano
cluster feeding	período de mamadas frecuentes
cradle position	acunar, posición para tomar al niño en brazos
cross cradle position	utilizar la mano para sostener al bebé y acomodarlo al pecho opuesto
exclusive breastfeeding	dar el pecho exclusivamente
feed your baby	déle pecho a su bebé
football hold	posición lateral debajo del brazo (sandía)
growth spurts	períodos de crecimiento acelerado
hand expression	sacar la leche usando presión manual
nipple shield	protectores flexibles para el pezón; pezonera
repositioning baby	reposicionar mejor el bebe al pecho
skin to skin	tener el bebé con sólo el pañal en contra de su piel; de piel a piel
supplemental feeding	alimentación suplementaria

▶ **QUESTIONS AND INSTRUCTIONS:**

How may I help you?	¿Cómo puedo ayudarla?
In a day, how many times do you breastfeed?	¿En un día, cuántas veces le da pecho a su bebé?
Describe a normal 24 hour day.	Descríbame un día de 24 horas.
How often does your baby nurse?	¿Cuán a menudo toma el pecho su bebé?
Can you hear your baby swallowing?	¿Puede oír los tragos de su bebé?
Does your breast feel softer after feeding?	¿Se ablanda el pecho después de una mamada?
How many wet diapers each day?	¿Cuántos pañales mojados cada día?
How many soiled diapers each day?	¿Cuántos pañales con evacuación cada día?
What color are the soiled diapers?	¿De qué color son las evacuaciones?
How much does your baby weigh?	¿Cuánto pesa su bebé ahora?
How much did your baby weigh at birth?	¿Cuánto pesó su bebé cuando nació?
Breastfeed at least 8 times each day.	Déle pecho por lo menos ocho (8) veces al día.
Do you feel pain when you breastfeed?	¿Siente dolor cuando da pecho?
Where?	¿Dónde?
When?	¿Cuándo?
At the beginning or during the whole feed?	¿Al comienzo o durante toda la toma?
If necessary, feed your baby by spoon or dropper.	Si es necesario, alimente a su bebé por cuchara o gotero.
If you think you need to give your baby formula call a lactation consultant first.	Si piensa que necesita darle fórmula a su bebé primero llameuna consejera de lactancia.

INDEX